OXFORD MEDICAL PUBLICATIONS

Tropical Neurology

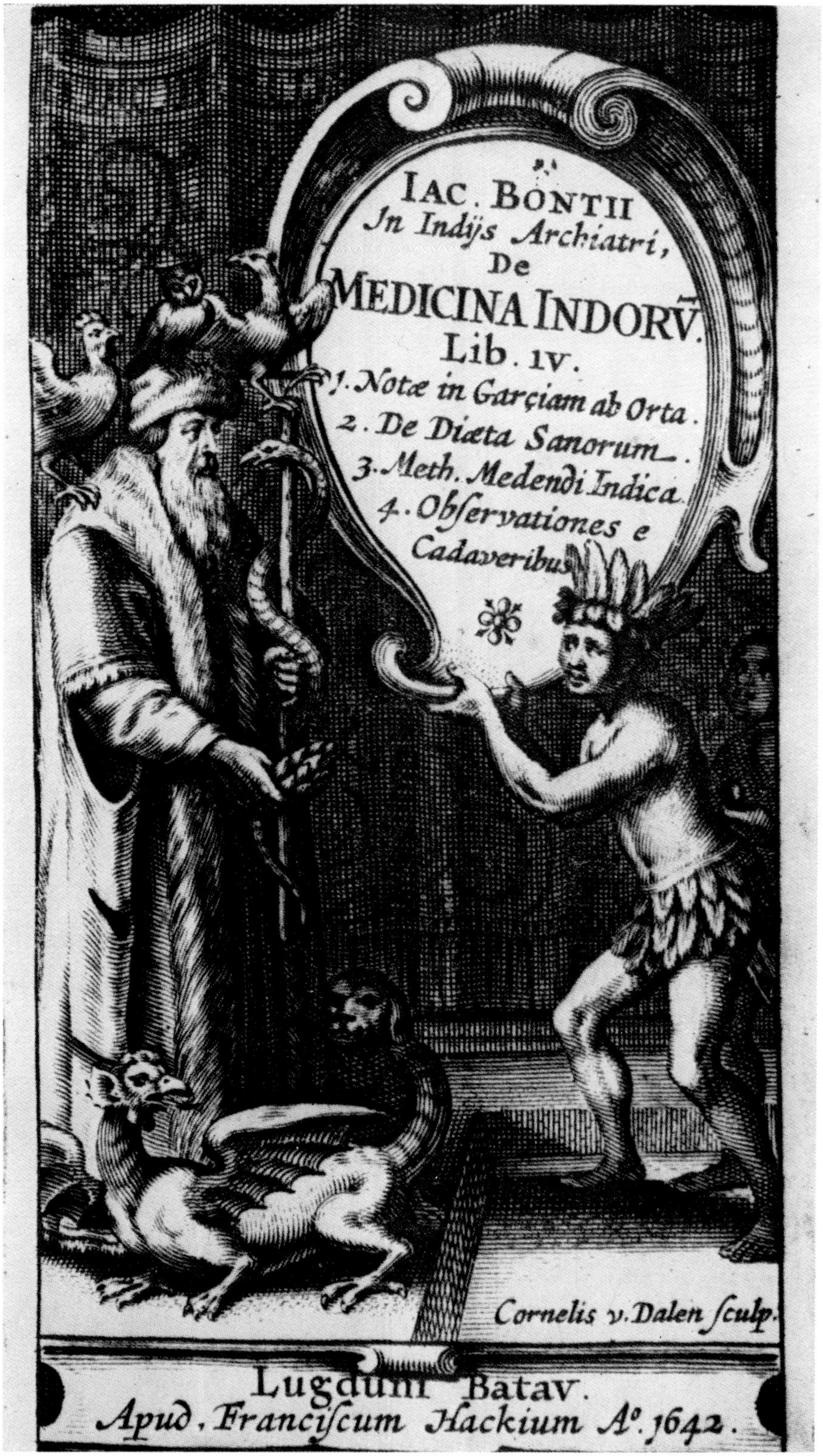

The frontispiece to the first book on tropical medicine by Jacob C. Bontius, *De Medicina Indorum*, 1642.

[Frontispiece]

Tropical Neurology

Edited by

JOHN D. SPILLANE M.D., F.R.C.P.

Consultant Neurologist, The University Hospital of Wales, Cardiff, and the Welsh Hospital Board

LONDON

OXFORD UNIVERSITY PRESS

NEW YORK TORONTO

1973

Oxford University Press, Ely House, London W.1
GLASGOW NEW YORK TORONTO MELBOURNE WELLINGTON
CAPE TOWN IBADAN NAIROBI DAR ES SALAAM LUSAKA ADDIS ABABA
DELHI BOMBAY CALCUTTA MADRAS KARACHI LAHORE DACCA
KUALA LUMPUR SINGAPORE HONG KONG TOKYO

ISBN 0 19 264154 9

Made in Great Britain at The Pitman Press, Bath

Contents

Preface vii

Acknowledgements ix

List of Contributors xi

List of Plates xiii

Introduction J. D. SPILLANE 3

Part One India

1. An Introduction to Neurology in India N. H. WADIA 25
2. Tuberculosis of the Central Nervous System P. N. TANDON and S. N. PATHAK 37
3. Radiculomyelopathy associated with Spinal Meningitides (Arachnoiditis) with Special Reference to the Spinal Tuberculous Variety N. H. WADIA 63
4. Neurological Complications in Tropical Sprue G. M. TAORI and G. V. IYER 73
5. Neurological Disease in South India K. S. MANI 78
6. Cerebrovascular Disorders in South India J. ABRAHAM 86
7. The Aortic Arch Syndrome P. M. DALAL 92
8. Congenital Atlanto-Axial Dislocation and its Manifestations due to Spinal Cord Compression N. H. WADIA 99
9. Anterior Encephaloceles P. N. TANDON 108
10. The Infantile Tremor Syndrome P. N. TANDON and P. C. BAJPAI 114
11. Painful Ophthalmoplegia N. T. MATHEW 120
12. Endemic Fluorosis in India A. H. SIDDIQUI 124
13. Juvenile Motor Neurone Disease K. JAGANNATHAN 127

Part Two Africa

14. Neurological Disorders in Senegal H. COLLOMB, M. DUMAS and P. L. GIRARD 133
15. Neurological Disorders in Ghana D. R. W. HADDOCK 143
16. Neurological Disorders in Nigeria B. O. OSUNTOKUN 161

17. Neurological Disorders in Uganda J. R. BILLINGHURST 191

18. Neurological Disorders in Kenya J. R. HARRIES 207

19. Neurosurgery in Rhodesia L. F. LEVY and J. AXTON 223

20. Neurological Disorders in Rhodesia I. RACHMAN 237

21. Neurological Complications of Parasitic Disease M. GELFAND 247

22. Neurological Disease in Natal J. E. COSNETT 259

23. Porphyria Variegata and Multiple Sclerosis in South Africa G. DEAN 273

Part Three South-East Asia

24. Neurological Disorders in Singapore A. L. GWEE and G. A. RANSOME 283

25. Neurological Disorders in Malaysia R. SELBY 299

26. Leprosy J. H. S. PETTIT 321

27. Neurology in Thailand A. VEJJAJIVA 335

Part Four Oceania

28. Amyotrophic Lateral Sclerosis and Parkinsonism-Dementia in Guam J. A. BRODY and L. T. KURLAND 355

29. Kuru in the New Guinea Highlands D. C. GAJDUSEK 376

Part Five Latin America

30. Neurological Disorders in Peru J. O. TRELLES 387

31. Chagas' Disease and the Nervous System A. SPINA-FRANÇA and L. C. MATTOSINHO-FRANÇA 397

32. Hydatid Echinococcosis of the Nervous System R. ARANA-IÑIGUEZ 408

Part Six West Indies

33. Neurological Disorders in Jamaica E. K. CRUICKSHANK 421

Index 435

Preface

My interest in neurology in a tropical environment was aroused during the Second World War, and I have managed to sustain and nourish it while practising in Wales by periodic forays into tropical territory. I have seen nearly all the disorders described in this book and have enjoyed discussions about them with many friends and colleagues overseas. An account of them, I thought, would be an interesting endeavour.

There was a time when tropical medicine and neurology were poles apart. It is still rare to find more about neurology in a textbook of tropical medicine than an account of encephalitis, running amok, latah, koro, and tropical neurasthenia. Yet no physician visiting a hospital in the tropics can fail to be struck by the number and variety of neurological disorders waiting to be unravelled. In the Western world we have completed a century of neurological nosography. Readers of the present volume may feel that a further century of study awaits us in the tropics. A disease cannot really be said to be known and understood if its manifestations in only one type of environment have been described.

It will be many years before a comprehensive account of tropical neurology can be undertaken. But this book should give some indication of the prospects for neurological research and practice in these countries. I wish to thank the contributors for their co-operation in this enterprise and I hope that they too will feel that it was worth while. At the Oxford University Press I am indebted to Dr. J. C. Gregory and my daughter, Mrs. Susan Meakin, for their expert advice.

Cardiff
November 1972

J.D.S.

Acknowledgements

The author of Chapter 1 would like to profusely thank Dr. S. K. Pandya, Neurosurgeon, Bombay, for much information regarding the history of early medicine in India.

He would also like to thank the many Indian neurologists who have freely discussed their findings at meetings and in other conversations about the unusual sleep disorder mentioned in the text. The author has drawn on their experiences and his own to give a cogent and, he hopes, useful account of the disease.

He thanks once again Dr. Roman Kocen of London, and his colleagues in the biochemical laboratories, for permission to quote their findings.

Finally, Dr. Meher Desai helped the author much with collection of the material and he acknowledges her help gratefully.

The authors of Chapter 2 wish to acknowledge their gratitude to Dr. H. D. Tandon, Professor and Head of the Department of Pathology, AIIMS, who kindly reviewed all the available material of tuberculous lesions of the central nervous system in the department, in order to provide an objective first-hand description of these lesions as encountered in the population.

Their colleague Dr. A. K. Banerji patiently read through the various manuscripts and made a number of valuable suggestions.

Their thanks are due to Dr. Dharam Paul Sharma and Dr. Stalin Ganji who helped them in collecting and analysing their data on tuberculous meningitis. Mr. P. Ganguli was responsible for providing the photographs.

Their special thanks are due to their secretary, Mr. C. P. Kumar, who painstakingly typed all the manuscripts.

The authors of Chapter 4 wish to thank Drs. V. I. Mathan and S. J. Baker for their assistance in the writing of this account.

The author of Chapter 16 wishes to acknowledge the permission of the Publishers and Editor of the *Journal of Neurological Sciences* to make extensive use of a paper submitted to the Journal for publication in 1971, on the picture of neurological practice in Nigeria. He wishes to acknowledge the kind permission of the following to reproduce the figures: Professor O. O. Akinkugbe, Professor of Medicine, University of Ibadan, for Fig. 16.1; the Editor of *Tropical and Geographical Medicine* for Plate 24c; Professor A. O. Williams, Professor of Pathology, University of Ibadan, for Plate 24e, and the Editor of the *West African Medical Journal* for Fig. 16.7.

The author's research on Nigerian tropical ataxic neuropathy has been generously supported by research grants from the Wellcome Trust of Great Britain, and to a lesser extent by Senate research grants of the University of Ibadan. The account of Nigerian tropical ataxic neuropathy is based in part on a paper read in London, in 1969, at a symposium on 'Cassava Diet, Chronic Cyanide Intoxication and Neuropathy', held under the auspices of the Wellcome Trust of Great Britain, and on a thesis submitted in part fulfilment for the requirements of the Ph.D. degree of the University of Ibadan, Nigeria.

The author thanks Mrs. C. A. Piper for secretarial assistance, and also the staff of the Medical Illustration Unit, University of Ibadan, for valuable assistance.

The author of Chapter 25 wishes to acknowledge his thanks to the Ministry of Health of Malaysia, the staff of the General Hospital, Kuala Lumpur, and in particular those of the Department of Neurosurgery, the Institute for Medical Research, the Arboviral

Laboratory of the Hooper Foundation of the University of California, the Medical Superintendent and staff of the Sungei Buloh Leprosy Hospital, Dr. Harry M. Zimmerman of Montefiore Hospital, New York, and many others throughout the world too numerous to mention.

The authors of CHAPTER 28 wish to acknowledge all their colleagues mentioned in the text for their enormous contributions to our present understanding of the conditions described. In addition, they wish to express their gratitude to the staff of the NINDS Research Centre on Guam and to the many physicians who have worked and are working on Guam throughout the years of the study, and to the people of Guam for their co-operation and forebearance.

List of Contributors

ABRAHAM, JACOB, M.S.(Gen.), M.S.(Neurol.), F.A.C.S., F.A.C.A. Professor of Neurosurgery, Department of Neurological Sciences, Christian Medical College Hospital, Vellore.

ARANA-IÑIGUEZ, ROMÁN, M.D. Professor of Neurology, and Director of the Neurological Institute, Facultad de Medicine, Hospital de Clinicas, Montevideo, Uruguay.

AXTON, JOHN H., M.B., M.R.C.P., D.C.H. Lecturer in Paediatrics, University College of Rhodesia. Late House Surgeon, Neurosurgical Unit, Harare Central Hospital, Salisbury, Rhodesia.

BAJPAI, PRAKASH C., M.D., M.R.C.P., D.C.H. Professor of Paediatrics, King George's Medical College, Lucknow.

BILLINGHURST, JOHN R., B.M., M.R.C.P. Senior Lecturer in Medicine, Makerere University College Hospital, Kampala, Uganda.

BRODY, JACOB A., M.D. Epidemiology Branch, C. and F. R. National Institute of Neurological Diseases and Stroke, National Institutes of Health, Bethesda, Maryland.

COLLOMB, HENRI, M. D. Professor of Neurology, Faculty of Medicine, University of Dakar, Dakar, Senegal.

COSNETT, JOHN E., B.Sc., M.D., M.R.C.P. Principal Physician and Head of Department of Medicine, Edendale Hospital, Pietermaritzburg, Natal.

CRUICKSHANK, ERIC K., O.B.E., M.D., F.R.C.P. (Lond. and Glas.), F.A.C.P. Professor and Dean of Postgraduate Medical Education, University of Glasgow.

DALAL, PRAFULCHANDRA, M., M.D. Professor of Neurology, T. N. Medical College, Bombay.

DEAN, GEOFFREY, M.D., F.R.C.P. Director, The Medico-Social Research Board, Dublin.

DUMAS, M., M.D. Department of Neurology, Faculty of Medicine, University of Dakar, Senegal.

GAJDUSEK, D. CARLETON, M.D. Department of Health, Education and Welfare, National Institutes of Health, Bethesda, Maryland.

GELFAND, MICHAEL, C.B.E., M.D., F.R.C.P. Professor of Medicine, Department of Medicine, University of Rhodesia, and Harare Central Hospital, Salisbury, Rhodesia.

GIRARD, P. L., M.D. Department of Neurology, Faculty of Medicine, University of Dakar, Senegal.

GWEE, AH. L., M.D., F.R.C.P. Consultant Physician, Outram Road General Hospital, Singapore.

HADDOCK, DAVID R. W., M.D., F.R.C.P. Formerly Associate Professor of Medicine, Ghana Medical School, University of Ghana, Accra. Professor of Medicine, Department of Medicine, University of Benin, Benin City, Nigeria.

HARRIES, JAMES R., O.B.E., M.D., F.R.C.P. Agip House Building, Nairobi, Kenya.

IYER, GOPALAKRISHNA V., M.D. Departments of Neurological Sciences and Wellcome Research Institute, Christian Medical College Hospital, Vellore.

JAGANNATHAN, KANTHIMATHINATHAN, M.D., D.T.M. Professor of Neurology, Madras Medical College, and Consultant Neurologist, Government General Hospital, Madras.

KURLAND, LEONARD, T., M.D. Department of Epidemiology, Medical Statistics and Population Genetics, The Mayo Clinic, Rochester, Minnesota.

LEVY, LAURENCE, F., M.B., B.S., M.Sc., F.R.C.S., F.A.C.S. Professor of Surgery and Neuro surgeon, Salisbury Hospitals Group and Department of Surgery, University of Rhodesia, Salisbury, Rhodesia.

MANI, KALYANASUNDARAM S., M.D. Professor of Neurology, All India Institute of Mental Health, Bangalore.

MATHEW, NINAN T., M.D., D.M. (Neurol.) Neurologist, Department of Neurological Sciences, Christian Medical College Hospital, Vellore.

MATTOSINHO-FRANÇA, L. C., M.D., F.C.A.P. Director, Division of Pathology, Hospital do Servidor Público, São Paulo.

OSUNTOKUN, BENJAMIN O., M.D., B.Sc., M.R.C.P., Ph.D. Professor of Neurology, Department of Medicine, University College Hospital, Ibadan, Nigeria.

PATHAK, SUMEDHA N., M.B., B.Sc., M.R.C.P., D.C.H. Professor and Head of Department of Neurology, All India Institute of Medical Sciences, New Delhi.

PETTIT, JOHN H. S., M.B., F.R.C.P. Consultant Dermatologist, 14 Jalan Damai, Kuala Lumpur.

RACHMAN, ISAAC, M.B., M.R.C.P. Consultant Physician, Mpilo Central Hospital, Bulawayo, Rhodesia.

RANSOME, SIR GORDON A., K.B.E., M.D., F.R.C.P. Professor Emeritus of Medicine, Faculty of Medicine, University of Singapore.

SELBY, ROY, M.D., Chairman, Department of Neurosurgery, Cook County Hospital; Associate Professor, Department of Neurosurgery, Abraham Lincoln School of Medicine, University of Illinois, Chicago; Visiting Associate Professor of Neurosurgery, Rush Medical College, Chicago. (Formerly of the Department of Neurosurgery, Kuala Lumpur.)

SIDDIQUI, ABUL HASAN, M.B., F.R.C.P. Specialist in Internal Medicine, King Abdel Azis Hospital, Mecca. (Formerly Professor of Principles and Practice of Medicine, Osmania Medical College, Hyderabad.)

SPILLANE, JOHN D., M.D., F.R.C.P. Consultant Neurologist, University Hospital of Wales, Cardiff.

SPINA-FRANÇA, A., M.D. Associate Professor of Clinical Neurology, Department of Neurology, Hospital das Clinicas, Faculdade de Medicina da Universidade de São Paulo, São Paulo.

TANDON, PRAKASH N., M.S., F.R.C.S. Professor and Head of Department of Neurosurgery, All India Institute of Medical Sciences, New Delhi.

TAORI, GIRDHARILAL M., M.D., F.R.C.P.(C). Departments of Neurological Sciences and Wellcome Research Institute, Christian Medical College Hospital, Vellore.

TRELLES, J. O., M.D. Professor of Neurology, Hospital Santo Toribio de Mogrovejo, Lima.

VEJJAJIVA, ATHASIT, M.B., B.Sc., M.R.C.P. Chief, Division of Neurology, Department of Medicine, Faculty of Medicine, Ramathibodi Hospital, Mahidol University, Bangkok.

WADIA, NOSHIR H., M.D., F.R.C.P. The Department of Neurology, J. J. Group of Hospitals, Byculla, Bombay.

List of Plates

FRONTISPIECE The frontispiece to the first book on tropical medicine by Jacob C. Bontius, *De Medicina Indorum*, 1642

PLATES between pp. 160 and 161

1a. *India*. The Sir J. J. Hospital, Bombay
b. *Thailand*. Siriraj Teaching Hospital, Bangkok
2a. *Uganda*. Mulago Hospital and Makerere Medical School, Kampala
b. *India*. The All India Institute of Medical Sciences, New Delhi
3a. *Nigeria*. Wood carving of native doctor
b. *Thailand*. Ancient physiotherapy
c. *India*. The Ross Commemoration tablet, Calcutta
d. *Brazil*. Window of Neurological Institute of Rio de Janeiro
4. Cassava preparation in Nigeria
5a. Tetanus in a Nigerian
b. Infantile tremor syndrome (*India*)
c. and d. Endemic fluorosis (*India*)
6a. *Bangkok*. Right third nerve palsy; encephalomyelitis due to antirabic vaccine
b. Rickets in an Indian child
c. and d. Pellagra in Hyderabad, India
7a. and c. Ataxic neuropathy of Nigeria
b. Lathyrism in Central India
d. Ataxic neuropathy of Nigeria
8a. Ataxic neuropathy of Nigeria
b. and c. Jamaican neuropathy
9a. Kwashiorkor in a Jamaican infant
b. Leprosy
c. The consequences of leprosy
10a. and b. Tuberculous meningitis (*India*)
c. and d. Microphotographs of characteristic tuberculous meningitis (*India*)
11a. and b. Tuberculomas of the brain (*India*)
c. and d. Microphotographs of tuberculoma of the brain (*India*)
12a. and b. Lumbar myelograms in Pott's paraplegia (*India*)
13a. and b. Radiculomyelopathy: lumbar myelograms (*India*)
c. Lower end of spinal cord
14a. Radiculomyelopathy: transverse section of cord (*India*)
b. and c. Microphotographs of exudate in radiculomyelopathy (*India*)
15a. to d. Painful ophthalmoplegia, before and after treatment (*India*)
16a. Aortic arch syndrome (*India*)
b. Cross-section of main vessels of the aortic arch (*India*)
c. Electronmicrophotograph of section through intimal and subintimal region (*India*)
d. High-power view of collagen fibres (*India*)

PLATES between pp. 160 and 161

17a. Congenital atlanto-axial dislocation: lateral tomogram (*India*)
b. Macerated specimen of Group I cases (*India*)
c. Attenuated upper cervical cord (*India*)
d. Tomogram of lateral view of cervical spine (*India*)
18a. and b. Anterior encephaloceles (*India*)
c. and d. Ventriculogram: brow-up AP and lateral views (*India*)
19a. to d. Fronto-ethmoidal encephalocele: pre- and post-operative photographs (*India*)
20a. and b. Infantile tremor syndrome (*India*)
c. Polygraphic record of tremors (*India*)
d. EEG showing short burst of poly spikes (*India*)
21a. and b. Infantile tremor syndrome (*India*)
c. and d. Endemic fluorosis (*India*)
22a. and b. Endemic fluorosis (*India*)
c. Radiograph of forearms (*India*)
d. Radiograph of lumbar spine (*India*)
23a. Endemic fluorosis (*India*)
b. and c. Juvenile motor neurone disease (*India*)
24a. 'Spider-web' clot in cerebrospinal fluid in tuberculous meningitis (*Nigeria*)
b. Severe contractures of hands from burns applied in epileptic coma (*Nigeria*)
c. Colloid cyst of third ventricle (*Nigeria*)
d. Ocular presentation of Burkitt's neoplasm (*Nigeria*)
e. Muscular dystrophy in a Nigerian youth
25a. *South Africa:* hand of a man with porphyria variegata
b. *Singapore:* clamp used in koro
c. *Kuala Lumpur:* tuberculoid lesion in a case of leprosy
26a. to c. *Kuala Lumpur:* classical borderline leprosy
d. Erythema nodosum leprosy
27a. *Kuala Lumpur:* severe nodular lepromatous leprosy
b. Tuberculoid leprosy
c. Facial paralysis in leprosy
d. Secondary xeroderma
28a. and b. *Kuala Lumpur:* interosseal wasting in tuberculoid leprosy
c. and d. Leprosy. Charcot arthropathy of ankle joint
29. *New Guinea:* groups of kuru patients in first and second stages of the disease
30. *New Guinea:* three child victims of kuru in stages 1, 2 and 3, respectively
31a. *New Guinea:* extensive loss of Purkinje cells and neurones in kuru
b. Status spongiosus of grey matter in kuru
c. Extensive astroglial hypertrophy and proliferation in kuru
32a. and b. *Peru:* verruga peruana
c. Meningeal and vascular cortical reactions in verruga peruana
d. Neuronal and glial alterations
e. Frontal cortex; glial infiltration and axonal alterations
33a. *Peru:* three phases of verruca formation in the brain
b. and c. Cystic cysticercosis

PLATES between pp. 160 and 161

34a. *Peru:* racemose form of cysticercosis
b. Subpial vesicle with scolex
c. Racemose vesicle in the cauda equina
d. Fibrovascular connective tissue reaction surrounding parasite
35a. and b. *Peru:* cystic cysticercosis. Spinal cord
36a. *Peru:* cystic cysticercosis. Deep fibrocanalicular layer
b. Schematic representation of reaction produced by cysticercus in brain tissues
37a. and b. *Brazil:* human Chagas' acute encephalitis
c. and d. Experimental Chagas' infection in mouse
38a. *Uruguay:* hydatid disease of the nervous system
b. and c. Schematic explanation of San Julián and Arana-Iñiguez's procedure
39. *Uruguay:* hydatid disease of the nervous system. Three stages in surgical procedure
40a. *Uruguay:* hydatid disease of the nervous system. Cranial hydatidosis
b. and c. Vertebral hydatidosis

INTRODUCTION

J. D. Spillane

See PLATES 1–9

Introduction

J. D. SPILLANE

When Thomas Willis, in his celebrated *Cerebri Anatome* (1664), coined the term *Neurologie,* to mean the 'doctrine of the nerves', his world was a small one and Western medicine was in its infancy. The continents of Africa, India, America and Australasia were virtually unexplored. More than a century was to pass before the structure and function of the nervous system were seriously examined.

It is not until the nineteenth century that we encounter the remarkable flowering of clinical neurology—and this was a European phenomenon. It was almost entirely in the medical schools of France, Germany, and Britain that the major classical disorders of the nervous system were identified and described. The first textbook of neurology was written by Romberg in 1846 when he was a Professor in Berlin; it was translated into English in 1853. The civilized world had expanded since Willis's day but Africa was still the 'Dark Continent' and India was not yet wholly under British rule. When the National Hospital for Nervous Diseases opened its doors in 1860 in London, work had just begun on cutting the Suez Canal. The year 1870 saw the completion of the canal, and the publication of two classics of neurological literature which marked a new era in the study of the brain. From Queen Square, London, came Hughlings Jackson's *A Study of Convulsions;* from Berlin, Fritsch and Hitzig's description of the *Electrical Excitability of the Cerebral Cortex.*

During the next two decades the publication of three renowned textbooks of neurology from France, England and Germany stand out clearly as landmarks in the history of neurology. In 1873 Charcot published his masterpiece *Leçons sur les Maladies du Système Nerveux Faites à la Salpêtrière.* In that year in Central Africa Dr. David Livingstone, missionary and explorer, still searching for the source of the Nile, was on his last fatal journey. The year 1888 saw the completion of Gowers's *Diseases of the Nervous System,* a work which came to be affectionately known as the 'Bible of Neurology'. We do not know whether Gowers ever read the account, published in that same year by Strachan, senior medical officer in Jamaica, of the 510 strange cases of peripheral neuropathy from Kingston Hospital, but we can be sure his curiosity would have been quickly roused. Then, in 1894, the year of the discovery of the plague bacillus in the pandemic of Hong Kong, Oppenheim's famous *Lehrbuch der Krankenheiten* appeared. At the end of the century European neurology was firmly established.

Meanwhile, another branch of medicine was emerging, not from the universities of Europe but from outposts of the colonial Empire of the day. This was tropical medicine. The ancient diseases of leprosy, plague, and cholera, known in Europe for centuries, had been retreating to tropical and subtropical regions of the world; but other scourges awaited the newcomer, and colonization brought medicine to the forefront of imperial planning. The famed Indian Medical Service had been established by the East India Company in 1764; hospitals had been built in Madras (1664), Bombay (1676) [PLATE 1a], and Calcutta (1708), and at the end of the nineteenth century there were a dozen or so medical schools in India. It is said that by then there were more than one and a half million British graves in the land. 'Two monsoons are the life of a man' ran an old Anglo-Indian saying.

The evil reputation of West Africa persisted. Mary Kingsley, in 1897, wrote: 'Remember, before you elect to cast your lot with the West Coasters, that 85 per cent of them die of fever or return home with their health permanently wrecked'. She herself died of typhoid fever while serving as a nurse in the Boer War. In East Africa things were better until sleeping sickness was introduced into Uganda from the Congo in 1891. It was a deadly disease, and had destroyed nearly two-thirds of the local population by 1897.

> Diseases were often spread by the energies of Empire. . . . Almost every year meningitis sallied from Calcutta with the coolie ships for the West Indies, and in return the jigger insect, indigenous to the Americas, found its way from Mombasa across the Indian Ocean to Bombay. Hookworm was taken all over the world by indentured labourers from India, British ships often took cholera to the Far East, hidden away in bottles of holy water from the well Zem Zem, one of the five holy places of the pilgrimage to Mecca. (*Pax Britannica*, 1968, by James Morris.)

The health of Army garrisons was appalling. The mortality rate in Jamaica was 130 per thousand; in Madras, 106 per thousand. There were more deaths from typhoid fever in the South African War at the turn of the century than there were men killed in action. In the Navy, the West African and West Indies stations were notorious for their high sickness and death rates. Throughout the tropics, moreover, the nineteenth-century builders of roads, railways, bridges, ports, and canals fell victim to many fevers and diverse ailments. The construction of the Kenya-Uganda railway from Mombasa to Lake Victoria, made famous by J. H. Patterson's book *The Man Eaters of Tsavo*, was an incredible feat of endurance in the face of famine and drought, plague, smallpox, and rinderpest, not to mention hostile tribesmen and man-eating lions. In India the larger trains carried coffins in case a passenger died suddenly of cholera or heat exhaustion. But it was the cutting of the Panama Canal that really drove home the lessons of preventive medicine in the tropics. The French had failed in 1888 after struggling for 8 years in jungles infested with malaria and yellow fever; the Americans succeeded, in 1904–12, losing some 4000 from disease where the French had lost 50 000.

It was these developments that led to the creation of schools of tropical medicine in the city ports of Liverpool and London in 1898.

The impact of races during the centuries of exploration and conquest in the tropics had far-reaching consequences for the health of mankind. It is generally believed that syphilis, even if it previously existed in pre-Columbian Europe, spread rapidly from Spain, the foremost colonizing country of the day, throughout the early sixteenth century. Yellow fever, endemic in the Spanish colonies in the Americas, first took hold in Europe in the maritime cities of Spain and Portugal. Smallpox, carried by the Spaniards, ravaged the Indians of Mexico and Peru and contributed to the conquests of Cortes and Pizarro. 'Between the years 1550 and 1850 at least three million Amerindians died from smallpox in the West Indies, Central and South America' (Stearn and Stearn, 1945.) Tuberculosis and smallpox decimated the Australian aborigines and the Polynesians. In the Africa of Livingstone's day, tuberculosis had not yet gained entry, but leprosy and trachoma had already been exported from the Continent to the Americas via the slave-trade.[1] French imperialism had been halted in Egypt and Syria as much by plague and trachoma as by defeat in battle, and in Haiti yellow fever had destroyed an army and created a republic.

The rise and growth of tropical medicine during the nineteenth century was assured by the new science of bacteriology. In 1800 the idea of the microbic origin of disease had not taken hold; scabies was the only malady then known to be due to a parasite. The first human disease shown to result from infection by a living organism was none other than leprosy, in 1870. It remains not only the commonest form of neuritis in the world but also the only one in which the responsible agent actually invades the nerves. By 1900 the causal organisms of a whole series of infectious diseases were known, and Robert Koch, who discovered the tubercle bacillus in 1882 and the cholera bacillus in 1884, was investigating plague in India, malaria in Java, and rinderpest in Africa.

The role played by insect vectors of micro-organisms was recognized with the discovery by Manson, in China in 1887, that filariae were introduced into the human body by mosquitoes. He was also responsible for showing Ross the parasites of malaria [PLATE 3c] that had been found in the blood by the French military doctor, Laveran, in Algiers in 1880. Moreover, it was Manson who promoted the founding of the medical school in Hong Kong and the London School of Tropical Medicine. He has been called the 'Father of Tropical Medicine'.

We see, then, that the achievements of the nineteenth century clinical neurologists in Europe took place at a time when scientific progress made tropical exploration and expansion inevitable. Sooner or later neurology itself would be influenced by medical experience in the tropics. There are already signs that a century of tropical neurology may well have repercussions in the whole field of medicine. Even from the point of view of purely descriptive neurology, which has characterized the past century, it is difficult to believe that experience in temperate climates is the beginning and end of the story. The processes of disease are exceedingly complex and the human nervous sytem which may succumb is the product of generations of influences wrought by heredity, race, diet, and climate. The late Lord Brain (1964) writing of clinical neurology today, thought that the descriptive era was by no means at an end:

> Where does clinical neurology stand today? People sometimes speak as though nosography in neurology was almost exhausted, but this is quite untrue. The discovery of new diseases or syndromes, and equally the elaboration of the clinical pictures of existing ones, are partly a matter of seeing differences in what was hitherto thought to be homogeneous.

In the past two decades the landscape of clinical neurology has been extended by the recognition of syndromes such as compression of the median nerve in the carpal tunnel, cervical spondylosis, the carcinomatous neuromyopathies, subacute encephalitis and subacute encephalopathy, progressive supranuclear palsy, multifocal leuco-encephalopathy, central pontine myelinosis, subacute necrotizing encephalopathy, neurogenic orthostatic hypotension, communicating hydrocephalus, and the neurological consequences of hepatic disease, collagen diseases, and various metabolic disorders. These developments were not primarily due to the arrival of new techniques, but were a continuation of the classical methods of clinico-pathological correlation which reaped such rich rewards in the past. Methods which, practised in new human environments, should further the notion of a world neurology.

TROPICAL MEDICINE

At this stage it is necessary to consider the term 'tropical medicine', of which tropical neurology is but a part. In his *A History of Tropical Medicine* (1939), Sir H.

[1] A modern pathologist in Africa writes that 'the Central African's first contact with tuberculosis is usually his last' (Davies, 1947*a*).

Harold Scott, recognized the difficulty inherent in the term:

> Another difficulty, and a very real one, consists in the fact that we have no definition of the term 'Tropical Medicine'. If we take its narrow interpretation as 'disease restricted to the tropics', i.e. to 23° 27′ of latitude on either side of the equator, we could with a close approximation to the truth say that it is non-existent. If we extend our limits to 'disease met with in wares climates', this apparently small extension in reality comes to include nearly all the ills that flesh is heir to, except, perhaps, frost-bite, and even that might occur on the mountain heights of a country generally regarded as among warm climates—Fujiyama, Kilimanjaro, Mount Kenya, for example.
>
> Yet again we encounter further difficulties if we cut the Gordian knot by deciding to study the prevailing diseases in warm climates, for we find curious changes in distribution when we try to trace their histories. Thus, there are several diseases which, though now they are almost confined to torrid zones, in former times were found in temperate climates also; among these we may mention malaria, cholera, plague, relapsing fever, leprosy, ankylostomiasis and other helminthic infestations, and, as regards British possessions at least, smallpox and typhoid fever.
>
> A second group would consist of diseases which have never become widespread beyond warm countries, though purely as a fortunate chance because the vectors had not been introduced from their original habitat, or, if they had, they had not succeeded in flourishing. As members of such a group we may enumerate yellow fever, human trypanosomiasis, leishmaniasis, melioidosis, clonorchiasis, paragonimiasis, onchocerciasis, filariasis, certain tick-borne infections, Japanese river fever, Rocky Mountain fever, some varieties of endemic typhus.
>
> A third group there is, comprising diseases which are often considered as tropical, but are in reality widespread; such, for example, as undulant fever, long regarded as limited to Malta and the Mediterranean, but now known, from inclusion of abortus fever, to be almost universally distributed. Another member of this group is amoebic dysentery which caused a serious epidemic in Chicago in 1935; also sprue, pellagra, alastrim, tularaemia and, again, varieties of typhus.

In the generally accepted connotation of the term, the first steps in tropical medicine were those taken to protect the health of traders, officials, and servicemen working in the torrid zones of the world.

Protecting the health of the native was not considered an official obligation until it was realized that his co-operation was to some extent determined by his health and general well-being. This in turn often influenced the survival of the white man in his midst, as, for example, in the case of native-born infections. Progress in a colony necessitated the introduction of those measures of public health and hygiene which had successfully banished many so-called tropical diseases from Europe. At first locally administered, these steps spread throughout the colony, services were organized, and the welfare of the native became paramount. At the same time religious and philanthropic sentiments were responsible for much of the propagation of Western medicine in these areas of the world. Some modern schools of medicine in the tropics started as humble mission hospitals, as in the cases of Vellore in South India and Makerere in Uganda [PLATE 2].

Education of the native was a natural consequence of accepting responsibility for his welfare. The gigantic tasks that had to be tackled explain the way in which tropical medicine grew. The prevention and control of infections and infestations, the introduction of hygiene, proper nutrition, and maternal and infant welfare were necessary preliminaries.

As time passed, the prevailing diseases and major health hazards in different tropical zones came to be recognized and studied [FIG. 1]. Many diseases were

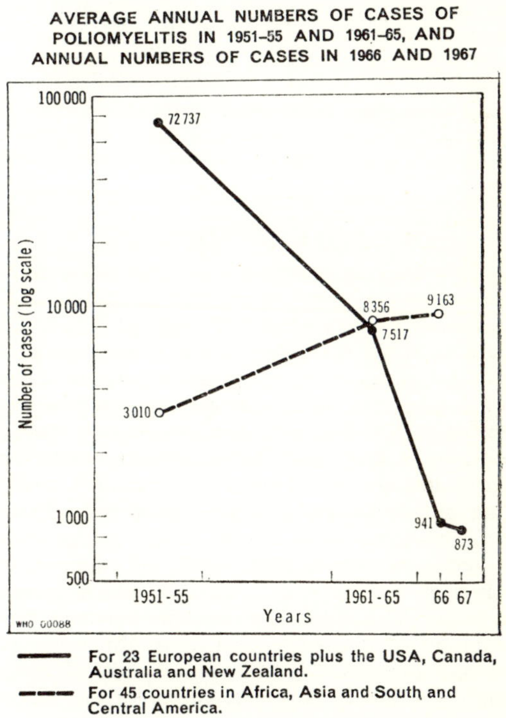

FIG. 1. Graph showing the world incidence of poliomyelitis. Declining in the West; increasing in the tropics. *Source:* Cockburn, W. C., and Drozelow, M. D. (1970) Poliomyelitis in the world, *Bull. Wld Hlth Org.*, 42, 405.

widespread in the tropics, others were concentrated in particular areas. There was bilharzia in Egypt, trypanosomiasis in Uganda, lathyrism in India [FIG. 2], beriberi in the Far East, and parasitic infestations in Latin America; there was a geography of tropical medicine.

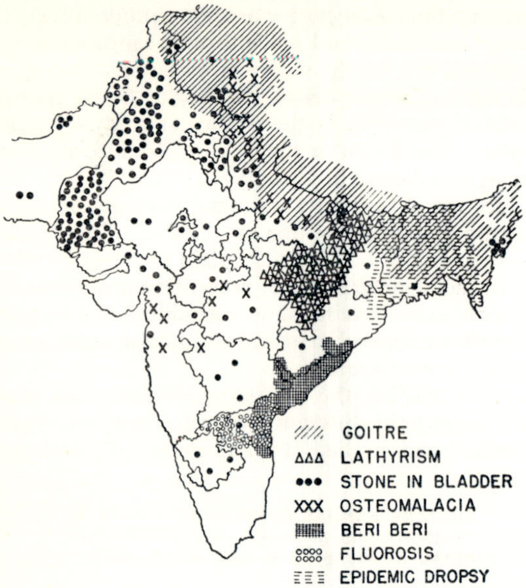

FIG. 2. The geographical distribution in India of some major disorders. (By courtesy of the late Professor V. N. Patwardhan, Coonor, and the Editor, *Indian Journal of Medical Sciences.*)

THE GEOGRAPHY OF MEDICINE

The geography of diseases was first recognized in ancient times with the observations of Hippocrates in the third century B.C. on *Airs, Waters and Places:* 'For if one knows all these things well, or at least the greater part of them, he cannot miss knowing, when he comes into a strange city, either the diseases peculiar to the place, or the particular nature of common diseases.' Hippocrates noted that in Thasos 'during winter paraplegia set in and attacked many and some died speedily'. He recognized lathyrism and recorded its association with the consumption of certain pulses: 'At Ainos those men and women who continually fed on pulse were attacked by a weakness of the legs which remained permanent.' The Hippocratic injunction to consider the topography of disease is evident in the writings of Sydenham in the seventeenth century and of his contemporary Charles Clermont, author of *On the Airs, Waters and Places of England.*

In the eighteenth and nineteenth centuries there were many accounts of the diseases encountered in particular regions or countries. Some of them contain the first major description of a disease.

Hillary's (1759) *Observations on the Changes of the Air and the Concomitant Epidemical Diseases in the Island of Barbados* includes a vivid account of tropical sprue: 'And I shall begin with the description of a disease which I think I may safely say is new, and has never yet been described by any author, neither ancient or modern.' Hillary described the afebrile, chronic, fluctuating, relapsing course of the illness which was characterized by glossitis, colic, diarrhoea, acrid stools, and anal excoriation which 'drains and exhausts the fluids of the body'.

Casal's (1762) *Natural and Medical History of the Principality of the Asturias* described pellagra; Rutty's (1770) *A Chronological History of the Weather and Seasons and of the Prevailing Diseases in Dublin,* described relapsing fever.

Winterbottom's (1803), *An Account of the Native Africans in the Neighbourhood of Sierra Leone* described sleeping sickness (African trypanosomiasis):

> The Africans are subject to a species of lethargy, which they are much afraid of, as it proves fatal in every instance . . . it is called sleepy sickness . . . the patient commonly has a ravenous appetite . . . squinting . . . convulsions . . . small glandular tumours in the neck . . . the disposition to sleep is so strong . . . even the repeated application of the whip is hardly sufficient to keep the poor wretch awake.[2]

The *history* of diseases, on the other hand, only began in the eighteenth century with studies of the plague, syphilis, smallpox and so on. But it is only by combining these two approaches, together, naturally, with clinical and laboratory data that knowledge of a disease may be perfected. Ackerknecht (1965) in his *History and Geography of the Most Important Diseases,* puts it thus:

> If any particular problem is viewed from the geographical viewpoint only, e.g. if one were to study a recent map showing the area of distribution of malaria, one might arrive at the erroneous conclusion that malaria is a tropical disease. As a matter of fact, only one hundred years ago malaria was still widespread in temperate climates as well. The study of the *history* of malaria would bring out such facts and would result, therefore, in a better and far more thorough understanding of the disease. The same may be said about other so-called 'tropical' diseases such as the plague, leprosy, cholera, etc. The study of the *history* of diseases is consequently a *conditio sine qua non* for the epidemiologist.

The first successful attempt to achieve such a synthesis was that of Hirsch in 1860–64 in his *Handbook of Historical and Geographical Pathology.* It was translated into English by Creighton, the author of the celebrated *History of Epidemics in Britain.* It would probably have made more impact, especially in tropical medicine, if the era of bacteriology had not so quickly dawned. Medical geography seemed unimportant at a time when, nearly every year, a new organism was identified as the cause of some human disease. Sigerist (1951) considered that medico-geographical studies also became somewhat discredited because 'previous work had in many ways been too ambitious, attempting a synthesis before the materials were available'. (A reminder which

[2] 'Winterbottom's Sign', enlargement of lymph nodes in the posterior cervical triangle, is still noted in current textbooks (e.g. *Pathology in the Tropics,* by Edington and Gilles, 1969, p. 33).

the present writer heeded when he conceived the idea of a book on tropical neurology.) Interest in medical geography did, however, increase after the First World War, and in 1929 the International Society of Geographical Pathology was founded, and symposia on cirrhosis of the liver (1931), gastric ulcer (1934), and anaemia (1937) brought pathologists together to compare their autopsy findings. In recent years there have been symposia on hepatitis, cancer, peptic ulcer, eclampsia, and myocardial infarction.

Several international organizations have begun the study of the distribution of diseases. At a meeting in 1957 under the auspices of UNESCO and WHO the Council for International Organizations of Medical Sciences published the report of a study group, *Methods of Geographical Pathology* (Doll, 1959). Geographical pathology was defined as 'the comparative study of the incidence of disease and the distribution of physiological traits in peoples belonging to different communities throughout the world and the correlation of these data, with features of the social and geographical environments'. It implied comparative studies between different ethnic, national, and social groups. Such studies should help in three ways. *First*, by defining communities which show a substantial difference in the frequency of a disease of unknown causation, for example multiple sclerosis, some light may be cast on aetiology. *Secondly*, the value of a hypothesis about the cause of a disease may be tested by examining the incidence of the disease in communities which are exposed to the suspected factor to different degrees, as in the possible relationship of congenital malformations of the nervous system with natural radiation or diet. *Thirdly*, it may help to unravel the relative effects of heredity and environment by studying the frequency of a disease among two races living in the same environment, or among each race separately under different conditions. Interesting data have already been obtained concerning the incidence of Parkinson's disease and cerebrovascular accidents among white and Negro populations in the United States, and we now require to know the incidence of these diseases in the African Negro for comparison with the American Negro.

The limitations of statistical studies of this kind are engendered by such factors as the difficulties in determining true prevalence and incidence rates, in comparing mortality rates, and in drawing trustworthy deductions. These methods are fraught with danger, they may never constitute final proof of a cause and effect relationship in a given disease, but they have already provided information of an intriguing nature in several diseases.

THE GEOGRAPHY OF NEUROLOGY

When we turn to the geographical aspects of neurology, we find that although data are meagre there are indications, especially from the past decade or two, that this is a promising field of research. Hirsch lamented the paucity of neurological data throughout the world:

> In the province of diseases of the nervous system, the inquiry into history and geography encounters a good many insuperable difficulties . . . most of all do we feel the want of statistics; for in the majority of the tables of mortality these diseases are either entered as causes of death under one class, or they figure as palsies, apoplexies and the like.

A hundred years later one reads that 'in few centres in the tropics has the study of neurology been pursued intensively; knowledge of diseases affecting the nervous system is therefore fragmentary' (Edington and Gilles, 1969). Hirsch had to confine himself to such illnesses as neuralgia, hysteria, chorea, epilepsy, apoplexy, 'hallucinations of the desert', cerebrospinal meningitis, tetanus and 'Negro lethargy'. Physicians in the tropics will not be surprised to read that concerning apoplexy Hirsch wrote that 'the tropics enjoy an exemption which, if not absolute, is at any rate very remarkable'. We now know that this is not true. Indeed, as the years pass, it is becoming clearer that the repeated assertion that many diseases of the nervous system are uncommon or actually rare in certain tropical zones is a premature generalization. There are notable exceptions like multiple sclerosis, tabes dorsalis and vitamin B_{12} neuropathy, it is true, and incidence rates of other diseases may vary, but we are nowhere near a position to make any broad and confident generalization about the distribution of diseases of the nervous system in the tropics.

In a symposium on geographical neurology held in Rome in 1961, mortality statistics from diseases of the nervous system in 33 countries were examined by Goldberg and Kurland (1962). Data were available from some tropical countries—India, Brazil, Burma, Egypt, Colombia, Mexico, the Philippines, Thailand, and Venezuela—on cerebral tumours, cerebrovascular accident, Parkinson's disease, epilepsy, multiple sclerosis, motor neurone disease and malformations of the nervous system. Age-adjusted mortality rates for these disorders were studied.

Cerebral tumours were evenly distributed apart from a higher rate in Israel and lower rates in Mexico, Chile, and Japan. Whether these were genuine or artefactual observations was very doubtful. There was a striking similarity in the rates for cerebrovascular accidents but with an exceptionally high rate for Japan. Paralysis agitans showed a wide range of mortality rates; eight times higher in Australia than in Mexico or Japan, and three times higher in whites than non-whites in the United States of America. For epilepsy there was no significant variation except for relatively higher rates in Columbia, Chile, Portugal, and Mexico. In the case of multiple sclerosis morbidity data have shown that countries in the temperate zone of the Northern Hemisphere tend to have higher rates than those in the tropics and subtropics [FIGS. 3 and 4]. The mortality data in this survey showed the lowest rates in the Philippines, Japan, Mexico, and Colombia; the highest rates were in Scotland and Ireland. Motor neurone disease showed a relatively wide range of variation, lowest in Mexico and highest in the Netherlands.

The interpretation of data of this kind is at present not possible. Differences in diagnosis and reporting methods are known to exist but it would be surprising if continuing analysis did not reveal differences that are genuine.

Cerebral Tumours

In Africa cerebral tumours are now being diagnosed more frequently. Gelfand (1957*a*) in *The Sick African* said that 'it is my experience, that glioma of the brain appears to be uncommon in the native'. Trowell (1960) in his book *Non-infective Disease in Africa* wrote that 'there is a curious but unexplained infrequency of gliomas among the Bantu in South Africa, so that meningiomas are actually more common'. But with the development of modern diagnostic facilities at university hospitals such as those in Makerere, Ibadan, Salisbury, and Dakar, there are indications that cerebral tumours may not be so uncommon in the African. At Makerere, Uganda, Billinghurst (1966) reported 57 intracranial tumours in the years 1953–65, of which 28 were primary neoplasms (gliomas 17; meningiomas 5). From Ibadan, Nigeria, Odeku and Janota (1967) analysed 46 intracranial space-occupying lesions in the years 1962–65. Primary neoplasms formed 80 per cent of the series; there were 20 gliomas and 11 meningiomas. In Dakar, Senegal, Collomb and his colleagues (1963) noted an increase in tumour diagnosis from 5 in 1959 to 16 in 1962. Levy, in Salisbury, Rhodesia, recounts his experiences as a neurosurgeon in CHAPTER 19 page 225. His figures clearly show that primary cerebral tumour in the East African native is not uncommon but that meningiomas comprise a higher percentage than in the European patients there. In Johannesburg, 20 years' experience of neurosurgical lesions led Froman and Lipschitz (1970) to conclude that cerebral gliomas were very rare in the African population. They found only 213 patients with primary intracranial tumours in the 20-year period 1949–68. Meningiomas comprised no less than 30 per cent and gliomas 16 per cent of the series. The rarest tumour was the acoustic neuroma; one case. They believe their figures indicate a true low incidence rate of cerebral tumours; it is not a matter of underdiagnosis.

From Bombay we have Dastur and his colleagues' (1968) 13-year analysis of 1000 intracranial space-occupying lesions of which 768 were tumours. Gliomas formed 48 per cent and meningiomas 13 per cent of the tumour series. Ramamurthi (1969 *a*), in Madras, gave an incidence of gliomas as 33 per cent, meningiomas 10 per cent. Neither of these series shows differences of any major character from those of the West, but when analysed on the basis of intracranial masses, rather than primary tumours, we find that there is a very high incidence of tuberculomata in Indian reports, usually 20 per cent to 25 per cent of all cases. Dastur and his colleagues interestingly comment that this high rate of tuberculomata is comparable to that in England half a century ago. In an industrial city like Leeds, for example, tuberculomata formed 34 per cent of intracranial masses found at post-mortem in the years 1910–31 (Garland and Armitage, 1933).

For the present it would be as well to defer judgement on international mortality rates such as those of Doll and his colleagues (1966). They reported low incidence rates for brain tumours in Uganda, Nigeria, Japan, among the Chinese in Singapore, among the Bantu in Johannesburg, and in the West Indies. A personal impression is that neurofibromatosis is commoner in Indian and African hospitals than in the United Kingdom.

Cerebrovascular Disorders

In general, geographical studies of atherosclerosis suggest that lesions appear to develop later in life in the cerebral arteries than in the aorta and coronary arteries (McGill, 1969). Hypertension is common in Africa and India. Cerebral atherosclerosis without hypertension is much less common in Africa than in temperate climates (Edington and Gilles, 1969). In India about 1 per cent of all admissions to large city hospitals are accounted for by cerebrovascular episodes; 75 per cent to 80 per cent of these are due to cerebral thrombosis and embolism (Dalal, 1969). In Bombay, Dalal and his colleagues (1968) found that acute strokes comprised only 4·5 per cent of all medical admissions. They thought that such a low hospital incidence of strokes might to some extent be due to the short life-span of Indians in general; the average is reported to be under 50 years. With increasing longevity the incidence of stroke may approach that of the West.

In Africa, India, and the Far East cerebral complications may arise in children and young adults afflicted with arteritis which mainly involves the aorta and its larger branches. This is an important cause of renovascular hypertension in Asian populations (Ooi, Chen, Toh, and Khoo, 1970). Whether they are of similar aetiology is not known but Edington and Gilles (1969) do not consider that Takayasu's disease and the idiopathic aortitis of the tropics can be distinguished on pathological evidence.

Multiple Sclerosis

A neurological traveller in an antique land will certainly find few cases of multiple sclerosis in hospitals. Although the disease undoubtedly occurs in tropical countries it is distinctly rarer [FIG. 3.] Gelfand (1957 *a*) wrote: 'In my experience it is not seen in the African

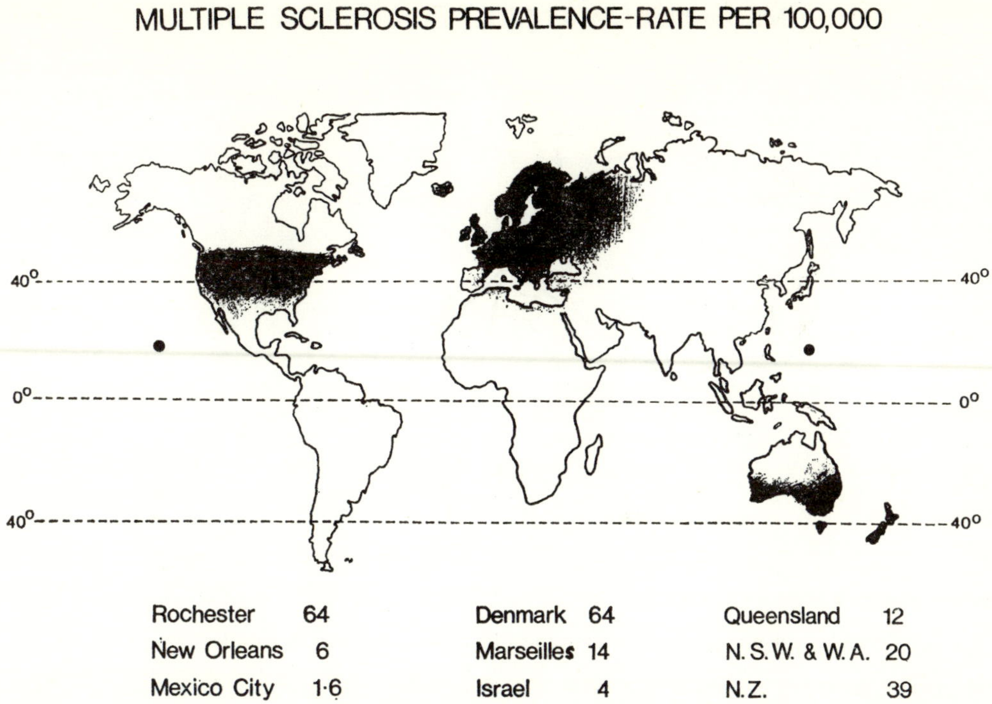

FIG. 3. Multiple sclerosis prevalence rate per 100 000. A high-risk zone is one with a prevalence rate of more than 40 per 100 000 population. There is no such zone between latitudes 40°N and 40°S. In the high-frequency band (30 to 60 per 100 000) are western Europe, the northern United States, and southern Canada. In the medium-frequency band (5 to 15 per 100 000) lie the southern United States, southern Europe and Australia. Low-frequency areas (0 to 4 per 100 000) include Israel, Africa, and Japan. In Hawaii (latitude 19°N) the rate is 8 to 10 per 100 000. In Guam, however (latitude 13°N), no case of multiple sclerosis has been discovered.

native'. No patient has yet been found among South Africa's 11 million Bantu (Dean, 1967). It is not seen in the Zulu (Cosnett, 1964) nor among the Maoris of New Zealand; only one Australian aborigine has been found to be affected (Sutherland, Tyrer, and Eadie, 1962). It is extremely rare in Jamaica; four cases among indigenous Jamaicans at the University College of the West Indies in 10 years (Cruickshank and Montgomery, 1961). In South Africa Dean has shown that the disease is virtually confined to European immigrants. He found that emigration from a high-risk area to South Africa, a low-risk area, does not apparently lessen the risk of developing the disease. In Israel, Alter and his colleagues (1962) and Antonovsky *et al.* (1967) found that Europeans have five to ten times as much multiple sclerosis as do the Afro-Asians living there. It made no difference to the course of the disease if the patient moved from a temperate to a tropical area. That immigrants retain the multiple sclerosis prevalence rate of the country of origin when moving to low-frequency areas is also attested by the studies of Moffie (1966) in the Dutch Antilles [FIG. 4]. In 11 years Moffie met only five cases of multiple sclerosis in Curaçaoan natives, an incidence of 2·86 per 100 000. The rate in Dutch immigrants was 59 per 100 000, similar to that in the Netherlands. Studies in Australia and Tasmania (Saint and Sadka, 1962; Rischbieth, 1966; Sutherland *et al.*, 1966; McCall *et al.*, 1968) and in New Zealand (Hornabrook, 1971) confirm the relationship between latitude and prevalence observed in the Northern Hemisphere but do not appear to indicate that European immigrants have higher rates than native-born Australians.

It will be of vital importance to learn what the immigrant carries with him to a tropical zone that determines his chance of developing the disease. I have seen classical examples of it in Bangkok, Kuala Lumpur, Singapore, in several centres in India, in Nigeria and Brazil, in Peru and Colombia, but everywhere the disease was rarely encountered even by physicians who had had training and experience in Europe or the United States which familiarized them with the features of the disease. Four cases in 6 years were seen in one teaching hospital in Delhi. Six cases in 20 years was the sole experience with the disease of one Calcutta professor.

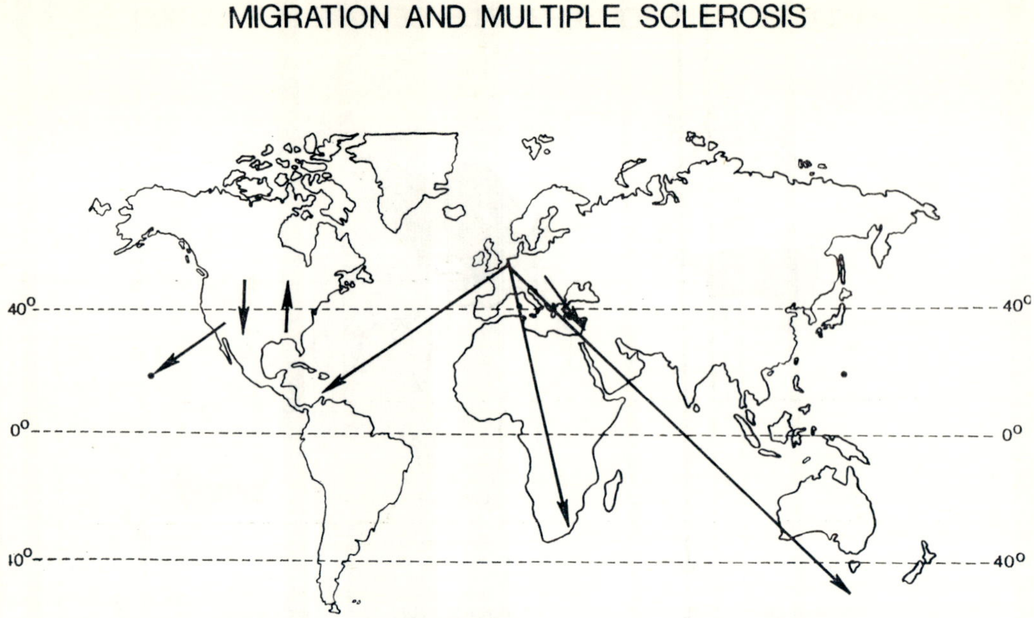

FIG. 4. Migration and multiple sclerosis. Studies in Hawaii, the Dutch Antilles, South Africa, and Israel show that immigrants tend to retain the prevalence rate of their country or state of origin. In Australia, Tasmania and New Zealand, however, it does not appear that European immigrants have higher rates than the native born.

Bharucha and Umarji (1961) were able to collect only 45 cases from three large teaching hospitals in Bombay in the years 1956–60. From 41 medical centres in India they collected a total of 151 accepted cases of the disease. Only 10 centres were able to report any cases.

There is very little published information about multiple sclerosis from Central and South America but from personal inquiries it seems to be much less common than in Europe. In Brazil the mortality rate is said to be only 0·2 per 100 000 as compared with 1·7 to 2·8 per 100 000 in Europe (Käfer and Poch, 1961). In Mexico the prevalence rate is 1·6 per 100 000, one of the lowest reported rates anywhere in the world (Alter and Olivares, 1970).

In the United States, with its climatic differences between north and south, its mixed racial population, and the migration of its citizens, observations of the prevalence of multiple sclerosis are of particular interest. For some time it has been known that rates are high for the northern states and low for the southern states. Death rates for immigrants are similar to those reported for natives of their homeland. Two recent studies may be mentioned. Kurtzke, Kurland, and Goldberg (1971) analysed the deaths attributed to multiple sclerosis for 1959–61 and found an average annual crude death rate of 0·8 per 100 000 population. The latitude 37° North separated the regions of high and low prevalence. This was true for place of birth and residence at death and for those who migrated only within the northern and southern tier. However, for those who were born in the north and died in the south or vice versa, the significant north-south difference in risk disappeared. A comparison of the mortality rates among migrants and non-migrants suggested that residence in the northern states is an important factor in the high risk of multiple sclerosis. The critical age for the acquisition of the disease may be near puberty.

In another study aimed at obtaining an idea when the disease might be acquired, Alter and colleagues (1971) examined the situation in Hawaii. In 1968 the population numbered 778 300 and included 72 per cent non-whites, the largest majority of whom were Orientals. A total of 521 461 were born in Hawaii and 43 per cent of these were Oriental, 16 per cent were Caucasian, 28 per cent were native and mixed Hawaiian, and 13 per cent were mixed Oriental-Caucasian. There were 77 cases of multiple sclerosis and the prevalence was more than five times higher among immigrants to Hawaii than among the Hawaiian born. Ninety-six per cent of the immigrants had migrated after 15 years of age. Again, we have the suggestion that the critical age for the development of the disease is about the time of puberty. As in the Far East, the clinical manifestations in the Orientals showed a higher frequency of retrobulbar neuritis and neuromyelitis optica than is seen in Caucasians.

It is not difficult to see why the concept of a slow virus infection in this disease must be entertained.

Neurosyphilis

With the declining incidence of syphilis in the tropics we may never learn whether the alleged rarity of general paresis and tabes dorsalis was genuine or spurious. Certainly most of the earlier writers on the subject believed that, although syphilis was widespread and that the acute and subacute meningovascular forms were common, the native appeared to be relatively immune from the parenchymatous forms of neurosyphilis which comprised so much of European neurology at the turn of the century. Osler (1909) noted that tabes was uncommon in the American Negro, and in 1930 Turner's analysis of 10 000 American cases showed that parenchymatous neurosyphilis was much less common in the Negro than in the white. General paresis comprised 13·4 per cent of the white and 2·3 per cent of the coloured cases; tabes formed 15·5 per cent of the white and 4·3 per cent of the coloured cases of neurosyphilis. Kinnier Wilson (1940) thought that many of the earlier claims that coloured people were in some way protected 'are proving visionary in the light of advancing knowledge'. He thought that 'native resistance to nervous syphilis is gradually undermined by factors incidental to "civilization" '.

It was Krafft-Ebing, of course, who held that general paresis was a product of 'syphilization and civilization'. There was a firm impression that there was something about modern Western civilization which rendered man especially liable to general paresis if he had acquired syphilis. A typical statement is that of Osler:

> An important predisposing cause is 'a life absorbed in ambitious projects with all its strongest mental effort, its long-sustained anxieties, deferred hopes, and straining expectation' (Mickle). The habits of life so frequently seen in active business men in our large cities, and well expressed by the phrase 'burning the candle at both ends', strongly predispose to the disease.

Pierre Marie (1895) was probably nearer the mark when, commenting on the higher incidence of parenchymatous neurosyphilis in the professional classes, he asked, 'Is it excessive use of the brain? Perhaps, but is it not more probably inconsiderate and indiscreet activity of the feelings?' Clergymen, he noted, were the only members of the professional classes who seemed rarely affected. Canadian lumberjacks were thought to be prone to tabes dorsalis and aortic aneurysm, rather than general paresis, because their labours were more physical than intellectual. Merritt, Adams, and Solomon (1946) referred to Edinger's stress theory which he formulated to explain why the spirochaete should in one case attack the frontal lobes and in another the posterior columns of the cord. It was suggested that excessive use might weaken a structure and so render it more liable to spirochaetal attack. The postman gets tabes and the thinker develops general paresis.

Kraepelin (1913) in his classic monograph on general paresis was puzzled by the lack of evidence of its existence in Europe in the eighteenth century, and by the manner in which syphilis itself had changed during the nineteenth century. He quoted Moebius' observation that no contemporary of the eighteenth century had described paretic symptoms in any prominent man, although, as a matter of fact, many of them had suffered from mental disease. By contrast, there were many well-known men of the nineteenth century who had succumbed to the disease—Schumann, Donizetti, Nietzsche, and Maupassant, for example. Kraepelin thought that during the ninteenth century syphilis had changed from an acute severe disease to a comparatively mild infection. He was aware of the 'extraordinary differences in its [general paresis] frequency in different countries. Paresis is apparently unknown in East Africa, Uganda, Zanzibar, Cameroon and certain Pacific islands whereas it was known in Cuba, Jamaica and British Guiana'. Kraepelin himself could not find a single case in Java.

He thought that if it were true that syphilis existed in a population for generations before the appearance of general paresis then 'it is still impending in the case of those nations in which syphilis has only appeared recently'.

It is possible that conceptions of this kind may have influenced opinion on the vulnerability of the native to parenchymatous neurosyphilis. Textbooks of tropical medicine have usually taught that general paresis and tabes are rare in natives. Thus, in 1966, it is said that 'tabes and general paresis are seldom observed in Central Africa and the Pacific islands and are excessively rare in West Africa and India' (Manson-Bahr, 1966). European textbooks of neurology teach likewise: 'In many tropical and subtropical countries where syphilis is rife general paresis is almost unknown amongst the natives' (Brain and Walton, 1969). How true is all this? If we turn to the writings of physicians and pathologists working in the tropics in recent times we find that there has never been any doubt about the frequency of the meningovascular forms, but that whereas general paresis does occur, tabes must be very rare.

Davies (1947 *b*), in Uganda, found evidence of syphilis in 11 per cent (338 cases) of a series of nearly 3000 autopsies. Eighty-four of these 338 cases had been patients in the Mulago Mental Hospital. There were 154 (44 per cent) who showed signs of neurosyphilis; 72 had general paresis; 28 a meningovascular form. There were no cases of tabes. Davies concluded that apart from the absence of tabes 'neurosyphilis in Africans fairly closely resembles neurosyphilis in Europeans, though the process is possibly more acute'.

Hutton (1956) analysed the medical admissions to the Mulago General Hospital, 1947–52, and found 727 neurological cases. Neurosyphilis was responsible for 166 of these; meningovascular 109; general paresis 57. There were no cases of tabes. Hutton commented on the acuteness and severity of many of the cases of paresis.

Gelfand (1957 *a*) recorded that the serum WR was negative in 81 per cent of 1500 consecutive adult admissions to Salisbury Hospital, Rhodesia. But 'neurosyphilis is by no means uncommon. . . . Although tabes and general paresis are encountered in the African, yet it is extraordinary how infrequent they are compared with the much higher incidence of meningovascular syphilis.' General paresis was 'uncommon'; tabes was 'rarely seen; some deny its existence'. Trowell (1960), after 30 years in Africa, thought that tabes was very rare in all parts of the continent but that general paresis accounted for some 20 per cent of admissions to one mental hospital.

Billington (1966) observed a striking decline in the role of syphilis in neurology from a study of the Mulago Hospital statistics. Neurosyphilis accounted for 0·3 per cent of admissions during 1937–41 and only 0·036 per cent during 1960–64. There were 111 cases of neurosyphilis (18 GPI) in the first period and only 19 (4 GPI) in the second period. There was only one case of tabes in the whole 10-year study. A modern statement from the pathology laboratory has it that 'there is nothing remarkable in its [syphilis] pathology in the tropics, apart from the fact that tabes dorsalis is said to be rare' (Edington and Gilles, 1969).

From India we read that 'there is an erroneous impression that dementia paralytica is very rare in the tropics. In a recent survey undertaken in a mental hospital in this country with over one thousand in-patients, this disease was found to constitute about 3 per cent of the in-patient population' (Mani, 1969). This writer gives a detailed account of tabes dorsalis but does not mention its incidence in India. Rao, Ranganathan, and Natarajan (1968) write that 'general paresis is quite prevalent in India . . . clinical studies by Indian workers have testified to its appreciable incidence among the mentally ill population'. Rao encountered 25 cases in the 3 years 1965–67 in a hospital in Madurai. Brain biopsy was performed in four of them; the characteristic histology was present in each and treponemes were found in three.

In my own travels in the tropics I have always been told that tabes dorsalis is virtually unknown.

It has often been suggested that some degree of immunity to neurosyphilis may result from exposure to febrile states such as malaria and relapsing fever. It was, after all, the observation that fever seemed to have a therapeutic benefit in neurosyphilis that induced Wagner-Jaurreg (1922) to try the effect of malaria 50 years ago. He found it much more effective than relapsing fever. Another theory was that some strains of spirochaete were not neurotropic. But nothing has come of these conjectures and general experience has been that the white man can acquire these diseases from spirochaetes resident in all climates. I have seen classical tabes with severe optic atrophy in a young white woman whose husband acquired syphilis in West Africa.

Subarachnoid Haemorrhage

During a ward round in the Prasat Neurological Hospital in Bangkok, some years ago, two out of three patients who had suffered an acute subarachnoid haemorrhage proved to have angiomas, not aneurysms, on angiography. I was informed that angiomas were more commonly found than aneurysms. No figures were available but subsequent inquiries in other Bangkok centres and in Malaya tended to confirm this evidence. Chitanondh (1965) thought that the ratio was about 4 angiomas to 1 aneurysm. Selby, at the Neurosurgical Unit in Kuala Lumpur, thought that his experience pointed to a ratio of 6 or 7 to 1, in favour of angiomas. Inquiries in Indian neurological centres did not disclose such a high proportion of angiomas, but in most centres subarachnoid haemorrhage appeared to be less common that in the West and angiomas were more frequently diagnosed. Ramamurthi (1969 *b*), from the neurosurgical centre in Madras, reports on the rarity of bleeding aneurysms in India. Between 1958 and 1969 there were only 39 cases of acute subarachnoid haemorrhage; 20 were due to aneurysms and 19 to angiomas. From his neurosurgical department in Bombay, Dastur (1970) reports that in the 13 years 1957–70 cerebral angiography in 89 patients, nearly all with subarachnoid haemorrhage, showed that in 33 there was an aneurysm and in 36 an angioma; in 20 the angiogram was normal. Only a few of these 89 cases presented with focal signs without haemorrhage. Over the same period there were 42 admissions because of primary intracerebral haemorrhage.

It does seem, therefore, that in these countries angiomata play a greater role in the aetiology of subarachnoid haemorrhage than they do in the West. In the United Kingdom aneurysm is nine or ten times as common as angioma in subarachnoid haemorrhage (Brain and Walton, 1969). More statistics are required to determine the incidence of subarachnoid haemorrhage in various areas of the tropics.

Anterior Encephaloceles

In recent years the varying geographical distribution of malformations of the nervous system has attracted attention. Hydrocephalus and spina bifida are seen in all tropical countries, but cranium bifidum may be commoner in some areas than spina bifida. In the West the ratio of spina bifida to cranium bifidum is about 7 to 1 (Schwidde, 1952). In South Wales the ratio of spinal to cranial dysraphic lesions is 14 to 1 (Laurence, 1970). There were 425 cases in the years 1956–62; 28 cranial and 397 spinal malformations.

Some years ago I was shown two children with anterior (fronto-ethmoidal) encephaloceles in a Bangkok hospital. It seemed to be commoner than spina bifida there. Suwanwela and Hongsaprabhas (1966) found that in their medical school they had had 25 cases of anterior encephalocele in 3 years, during which period there were ten spinal and three occipital meningoceles. Suwanwela (1969) believes that there is an unusually high incidence of anterior encephaloceles in South-East Asia, including Thailand, Malaysia, and Indonesia. A less marked incidence was reported from North Africa and Northern India. It is rare in the West, Japan, China, and Southern India. Suwanwela has now collected 72 cases in Bangkok; blood group and chromosome studies showed no unusual deviation. In a population survey in a limited area in Northern Thailand an incidence of nine cases of anterior encephalocele were found in a total population of 31 582, i.e. approximately 1:3500 (Flatz and Sukthomya, 1970).

From Delhi, Tandon (1970) reports 40 encephaloceles of which 11 were of the anterior and 24 of the posterior variety. In Casablanca, Acquaviva and colleagues (1965) also found a higher incidence of anterior encephaloceles than in Europe and North America.

These observations suggest that there is a genuine variation in the geographical distribution of these congenital malformations, and both genetic and environmental factors may play a role.

MALNUTRITION

In the Western world defective diet no longer plays any significant role in the aetiology of disorders of the nervous system. The outbreaks of beriberi and pellagra in the asylums and institutions at the turn of the century actually subsided before the precise causes of these disorders were discovered. Takaki in the Japanese naval training ship *Ringio*, and Goldberger in the Rankin prison farm in Mississippi eradicated beriberi and pellagra respectively because they did not accept the evidence of contagion, a theory which was an almost inevitable reflection of the golden years of bacteriology. With their own eyes they saw that 'official' rations were poor. They were field naturalists with an ecological approach; one that remains so important today. Fraser Darling (1970) writes: 'I have a feeling that the microscope and the discovery of bacterial and protozoal infections sent medicine into the laboratory to the detriment of that special medical capacity of grasping the larger field of the environment.'

Beriberi, a disease which could be wiped out, remains a major health hazard in the Far East (Williams, 1961). In the Philippines it still ranks as the fourth leading cause of death, exceeded only by pneumonia, tuberculosis, and bronchitis. Yet, writes Salcedo (1962), 'It is rare for a medical student to see a case of beriberi in hospital wards in Manila and other metropolitan centres . . . beriberi is not disappearing, nor is its severity diminishing'. What has changed in the Philippines is the pattern of distribution of the disease; 84 per cent of the population is rural.

The dementing pellagrin is seen in maize-eating populations of Africa, India and South America [PLATE 6c and d]. Over 30 years ago Kinnier Wilson (1940) wrote of pellagra: 'Someone has asked what can be the common factor when a woman in the Orkney islands, an Egyptian peasant, a small boy in London, a lunatic in an English asylum, a native in Nyasaland, and a governess in a well-to-do family in the southern United States, all suffer from Pellagra?' We now know that the answer is a deficiency of nicotinic acid, which serves to recall the words of Herbert Spencer that 'it is a truth perpetually that accumulated facts lying in disorder begin to assume some order when an hypothesis is thrown among them'.

Lathyrism, epidemic spastic paraplegia, is still common in parts of India. It results from excessive consumption of *Lathyrus sativus*. No better account of the ravages of this ancient disease can be found than that by Sleeman (1844) in his *Rambles and Recollections of an Indian Official:*

> In 1829 the wheat and other spring crops in this and the surrounding villages were destroyed by a severe hailstorm; in 1830 they were deficient from the want of seasonable rains: and in 1831 they were destroyed by blight. During these three years the 'teori' or what in other parts of India is called 'kesari' (*L. sativus*) a kind of wild vetch which, though not sown itself, is left carelessly to grow among the wheat and other grain, and given in the green and dry state to cattle, remained uninjured and thrived with great luxuriance. In 1831 they reaped a rich crop of it from the blighted wheat fields and subsisted upon its grain during that and the following years, giving the stalks and leaves only to their cattle. In 1833 the sad effects of this food began to manifest themselves. The younger part of the population of this and the surrounding villages, from the age of thirty downwards, began to be deprived of the use of their limbs below the waist by paralytic strokes, in all cases sudden, but in some cases more severe than in others. About half the youth of this village of both sexes became affected during the years 1833 and 1834 and many of them have lost the use of their lower limbs entirely, and are unable to move. . . . Since the year 1834 no new case has occurred; but no person once attacked has been found to recover the use of limbs affected; and my tent was surrounded by great numbers of the youth in different stages of the disease, imploring my advice and assistance under this dreadful visitation.

In some parts of Central India 4 per cent of the rural population is affected by lathyrism (Berry, 1969) [PLATE 7b]; a poor monsoon is usually followed by an epidemic. 'All individuals who obtain more than one-quarter of their calorie intake from *Lathyrus sativus*, are liable to get lathyrism.'

These diseases, and perhaps others, would disappear if the new high-yielding varieties of wheat, corn, rice, sorghum and millets, in association with modern farming and distribution techniques, became generally available in the overpopulated areas of the world. Such activities are beyond the province of a neurologist working in the tropics, but the role of malnutrition in the growth and development of the nervous system, and its relationship to the obscure spinal cord disorders which have been described in many tropical countries, are well within his field of study.

In tropical Africa the main crops are banana, cassava, sweet potato, maize, pawpaw, and beans. These crops are not indigenous to Africa; they come from South America and Asia. Indeed, the tropical forests of Africa have not produced a single important plant that can be cultivated for food. In Central India 94 per cent of female patients and 74 per cent of male patients attending a teaching hospital had total plasma proteins of less than 69 per 100 ml (Madan and Berry, 1964). Protein deficiency is the main cause of malnutrition in the tropics, and in kwashiorkor we have a disease of infants which is so widespread that one wonders what effect it may have on the potential of communities [Plate 9a].

The Infant

Kwashiorkor [Plate 9a], all observers agree, not only retards growth but exerts a profound effect on the mental state of the infant or child. There is abject misery and apathy; 'a smile may be the first sign of improvement'. There are no frank neurological signs or sequelae and at autopsy the cardinal changes are seen in the liver, intestines, pancreas, and muscles. But what of the brain? Its growth is normally ahead of most other organs of the body. Synthesis of new proteins continues during the first few years of life at a rate corresponding to the rapid increase in weight of the brain. It is not difficult to believe that severe protein-calorie malnutrition in the first year of life may limit the potential of mental development. But malnutrition of the human foetus and infant is usually found in circumstances where other adverse factors are at work, so that it becomes exceedingly difficult to determine the consequences of one particular disturbance. A stunted schoolchild of poor intelligence may have had infantile malnutrition, but he may also have parents who are poorly endowed, he may be anaemic or infected, and he has probably grown up in an environment where full mental development is improbable. To isolate these influences so that they may be analysed is wellnigh impossible, although interesting attempts continue to be made. It is here that one envies the position of the animal experimentalist, for he can study the effects of malnutrition on the developing nervous system of the suckling rat or pig and compare the results with normally nourished members of the litter. But whereas the animal experimentalist can use very elaborate methods to study the effects of malnutrition on the biochemistry of brain, the techniques for examining the behavioural consequences are much less precise. On the other hand, the field worker among malnourished children is in the opposite position.

Two important reviews on the possible late effects of infantile malnutrition on the development of the human nervous system are those of Winick (1969) and Eichenwald and Fry (1969). Recent experimental studies in rats on the effect of neonatal malnutrition on the developing cerebrum are reported by Bass, Netsky, and Young (1970). The Ciba Foundation Symposium, *Lipids, Malnutrition and the Developing Brain* (1972), is an authoritative statement of one aspect of this vital subject.

In all mammalian species the brain approaches its adult weight long before growth has ceased. In the rat and pig it has been shown that early malnutrition reduces the brain weight (Widdowson, Dickerson, and McCance, 1960; Dobing, 1964). The earlier the malnutrition, the more severe the effect and the less likely recovery. Does this happen in the malnourished human infant? There is some evidence that it does. In Uganda, Brown (1965) found that malnutrition in infancy and early chilhood does lead to a decreased brain weight. His conclusion was based on an analysis of 1100 autopsies in children from birth to 15 years of age. The mean brain weights were significantly lower in malnutrition.

Moreover, Stoch and Smythe (1968) found a reduced head circumference in Cape-coloured children in South Africa when there had been gross malnutrition in the first year of life. Their investigations included the study of a matched control group. Does head growth normally reflect brain growth? The studies of Winick and Rosso (1969 *a* and *b*) show that during the first year of life increase in head circumference is a good measure of brain growth. They found that it accurately reflects the growth pattern (weight, protein synthesis and DNA content) during this time and that, moreover, severe malnutrition retards this growth. Their malnourished brains were from Chilean infants. Here, then, is a useful clinical tool which, if generally confirmed, would aid in the recognition and assessment of nutritional deprivation of the brain. (Crounce, Bollet, and Owens (1970) find that a simple DNA test of human hair will detect early protein deficiency.)

It has recently been observed that cranial suture diastasis may occur, apparently as a result of rapid brain growth, in marasmic infants and children when treatment is undertaken (Capitanio and Kirkpatrick, 1969; Sondheimer, Grossman, and Winchester, 1970). It is thought that the sutures spread because the skull growth or ossification is not commensurate with the rapid brain growth.

In the adult human brain, one-half of the lipids are built into myelin, with a preponderance of cerebrosides and cholesterol. Gangliosides occur mainly in the neuronal and synaptic structures. The normal processes of myelination in the nervous system of the experimental animal are disturbed by malnutrition. Myelin is a complex lipid made up of a number of components: some 70 per cent of total rat brain cholesterol sulphatides and sphingomyelin is present in myelin (Winick, 1969). Nearly all cerebroside in the rat brain appears to be located in myelin. Analysis of these substances will reflect the amount of myelin in brain. The period of myelination varies in different species and indeed in different parts of the nervous system. Once formed and laid down myelin is a relatively stable substance metabolically, although some recycling of sterols does seem to occur. About 70 per cent of the dry weight of separated myelin is lipid; 30 per cent is protein. The stability of myelin increases with age.

The myelin content of the brain may be reduced only during the period of myelination. It has been shown that malnutrition of the suckling rat or pig impairs myelination if it occurs at the critical time of rapid myelination (Dobbing and Widdowson, 1965; Davison and Dobbing, 1966). Thus, there is a 'vulnerable' or 'sensitive' period when brain development, as measured by myelination, may be seriously impaired by malnutrition. Chase, Dorsey, and McKhann (1967) have used the synthesis of sulphatides as a biochemical marker for myelin formation. Early malnutrition of the rat reduced its formation; it could not be corrected by refeeding.

Whether myelination is reduced in early human malnutrition is not known. Winick (1969) believes it is, because the brain weight is reduced and because other animal studies have shown that not only myelin content but also cell number and DNA content are affected by early malnutrition.

The formation of myelin and the insults which may disturb it are only one aspect of the problem of retarded development of the human brain. Dobbing (1971) points out that formation of nerve cells is essentially a prenatal process, whereas multiplication of glia is perinatal. The ramification of dendrites, establishment of synaptic connexions and the process of myelination are postnatal growths. Infantile malnutrition may have more subtle effects than amyelination. A deficiency of synaptic growth may, in the end, be more important than slightly fewer layers of insulating sheath.

These morphological and biochemical studies of the malnourished developing brain have been supported by investigations of the physical and mental activity of animals and children who were malnourished in infancy. The studies of Cravioto, de Licardie, and Birch (1966) in Mexico and Guatemala, and those of Cobos (1972) in Colombia, suggest that malnutrition can be identified as one factor in the aetiology of human retardation. Malnutrition before the age of 6 months may result in damage to the intellect which may be permanent (Cravioto and Robles, 1965). The clinical estimates in these studies of native children in Central America have included the use of the Gesell and Griffiths Infant Scales of mental development and the André-Thomas techniques for neuromotor assessment. The evidence is impressive.

Commenting on the whole question of malnutrition and brain development, Winick (1969), reviewing his own experience and that of others, both animal and human, writes: 'The evidence is becoming more and more weighty that malnutrition in infancy permanently affects the minds of the children who have been afflicted'. If it can be shown that the educability of such children has been impaired, then certainly malnutrition has left its mark on the brain.

The complexity of the problem has been stressed by many, including the geneticist. In a symposium entitled 'Relation of Nutrition to Central Nervous System Development and Function', Witkop (1967) commented on the slight build of the Vietnamese and wondered whether this phenotype had been selected as the most efficient under periods of starvation. There is a genetic regulation of protein synthesis. Many, including Graham (1967), have commented on the physical growth of the Japanese race which has taken place in recent decades; it has far outstripped their supposed genetic potential. Their environment has changed as much in a nutritional way as in any other.

When we learn that two-thirds of the children under 5 years of age in Colombia, some 2 million children, are malnourished (Cobos, 1972) the immensity of this problem throughout the third world can be envisaged.

The Adult

Whether malnutrition plays a role in the ataxic and spastic paraplegias which have been described in tropical countries in recent years is another intriguing question (Spillane, 1969). There is little doubt that the syndromes described and reviewed by Stannus (1936) from Africa, India and the Far East were manifestations of malnutrition [PLATES 7a, c and d, 8a]. So also were the disorders that arose in prisoner-of-war camps during the Second World War (Spillane, 1947). Cruickshank (1956), in Jamaica, considered that the cases he encountered there were 'virtually the same' as he had previously encountered in Changi prisoner-of-war camp in Singapore [PLATE 8b and c]. Collomb and his colleagues (1967), in Senegal, believe their cases are due to defective nutrition. Osuntokun (1968) has presented evidence that the Nigerian neuropathies are related to the high consumption of cassava (manioc). Moore (1934 *a* and *b*) had come to the opinion that retrobulbar neuropathy in Nigerian children was related to the cassava in their diet. Gelfand (1957*b*) noted that Livingstone, travelling in Angola in 1855, mentioned deterioration of vision in natives living on a predominantly cereal diet. I was interested to discover that Livingstone (1857) actually incriminated cassava [PLATE 4]. He wrote:

> The chief vegetable food is the manioc and lotsa meal. These contain a very large proportion of starch, and when eaten alone for any length of time, produce most distressing heartburn. As we ourselves experienced in coming north, they also cause a weakness of vision, which occurs in the case of animals fed on pure gluten or amylaceous material. I now discovered that when these starchy substances are eaten along with a proportion of

> groundnuts, which contain a considerable quantity of oil, no injurious effects follow.

The neurometabolic consequences of a primitive diet may be a question of deficiency or toxicity or both. The biochemical lesion responsible for the neurological complaint may be the outcome of several factors. The distinction between deficiency and toxicity is not a fundamental one. What Peters (1963) has described as 'lethal synthesis' may well be relevant to the aetiology of some of these disorders. He coined the term when he discovered that the fluoroacetate of a plant that poisons cattle in the Transvaal makes use of the enzyme machinery of the body to convert itself by synthesis into a very toxic fluorocitric acid. The example of lathyrism is so striking that it may prove to be a key problem; its solution may lead to other things.

The lesson of beriberi must not be forgotten. In recent decades I doubt whether there has been a concept more fundamental or rewarding than that formulated by Peters in 1963, which he entitled the 'biochemical lesion'. It gave a new impetus to medical research and was a catalyst of neurochemical thought. Yet this chapter of medical history really began in the Dutch East Indies with the struggle against beriberi. The gist of it is recounted here as it so well illustrates my theme.

It was Jacob Bontius (1592–1631), dying in Java after 4 years' service there, who made known the disease of beriberi to the physicians of the Western Hemisphere. His *De Medicina Indorum* may be taken as the first book on tropical medicine. He suffered from the disease himself and he may well have also described nutritional amblyopia.

Although there were suggestions that a poor diet was in some way associated with beriberi it was not until the studies of Eijkman, in the 1890s, that a connexion with rice was appreciated. He was the first director of the Batavian Institute of Pathology founded in 1887 and 10 years later he published his famous paper 'A Beri-Beri-like Disease,' proving that the paralysis which afflicted fowls in his laboratory, and in local prisons and hospitals, was identical with human beriberi. Many modern references to his work imply that he first observed that fowls fed on refuse rice developed paralysis. This way of putting it is not only inaccurate but, tersely and unimaginatively, devalues the lesson that is there. His first studies on the fowl paralysis were directed at its nature. He proved that the fundamental pathology was a polyneuritis and that the cardiac musculature was often involved. He eventually recognized that the disease, clinically and pathologically, was the same as human beriberi.

Eijkman searched for a cause—bacteria or parasite—and found none. Then, he wrote, 'a chance circumstance' threw suspicion on the fowls' feed. The onset and cessation of the epidemic in the fowls, which lasted 6 months, coincided respectively with the introduction of refuse, cooked, polished rice and its subsequent replacement with raw whole grain. Next came the experiments which proved that the polishings contained a substance which cured the fowls. Eijkman's work indicated how beriberi could be prevented and cured.

No less instructive in this narrative is the nature of medical reaction to his studies, for they were doubted and questioned for a decade. It was the hey-day of the infective origin of disease. This new work did not fit in with any current concept of pathogenesis. The germ and toxic theory of the origin of beriberi was entrenched; it was affirmed by many notable authorities of the day. Manson, in his presidential address to the Epidemiological Society of London in 1901, entitled 'The Aetiology of Beriberi' was not impressed by Eijkman's theory. 'The disease', he said, 'is purely an intoxication produced by a toxin elaborated by a germ.' In Osler's *Principles and Practice of Medicine* of 1909 (7th ed.) the germ and food theories received equal notice, and the latter offered no hint that something might be *wanting* in a rice diet; toxins, organismal or hypothetical, were the supposed alternatives.

Today, in the old Government Institute of Medical Research, in Kuala Lumpur, there is a plaque commemorating the work of Fraser and Stanton there in 1909, which finally showed that human beriberi responded in the same way as that of Eijkman's birds.

From that time it was the turn of the biochemists. In 1911, Funk, who died in 1967, prepared an extract from rice pericarp which was therapeutically active and he coined the word 'vitamines' for those substances which, by their absence, were responsible for the diseases of beriberi, scurvy, rickets and pellagra. The antiberiberi factor was subsequently isolated in 1926, synthesized in 1936 and named thiamine.

Thiamine-deficient pigeons developed head retraction and opisthotonus, and Peters, writing in 1969, said:

> Like others, I tried, fruitlessly, various procedures in the attempt to show up biochemical changes in the muscles of the avitaminous pigeons. The problem did not progress until I decided that the head retraction might be central in origin, and that the proper course was to study the brain and to take no notice of the usual description of the condition as 'avian polyneuritis'.

From these studies he conceived of the *biochemical lesion*—the 'biochemical change or defect which directly precedes pathological change or dysfunction'. In this instance the change was in pyruvate metabolism. This metabolite accumulated in the avitaminous pigeon brain and in the serum of patients with beriberi and Wernicke's encephalopathy; it disappeared on the administration of thiamine. 'This was the first time that an action of a vitamin *in vitro* had been discovered' (Peters, 1963). 'It was a lucky circumstance that this work developed with thiamine and the pigeon's brain, as this vitamin and tissue show the biochemical lesion better than any other yet found' (Peters, 1962). Perhaps so. 'The casual felicity of particular events' is not to be relied upon but, as Medawar has stated, 'an episode or scientific discovery begins with the plain and unembroidered evidence of the senses—with innocent, unprejudiced observation'.

Wernicke's encephalopathy may be cited as another example of a disorder whose aetiology was unravelled following an observation on a 'tropical' disease. The clinical and pathological features of Wernicke's encephalopathy were described in 1881. It was usually encountered in chronic alcoholics and occasionally in hyperemesis gravidarum and in terminal cachectic states. It was not until 1934 that the first aetiological clue was reported. There was a disease of Japanese and Philippine infants called 'breast-milk intoxication' about which opinions differed widely. Some thought it was a distinct disease, others that it was a form of infantile beriberi. Tanaka (1934) noted that in addition to gastrointestinal symptoms and stupor many infants showed signs of brain-stem lesions. These were crossed paralyses, ocular palsies, nystagmus, ataxia, and opisthotonus. Post-mortem on one case revealed vascular lesions in the brain stem which Tanaka recognized as similar to those of Wernicke's encephalopathy. The curious thing is that in the literature of Oriental beriberi, Wernicke's encephalopathy is the missing witness.

In that same year, 1934, Prickett observed that rats made deficient of vitamin B_1 developed focal vascular lesions in the brain stem. He did not notice any similarity to the Wernicke lesions. This splendid observation was made 4 years later by Alexander, Pijoan, and Myerson (1938) and they were quickly able to produce the characteristic Wernicke lesions in thiamine-deficient pigeons.[3] Subsequent studies confirmed the value of thiamine in the treatment of the disorder, and after the Second World War, with its grim Far East prisoner-of-war experience, Wernicke's encephalopathy came to be regarded as cerebral beriberi.

NEUROLOGY IN THE TROPICS

In the foregoing pages I have outlined the ways in which clinical experience in tropical zones has contributed to general medical knowledge and how neurological studies are beginning to suggest lines of research. This Introduction is a personal one, based mainly on observations and impressions gleaned on tropical forays, on reading, and influenced by the belief that the subject is one which lends itself to the historical and ecological approach.

I am conscious that this chapter could be written in other ways and indeed the whole book organized in a different fashion. But I wished to portray, as far as possible, the neurological scene in the tropics and to indicate some of its fascinations. The modern periodeutas knows only too well how descent on a medical centre too frequently deteriorates into an inspection of the latest facilities, architectural and electronic, with a retina-detaching nocturnal examination of a bundle of reprints. I once spent several days in a teaching hospital in a tropical country and saw not one patient. And yet the ward remains the place of greatest interest and what one sees there is the very warp and woof of medicine. The symptoms and signs of paraplegia, tetraplegia, ophthalmoplegia, stupor, fits and coma may be substantially similar everywhere, but their causes vary widely in different parts of the world. The so-called tropical paraplegias are already presenting formidable problems to the nosographer and researcher.

Lest my fascination with the subject should tire the reader, let me here say what I believe should be the aims of the neurologist in the tropics. (Napoleon Bonaparte said that he always 'measured his dreams with the calipers of reason'.) There are three main aims. *First*, we need to learn the incidence of all those well-known diseases of the nervous system described in the classical literature. *Secondly*, we need to learn their natural history. Are there differences in their modes of onset and course? What are the possible effects of climate, diet, infection, customs, and genetic factors? *Thirdly*, any new, or apparently new, neurological syndrome or disease should be documented in the classical manner of earlier nosographers using the method of clinico-pathological correlation which has served so well in the past.

Is trigeminal neuralgia uncommon in the African? And migraine and Ménière's syndrome? What is the explanation for recurrent painful ophthalmoplegia in the Indian? (In South Wales I have only seen it in an Indian doctor and a Hong Kong cook.) What is the nature of the so-called infantile tremor syndrome in India [PLATE 5b], a striking and unmistakable clinical picture which I have never seen nor heard described in the West? Why is congenital atlanto-axial dislocation so often observed as a cause of myelopathy in Bombay? Why does the pineal gland calcify less frequently in Thailand and Malaya than in the West? What is the real distribution of gliomas and meningiomas in the tropics? Are intracranial angiomata commoner in Asia? Are bleeding intracranial aneurysms rarer in India? Why is tabes dorsalis so rare in areas where syphilis is common? Why is subacute combined degeneration so rare in the tropics? And, most puzzling of all, why the rarity of multiple sclerosis in Africa, India, South-East Asia, and Latin America?

Then there are the foci of neurological disorders throughout the tropics—myelopathies of mysterious origin in Jamaica, Nigeria, Senegal, and South India; amyotrophic lateral sclerosis and parkinsonism-dementia syndromes in Guam, and kuru in New Guinea.

[3]This historical paper was read at a meeting of the American Neurological Association in Atlantic City, New Jersey, in May, 1938. The writer was present and can recall the brief, dry nature of the presentation and the almost complete lack of discussion.

Who would have imagined, 10 years ago, that a fatal form of cerebellar degeneration, kuru, would be linked with cannibalism?[4] Is this disease, virtually confined to one tribe in a remote location and already disappearing, only going to be of historical interest—a 'virus' that came and went? What will be the outcome of the discovery of its transmissibility to the ape? Will there be other human brain 'degenerations', like the Creutzfeldt-Jakob disease, which will be transmissible? Is the concept of the 'slow virus' going to be as important to neurology as was the 'biochemical lesion'? Is the virus of Burkitt's lymphoma going to be, in Himsworth's words, a 'Rosetta stone for cancer research'?

It is as well to recall that it was the Health Section of the ill-fated League of Nations which was the most successful and non-controversial part of that organization. Evang (1967) has reminded us that health was 'forgotten' when the Covenant of the League was drafted after the First World War. Only at the last moment was world health brought in. The United Nations Organization, the League's successor, has designated the seventies as the 'Second Development Decade'. Medicine has a role in the developing world of immeasurable consequence and neurology, by its very nature, is in a unique position to contribute. As the late Lord Brain once wrote, 'In one important respect neurology differs from all other branches of physiology and of medicine; it is concerned with that part of the human organism which is most distinctively human.'

References

ACKERKNECHT, E. W. (1965) *History and Geography of the Most Important Diseases*, New York.

ACQUAVIVA, K., TAMIC, P. M., BRU, P., LEBASCLE, J., and KERDOUDI, H. (1965) Anterior basal meningoencephaloceles: observations on 39 personal cases, *Excerpta Medi. (Amst.), Int. Cong. Ser.*, 93, 165.

[4] It was a social anthropologist (Glasse, 1967) who first suggested that cannibalism was the mode of transmission of the disease kuru. Cannibalism has a long history and the observations of De Rochefort in 1658, in *Histoire Naturelle des Antilles de l'Amerique*, are of interest. The following quotation is taken from P. L. Fermor's *The Traveller's Tree*, p. 114:

> 'De Rochefort reports that a Carib prisoner, while being made ready, would jeer at his captors, saying that, although they would soon be eating him, he had already swallowed so many of their family and tribe, and was so thoroughly nourished on their neighbours and kin, that they would virtually be eating one of their own people. This kind of language would continue until the final blow was delivered. It never failed to exasperate the company, and to cast an atmosphere of dejection over the whole meal.'

No doubt the victim would be further cheered if he knew that his fate might also determine that of his captors.

ALEXANDER, L., PIJOAN, M., and MYERSON, A. (1938) Beriberi and scurvy, *Trans. Amer. neurol. Ass.*, **64**, 135.

ALTER, M., HALPERN, L., KURLAND, L. T., BORNSTEIN, B., LEIBOWITZ, U., and SILBERSTEIN, J. (1962) Multiple sclerosis in Israel: prevalence among immigrants and native inhabitants, *Arch. Neurol. (Chic.)*, **7**, 253.

ALTER, M., OKIHORO, M., ROWLEY, W., and MORRIS, T. (1971) Multiple sclerosis among Orientals and Caucasians in Hawaii, *Neurology (Minneap.)*, 21, 122.

ALTER, M., and OLIVARES, L. (1970) Multiple sclerosis in Mexico, *Arch. Neurol. (Chic.)*, 23, 451.

ANTONOVSKY, A., LEIBOWITZ, V., MEDALIE, J. M., SMITH, H. A., HALPERN, L., and ALTER, M. (1967) Epidemiological study of multiple sclerosis in Israel, *J. Neurol. Psychiat.*, 30, 1.

ASHBURN, P. M. (1947) *The Ranks of Death: A Medical History of the Discovery of America*, Crosby, New York.

BAILEY, O. T., and SMITH, D. E., eds. (1968) *The Central Nervous System; Some Experimental Models of Neurological Diseases*, Baltimore, Md.

BASS, N. H., NETSKY, M. G., and YOUNG, E. (1970) Effect of neonatal malnutrition on developing cerebrum, *Arch. Neurol. (Chic.)*, 23, 289, 303.

BERRY, J. N. (1969) in *Textbook of Medicine*, ed. Vakil, R. J., Association of Physicians of India, Bombay.

BHARUCHA, E. P., and UMARJI, R. M. (1961) *Multiple Sclerosis in India*, paper presented at the Seventh International Congress of Neurology, Rome; quoted by Bharucha, E. P. (1970) *J. Ass. Phycns India*, 18, 43.

BILLINGHURST, J. R., (1966) Intracranial space-occupying lesions in African patients at Mulago Hospital, Kampala, *E. Afr. med. J.*, 43, 385.

BILLINGTON, N. E. (1966) Neurosyphilis in Uganda: a comparison of two five-year periods, *E. Afr. med. J.*, 43, 469.

BRAIN, LORD (1964) in *Doctors Past and Present*, London, p. 139.

BRAIN, LORD, and WALTON, J. N., eds. (1969) *Brain's Diseases of the Nervous System*, 7th ed., London, p. 315.

BROWN, R. E. (1965) Decreased brain weight in malnutrition and its implications, *E. Afr. med. J.*, 11, 584.

BRYANT, J. (1970) *Health and the Developing World*, Cornell University, Ithaca, N.Y.

CAPITANIO, M. A., and KIRKPATRICK, J. A. (1969) Widening of the cranial sutures; a roentgen observation during periods of accelerated growth in patients treated for deprivation dwarfism, *Radiology*, 92, 53.

CHASE, H. P., DORSEY, J., and MCKHANN, G. M. (1967) The effect of malnutrition on the synthesis of a myelin lipid, *Pediatrics*, 40, 551.

CHITANONDH, H. (1965) Personal communication.

COBOS, F. (1972) Malnutrition and mental retardation; conceptual issues, in *Lipids, Malnutrition, and the Developing Brain*, Ciba Foundation Symposium, Amsterdam, p. 227.

COCKBURN, W. C., and DROZELOW, M. D. (1970) Poliomyelitis in the world, *Bull. Wld Hlth Org.*, 42, 405.

COLLOMB, H., COURSON, B., PHILLIPPE, Y., CARAYON, A., CAMAIN, R., and DUMAS, M. (1963) Tumeurs cérébrales chez l' Africain, *Bull. Soc. méd. Afr. noire Langue franç.*, 8, 261.

COLLOMB, H., QUERRE, M. A., CROS, J., and GIORDANO, C. (1967) The nutritional neuropathies of Senegal, *J. neurol. Sci.*, 5, 159.

COSNETT, J. E. (1964) Neurological disorders in the Zulu, *Neurology (Minneap.)*, **14**, 443.

CRAVIOTO, J., LICARDIE, E. R. DE, and BIRCH, H. G. (1966) Nutrition, growth and neurointegrative development: an experimental and ecologic study, *Pediatrics*, 38 (Suppl.), 2, II.

CRAVIOTO, J., and ROBLES, B. (1965) Evolution of adaptive and motor behaviour during rehabilitation from kwashiorkor, *Amer. J. Orthopsychiat.*, **35**, 449.

CROUNCE, R. G., BOLLET, A. J., and OWENS, S. (1970) Quantitative tissue of human malnutrition using scalp hair roots, *Nature (Lond.)*, **228**, 465.

CRUICKSHANK, E. K. (1956) A neuropathic syndrome of uncertain origin, *W. Indian med. J.*, **5**, 147.

CRUICKSHANK, E. K., and MONTGOMERY, R. D. (1961) Multiple sclerosis in Jamaica, *W. Indian med. J.*, **10**, 211.

DALAL, P. M. (1969) in *Textbook of Medicine*, ed. Vakil, R. J., Association of Physicians of India, Bombay, p. 1135.

DALAL, P. M., SHAH, P. M., AIYAR, R. R., and KIKANI, B. J. (1968) Cerebrovascular diseases in West Central India. A report on angiographic findings from a prospective study, *Brit. med. J.*, **3**, 769.

DARLING, FRASER, F. (1970) Borderlands of medicine and ecology, *Proc. roy. Soc. Med.*, **63**, 1164.

DASTUR, H. M. (1970) Personal communication.

DASTUR, D. K., LALITHA, V. S., and PRABHAKAR, V. (1968) Pathological analysis of intracranial space-occupying lesions in 1000 cases including children, Part I. Age, sex and pattern of the tuberculomas, *J. neurol. Sci.*, **6**, 575.

DAVIES, J. N. P. (1947 *a*) Pathology of Central African natives, *E. Afr. med. J.*, **24**, 352.

DAVIES, J. N. P. (1947 *b*) Pathology of Central African natives; spirochaetal diseases in Uganda, *E. Afr. med. J.*, **24**, 437.

DAVISON, A. N., and DOBBING, J. (1966) Myelination as a vulnerable period in brain development, *Brit. med. Bull.*, **22**, 1.

DEAN, G. (1967) Annual incidence, and mortality of multiple sclerosis in white South African-born and in white immigrants to South Africa, *Brit. med. J.*, **1**, 724.

DICKERSON, J. W. T., and DOBBING, J. (1967) Prenatal and postnatal growth and development of the central nervous system of the pig, *Proc. roy. Soc. B*, **166**, 384.

DOBBING, J. (1964) The influence of early nutrition on the development and myelinations of the brain, *Proc. roy. Soc. B*, **159**, 503.

DOBBING, J. (1971) in *Chemistry and Brain Development*, eds. Paoletti, R., and Davison, A. N., New York, p. 399.

DOBBING, J., and WIDDOWSON, E. M. (1965) The effect of undernutrition and subsequent rehabilitation on myelination of rat brain as measured by its composition, *Brain*, 88, 357.

DOLL, R. (1959) in *Methods of Geographical Pathology*, Oxford, p. 11.

DOLL, R., PAYNE, P., and WATERHOUSE, J. (1966) *Cancer Incidence in Five Continents: A Technical Report*, International Union against Cancer, Berlin.

EDINGTON, G. M., and GILLES, H. M. (1969) in *Pathology in the Tropics*, London.

EICHENWALD, H. F., and FRY, P. C. (1969) Nutrition and learning, *Science*, **163**, 644.

EVANG, K. (1967) *Health of Mankind*, Ciba Foundation Hundredth Symposium, eds. Wolstenholme, G., and O'Connor, M., London.

FLATZ, G., and SUKTHOMYA, C. (1970) Fronto-ethmoidal encophalomeningoceles in the population of Northern Thailand, *Hum. Genet.*, **11**, 1.

FROMAN, C., AND LIPSCHITZ, R. (1970) Demography of tumours of the central nervous system among the Bantu population of the Transvaal, South Africa, *J. Neurosurg.*, **32**, 660.

GARLAND, H. G., and ARMITAGE, J. (1933) Intracranial tuberculosis, *J. Path. Bact.*, **37**, 461.

GELFAND, M. (1957 *a*) *The Sick African*, 3rd ed., Capetown, pp. 565, 583.

GELFAND, M. (1957 *b*) *Livingstone the Doctor: A Study in Medical History*, Oxford, pp. 10, 96.

GLASSE, R. (1967) Cannibalism in the Kuru region of New Guinea, *Trans. N. Y. Acad. Sci.*, **29**, 748.

GOLDBERG, I. D., and KURLAND, L. T. (1962) Mortality in 33 countries from diseases of the nervous system, *Wld Neurol.*, **3**, 444.

GRAHAM, G. G. (1967) Effect of infantile malnutrition on growth, *Fed. Proc.*, **26**, 139.

HIRSCH, A. (1886) in *Geographical and Historical Pathology*, New Sydenham Society, London.

HORNABROOK, R. W. (1971) The prevalence of multiple sclerosis in New Zealand, *Acta neurol. scand.*, **47**, 426.

HORNABROOK, R. W., and MOIR, D. J. (1970) Kuru. Epidemiological trends, *Lancet*, ii, 1175.

HUTTON, P. W. (1956) Neurological disease in Uganda, *E. Afr. med. J.*, **33**, 209.

KÄFER, J. P., and POCH, G. F. (1961) *Neurologia*, Buenos Aires, p. 479.

KINGSLEY, M. H. (1897) *Travels in West Africa*, London, 1965, p. 690.

KRAEPELIN, E. (1913) *General Paresis*, Nervous and Mental Disease Monograph Series No. 14, New York, pp. 141, 163.

KURTZKE, J. F., KURLAND, L. T., and GOLDBERG, I. (1971) Mortality and migration in multiple sclerosis, *Neurology (Minneap.)*, **21**, 438.

LAURENCE, K. M. (1970) Personal communication.

LIVINGSTONE, D. (1857) *Missionary Travels and Researches in South Africa*, London, p. 455.

MADAN, M. S., and BERRY, J. N. (1964) Incidence of malnutrition in patients admitted in a teaching hospital in Central India, *J. Ass. Phycns India*, **12**, 465.

MANI, K. S. (1969) in *A Textbook of Medicine*, ed. Vakil, R. J., Association of Physicians of India, Bombay, p. 1121.

MANI, K. S., MANI, A. J., and MONTGOMERY, R. D. (1969) A spastic paraplegia syndrome in South India, *J. neurol. Sci.*, **9**, 179.

MANSON, P. (1901) The aetiology of beriberi, *Lancet*, ii, 1391.

MANSON-BAHR, P. E. C. (1966) *Manson's Tropical Diseases; A Manual of the Diseases of Warm Climates*, 16th ed., London, p. 454.

MARIE, P. (1895) *Lectures on Diseases of the Spinal Cord*, New Sydenham Society, London, p. 308.

MCCALL, M. G., BRERETON, T. LE G., DAWSON, A., MILLINGEN, K., SUTHERLAND, J. M., and ACHESON, E. D. (1968) Frequency of multiple sclerosis in three Australian cities; Perth, Newcastle, Hobart, *J. Neurol. Neurosurg. Psychiat.*, **31**, 1.

McGill, H. C., Jr., ed. (1969) *The Geographic Pathology of Atherosclerosis*, Edinburgh.

Medawar, P. B. (1969) *The Art of the Soluble*, Harmondsworth, p. 147.

Merritt, H. H., Adams, R. D., and Solomon, H. C. (1946) *Neurosyphilis*, New York.

Moffie, D. (1966) De geografische verbreiding van multipele sclerose, *Ned. T. Geneesk.*, **110**, 1454.

Montgomery, R. D., Cruickshank, E. K., Robertson, W. B., and McMenemey, W. H. (1964) Clinical and pathological observations on Jamaican neuropathy, a report on 206 cases, *Brain*, 87, 425.

Moore, D. F. (1934 *a*) Retrobulbar neuritis and partial optic atrophy as sequelae of avitaminosis. *Ann. trop. Med. Parasit.*, 28, 295.

Moore, D. F. (1934 *b*) Manioc (cassava) as native food in Nigeria *W. Afr. med. J.*, 7, 97.

Odeku, E. L. (1967) Congenital malformations of the cerebrospinal axis seen in Western Nigeria: the African child with 'encephalocele', *Int. Surg.*, 48, 52.

Odeku, E. L., Grant, I. H., and Ekop, A. C. (1967) Congenital malformations of the cerebrospinal axis seen in Western Nigeria: the spinal meningoceles, *Int. Surg.*, 47, 580.

Odeku, E. L., and Janota, I. (1967) Analysis of 46 intracranial space-occupying lesions, *W. Afr. med. J.*, **16**, 31.

Okinaka, S., Reese, H. H., Natsupi, S., Ueki, K., Kuroiwa, Y., Araki, S., Shiraki, H., and Kurland, L. T. (1966) The prevalence of multiple sclerosis and other neurological diseases in Japan, *Acta neurol. scand.*, 42, Suppl. 19, 68.

Ooi, B. S., Chen, B. T. M., Toh, C. C. S., and Khoo, O. T. (1970) Causes of hypertension in the young, *Brit. med. J.*, 2, 744.

Osler, W. (1909) *Principles and Practice of Medicine*, 7th ed., London, p. 886.

Osuntokun, B. O. (1968) An ataxic neuropathy in Nigeria: a clinical, biochemical and electrophysiological study, *Brain*, 91, 215.

Peters, R. A. (1962) Significance of thiamine in brain metabolism and function, in *Neurochemistry*, 2nd ed., eds. Elliott, K. A. C., Page, I. H., and Quastell, J. H., Springfield, Ill., p. 268.

Peters, R. A. (1963) *Biochemical Lesions and Lethal Synthesis*, Oxford, p. 3.

Peters, R. A. (1969) The biochemical lesion and its historical development, *Brit. med. Bull.*, 25, No. 3.

Prickett, C. O. (1934) Effect of deficiency of vitamin B upon central and peripheral nervous system of rat, *Amer. J. Physiol.*, 107, 459.

Ramamurthi, B. (1969 *a*) in *Textbook of Medicine*, ed. Vakil, R. J., Association of Physicians of India, Bombay, p. 1100.

Ramamurthi, B. (1969 *b*) The rarity of bleeding aneurysms in India, *Excerpta Med.* (*Amst.*), *Int. Cong. Ser.*, **193**, 149; and personal communication.

Rao, A. V., Ranganathan, P. S., and Natarajan, M. (1968) Report on a study of cerebral biopsy in general paretics, *Neurology* (*Bombay*), **16**, 26.

Rischbieth, R. H. (1960) The prevalence of disseminated sclerosis in South Australia, *Med. J. Aust.*, **1**, 774.

Royal Society of Medicine (1970) Problems of world medicine, Symposium No. 12, *Proc. roy. Soc. Med.*, **63**, 1163.

Saint, E. G., and Sadka, M. (1962) The incidence of multiple sclerosis in Western Australia, *Med. J. Aust.*, 2, 249.

Salcedo, J. J. (1962) Experience in the aetiology and prevention of thiamine deficiency in the Philippine Islands, *Ann. N.Y. Acad. Sci.*, 98, 568.

Schwidde, J. T. (1952) Spina bifida; survey of 225 encephaloceles, meningoceles and myelomeningoceles, *Amer. J. Dis. Child.*, 84, 35.

Scott, Sir H. (1939) *A History of Tropical Medicine*, Vol. I, New York, p. vi.

Sigerist, H. E. (1951) in *A History of Medicine*, Vol. I, New York, p. 78.

Sondheimer, F. K., Grossman, H., and Winchester, P. (1970) Suture diastasis following rapid weight gain, *Arch. Neurol.* (*Chic.*), 23, 314.

Spillane, J. D. (1947) *Nutritional Disorders of the Nervous System*, Edinburgh.

Spillane, J. D. (1969) Tropical neurology, *Proc. roy. Soc. Med.*, 62, 403.

Stannus, H. S. (1936) Pellagra and pellagra-like conditions in warm climates, *Trop. Dis. Bull.*, 33, 729, 815, 885.

Stearn, E. W., and Stearn, A. E. (1945) *The Effect of Smallpox on the Destiny of the Amerindian*, Boston, p. 14.

Stoch, M. B., and Smythe, P. M. (1968) Does undernutrition during infancy inhibit brain growth and subsequent intellectual development?, *Arch. Dis. Childh.*, 38, 546.

Sutherland, J. M., Tyrer, J. H., and Eadie, M. J. (1962) The prevalence of multiple sclerosis in Australia, *Brain*, 85, 149.

Sutherland, J. M., Tyrer, J. H., Eadie, M. J., Casey, J. H., and Kurland, L. T. (1966) The prevalence of multiple sclerosis in Queensland, Australia, *Acta neurol. scand.*, 42, Suppl. 19, 57.

Suwanwela, C. (1969) Sincipital encephalomeningocele. A geographical, genetic and pneumoencephalographic study in 72 patients, *Excerpta Med.*, *Int. Cong. Ser.*, **193**, p. 158.

Suwanwela, C., and Hongsaprabhas, C. (1966) Fronto-ethmoidal encephalomeningocele, *J. Neurosurg.*, 25, 172.

Tanaka, T. (1934) So-called breast-milk intoxication, *Amer. J. Dis. Child.*, 47, 1286.

Tandon, P. N., (1970) Meningoencephaloceles, *Acta neurol. scand.*, 46, 369.

Trowell, H. C. (1960) *Non-infective Disease in Africa*, London, p. 243.

Turner, T. B. (1930) The race and sex distribution of the lesions of syphilis in 10 000 cases, *Bull. Johns Hopk. Hosp.*, 46, 159.

Wagner-Jauregg, J. (1922) The treatment of general paresis by inoculation malaria, *J. nerv. ment Dis.*, **55**, 369.

Widdowson, E. M., Dickerson, J. W., and McCance, R. A. (1960) Severe undernutrition in growing animals, *Brit. J. Nutr.*, 14, 457.

Williams, R. R. (1961) *Towards the Conquest of Beriberi*, Cambridge, Mass.

Wilson, S. A. Kinnier (1940) *Neurology*, Vol. 1, p. 462, Vol. 2, p. 1365, London.

Winick, M., (1969) Malnutrition and brain development, *J. Pediat.*, 74, 667.

WINICK, M., and ROSSO, P. (1969 *a*). Effects of severe early malnutrition on cellular growth of human brain, *Pediat. Res.*, 3, 181.

WINICK, M., and ROSSO, P. (1969 *b*) Head circumference and cellular growth of the brain in normal and marasmic children, *J. Pediat.*, 74, 774.

WITKOP, P. (1967) Relation of nutrition to central nervous system development and function, *Fed. Proc.*, 26, 148.

WORLD FEDERATION OF NEUROLOGY (1961) *Tropical Neurology; Proceedings of the First International Symposium, Buenos Aires*, eds. Bogaert, L. Van, Köfer J. P., and Poch, G. F., Buenos Aires.

Part One

INDIA

See PLATES 10–23

I An Introduction to Neurology in India

N. H. WADIA

Sealed off from the rest of the world to the north by the towering great wall of the Himalayas, India juts into the sea, forming a huge triangle stretching from longitude 66° to 97°E. India lies well within the tropics and this vast land is a mosaic of cloud-piercing mountains, rolling plains, hot desert, flowing rivers and placid lakes. As it is surrounded on all sides except the north by sea, it has a long coast-line. All this leads to climatic conditions which vary considerably, from the cold snow-bound Kashmir to the warm southern tip of India. Unlike Europe or America, except in the very north, there is no sharp contrast between winter and spring, but the variation in seasons is dominated by the arrival of the monsoon, which is nowhere in the world as well developed as it is in India. Once again the intensity of the rains and the contrast of the seasons will vary according to where one lives.

The population of India is rapidly approaching 560 million today. As a result of centuries of peaceful immigration and forceful invasion, a more variegated group of people living on one soil would be hard to find anywhere else. By 1500 B.C., a long series of conquests had got under way. From the North and West came Aryans, Persians, Greeks, Synthians, Parthians, Huns, Arabs, and Mongols to conquer India for its riches, but they often remained to settle among and integrate with the local population. More recent days saw the arrival of the Moguls, Portuguese, French and finally the British. All this has left India with a rich heritage of many languages and many forms of art, drama, literature and dance which have not yet yielded to the harsh levelling effects of modernization and industrialization, at least in the villages where the majority of Indians reside and where the all-pervading television and telephone have, blissfully, not yet penetrated. Hence, the 25-year-old Republic of India is comprised of 21 states on the basis of their distinct language and culture. For example, the hardy Jats of the Punjab are in so many ways diametrically opposite to the peoples of Bengal or Kerala, that it is indeed remarkable that they can live peacefully under one rule. But as Jawaharlal Nehru once said, the genius of India consists of its synthesis. The mellow and all-encompassing religious philosophy of Hinduism, which dominates India, teaches its people immense tolerance and an ability to absorb all who come to its door. Besides the Hindus, the Muslims and Sikhs form a fairly large minority population of the country. Christians, Buddhists, Jews, Zoroastrians (Parsees) and many other smaller groups practise their own religions and speak their own languages unfettered.

The majority of Indians are vegetarians. Rice, with wheat in some parts, is the staple diet. Fish from the vast coast-line is popular and meats and innumerable varieties of fruits and vegetables are available for those who can afford them. Tea, and coffee in the South, are the drinks most enjoyed. Alcoholism is not the problem it is in the West, because alcohol is not a social drink in most Indian households. Tobacco in various forms has, however, pervaded society down to the village level.

Medicine in India has been traditionally practised by the local doctor, the Vaidya, for centuries, and Ayurveda is still taught and practised extensively, especially in the villages. With the arrival of the Muslims in India, the Unani physician, called the Hakim, also appeared, bringing one more system of medicine to India, which still flourishes. Western or allopathic medicine only arrived with the Portuguese in their small enclaves as late as the sixteenth century and then later with the British. Apart from imparting elementary knowledge about the application of dressings, compounding of drugs and other such mundane practical tasks to their Indian assistants, no attempt at formal medical training of Indians was made until 1822, when a school was set up at Calcutta to train Indians in the art and practice of medicine. Even so, the aim was to create a cadre of assistants to the English doctors. In 1835, the first medical college was set up in Calcutta with the aim of training fully-fledged doctors. The curriculum, however, was spread out over 3½ years only and the standards of education were not up to those in English medical colleges. The Madras medical college, established soon after, was also beset by similar limitations. It was only after Sir Robert Grant, the Governor of Bombay, proposed in 1837 the first moves to provide modern medical education for the first time to the native born on his own soil, that the beginnings of allopathic medicine were made in India. His aim was to found a medical college equal to the best anywhere in England. Unfortunately, he did not live to see his dreams realized as he succumbed to apoplexy in 1838. The citizens of Bombay, with the encouragement of Nana Sankershett, collected funds to honour the memory of this great friend of Bombay and founded the Grant Medical College in 1845. Sir Jamshetjee Jeejeebhoy, a philanthropic Indian came forward with a donation of Rs. 1 00 000/-, a munificent amount by the standards of that era, to found the affiliated J. J. Hospital. From the very beginning, the highest standards of medical education were enforced here by Dr. Charles Morehead, the first principal and professor of medicine.

From these small beginnings, allopathic medicine expanded its scope and today there are 91 medical colleges, most of them founded after the Independence of India in 1947.

Despite this development over nearly 100 years, specialization in neurology only began after the Second World War. It was perhaps a part of the general upsurge in medical education which followed the Independence of the country, but it is as likely that it would have occurred anyway as it was long overdue. The teaching hospitals were naturally at the forefront. The Christian Medical College, Vellore, gave the lead in neurosurgery and within the next 3 years Madras, Bombay and Calcutta followed suit and neurology, neurosurgery and even neuropathology Units were established. The Neurological Society of India was formed in 1951 with a handful of members, but as these early centres began training specialists, and more trained Indians returned home, the membership (which includes all branches of the Neurological Sciences) rapidly grew and today stands at 208.

There are now well-run neurological departments in many of the larger cities of India and several in Madras, Bombay, Calcutta and New Delhi, totalling approximately 25. It is obvious that for a population nearing 560 million these facilities are far from adequate and many large areas of rural India go unattended. Institutes of Neurology have been established in Madras and Calcutta, and are planned in Bangalore and New Delhi.

It would be pointless and invidious to give details of some of these departments to the exclusion of others, as but for their size and organization the pattern would remain the same, wherever one travelled. All these departments have adequate service facilities for the day-to-day practice of neurology and neurosurgery. Neuropathology material is mostly reported on by the general pathologist interested in neuropathology, or by a neuropathologist within the Department of Pathology, but at the J. J. Group of Hospitals, Bombay, a full-time Professor of Neuropathology has been appointed. In Vellore, a well-equipped separate neurochemistry section exists. Neuroradiological examinations are usually performed by the staff of the clinical departments with the help of a general radiologist, who has an extra interest in neuroradiology. Entirely specialized neuroradiologists have not yet appeared in India, except at the Institute in Madras. There is a fairly closed liaison between these neurological disciplines, and although in many places neurology falls within the sphere of the Department of Medicine, and neurosurgery with surgery, there is an increasing tendency to form a separate group of the neurologically orientated disciplines under one department, as for example at the Institute of Neurology, Madras. In most hospitals, outpatients are seen in a separate clinic or are referred by the staff of the hospital itself, or by the practitioners within the city and State. As most of the departments are within a free public teaching hospital, the clinics are 'open house' and no prior appointments are made; among other reasons, this is because many patients travel long distances to reach the hospitals and cannot afford the time or money to await a fixed appointment, which would only be possible on arrival. To the neurologists of the West, used to their fixed number of patients at appointed times, these over-burdened clinics would indeed be a new experience in diagnostic medicine.

The staff of these departments is usually full-time, but part-time and honorary appointments still exist in many hospitals. Whereas the teaching hospitals cater for the bulk of the patients, in the bigger cities private consulting practice thrives within private hospitals and nursing homes, attending to the relatively more affluent.

So large is the service load that much of the Indian neurologist's time is taken up with his patients. Some time is spent in teaching medical students, but this varies considerably from one medical school to another. At some places, the neurologist is purposefully brought in to participate in the undergraduate teaching programme, while in others he is zealously kept out as one too specialized in his art to be capable of teaching simple neurology to undergraduates. At a postgraduate level several Indian universities have a special doctorate in neurology (DM) and neurosurgery (M.Ch.) at the end of a 5-year course after obtaining the basic qualification, the M.B. B.S. The training of these students is the neurologist's main responsibility, but he also participates in many ways in the courses laid down for postgraduate degrees in general medicine, psychiatry and paediatrics. As most of the departments are manned by a 3- to 5-member consultant staff, little time is left for research, which is largely clinically and epidemiologically orientated. Many Indian neurologists feel that this is as it should be, because neurology is in its infancy in India and the time spent on studying local diseases and cataloguing the prevalence of such diseases in India is more fruitful in the longer run, than time spent in fundamental research with the limited resources available in India, which can be done better in the more affluent countries which have at their command vast resources of money and man-power to do such work. However, this does not detract from the fact that some very worthwhile fundamental or applied research in neurophysiology, neuropathology, and neurochemistry is being carried out in India in a few centres, where laboratory orientated research and animal experimentation are strongly encouraged.

The common diseases of the nervous system are seen in India as anywhere else, yet the Western-trained Indian neurologist, on returning home, is at once struck by *the contrast in the general disease pattern* from that which he has seen abroad.

For many reasons, it would be inaccurate to use the

inpatient records statistics of any one department of neurology to draw conclusions about this disease pattern; e.g. leprosy is by far the commonest disorder of the peripheral nervous sytem, yet except in a few places such patients are seen and treated in other departments (especially dermatology) or in special institutions. Once again, cases of acute cerebrovascular disease are admitted most often to the general medical wards, while the patients with milder strokes rarely visit a hospital, completely distorting the statistics. As very few epidemiological surveys, especially on a national scale, have been conducted such information is also wanting. Hence, the variations in neurological practice can only be pointed out from the individual, and sometimes collective, experience of the few active neurologists practising in the far-distant major cities of India. TABLE 1.1 gives some idea of such diseases at a glance.

Table 1.1
Some Neurological Disorders Found in India

1. Leprosy	8. Lathyrism
2. Neurotuberculosis	9. Fluorosis (neurological complications)
3. Tetanus	10. Juvenile motor neurone disease
4. Nutritional disorders of the nervous system	11. Tropical spastic paraplegia
5. Strokes in the young	12. Spinal meningitis
6. Craniovertebral anomalies (atlanto-axial dislocation)	13. Oculomotor neuritis
7. Spinocerebellar degeneration with slow eye movements	14. Infantile tremor syndrome

INFECTIONS

Infections of the nervous system unfortunately still cripple and kill a large number of Indians every year. Leprosy, tuberculosis, and tetanus head the list.

There are 2·5 million known *leprosy* patients in India today, and it is believed that as new cases of leprosy are not compulsorily registered this figure is much smaller than the actual number. According to the *Annual Report* of the Ackworth Leprosy Hospital (1970), the number of new leprosy cases registered at that hospital was 3163 in 1962, and 4039 in 1970.

Tuberculous meningitis and other forms of neurotuberculosis are still rampant and the figures are reminiscent of the first four decades of this century in Europe and North America. At the Institute of Child Health in our hospital, it has been noted that tuberculosis of the nervous system formed 2·5 per cent of an average of 4200 total admissions every year from 1963 to 1967 (Udani, Parekh, and Dastur, 1971), and 45 per cent of all forms of tuberculosis in children below the age of 12 years (Parekh, 1968). It has also been found that tuberculous meningitis formed 82 per cent of 500 cases of neurotuberculosis (Udani, Parekh, and Dastur, 1971). Fortunately, tuberculous meningitis does not cause so much havoc among adults, yet at any one time in our 45-bedded unit two or more patients would be under treatment for this disease. A similar high incidence has been reported from all over India as mentioned by Tandon and Pathak in their chapter in this book [p. 39].

Whereas *tuberculomas* formed a large proportion of 'brain tumours' in some series as recently analysed as those of Dastur and Desai (1965) and Ramamurthi (1966), which mention figures of 30·5 and 24·3 per cent respectively, the subsequent years have shown a decline in tuberculomas, especially among adults. Even in the paper of Dastur and Desai there was no case of tuberculoma in a male over 25 years. Dastur and Lalitha (1972), from Bombay, found that in the past 3½ years, tuberculomas formed only 12 per cent of all brain tumours, while Tandon and Pathak from Delhi [CHAPTER 2] found the figure as low as 4·2 per cent. However, D. K. Dastur (personal communication) maintains that even today 46 per cent of tumours in children below 15 years are tuberculomas. H. M. Dastur's informative and current tuberculoma review (1972) is recommended reading for all interested in this subject.

The clinical features, pathology and diagnosis of *primary spinal tuberculous meningitis* causing radiculomyelopathy have now been carefully described (Wadia and Dastur, 1969; Dastur and Wadia, 1969; and CHAPTER 3). As this condition is not uncommon and is eminently treatable in the early stages, it requires the close attention of neurologists who often misdiagnose it as transverse myelitis.

Tetanus, although clearly a disease of the nervous system, is rarely managed by neurologists, yet it should form an important chapter in Indian neurology even today. During 1971, 227 patients were diagnosed as suffering from tetanus at the J. J. Group of Hospitals, Bombay. Seventy of them died from the disease.

MALNUTRITION

Most Indians are vegetarians (animal food is never touched, or may be taken once in a while) either from choice or financial necessity. Malnutrition, in its overt and covert forms, is still widespread in India, and neurological complications resulting from it are frequently seen, although the exact prevalence or forms of this nervous system involvement have not been studied. However, its extent can be gauged by Gopalan's remarks (1969) about the incidence of pellagra in the Deccan plateau of India. He maintained that in Hyderabad, South India, 'nearly 1 per cent of admissions to general hospitals and (in certain seasons) 8 to 10 per cent of admissions to mental hospitals are cases of pellagra'. A similar problem exists in certain famine areas of Rajasthan, North-west India (Shah, Singh, and Jain, 1971).

Another example of the widespread nature of

malnutrition is the probable damaging effect of protein-calorie deficiency (kwashiorkor) in early childhood on brain growth and subsequent mental development. Gopalan (1970) reported that nearly 2 per cent of children between the ages of 1 and 5 years, belonging to the poor socio-economic group, were suffering from frank protein-calorie malnutrition (kwashiorkor or marasmus). And even this, he admitted, was a gross underestimate of the real dimensions of the problem. If the association between intellectual capacity in adult life and the intake of proper nutrition in early childhood (albeit as one of the several factors) is finally substantiated by longitudinal studies, then the magnitude of the problem would be such that it would require steps at the highest national level to solve it.

Finally, Wadia and Swami (1970) studied the pattern of nutritional deficiency disorders of the nervous system in adults in Bombay. They found them related either to the vitamin D or to the B-complex group. They pointed out that *nutritional osteomalacia* with proximal pelvic, and at times shoulder girdle, weakness was seen only in women, most of whom were undernourished, young and multiparous with a history of almost continuous breast-feeding from one child to another over a number of years. They found that the vitamin B-complex deficiency caused three distinct syndromes:

1. Most of the cases of *vitamin B_{12} neuromyelopathy* presented with the usual features, but difficulty in diagnosis was experienced when the disease presented with or was predominated by cerebellar ataxia, precipitate micturition, proximal pelvic girdle weakness, or cutaneous sensory loss up to a level on the trunk in some patients. Although megaloblastic bone-marrow changes were seen in all, the haemoglobin was most often above 10g per cent and the average red blood cell count was 4 million/cmm. Classical Addisonian pernicious anaemia, or its accompanying subacute combined degeneration is rare in India, but this was carefully excluded before a diagnosis of nutritional ceuromyelopathy was made.

2. *Sensory ataxia—optic atrophy syndrome:* this group of patients complained of burning and tingling in the palms and soles, and difficulty in balancing. They had a glove and stocking anaesthesia and remarkable sensory ataxia with loss of vibration and postural sense in the lower limbs. Some also had optic atrophy. Some improved on a wholesome hospital diet, while others only did so after parenteral vitamin B-complex, having failed to respond to injections of thiamine, nicotinic acid, pyridoxine or vitamin B_{12} alone, when given sequentially.

3. In their largest group of 28 patients, the majority were alcoholic and showed dermal pellagra; their nervous symptoms of burning acral paraesthesiae, with cutaneous peripheral sensory loss and absent ankle jerks with preservation of balance, vibration and postural sense, suggested a *cutaneous peripheral sensory neuropathy*. Six of them had additional optic atrophy. Diarrhoea was frequently complained of, but psychosis was seen only in three patients.

Whereas dermal pellagra and peripheral sensory neuropathy had clinically suggested a deficiency of nicotinic acid only, further work on a collaborative basis on similar cases has shown a reduction in the serum levels of vitamins B_1, B_2, B_3, B_5, and B_6, leaving the question wide open as to which vitamin or vitamins are responsible for the neuropathy (*Studies on Nutritional Disorders of the Nervous System*, 1972). A nourishing hospital diet and a temporary withdrawal from alcohol in some patients rapidly cleared the skin condition and also somewhat improved the neuropathy, which was quickly relieved by injections of nicotinic acid or thiamine. One other point of interest was that, on administration of nicotinic acid or thiamine, the serum levels not only of these two vitamins rapidly rose, but also those of the other B-vitamins mentioned above, suggesting a curious interrelationship between these vitamins, although the adequate hospital diet may also have been responsible for the rise in these levels. The rapid improvement in spite of continuing to take alcohol at times, suggested the role of nutrition rather than alcohol itself.

CEREBROVASCULAR DISEASES

Cerebrovascular diseases complicating atherosclerosis, hypertension and diabetes are not uncommon in the cities of India. However, as Abraham points out in a later chapter [p. 86], hospital-based statistics on which this statement is based may not be a true reflection of the exact incidence of the illness. Its rural prevalence is also not known. To the neurologist practising in India, three interesting differences appear as outstanding:

1. The higher incidence of 'strokes' in the young (below 40 years of age).
2. Pulseless disease with neurological complications.
3. The lower incidence of subarachnoid haemorrhage and berry aneurysms.

Strokes

Abraham, in his chapter on cerebrovascular disorders in India [p. 86], discusses the first problem well. In 407 consecutive cases of cerebrovascular disease, 127 (32 per cent) were in the 11- to 40-year age-group. This appears to be equally true of other parts of India, and I have always been impressed by this higher incidence in my practice.

Abraham found cerebral (thrombosis) infarction to be the cause in as large a percentage as 49 of these 127 patients. He has postulated that in view of the relative absence of evidence of atheroma in the aorta and main neck arteries, hypertension, hypercholesterolaemia, and diabetes, the cause is most likely to be found in the smaller cerebral vessels. He is unable to decide the exact nature of this small vessel disease, but has conjectured that it may be an arteritis or an autoimmune process secondary to common tropical diseases.

Pulseless Disease

Hemiplegia, blindness and other neurological complications following diseases of the aorta and the main arterial trunks which arise from it, have been named by Dalal the 'aortic arch syndrome' [CHAPTER 7]. This is a common disease in India and elsewhere has been called, among other things, the pulseless disease or Takayasu's disease. Whereas most authors, including Indians (Rose and McKusick, 1953; Pahwa, Pandey, and Gupta, 1959; Sen, Kinare, Kulkarni, and Parulkar, 1962) believe that this is due to some form of arteritis, Dalal contends that, at least in India, a good proportion of these cases, especially in the male, are due to a non-inflammatory subintimal proliferation of connective tissue and rupture of the internal elastic lamina, causing diffuse thickening, irregularity and narrowing of the ostium of the large arteries arising from the arch of the aorta. He is unable to define the aetiological agent but has suggested the possibility of juvenile or premature atherosclerosis. It thus appears that there are two main groups within the aortic arch syndrome, the arteritic group, predominant in the young female and increasing the incidence of young hemiplegics, and the non-arteritic variety more predominant in the slightly older male, between 35 and 55 years.

Subarachnoid Haemorrhage and Berry Aneurysms

Most of us in India have noted the relative infrequency of subarachnoid haemorrhage and intracranial aneurysms, but the reason is not known and the suggestion that the less severe cases of subarachnoid haemorrhage are missed is not satisfactory. An isolated acute paralysis of the third nerve, which would elsewhere frequently be found on angiography to be due to an intracranial aneurysm, rarely turns out to be so here.

Such is the interest in this relative infrequency, that a multicentred collaborative national research group has begun to look at the veracity of this impression and also all other aspects of this problem. Ramamurthi (1965), from Madras, in his paper on 'Are Subarachnoid Haemorrhages Uncommon in India ?', mentioned that over a period of 14 years (1950 to 1964) he saw only 62 intracranial aneurysms, the highest figure being 9 in 1960. As against this, he found 36 angiomas in the same period of time. He did not mention how many of either group presented with subarachnoid haemorrhage, but the rarity of the haemorrhage can be clearly envisaged. Quoting other Indian authors and others from Iran and Japan, he has maintained that aneurysms are relatively uncommon in the 'Eastern countries'. Like Ramamurthi (1969), H. M. Dastur, from Bombay (personal communication), also found an equal proportion of aneurysms and angiomas over a 13-year period.

CRANIOVERTEBRAL ANOMALIES

Craniovertebral anomalies are seen all over the world (Spillane, Pallis, and Jones 1957; McRae, 1953; McRae and Barnum, 1953) but are much commoner in India. After Wadia (1960) first pointed this out, a large number of cases were seen all over the country, and in any of the bigger departments it would be easy to see 80 to 100 such patients in a 10-year period. Bharucha and Dastur (1964); and Wadia (1967) have pointed out many features of clinical, radiological and diagnostic interest. In CHAPTER 8 of this book, Wadia stresses the importance of separating out the congenital atlanto-axial dislocation and the compressive myelopathy caused by it from other craniovertebral anomalies. He points out distinctive clinical and radiological features, and maintains that the ultimate prognosis following successful surgery depends on distinguishing atlanto-axial dislocation from basilar invagination. This is because the usual operation of removing the posterior rim of the foramen magnum or the occipitalized atlas, while curative for invagination, is most often disastrous for atlanto-axial dislocation, resulting in haematomyelia, transection ofthe cord, and death. An alternative surgical approach for atlanto-axial dislocation was proposed from our department (Sinh and Pandya, 1968).

The pathology of the myelopathy (medullospinal compression) and the complicating haematomyelia have also been discussed by us (Dastur, Wadia, Desai, and Sinh, 1965).

SPINOCEREBELLAR DEGENERATION

An entirely indigenous variety of *heredofamilial spinocerebellar ataxia* has been described by Wadia and Swami (1971) and Wadia (1972). In all, 36 members of 12 families collected over 10 years have been examined. Severe progressive cerebellar and milder spinal cord and peripheral nervous signs are accompanied by a disorder of eye movements [FIG. 1.1]. This disease appears to have an autosomal dominant trait with some male preponderance [FIG. 1.2]. There is no paralysis of muscles, but a slowing down of movements of the eyes in all directions, whether performed randomly while scanning, on command, or while following an object. The word 'viscous' has been used for these movements, which are somewhat similar to those sometimes seen in the rigid variety of Huntington's chorea (Starr, 1967). Abnormal, jerky compensatory head and neck movements were seen and abnormal oculolabyrinthine reflex responses were elicited. Wadia and Kulkarni (1972) found that in these patients there is a total absence of the fast saccadic movements of the eyes, leaving the slower movements with a heightened fixation reflex to carry on the oculomotor function. Wadia and Swami (1971) mentioned that only five families with Friedreich's ataxia were seen in the same period of time and they maintained that, on ethnological grounds, it was not surprising to see a different and more common variety of indigenous ataxia.

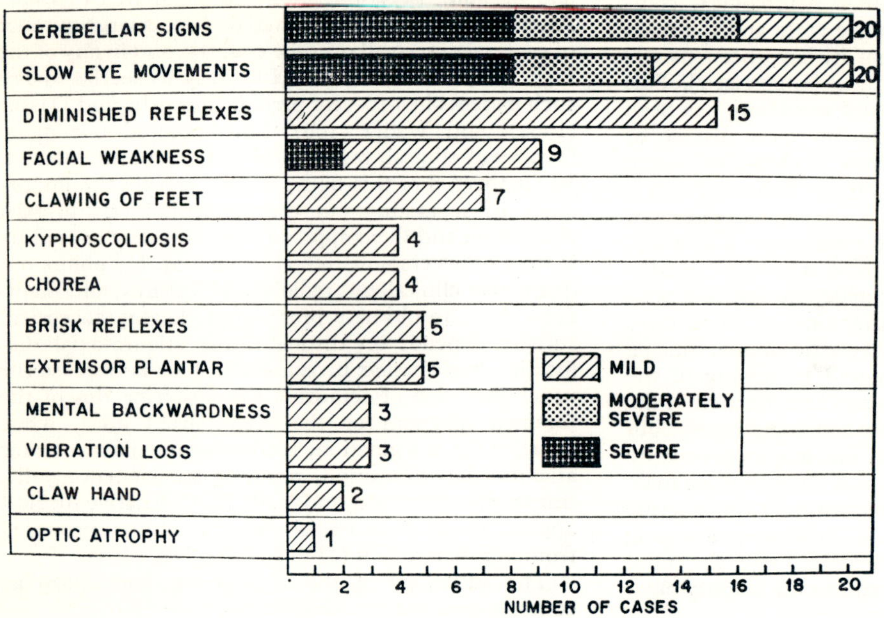

FIG. 1.1. The frequency of various symptoms and signs of heredofamilial spinocerebellar degeneration (indigenous variety).

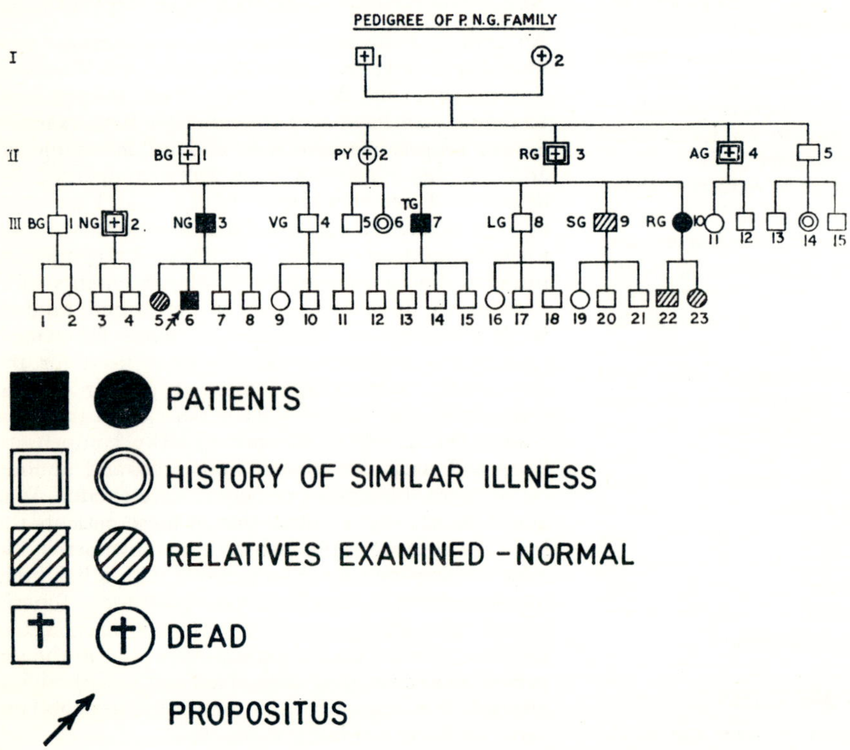

FIG. 1.2. Pedigree of one family of the above disorder showing the autosomal dominant trait.

DISORDERS OF THE SPINAL CORD

Five disorders of the spinal cord common in India but rarer elsewhere must be mentioned here:

1. Lathyrism.
2. Neurological complications of fluorosis.
3. Juvenile motor neurone disease.
4. Tropical spastic (South Indian) paraplegia.
5. Spinal meningitis causing radiculomyelopathy.

While the first two conditions are truly regional and related to intoxication through food and water, the third and fourth, though described from South India, are seen in many other parts of the country, though unreported.

Lathyrism

This has been a major public health problem in Central India, where the disease is endemic but periodically assumes epidemic proportions (Gopalan, 1970). The disease has been known for over a century and causes a spastic paraplegia. In the majority of patients, the onset is acute or subacute, beginning with severe muscle cramps, weakness, stiffness and heaviness of the lower limbs. The acute onset is often precipitated by exposure to rain or cold. The severity of the paralysis varies and it is not uncommon to see, in certain villages, patients of all ages either confined to bed or walking around with a classical gait with the support of one or two sticks. Spasticity is often a greater handicap than weakness. The lower limb reflexes are always exaggerated and the plantar responses extensor. Except for brisk reflexes, the arms are spared. Sensory and bladder functions remain unimpaired. It has been known for many years that the disease is caused by the ingestion of the seed of *Lathyrus sativus*, a hardy crop (which grows where other crops fail) used as food for humans and cattle and deeply entrenched in the rural economy; but it is only recently that the toxic factor in the seed has been identified (Nagarajan, Roy, Mohan, and Gopalan, 1963; Adiga, Rao, and Sarma, 1963). The toxic agent is known as B-(N)-oxalyl aminoalanine (BOAA), and its discovery has brought closer the solution of the problem of this disease. Whereas it was found impossible to ban the growth of the crop because of its economic implications, methods have been found to detoxicate the seed of its noxious chemical (BOAA) by steeping the pulse in a large volume of hot water, or by parboiling it before cooking.

Fluorosis

The excessive content of fluorine in the water of certain areas of Andhra Pradesh and the Punjab causes a severe osteosclerosis to which the name *fluorosis* is given. The vertebral column is often affected, and the narrowing of the spinal canal and intervertebral foramina results in a variety of compressive symptoms, discussed by Siddiqui in CHAPTER 12. Prevention seems to be more effective than cure.

Motor Neurone Disease

Classical motor neurone disease is as common in India as elsewhere, but I have been impressed by the frequency of a *non-familial, progressive, often asymmetrical amyotrophy of the upper limbs*, which begins in the second or third decade of life and slowly worsens. Spasticity is uncommon, though the deep reflexes are often exaggerated and the plantar responses may be extensor. No cases have come to autopsy, but electromyography and muscle biopsy have indicated the lesion to be at the anterior horn-cell level principally in the cervical cord. In our cases bulbar involvement has been rarely seen. Jagannathan [CHAPTER 13] describes a personally observed series of 14 young patients from Madras over 4 years, in whom a somewhat similar progressive amyotrophy was seen, but additionally 10 of these 14 patients had bulbar and facial paralysis or deafness. These cases formed 10 per cent of all motor neurone disease seen in his department at the same time. It is possible that these two groups of patients form variants of the same disease in two far-apart regions of India, but it is also as likely, especially in view of the perceptive deafness, that they are different diseases.

Tropical Spastic Paraplegia

Myelopathy of unknown aetiology, often presenting as posterolateral sclerosis at the thoracic or cervical level appears to be somewhat more prevalent in South India, although seen in other parts too. Mani [CHAPTER 5], analysing a total series of 250 cases of non-compressive paraplegia, found a group of 47 patients with a common presentation, in which he was unable to identify the exact causative agent. He maintains that after the exclusion of paraplegia due to compression of the spinal cord, this group forms 18·8 per cent of the total number and is the largest group of 'medical' paraplegias admitted to his hospital in Bangalore. He has designated the condition as 'tropical spastic paraplegia' because of its wider prevalence, although he had earlier called it South Indian paraplegia. A progressive paraplegia, appearing usually within 4 weeks and leaving behind a partially or severely handicapped person, spasticity, and postural and vibration loss in the lower limbs appear to be the predominant features, but distal paraesthesiae, bladder disturbance, and wasting of hands and feet of a much lesser degree and frequency were also seen. The autopsy examinations of two rather atypical cases have not clarified matters except to show posterolateral column demyelination.

Spinal Meningitis

The condition of *spinal meningitis*, especially of the tuberculous variety causing a radiculomyelopathy, is a common spinal cord disorder and has been fully described earlier (Dastur and Wadia, 1969; Wadia and Dastur, 1969), and in CHAPTER 3 by Wadia; the acute form of the disease presents with a rapidly ascending paralysis simulating transverse myelitis or the Guillain-Barré syndrome, but the often severe backache and root pains, the CSF changes of an inflammatory spinal block, the classical myelographic appearance, and the good response to antituberculous therapy clarifies the diagnosis. The chronic form closely apes a spinal cord tumour but can most often be distinguished by myelography.

OCULOMOTOR NEURITIS (CRANIAL POLYNEURITIS)

This is a fairly common condition seen by neurologists and ophthalmologists throughout India. Over 100 cases of this disease have been seen in our department over the last 15 years. It presents with an acute paralysis of a single or all oculomotor nerves of one side, immediately preceded or accompanied by often severe pain over the forehead or temple. There is no fever, vomiting or neck stiffness. The third nerve is most commonly involved, followed by the sixth and fourth; a total internal and external ophthalmoplegia may be seen, though not infrequently the pupil is spared. The pain disappears in a few days, but the paralysis may take several weeks to clear, frequently resulting in complete recovery. Recurrent attacks are seen, and may involve a different cranial nerve, once again confined to the oculomotor group, but I have seen facial paralysis indistinguishable from the classical Bell's palsy as a part of this disease. More rarely, a reversible sensory or motor paralysis of the fifth nerve, or retrobulbar neuritis has been noted. Keeping in mind Symonds' paper on 'Recurrent Multiple Cranial Nerve Palsies' (1958), extensive investigations, including CSF examination, blood VDRL, systemic investigations for infections, immunological disorders and parasitic diseases have revealed no definite clue to the aetiology. Appropriate angiography has always been normal. In fact, on seeing an acute, isolated, painful third nerve palsy, the Western-trained neurologist anticipates the diagnosis of an aneurysm, orders angiography, and most often finds himself wrong. I am struck by the similarity of this isolated third nerve palsy to Bell's palsy, and I am not talking of the facial palsy due to diabetes, syphilis, etc. Sudden onset, accompanying local pain, good recovery in the majority of patients, and indefinite aetiology are common to both. Mathew, in his chapter on 'Painful Ophthalmoplegia' [p. 120], describes a similar condition from Vellore, although it appears that in his patients pain preceded the ophthalmoplegia for weeks and was more severe, while the recovery of oculomotor function took longer. The fifth nerve involvement appears to occur more frequently in his cases than in mine. Mathew postulates immuno-allergic mechanisms to explain this disease and strongly recommends administration of corticosteroids. Krishna (1972) has also reported such cases from Bangalore and, in fact, the condition is commonly seen all over India. In neighbouring Ceylon, Ratnavale (1968) has seen a similar condition of uncertain aetiology in which all the cranial nerves except the olfactory and auditory may be involved. As in some of Mathew's cases, the ESR was consistently high, but unlike our experience in India, he found pleocytosis and raised protein in the CSF. He also noted dramatic response on administering cortiocosteroids to his patients.

PAEDIATRIC NEUROLOGY

Infantile Tremor Syndrome

The realm of paediatric neurology has still to be explored in India, yet a few interesting observations can be mentioned here. The 'infantile tremor syndrome' discussed by Tandon and Bajpai in this book [CHAPTER 10] and initially recognized in India by Pohowalla, Kaul, Bhandari, and Singh (1960), is one such example. Tandon and Bajpai draw on their experience of 212 cases seen over a period of 10 years, and mention that it essentially affects children in the first 30 months of life, causing a rapid high-intensity tremor usually affecting the whole body, though some parts are more affected than others. An open mouth, vacant expressionless look, light-coloured sparse silky hair, pallor and plumpness of the face have been noted by them as other characteristics of the syndrome, which spontaneously recovers with a gradual subsidence of the tremor in an average of 43 days. The aetiology of this disease still remains uncertain, though Jadhav, Webb, Vaishnaya, and Baker (1962) claim that it is due to vitamin B_{12} deficiency. This view is vigorously opposed elsewhere and the possibility of a meningo-encephalitis is raised on some post-mortem evidence.

Skilled obstetric aid to the pregnant mother is far from universal and difficult labour with resulting *cerebral palsy* is still fairly common to see, swelling the ranks of the epileptics and young hemiplegics among the population. Abraham [CHAPTER 6] found infantile hemiplegia to form 7·9 per cent of a total of 127 young hemiplegics whom he examined in the area around Vellore city.

Inborn Errors of Metabolism

Many of the already known *inborn errors of metabolism* are also seen in India, but have not yet been extensively studied. When this has been done in some instances, variation in the frequency or pattern of the diseases has emerged. An example of each may be quoted:

1. Centerwall and Itteyrah (1966) conducted a survey of 1123 individuals in 24 of the 26 institutions for the *mentally retarded* scattered all over India, and found only two cases of phenylketonuria originating from Mysore State; they concluded that the disease is 'significantly less common in India than in the West'. From the then existing literature of the Indian sub-continent (India and Pakistan) they found only five other cases, and noted that all of them came from Mysore State or West Pakistan, where consanguineous marriages are frequent. Interestingly enough, Sridhara

Rama Rao, Narayanan, and Narayana Reddy (1970) have subsequently detected five more cases also from Mysore State and all from consanguineous marriages, and mentioned two other reported cases again from South India (Madras and Andhra Pradesh), bringing the total to 12 cases in this country up to 1970.

2. Wadia and Dastur (1963) reported the first seven biochemically proven cases of *Wilson's disease* in India from four families in 5 years. No unusual clinical features were then noted, but by 1967 they had seen 25 patients in 18 families and a possible new variant had emerged (Dastur, Manghani, and Wadia, 1967, 1968). Eight of these 25 patients presented with the predominant complaint of difficulty in getting up from the squatting position, climbing stairs and running. Lumbar lordosis, waddling gait and a typical method of climbing up one's legs to get up from the ground gave the clinician the impression of myopathy. In fact, that was the diagnosis with which some of these cases were referred. In five of the eight patients, after several years of the disease, the neurological illness had remained negligible, consisting of mild tremors or slurred speech in three, tremors and incoordination in one, and motor rigidity and dysarthria in one. The remaining three had no neurological signs. All had renal rickets and a non-progressive disease of the liver: we called this an osseo-muscular variant. The muscular weakness improved considerably in those who could be given penicillamine, and even without treatment the course of the disease was slower and more benign than in the predominantly neurological variety of the disease. No deaths were reported from this group as opposed to five from the predominantly neurological cases in the same period of time.

The above two examples also show the disastrous effects of consanguineous marriage which is the accepted custom in certain parts of India and in certain communities where it is positively encouraged. I have often wondered what pattern of mental retardation (often in more than one sib) and what forms and variants of the already known aminoacidurias may exist within these closely in-bred communities.

A recently noted, though yet unreported and rare, example of such a genetic (probably metabolic) familial defect may be mentioned here. In the last few years, neurologists from Bombay and Madras have noticed a *disorder of sleep* afflicting more than one member of a sibship usually starting in the first, or at most the second, decade of life. An otherwise normal child in every way is seized by recurrent attacks of overpowering sleep. The attack is preceded at times by a feeling of dizziness or nausea. The sleep overtakes the child within minutes and continues for several hours to a few days. The child can be woken up from some attacks as from normal sleep, and fed or taken to the toilet but is usually very irritable, while during other attacks the sleep is deep. No specific pupillary or other abnormalities have been consistently noted. The child wakes up from an attack spontaneously, when some nystagmus and broad-based gait may be noticed. In some individuals, extreme irritability and aggressiveness briefly appear, and a desire to eat and drink at times excessively and abnormally as for example, a desire to suck pieces of ice. Within an hour or so, the child returns to complete normality. No mental or physical abnormality has been found between the attacks. The frequency and duration of the attacks have varied. In three of the five families (including the one personally studied by me) that have been brought to my notice, a child has died during a bout of deep irreversible sleep, apparently from asphyxia due to aspiration. The condition superficially resembles the Kleine-Levine syndrome, but there are obvious differences. Pneumoencephalography has always been normal. Extensive EEG examinations have been on some occasions normal, and at other times have shown striking abnormalities, both interictally and during the attack, and during normal sleep. Detailed reports of these families seen by individual neurologists should soon be expected from India.

One of my patients, originally seen by my colleagues from Madras, was admitted recently under the care of Dr. Roman Kocen to the National Hospital for Nervous Diseases, Queen Square, London. Biochemical investigations by Dr. P. T. Lascelles and by Dr. D. Gompertz of the Royal Postgraduate Medical School showed that the child was ketotic and large amounts of lactic acid were found in the urine. Trace amounts of other interesting metabolites were also found. The pattern of these other metabolites varied from attack to attack and no consistent pattern could be found or a definite biochemical diagnosis made.

EPILEPSY

Epilepsy has been known to Indians since the dawn of civilization. An extensive survey of the rural and urban population of a part of South India, conducted by a team headed by Dr. K. V. Mathai from the Christian Medical College, Vellore, showed that the prevalence rate of afebrile, active and recurrent cases was about nine per thousand population (Christian Medical College, Vellore, 1971). If this figure is accepted for the rest of India, one would expect a little over 6 million epileptics in this country. Whereas hospital-based statistics are available from other parts of India, their obvious bias has prevented me from comparing the figures. For example, at the Christian Medical College, Vellore, epilepsy formed 14·4 per cent of all neurological disorders during an annual survey, while at the All India Institute of Mental Health, Bangalore, 41·5 per cent of all new neurological consultations were for epilepsy (Mani, CHAPTER 5). A five-centre collaborative project between various neurological departments is now under way which should supply much useful and interesting information on many epidemiological and other aspects of epilepsy.

Again, some variations on the broad theme of

epilepsy as seen elsewhere in the world are to be expected. Birth injury and childhood infective illness such as tuberculous meningitis and encephalitis, where survival is now common, will push the figures upwards in the very young. One would also expect some new examples of reflex excitation and inhibition of epilepsy. One such disorder has already emerged from South India. Mani, Gopalakrishnan, Vyas, and Pillai (1968) reported 42 cases from Bangalore of what they called '*hot-water epilepsy*'. The attacks occurred after pouring hot water on the body, especially on the head while bathing. The attacks were largely of the temporal lobe variety, but in a third grand mal seizures were seen. Twenty per cent of these patients had epileptic attacks at other times also. Subsequently, more cases have been reported, confirming these initial observations (Mani, Mani, Ramesh, and Ahuja, 1972; Subrahmanyam, 1972).

MYOPATHY

Myopathy as a disease is as common in India as elsewhere, and the well-known heredofamilial muscular dystrophies have now been carefully identified and studied here. However, a wealth of unidentified and hard-to-label clinical material awaits the eager young neurologist armed with clinical commonsense and well-learnt electrophysiological and laboratory techniques, in the field of acquired myopathy of onset beyond the age of 20 years and familial or non-familial myopathy in children below 5 years of age. Once again, even when the association between the 'myopathy' and the principal disease is established their physiopathological basis has not been worked out. For example, the nature of the proximal muscle weakness in the lower limbs in osteomalacia, pellagra, vitamin B_{12} deficiency, and Wilson's disease, which we have often seen, has never been clearly explained.

NEUROLOGICAL DISORDERS RARE IN INDIA

I have so far mentioned the neurological diseases commoner in India than elsewhere, but except for subarachnoid haemorrhage I have not mentioned those which are strikingly rare. One such example is *multiple sclerosis*. Although not a single published autopsy report of this disease is available in India, we have all seen clinically unimpeachable cases of multiple sclerosis here. Bharucha and Umarji (1961), after a nationwide inquiry for cases seen between 1956 to 1960 (5 years) found only 151 cases, including 17 cases of Devic's disease. Out of 41 medical centres written to, only 10 had cases to report. From five large hospitals in Bombay only 30 cases could be found. Over the last 15 years, I have personally treated only 30 patients with this disorder; these figures merely show that our problem is negligible compared to that in the West. Two personal impressions may be permitted here:

1. Whereas Bharucha and Umarji (1961) found an even scatter of cases from all over the country, in the ethnological melting pot of Bombay I have found, surprisingly, many more patients with fair complexion and even light eyes (uncommon in India except among certain sects of Brahmins and other persons of Aryan extraction).
2. The disease takes a relatively more atypical and benign course than that reported from the West, and only a few of my patients have become bed-ridden.

Cysticercosis and *hydatid disease* of the nervous system are occasionally seen and the frequency of the former seems to be far higher in the North-western States of Punjab and Hariyana than elsewhere, although the incidence of parasitic infestation of the nervous system is much less than is reported from South America or Thailand [CHAPTER 27]. It may be mentioned here that cysticercosis has even been seen among strict vegetarians.

I have not seen a single case of temporal arteritis or of neurosarcoidosis in India, and carcinomatous neuromyopathy has rarely been seen, although I had been well acquainted with these diseases earlier. Much has been written recently about SMON (Kono, 1971; Shiraki, 1971; and Tsubaki, 1971), but against nearly 8000 cases from Japan, only a handful of cases have been reported from elsewhere (Osterman, 1971; Selby, 1972). The relationship between the intake of clioquinol and the disease seems to be well established, but the ethnic differences have not yet been explained. Amoebiasis is rampant in India and repeated courses of self-administered or prescribed clioquinol are commonly taken and millions of tablets swallowed. It is not uncommon to prescribe 1·5 to 1·8 G of clioquinol per day for 3 weeks, to be repeated later after an interval. In fact, a quick outpatients' survey of our hospital over a period of a month showed that 54 patients had taken a dose of 20 G clioquinol or more, half of them having taken over 30 G with a maximum of 60 G in 60 days. Once again, clioquinol in doses of 300 to 500 mg daily has been taken for months or years by many Indians as a part of digestive pills or to ensure smooth bowel action, and by Europeans here as a prevention for gastrointestinal infection. Against this background, I have seen only three patients with subacute myelopathy who had taken clioquinol intermittently for 2 years or so. In two, the relationship between the drug and the disease was retrospectively realized when we recalled some of our patients with 'myelopathy of unknown aetiology' on hearing of SMON; in the third, the diagnosis was clear from the beginning. It appears that in most of the non-Japanese cases, including our own, the preceding severe abdominal pain is absent, and in our cases spasticity and paralysis seem to be as predominant as the sensory ataxia; the disturbing paraesthesiae in the lower limbs were complained of just as much by our patients.

Despite 20 years of specialization in neurological practice in India, much remains to be identified, investigated, classified and explained. One has only to look at the vast untapped fields of paediatric neurology, mental retardation, 'myelopathies', and muscle disorders, to give only four examples, to see the magnitude of the problems awaiting solution; the young neurologist, often fresh from the West, rightly baulks at the challenge for want of sophisticated methods of investigation, but he need not entirely despair, for there is much that his eyes can see and his hands can feel which his pen may describe.

References

ACKWORTH LEPROSY HOSPITAL AND CLINIC, AND THE GREATER BOMBAY LEPROSY CONTROL SCHEME (1970) *Annual Report*, Bombay.

ADIGA, P. R., RAO, S. L. N., and SARMA, P. S. (1963) Some structural features and neurotoxic action of a compound from *L. sativus* seeds, *Curr. Sci.*, 32, 153.

BHARUCHA, E. P., and DASTUR, H. M. (1964) Craniovertebral anomalies, *Brain*, 87, 469.

BHARUCHA, E. P., and UMARJI, R. M. (1961) *Disseminated Sclerosis in India*, paper presented at Seventh World Congress of Neurology, Rome.

CENTERWALL, W. R., and ITTEYRAH, T. R. (1966) Phenylketonuria among the mentally retarded in India, *Lancet*, ii, 193.

CHRISTIAN MEDICAL COLLEGE, VELLORE (1971) *Investigation into Methods for the Rehabilitation of Persons Disabled by Convulsive Disorder, Final Report*, SRS Project No. 19-P-58113-F-01, Department of Neurological Sciences, Christian Medical College and Hospital, Vellore.

DASTUR, D. K., and LALITHA, V. S. (1972) Many facets of neuropathology of neurotuberculosis, in *Progress in Neuropathology*, ed. Zimmerman, H., New York (in press).

DASTUR, D. K., MANGHANI, D. K., and WADIA, N. H. (1967) Wilson's disease in India; geographic and genetic aspects and a possible new variant, *Excerpta med. (Amst.)*, *Int. Cong. Ser.*, 175, 615.

DASTUR, D. K., MANGHANI, D. K., and WADIA, N. H. (1968) Wilson's disease in India: I. Geographic, genetic and clinical aspects in 16 families, *Neurology (Minneap.)*, 18,21.

DASTUR, D. K., and WADIA, N. H. (1969) Spinal meningitides with radiculomyelopathy: Part 2. Pathology and pathogenesis, *J. neurol. Sci.*, 8, 261.

DASTUR, D. K., WADIA, N. H., DESAI, A. D., and SINH, G. (1965) Medullospinal compression due to atlanto-axial dislocation and sudden hematomyelia during decompression, *Brain*, 88, 897.

DASTUR, H. M. (1972) A tuberculoma review with some personal experiences, *Neurology (India)*, **20**, 111.

DASTUR, H. M., and DESAI, A. D. (1965) A comparative study of brain tuberculomas and gliomas based upon 107 case records of each, *Brain*, 88, 375.

GOPALAN, C. (1969) Possible role for dietary leucine in the pathogenesis of pellagra, *Lancet*, i, 197.

GOPALAN, C. (1970) Some recent studies in the Nutrition Research Laboratories, Hyderabad, *Amer. J. clin. Nutr.*, 23, 35.

JADHAV, M., WEBB, J. K. G., VAISHNAYA, S., and BAKER, S. J. (1962) Vitamin B_{12} deficiency in Indian infants: a clinical syndrome, *Lancet*, ii, 903.

KONO, R. (1971) Subacute myelo-optico-neuropathy, a new neurological disease prevailing in Japan, *Jap. J. med. Sci. Biol.*, 24, 195.

KRISHNA, A. G. (1972) Ophthalmoplegia: a clinical analysis of 180 cases, *Neurology, (India)*, **20**, Suppl. 3 (in press).

MCRAE, D. L. (1953) Bony abnormalities in the region of the foramen magnum, *Acta radiol. (Stockh.)*, **40**, 335.

MCRAE, D. L., and BARNUM, A. S. (1953) Occipitalization of the atlas, *Amer. J. Roentgenol.*, **70**, 23.

MANI, K. S., GOPALAKRISHNAN, P. N., VYAS, J. N., and PILLAI, M. S. (1968) 'Hot-water epilepsy': a peculiar type of reflex epilepsy. A preliminary report, *Neurology (India)*, **16**, 107.

MANI, K. S., MANI, A. J., RAMESH, C. K., and AHUJA, G. K. (1972)Hot-water epilepsy: clinical and electroencephalographic features, *Neurology (India)*, 20, Suppl. 4 (in press).

NAGARAJAN, V., ROY, D. N., MOHAN, V. S., and GOPALAN, C. (1963) *Ann. Rep. Nutr. Res. Lab., Hyderabad*, p. 39.

OSTERMAN, P. O. (1971) Myelopathy after clioquinol treatment, *Lancet*, ii, 544.

PAHWA, J. M., PANDEY, M. P. N., and GUPTA, D. P. (1959) Pulseless disease or Takayasu's disease, *Brit. med. J.*, **2**, 1439.

PAREKH, U. C. (1968) *Tuberculosis of the CNS in Children*, dissertation submitted to the University of Bombay in part fulfilment of M.D., p. 95.

POHOWALLA, J. N., KAUL, K. K., BHANDARI, N. R., and SINGH, S. D. (1960) Infantile meningoencephalitic syndrome, *Indian J. Pediat.*, 27, 49.

RAMAMURTHI, B. (1965) Are subarachnoid haemorrhages uncommon in India?, *Neurology (India)*, 13, 42.

RAMAMURTHI, B. (1966) Quoted by Dastur, D. K., Lalitha, V. S., and Prabhakar, V. (1968) Pathological analysis of intracranial space-occupying lesions in 1000 cases including children, *J. neurol. Sci.*, **6**, 575.

RAMAMURTHI, B. (1969) The rarity of bleeding aneurysms in India, *Excerpta med. (Amst.)*, *Int. Cong. Ser.*, **193**, 149.

RATNAVALE, G. S. (1968) Cranial polyneuritis: a distinct clinical entity, *Proc. Aust. Ass. Neurol.*, **5**, 527.

ROSS, R. S., and MCKUSICK, V. A. (1953) Aortic arch syndromes; diminished or absent pulses in arteries arising from arch of aorta, *Arch. intern. Med.*, **92**, 701.

SELBY, R. (1972) Subacute myelo-optico neuropathy in Australia, *Lancet*, i, 123.

SEN, P. K., KINARE, S. G., KULKARNI, T. P., and PARULKAR, G. B. (1962) Stenosing aortitis of unknown etiology, *Surgery*, **51**, 317.

SHAH, D. R., SINGH, S. V., and JAIN, I. L. (1971) Neurological manifestations in pellagra, *J. Ass. Phycns India*, **19**, 443.

SHIRAKI, H. (1971) Neuropathology of subacute myelo-optico-neuropathy, 'SMON', *Jap. J. med. Sci. Biol.*, **24**, 217.

SINH, G., and PANDYA, S. K. (1968) Treatment of congenital atlanto-axial dislocations, *Proc. Aust. Ass. Neurol.*, **5**, 507.

SPILLANE, J. D., PALLIS, C. A., and JONES, A. M. (1957) Developmental abnormalities in the region of the foramen magnum, *Brain*, **80**, 11.

SRIDHARA RAMA RAO, B. S., NARAYANAN, H. S., and NARAYANA REDDY, G. N. (1970) Biochemical investigations in five patients with phenylketonuria, *Indian J. med. Res.*, 58, 1753.

STARR, A. (1967) A disorder of rapid eye movements in Huntington's chorea, *Brain*, **90**, 545.

STUDIES ON NUTRITIONAL DISORDERS OF THE NERVOUS SYSTEM (1972) *Interim Report*, NIH Project No. 01-011-1, Bombay.

SUBRAHMANYAM, H. S. (1972) Hot-water epilepsy, *Neurology* (*India*), **20**, Suppl. 4 (in press).

SYMONDS, C. P. (1958) Recurrent multiple cranial nerve palsies, *J. Neurol. Neurosurg. Psychiat.*, **21**, 95.

TSUBAKI, T. (1971) Neurological syndrome associated with clioquinol, *Lancet*, **i**, 696.

UDANI, P. M., PAREKH, U. C., and DASTUR, D. K. (1971) Neurological and related syndromes in CNS tuberculosis: clinical features and pathogenesis, *J. neurol. Sci.*, **14**, 341.

WADIA, N. H. (1960) Chronic progressive myelopathy complicating atlanto-axial dislocation due to congenital abnormality, *Neurology* (*Bombay*), **8**, 81.

ADIA, N. H. (1967) Myelopathy complicating congenital Watlanto-axial dislocation, *Brain*, **90**, 449.

WADIA, N. H. (1972) An indigenous form of heredo-familial spino-cerebellar degeneration with slow eye movements, *Neurology* (*India*), **20**, Suppl. 4 (in press).

WADIA, N. H., and DASTUR, D. K. (1963) Wilson's disease in four Indian families (clinical, genetical and biochemical aspects), *Neurology* (*Bombay*), **11**, 1.

WADIA, N. H., and DASTUR, D. K. (1969) Spinal lepto-meningitides with radiculo-myelopathy; Part I. Clinical and radiological features, *J. neurol. Sci.*, **8**, 239.

WADIA, N. H., and KULKARNI, S. A. (1972) Unpublished data.

WADIA, N. H., and SWAMI, R. K. (1970) Pattern of nutritional deficiency disorders of the nervous system in Bombay, *Neurology* (*India*), **18**, 203.

WADIA, N. H., and SWAMI, R. K. (1971) A new form of heredo-familial spino-cerebellar degeneration with slow eye movements (nine families), *Brain*, **94**, 359.

2 Tuberculosis of the Central Nervous System

P. N. TANDON and S. N. PATHAK

INTRODUCTION

The All India Institute of Medical Sciences, New Delhi, was established as an autonomous institute by Act of Parliament in 1956. The prime concern of the Institute is to develop patterns of teaching in undergraduate and postgraduate medical education in all branches, so as to demonstrate a high standard of medical education to all medical colleges and other allied institutions in India. This educational experience is to be imparted in an atmosphere of research. The Institute consists of a complex of buildings housing the teaching unit, research laboratories, a 750-bed hospital, outpatient clinics, library, animal house, and assembly hall. It functions as a residential university where faculty and students live on the campus. It awards its own degree in medical sciences both undergraduate and postgraduate.

Besides those from Delhi, the Institute Hospital sees patients from the neighbouring states of Uttar Pradesh, Hariana, Rajasthan, Himachal Pradesh, Punjab, Jammu, and Kashmir and occasionally from neighbouring countries, e.g. Nepal and Afghanistan. TABLE 2.1 shows the domicile of patients admitted to the Neurosurgery Unit during the year 1970. In short, we drain an area of nearly 40 000 square miles. Outside Delhi there are only four neurosurgery units in the surroundings states.

The medical services in Delhi comprise five large hospitals where 90 per cent of the beds and medical aid are free of charge. Besides the hospital services, free medical services are provided in the various dispensaries (outpatient clinics) through the Central Government Health Scheme and Employees State Insurance Scheme. In the rural area, medical health services are provided by primary health centres which provide prophylactic and therapeutic services.

An analysis of patients admitted to the Neurology and Neurosurgery Units of the Institute during the year 1970 provides a profile of neurological disorders seen in this part of the world [TABLES 2.2 and 2.3]. As the Institute Hospital serves primarily as a referral centre, the number of patients with acute traumatic lesions as well as some routine neurological disorders is usually much less than in a general service.

Table 2.1

Domicile of Patients Admitted to the Department of Neurosurgery, AIIMS Hospital during 1970

State	*No.*
Delhi	133
Uttar Pradesh	127
Hariana	20
Rajasthan	20
Jammu and Kashmir	15
Punjab	7
Madhya Pradesh	6
Himachal Pradesh	6
Bihar	4
Assam	2
Gujerat	1
Mysore	1
Not recorded	3
Total	345
Nepal	3
Afghanistan	2

Table 2.2

Diagnosis of Patients Admitted to Neurological Service, AIIMS Hospital, New Delhi (Year 1970)
(Total No. 368)

Disorder	*No. of Cases*	*Percentage*
Cerebrovascular accidents	103	27.8
Intracranial tumours	38	10.3
Spinal cord compression	40	10.9
Subdural haematoma	7	1.9
Cerebral seizures	39	10.6
INFECTIONS		
Tuberculous meningitis	29	7.9
Pyogenic meningitis	10	2.7
Encephalitis	16	4·4
SSLE	3	0·8
DEGENERATIVE DISORDERS		
Motor neurone disease	13	3·5
Diseases of basal ganglia	8	2·2
Presenile dementia	5	1·4
Cerebellar ataxia	5	1·4
Diseases of muscle	13	3·5
Peripheral neuropathy	16	4·4
Myelopathy	8	2·2
Functional disorders	12	3·3
Congenital anomalies	3	0·8
Totals	368	100·0

Table 2.3

Diagnosis of Patients Admitted to Neurosurgical Service, AIIMS Hospital, New Delhi (Year 1970)
(Total No. 351)

Disorder	*No. of Cases*	*Percentage*
Brain tumour	122	34·57
Space-occupying lesions of inflammatory origin	15	4·29
Tuberculous meningitis	9	2·86
Raised intracranial pressure without tumour	12	3·43
Head injury and its sequelae	70	20·00
Cerebrosvascular lesions	16	4·57
Spine and spinal cord	39	11·14
Congenital malformations	13	3·71
Nerve lesions	2	0·57
Miscellaneous	41	11·43
Undiagnosed	12	3·43
Totals	351	100·00

Table 2.4

Classification of Intracranial Space-Occupying Lesions
(Surgically verified between June 1965–December 1969)

	Supratentorial	*Infratentorial*	*Midline*
Glioma	109	17	4
Meningioma	38	—	—
Haematoma	34	1	—
Abscess	26	5	—
Pituitary tumours and cranio-pharyngiomas	—	—	32
Neurofibroma	—	21	—
Tuberculoma	10	6	1
Sarcoma	5	6	—
Haemangioblastoma	—	6	—
Miscellaneous	23	20	18
Total	245	82	55

The commonest cause of admission to the neurology service in 1970 was cerebrovascular accident accounting for 27·8 per cent of all admissions. Tumours of the central nervous system were responsible for about 35 per cent of the neurosurgical patients. Inflammatory lesions constituted approximately 20 per cent of the patients admitted to the two units. Degenerative disorders are represented much less among those admitted. This may not, however, reflect the true incidence of these lesions. The priority for admission to the restricted number of beds available in our hospital is dictated very often by the therapeutic possibilities in an individual case. However, it may be mentioned that while multiple sclerosis is not unknown, it is seen only very infrequently. Nearly one-half of the patients attending the Neurology Outpatient Department are suffering from cerebral seizures. Fluorosis, frequently seen in Punjab and Hyderabad, is encountered only as a stray case in Delhi. Lathyrism, which is responsible for a large number of paraplegics in Madhya Pradesh and eastern Uttar Pradesh, is hardly ever seen. Among the cases of cerebrovascular accidents intracranial aneurysms are relatively infrequent. An impression is gained that occlusive lesions are more frequently seen at an early age. The incidence of intracranial tumours is more or less the same as that reported from most Western countries [Table 2.4]. Intracranial space-occupying lesions of inflammatory origin, e.g. tuberculoma, abscess, cysticercosis and fungus granuloma are not uncommon. As mentioned later, the incidence of tuberculoma in the north is much less than that in the south. Cysticercosis, though seen occasionally, is not as common as reported from Mexico. Among spinal lesions arachnoiditis is much more frequently seen in India than reported from elsewhere.

TUBERCULOSIS AFFECTING THE CENTRAL NERVOUS SYSTEM

Tuberculosis still remains a major health problem in India. A sample survey made by the Indian Medical Research Council (1959) in various parts of the country revealed that 13 to 25 of every 1000 persons had radiologically detectable lung lesions and in 2 to 8 of these bacteriological evidence of tuberculosis was present. A survey in Bombay revealed that as much as 5·5 per cent of the population in some areas had pulmonary tuberculosis. This incidence increased to 7 per cent among the industrial workers of the city. Nayak *et al.* (1970) encountered active pulmonary lesions in 17 per cent of 1680 consecutive medico-legal autopsy cases in Delhi. It is therefore not surprising that a significant percentage of patients admitted to any neurology and neurosurgery unit in our country are afflicted with a tuberculous lesion of the central nervous system. One must be alert to recognize any one of its protean manifestations, as it can mimic most of the common neurological diseases.

Recent years have witnessed a renewed interest in the study of various aspects of this disease by a number of workers all over the country. This has brought to light some changing patterns in the clinical manifestations of various tuberculous lesions of the central nervous system; some uncommonly recognized syndromes have been delineated. Experience in the management of large series of such cases has accumulated. In presenting a comprehensive account of these lesions an attempt will be made to highlight these recent studies.

The subject will be considered under the following headings:

1. Tuberculous meningitis.
2. Intracranial tuberculomas.
3. Pott's paraplegia.
4. Intraspinal tuberculous granulomas.

TUBERCULOUS MENINGITIS

Incidence

The incidence of tuberculous meningitis in a given community is directly proportional to the prevalence of tuberculous infection in general, which to a great extent is dependent upon the socio-economic and hygienic conditions of that community. Not surprisingly, tuberculous meningitis has become a rare condition in most of the affluent countries. The already low incidence in these countries declined remarkably with the introduction of antitubercular chemotherapy, permitting prompt treatment of the primary infection. In Cleveland Metropolitan General Hospital, for instance, during the years 1948–54, the incidence of tuberculous meningitis was reported to vary from 5·8 to 12·9 per 10 000 admissions. It declined to 4·4 to 8·4 per 10 000 admissions during 1959–63 (Hinman, 1966).

Auerbach (1951), also in the United States found tuberculous meningitis to be the cause of death in 4·6 per cent of all autopsies from a general hospital. It accounted for 42·2 per cent of all cases of tuberculosis in the paediatric age-group, but only 2·9 per cent in adults. Mackay (1967), from Wellington, New Zealand, reported a fall of 80 per cent in the incidence of tuberculous meningitis in that area during the last 25 years. The rate of the disease in the native Maori was approximately 40 times that in the Europeans.

In spite of some reduction in the overall incidence of tuberculosis in India also, tuberculous meningitis is still a very common disease. The admission rate for all cases of tuberculosis to a paediatric hospital in Bombay fell from 15 per cent in 1953 to 9 per cent in 1960 (Udani, 1961). Forty-two per cent of these cases were suffering from tuberculous meningitis. Bharucha and Potdar (1967) reported that 4·1 per cent of all paediatric admissions were victims of tuberculous meningitis. More or less identical figures have been reported from other centres in India (Sheth, 1961; Khatua, 1961; Prasad, 1963).

The incidence of tuberculous meningitis in patients with tuberculosis has been reported to vary from 7·4 to 11·8 per cent from various centres in India (Webb, 1956; Khandelwal, 1960; Ramchandaran and Purnayyan, 1966).

Negroes are reported to be more susceptible to tuberculous meningitis than whites (Auerbach, 1951; Coetzee, 1953; Falk, 1965). This has been attributed to the tendency for a large progressive primary complex to form, increasing the chances of haematogenous spread.

The incidence of miliary and meningeal tuberculosis has been reported to be higher in the spring season (Coetzee, 1953, Khatua, 1961).

Aetiology

As with most other tuberculous lesions in India, it is nearly always the human type of tubercle bacilli which is responsible for meningitis. Coetzee (1953) from the Western Province of the Cape of Good Hope found the bovine type of organism in only two out of 200 cases of tuberculous meningitis.

In recent years a number of stray reports of tuberculous meningitis due to atypical mycobacteria have appeared in the literature (Wood, Buhier, and Pollak, 1956; Chan and Pathmanathen, 1961; Huempfner, Kinglover, and Deuschle, 1966). Joishy and Sant (1969) from Bombay isolated 12 strains of rapidly growing (Group IV) atypical mycobacteria from a total of 100 cases of tuberculous meningitis in children.

Pathogenesis

Tuberculosis of the central nervous system is always secondary to tuberculosis elsewhere in the body. A high incidence of meningitis in patients dying of miliary tuberculosis led to the belief that tuberculous meningitis was simply miliary tuberculosis of the meninges. This view was challenged by Rich (Rich and McCordock, 1933; Rich, 1951), who produced evidence to show that the meningitis develops in two stages. First, during a stage of bacteraemia, tuberculous lesions—the so-called Rich's foci—are seeded in the brain or the meninges and, later, one or more of these rupture, resulting in discharge of *Mycobacterium tuberculosis* into the subarachnoid space. This hypothesis was supported by Schwarz (1949) and Auerbach (1951), and more recently by Dastur *et al.* (1970), who found tuberculomata of the brain substance or of the meninges in a large percentage of the cases studied by them at autopsy. Failure to produce tuberculous meningitis in experimental animals by haematogenous challenge and the ease with which it results from injection of tubercle bacilli directly into the subarachnoid space would also favour such a view.

The type and extent of the lesions following subarachnoid injection of tubercle bacilli depend upon the state of immunity or allergy of the animal at the time of insult. In an unimmunized animal such a challenge results in diffuse meningitis while in a BCG-vaccinated animal, the meningitis is localized to the site of injection. A hypersensitized animal reacts with much greater oedema and necrosis (Tandon *et al.*, 1970 *c*).

Infrequently the meninges become infected by direct spread from a neighbouring tuberculous focus, notably otitis media or spinal caries (Smith, 1963).

A number of reports on spinal tuberculous meningitis mostly from India, have raised the possibility of a secondary involvement of the intracranial subarachnoid space from such a lesion (Singh, Jolly, and Goyal, 1959; Ghosh, 1963; Bawa and Wahi, 1961; Dastur and Wadia, 1969).

Pathology

Rich (1951) classified meningeal tuberculosis into:

1. Disseminated miliary tubercles.
2. Focal caseous plaques.

3. Acute inflammatory caseous meningitis: (*a*) localized, (*b*) diffuse.
4. Proliferative meningitis: (*a*) localized, (*b*) diffuse.

While these lesions are all pathologically important, the acute inflammatory caseous meningitis is the one which clinically manifests as tuberculous meningitis, and hence is of maximum interest to the clinicians. The description that follows, therefore, primarily refers to this variety.

The brunt of disease in tuberculous meningitis undoubtedly falls on the basal meninges. However, the secondary vascular changes and the parenchymatous lesions of the brain are equally characteristic and probably of much greater significance clinically. Each one of these will, therefore, be described separately.

Meninges

There is a diffuse greyish opacity of the meninges, most characteristically seen in the basal regions. At the base of the brain a mass of gelatinous exudate is seen obliterating the cisterna pontis and interpeduncularis, extending anteriorly along the floor of the third ventricle, to cover the optic chiasma and the distal ends of the internal carotid arteries [PLATE 10a and b]. From the base, the exudate preferentially spreads along the Sylvian fissures, the cerebellopontine and ambiens cisterns. In most cases the posterior portion of the basal cisterns is relatively free from the exudate. The meninges over the convexity of the hemispheres are by comparison far less involved. The predominantly basal location of the exudate is attributed to the presence of tubercles or small tuberculomata (Rich's foci) just within the brain surface in the tissues around the interpeduncular fossa, notably the subthalamic region, the floor of the third ventricle, and the temporal poles (Dastur *et al.*, 1970).

Apart from other factors, the nature of the exudate varies with the duration of the illness and the treatment received. Cases with a short duration have mild to moderate basal exudate, which in cases of longer duration may become plaque-like or thick, fibrous, or even 'woody'.

Microscopic Examination. The leptomeningeal reaction is characterized by a profound laying down of fibrin accompanied by a marked vasodilatation and large areas of caseous necrosis with serpiginous outlines [PLATE 10c]. In contrast to the tuberculomas of the brain, the characteristic cell response is not seen as frequently in this region. The epithelioid cell reaction, for example, is on the whole poor, and giant cells distinctly infrequent. The unusually large giant cells so frequently seen in tuberculomas are not seen at all. The cellular exudate consists predominantly of lymphocytes and plasma cells. Often the inflammatory exudate abounds in polymorphonuclear leucocytes in aggregates or diffusely enmeshed in fibrin. The degree of cellular exudate and of caseation varies from case to case. In a given case, the changes of both healing and active lesions may be seen in two separate areas. In one of our patients with a large tuberculoma in the cerebellum, the basal meninges showed a characteristic granulomatous meningitis, while the meninges over the upper cervical cord manifested a non-specific arachnoiditis. In another patient, who presented with a blocked fourth ventricle, histopathological examination of the thickened arachnoid showed a non-specific chronic inflammatory lesion, but tubercle bacilli could be seen in the smear and grown in culture.

Ependyma and Choroid Plexus

Ependymitis and choroid plexus involvement is a frequent finding in cases of tuberculous meningitis. Frank tubercles may be seen on the ventricular ependyma, subependymal region and the choroid plexus. The histological picture of these lesions is identical to that seen in the leptomeninges.

The Vascular Changes

Arteritis is a prominent feature of tuberculous meningitis and, according to Doniach (1949), was first described in 1881 by Baumgarten. Most pathologists are in agreement with Rich and McCordock (1933) in believing that the arteries are altered chiefly from without in their passage through the subarachnoid exudate. The terminal portion of the internal carotid artery and the proximal 2 cm of the middle cerebral artery in the Sylvian fissure are the most frequently involved vessels, while the basilar system usually escapes. The grosser the exudate the more profound is the arteritis. Arteries traversing the sulci of the vertex where there is little or no exudate are unaffected.

The microscopic changes in the blood vessels consist of cellular accumulation in the subendothelial region of the intima, nodular formation in the adventitia and fibrinoid changes in the media. The infiltrating cells consisting of endothelial cells intermingled with lymphocytes are generally limited to the intima, but occasionally they may extend to the media. Within the adventitia are circumscribed tubercles which have the cellular characteristics of the surrounding meninges. At times it may show a typical tuberculous granuloma or a complete caseous necrosis. Occasionally, thrombi in various stages of organization, in some cases completely occluding the lumen, are seen in the meningeal vessels.

The pial veins traversing the exudate show an intense phlebitis. In the border zones between the normal and infected pia-arachnoid, phlebitis precedes arteritis (Doniach, 1949).

Dastur and Udani (1966) illustrated the changes at the capillary and venular levels in tuberculous encephalopathy without significant ischaemic lesions.

Soon after the introduction of streptomycin a number of workers reported on the evolution of pathological changes in tuberculous meningitis under chemotherapy (Medical Research Council, 1948; Smith, Vollum, and Cairns, 1948; De, 1949; Doniach, 1949;

Auerbach, 1951; Terplan, 1953). There were characteristic changes which occurred in meningitis under prolonged streptomycin therapy. The gelatinous character of the exudate had given way to a thickened dull grey mass, at times measuring 1–2 cm in thickness and obliterating the subarachnoid space. Fibrous and caseous tubercles up to 0·5 cm in diameter were seen along the major vessels. Terplan (1953) observed huge meningeal tuberculomas of a size rarely observed in untreated cases. Dastur *et al.* (1970) observed a higher incidence of infarction and internal hydrocephalus in treated than in untreated cases. However, they considered the organization and hardening of the basal exudate responsible for these parenchymal lesions to be more a result of longer duration of survival than of the therapy itself.

Microscopically, there are two characteristic changes in the fibrinocellular exudate in cases treated with streptomycin (Auerbach, 1951). He observed a degree of caseation far in excess of that noted in untreated cases, and marked proliferation of granulation tissue. As the treatment continues, the collagen fibrils apparently increase until the granulation tissue is replaced by hyalinized connective tissue.

Grumbach (1966) studied the evolution of infiltration in 120 treated cases and reported the changes to be necrotic during the first month, granulomatous from the first to the third month, and resolvent after the third month of treatment.

Studying the pathological changes in untreated and treated cases of tuberculous meningitis, Terplan (1953) was impressed by the necrotizing panarteritis in the former and the endarteritic protrusions, which he described as 'pillow-formation', in the latter. In the treated cases the adventitia is replaced by a thick ring of hyalinized collagen, and the intima is thickened by fibrous tissue usually lunate but sometimes concentric.

The Brain

Involvement of the brain parenchyma is the rule rather than the exception in cases of tuberculous meningitis. As a matter of fact, pathologically the disease is a meningo-encephalitis, rather than a pure meningitis. The degree and extent of involvement of the brain vary from case to case.

Border-zone Parenchymal Reaction. In the region of the meningeal exudate, the underlying brain is invariably involved. The border-zone often participates in the inflammatory and necrotic process [PLATE 10d]. Surrounding this area for a variable distance one finds oedema, gliosis, and perivascular inflammatory response.

Tuberculous Encephalopathy. In recent years Dastur and Udani from India (Dastur and Udani, 1965, 1966; Udani and Dastur, 1970) have focused attention on a comparatively lesser known feature of tuberculous meningitis, i.e. the tuberculous encephalopathy. This condition is commonly characterized by diffuse brain damage due to oedema in the absence of overt infarction, tuberculoma or severe hydrocephalus. Less frequently these workers have observed perivascular myelin loss, and, rarely, a picture identical to that of haemorrhagic leuco-encephalopathy. They have attributed these changes to hypersensitivity reaction. In our restricted experience we have not encountered this type of lesion in human cases. However, our experimental study in monkeys has revealed excessive brain oedema and necrosis in hypersensitized animals as opposed to the BCG-vaccinated ones (Tandon *et al.*, 1970c).

Infarcts and Ischaemic Lesions. In the presence of such marked vascular changes, as already described, it is not surprising to find ischaemic lesions and frank infarcts in the brain in cases of tuberculous meningitis [PLATE 10d].

The majority of infarcts are in the territory of the middle cerebral artery. Like the vascular changes, these are uncommon in the territory of the vertebrobasilar system. We have, however, encountered minute and even macroscopic infarcts in the brain stem both in human and experimental material.

Hydrocephalus. Some degree of hydrocephalus is nearly always present in cases of tuberculous meningitis who have survived more than 4–6 weeks. This hydrocephalus is mostly of the communicating variety (Wright and Rees, 1948; Smith, Vollum, and Cairns, 1948; Medical Research Council, 1948). Blockage of the cisterna pontis and interpeduncularis by the tuberculous exudate or granulation tissue is primarily responsible (De, 1949). Our recent studies on RHISA (radioactive human iodinated serum albumen) cisternography in these cases, however, suggest that in some cases at least lack of absorption of CSF over the surface of the hemisphere is an important factor (Tandon *et al.*, 1970*b*). Similarly, we have encountered a number of cases of obstructive hydrocephalus due to blocked fourth ventricle. Smith (1963) and Dastur *et al.* (1970) have reported obstructive hydrocephalus due to narrowing or blockage of the aqueduct. Exudate completely surrounding and compressing the brain stem, a tuberculoma of the vermis or the brain stem, a plug of ependymal exudate, or mesencephalic oedema alone have been held responsible for it. It is thus important to appreciate that in a given case more than one factor may be responsible for the hydrocephalus.

In summary, the basis of symptoms and signs in tuberculous meningitis may be any one or more of the following factors:

1. The meningeal exudate, causing meningeal signs, cranial nerve involvement and hydrocephalus.
2. Extension of the infection to the brain parenchyma, resulting in clouding of consciousness, seizures, hypothalamic and brain stem signs.
3. Arteritis and vascular obstruction, responsible for the focal neurological deficit.
4. Allergic or hypersensitivity response, producing

massive brain oedema and raised intracranial pressure in the absence of hydrocephalus.

Clinical Features

The classical clinical picture of tuberculous meningitis is well known, and while reference will be made to it in the description that follows, we shall also try to highlight the variants of the classical picture, which are so frequently seen in our country. While atypical presentations have been mentioned in most large series of cases reported from all over the world, their frequency is not mentioned. It is therefore difficult to compare the incidence of atypical cases in various geographical areas. The difficulty of diagnosis in the early stages, even in the typical cases, is well known and atypical presentations add to this difficulty. This is the reason for emphasizing the atypical or unusual presentations. The high incidence of the so-called atypical cases seen by us may be the result of a variety of factors. Manchanda and Lal (1966) pointed out the role of pre-existing malnutrition in modifying the course of illness and in creating confusion in early diagnosis. The uncontrolled use of 'penicillin—streptomycin' for all kinds of illnesses, febrile or even non-febrile, practised by a large number of unqualified and qualified medical practitioners, modifies the course and the clinical presentation before the patient seeks proper medical attention. Apart from these iatrogenic factors there are probably others inherent in the soil and the seed. A number of bacteriological studies have emphasized the low virulence of the tubercle bacilli isolated from Indian patients (Frimodt-Moller, 1957; Mitchison *et al.*, 1960; Bhatia *et al.*, 1961, 1963; Singh, 1964).

Age Incidence

Tuberculous meningitis is generally considered a disease of childhood, commonly arising as a complication of the primary infection. It must be emphasized, however, that it may arise at any time during the course of chronic tuberculosis. In our experience such cases are not uncommon. As a matter of fact, in our series the child/adult ration is nearly 1:1. Twenty-two per cent of autopsy-proved cases reported by Dastur *et al.* (1970), who are closely associated with an active paediatric unit, were above the age of 14 years.

A shift to increasing incidence in older age-groups has also been reported from the United Kingdom (Lorber, 1956; Smith, 1963) and the United States (Hinman, 1966). Falk (1965) reported 365 cases of tuberculous meningitis among war veterans, 67 per cent between 20 and 40 years of age and 22 per cent between 51 and 70.

Onset

Classically, the onset is insidious, characterized by a vague illness, lasting for 1 to 3 weeks before meningeal symptoms and signs appear. Listlessness, apathy, irritability, lack of appetitie, nausea, sometimes vomiting and abdominal pain are the common features. Unfortunately, these are not uncommon symptoms in protein-calorie malnutrition as well as a host of other diseases prevalent in our country. Some degree of fever is the rule, but it may be of low grade and remain unobserved. In approximately 10–15 per cent of children and 25–30 per cent of adults there may be no history of fever. This is particularly so in patients in poor general condition, in a state of 'anergy', and in some cases of low-grade infection. Thus, until the meningeal signs appear, the correct diagnosis may not be suspected. Even the meningeal signs may develop very late in the course of the disease or may never appear. It is often not realized that in infants the cardinal sign of meningitis is not stiffness of the neck but fullness of the fontanelle (Smith, 1963). In children, vomiting is a much more frequent symptom than headache, at least in the initial stages.

Instead of the usual subacute onset, tuberculous meningitis may present acutely, or the prodromal stage may be unduly prolonged. Dastur *et al.* (1970), in their autopsy-proved cases, reported an acute or fulminant onset in 51 per cent of the children and only 14 per cent of the adults. This is in contrast to the incidence of acute onset (4 per cent) reported by Taylor, Smith, and Vollum (1955) from Oxford in 200 unselected consecutive cases. Once again the poor general condition and malnourishment of the Indian patients may be responsible for this difference.

Focal or generalized epileptic fits may herald the onset of tuberculous meningitis in children, while in adults behaviour or personality change may be the first symptom. We have thus diagnosed a number of cases of tuberculous meningitis from our psychiatric ward, at a time when no evidence of meningeal irritation or focal neurological deficit was observed. Lincoln, Sordillo, and Davies (1960) described convulsions at the onset in 9·5 per cent of 241 cases. These were restricted to children under 5 years of age. Among children below 2 years, 17 per cent presented with convulsions.

Abrupt onset of focal neurological deficit as the presenting feature is equally frequently seen both in children and adults. Thus, sudden onset of hemiparesis or monoparesis during the course of tuberculous meningitis is commonly recognized, but occasionally it may be the initial symptom. Similarly, we have seen a number of adult patients presenting with painful ophthalmoplegia as the only manifestation of tuberculous meningitis (Tandon *et al.*, 1970 c).

Not infrequently symptoms and signs of raised intracranial pressure may be the most conspicuous presenting features. One or two such cases presenting as hydrocephalus in infancy and childhood, and as a 'tumour syndrome' in adults, ultimately proving to be tuberculous meningitis, are seen by us every month. Bhagwati and Singhal (1967), and Mathai and Chandy (1967) have also reported identical cases.

Yet another mode of presentation is the so-called spinal form which is discussed in detail by Wadia [CHAPTER 3].

Udani and Dastur (1970) have described a series of

cases in childhood who, following an initial episode of tuberculous meningitis of varying severity, presented with the clinical picture of progressive spasticity, decerebration, convulsions and coma. In such cases the symptoms and signs of diffuse brain involvement may predominate. The classical features and cerebrospinal fluid changes of tuberculous meningitis may not be present at the time of examination. At autopsy, they are found to have diffuse oedematous encephalopathy with or without meningitis.

A clinico-pathological study of fatal cases, 24 children (Bharucha *et al.*, 1969) and 18 adults (Deshpande, Bharucha, and Mondkar, 1969), revelaed some interesting differences between the two groups. There was a low incidence of hydrocephalus in adults (2/18) compared with gross degrees of ventricular dilatation (16/24), with or without tentorial herniation in children. Convulsions and brain stem signs with decerebration were much more frequent in the children than in the adults. The high incidence of atypical presentations in adults was attributed to the frequent finding of well-circumscribed, dense, tough, thick, fibrous exudate (tuberculoma-en-plaque) in atypical situations, not seen in any of the children's series.

As mentioned earlier, variability of clinical presentation has also been commented upon by others from outside India (Kocen and Parsons, 1970; Smith and Daniel, 1947; Joseph, Job, and Defranoux, 1962). Smith (1963) briefly mentioned the anomalies of onset referred to above. Sahs and Joynt (1962) described the symptomatology of tuberculous meningitis to be variable. They pointed out that occasionally the clinical manifestations of the infection may be minimal almost to the time of death. Medovaya (1964) observed atypical signs in 40 out of 379 patients, most of these in patients between 16 and 30 years of age. Norris, Garvey, and Swalback (1964) reported a mild form of tuberculous meningitis, while Meyer *et al.* (1960) observed that a mild case may be ignored as viral meningitis.

Course

In an untreated case sooner or later the picture of indefinite ill health gives way to one of definite meningitis. By this time the patient is obviously seriously ill. Drowsiness, irritability, mental confusion and clouding of consciousness are invariably associated with meningeal signs. The problem at this stage is not one of diagnosis of meningitis but of establishing its nature. Signs and symptoms of raised intracranial pressure, cranial nerve palsies, pupillary abnormalities, and focal neurological deficit soon appear. The patient lapses into coma, develops decerebrate spasms, irregularity of pulse and respiration, and untreated cases will die in 4–6 weeks from the onset of illness.

The simple clinical classification suggested by Lincoln, Sordillo, and Davies (1960) divides the clinical course into three stages:

Stage 1: patients with meningeal signs but without neurological involvement.
Stage 2: patients with evidence of neurological involvement but without impairment of sensorium.
Stage 3: the advanced cases with marked neurological and sensorial involvement.
Unfortunately, in our country we still see a large majority of patients at stages 2 and 3.

Institution of antitubercular chemotherapy will modify the course of illness. If the treatment is started in the early stage of the illness, prompt and complete remission of the signs and symptoms occurs in most of the cases. In contrast, treatment is of no avail in the large majority of patients who are already in deep coma. Even after an initial satisfactory response to treatment, the course of illness may be punctuated with secondary complications due to organization of the inflammatory exudate, arteritis, or drug resistance. Thus, hydrocephalus, optic atrophy, cranial nerve palsies due to basal exudate, paraplegia due to spinal block, or hemiplegia due to arteritis may suddenly appear in a patient who is otherwise responding satisfactorily. Intermittent exacerbations may occur even on continued treatment. Recurrence of symptoms, after adequate control for more than a month, are occasionally seen. This is usually due to inadequate therapy.

Laboratory Investigations

Routine laboratory investigations of blood and urine are not of much help. Slight leucocytosis in peripheral blood (TLC—total leucocyte count—10 000–20 000/c mm) with relative increase in polymorphonuclear cells, particularly in early stages of the disease, may mistakenly suggest a pyogenic infection. Raised erythrocyte rate is observed in nearly two-thirds to three-quarters of these patients.

A tuberculin test, which is positive in 75 to 80 per cent of cases, is of some help in diagnosis in the paediatric age-group. The important fact to realize is that in various reported series there are 10 to 30 per cent of cases of tuberculous meningitis with a negative tuberculin test.

Roentgen examination of the chest is an essential investigation in all cases of suspected tuberculous meningitis as an associated tuberculous lesion of the lung is a frequent finding.

Cerebrospinal Fluid Examination

In every suspected case of meningitis, a diagnostic lumbar puncture should be performed before the patient is administered any antibiotics. Even a few days of treatment may alter the findings sufficiently to create confusion in diagnosis.

Typically, in tuberculous meningitis the CSF is under pressure, usually clear, infrequently somewhat opalescent. In late cases it may be xanthochromic. The appearance of a fine flocculent lot—the 'cobweb'—on allowing the CSF to stand in the tube for some time is neither a constant nor a diagnostic feature. There is a moderate degree of pleocytosis (usually less than 500 cells), with a predominant lymphocytic response. Occasionally in the early stages and sometimes during the course of treatment, there may be brief periods of polymorphonuclear reaction.

Biochemical examination reveals raised protein, usually below 200 mg per cent. But in late cases and particularly when a spinal block develops the protein content may be as high as 1 to 1·5 g per cent. Sugar is reduced to 40 mg per cent or below, but unlike pyogenic meningitis it is never absent. Too much emphasis has been given to lowering of CSF chlorides. In our experience this is an inconstant finding of no diagnostic or prognostic significance.

Like the atypical presentations of clinical features, the CSF findings may also manifest wide departures from the characteristic picture. The characteristic CSF responses may be either diminished or exaggerated as pointed out by Smith (1963). Thus, very early in the illness and sometimes even in advanced cases there may be only a very mild pleocytosis, less than 30 or even 20 cells per c mm and the protein content may also be low. A completely normal CSF was reported in three cases by Bharucha *et al.* (1969) in a small series of autopsy-proved cases. An initially normal CSF, showing typical changes later on, has been documented by Kocen and Parsons (1970). In contrast, in some cases the cell count may be well above the 1000 per c mm usually considered the upper limit; a large number of these may be polymorphonuclear leucocytes.

Demonstration of tubercle bacilli in smear, culture, or by guinea-pig inoculation of the CSF is the only positive proof of the tuberculous nature of the meningitis. The incidence of such proof varies in different reports. Surprisingly, in most series reported from India there is a very low incidence of bacteriological verification. Most workers in this field are baffled by this problem. The various reasons attributed are technical faults, high incidence of pretreatment before CSF examination and low virulence of tubercle bacilli in India. A number of techniques have been advocated to improve the detection rate. Udani (1963), and Thapar (1967) recommended the use of a special floatation hydrocarban technique. Smith (1963) pointed out that *Myco. tuberculosis* is more frequently found in ventricular than in lumbar CSF. Whenever there is any opportunity to do a ventricular puncture, CSF obtained should be submitted to bacteriological investigations.

The permeability of blood-CSF barrier to bromide is greatly increased, so that the ratio of serum-bromide to CSF-bromide, which is normally between 0·3 and 0·5, is increased to 0·6 or even 1 (Taylor, Smith, and Hunter, 1954).

Ching-Tsai Kuo (1969), from Taiwan, has described an immunological reaction of CSF utilizing a modified haemagglutination reaction. He considers it specific for tuberculous meningitis, and suggests that it has a prognostic value.

Chick (1965) described a complement-fixation test for the diagnosis of tuberculous meningitis. It was positive in all his 60 cases.

We have no experience with the above investigations.

Electroencephalography

More EEG abnormalities occur in tuberculous meningitis than in other types of meningitis, but findings vary with the age of the patient, the extent and duration of the meningitis, and the severity of associated symptoms. These abnormalities are most frequent in patients below 3 years of age. To start with the abnormality consists of diffuse slowing of the record. A child with a lymphocytic meningitis who has a very slow record in the initial stages of illness is very likely to be suffering from tuberculous meningitis (Turrell *et al.*, 1953). During the course of the illness spike discharges and focal abnormalities may appear. With the control of the disease the EEG changes also show a tendency to revert to normal. However, minor EEG changes persist in more than half the surviving patients during follow-up, while 10 to 15 per cent are left with major abnormalities. Even in those whose EEG becomes normal, it takes 2 years to do so. This occurs mostly in those with severe neurological deficits.

Pneumoencephalography or Ventriculography

These may be required for patients presenting with hydrocephalus, raised intracranial pressure, or focal neurological deficits. These investigations are quite safe, even in acute cases, and we have observed no significant exacerbation of symptoms following them. Some degree of hydrocephalus is observed in a large majority of patients in the paediatric age-group, especially in cases with late diagnosis. The hydrocephalus is usually of the communicating variety, with only 10 to 15 per cent due to blockage of the foramina of the fourth ventricle. The classical appearance is that of a block at the tentorial opening, as demonstrated by hold-up of the air bubble in the cisterna pontis. In adults, presenting with raised intracranial pressure, hydrocephalus is infrequent, and the pneumoencephalographic appearance is consistent with that of pseudo-tumour.

In patients with focal neurological deficits, especially adults, cerebral atrophy is a more frequent finding than hydrocephalus (Foltz and Sheehy, 1956).

Angiography

Greitz (1964), Lehrer (1966), Wadia and Singhal (1967) and Mathew, Abraham, and Chandy (1970) have reported abnormalities in carotid angiography in one-half to two-thirds of cases of tuberculous meningitis submitted to this investigation. Narrowing of the intracranial portion of the carotid artery involving the siphon and occasionally extending to the proximal segments of the anterior and middle cerebral arteries is the commonest abnormality reported. Lehrer (1966) described a triad in the angiographic pattern consisting of an abnormal course of the anterior cerebral artery or thalamostriate vein due to hydrocephalus, narrowing of major arteries at the base, and occlusive disease of medium to smaller arteries. While Greitz (1964) suggested that vasculitis combined with vasospasm is responsible for narrowing of the vessels, Wadia and Singhal (1967) attributed this to structural changes alone. There is good correlation between the extent of angiographic abnormality and the clinical state of the patient. Angiographic abnormalities are more frequent in patients with neurological deficit and in those who are seriously ill.

Lehrer (1966) commented upon the paucity of collaterals in cases of arterial blocks in tuberculous meningitis. However, Mathew, Abraham, and Chandy (1970) demonstrated in them a variety of collateral circulation as seen in cases of carotid occlusion due to other causes.

Treatment

Before the introduction of streptomycin in 1944, tuberculous meningitis was invariably fatal within 3 to 8 weeks of the onset of symptoms. The 1948 report of the Medical Research Council of the United Kingdom unequivocally established the benefit derived from streptomycin in the treatment of this malady. However, the mortality rate was still 70 per cent in those treated with intramuscular streptomycin and 58 per cent if intrathecal therapy was added. Addition of para-amino-salicylic acid (PAS) improved the results slightly but the next real advance came with the introduction of isoniazid hydrazide (INH) in 1952. Unlike streptomycin and PAS, INH has a good diffusibility in the CSF, it penetrates the cell membrane and thus reaches the intracellular organisms. It is known to open up new vascular channels in the relatively avascular tuberculous granulation tissue. The only significant side-effect of INH is the development of peripheral neuropathy. The risk of this complication is minimized by the simultaneous administration of pyridoxine in the dosage of 50 mg daily.

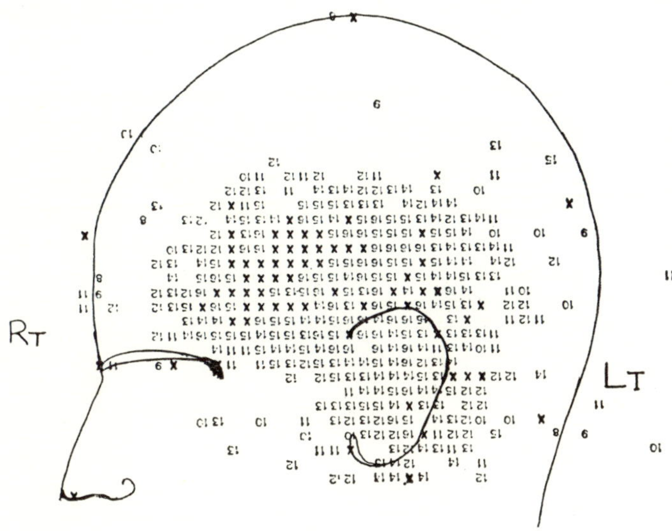

FIG. 2.1. RHISA cisternogram 3 hours after injection of the isotope in lumbar theca.

Isotope Cisternography

DiChiro, Reames and Matthews (1964) described the technique of isotope cisternography as a means of studying CSF circulation. In some respects this is superior to air-study. A few cases studied by us using this technique reveal that the abnormality in CSF circulation in cases of tuberculous meningitis may be multifocal [FIGS. 2.1, 2.2, and 2.3]. The hold-up of the isotope in the basal cistern, even after 24 hours, suggests a tentorial block. This block is evidently partial as the isotope has reached the supratentorial subarachnoid space. However, persistence of significant radioactivity after 96 hours indicates delayed absorption from the surface also.

Thiacetazone, a compound belonging to the group of thiosemicarbazones, has been shown to have a definite therapeutic value as a companion drug to INH. A combination of thiacetazone in a dosage of 150 mg per day and INH has been found to be comparable to INH + PAS as regards clinical, radiological, and bacteriological results, and also the incidence of toxic manifestations (Menon, 1966). The former combination, as it is cheaper, is more readily acceptable to our poor population. After the initial 6 months, when streptomycin and PAS are omitted, the patient is given INH + thiacetazone. The side-effects commonly met with are nausea, vomiting, giddiness, cutaneous hypersensitivity reaction, jaundice, and psychosis. The patient

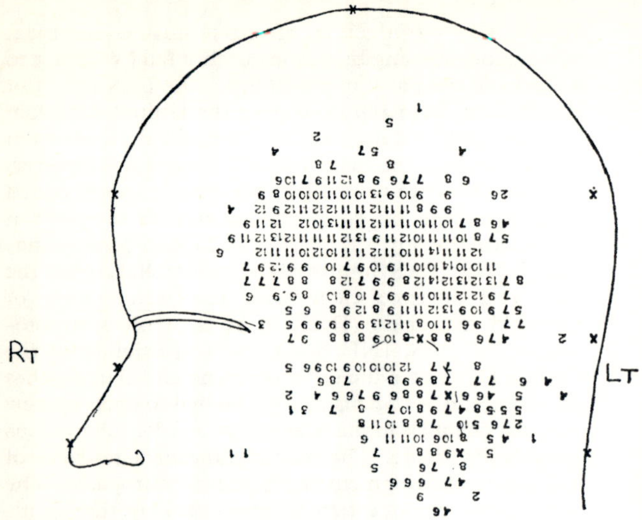

FIG. 2.2. RHISA cisternogram 24 hours after injection of the isotope in lumbar theca. Persistence of such marked radioactivity in the basal region after 24 hours indicates obstruction to CSF flow in the basal cisterns.

is advised to discontinue thiacetazone if any of the last three symptoms appears. The drug is poorly tolerated by elderly patients or those in poor general condition.

With the use of the therapy mentioned above, it is now possible to reduce the mortality of tuberculous meningitis to less than 20 per cent. If the treatment is started in the initial stage of the illness (stage 1), a complete cure should be possible in nearly all cases.

With minor modifications the therapeutic regimen generally recommended and followed by us is that give in TABLE 2.5.

Table 2.5
Therapeutic Regimen in Tuberculous Meningitis

Drug	*Dosage* *Children*	*Adult*	*Duration*
1. Streptomycin	40 mg/kg	1 G OD	3 months
	40 mg/kg	1 G alt. day	3 months
2. INH	15 mg/kg	300–400 mg/day	18 months
3. PAS	0·2 G/kg	10–12 G/day	18 months
4. Thiacetazone	3·4 mg/kg	150 mg/day	As an alternative to PAS during last 12 months
5. Pyridoxine	5 mg BD	10 mg BD	18 months

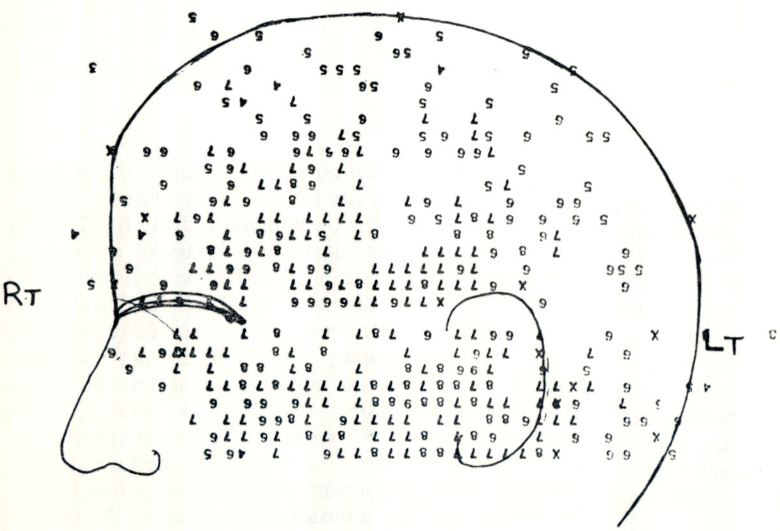

FIG. 2.3. RHISA cisternogram 96 hours after injection of the isotope in lumbar theca. Lack of complete clearance even after 96 hours suggests defective absorption.

Smith and Vollum (1950) advocated the use of intrathecal tuberculin in patients who made poor progress on standard treatment. It produced an allergic response which helped to increase the concentration of streptomycin reaching the basal exudate. In spite of occasional excellent results, however, this treatment has been generally abandoned as it is an ordeal for the children and not without risk.

Among the newer antitubercular drugs, cycloserine and ethionamide behave similarly to INH as regards free diffusion across the blood-brain barrier. On the other hand, ethambutol, like streptomycin, appears in the CSF only when the meninges are inflamed. These medicines are used only if there is evidence of resistance to the primary drugs. Place, Marjorie, and Huerger (1969) reported satisfactory response in all cases treated with ethambutol.

Starting in 1952, a number of workers advocated the use of corticosteroids as an adjunct to the antitubercular drugs (Shane, Clowater, and Riley 1952; Barnard, 1953; Bulkeley, 1953; Wasz-Hockert, 1954; Ashby and Grant, 1955). By reducing the inflammatory and exudative reaction, the steroids tend to reduce the incidence of complication resulting from the dense basal exudate. Generally, it reduces the toxicity and creates a feeling of well-being in the patient. The experimental work by Feldman and his co-workers (1955) and Oppenheimer and Reister (1953) confirmed its utility in reducing pia-arachnoid adhesions. However, Weiss and Flippin (1961) did not find any significant change in the survival rate following use of steroids. Wasz-Hockert and Donner (1962 *b*) reiterated its utility, especially in severe cases. Their primary mortality fell from 30 per cent to 11 per cent with the addition of steroids. Nevertheless, overall mortality remained 24 per cent. In spite of controversial opinions regarding the advisability of routine use of corticosteroids (Hockaday and Smith 1966), it is generally accepted that it is a useful adjunct in children below 1 year, in severely ill patients, and in those with threatened spinal block. We restrict the use of steroids to these groups of patients.

We prefer to continue the treatment for at least 18 months. Most patients will show a satisfactory response within 2 to 3 weeks of starting the therapy. Failure to observe perceptible improvement should arouse the suspicion of wrong diagnosis or the existence of some associated complication such as hydrocephalus or tuberculoma.

Management of Complications

The two important complications, hydrocephalus and spinal block, require additional management.

Hydrocephalus. Cairns (1949) advocated the use of burr-holes and repeated tapping of the ventricles to tide over the acute stage of the illness. In patients with established hydrocephalus, especially when the disease is otherwise under control, Ginde (1962) advocated anterior third ventriculostomy. We have observed some dramatic successes following this operation. It may be successful if the block is in the roof of the fourth ventricle or even up to the tentorial opening. If, however, the anterior basal cisterns are obliterated or the absorption from the surface of the cerebral hemispheres is also defective, third ventriculostomy will be unsuccessful. For the same reason de-roofing of the fourth ventricle in cases of obstructive hydrocephalus secondary to blocking of the outlet foramina is seldom successful. Ventriculo-atrial shunt is, therefore, the operation of choice. Slight pleocytosis or increased protein in the CSF is not a contra-indication to this operation provided the disease is otherwise responding to chemotherapy (Bhagwati, 1968). Intrathecal or intraventricular corticosteroids are of no use in cases of established hydrocephalus.

Spinal Block. In a large majority of cases the suspected partial block indicated by rising CSF protein, xanthochromia, and defective manometry on jugular compression, will clear up during the course of therapy. In some cases, in spite of adequate treatment including oral corticosteroids, the spinal block progresses and produces varying degrees of paraparesis. Intrathecal corticosteroids (hydrocortisone 50 mg daily for 5 days and on alternate days for another five to ten injections) has been found to be helpful in a number of these cases (Tandon, Misra, and Singh, 1968). Intrathecal streptokinase—streptodornase (Hazlehurst, 1955) and crystalline pancreatic desoxyribonuclease (Johnson, Ayvazian, and Tillett, 1959) have been tried to resolve the subarachnoid block, but with indifferent results. When infection has burnt out and dense fibrous adhesions have formed such treatment is unlikely to be of avail. If the residual arachnoiditis is restricted to a small segment surgical decompression may be helpful. However, a number of these patients are left with extensive dense arachnoiditis with secondary changes in the spinal cord. No medical or surgical treatment is then of any avail.

Prognosis

The mortality of tuberculous meningitis, a uniformly fatal disease two decades ago, has been reduced to as low as 4 per cent (Wasz-Hockert and Donner, 1962 *a*). In India the mortality is still high; the lowest figure (16·7 per cent) is reported by Rao, Bharucha, and Bharucha (1970) and the highest (71·9 per cent) by Manchanda and Lall (1966).

There has been a progressive improvement in the survival rate with the availability of potent antituberculous drugs (Lorber, 1960; Wasz-Hockert and Donner, 1962 *a*). TABLE 2·6 summarizes the results of two well-controlled series.

The mortality depends upon the age of the patient, the stage of disease at the time of diagnosis, and the presence of raised intracranial pressure or hydrocephalus. Undoubtedly, the general state of nutrition

Table 2.6
Results of Treatment with Antituberculous Drugs

Therapy	Lorber, 1960 Total No. of Cases	Lorber, 1960 % Survival	Wasz-Hockert and Donner, 1962 a Total	Wasz-Hockert and Donner, 1962 a % Survival
Streptomycin	82	36	16	25
Streptomycin + PAS	48	73	101	51*
Streptomycin, INH + PAS	80	83	33	70
Streptomycin + INH + PAS + cortisone	—	—	37	89*

* Additional secondary mortality of 3 and 13 per cent respectively in these groups.

of the patient and presence or absence of associated lesions elsewhere influences the outcome. Mortality is high in children below 3 years of age, and in those admitted in late stages of the disease, especially those in coma and manifesting gross neurological deficit. Development of hydrocephalus affects the prognosis adversely; survival is unlikely if gross hydrocephalus already exists when the treatment is started.

While the survival rate has improved, the incidence of sequelae has increased. This is partly due to the therapy, but in great measure due to the disease itself. The incidence of late sequelae varies from approximately 10 per cent (Rao, Bharucha, and Bharucha, 1970) to nearly 90 per cent (Erdos, Szaba, and Hodosi, 1966). In most large series, however, 20 to 30 per cent of survivors manifest a variety of physical and mental abnormalities. Readers are referred to a very detailed and painstaking study of late sequelae of tuberculous meningitis by Wasz-Hockert and Donner (1962 *a*).

Mental Subnormality and Psychiatric Disturbances

Patients below 3 years of age are most prone to these sequelae. All factors which adversely affect the survival rate also predispose to a higher incidence of mental subnormality in the survivors. The functions found to be lost or altered are the same as those affected by other types of brain injury, i.e. attention, concentration, memory, abstraction, and synthesis. Pentti *et al.* (1962) reported profound mental retardation in only 6 out of 100 survivors, Lincoln, Sordillo, and Davies (1960) in 9 out of 50, and Todd and Neville (1964) in 12 out of 65. Progressive mental deterioration is generally not observed in older children. They develop mental disturbances, emotional liability, irritability, affective hyperaesthesia, and paroxysmal depression.

Neurological Deficit

Gross neurological deficits, e.g., hemiplegia, tetraplegia or paraplegia, are observed in approximately 10 to 15 per cent of survivors. Minor neurological deficits such as cranial nerve palsies, incoordination, and nystagmus are seen in an additional 10 to 15 per cent of cases. Monoplegia, hemiplegia, and dysphasia are due to ischaemic lesions secondary to arteritis, while paraplegia and tetraplegia are usually due to compression of the brain stem or the spinal cord by the granulomatous exudate and secondary arachnoiditis.

Visual Defects. Blindness, due to direct involvement of the optic nerves in the tuberculous process, or strangulation of the chiasma by the inflammatory exudate or arachnoiditis or, rarely, secondary to papilloedema, is reported in a small number of cases (2 to 5 per cent) by Pentti *et al* (1962) and Lorber (1961). A surprisingly low incidence (0·8 per cent) has been reported by Rao, Bharucha, and Bharucha (1970) from Bombay. In our experience, blindness is much more frequently observed; a number of the children, affected however, do not survive.

Otological Sequelae. Deafness or significant impairment of hearing is observed in 5 to 10 per cent of the survivors. In all likelihood this is due to drug toxicity rather than the disease *per se*.

Spinal Block. A partial spinal block occurs frequently during the course of illness. It may occasionally present for the first time several years after the arrest of the disease (Rao and Subrahmanyam, 1962; Kozlowksi, 1963; Tandon, Misra, and Singh, 1968). While intrathecal streptomycin therapy may have been responsible for some of the reported cases, spinal block is observed in a significant number of cases not submitted to such treatment. Kaminska and Kulczynskak (1964) encountered this complication in 6·6 per cent of 685 cases studied. In most cases the spinal block clears up during treatment but in a few it may lead to severe spinal cord compression and paraplegia.

Hydrocephalus

As already described, hydrocephalus is a frequent feature during the acute stage of the illness in children. In a small number of cases it may manifest for the first time when the disease is otherwise under control. It may be responsible for blindness and delayed death. Arrested hydrocephalus or hydrocephalus secondary to cerebral atrophy are observed as late sequelae in patients left with severe neurological deficits.

Convulsions

While convulsions are a frequent feature during the acute stage of the illness, the overall incidence of seizures in survivors varies from 8 to 12 per cent. The frequency of convulsions is higher in those with gross neurological deficits, but it may be the only sequel.

Intracranial Calcification

The longer the duration of follow-up, the higher the incidence of intracranial calcification. In patients followed up for more than 5 years, patchy calcification in the meninges or the brain parenchyma is observed in 30 to 50 per cent of cases.

Abnormal Electroencephalogram

Varying degrees of EEG abnormalities are observed in 30 to 40 per cent of the survivors. Gross abnormalities are, however, observed in those with severe neurological or mental deficits.

Other Sequelae

Endocrine disturbances, obesity, sexual precocity and other hypothalamic syndromes, subdural effusion (Kumbhat, 1960), and ectopic ossification of hip joints (Lorber, 1961) are occasionally observed during the follow-up.

A description of the various sequelae tends to depict a very dismal picture of the survivors. Nevertheless, it must be pointed out that approximately 70 per cent of them are able to lead a normal or near normal life with or without minimal sequelae. Only a small percentage (5 to 10 per cent) are left as complete cripples. Early diagnosis, prompt institution of therapy, and continued supervision will no doubt reduce the incidence of permanent residual damage.

References

ASHBY, M., and GRANT, H. (1955) Tuberculous meningitis treated with cortisone, *Lancet*, i, 65.

AUERBACH, O. (1951) Tuberculous meningitis: correlation of therapeutic results with the pathogenesis and pathologic changes. I. General considerations and pathogenesis, *Amer. Rev. Tuberc.*, **64**, 408.

BARNARD, C. (1953) Tuberculous meningitis: cortisone treatment as an adjunct to the antibiotics, *S. Afr. med. J.*, 27, 219.

BAWA, T. S., and WAHI, P. L. (1961) Spinal tuberculous meningitis, *J. Indian med. Ass.*, 37, 449.

BHAGWATI, S. N. (1968) *Ventriculo-atrial Shunt in Meningitis*, Paper presented at the Eighteenth Annual Conference of the Neurological Society of India, Calcutta, December 1968.

BHAGWATI, S. N., and SINGHAL, B. S. (1967) *Raised Intracranial Pressure as a Primary Manifestation in Tuberculous Meningitis*, Paper presented at the Seventeenth Annual Conference of the Neurological Society of India, New Delhi, December 1967.

BHARUCHA, P. E., IYER, C. G. S., BHARUCHA, E. P., and DESHPANDE, D. H. (1969) Tuberculous meningitis in children. A clinico-pathological evaluation of 24 cases, *Indian Pediat.*, **6**, 282, 1969.

BHARUCHA, P. E., and POTDAR, R. D. (1967) An analysis of patients treated at K.E.M. Hospital, Bombay, during a 4-year period 1961–64, *Indian Pediat.*, 4, 341.

BHATIA, A. L., CSILLAQ, A., MITCHISON, D. A., SELKON, J. B., SOMASUNDARAM, P. R., and SUBBAIAH, T. V. (1961) The virulence in the guinea-pig of tubercle bacilli isolated before treatment from South Indian patients with pulmonary tuberculosis: comparison with virulence of tubercle bacilli from British patients, *Bull. Wld Hlth Org.*, 25, 313.

BULKELEY, W. C. M. (1953) Tuberculous meningitis treated with ACTH and isoniazid. Comparison with intrathecal streptomycin, *Brit. med. J.*, 2, 1127.

CAIRNS, H. (1949) Surgical aspects of meningitis, *Brit. med. J.*, 1, 969.

CHAN, K. E., and PATHMANATHEN, T. (1961) Meningitis due to atypical mycobacteria, *Med. J. Malaya*, 15, 113.

CHICK, L. F. (1965) Detection of specific antibodies in the cerebrospinal fluid as a method of early diagnosis of tuberculous meningitis in adults, *Excerpta med.* (*Amst.*), (*Sect. VIII*), 18, 519.

COETZEE, J. N. (1953) An epidemiological investigation of tuberculous meningitis in the Western Province of the Cape of Good Hope. *S. Afr. med. J.*, 27, 441.

DASTUR, D. K., LALITHA, V. S., UDANI, P. M., and PAREKH, U. (1970) The brain and meninges in tuberculous meningitis. Gross pathology in 100 cases and pathogenesis, *Neurology* (*India*), 18, 86.

DASTUR, D. K., and UDANI, P. M. (1965) Pathology and pathogenesis of tuberculous encephalopathy, *Excerpta med.* (*Amst.*), *Int. Cong. Ser.*, **100**, 1006.

DASTUR, D. K., and UDANI, P. M. (1966) Pathology and pathogenesis of tuberculous encephalopathy, *Acta neuropath.* (*Berl.*), 6, 311.

DASTUR, D. K., and WADIA, N. H. (1969), Spinal meningitides with radiculo-myelopathy: Part 2 Pathology and pathogenesis, *J. neurol. Sci.*, 8, 261.

DE, S. N. (1949) Streptomycin in development of hydrocephalus in tuberculous meningitis, *Brit. med. J.*, 2, 214.

DESHPANDE, D. H., BHARUCHA, E. P., and MONDKAR, V. P. (1969) Tuberculous meningitis in adults. A clinico-pathological study of 18 cases, *Neurology* (*India*), 17, 28.

DICHIRO, G., REAMES, P. M., and MATTHEWS, W. B. (1964) RISA-ventriculography and RISA-cisternography, *Neurology* (*Minneap.*), 14, 185.

DONIACH, I. (1949) Changes in meningeal vessels in acute and chronic (streptomycin treated) tuberculous meningitis, *J. Path. Bact.*, **62**, 253.

ERDOS, Z., SZABO, J., and HODOSI, R. (1966) Follow up of tuberculous meningitis, *Lancet*, i, 1106.

FALK, A. (1965) Co-operative study on the chemotherapy of tuberculosis. XIII. Tuberculous meningitis in adults with special reference to survival, neurologic residuals and work status, *Amer. Rev. resp. Dis.*, **91**, 823.

FELDMAN, S., BEHAR, A. J., and SAMUELOFF, M. (1955) Effect of cortisone and hydrocortisone on pia-arachnoid adhesions, an experimental study, *Arch. Neurol. Psychiat.* (*Chic.*), 74, 681.

FOLTZ, E. L., and SHEEHY, T. F. (1956) Pneumoencephalography in tuberculous meningitis, *Amer. Rev. Tuberc.*, 74, 835.

FRIMODT-MOLLER, K. (1957) in *Technical Report of the Scientific Advisory Board*, Indian Council of Medical Research, New Delhi, p. 153.

GHOSH, S. (1963) Tuberculous meningitis—pathological observations, *J. Indian. med. Ass.*, 41, 538.

GINDE, R. G. (1962) *Visual Failure in Tuberculous Meningitis*, Paper presented at the First Asian and Australian Conference of Neurologistis and Neurosurgeons, Tokyo, 1962.

GREITZ, T. (1964) Angiography in tuberculous meningitis, *Acta radiol. Diagn.*, **2**, 369.

GRUMBACH, R. (1966) Evaluation anatomique de la meningite tuberculeuse, *Sem. Hôp. Paris.*, **42**, 2537.

GUPTA, B., and WEBB, J. K. G. (1962) Tuberculous meningitis in South Indian children. A review of 117 cases, *Indian J. Child Hlth*, **11**, 93.

HAZLEHURST, G. N. (1955) Studies on the intrathecal use of streptokinase-streptodornase in tuberculous and other types of bacterial meningitis, *Amer. Rev. Tuberc.*, **71**, 12.

HINMAN, A. R. (1966) Tuberculous meningitis at Cleveland Metropolitan General Hospital, *Amer. Rev. resp. Dis.*, **94**, 465.

HOCKADAY, J. M., and SMITH, H. M. (1966) Corticosteroids as an adjuvant to the chemotherapy of tuberculous meningitis, *Tuberculosis (Habana)*, **47**, 75.

HUEMPFNER, H. R., KINGLOVER, W. R., and DEUSCHLE, K. W. (1966) Tuberculous meningitis caused by both *M. tuberculosis* and atypical mycobacteria, *Amer. Rev. resp. Dis.*, **94**, 612.

INDIAN MEDICAL RESEARCH COUNCIL (1959) *Tuberculosis in India. A sample survey* (1955–1958), New Delhi.

JOHNSON, A. J., AYVAZIAN, J. H., and TILLETT, W. S. (1959) Crystalline pancreatic desoxyribonuclease as an adjunct to the treatment of pneumococcal meningitis, *New Engl. J. Med.*, **260**, 893.

JOISHY, K. N., and SANT, M. V. (1969) Some observations on atypical mycobacteria from tuberculous meningitis in children. Part I, *Indian J. Tuberc.*, **16**, 106.

JOSEPH, R., JOB, J. C., and DEFRANOUX A. (1962) Quoted by Kocen and Parsons (1970).

KAMINSKA, M., and KULCZYNSKAK, K. (1964) The incidence of spinal block in tuberculous meningo-encephalitis, *Pediat. pol.*, **39**, 163.

KHANDELWAL, M. K. (1960) Quoted by Prasad (1963).

KHATUA, S. P. (1961) Tuberculous meningitis in children. Analysis of 213 cases, *J. Indian med. Ass.* **37**, 332.

KOCEN, R. S., and PARSONS, M. (1970) Neurological complications of tuberculosis: some unusual manifestations, *Quart. J. Med.*, **39**, 17.

KOZLOWSKI, K. (1963) Late spinal block after tuberculous meningitis, *Amer. J. Roentgenol.*, **90**, 1220.

KUMBHAT, M. M. (1960) Subdural effusion in tuberculous meningitis, *Indian J. Child Hlth*, **5**, 4.

KUO, CHING-TSAI (1969) The diagnosis of tuberculous meningitis by immunologic reaction of cerebrospinal fluid, *Amer. Rev. resp. Dis.*, **100**, 565.

LEHRER, H. (1966) The angiographic triad in tuberculous meningitis, *Radiology*, **87**, 829.

LINCOLN, E. M., SORDILLO, S. V. R., and DAVIES, P. A. (1960) Tuberculous meningitis in children, *J. Pediat.*, **57**, 807.

LORBER, J. (1956) Tuberculous meningitis, *Practitioner*, **176**, 150.

LORBER, J. (1960) Treatment of tuberculous meningitis, *Brit. med. J.*, **1**, 1309.

LORBER, J. (1961) Long-term follow-up of 100 children who recovered from tuberculous meningitis, *Pediatrics*, **28**, 778.

MACKAY, J. B. (1967) Tuberculous meningitis. A 25-year survey in the Wellington area, *N.Z. med. J.*, **66**, 82.

MANCHANDA, S. S., and LAL, H. (1966) Tuberculous meningitis in children—a problem unsolved in India, *Indian Pediat.*, **3**, 167.

MATHAI, K. V., and CHANDY, J. (1967) Tuberculous infections of the nervous system, *Clin. Neurosurg.*, **14**, 145.

MATHEW, N. T., ABRAHAM, J., and CHANDY, J. (1970) Cerebral angiographic features in tuberculous meningitis, *Neurology (Minneap.)*, **20**, 1015.

MEDICAL RESEARCH COUNCIL (1948) Streptomycin treatment of tuberculous meningitis, report of the Committee on Streptomycin in Tuberculosis Trial, *Lancet*, **i**, 582.

MEDOVAYA, T. N. (1964) Atypical signs in tuberculous meningitis in adults, *Probl. Tuberk.*, **42**, 50.

MENON, N. K. (1966) Scientific contributions of the tuberculosis chemotherapy centre, Madras, *J. Indian med. Ass.*, **47**, 82.

MEYER, H. M., JOHNSON, R. T., CRAWFORD, I. P., and DASCOMB ROGERS, N. G. (1960) Central nervous system syndromes of 'viral' etiology, *Amer. J. Med.*, **29**, 334.

MITCHISON, D. A., WALLACE, G. J., BHATIA, A. L., and SELKON, J. B. (1960) A comparison of the virulence in guinea-pigs of South Indian and British tubercle bacilli, *Tuberculosis (Habana)*, **41**, 1.

NAYAK, N. C., SABHARWAL, B. D., BHATHENA, D., MITAL, G. S., and RAMALINGASWAMI, V. (1970) The pulmonary tuberculous lesion in North India: a study in medico-legal autopsies. 1. Incidence, nature and evolution, *Amer. Rev. resp. Dis.*, **101**, 1.

NORRIS, F. H., GARVEY, P. H., and SWALBACK, G. W. (1964) A mild form of tuberculous meningitis, *Arch. Neurol. (Chic.)* **10**, 398.

OPPENHEIMER, J. H., and REISTER, W. H. (1953) Influence of cortisone on leptomeningeal reaction produced by talc, *Proc. Soc. exp. Biol. (N.Y.)*, **83**, 844.

PENTTI, R., DONNER, M., VALANNE, E., and WASZ-HOCKERT, O. (1962) Late psychological and psychiatric sequelae of tuberculous meningitis, *Acta paediat. (Uppsala)*, **51**, Suppl. 141, 65.

PLACE, A. V., MARJORIE, M. P., and HUERGER, J. D. L. (1969) Ethambutol in tuberculous meningitis, *Amer. Rev. resp. Dis.*, **99**, 783.

PRASAD, S. (1963) Etio-epidemiology of tuberculous meningitis in children, *Indian J. Child Hlth*, **12**, 110.

RAMCHANDARAN, R. S., and PURNAYYAN, S. (1966) Tuberculosis in children, *Indian Pediat.*, **3**, 218.

RAO, B. D., and SUBRAHMANYAM, M. V. (1962) Spinal cord complications of tuberculous meningitis, *Neurology (Bombay)*, **10**, 62.

RAO, S., BHARUCHA, P. E., and BHARUCHA, E. P. (1970) Prognosis in tuberculous meningitis, *Indian Pediat.*, **7**, 257.

RICH, A. (1951) *The Pathogenesis of Tuberculosis*, 2nd ed., Springfield, Ill.

RICH, A., and MCCORDOCK, H. A. (1933) The pathogenesis of tuberculous meningitis, *Bull. Johns Hopk. Hosp.*, **5**, 52.

SAHS, A. L., and JOYNT, R. J. (1962) in *Clinical Neurology* Vol. 2, 2nd ed., ed. Baker, A. B., New York.

SCHWARZ., J. (1949) Tuberculoma and meningitis, *Tuberculology*, **10**, 80.

SHAH, J. R., WARAWADEKAR, M. S., MEHTA, R. H., and DESHMUKH, P. A. (1961) Prevalence of pulmonary tuberculosis in Bombay, *Bombay Hosp. J.*, **3**, 140.

SHANE, S. J., CLOWATER, R. A., and RILEY, C. (1952) Treatment of tuberculous meningitis with cortisone and streptomycin, *Canad. med. Ass. J.*, **67**, 13–15.

SHETH, S. C. (1961) Extrapulmonary tuberculosis, *J. Indian med. Ass.*, **37**, 443.

SINGH, A., JOLLY, S. S., and GOYAL, A. C. (1959) Spinal tuberculous meningitis, *Neurology (India)*, 7, 74–5.

SINGH, B. (1964) The guinea-pig virulence of Indian tubercle bacilli, *Amer. Rev. resp. Dis.*, 89, 1.

SMITH, H. V. (1963) Tuberculous meningitis, *Int. J. Neurol. (Montevideo)*, 4, 134.

SMITH, H. V., and Daniel, P. M. (1947) Some clinical and pathological aspects of tuberculosis of the central nervous system, *Tuberculosis (Habana)*, 28, 64.

SMITH, H. V., and VOLLUM, R. L. (1950) Effects of intrathecal tuberculin and streptomycin in tuberculous meningitis—interim report, *Lancet*, ii, 275.

SMITH, H. V., VOLLUM, R. L., and CAIRNS, H. (1948) Treatment of tuberculous meningitis with streptomycin (a report of the Medical Research Council), *Lancet*, i, 627.

TANDON, P. N., BANERJI, A. K., PRAKASH, B., and GHOSH, S. K. (1970 *a*) Superior orbital fissure syndrome of inflammatory origin, *Bull. All-India Inst. med. Sci.*, 4, 7.

TANDON, P. N., MISRA, R. N., and SINGH, B. (1968) Post-meningitic spinal arachnoiditis, *Bull. All-India Inst. med. Sci.*, 2, 88.

TANDON, P. N., RAO, M. A. P., PATHAK, S. N., and DAS, B. S. (1970 *b*) *Use of* ^{131}*I-labelled Human Serum Albumin in the Scanning of CSF Pathways*, paper presented at the Second Annual Conference of the Society of Nuclear Medicine, 23 October, New Delhi.

TANDON, P. N., SINGH, B., MOHAPATRA, L. N., KUMAR, M., and DAS, S. (1970 *c*) Experimental tuberculosis of the central nervous system, *Neurology (India)*, 18, 81.

TAYLOR, L. M., SMITH, H. V., and HUNTER, C. (1954) Quoted by Smith (1963).

TAYLOR, L. M., SMITH, H. V., and VOLLUM, R. L. (1955) Quoted by Smith (1963).

TERPLAN, K. (1953) The effects of streptomycin on the gross and histologic picture of tuberculous meningitis, *Amer. J. Path.*, 29, 616.

THAPER, R. K. (1967) Incidence of positive bacteriology in cases of tuberculous meningitis in children, *Indian I. Pediat.*, 4, 169.

TODD, R. M., and NEVILLE, J. G. (1964) The sequelae of tuberculous meningitis, *Arch. Dis. Childh.*, 39, 213.

TURELL, R. C., SHAW, W., SCHMIDT, R. P., LEVY, L. L., and ROSEMAN, E. (1953) Electroencephalographic studies of encephalopathies, II. Serial studies in tuberculous meningitis. *Electroenceph. clin. Neurophysiol.*, 5, 53.

UDANI, P. M. (1961) Incidence of tuberculosis in children, *Indian J. Child Hlth*, 10, 515.

UDANI, P. M. (1963) Quoted by Thapar (1967).

UDANI, P. M., and DASTUR, D. K. (1970) Tuberculous encephalopathy with and without meningitis. Clinical features and pathological correlations, *J. neurol. Sci.*, 10, 543.

WADIA, N. H., and DASTUR, D. K. (1969) Spinal meningitides with radiculomyelopathy: Part 1. Clinical and radiological features, *J. neurol. Sci.*, 8, 239.

WADIA, N. H., and SINGHAL, B. S. (1967) Cerebral arteriography in tuberculous meningitis (a study of 33 cases), *Neurology (India)*, 15, 127.

WASZ-HOCKERT, O. (1954) Cortisone in tuberculous meningitis, *Nord. Med.*, 51, 101.

WASZ-HOCKERT, O., and DONNER, M. (1962 *a*) Late prognosis in tuberculous meningitis, *Acta paediat. (Uppsala)*, 51, Suppl. 141.

WASZ-HOCKERT, O., and DONNER, M. (1962 *b*) Results of the treatment of 191 children with tuberculous meningitis, *Acta paediat. (Uppsala)*, 51, Suppl. 141, 7.

WEBB, J. K. G. (1956) Quoted by Prasad (1963).

WEISS, W., and FLIPPIN, H. F. (1961) Prognosis of tuberculous meningitis in the isoniazid area. *Amer. J. med. Sci.*, 242, 423.

WOOD, L. E., BUHIER, V. B., and POLLAK, A. (1956) Human infection with the 'yellow' acid-fast bacillus. A report of fifteen additional cases, *Amer. Rev. Tuberc.*, 73, 917.

WRIGHT, G. P., and REES, R. J. W. (1948) Brains from streptomycin-treated cases of tuberculous meningitis, *Proc. roy. Soc. Med.*, 41, 456.

INTRACRANIAL TUBERCULOMAS

Tuberculous lesions primarily involving the parenchyma of the brain may manifest as miliary tubercles, tuberculomas, or rarely as diffuse oedematous encephalopathy.

The term tuberculoma is often likely to be interpreted differently by clinicians and pathologists. Conventionally, to a clinician a tuberculoma constitutes a lesion, single or multiple, or a tumour-like mass of characteristic granulomatous tissue which produces symptoms of a space-occupying lesion. The size of the lesion which becomes clinically manifest may vary from a few millimetres in the periaqueductal region to one occupying a large portion of a hemisphere.

Incidence

Intracranial tuberculomas, which have become a rare lesion in most of the developed countries, still constitute a significant percentage of intracranial space-occupying lesions (ICSOL) in developing countries. A high incidence is reported not only from tropical countries but also from several other regions of the world. It is not so much the tropical climate, but perhaps the socio-economic conditions prevalent in these countries that determine the incidence [TABLE 2.7].

Intracranial tuberculomas constitute less than 1 per cent of all ICSOL in any large series reported from the United Kingdom, the United States, or Scandinavia (Dott and Levin, 1939; Grant, 1956; Hoessly and Olivecrona, 1956). Their incidence is somewhat higher in Southern and Eastern Europe. Obrador (1959), from Spain, reported an incidence of 4 per cent, while Arseni (1958), from Rumania, encountered 201 tuberculomas in a series of 2757 ICSOL, i.e., an incidence of 7·3 per cent. Reports from South America indicate an even higher incidence; 8 per cent in Panama (Gonsalez-Revilla, 1952) and 15·9 per cent in Chile (Asenjo, Valladares, and Fierro, 1951).

Cabraal (1966), from Ceylon, reported an incidence of 9·1 per cent, and the latest figures are 7·2 per cent (Cabraal and Weinman, 1970). Descuns, Garre, and Pheline (1954) and Roedenbeck (1962) have reported 'high incidence' of this lesion in Algeria and Peru respectively, but the actual figures are not provided.

Table 2.7
Incidence of Intracranial Tuberculomas

Author	*Country or Town*	*Year*	*No. of Tumours*	*No. of Tuberculomas*	*Percentage*
Starr	Great Britain	1889	300	152	50·0
Kinnier Wilson	Great Britain	1954	2190	78	3·6
Cushing	America	1932	2023	33	1·6
Gonsalez-Revilla	Panama	1952	—	—	8·0
Asenjo	Chile	1951	610	97	15·9
Grant	America	1956	2326	18	0·77
Katsura *et al.*	Japan	1959	3312	80	2·4
Obrador	Spain	1959	—	—	4·0
Arseni	Rumania	1958	2757	201	7·3
Cabrall	Ceylon	1966	559	51	9·1
Bagchi	Calcutta	1961	183	16	8·7
Ramamurthi	Madras	1956	—	—	19·4
Dastur, H. M. and Desai	Bombay	1965	373	114	30·5
Sinh *et al.*	Bombay	1968	386	70	18·0
Dastur, D. K., *et al.*	Bombay	1968	1000	211	21·1
Tandon *et al.*	New Delhi	1970	382	16	4·2
Reddy	Madras				10·5
	Andhra	1951	—	—	14·5
Rath *et al.*	Vellore	1967	1492	139	8·1

The incidence of intracranial tuberculomas in Japan was reported to be 6 per cent in 1949. However, Katsura, Suzuki, and Wada (1959) could find only 80 well-documented cases among 3312 ICSOL collected from 23 neurosurgical clinics.

The highest incidence of this lesion has been reported from India. However, there is a distinct regional variation in the country. Dastur and Desai (1965), Dastur, Lalitha, and Prabhakar and Sinh, Pandya, and Dastur (1968), all from Bombay (western coast of India), reported an incidence varying from 18 to 30·5 per cent. The incidence in Madras and Andhra (South India) is nearly as high, at 19·4 per cent (Ramamurthi, 1956) and 14·5 per cent (Reddy, 1951). Rath, Mathai, and Chandy (1967), from Vellore also in South India, reported an incidence of 8·1 out of a total of 1492 ICSOL. In contrast, Bagchi (1961), from Calcutta encountered only 16 tuberculomas among 183 ICSOL (8·7 per cent). The incidence in Northern India appears to be even lower. In Delhi we have observed an incidence of 4·1 per cent in a series of 382 verified ICSOL (Tandon *et al.*, 1970), and this trend remains unchanged in another 100 cases of ICSOL operated upon since the publication of this data. Experience of other neurosurgeons in this part of the country is reported to be identical. Reports from all over India indicate a definite tendency towards lowering of the incidence in recent years.

Aetiology

In all except one of our cases the organisms recovered from the tuberculomas were of the human type. The exception was an atypical tubercle bacillus (Scotochromogen) which is known to produce pathological lesions identical with those produced by the human or bovine type of bacilli. In our experimental study, too, in spite of the variety of pathological responses, we did not observe any alteration in cultural or biochemical characteristics or in the virulence of organisms recovered from such lesions.

Pathogenesis

Precise pathogenesis of the intracranial tuberculomas is not understood. An experimental model of this condition, as encountered in human beings, has not been developed so far, although spontaneous occurrence of this lesion is well documented in a variety of animals including monkeys and cattle (Tandon, Singh, Mohapatra, Kumar, and Das, 1970; Jungherr, 1963; Ruch, 1959). The so-called Rich's foci are really not identical with the human tuberculoma. The views expressed here are based upon a review of the literature, a detailed study of our pathological material, consisting of both surgical and autopsy specimens, as well as the knowledge gained from our experimental studies.

Intracranial tuberculomas result from a haematogenous spread of infection from elsewhere in the body, the commonest site of the primary lesion being the lungs. The primary site of infection may not be apparent when the intracranial lesion is discovered. In a series of 107 cases of tuberculomas of the brain, Dastur and Desai (1965) found associated tuberculous lesions elsewhere in the body in 47 patients, the commonest site being the lungs, with the lymph nodes next in frequency. In isolated cases the associated lesion was peritoneal, renal, ophthalmic, cutaneous, or osseous, etc. Arseni

(1958) reported a nearly identical incidence of associated extracranial lesions.

It may be mentioned that the possibility of a patient with active tuberculosis developing intracranial tuberculoma is rather small. Thus, Lewison, Freilick, and Ragins (1934) found only 20 cases of brain tuberculomas in a consecutive series of 757 autopsies on patients afflicted with tuberculosis—an incidence of less than 3 per cent.

Once the tubercle bacilli have lodged in the brain, the lesion appears to develop in the following manner. The early lesion, the tubercle, generally appears in the cortex or the subcortical region and consists of a central area of incipient or frank necrosis surrounded by a characteristic epithelioid and giant cell reaction. In some cases it contains a dense collection of polymorphonuclear leucocytes in the centre. To start with such microscopic foci are multiple and are usually perivascular [Plate 11c]. The lesion enlarges through expansion of the individual foci and later by means of their conglomeration [Plate 11d]. This results in multiple small macroscopic tuberculomas which may remain isolated from each other or merge together to form a solitary mass [Plates 11a and b]. The ultimate evolution of the lesion appears to depend upon the interplay of hypersensitivity and immune responses. The former is characterized by profound vasodilatation, oedema, and a polymorphonuclear exudation, whereas in the latter there is an abundance of epithelioid cells, giant cells, lymphocytes, and plasma cells. Endarteritic changes in the blood vessels are observed but infrequently, and it seems that ischaemia *per se* does not play a significant role in the progression of the disease.

Healing in tuberculosis takes place predominantly by means of fibrosis, which is thought to impair the oxygen supply to the organisms by obliterating the vascular channels. In our experience fibrous encapsulation is seen very infrequently. There is little participation by fibroblasts except where the lesion reaches the surface meninges. This is not surprising in view of the inherent architecture of the brain tissue. Therefore, for all practical purposes most of these lesions should be considered active. When, however, healing sets in fibrosis and even calcification develop.

Pathology

Macroscopic Examination

Grossly, a tuberculoma is a well-circumscribed, greyish-white, firm nodular or lobulated mass with a granular surface, measuring from a few millimetres to 3–4 cm or even more in diameter [Plates 11a and b]. The largest one reported occupied an entire half of the hemisphere (Ramamurthi, Varadarajan, and Vedachalam, 1961). We have encountered one virtually replacing a cerebellar hemisphere. It may be solitary or multiple. The incidence of multiple tuberculomas, not surprisingly, is higher in autopsy series than in surgical reports. Multiple tuberculomas may be in the form of a large mass, surrounded by small satellites in the immediate vicinity which are separated by intervening gliosed tissue, or perhaps widely scattered throughout the brain. There is another variety that we have recently encountered, which had the appearance of a cluster of grapes, each individual tuberculoma being no bigger than 0·5 cm in diameter although combined together they produced a sizeable mass in the parietal lobe. Multiple lesions such as this were also found scattered in the brain stem.

Instead of a well-circumscribed mass, less frequently a tuberculoma may occur as a diffuse infiltrating lesion. This variety involves the cortex and the overlying dura. It is sometimes difficult to say whether it represents a primary meningeal lesion, as described by Rich (1951) under the title 'focal caseous plaque,' or a truly parenchymatous lesion. This type of lesion has been commonly designated as 'tuberculoma-en-plaque' (Ramamurthi, Varadarajan, and Vedachalam, 1961; Ferris, Lehrer, and Shapiro, 1967). Owing to involvement of the overlying meninges the periphery of this lesion tends to be quite vascular. This is the type of lesion which on angiography may show a 'tumour blush' or 'tumour circulation'. A slight variant of this lesion was encountered by us in a young female, who had an 'en-plaque' type of lesion on the surface in the parietal parasagittal region, separated by a layer of gliosed brain from a well-circumscribed, lobulated, avascular mass in the depth. Still more rarely, a tuberculoma may spread through the overlying dura to involve the calvarium.

On cut-section the centre is necrotic but firm and presents the typical creamish-white appearance of caseation. Rarely, it may become cystic as a result of liquefying necrosis of the central caseous material (Sinh, Pandya, and Dastur, 1968; Dastur, Desai, and Dastur, 1962; Rao, Subrahmanyam, and Sathe, 1963) or present as a tuberculous abscess (Courville, 1945; Arseni, 1958; Sinh, Pandya, and Dastur, 1968).

Microscopic Examination

The core of the lesion is made up of a massive coagulative necrosis, often scattered with shadows of cells or a variable amount of cellular debris, as described in classical caseation. This is surrounded by epithelioid cells with an admixture of lymphocytes, plasma cells, histiocytes and numerous giant cells of Langhans type. The Langhans giant cells are much more conspicuous here than in the leptomeninges in cases of tuberculous meningitis. Another notable feature, in the material studied by us, was the presence of unusually large giant cells, many resembling the foreign body type, most unlike the giant cells seen in tuberculous lesions elsewhere in the body.

The surrounding cellular reaction is not always as classically described in other organs. Not infrequently one encounters a lesion with a sharply punched out focus of necrosis with scant epithelioid cell reaction and only a thin rim of lymphocytes, plasma cells and stray giant cells of Langhans type. On the other hand, in some tuberculomas a significant feature is the presence of an appreciable, often conspicuous, number of polymorphonuclear leucocytes participating in the inflammatory cell reaction. Indeed, in some places they resemble micro-abscesses as observed in acute pyogenic infections.

Arranged around the central lesion are numerous granulomas in various stages of evolution, ranging from sharply outlined, predominantly epithelioid cell foci with scattered giant cells, to those with incipient or established caseation and the usual range of cellular reaction.

In the cases which we reviewed microscopic examination confirmed the lack of a well-formed fibrous capsule. At most in a few cases the lesion appeared to have a thin, generally incomplete, pseudo-capsule made up of compressed gliosed surrounding brain tissue. Where the lesion approached the surface, there was attempted collagenization in the area, rarely accompanied by what looked like hyalinized granulomas. It may, however, be emphasized that such a reaction was patchy and rarely observed in lesions occupying the deeper portions of the brain tissue.

A tuberculoma is generally described as an avascular lesion. The central core of the lesion is, of course, avascular, but the same cannot be said of the periphery. Vastly dilated, thin-walled blood vessels are encountered with striking frequency in this region. A variety of other vascular changes are observed in this area. These consist of a variable degree of fibrous thickening of the intima, sometimes eccentric, resulting in appreciable narrowing of the lumen in the medium-sized vessels. Classical changes of endarteritis obliterans affecting smaller vessels are, however, not frequent.

The surrounding brain tissue shows a variable degree of gliosis and oedema. The blood vessels often show a prominent cuffing with non-specific, predominantly lymphocytic infiltration, extending to variable depths around the central lesion. In an occasional case there are distinct freshly formed granulomas in the perivascular spaces constituting numerous satellite foci. Generally, the oedema of the surrounding brain tissue is much less here than it is in a pyogenic abscess. However, very occasionally a small tuberculoma may be surrounded by an enormous amount of brain oedema, which may dominate the clinical as well as the pathological picture. This oedema is not just peritumoural and a consequence of the inflammatory nature of the lesion, but is postulated to be an expression of allergic response (Sinh, Pandya, and Dastur, 1968).

The meningeal reaction is also variable, chiefly depending upon the location of the parent lesion. Where the lesion approaches the surface, the meninges show a characteristic granulomatous reaction spreading over an area much wider than that constituting the immediate periphery of the lesion. In some cases we have seen, the leptomeningeal granulomas were active and caseating. In most cases, however, the meninges show only a non-specific inflammatory reaction with or without diffuse fibrous thickening. In a small number of cases, frank acute tuberculous meningitis and a brain tuberculoma may co-exist.

Clinical Picture

Age Incidence

The disease primarily affects younger subjects, nearly one-third being below 10 years of age in any large series reported. The incidence remains high in the second and third decades, and suddenly declines in the fourth decade, being rare above 40 years of age. The youngest reported case was 3 months old and the oldest 68 years (Arseni, 1958). Cabrall (1966) had no case above 40 years of age and Ramamurthi, Varadarajan, and Vedachalam (1961) had only two in a series of 175 cases.

Sex Incidence

There appears to be no significant difference in the incidence among the two sexes. However, Dastur and Desai (1965) concluded that a male above 25 years of age has a very slender chance of developing a supratentorial tuberculoma. Among their 11 cases above the age of 30 years, there were 10 females and only one male.

Site

In the paediatric age-group, intracranial tuberculomas are encountered more frequently in the posterior fossa than supratentorially, with nearly 60 per cent located in the cerebellar hemispheres. However, in adults supratentorial lesions are much more frequent. In the cerebral hemispheres the commonest site is the fronto-parietal region. The temporal lobes, centrum semi-ovale, and basal ganglia are less often involved. Approximately 4 to 5 per cent of intracranial tuberculomas are located in the brain stem. Roedenbeck (1962), from Peru, has reported a surprisingly high incidence of tuberculomas of the brain stem; out of a total of 57 cases, 10 were in a cerebral peduncle, 4 in the 'bulbar protuberance' (? pons) and 2 in the medulla. Another infrequent site is the lateral ventricle. We have encountered intraventricular tuberculomas in three cases, while Bagchi (1961) reported one such case.

Intracranial extradural tuberculomas are extremely rare. We have seen only one such case (Tandon, Banerji, Das, and Dar, 1970). Sinh, Pandya, and Dastur (1968) reported transdural spread of an intracranial lesion to involve the calvaria. Isolated tuberculomas of the meninges are also reported (Rich, 1951). The lesions are multiple in 6 to 10 per cent of cases.

Symptoms and Signs

The clinical presentations of intracranial tuberculoma are similar to those of any other intracranial space-occupying lesion. The duration of symptoms varies from 1 month to 3 years or even more. As in other brain tumours, depending upon the site of the lesion, the presenting symptoms and signs are those of raised intracranial pressure, focal or generalized seizures, and focal neurological deficit. Dastur and Desai (1965) pointed out the higher incidence of false localizing signs and symptoms in cases of tuberculomas of the brain as compared with gliomas. This is mainly the result of the multiplicity of lesions in the former, the predominant signs being due to the larger mass, while a smaller lesion elsewhere is responsible for the false localizing sign. Strictly speaking, these are not false localizing signs. For example, one of our patients with a conglomeration of multiple tuberculomas in the parietal region had marked cerebellar signs besides the parietal lobe signs. Radiological investigations revealed only the parietal lobe mass. The explanation of the cerebellar signs was apparent 4 months later at autopsy which revealed multiple small tuberculomas in the brain stem which had produced no detectable abnormality in the ventriculogram.

On the basis of clinical, radiological and pathological findings Ramamurthi, Varadarajan, and Vedachalam (1961) classified their cases into two groups. The major group consisted of large, discrete, tuberculomatous masses, usually occurring in the subcortical area or the deeper regions of the brain, and often presented with raised intracranial pressure. Less frequently the lesion may be of the infiltrating variety, designated as 'diffuse tuberculoma', which occurs in the cortex and the subcortical regions of the cerebrum or the cerebellum. These patients present with a progressive neurological disability with concomitant tuberculous infection elsewhere in the body. The intracranial pressure in such cases is usually not elevated. Angiographically, they show increased vascularity, in contrast to the former group which tends to present with avascular lesions. The existence of these two groups, radiologically and pathologically, is well documented, but along with others, we do not think it possible to distinguish them on clinical grounds alone. Contrary to general expectation, fever is only rarely a feature of tuberculomas of the brain. However, evidence of tuberculosis elsewhere in the body is an indication of such a possibility. Associated active, chronic, or healed tuberculous lesions, mostly in the lungs but occasionally in other organs, have been reported in 30 to 60 per cent of these patients. In a country where tuberculosis is still a common disease, the discovery of a tuberculous lesion elsewhere in the body does not necessarily imply that the intracranial lesion is of the same aetiology. Approximately 4·5 per cent of neoplastic lesions of the brain have an associated extracranial tuberculous lesion. Concomitant evidence of meningitis is also infrequent, even though tuberculomas are so frequently found at autopsy in cases of tuberculous meningitis.

Laboratory Investigations

Routine laboratory investigations are not very helpful in the diagnosis of intracranial tuberculomas. The erythrocyte sedimentation rate is raised in a small percentage of cases only. A strongly positive tuberculin test in a child with evidence of ICSOL may suggest the possibility of its being a tuberculoma, but this is not of much value in adults. As mentioned earlier, evidence of a tuberculous lesion in a plain chest X-ray increases the chances of an intracranial lesion being tubercular.

Plain skull X-ray usually shows signs of raised intracranial pressure. Calcification is not commonly seen. In most large series the incidence of calcification is not more than 4 to 6 per cent. However, in a small series Armstrong and Edwards (1963) reported calcification in 60 per cent of their patients who were mostly Indians and Eskimos from Alberta, Canada.

Calcification represents healing of the tuberculoma but it is not an indication of continued quiescence. Berlin (1963) considers an irregular, broken, calcareous shell as characteristic of a tuberculoma. Mascherpa and Valentino (1959) described a 'lobulated' and a 'nodular' type of calcified lesion. The former is usually 1–3 cm in diameter, the calcification being dense and jagged at the periphery and radiolucent in the centre. The nodular variety, which is less common, is composed of multiple calcareous concretions grouped together. We feel that it is seldom possible to diagnose a tuberculoma confidently from the pattern of calcification seen in the roentgenogram of the skull.

Angiography

Generally there is no pattern specific for tuberculomas, the radiological picture being that of a relatively avascular space-occupying lesion. Two features, however, need special mention. Occasionally, a sudden reduction in the calibre of the blood vessels traversing the tumour or in its vicinity has been reported (Dastur and Desai, 1965). Davis and Taveras (1967) suggested that the presence of a mass in the parasagittal region, a common site for tuberculomas, in association with evidence of arterial narrowing, indicating arterial spasm, should arouse suspicion of an infectious process. Secondly, still more uncommonly the angiogram may reveal increased vascularity which may be prominent enough to suggest a 'tumour blush' or a 'tumour circulation'. The angiogram of one of our patients was scarcely distinguishable from that of a meningioma, a diagnosis confidently made by a number of independent observers fully acquainted with tuberculomas. Similar cases have been reported by Ramamurthi, Varadarajan, and Vedachalam (1961).

Posterior fossa tuberculomas, commonly diagnosed by air or *Myodil* ventriculography, have no characteristic features which help to differentiate them from other space-occupying lesions in this region.

Treatment

As recently as 1932, Cushing advocated decompression as the only surgical procedure for these lesions. Surgical results remained poor and medical therapy non-existent until the introduction of antitubercular chemotherapy. Among 60 cases operated upon by Arseni (1958) before the advent of streptomycin, the operative mortality was 10 per cent but an additional 40 per cent died of tuberculous meningitis.

A pre-operative course of antitubercular drugs for approximately 2 weeks is advisable when tuberculoma is suspected. Owing to its high incidence in some regions of India, routine antitubercular chemotherapy is administered to all patients below the age of 30 years waiting for surgery for a suspected intracranial tumour. The treatment is, of course, discontinued as soon as the lesion is proved to be non-tubercular. In Delhi we have not followed this practice unless a tuberculous lesion is discovered elsewhere in the body, or if the patient has a strong family history of tuberculosis, or if he is pyrexial. The risk of postoperative tuberculous meningitis is negligible if chemotherapy is started immediately after the operative confirmation of the diagnosis.

There is still some controversy regarding the possibility of curing intracranial tuberculoma by medical treatment alone. Ramamurthi, Varadarajan, and Vedachalam (1961) believe that the so-called infiltrating variety of tuberculoma, which could be reasonably diagnosed by angiography, is treatable by antitubercular drugs alone. Roedenbeck (1962) concluded that 'in tuberculomas of the nervous system, even when there is a well-developed syndrome of endocranial hypertension, therapeutic benefits from medical treatment based on streptomycin and isoniazid are much superior to those from surgical intervention'. Lack of histological verification of the lesion in these workers' patients makes it difficult to assess the reliability of this conclusion. The circumstantial evidence in some of the patients prevents an outright dismissal of such claims. Many of us have observed a dramatic improvement in the condition of an occasional patient with an undoubted clinical picture of an intracranial space-occupying lesion, following administration of antitubercular drugs, such that eventual surgery is not required. In most such cases, however, objective proof of the presence of a tuberculoma has been lacking. In this connexion it may be worth mentioning two of our own patients. One, a young lady of 28 years with a well-documented history of pleural effusion 6 months earlier, was admitted with low-grade pyrexia (99–100·5°F), severe headache, vomiting and progressive right hemiparesis. On examination she was found to have bilateral papilloedema. A left carotid angiogram revealed a mass in the frontal region. She was put on antitubercular drugs which resulted in complete remission of her signs and symptoms. A repeat angiogram 2 years later was normal. The patient has been followed up now for 7 years without any evidence of recurrence. The second patient, a young man of 25 years with three tuberculomas in the right cerebellar hemisphere, surgically excised and verified, had a right-sided supranuclear facial palsy which had prompted a left carotid angiogram pre-operatively. This revealed a left to right shift of the anterior cererbal artery which was confirmed on ventriculography. This supratentorial lesion was not explored, as the cerebellar lesion was judged to be predominantly responsible for his clinical condition. He was given antitubercular chemotherapy postoperatively and after 1 year, while he was asymptomatic, a repeat carotid angiogram showed no abnormality. Identical cases have been reported by Cabrall (1966) and Ramamurthi (1970).

The majority of patients with intracranial tuberculomas require surgical treatment even if the lesions are calcified. As far as possible an attempt is made to excise the lesion totally, which is usually not difficult as it tends to shell out from the surrounding brain. For extensive lesions or those situated strategically subtotal removal and adequate internal decompression may be satisfactory.

Postoperatively, all patients are given chemotherapy for 1½ years. We generally give streptomycin 1 G OD, isonicotinic acid hydrazide (INH) 300–400 mg per day and para-aminosalicylic acid (PAS) 12 G per day, all three for the first 3 months, followed by INH and PAS, or INH and thiacetazone, for the remaining 15 months. Pyridoxine or vitamin B-complex is always given along with INH.

Prognosis

With the routine use of antitubercular drugs, mortality from tuberculoma of the brain has been reduced to less than 10 per cent. One of the causes of postoperative death observed by us is associated basal meningitis, which may prevent adequate relief of raised intracranial pressure even after the successful excision of a large tuberculoma in the posterior fossa. In such cases a complete excision of a cerebellar tuberculoma was performed. Autopsy revealed a dense basal meningitis which was responsible for persistent raised intracranial pressure. The incidence of postoperative tuberculous meningitis is less than 5 per cent and in most cases this is readily controlled. Late deaths may result from inadequate postoperative treatment or overlooked tuberculomas.

Apart from mortality, postoperative morbidity is still very disheartening. In the advanced cases that are generally encountered in India, blindness is a frequent cause of morbidity in 10 to 15 per cent of cases. Residual hemiparesis, ataxia, and convulsions account for an additional 10 per cent of cases. On the whole, nearly 60 to 70 per cent of patients return to normal life.

References

Armstrong, F. B., and Edwards, A. M. (1963) Quoted by Cabrall (1966).

Arseni, C. (1958) Two hundred and one cases of intracranial tuberculomas treated surgically, *J. Neurol. Neurosurg. Psychiat.*, **21**, 308.

ASENJO, A., VALLADARES, H., and FIERRO, J. (1951) Tuberculomas of the brain. (Report of one hundred and fifty-nine cases.), *Arch. Neurol. Psychiat.* (*Chic.*), 65, 146.
BAGCHI, A. (1961) The intracranial tuberculomas, *J. Indian med. Ass.*, 37, 429.
BERLIN, L. (1963) Tuberculoma of the brain, *Amer. J. Roentgenol.*, 90, 1185.
CABRALL, S. A. (1966) Tuberculoma of the brain, *Ceylon med. J.*, 11, 87.
CABRALL, S. A., and WEINMAN, D. (1970) Personal communication.
COURVILLE, C. B. (1945) *Pathology of the Central Nervous System*, 2nd ed., California.
CUSHING, H. (1932) *Intracranial Tumours. Notes upon a Series of Two-thousand Verified Cases with Surgical Mortality Percentages Pertaining Thereto*, Springfield, Ill.
DASTUR, D. K., LALITHA, V. S., and PRABHAKAR, V. (1968) Pathological analysis of intracranial space-occupying lesions in 1000 cases including children, Part 1. Age, sex and pattern of the tuberculomas, *J. neurol. Sci.*, 6, 575.
DASTUR, H. M., and DESAI, A. D. (1965) A comparative study of brain tuberculomas and gliomas based upon 107 case records of each, *Brain*, 88, 375.
DASTUR, H. M., DESAI, A. D., and DASTUR, D. K. (1962) A cystic cerebral tuberculoma treated surgically, *J. Neurol. Neurosurg. Psychiat.*, 25, 370.
DAVIS, D. O., and TAVERAS, J. M. (1967) Radiological aspects of inflammatory conditions affecting the central nervous system, *Clin. Neurosurg.*, 14, 192.
DESCUNS, P., GARRE, H., and PHELINE, C. (1954) Tuberculomas of the brain and cerebellum, *J. Neurosurg.*, 11, 243.
DOTT, N. M., and LEVIN, E. (1939) Intracranial tuberculoma, *Edinb. med. J.*, 46, 36.
EVANS, H. S., and COURVILLE, C. B. (1938) Calcification and ossification in tuberculomas of brain, *Arch. Surg.*, 36, 637.
FERRIS, E. J., LEHRER, H., and SHAPIRO, J. H. (1967) Pseudo-subdural hematoma, *Radiology*, 88, 75.
GONSALEZ-REVILLA, A. (1952) Intracranial tuberculomas; experience with 10 consecutive cases, *J. Neurosurg.*, 9, 555.
GRANT, F. C. (1956) A study of the results of surgical treatment in 2326 consecutive patients with brain tumour, *J. Neurosurg.*, 12, 479.
HOESSLY, G. F., and OLIVECRONA, H. (1956) Report on 280 cases of verified parasagittal meningioma, *J. Neurosurg.*, 12, 614.
JUNGHERR, E. (1963) Tumours and tumour-like conditions in monkeys, *Ann. N.Y. Acad. Sci.*, 108, 777.
JUUL-JENSEN, P., and DENNY-BROWN, D. (1966) Epilepsia partialis continua: a clinical electrographic and neuropathological study of nine cases, *Arch. Neurol.* (*Chic.*), 15, 563.
KATSURA, S., SUZUKI, J., and WADA, T. (1959) A statistical study of brain tumours in the Neurosurgical Clinics in Japan, *J. Neurosurg.*, 16, 570.
LEWISON, M., FREILICK, E. B., and RAGINS, O. D. (1934) Tuberculoma of brain, *Ann. intern. Med.*, 7, 1141.
MASCHERPA, F., and VALENTINO, V. (1959) *Intracranial Calcification*, Springfield, Ill., p. 52.
OBRADOR, S. (1959) Intracranial tuberculomas; review of 47 cases, *Neurochirurgia.* (*Stuttg.*), 1, 150.
RAMAMURTHI, B. (1956) Tuberculoma of the brain, *Indian J. Surg.*, 18, 452.
RAMAMURTHI, B. (1970) *Contributions to Knowledge*, Souvenir published on the occasion of the Twentieth Anniversary celebrations of the Department of Neurology and Neurosurgery, Madras Medical College. (Personal communication.)
RAMAMURTHI, B., VARADARAJAN, M. G., and VEDACHALAM, S. P. (1961) Tuberculoma of the brain. (Pathologic picture and diagnosis.), *J. int. Coll. Surg.*, 35, 605.
RAO, B. D., SUBRAHMANYAM, M. V., and SATHE, N.M. (1963) Cerebral tuberculoma simulating a cystic glioma. A case report, *J. Neurosurg.*, 20, 172.
RATH, S., MATHAI, K. V., and CHANDY, J. (1967) Intracranial space-occupying lesions. (An analysis of incidence.), *Neurology* (*India*), 15, 169.
REDDY, D. J. (1951) Tuberculoma of the brain, *Indian J. Surg.*, 13, 138.
RICH, A. R. (1951) *The Pathogenesis of Tuberculosis*, 2nd ed., Springfield, Ill., p. 882.
ROEDENBECK, S. D. (1962) Tuberculomas of the nervous system in children. (A report of 32 cases.), *Wld Neurol.*, 3, 54.
RUCH, T. C. (1959) *Diseases of Laboratory Primates*, Philadelphia.
SINH, G., PANDYA, S. K., and DASTUR, D. K. (1968) The pathogenesis of unusual intracranial tuberculomas and tuberculous space-occupying lesions, *J. Neurosurg.*, 29, 149.
TANDON, P. N., BANERJI, A. K., DAS, B. S., and DAR, J. (1970) Intracranial space-occupying lesions. A five-year survey at the *AIIMS, Bull. AIIMS*, 4, 119.
TANDON, P. N., SINGH, B., MOHAPATRA, L. N., KUMAR, M., and DAS, S. (1970) Experimental tuberculosis of the central nervous system, *Neurology* (*India*), 18, 81.
WAGENEN, W. P. VAN (1927) Tuberculoma of brain, its incidence among intracranial tumours and its surgical aspect, *Arch. Neurol. Psychiat.* (*Chic.*), 17, 57.

POTT'S PARAPLEGIA

The association of paraplegia with disease of the spinal column was classically described by Percivall Pott (1779) in his paper entitled 'Remarks on That Kind of Palsy of the Lower Limbs Which is Frequently Found to Accompany a Curvature of the Spine, and is Supposed to be Caused by It, Together with the Method of Cure'. The tuberculous nature of the spinal lesion was, of course, not known at that time. It is claimed that Diechamp had described a similar condition as early as 1517. According to Professor Keshwani (1967), the disease is mentioned in a number of hymns in *Atharva Veda* (approximately 1500 BC). The term 'Pott's paraplegia' is now, however, generally used for all cases of paraplegia due to tuberculosis of the spine.

Incidence

Spinal tuberculosis accounts for more than 50 per cent of all bone and joint tuberculosis (Mukhopadhaya and Mishra, 1957; Ohri and Krishnamoorthy, 1954; Roaf, Kirkaldy-Willis, and Cathro, 1959). The incidence of paraplegia in cases of spinal tuberculosis has been reported to vary from approximately 10 to 40 per cent;

Butler (1935) reported 11·4 per cent; Ohri and Krishnamoorthy (1954) 15·7 per cent; Mukhopadhaya and Mishra (1957) 24 per cent; Jones (1958) 41 per cent. In the developing countries, tuberculosis of the spine is probably the commonest cause of compression paraplegia (Misra, Tandon, and Lahiri, 1964; Roaf, Kirkaldy-Willis, and Cathro, 1959).

The site of the lesion in 100 cases of Pott's paraplegia was found to be cervical in 7 per cent, cervicodorsal in 16 per cent, mid-dorsal in 47 per cent, lower dorsal and upper lumbar in 35 per cent, with double lesions in 5 per cent. However, if one considers the risk of paraplegia in relation to the frequency of tuberculosis at a particular level, the highest incidence is reported in cervicodorsal lesions (approximately 60 per cent); mid-dorsal lesions are likely to result in paraplegia in nearly 40 per cent of cases.

Age

The disease can occur at any age. While the overall incidence of spinal tuberculosis may be higher below 12 years of age, the relative incidence of paraplegia is higher above this age. In contrast to the 9 per cent out of a total of 360 cases of spinal tuberculosis in children below the age of 12 years who developed paraplegia, 17·4 per cent of 155 adults developed this complication (Mukhopadhaya, 1954). It is our impression that there is a general shift in the incidence of this disease towards older age-groups, so that we now see a greater percentage of adults than children.

Aetiopathogenesis

Before discussing the aetiopathogenesis of paraplegia in cases of spinal tuberculosis it may be worth considering the well-established clinico-pathological classification of paraplegia into that of early onset and late onset, initially proposed by Sorrel-Dejerine (1925) and later elaborated by Butler (1935) and Seddon (1935). They considered it important in relation to both pathology and prognosis. This classification was based upon a clinico-pathological study of a large series of cases long before the introduction of antitubercular chemotherapy. This gives an insight into the natural history of the disease. In our opinion it has served its purpose and has outlived its utility. It contains inconsistencies and contradictions of statements with regard to aetiopathogenesis, and cannot be considered a guide to therapy or prognosis under modern circumstances. At least one of the proponents of this classification, Seddon, in a comparatively recent publication, has commented upon its 'irritating vagueness' (Griffiths, Seddon, and Roaf, 1956). Roaf, Kirkaldy-Willis, and Cathro (1959) were unable to classify their cases according to this classification.

The cause of paraplegia in the vast majority of cases of caries of the spine is compression of the spinal cord (Rao and Dinkar, 1970). There is no proof that the paraplegia is ever due to toxic and vascular reactions in the cord secondary to the presence of active tuberculosis in immediate relationship to the dura mater, as proposed by Butler (1935) for his type 1 cases. Whenever neurological deficit, however minimal, has been observed by us in a case of tuberculosis of the spine, myelography has revealed unequivocal evidence of spinal compression. One such patient was investigated for backache. Initially he had no neurological deficit. A few days before the myelogram he developed minimal weakness in one leg with slight sensory and reflex changes. The myelogram clearly demonstrated a partial block. After 6 weeks of conservative treatment, including antitubercular chemotherapy, the neurological signs regressed. Rescreening of the spine revealed normal filling.

The compression may be caused by:

1. Fluid abscess in the spinal canal.
2. Paraspinal abscess invading the spinal canal.
3. Granulation tissue encircling the dura.
4. Sequestrated bone or intervertebral disc.
5. Dislocated vertebra.
6. In very chronic cases a thick transverse ridge of fibrous tissue pressing anteriorly on the dura and causing indentation or even acute angulation of the spinal cord with localized ischaemia (Hodgson *et al.*, 1960).
7. A combination of any of the above.

While Sorrel-Dejerine attributed the cases of paraplegia of late onset to pachymeningitis, later studies could not substantiate its existence. However, in recent years Hodgson *et al.* (1960) have demonstrated that on rare occasions the tuberculous process may involve the dura, pia-arachnoid and even the spinal cord. Frank meningitis is, of course, extremely uncommon.

Apart from compression, the only other cause of paraplegia in cases of spinal caries is thrombosis of a radicular artery. The artery may be compressed in an intervertebral foramen or it may be the seat of tuberculous arteritis. The incidence of this complication is uncertain, but it probably accounts for an occasional case of severe paraplegia of rapid onset.

Clinical Picture

It is probably best to consider the clinical picture of Pott's paraplegia in the following four groups:

1. Paraplegia arising in a known case of spinal tuberculosis.
2. Paraplegia as the presenting symptom of spinal tuberculosis.
3. 'Spinal tumour' syndrome.
4. Paraplegia due to tuberculosis of the posterior neural arch.

Paraplegia Arising in a Known Case of Spinal Tuberculosis

It is generally recognized now that paralysis can begin at any time and during any phase or stage of the vertebral disease, even after apparently sound healing. As mentioned earlier, it serves no useful purpose to speak of paraplegia of early or late onset. This is the commonest mode of presentation and diagnosis is not difficult. It is advisable for all cases of spinal tuberculosis to have a periodic, detailed neurological examination.

Paraplegia as the Presenting Symptom

A patient with tuberculosis of the spine may present for the first time when paralysis has already set in. This is, unfortunately, not an uncommon presentation in our country, where patients often fail to seek medical advice until very late. Pain and tenderness in the affected part, muscle spasm with restricted spinal movements, a varying degree of gibbus, and frequently a palpable cold abscess point to the diagnosis. Plain X-ray of the spine will confirm it.

These two groups of patients are not of particular interest to neurosurgeons; they are generally looked after by orthopaedic surgeons.

Spinal Tumour Syndrome

These patients, who have obvious signs of spinal compression but without clinical or radiological evidence of disease of the spine, are generally referred to neurosurgeons. The true nature of their disease is disclosed only after surgery. In our experience a retrospective review of the roentgenograms reveals the bony lesion in the majority of these cases. It is often very restricted but exuberant granulation tissue may spread for a varying extent extradurally and compress the cord. The exact site of compression may thus be at some distance from the site of the bony lesion, as illustrated by the following case.

A 14-year-old girl was admitted with rapidly developing paraplegia of 6 weeks' duration. Clinical examination localized the lesion to the level of the third dorsal vertebra. Plain X-ray of the spine at this level revealed no abnormality. A cisternal myelogram showed a block at the expected site [PLATE 12a]. A lumbar myelogram demonstrated the lower limit of the block opposite the twelfth dorsal vertebra [PLATE 12b]. Laminectomy from D3-D12 revealed extensive tuberculous granulation tissue completely encircling the cord. The unequivocal narrowing of the D11-D12 intervertebral disc space with fuzziness of the margins of the adjacent vertebrae was only discovered retrospectively.

A tiny area of radiolucency at the posterior-inferior angle of the seventh cervical vertebra was overlooked in another patient with tetraparesis until after surgical exposure of a small sequestrum and tuberculous debris.

Improved radiological techniques, especially the use of tomography, will no doubt increase the chances of correct pre-operative diagnosis. There will still be a few cases in which the bony lesion cannot be demonstrated. These are described separately under intraspinal tuberculous granulomas.

Paraplegia due to Tuberculosis of the Posterior Neural Arch

This is reported to be an extremely rare condition. However, we have encountered a number of cases of paraplegia due to lesions of the pedicle and/or lamina. The majority of these patients are adults between 30 and 50 years of age. They present with the usual history of local pain and progressive paraplegia of varying duration. Clinically, there is generally no indication of the tuberculous nature of the disease. Radiologically, the destruction of the affected part is apparent, but there is nothing characteristic of its nature. The association of a paravertebral soft tissue shadow may point to the correct diagnosis, as also the presence of a tuberculous lesion elsewhere in the body.

Laboratory Investigations

Routine laboratory investigations are of little help. The ESR is generally raised. The tuberculin test is usually positive. A careful roentgenographic examination provides the most useful information, however. The classical radiological features are well documented in textbooks of radiology and orthopaedics and need not be enumerated here. However, in countries where this disease is still very prevalent, one has to be aware of the uncommon and atypical presentations.

Treatment

As soon as the diagnosis is suspected, the patient is put on antitubercular chemotherapy. Streptomycin, isonicotinic acid hydrazide (INH), and para-aminosalicylic acid (PAS) are administered in adequate doses. If a definite favourable response is observed within a couple of weeks, medical treatment with bed rest and later external immobilization may be continued for the first two groups of patients. However, there is already enough evidence in favour of surgical excision of the tuberculous focus in all cases, after a preliminary course of chemotherapy. The operative mortality has been reduced to less than 5 per cent in all large series of cases (Hodgson *et al.*, 1960; Goel, 1967; Roaf, Kirkaldy-Willis, and Cathro, 1959). Recovery from paraplegia is achieved in 70 to 80 per cent of cases. The speed of recovery is enhanced and the chances of recurrence definitely reduced.

Even if every patient is not submitted to surgery, the following would generally be accepted as indications for surgery:

1. Paraplegia arising while the patient is under adequate conservative treatment for spinal tuberculosis.
2. Paraplegia deteriorating despite conservative treatment.
3. Paraplegia of rapid onset.
4. Severe or complete paraplegia.
5. Recurrent paraplegia.

6. Paraplegia due to disease of the posterior neural arch.
7. Spinal tumour syndrome—where diagnosis is in doubt.
8. In cases where conservative treatment is unduly hazardous or impossible; severe spasms or spasticity or bed sores making immobilization difficult; paraplegia in old age, when immobilization may result in dangerous complications.

There are a variety of surgical approaches to a tuberculous lesion of the spine associated with paraplegia, and each has advantages for special circumstances and particular areas. For practical purposes these may be divided into four groups:

1. *Costotransversectomy:* this operation was first advocated by Menard in 1894. It aims at evacuation of a paraspinal abscess without exposing the spinal canal. It is not a reliable operation, and cannot deal with the intraspinal causes of paraplegia. However, it may be useful for poor-risk patients whose X-rays show a tense paraspinal abscess (Mukhopadhaya and Mishra, 1957).

2. *Anterolateral decompression:* this is really a modification of the operation described above. The aim is to expose the spinal canal through a lateral extrapleural approach and remove the intraspinal abscess, granulations, or debris anterior to the spinal cord. The operation was first described by Alexander (1946). Some modifications of the same operation have been described by Capener (1954, 1967) and Goel (1967). This operation is best suited to disease of the dorsal spine.

3. *Anterior approach:* this approach has been recently popularized by Hodgson and his colleagues from Hong Kong (1956, 1960). The object of this operation is to allow full visualization of the lesion by a wider anterior exposure, to facilitate complete excision of all diseased and devitalized tissue and to provide for immediate fusion by means of a strut graft in compression between adjacent healthy vertebral bodies. Operation on the first 100 cases reported by the authors achieved a fusion rate of 93 per cent, complete recovery from paraplegia in 74 per cent and a mortality rate of 4 per cent. There was only one relapse of the disease within the period of follow-up. The operation can be utilized for disease at all levels.

4. *Laminectomy:* this operation is contra-indicated in cases of tuberculosis of the body of vertebra. However, this is the only correct approach in cases of spinal tumour syndrome. It also provides for complete excision of the lesion in cases with posterior neural arch involvement.

Irrespective of the type of surgical approach, antitubercular chemotherapy is continued for at least 1½ years.

Prognosis

With modern treatment, the prognosis of Pott's paraplegia has radically changed. If the correct treatment is instituted early in the course of disease, complete recovery can be expected in the majority of cases. Taking all types of cases together, early and advanced, most large series record complete recovery in 70 to 75 per cent of cases and partial recovery in an additional 10 to 15 per cent. Cases of spinal tumour syndrome and posterior neural arch disease have been reported to have a bad prognosis (Seddon, 1935, 1949). However, in our experience these cases have provided no special problem in management except that the diagnosis may not be apparent until late. Satisfactory results have also been reported by Ramamurthi and Thayumanaswami (1954) and Rao, Rao, Subrahmanyam, and Reddy (1965).

References

ALEXANDER, G. L. (1949) Neurological complications of spinal tuberculosis, *Proc. roy. Soc. Med.*, **39**, 730.

BUTLER, R. W. (1935) Paraplegia in Pott's disease with special reference to the pathology and aetiology, *Brit. J. Surg.*, 22, 738–68.

CAPENER, N. (1954) The evolution of lateral rhachotomy, *J. Bone Jt Surg.*, **36B**, 173–9.

CAPENER, N. (1967) Vertebral tuberculosis and paraplegia, Editorial, *J. Bone Jt Surg.*, **49B**, 605–6.

GOEL, M. K. (1967) Treatment of Pott's paraplegia by operation, *J. Bone Jt Surg.*, **49B**, 674–81.

GRIFFITHS, D. LL., SEDDON, H. J., and ROAF, R., (1956) *Pott's Paraplegia*, London.

HODGSON, A. R., and STOCK, F. E. (1956) Anterior spinal fusion: a preliminary communication on the radical treatment of Pott's disease and Pott's paraplegia, *Brit. J. Surg.*, 44, 266–75.

HODGSON, A. R., STOCK, F. E., FANG, H. S. Y., and ONG, G. B. (1960) Anterior spinal fusion: the operative approach and pathological findings in 412 cases with Pott's disease of the spine, *Brit. J. Surg.*, 48, 172–8.

JONES, B. S. (1958) Pott's paraplegia in the Nigerian, *J. Bone Jt Surg.*, **40B**, 16–32.

KESHWANI, N. H. (1967) Ancient Hindu orthopaedic surgery, *Indian J. Orthop.*, **1**, 76.

MISRA, R. N., TANDON, P. N., and LAHIRI, A. K. (1964) Etiological survey of paraplegia, *Neurology* (*India*), **12**, 50–3.

MUKHOPADHAYA, B. (1954) Pott's paraplegia. A study of 41 cases, *Indian J. Surg.*, **16**, 40–7.

MUKHOPADHAYA, B., and MISHRA, N. K. (1957) Tuberculosis of the spine, *Indian J. Surg.*, **19**, 59–81.

OHRI, B. B., and KRISHNAMOORTHY, R. (1954) Tuberculosis of the spine, *Indian J. Surg.*, **16**, 232–41.

POTT, P. (1779) Remarks on that kind of palsy of the lower limbs which is frequently found to accompany a curvature of the spine, and is supposed to be caused by it, together with the method of cure, London; reprinted in *Medical Classics 1*, No. 4 (1936), Baltimore, Md.

RAMAMURTHI, B., and THAYUMANASWAMI, V. R. (1954) Laminectomy in Pott's paraplegia, *Indian J. Surg.*, **16**, 242–5.

RAO, B. D., RAO, K. S., SUBRAHMANYAM, M. V., and REDDY, M. V. R. (1965) Granulomatous lesions of the spinal epidural space, *Neurology* (*India*), **13**, 89–92.

RAO, B. S., and DINKAR, I. (1970) Epidural spinal compression, *J. postgrad. Med.*, **16**, 128–31.

ROAF, R., KIRKALDY-WILLIS, W. H., and CATHRO, A. J. M. (1959) *Surgical Treatment of Bone and Joint Tuberculosis*, Edinburgh.

SEDDON, H. J. (1935) Pott's Paraplegia: prognosis and treatment, *Brit. J. Surg.*, 22, 769–99.

SEDDON, H. J. (1949) Discussion on spinal caries with paraplegia, *Proc. roy. Soc. Med.*, 39, 723–30.

SORREL-DEJERINE, J. (1925) Quoted by Butler, (1935).

INTRASPINAL TUBERCULOUS GRANULOMAS

Intraspinal tuberculous granuloma, unassociated with spinal caries, is an uncommon lesion. Dibble and Cascino (1956) found only 171 cases reported in the literature up to that time. A detailed review of the subject has fairly recently been provided by Parsons and Pallis (1965).

Intraspinal tuberculomas may be extradural, intradural, extramedullary and intramedullary. These lesions are briefly described below. Another intraspinal tuberculous lesion, i.e. spinal meningitis and radiculomyelopathy is described on page 63.

Extradural Spinal Tuberculoma

The majority of extradural tuberculous granulomas are in fact secondary to extension of the vertebral disease. However, a number of cases have been reported in which no evidence of an associated bony lesion could be detected (Arseni and Samitca, 1960; Rao *et al.*, 1965; Natrajan, Vedachalam, and Ramamurthi, 1962; Shenkin, Horn, and Grant, 1945; Johnston, Ashbell, and Rosomoff, 1962). In the majority of these cases, during the follow-up period and often after several years, a tuberculous lesion of the spine appears at the same level. As mentioned earlier [see p. 59] we are inclined to think that most, if not all of these cases, are secondary to an undetected bony lesion. However, the possibility of haematogenous spread resulting in a granulomatous lesion of the extradural adipose tissue cannot be completely excluded.

We should mention that a number of cases of extradural compression due to a chronic inflammatory lesion have been reported from South India. Their true aetiology is not known; most probably they are not tuberculous in nature (Ramamurthi, 1952, 1970; Rao, Rao, Subramanyam, and Reddy, 1965).

There is nothing typical about the clinical picture of this condition. Diagnosis is established only after surgical exploration for spinal compression. Treatment consists of decompressive laminectomy and excision of as much as possible of the granuloma, which can be scraped off the dura. The granuloma usually encircles the spinal dura and no attempt is made to excise it totally; the anteriorly situated part can be safely left if the decompression is otherwise satisfactory. Antitubercular chemotherapy is instituted and continued for at least 1½ years.

Intradural Spinal Tuberculoma

Only a few isolated cases of intradural spinal tuberculoma have been reported in the literature (Bucy and Oberhill, 1950; Arseni and Samitca, 1960; Parsons and Pallis, 1965; Jenkins and Hill, 1963; Slade and Glazer, 1955; Dibble and Cascino, 1956).

The lesion may present either as a hard, round- or oval-shaped mass densely adherent to the inner aspect of the dura and the spinal cord, in which it digs a crater (Arseni and Samitca, 1960), or as a diffuse granulomatous mass encasing the cord (Bucy and Oberhill, 1950). The only case of this type seen by us belonged to the second category. Either the granuloma itself or the associated arachnoiditis may extend over several segments.

Intramedullary Tuberculoma of the Spinal Cord

Incidence

Arseni and Samitca (1960) encountered five such cases among 38,500 neurosurgical patients consisting of 421 spinal tumours of other types and 201 intracranial tuberculomas. Lin (1960) could find only 104 cases reported in the literature. In recent years isolated cases have been reported from India also (Sarin and Chandy, 1960; Rao and Subrahamnyam, 1962; Natrajan, Vedachalam, and Ramamurthi, 1962; Dastur and Shah, 1968).

Pathogenesis and Pathology

The pathogenesis and pathology of intramedullary tuberculomas of the spinal cord are the same as in the brain. The lesion is usually a single, hard, circumscribed mass measuring 7–10 mm in diameter and often associated with more or less intense localized arachnoiditis. Microscopically, it consists of a central area of necrosis surrounded by typical tuberculous granulation tissue.

Clinical Picture

Most of the patients reported in the literature had evidence of pulmonary tuberculosis prior to the onset of symptoms indicating spinal cord dysfunction. The neurological symptoms are insidious in onset and slowly progressive. There is nothing characteristic about the neurological picture and the only indication of its nature may be the presence of an associated tuberculous lesion elsewhere in the body.

Laboratory Investigations

These are of little help in diagnosing the nature of the lesion. Plain X-ray of the spine is normal. The cerebrospinal fluid protein is raised and it is frequently xanthochromic.

Treatment

Intramedullary tuberculoma can be easily enucleated. The treatment of choice is, therefore, excision.

Prognosis

The majority of cases reported in the literature were post-mortem findings. However, among the 16 surgically treated cases collected by Lin (1960) a successful result was recorded in 7. Most of the cases subsequently reported were treated surgically with good results.

References

ARSENI, C., and SAMITCA, D. C. (1960) Intraspinal tuberculous granuloma, *Brain*, 83, 295.

BUCY, P. C., and OBERHILL, H. R. (1950) Intradural spinal granulomas, *J. Neurosurg.*, 7, 1.

DASTUR, H. M., and SHAH, M. D. (1968) Intramedullary tuberculoma of the spinal cord, *Indian J. Pediat.*, **10**, 468.

DIBBLE, J. B., and CASCINO, J. (1956) Tuberculoma of the spinal cord, *J. Amer. med. Ass.*, 162, 461.

JENKINS, R. B., and HILL, C. (1963) Intradural spinal tuberculoma with genito-urinary symptoms, *Arch. Neurol. (Chic.)*, 8, 539.

JOHNSTON, J. D. H., ASHBELL, T. S., and ROSOMOFF, H. L. (1962) Isolated intraspinal extradural tuberculosis, *New Engl. J. Med.*, **266**, 703.

LIN, T. H. (1960) Intramedullary tuberculoma of the spinal cord, *J. Neurosurg.*, 17, 497.

NATARAJAN, M., VEDACHALAM, S. P., and RAMAMURTHI, B. (1962) Intramedullary tuberculoma of the spinal cord (a case report), *Indian J. Surg.*, 24, 727.

PARSONS, M., and PALLIS, C. A. (1965) Intradural spinal tuberculomas, *Neurology (Minneap.)*, 15, 1018.

RAMAMURTHI, B. (1952) Chronic spinal extradural inflammation, *Indian J. Surg.*, 14, 354.

RAMAMURTHI, B. (1970) *Contributions to Knowledge*, Souvenir published on the occasion of the Twentieth Anniversary celebrations of the Department of Neurology and Neurosurgery, Madras Medical College. (Personal communication.)

RAO, B. D., RAO, K. S., SUBRAHMAYAM, M. V., and REDDY, M. V. R. (1965) Granulomatous lesions of the spinal epidural space, *Neurology (India)*, **13**, 89.

RAO, B. D., and SUBRAHMANYAM, M. V. (1962) Spinal cord complications of tuberculous meningitis, *Neurology (India)*, **10**, 62.

SARIN, M. G., and CHANDY, J. (1961) Intramedullary tuberculoma of the spinal cord, *Neurology (India)*, **9**, 103.

SHENKIN, H. A., HORN, R. C., and GRANT, F. C. (1945) Lesions of the spinal epidural space producing cord compression, *Arch. Surg.*, 51, 125.

SLADE, H. W., and GLAZER, N. (1955) Extramedullary spinal tuberculoma, report of a case with unusual clinical and laboratory findings, *J. Pediat.*, **46**, 288.

3 Radiculomyelopathy associated with Spinal Meningitides (Arachnoiditis) with Special Reference to the Spinal Tuberculous Variety

N. H. WADIA

The famous British neurosurgeon, Sir Victor Horsley, was the first person to give a composite account of this condition in 1909 under the title of 'chronic spinal meningitis', a designation more appropriate than several others subsequently suggested. Howell (1936) called it 'arachnoiditis' and stressed the use of lipiodol in diagnosis. In the same year Elkington analysed the clinical and operative features of 'meningitis circumscripta spinalis', a subject which he later reviewed at length under the different title of 'spinal arachnoiditis', as a form of arachnoiditis generally evident in the nervous system (1951). Ransome and Monteiro (1947), in Singapore, were the first to draw attention to the tuberculous aetiology of some cases, as a variant of tuberculous meningitis presenting principally with rapidly developing spinal cord symptoms.

It becomes clear from a perusal of the subsequent literature that whereas spinal meningitis (arachnoiditis) as described by Elkington (1951) seems to be disappearing from the West and receiving diminishing attention in Western textbooks, the condition is still common in tropical countries such as India (Ramamurthi, 1961; Arjundas, 1961; Wadia and Dastur, 1969; Mani, Mani and Montgomery, 1969; Siddiqui, 1968), Ceylon (Cabrall, 1961), West Indies, (Cruickshank, 1962), South America and Africa. Ramamurthi found that 'arachnoiditis' was the commonest cause of spinal cord compression in the patients admitted to the Department of Neurosurgery at Madras, where out of a total of 123 operated cases of spinal cord compression (1951 to 1959), 43 were cases of arachnoiditis, followed well behind by 28 neurofibromas. He did not include compression from Pott's spine in this series. Mani, Mani, and Montgomery (1969) examined 170 cases of spastic paraplegia in Bangalore and found that, after a condition described by them as South Indian paraplegia [page 81], arachnoiditis formed the second largest group of cases. Elkington (1951), in his oft-quoted chapter, either failed to take note of the cases described by Ransome and Monteiro (1947) or did not mention them because he may have believed that the rapidly progressive spinal tuberculous condition described by them was different from the slowly developing form of the disease he had studied, in which either the aetiological agents were different or else no cause was found to explain the disease.

Unfortunately, the reports from tropical countries mentioned earlier, except that of Wadia and Dastur (1969), have followed suit. Acute or chronic arachnoiditis (meningitis) is not usually considered to be a possible primary expression of tuberculosis in the CNS.

On the other hand, reports have appeared, some from India, of patients similarly afflicted as those of Ransome and Monteiro, but under different titles (Bucy and Oberhill, 1950; Singh, Jolly, and Goyal, 1959; Arseni and Samitca, 1960; Bawa and Wahi, 1961; Jenkins and Hill, 1963; Parsons and Pallis, 1965). Except the last authors, none referred to the paper of Ransome and Monteiro; Parsons and Pallis in their turn did not realize that what they were dealing with was a form of 'arachnoiditis' (meningitis) similar to that described by Ransome and Monteiro, and different only from that reported by Elkington in its tempo and aetiology. The common basic pathology of inflammation of the meninges was not used to bring them all together in one large group.

Wadia and Dastur (1969) mentioned that, like others in India and elsewhere, they were not aware of the entity described by Ransome and Monteiro when their study of arachnoiditis in India first began in 1958. However, as it progressed they found that there was a distinct subgroup of patients with a rapidly developing radiculomyelopathy, due to an extensive spinal meningitis which was the first expression of tuberculosis of the nervous system. They came to this conclusion because:

1. Most of these patients at one time or another had had tuberculosis elsewhere in the body.
2. Untreated, a number of them later showed manifestations of tuberculous basal meningitis and died from that complication.
3. Biopsy of the spinal meninges showed a clear tuberculous pathology.
4. At autopsy not only were the biopsy findings confirmed but similar changes were found in the basal meninges, whether the patient had cranial symptoms during life or not. Moreover, small and large tuberculomata were seen in the brain and spinal cord, and tubercle bacilli were isolated from the basal meninges in occasional patients.
5. Early treatment with antituberculous drugs was beneficial; no intracranial extension of the meningitis occurred and recovery was observed.

They then realized that the term 'arachnoiditis' was a narrow one, encompassing only one group of chronic cases but leaving out another whole group similar in its basic symptomatology and pathology, though perhaps variable in the tempo of the disease, the aetiology, and the details of the pathology. They pointed out that whether the arachnoid alone or all three meninges were inflamed, whether the inflammation was due to infection or otherwise (trauma, etc.), whether it was acute or chronic, mild or severe, localized or extensive, nevertheless the end-result was always a cellular, vascular, and fibrous reaction of varying degree and extent in all cases. They therefore felt that all these cases should be considered under one generic title and then classified according to the various aetiological agents. Thus, the titles chronic spinal meningitis (Horsley, 1909), arachnoiditis (Howell, 1936), meningitis circumscripta spinalis, and spinal arachnoiditis (Elkington, 1936, 1951), a rare form of tuberculous meningitis (Ransome and Monteiro, 1947), intradural spinal granuloma (Bucy and Oberhill, 1950), spinal cord complications of tuberculous meningitis (Brooks, Fletcher, and Wilson, 1954), tuberculoma of the spinal cord (Dibble and Cascino, 1956), spinal tuberculous meningitis (Singh, Jolly, and Goyal, 1959; Bawa and Wahi, 1961), intraspinal tuberculous granuloma (Arseni and Samitca, 1960), intraspinal arachnoiditis (Ramamurthi, 1961), spinal arachnoiditis and arachnoid cysts (Cabrall, 1961), pantopaque arachnoiditis (Sehgal, Gardner, and Dohn, 1962), intradural spinal tuberculoma (Jenkins and Hill, 1963; Parsons and Pallis, 1965), and crytococcal spinal arachnoiditis (Davidson, 1968) serve to confuse the essential picture of acute or chronic inflammation of the spinal meninges from various known and unknown agents with neurological manifestations due to root and cord involvement. The title 'radiculomyelopathy associated with spinal meningitides' seems to be the most accurate and descriptive one for this discussion.

In the Department of Neurology of the J. J. Hospital, 94 such patients have been seen between 1958 and 1970. In twin papers, Wadia and Dastur (1969), and Dastur and Wadia (1969), made a 10-year report (1958 to 1968) of their experience of this disease.

Table 3.1
Aetiology

I. INFECTIVE
- 1. Tuberculous:
  - (a) Primary spinal variety
  - (b) Secondary to tuberculous basal meningitis (intracranial)
  - (c) Secondary to tuberculous vertebral caries
- 2. Syphilis
- 3. Pyogenic (coccal)
- 4. *Cryptococcus neoformans*

II. NON-INFECTIVE
- 1. Prolapsed lumbar intervertebral discs
- 2. Trauma
- 3. Cervical spondylosis
- 4. Rheumatoid and other spinal arthritis
- 5. Postoperative (laminectomy)
- 6. Chemical:
  - (a) Penicillin
  - (b) Streptomycin
  - (c) Anaesthetics
- 7. Intraspinal tumours, spinal angioma, disseminated sclerosis

III. IDIOPATHIC

AETIOPATHOLOGY

TABLE 3.1 shows the numerous agents so far known to cause the disease, organized into three groups. The third, idiopathic, group still remains to be assessed, especially in the chronic form.

Infective Agents

Tuberculosis

Tuberculosis is still rife in India, and this seems to be the commonest cause of spinal meningitis in our practice today; it originates in three ways:

1. A tuberculous lesion starting primarily in the spinal structures, as the first expression of tuberculosis of the central nervous system.
2. Secondary extension downwards of an already established intracranial tuberculous basal meningitis.
3. Secondary extension from caries of the vertebrae.

The Primary Spinal Variety. This has been quite frequently seen by us, and comprised 20 of the 70 cases reported by Wadia and Dastur (1969), forming the largest group among the aetiological agents. The insufficiently heeded report of Ransome and Monteiro (1947) mentioned a Sikh, a white man, and two Chinese, who presented with a rapid clinical picture of widespread cord disturbance simulating ascending myelitis. Lumbar puncture and CSF examination pointed to a subarachnoid block; the patients died in coma from what was seen at autopsy to be a later spread of the tuberculosis to the basal meninges from the spinal canal. They vividly described the autopsy observation of an extensive spinal meningeal exudate, 'as if a yellow jelly had been poured into the subarachnoid space and allowed to set'. They found the tubercle bacilli in the basal meninges.

The clinical presentation which both they and we saw was of the subacute progressive variety, simulating myelitis, but Bucy and Oberhill (1950) from the United States, and Arseni and Samitca (1960) from Rumania, have reported a much slower clinical form, which was clinically indistinguishable from a spinal cord tumour, and in which the presentation of the disease had been made over months. The diagnosis in all their cases was made after operation and biopsy, from which Bucy and Oberhill grew tubercle bacilli. Singh, Jolly, and Goyal (1959), and Bawa and Wahi (1961), from India, Jenkins (1963), from the United States, and Parsons and Pallis (1965), from the United Kingdom, have all drawn attention to this either acute or slow progressive form of spinal tuberculosis by short case-reports, and the paper of Kocen and Parsons (1970) shows the renewed awareness of the presence of this condition among the non-European immigrants to the United Kingdom, most of whom have arrived from tropical countries over the last decade. Elkington (1951), however, largely reviewing the pre-streptomycin era, when tuberculosis was still common in the West, came across no example of it.

Dastur and Wadia (1969) believed that the meningitis arises probably from a flare-up of a local parenchymal (Rich, 1951) focus on the surface of the spinal cord, pathogenetically somewhat similar to what happens intracranially in tuberculous basal meningitis. They felt that the meningeal reaction varies in different cases, and depending on the interpretation of what is visualized at operation, autopsy, and microscopically, the words meningitis, arachnoiditis, granuloma, and tuberculoma are variously used by different authors. The rapidity or otherwise of the nervous system involvement would determine the clinical course.

Secondary Involvement of the Spinal Meninges. Secondary involvement spread from a tuberculous basal meningitis (TBM) is commoner and more often recognized than the first variety. Although Wadia and Dastur had fewer (18) cases of this variety, it is known that the majority of cases of tuberculous basal meningitis are admitted to paediatric and general medical wards of their hospital, while those with a spinal presentation go to the neurologists. Brooks, Fletcher, and Wilson (1954), Dibble and Cascino (1956), Arseni and Samitca (1960), and Rao and Subrahmanyam (1961) have all added to the literature on this subject, which contained some earlier mention of this variety, particularly in the form of single case-reports (Wilson, 1940). The patients of Brooks, Fletcher, and Wilson had all been given intrathecal streptomycin, and while accepting its pathogenetic role it should be pointed out that even though the practice of administration of intrathecal streptomycin has practically ceased for over a decade, we still encounter this spinal complication of TBM.

Secondary Extension from Caries of the Vertebrae. Finally, while tuberculous vertebral caries, cold abscesses and extradural granulomas are very common in India, spread of infection to the intradural tissues is rare. In the first of their twin papers (1969). Wadia and Dastur had come across no example of it, but later they found three such cases out of the 50 that they histopathologically examined (Dastur and Wadia, 1969). Elkington (1951), however, mentioned that 'in the past tuberculous arachnoiditis has been confined to cases of tuberculous spinal caries'.

Syphilis

At one time syphilis was believed to be a very common cause of arachnoiditis; in fact Horsley (1909) thought it to be the commonest. Siddiqui (1968) has still found it common in India, although Wadia and Dastur (1969) have reported only four such cases out of 70. Elkington (1951) had also not been fully impressed by its role in the causation of arachnoiditis.

Pyogenic (Coccal) Meningitis

Acute or chronic infection of the spinal subarachnoid space following *meningococcal and other pyogenic meningitis*, either primarily cranial or spinal, and giving rise to a radiculomyelopathy, is now rare. One only comes across an occasional case following an improperly performed diagnostic lumbar puncture, where the complicating meningitis has been inadequately treated.

Cryptococcus Neoformans

Cryptococcal spinal granuloma and 'arachnoiditis' are still a rarity. Davidson (1968) mentioned that there were only 11 cases in the literature and added a twelfth. He pointed out, however, that there was an increase in the infection rate by *Cryptococcus neoformans* generally in the United States, especially in chronically ill patients with malignancy and sarcoidosis. He hinted that more cases of cryptococcosis might be expected. As *Cryptococcus neoformans* also secondarily infects tuberculous patients, the possibility of spinal meningitis from this fungus must always be excluded even in patients with systemic tuberculosis.

Non-infective Agents

Prolapsed Lumbar Intervertebral Disc

Localized spinal arachnoiditis is seen to accompany a long-standing *prolapsed lumbar or cervical intervertebral disc.* The neurological symptoms in such patients are produded by the combined effects of both these conditions and are hard to separate clinically. Wadia and Dastur (1969) found 12 such examples in the lumbar region in their series. Most of these patients had bilateral sciatica and considerable neurological deficit.

Trauma

Spinal trauma as a cause has been mentioned by previous authors, but its role is very questionable.

Cervical Spondylosis, Rheumatoid Arthritis and Other Forms of Chronic Spinal Arthritis

These may be occasionally accompanied by localized arachnoiditis with neurological involvement (Ramamurthi, 1961).

Postoperative Laminectomy

Laminectomy performed for a prolapsed lumbar intervertebral disc or spinal cord tumour, may be followed by spinal meningitis of a chronic, adhesive, localized form, where none existed previously. Calcification and even ossification in such a fibrous mass has been seen by us and reported by others (Cabrall, 1961). Postoperative infection adds to the danger.

Chemical Agents

Chemical spinal meningitis with a rapidly developing ascending form of permanent paralysis has been observed by this author more than once, following spinal anaesthesia which is still being used extensively in India. Delayed-onset chronic meningitis has also been reported. Intrathecal introduction of myodil, *Pantopaque*, penicillin, and streptomycin have also been incriminated.

Intraspinal Tumours

Local adhesive arachnoiditis has been reported by surgeons operating on spinal cord tumours, and the pre-operative myelogram may cause confusion, because it may clearly reveal the leptomeningitis allowing the tumour to go undetected, even at operation. Repeated small or large spinal subarachnoid haemorrhages also lead to an irritative phenomenon of fibrosis in the meninges (Henson and Croft, 1956).

Idiopathic Agents

There remains the idiopathic group which varies in every series depending on what types of cases have been included under the title of 'arachnoiditis' or 'meningitis', and what efforts have been made to hunt for the aetiological agent. Wadia and Dastur (1969) had only 13 such patients out of the 70 seen by them. This is a very modest figure compared to other series where a large idiopathic group remained (Elkington, 1951; Ramamurthi, 1961; Siddiqui, 1968). It is possible that in tropical countries where tuberculosis is still rife, a reassessment of the so-called 'idiopathic' cases may show that a number of them are of tuberculous aetiology. While this would be more true of the subacute cases, a slow symptomatology does not rule out tuberculosis.

CLINICAL FEATURES

The majority of symptoms arise because of cord and root involvement by the meningitis which by itself, especially in the less acute cases, can be entirely symptomless. We have all seen at post-mortem cases of TBM that a widespread extension of the process into the spinal canal has remained symptomless because the cord or roots wrapped with the exudate have somehow not been sufficiently disturbed in their functioning.

Hence, the essential clinical picture is one of either a rapid or a slow (subacute or chronic), single- or multiple-level, ascending or transverse radiculomyelopathy. The predominance and extent of the root and cord symptoms depend on the site of maximal affection of these structures; thus, in the cauda equina the symptoms are principally those of a radiculopathy, while the cord is more involved in a single-level lesion at a higher level. Even if the meningitis is widespread, symptoms may arise from a single lesion in the spinal cord anywhere along its length, although more often a multifocal radiculomyelopathy is seen.

The age and sex of these patients vary with the aetiological agent; thus, because tuberculosis is much commoner in poor young females, who inhabit the area around our hospital, the spinal complications follow suit; on the other hand, traumatic arachnoiditis is commoner in older males. Except the very young and the very old, no age-group is exempt from the disease, which we have seen to affect those from the age of 5 to 65 years.

The clinical course of the disease may be subacute or chronic.

The Subacute Form

In this form, the clinical picture develops on average in 2 months, although maximal severity is often reached within 2 to 5 days, and the condition then remains stationary.

The symptoms include root pains, paralysis, paraesthesiae, bladder disturbance, and wasting of muscles. Fever, often low, malaise, asthenia, and anorexia may precede these symptoms. The root pains of lancinating character are severe and often unrelieved by analgesics. They may arise from a single root, or a bunch of roots at one segmental level, or in the more severe form the pains are widespread. At times, the disease presents with severe sciatica, often bilateral, and then the root pains appear in an ascending sequence up the body. Pain and stiffness of the spine, although not so remarkable, often accompany the root pains, usually over the segments of origin of the roots.

Paralysis of the limbs is mostly severe and takes the form of a paraplegia or tetraplegia of the upper or lower motor neurone or a mixed variety, depending on the extent of the radiculomyelopathy. It is not uncommon to find deep reflexes absent in the lower limbs with flaccidity in the presence of extensor plantar responses. Acute retention of urine often accompanies the paralytic symptoms or can be a presenting feature at the onset. Tingling and numbness often follow the root pains, and loss of sensation up to a segmental level on the trunk is often complained of, and found on examination. Vibration and postural loss in the limbs has been constantly seen.

There are three modes of development of the natural history of this form of the disease:

1. A single-level neurological lesion.
2. A multifocal radiculomyelopathy.
3. An ascending variety.

In all cases the onset is sudden, the patient looks ill and there may be a low fever. The most striking and often the first symptom is pain in the spine and severe root pains. This is soon followed by paralysis of motor, sensory and bladder functions. When the neurological deficit is confined to a single level of the cord, a picture of *acute or subacute transection* at any level of the cord occurs, closely simulating an acute transverse myelitis. If the level of the lesion is confined to the conus medullaris, a flaccid, areflexic, hypotonic paraplegia with urinary retention results. If the level is somewhat higher, after the initial stage of acute spinal shock is over the legs become spastic and show evidence of pyramidal tract disturbance. The motor, sensory and root involvement all point to a single level of damage in the spinal cord.

When the root pains, paraesthesia, sensory level, motor disturbance and areflexia do not coincide at a single level, a *multifocal radiculomyelopathy* results, and it is not uncommon to see a patient with severe root pains in the upper limbs, whose sensory loss is as low as D10 but who also complains of severe sciatica and has flaccid ankles, absent ankle jerks and extensor plantar responses.

Finally, in *the ascending variety*, the lumbosacral roots are affected first and severe sciatica is followed by an areflexic, hypotonic, limb and bladder paralysis, and sensory loss. Soon the sensory loss, the root pains and paralysis ascend to involve all the four limbs, and at times the intercostal muscles and the diaphragm, even leading to respiratory paralysis and death. This variety is often mistaken for the Landry-Guillain-Barré syndrome or ascending myelitis.

The majority of cases of this acute form of the disease result from tuberculosis, and hence, a past or present history of pulmonary or glandular tuberculosis is often forthcoming and clinical examination may show evidence of systemic tuberculosis. The fever which often precedes this acute illness is mostly produced by the systemic tuberculosis rather than by the spinal meningitis. In some of these patients the meningitis, having started in the spinal canal, spreads intracranially in a matter of days to weeks, causing drowsiness, confusion, neck stiffness, and other clinical signs of classical tuberculous basal meningitis. This happened in some of our earlier cases when we had not realized the value of antituberculous treatment.

Spinal extension of a tuberculous basal meningitis usually appears within weeks, in an inadequately or improperly treated case, but we have also seen it develop in the face of an improving, well-treated case of intracranial condition after several months. In none of our cases had streptomycin been introduced intrathecally, as reported by Brooks, Fletcher, and Wilson (1954) in their patients.

If the condition is caused by syphilis, other clinical evidence of syphilis, like the Argyll Robertson pupils, must be looked for, although very often the search is fruitless. The same may be said for cryptococcosis, where abnormal lung signs may or may not be detected. If the condition follows the intrathecal administration of a spinal anaesthetic the course may be fulminating.

The Chronic Form

This may progress slowly over months or years, and is often indistinguishable from other varieties of spinal cord compression, especially tumours, where the neurological lesion is localized to a single level. It may only be suspected when the root pains (not as often present as in the acute form) are scattered, persistent or severe, or when one comes across lower motor neurone signs, like absent lower limb deep reflexes or wasting, or sciatica in a patient whose principal signs point to a much higher level of lesion. Chronic spinal meningitis should always be considered in such multifocal spinal cord lesions, particularly in patients who live or have lived in the tropics.

INVESTIGATIONS

In the acute form of the disease radiographs of the whole spine should be taken, regardless of the level of the lesion, to rule out tuberculous caries. It is only when this has been excluded that primary spinal meningitis is considered.

Lumbar Puncture

In the acute form of the disease, there is often a partial or complete subarachnoid block on manometric examination, with a positive Queckenstedt test. At times there is a dry tap. The fluid may be clear, but more often it is various shades of yellow. In severe cases only a few drops of deep yellow fluid may be obtained. The protein level was elevated in all but two of the 24 patients of Wadia and Dastur (1969), 12 showing a level above 1 g/100 ml. The cellular response was lymphocytic and not so remarkable, with more than 8 cells/mm^3 in 13 of them, and a maximum of 670 cells/mm^3. The sugar content was reduced only in some of the cases of the tuberculous variety. The VDRL or WR may be positive in the syphilitic cases. A rising CSF protein content, in a patient under treatment for basal tuberculous meningitis, should make one suspect a developing subarachnoid block, which is often, though not always, followed by paralysis. Such a timely warning may be useful for prophylactic treatment.

Besides the routine examination, the CSF should be appropriately stained, cultured, and inoculated into animals, to identify, if possible, the infective agent.

In the more localized or more chronic forms of the disease, the CSF, according to Elkington, may show no abnormalities in the majority. We have found that although there is very little cell rise, the protein content is often high. When the CSF of a case of a chronic prolapsed lumbar intervertebral disc shows a very high protein or yellow fluid, it should make one suspect an associated arachnoiditis and the myelogram should be carefully assessed.

The cisternal CSF is normal in chronic cases. In the primarily spinal tuberculous cases only a slight rise of protein and increased cells are found, as long as the condition remains confined to the spinal canal, but when the meningitis spreads intracranially, the classical CSF changes of tuberculous meningitis are seen. Sometimes, under these circumstances, a previously easy cisternal puncture may yield a dry tap.

The blood VDRL and WR should always be done. Chest X-ray and ESR and other necessary examinations should be undertaken for detection of tuberculosis, cryptococcosis, etc., elsewhere in the body, whenever indicated.

Myelography

Myelography is essential. It should be performed by the lumbar route except in the case of a dry tap, when the cisternal one is necessary. Additionally, cisternal myelography is sometimes necessary to see the extent of the leptomeningitis in case of a low total block via the lumbar route. Myelography shows many diagnostic features of this condition (Lombardi, Passerini, and Migliavacca, 1962; Sidhva, 1963; Teng and Papathedorau, 1967; Wadia and Dastur, 1969):

1. On screening, the dye moves very slowly, often showing filling defects and fragmentation of the column.
2. Often there is a total block, with a ragged edge, or one extending obliquely over 2 or more vertebral levels [PLATE 13a]. At times, a pitchfork appearance may be seen. There is rarely a single distinct cut-out, such as the concave edge of the block as seen with spinal tumours.
3. The *Myodil* column, with or without a block, may show: (a) multiple filling defects, which are usually small and spotty [PLATE 13b]; (b) large areas of candle guttering over a long length of the spinal canal, which may be pronounced to show a fluffy effect; (c) in the cauda equina region, the presence of exudate around the roots may give an appearance of a 'bundle of faggot sticks', or the lower end may taper to a 'rat-tail'; (d) in a few cases, multiple, small, round, clear areas or a single large one, may point to cyst formation.
4. In those cases in which both the lumbar and cisternal myelograms show a block, the unfilled area in-between, often over many segments, together with the irregular columns below and above shows the extent of the affected area. PLATE 13c illustrates this fact clearly.

Finally, whereas in spinal cord compression due to tumour the myelogram shows a block at or near the site indicated clinically, in this condition the correlation between the two is often wanting. We have frequently seen a total block at L3 or L4 level via the lumbar route, when the highest or the only level revealed on clinical examination was in the cervical segments. The same has been seen with a high cervical block via the cisternal route in a patient with a clinical level at D10. This absence of correlation is seen more often with the acute form of this disease and is a very useful criterion for differentiating diffused meningitis from other cases of cord compression. When spinal meningitis complicates an already present spinal condition, like a spinal cord tumour or a prolapsed disc, the myelographic features of both conditions should be assiduously looked for, and extra care taken on examining the radiographs. Quite often the presence of one masks the other and the final diagnosis may only be made at operation.

Differential Diagnosis

The diagnosis of spinal meningitis can quite often be made on the pattern of its symptomatology, the signs of diffuse (multifocal) involvement of the root and spinal cord, the CSF findings, and the distinctive myelographic features. The history of widespread root pains is most useful. The presence of conditions known to be associated with either the acute or chronic form of the disease further acts as a pointer to the diagnosis. In the Landry-Guillain-Barré syndrome, root pains and pyramidal tract signs are rare, bladder disturbance occasional, and segmental sensory loss up to a level on the trunk never found on examination, while all these are the hallmarks of the radiculomyelopathy complicating acute spinal meningitis. The subarachnoid block, the yellow CSF, the high CSF protein with a cellular response, are quite distinctive features from the mere rise of protein in the Guillain-Barré syndrome. Once clinically suspected, the myelogram usually enables the distinction to be made.

When root pains are not marked, the differentiation between transverse or ascending myelitis and acute spinal meningitis is difficult, especially where the neurological lesion is restricted to one level. In the milder cases of meningitis, the subarachnoid block may be missed unless sophisticated manometry is carried out and even the CSF may not show the marked rise in protein which often helps in diagnosis. In such cases, myelography will not show a total block and it is only the discerning who will detect the slowing and irregularity of the *Myodil* column on screening and identify the filling defects in the column on the radiographs.

Repeatedly, patients have been referred with a diagnosis of transverse or ascending myelitis, where the clinical differentiation has been very slight, but where an associated history of tuberculosis has made us carry out a myelogram; on finding small filling defects, we have advised exploratory laminectomy and biopsy to arrive at the diagnosis. We feel that in such borderline cases, even a diagnostic surgical procedure is justified because treatment completely changes the prognosis. We believe that in the past many of these patients were diagnosed on mere clinical grounds as 'viral myelitis' and left to lead a paraplegic life or even die. Today, appropriate, and what is more important, timely diagnosis, and treatment at least in the infective (tuberculous and others) cases may result in full recovery.

The differential diagnosis between subacute and chronic compressions of other aetiology and spinal meningitis is not always easy even after myelography; the latter may not always show the classical pattern and very occasionally the picture is simulated by certain varieties of long tumours and spinal angiomata.

An intramedullary glioma extending over several spinal segments and protruding out of the cord, a long intradural, extramedullary malignant deposit, especially of reticulosis or multiple secondaries, and a spinal angioma may closely ape the clinical and even the myelographic features of both subacute and chronic spinal meningitis and make pre-operative diagnosis impossible. Once in a while, the surgeon is unable to differentiate a chronic granulomatous form of spinal meningitis from a reticulosis even on inspection at operation, and a biopsy report has to be awaited to settle the diagnosis. In slow, progressive cases with a single-level lesion, if the myelogram is not typical, diagnosis even from a neurofibroma can be made only after laminectomy. Finally, the tropical and nutritional myelopathies should pose no great problem in differential diagnosis if careful assessment of a case is made.

PATHOLOGY

Dastur and Wadia (1969) have made a thorough histopathological study of the meninges, roots and spinal cord in this disorder, although a large part of their material was collected from tuberculous cases. The pathological tissue was made available from 50 cases, 30 of whom had been clinically assessed personally by them. Their material comprised 32 biopsies of the leptomeninges taken at operation, and 18 autopsies where the full length of the spinal cord was available for study. A large part of the description given here is taken from their report.

Tuberculosis

The following description is common to all three varieties of tuberculous spinal meningitis mentioned under aetiology. At surgical operation the exudate is seen to surround the spinal cord throughout the whole exposed area and going beyond the operating field. Increased vascularity, difficulty in haemostasis especially after resection for biopsy, and compressed or atrophied roots and/or cord are reported by the surgeon.

The naked eye examination of the transverse slices of the spinal cord shows a thick collar of exudate surrounding the spinal cord, often more over its posterior than anterior surface in the more florid cases. The meninges look thick, opaque and lustreless. In many cases the thickness is of several millimetres, giving the appearance of a granuloma. Discrete and conglomerate tubercles with a caseating centre may be seen in the exudate [PLATE 14a]. The dura, though not as much affected as the pia and arachnoid which become separately unidentifiable, is often adherent and cannot be easily separated from the structures within it. Considerable atrophy of the spinal cord is seen in most specimens, when the patient has lived a long time with the disease. From the naked eye examination it is impossible to say whether the inflammatory changes started primarily in the spinal meninges, or are an extension of a tuberculous basal meningitis, or are accompanying a tuberculous spine.

Histopathology

The *exudate* surrounds but does not generally infiltrate the roots, posterior root ganglia, and the cord. Within a rich network of reticulin fibrils, frank tubercles are seen [PLATE 14b]. The tubercles are similar to those seen with any granulomatous reaction, and are made up of central giant cells or epithelioid cells surrounded by small monoculear cells. The other common histological changes are an occlusive thrombosis of small vessels, and occasional periarteritis and subintimal fibrosis of medium-sized arteries.

As the granulomatous reaction becomes more organized and reaches a more chronic stage of the disease, either microcysts [PLATE 14c] or more commonly large arachnoidal cysts within a fibrous matrix are seen. The subacute inflammation and chronic fibrotic changes may be seen side by side in certain specimens, so it is conceivable that a small biopsy of the leptomeninges may show only a chronic fibrotic reaction, missing the giant cell systems in a patient, the clinical course of whose disease was subacute. Thus, the clinico-pathological correlation which is mostly quite clear at postmortem may not be so evident when a small biopsy is taken.

The roots do not show histopathological changes of axon or even myelin degeneration, unless the condition has been of long standing when even a total loss of myelin of the compressed roots is seen.

The spinal cord shows four main types of changes:

1. The most frequent finding is that of a border-zone of rarefaction and sponginess of the cord, which though essentially circumferential has a greater tendency to involve the lateral white columns

including the corticospinal tracts, with resulting demyelination and axonal degeneration. This is probably due to parenchymal oedema resulting from venous congestion following compression of the cord. An occasional perivascular collar of small mononuclear cells may be seen.

2. Extensive atrophy and circumscribed central necrosis of the cord, with almost total disappearance of the grey horns is seen less often.
3. A more florid ischaemic myelopathy is seen still less often and is the result of involvement of almost all the blood vessels, except the main anterior spinal artery, in the meningeal exudative reaction. This is, therefore, a more severe stage of the process described under (2), above. At this stage, the cord is reduced to a mass of glial cells, with almost no recognizable parenchymal tissue.
4. Rarely, an intramedullary tuberculoma is seen. Dastur and Wadia came across one such case at autopsy.

Syphilis

As this spinal condition is becoming rare, even in India, we have no first-hand experience of its histology. Greenfield (1963) mentioned strangling of nerve roots by local thickening of meninges and their enclosure within small gummata. Loculation of subarachnoid fluid causes cyst formation pressing on the roots and spinal cord.

Cryptococcosis

On clinical examination, and even at operation and autopsy, it may be impossible to differentiate the tuberculous from the cryptococcal infection. Histopathological examination, especially of a biopsy specimen, unless carefully done may also be misleading, as happened in one of our cases where an initial diagnosis of tuberculous spinal meningitis was made by visualization of small 'tubercles' at operation. At autopsy the macroscopic examination of the spinal cord showed a 'tuberculoma' and spinal meningitis. It was only on staining the exudate with PAS that cryptococci were detected. These were also found in sections of the lungs; the intramedullary mass was a cryptococcoma and not a tuberculoma. The histopathology of this leptomeningitis shows multinucleated giant cells, lymphocytes and plasma cells.

PROGNOSIS

Although Elkington (1951) gave a rather unfavourable prognosis, this depends upon the cause and extent of the meningitis. We believe that early and adequate treatment of those patients belonging to the tuberculous group, whether primary or secondary, is rewarding. On the other hand, delay in diagnosis and treatment lead to irreparable damage to the blood vessels and the cord. Of the 13 patients with primary tuberculous spinal meningitis treated by Wadia and Dastur (1969) with antituberculous and corticoid therapy, seven made excellent recovery from an initially bed-ridden state, two others improved, but relapsed as they stopped the treatment too soon, while the rest showed no improvement. Brooks, Fletcher, and Wilson (1954) similarly mention good results from treatment of patients with spinal cord involvement secondary to a tuberculous basal meningitis. We have found that in these patients, on the first indication of an oncoming spinal block noted by manometry and of a rising protein content, intrathecal hydrocortisone often arrests the increasing neurological signs of cord involvement or even aborts their onset. Syphilis and even the cryptococcal infection of the spinal meninges respond well to appropriate therapy.

In the more chronic forms of the disease, a localized area of arachnoiditis, or cord compression from a cyst can be surgically treated with good results (Elkington, 1951; Ramamurthi, 1961), but the more extensive adhesive idiopathic variety usually progresses. Spontaneous arrest after a certain stage of worsening has been witnessed but no spontaneous cure has been recorded.

TREATMENT

Medical

In all rapidly developing cases of ascending or transverse radiculomyelopathy, with a diffuse subarachnoid block as seen by high protein, manometry and myelography, it would be entirely justifiable to quickly administer full antituberculous therapy along with corticosteroids because delay in its implementation can be disastrous. Where there is known association with present or past tuberculosis, or where tubercle bacilli are found in the CSF, or a quick laminectomy and meningeal biopsy show a tuberculous process, one's hand is further strengthened. CSF culture and guinea-pig inoculation of the CSF and tissue obtained should be undertaken to show the tubercle bacilli, but no valuable time must be wasted in starting therapy, pending results of these tests. Streptomycin, 1 G (or even 2 G initially) a day, intramuscularly, isonicotinic acid hydrazide 400 to 600 mg/day and PAS, 12 to 16 G/day must be given. The latter two are continued for anything up to 18 months, depending on the effectiveness of the therapy. Streptomycin is usually stopped after 90 to 120 G have been taken in all. Oral prednisolone 60 mg/day for at least a month and then in lesser doses up to 2 to 3 months seems necessary, although no control trial has been undertaken to establish its efficacy. This regime is for adults and should be adjusted for younger persons according to the weight and age. Toxic effects of the drugs may require adjustment of dose or use of other antituberculous drugs as in any other form of tuberculosis. We recommend twice weekly intrathecal, or failing this, intracisternal administration of 50 mg hydrocortisone. The total number of such injections depends on the response to treatment and the ease with which this procedure can be carried out, but usually 10 to 15 would give the optimum result.

In patients with basal tuberculous meningitis who are already under treatment, a rising protein content on repeated lumbar punctures, and a manometric block, should make one watchful of spinal complications which may follow in some patients. Hydrocortisone intrathecally as mentioned previously, should be started.

Cryptococcal spinal meningitis responding admirably to amphotericin B given intravenously has been reported by Davidson (1968).

He administered 0·25 mg/kg initially and later 1 mg/kg It was given 6 days a week for a total of 892 mg. Side-effects such as nausea, vomiting, and headache caused short breaks of a few days in the therapy. The treatment for syphilis and chronic pyogenic infections requires thorough and appropriate antibiotic therapy.

Corticosteroids seem to be of no great value in the more chronic cases of either the symptomatic or the idiopathic variety, although prednisolone by mouth, over prolonged periods in doses of more than 40 mg daily, has occasionally been followed by substantial improvement. Intrathecal hydrocortisone may also yield similar responses of a doubtful kind.

Surgical

The scope of surgery is limited. When the lesion is seen to be clinically and myelographically extensive, it becomes impossible to deal with it surgically. Surgery is performed for biopsy purposes and to confirm the diagnosis and detect the causative agent so that therapy is more accurate. If a large cyst is seen on the myelogram and its level coincides with the clinical level, surgical removal may help. Where meningitis is extensive the block may be well above or below the clinical level of the lesion, and as the *Myodil* cannot be taken to the clinically suspected area, it is difficult to decide where the laminectomy should be done—at the clinical (myelopathic) or the myelographic level. We advise that if decompression is contemplated the clinical level should be favoured, but for biopsy any convenient level for the surgeon will do.

As opposed to the ineffectiveness of surgery in extensive acute or chronic meningeal involvement, it has been reported to yield good results in the localized chronic form (Ramamurthi, 1961). Mere laminectomy and decompression do not help, but actual removal of the inflamed meninges and excision of cysts should be carried out. Great surgical skill is required not to tear the closely adherent roots or cord. The advent of microneurosurgery should assist matters.

References

ARJUNDAS, G. (1961) Intraspinal compressions, *Neurology (Bombay)* 9, 164.

ARSENI, C., and SAMITCA, D. C. (1960) Intraspinal tuberculous granuloma, *Brain*, 83, 285.

BAWA, Y. S., and WAHI, P. L. (1961) Spinal tuberculous meningitis, *J. Indian med. Ass.*, 37, 449.

BROOKS, W. D. W., FLETCHER, A. P., and WILSON, R. R. (1954) Spinal cord complications of tuberculous meningitis, *Quart. J. Med.*, 23, 275.

BUCY, P. C., and OBERHILL, H. R. (1950) Intradural spinal granulomas, *J. Neurosurg.*, 7, 1.

CABRALL, S. A. (1961) Spinal arachnoiditis and arachnoid cysts, *Neurology (Bombay)*, 9, 91.

CRUICKSHANK, E. K. (1962) Neurological disorders in the tropics, in *Modern Trends in Neurology*, Vol. 3, ed. Williams, D., London, p. 200.

DASTUR, D. K., and WADIA, N. H. (1969) Spinal meningitides with radiculo-myelopathy: Part 2. Pathology and pathogenesis, *J. neurol. Sci.*, 8, 261.

DAVIDSON, S. (1968) Cryptococcal spinal arachnoiditis, *J. Neurol. Neurosurg. Psychiat.*, 31, 76.

DIBBLE, J. B., and CASCINO, J. (1956) Tuberculoma of the spinal cord, *J. Amer. med. Ass.*, 162, 461.

ELKINGTON, J. ST C. (1951) Arachnoiditis, in *Modern Trends in Neurology*, Vol. 1, ed. Feiling, A., London, p. 149.

ELKINGTON, J. ST C. (1936) Meningitis circumscripta spinalis, *Brain*, 59, 181.

GREENFIELD, J. G. (1963) System degeneration of the cerebellum, brain stem and spinal cord, in *Greenfield's Neuropathology*, eds. Blackwood, W., McMenemey, W. H., Meyer, A., Norman, R. M., and Russell, D. S., London, p. 581.

HENSON, R. A., and CROFT, P. B. (1956) Spontaneous spinal subarachnoid haemorrhage, *Quart. J. Med.*, 25, 53.

HORSLEY, V. (1909) Chronic spinal meningitis, *Brit. med. J.*, 1, 513.

HOWELL, C. M. H. (1936) Arachnoiditis, *Proc. roy. Soc. Med.*, 30, 33.

JENKINS, R. B., and HILL, C. (1963) Intradural spinal tuberculoma with genito-urinary symptoms, *Arch. Neurol. (Chic.)*, 8, 539.

KOCEN, R. S., and PARSONS, M. (1970) Neurological complications of tuberculosis: some unusual manifestations, *Quart. J. Med.*, 39, 17.

LOMBARDI, G., PASSERINI, A., and MIGLIAVACCA, F. (1962) Spinal arachnoiditis, *Brit. J. Radiol.*, 35, 314.

MANI, K. S., MANI, A. J., and MONTGOMERY, R. D. (1969) A spastic paraplegia syndrome in South India, *J. neurol. Sci.*, 9, 179.

PARSONS, M., and PALLIS, C. A. (1965) Intradural spinal tuberculomas, *Neurology (Minneap.)*, 15, 1018.

RAMAMURTHI, B. (1961) Intraspinal arachnoiditis, *Indian J. med. Sci.*, 15, 776.

RANSOME, G. A., and MONTEIRO, E. S. (1947) A rare form of tuberculous meningitis, *Brit. med. J.*, 1, 413.

RAO, B. D., and SUBRAHMANYAM, M. V. (1962) Spinal cord complications of tuberculous meningitis, *Neurology (Bombay)*, 10, 62.

RICH, A. R. (1951) *The Pathogenesis of Tuberculosis*, 2nd ed. Oxford.

SEHGAL, A. D., GARDNER, W. J., and DOHN, D. F. (1962)

Pantopaque 'Arachnoiditis', *Cleveland Clin. Quart.*, **29**, 177.
SIDDIQUI, N. A. (1968) Spinal arachnoiditis, *Neurology (India)*, **16**, 131.
SIDHVA, J. N. (1963) The radiology of spinal arachnoiditis, *Neurology (Bombay)*, **11**, 59.
SINGH, A., JOLLY, S. S., and GOYAL, A. C. (1959) Spinal tuberculous meningitis, *Neurology (Bombay)*, **7**, 74.
TENG, P., and PAPATHEDORAU (1967) Myelographic findings in adhesive spinal arachnoiditis, *Brit. J. Radiol.*, **40**, 201.
WADIA, N. H., and DASTUR, D. K. (1969) Spinal meningitides with radiculo-myelopathy: Part I. Clinical and radiological features, *J. neurol. Sci.*, **8**, 239.
WILSON, S. A. K. (1940) Tuberculous encephalitis and myelitis, in *Neurology*, Vol. 1, London, 596.

4 Neurological Complications in Tropical Sprue

G. M. TAORI and G. V. IYER

Neurological complications in malabsorptive disorders usually result from deficiency of various nutrients. Tropical sprue is one example of this group of disorders. It is a disease of unknown aetiology which occurs in people who are or who have been resident in the tropics and in whom known aetiological factors, such as gluten sensitivity, have been excluded.

Tropical sprue has long been considered to have a peculiar geographical distribution (Manson-Bahr, 1953). Although it is present in most parts of the tropics, it has been thought to be very rare in East, Central and West Africa (Banwell *et al.*, 1967). However, there are occasional case-reports suggestive of tropical sprue from East Africa (Harries, 1964). Similarly, in South Africa some patients with megaloblastic anaemia have been found to have intestinal malabsorption of vitamin B_{12} of unknown aetiology (Hift and Adams, 1963).

The disease appears to have been present in India for many centuries. There is a good description of what is known as 'Grahani Vyadhi' or intestinal disease in the collected writings of Caraka compiled some time between the thirteenth and sixth centuries BC. The clinical description of this disorder in these writings is very similar to that of tropical sprue.

Early publications were concerned mainly with endemic and epidemic forms of this disease among British military personnel in India. However, Moorehead (1860) described the disease in Indians in Bombay. Since then there have been several publications from various parts of India describing the disease in Indians (Crombie, 1880; Megaw and Gupta, 1927; Cook, 1944; Chaudhuri and Chaudhuri, 1944).

More recently, the disease was found to be prevalent in South India (Baker, 1957) and subsequently it has been reported from other parts of the country by various authors (Jain and Sepaha, 1961; Jeejeebhoy *et al.*, 1966; Tandon, Iyenger, Deo, and Saraya, 1966; Misra, Krishnan, Ramalingaswamy, and Chuttani, 1967; Chuttani, Kasthuri, and Misra, 1968; Cowen, Satija, and Zacharia, 1968; Mehta, Mehta, and Wadhwa, 1968).

The disorder occurs in endemic as well as epidemic forms. Almost all reports of epidemics of tropical sprue are confined to India, Pakistan and Burma (Baker and Mathan, 1968*b*). Many of the epidemics described in the literature occurred in military personnel and mainly affected adult males. In civilian populations, however, the overall sex incidence is equal and all age-groups are affected, although the attack rate is higher in adults (Baker, Mathan, and Joseph, 1963).

Attempts to define the aetiological agent have so far been unsuccessful (Mathan and Baker, 1968 *a*). There is no relationship between case incidence and diet, source of water supply, wealth, housing, occupation or environmental sanitation. However, there is circumstantial evidence to suggest that the epidemics may be infective in origin (Baker and Mathan, 1970).

There have been several studies on the neurological manifestations of malabsorption syndromes (Snell, 1939; Cooke, 1952; Green and Wollaeger, 1960; Sencer, 1957; Cooke and Smith, 1966), but where patients with tropical sprue were included a clear distinction between tropical and non-tropical sprue has not always been made. Therefore, the actual prevalence and type of neurological disturbance in tropical sprue has not been established. Moreover, as Cooke and Smith (1966) pointed out, in most of the previous studies there is neither verification of steatorrhoea nor adequate neurological details. We have, therefore, made a prospective study of 25 consecutive cases of proven tropical sprue with steatorrhoea, xylose malabsorption, changes in barium-meal and jejunal biopsy, to determine the prevalence and nature of any neurological complications. In addition to the clinical neurological examination, electrodiagnostic tests such as determination of peripheral nerve conduction velocity, needle electromyography and electroencephalography were carried out (Iyer *et al.*, 1973).

NEUROLOGICAL COMPLICATIONS

Incidence

Mackie and Fairley (1929) stated that in their clinical experience there were no symptoms or signs of central or peripheral nervous system involvement in tropical sprue. Stefanini (1948) in his review of 1069 cases of tropical sprue in Italian prisoners of war in India observed that, although 17 per cent complained of paraesthesiae and a few had exaggerated tendon reflexes, as a rule neurological examination was negative. In 100 cases of sprue in Puerto Rico, Rodriguez-Molina (1954) noted that 14 per cent complained of numbness of the toes and fingers, formication and paraesthesiae; 10 per cent had decreased or absent deep tendon reflexes and decreased or absent vibration sense below the iliac crest. Green and Wollaeger (1960) encountered neurological complications in six out of 124 cases of non-tropical sprue. Only Sencer (1957) noted a high incidence of 52 per cent of neurological complications in a study of 94 cases of various types of malabsorption syndrome. However, all these authors noted the rarity of serious neurological complications in malabsorption states. In the present study 20 out of 25 cases of tropical sprue showed one or more neurological complications but serious ones were noted only in two [TABLE 4.1].

Table 4.1
Neurological Complications in Tropical Sprue (25 Cases): Clinical Features

Clinical Features	*No. of Cases*
Muscle weakness:	16
Proximal only	*8*
Generalized but predominating proximally	*8*
Paraesthesiae	7
Sensory impairment (glove and stocking type) with loss of ankle jerks	2
Myelopathy (subacute combined degeneration)	2
Loss of recent memory, bradyphrenia	3
Tetany	1
Night blindness	5
Coma	—

Proximal Muscle Weakness and Wasting

This has been described previously in conditions like cachexia (Harriman, 1965; Tomilson, Walton, and Rebeiz, 1969), senility (Serratrice, Ronx, and Aquaron, 1968), kwashiorkor (Sachdev, Taori, and Pereira, 1971) and metabolic bone diseases due to various causes including the osteomalacia of malabsorption syndrome (Prineas, Mason, and Henson, 1965; Smith and Stern, 1967).

Out of 25 cases studied, eight showed only proximal muscle weakness, while in another eight this was a significant finding in association with other manifestations, giving a total prevalence of 64 per cent. In 11 of these 16 cases needle electromyography studies showed low-voltage, short-duration potentials as seen in myopathies. In six of these, in addition to this myopathic pattern, there was pseudomyotonia on needle EMG from proximal as well as distal muscles. This improved in a few weeks on hospital treatment. Serum electrolytes were studied in five of these six cases and the abnormalities noted were hypokalaemia in two and hypocalcaemia in another two. This suggests that in the majority of these cases this feature of pseudomyotonia is related to electrolyte disturbance. The other features of myopathy improved with the general condition of the patients. It is possible that in the majority proximal muscle weakness and wasting was related to the hypoproteinaemia which was present in 15 out of 16 cases [TABLE 4.2]. In some it was probably related to deficiency of calcium and other electrolytes (Haddock, 1965; Klipstein, Samloff, and Schenk, 1966; Baker, 1957; Baker and Mathan, 1968 *a* and *c*).

Tetany

Sencer (1957) reported tetany in 17 per cent of patients with malabsorptive states. We noticed this complication in only one case. The serum calcium value was 6·7 mg per cent. It has been shown that calcium absorption is impaired in sprue (Schaaf, 1964) and serum calcium levels may be low (Haddock, 1965; Klipstein, Samloff, and Schenk, 1966). However, tetany is rare (Rodriguez-Molina, 1955) and is only seen in about 1 per cent of patients in South India (Baker, personal communication).

Peripheral Neuropathy

Subjective sensory disturbances suggestive of peripheral neuropathy were present in seven cases (28 per cent) but the objective evidence such as the glove and stocking type of anaesthesia, impaired vibration sense, and loss of ankle jerks were present only in two (8 per cent).

Table 4.2
Correlation of Neurological Manifestations with Serum Vitamin B_{12}, Folic Acid, Proteins, and Anaemia

Neurological Manifestations	*No. of Cases*	*Low Serum B_{12}* (Below 80 pg/ml)	*Low Serum Folate* (Below 6 ng/ml)	*Low Serum Proteins* (Below 6 g%)	*Anaemia* (*Hb* below 12 g%)
Muscle weakness	16	—	8	15	16
Objective peripheral neuropathy (clinical and/or nerve conduction slowing)	9	2	6	9	9
Myelopathy	2	2	1	2	2
Paraesthesiae only	4	—	2	3	4
Bradyphrenia, loss of recent memory	3	—	2	2	3
Abnormal EEG	6	1	3	5	6
No abnormality	5	—	1	3	2

These two cases also showed clinical features of subacute combined degeneration. Three cases from this group and six other cases who did not have peripheral neuropathy clinically, showed diminished conduction velocities in the peripheral nerves, either motor or sensory or both. Thus, nine cases (36 per cent) had definite evidence of peripheral neuropathy and another four (16 per cent) had only subjective paraesthesiae. Out of the former nine cases one had only low serum vitamin B_{12}, five had low serum folic acid and one had both low vitamin B_{12} and folic acid. Two of the latter group of four cases had low serum folate but normal vitamin B_{12} [TABLE 4.2]. Thus, it is obvious that folate deficiency was common but not always present in this group of cases. Six out of 12 who did not show any evidence of peripheral neuropathy had low serum folic acid. It is clear therefore, that deficiencies of folic acid and vitamin B_{12} cannot be the only causative factors in this peripheral neuropathy. Often these patients have clinical evidence of other vitamin deficiencies and it is quite likely that these are contributing to the causation of this complication.

Subacute Combined Degeneration

The rarity of this neurological manifestation in tropical sprue and other malabsorption syndromes has been commented upon by various authors (Fairley, 1934; Snell, 1939; Baker, 1957; Cooke, 1952; Richmond and Davidson, 1958; Sencer, 1957). Jeejeebhoy, Wadia, and Desai (1967), in their study of nutritional neuromyelopathy of obscure origin, noted deficiency of vitamin B_{12} associated with malabsorption of this vitamin in eight out of 12 cases. The pattern of malabsorption was similar to that of tropical sprue. In the present study of 25 cases subacute combined degeneration was noted in two. Only these two cases had serum vitamin B_{12} levels below 80 pg/ml [TABLE 4.2] In a recent review of 307 cases of tropical sprue, Baker and Mathan (1971) noted only two cases of subacute combined degeneration even though 20 per cent had serum vitamin B_{12} levels below 80 pg/ml. Thus the occurrence of this complication in 2 of the 25 cases in the present series is high, but this could be purely due to chance occurrence and does not reflect the true incidence of this complication in tropical sprue.

Grant, Hoffbrand, and Wells (1965) have reported subacute combined degeneration in folate deficiency, but Baker and Mathan (1971) did not observe it although folate deficiency was present in 71 per cent of 307 cases of tropical sprue. In the present study 13 cases had folate deficiency unassociated with low serum vitamin B_{12} but none had subacute combined degeneration although in three the serum folate levels were below 4 ng/ml.

Night Blindness

Baker and Mathan (1971) noted this complication in 20 per cent of their 307 cases. In the present series there were five cases. Baker and Mathan (1968 *b*) observed that in South India where vitamin A intake is marginal, the onset of tropical sprue may precipitate the appearance of signs of overt vitamin A deficiency.

Disturbance of Higher Cerebral Functions

Disturbances of higher cerebral functions in the form of loss of recent memory, bradyphrenia and emotional lability were observed in three cases (12 per cent). Slow dysrhythmia in frontal and temporal regions was noted in electroencephalographic studies of six out of 22 cases. Various factors such as electrolyte disturbances, anaemia, and vitamin deficiency were probably responsible for these changes.

Coma

No patient in this series either presented with or developed coma. However, this complication has been encountered by Baker (personal communication). The factors contributing to the development of this coma are severe dehydration, hyponatraemia, hypokalaemia and metabolic acidosis. One-fourth of the markedly dehydrated, hyponatraemic, hypokalaemic and acidotic patients have been reported to become drowsy or comatose on parenteral fluid and electrolyte therapy, in spite of apparent correction of fluid and electrolytes (Baker and Mathan, 1971). This may be due to the natural course of the illness or to disequilibrium created between brain and vascular system consequent on the rapid correction of fluid and electrolytes in the blood; the brain is unable to correct as rapidly because of the blood-brain-CSF barrier.

PROGNOSIS AND TREATMENT OF NEUROLOGICAL COMPLICATIONS

In the present series, the prevalence of neurological complications is high. This is probably due to greater awareness and to the use of electrodiagnostic methods. Neurological complications occur more frequently in those cases with overt deficiency of various nutrients. Serious neurological complications such as subacute combined degeneration are rare. Sencer (1957) commented that serious neurological complication such as a 'progressive crippling myeloradiculopathy' is rare in patients with malabsorption, but when it occurs it is refractory to all known medication. However, the only two cases of subacute combined degeneration noted in 307 cases of tropical sprue by Baker and Mathan (1971) responded well to replacement therapy with vitamin B_{12}. Jeejeebhoy, Wadia and Desai (1967) reported improvement in eight cases of nutritional neuromyelopathy on replacement therapy. Of our two cases of subacute combined degeneration the one with deficiency of vitamin B_{12} and folic acid responded well to replacement therapy, whereas the other with only vitamin B_{12} deficiency, failed to show any improvement either clinically or electrodiagnostically in spite of parenteral and intrathecal administration of vitamin B_{12}. The possibility of this case suffering from 'tropical ataxic neuromyelopathy' unrelated to vitamin B_{12} and folic acid deficiencies cannot be ruled out.

The other neurological complications such as proximal myopathy with or without pseudomyotonia, peripheral neuropathy, tetany, night blindness and mental changes, responded well to hospital diet, control of diarrhoea and, where necessary, replacement therapy with calcium and other electrolytes and vitamins.

As the causative factors for coma are severe dehydration, hyponatraemia, hypokalaemia, and metabolic acidosis, the correction of these forms the main line of treatment. The prevention of this complication is by prompt control of diarrhoea with bowel-binding mixtures and oral administration of fluids and electrolytes (Mathan and Baker, 1968).

References

BAKER, S. J. (1957) Tropical megaloblastic anaemias in South India, *Indian J. med. Sci.*, **11**, 687.

BAKER, S. J., MATHAN, V. I., and JOSEPH, I. (1963) *Malabsorption Syndromes*, ed. Schon, H., New York, p. 4.

BAKER, S. J., and MATHAN, V. I. (1968 *a*) Syndrome of tropical sprue in South India, *Amer. J. clin. Nutr.*, **21**, 984.

BAKER, S. J., and MATHAN, V. I. (1968 *b*) in *Proceedings of the* 1967 *Tropical Medicine Conference, Royal College of Physicians*, ed. Walters, J. H., London, pp. 65.

BAKER, S. J., and MATHAN, V. I. (1968 *c*) Unpublished observations.

BAKER, S. J., and MATHAN, V. I. (1970) Tropical sprue, in *Modern Trends in Gastroenterology*, Vol. 4, eds. Card, W. I., and Creamer, B., London, p. 198.

BAKER, S. J., and MATHAN, V. I. (1971) Tropical sprue in Southern India, in *Tropical Sprue and Megaloblastic Anaemia; A Wellcome Trust Collaborative Study*, London.

BANWELL, J. G., HUTT, M. S. R., LEONARD, P. J., BLACKMAN, V., CONNOR, D. W., MARSDEN, P. D., and CAMPBELL, J. (1967) Exocrine pancreatic disease and the malabsorption syndrome in tropical Africa, *Gut*, 8, 388.

CARAKA: Quoted by Baker and Mathan (1971)

CHAUDHURI, R. N., and RAI CHAUDHURI, M. N. (1944) Parasprue, *Indian med. Gaz.*, **79**, 404.

COOK, B. A. (1944) A vitamin B deficiency syndrome allied to sprue, *Indian med. Gaz.*, 79, 429.

COOKE, W. T. (1952) in *Modern Trends in Gastroenterology*, ed. Avery Jones, London, p. 495.

COOKE, W. T., and SMITH, W. T. (1966) Neurological disorders associated with adult coeliac disease, *Brain*, **89**, 683.

COWEN, B., SATIJA, V. K., and ZACHARIA, A. (1968) The small intestine in anaemia in Punjabis, *J. Ass. Phycns India*, **16**, 605.

CROMBIE, A. (1880) Particulars regarding the prevalence of diarrhoea at Simla in 1880, *Indian med. Gaz.*, **15**, 313.

FAIRLEY, N. H. (1934) Tropical sprue and its modern treatment, *Brit. med. J.*, **2**, 1192.

GRANT, H. C., HOFFBRAND, A. V., and WELLS, D. G. (1965) Folate deficiency and neurological disease, *Lancet*, ii, 763.

GREEN, P. A., and WOLLAEGER, A. E. (1960) Clinical behaviour of sprue in United States, *Gastroenterology*, **38**, 399.

HADDOCK, L. (1965) Quoted by Baker, S. J., and Mathan, V. I. (1970).

HARRIES, J. R. (1964) Quoted by Baker, S. J., and Mathan, V. I. (1970).

HARRIMAN, D. G. F. (1965) Muscle cachexia, in Proceedings of the Fifth International Congress of Neuropathology, Amsterdam, eds. Luthy, F., and Bischoff, A., *Excerpta med.* (*Aust.*), *Int. Cong. Ser.*, **100**, 677.

HIFT, W., and ADAMS, E. B. (1963) Malabsorption of vitamin B_{12} in megaloblastic anaemia among Africans and Indians in Durban, *Trans. roy. Soc. trop. Med. Hyg.*, **57**, 445.

IYER, G. V., TAORI, G. M., KAPADIA, C. R., MATHAN, V. I., and BAKER, S. J. (1973) Neurological complications in tropical sprue, *Neurology* (*Minneap.*).

JAIN, S. R., and SEPAHA, G. C. (1961) Parasprue, a malabsorption syndrome, *Indian J. med. Sci.*, **15**, 1.

JEEJEEBHOY, K. N., DESAI, H. G., NORONHA, S. M., ANTIA, F. P., and PAREKH, D. V. (1966) Idiopathic tropical diarrhoea with or without steatorrhea (tropical malabsorption syndrome), *Gastroenterology*, **51**, 333.

JEEJEEBHOY, K. N., WADIA, N. H., and DESAI, H. G. (1967) Role of vitamin B_{12} deficiency in tropical 'nutritional neuromyelopathy', *J. Neurol. Neurosurg. Psychiat.*, **30**, 7.

KLIPSTEIN, F. A., SAMLOFF, I. M., and SCHENK, E. A. (1966) Folate depletion associated with oral tetracyline therapy in tropical sprue, *Gastroenterology*, **51**, 317.

MACKIE, F. P., and FAIRLEY, N. H. (1929) The morbid anatomy of sprue, *Indian J. med. Res.*, **16**, 749.

MANSON-BAHR, P. E. C. (1953) The causation of tropical sprue, *Lancet*, ii, 389.

MATHAN, V. I., and BAKER, S. J. (1968) Epidemic tropical sprue and other epidemics of diarrhoea in South Indian villages. A comparative study, *Amer. J. clin. Nutr.*, **21**, 1077.

MEGAW, J. W. D., and GUPTA, J. C. (1927) Geographical distribution of some diseases in India, *Indian med. Gaz.*, **62**, 299.

MEHTA, S., MEHTA, S. K., and WADHWA, U. N. (1968) Tropical sprue in a child, *Indian Pediat.*, **5**, 170.

MISRA, R. C., KASTHURI, D., and CHUTTANI, H. K. (1966) Adult coeliac disease in the tropics, *Brit. med. J.*, **2**, 1230.

MISRA, R. C., KRISHNAN, N., RAMALINGASWAMY, V. and CHUTTANI, H. K. (1967) Tropical sprue in Northern India, *Scand. J. Gastroent.*, **2**, 192.

MOOREHEAD, C. (1860) *Researches on Disease in India*, 2nd ed., London.

PRINEAS, J. W., MASON, A. S., and HENSON, R. A. (1965) Myopathy in metabolic bone disease, *Brit. med. J.*, **1**, 1034.

RICHMOND, J., and DAVIDSON, S. (1958) Subacute combined degeneration of spinal cord in non-Addisonian megabloblastic anaemia, *Quart. J. Med.* (N.S.), **27**, 517.

RODRIGUEZ-MOLINA, R. (1954) Fundamental concepts in the diagnosis of sprue, *Ann. intern. Med.*, **40**, 33.

RODRIGUEZ-MOLINA, R. (1955) in *Tropical Sprue. Studies of the U.S. Army's Sprue Team in Puerto Rico*, Walter Reed Army Institute of Research, Washington, D.C., p. 24.

SACHDEV, K. K., TAORI, G. M., and PEREIRA, S. M. (1971) Neuromuscular status in protein-calorie malnutrition, *Neurology* (*Minneap.*), **21**, 801.

SCHAFF, M. (1964) Oral CA-47 absorption in normal subjects and in patients with tropical sprue, *Amer. J. dig. Dis.*, **9**, 795.

SENCER, W. (1957) Neurological manifestations in malabsorption syndrome, *J. Mt Sinai Hosp.*, 24, 331.

SERRATRICE, G., RONX, H., and AQUARON, R. (1968) Proximal muscle weakness in elderly subjects, *J. neurol. Sci.*, 7, 275.

SMITH, R., and STERN, G. (1967) Myopathy, osteomalacia and hyperparathyroidism, *Brain*, 90, 593.

SNELL, A. M. (1939): Tropical and non-tropical sprue. Their probable interrelationship, *Ann. intern. Med.*, 12, 1632.

STEFANINI, M. (1948) Clinical features and pathogenesis of tropical sprue, *Medicine (Baltimore)*, 27, 379.

TANDON, P. N., IYENGER, K. P., DEO, M. G. and SARAYA, A. K. (1966) A study of sprue syndrome in adults in Northern India, *J. Ass. Phycns India*, 14, 197.

TOMILSON, B. E., WALTON, J. N., and REBEIZ, J. J. (1969) The effect of ageing and of cachexia upon skeletal muscles. A histological study, *J. neurol. Sci.*, 9, 321.

5 Neurological Disease in South India

K. S. MANI

INTRODUCTION

The staple food of South India is cereal, usually rice, ragi, or sorghum. The diet of an agricultural labourer consists mainly of a thin or thick gruel, solid balls, grains or pancakes made up of the stock cereal of the region. This may be consumed as such or occasionally with thin red gram (*Cajanus cajan*) soup. This alone constitutes a meal and may be consumed twice or three times daily. The intake of vegetables and pulses is grossly inadequate. Milk, milk products and eggs are practically unknown. Fish is seldome eaten, except in the coastal districts. Meat is consumed in negligible amounts, perhaps once a month. Groundnut oil is used as a cooking medium. The diet is thus grossly deficient in calories, fats, proteins (except among fish-eaters), calcium, iron, vitamin A, riboflavine, nicotinamide, and ascorbic acid. But the diet even of a poor villager appears to have enough folates, about 300 μg. a day.

The dietary pattern of high socio-economic groups is better. The staple cereal is rice, generally of the milled variety, and wheat, the latter especially in the northern regions. Dhal soup made from red gram, and pancakes from a dozen other pulses are eaten. Variable amounts of vegetables are taken and include gourds, pumpkins, tubers, unripe plantains, nuts and leafy vegetables, especially greens, egg-plant and ochra. Milk and milk products are consumed in coffee or tea, and also as butter-milk, curds (yoghurt) and ghee (butter-fat). Fresh fruits are used in variable amounts. Cooking is done in sesame or groundnut oil; coconut oil is preferred in the coastal districts. About 10 per cent of the families of a town population never consume meat. About half take meat once or twice a week and about a third once or twice a month. Barely 1 per cent of town families take meat daily.

Villagers generally tend to show signs of protein-calorie malnutrition and vitamin A deficiency (except among the fish-eaters), and in about 14 per cent of the population vitamin B complex deficiency—cheilosis, angular stomatitis or glossitis.

Parasitic infestations of the alimentary tract occur in 80 per cent of the village population. Ankylostomiasis is widespread. This is far from surprising considering that people seldom wear shoes, especially while working in the fields. Nearly a third to one-half of a village population have a haemoglobin of less than 11 g per 100 ml. The anaemia is almost always microcytic, hypochromic, iron-deficiency type. Curiously enough, true nutritional megaloblastic anaemia without any evidence of malabsorption is extremely uncommon in the male in South India. Baker and Mathan (1971) could detect only seven such cases during a 7-year period in the Department of Haematology of the Christian Medical College Hospital, Vellore. It has also been observed that nutritional megaloblastic anaemia of pregnancy is much rarer in South India than in the developed countries (Baker, 1970). This is probably due to the high intake of folates in the diet.

Until two decades ago, malaria used to be the greatest health hazard in Mysore state. This has now been practically wiped out. Dysentery and diarrhoea followed by tuberculosis are the giant killers in the state and country today.

Medical Services

There are three general hospitals in Bangalore city, which has a population of just over 1·5 million. The daily turnover in each of the outpatient departments of the two government hospitals is about 2000. Taluk hospitals are present in most of the towns in the districts, while primary health centres cover an area of 80 to 100 square miles each and cater to a population of 60 000 to 100 000. The medical officer in charge of a primary health centre would see about 100 to 150 outpatients daily and has small inpatient premises with a microscope. He is expected to look after therapy, sanitation, maternity and child welfare and family planning.

The first hospital in the state was established in 1868, the Bowring and Lady Curzon Hospital, Bangalore, and the first medical school was opened in 1917 for the licentiate course. It was upgraded to a degree course in 1924, but moved to Mysore in 1930. Two more medical colleges were created in Bangalore in 1955 and 1963. At present the state has nine medical colleges, two of which are in Bangalore. The licentiate course was abolished a decade ago.

NEUROLOGICAL PRACTICE

The All India Institute of Mental Health, Bangalore, was established by the Government of India in 1955. It offers postgraduate training in psychiatry, clinical psychology, neurosurgery, neurology and psychiatric social work. The hospital facilities are provided in the attached Mental Hospital. There are 20 beds each for neurology and neurosurgery.

There is a tendency in the country as a whole for patients, particularly those with chronic ailments, to drift from doctor to doctor in search of a permanent cure. The referral system is practically non-existent. However, nearly a third of all patients seen in the department are referred by private practitioners or from other hospitals.

During the year 1966, 72 per cent of the outpatients came from urban, and 28 per cent from rural, areas; 63 per cent were residents of Bangalore city.

As the Departments of Neurology and Neurosurgery are located away from a general hospital, patients suffering from acute neurological disorders such as strokes, meningitis, and encephalitis are seldom seen. In a government hospital outpatient consultation is free but those with a monthly income of over Rs200 are charged for investigation. The cost of drug treatment for all outpatients is met by the patient himself. Very few can afford prolonged drug treatment.

Statistics for the year 1966

New cases	1917
Neurology clinic	949
Neurosurgical clinic	968

Table 5.1
Disorders Affecting the Brain or Spinal Cord 1966, *Bangalore*
(1632 cases)

Diagnostic Group	*Disorders involving exclusively/mainly*			
	Brain		*Spinal Cord*	
	No. of Cases	*Percentage*	*No. of Cases*	*Percentage*
Congenital disorders	44	2·69	16	0·98
Traumatic disorders	68	4·17	10	0·61
Inflammatory disorders	97	5·94	18	1·10
Vascular disorders	70	4·29	2	0·12
Neoplasms	85	5·21	8	0·49
Demyelinating disorders	—	—	4	0·25
Degenerative disorders	62	3·80	9	0·55
Toxic/metabolic disorders	3	0·18	—	—
Allergic/auto-immune disorders	7	0·43	1	0·06
Deficiency disorders	—	—	—	—
Paroxysmal disorders	815	49·94	NA	NA
Cerebral palsy and mental retardation and behaviour disorder	108	6·62	NA	NA
Miscellaneous group	2	0·12	1	0·06
Disorders of unknown aetiology	—	—	8	0·49
Total	*1361*	*83·39*	*77*	*4·71*

Of the 1917 cases seen in 1966, there was no evidence of any neurological disorder in 94 and 191 were judged to be suffering from some form of neurosis, 57 were undiagnosed and data were incomplete in 46. Analysis of this 1966 experience is outlined in TABLE 5.1.

Disorders involving mainly the brain and/or its coverings accounted for 83·4 per cent of all cases, while those affecting the spinal cord and/or its coverings amounted to 4·7 per cent of all cases.

By far the commonest neurological disorder for which help was sought was *epilepsy;* 678 new cases or 41·54 per cent of all neurological consultations. Grand mal epilepsy accounts for just under 50 per cent of all epilepsies and temporal lobe epilepsy for roughly a quarter. Mani *et al.* (1968) have described 42 instances of a peculiar type of reflex epilepsy—'hot-water epilepsy'—which was reported to occur after pouring hot water, especially on the head, while bathing. (The Indian is very rarely accustomed to a tub-bath. Water, hot or cold, is collected in a large vessel and poured on the body and/or the head with a mug.) This malady is commonly seen in the age-groups 6–15 years. *Migraine* and tension headache accounted for 75 and 17 cases respectively. Twenty-seven instances of trigeminal neuralgia were encountered.

Table 5.2
Intracranial Neoplasms in 85 *Cases*

Disorder	*No. of Cases*
Gliomas	21
Meningioma	6
Schwannoma (acoustic)	8
Pituitary tumour	3
Craniopharyngioma	2
Pinealoma	1
Metastases including lymphoma	4
Other types	5
Intracranial tumour: pathological type unknown	20
Increased intracranial tension: cause unknown	15
Total	*85*

There were 85 instances of verified or probable *intracranial neoplasms* in the year under review. The various subtypes are given in TABLE 5.2. These figures should be contrasted with those available for verified examples of *intracranial abscess* (11 cases), *intracranial tuberculoma* (12 cases), and 16 instances of *intracranial arachnoiditis*, mostly in the posterior fossa. It is interesting that the incidence of intracranial infections requiring neurosurgical treatment was nearly 40 as against 70 verified intracranial neoplasms.

There was only one case of *general paresis* and none of *cerebral syphilis* or *tabes dorsalis.* No instance of *luetic optic atrophy* was encountered in 1966. There were two instances of *subacute sclerosing panencephalitis* in children. The writer saw nine cases up to the end of 1966, of which four have been reported (Mani, Sriramachari, and Kishore, 1964). One patient had a remission and survived, though as an imbecile, for 8 years.

A diagnosis of *cysticercosis* of the brain has been made in only three cases up to 1966. Spillane (1969) has commented on the rarity in Malaysia and Thailand of calcification in the thighs in cysticercosis. In this connexion it may be interesting to refer to a paper by Pillai (1968) on *pineal gland calcification* in India. He analysed 1190 radiographs of the skull in Bangalore, and found evidence of pineal gland calcification in 23·51 per cent. This incidence reaches a peak in the fourth decade and then tends to subside. A similar incidence seems to be present in Japan (Kuwabara and Tsukamoto, 1967). Charas, Thomnoon, and Sillawat (1966), quoted by Spillane (1969), give an overall incidence of 8 per cent for pineal gland calcification in Thailand.

The low incidence of *intracranial aneurysms and angiomas* in this series appears to be real and this experience is shared by other neurologists and neurosurgeons in India (Jagannathan, Arjun Das, and Ramamurthi, 1965; Mathai and Chandy, 1965; Ramamurthi, 1965). From its very inception, this department has encountered only two verified examples of intracranial aneurysm and four of angioma in 5273 cases up to 1966.

Cerebral palsy or *mental retardation* with or without behaviour disorder forms 6·62 per cent of all neurological disorders. This hardly reflects the true incidence since these cases may go to the psychiatric outpatient department. A survey of the urinary amino acid pattern in 1200 of these patients from both psychiatry and neurology outpatient departments by Sridhara Rama Rao (1970) has revealed seven instances of phenylketonuria, three of homocystinuria and one of Hartnup's syndrome. Twenty-six cases of *hydrocephalus* were seen during this period, eight cases of spina bifida manifesta (meningocele) and four of spina bifida occulta, but no instance of frontal encephalomeningocele was encountered.

In 1966 there was no example of any cerebral demyelinating disorder but there were four cases of cord involvement. The rarity of primary demyelinating disease in the tropics is well recognized. During a 9½-year period, the writer has seen only four, five, and three cases respectively of multiple sclerosis, neuromyelitis optica, and Schilder's diffuse sclerosis. One of the cases of paraplegia seen in 1967 turned out at autopsy to be a classical case of multiple sclerosis. The only other autopsy-proven case of multiple sclerosis in India was seen in Hyderabad (Prabhakar, 1968).

Forty-nine cases of parkinsonism were seen during this year; most of them were in young adults presenting with unilateral tremor.

In view of the high incidence of parental consanguinity, heredofamilial degenerative disorders of the nervous system might be expected to occur quite frequently. But this does not appear to be the case and the explanation is obscure.

In TABLE 5.3 are listed the number of *heredofamilial disorders* seen in the past 9½ years. The commonest cause of *dementia* appears to be the arteriosclerotic variety. There were 13 cases of *motor neurone disease* in that period.

Table 5.3

Incidence of Certain Heredofamilial Disorders (in a Total of 5273 Neurological Cases)

Disorder	*No. of Cases*
Spinocerebellar degeneration	31
Lipidoses	14
Other types of progressive cerebral degenerations of infancy and childhood	16
Presenile dementia	25
Total	*86*

Compression of the median nerve at the *carpal tunnel* is extremely rare in Bangalore and only four cases were seen in the department up to the end of 1966. By far the commonest cause of peripheral neuropathy and indeed one of the commonest neurological disorders in Mysore state is leprosy, but patients with leprosy seldom come to a neurology clinic. There were six instances of Landry-Guillain-Barré syndrome.

Fifteen instances of *myopathy* were seen in 1966—six of them were *muscular dystrophy*, three probable polymyositis, and one myasthenia.

Unexplained optic atrophy and ocular palsies are common in South India. We saw 43 cases in 1966 [TABLE 5.4].

Table 5.4

Unexplained Cranial Nerve Palsies (43 Cases)

Disorder	*No. of Cases*
Optic atrophy	11
Oculomotor palsies	20
Lower cranial nerve palsies	6
Proptosis	3
Other types	3
Total	*43*

SPASTIC PARAPLEGIA IN SOUTH INDIA

An analysis of 249 cases of spastic paraplegia seen in the 5-year period 1963–68 is outlined in TABLES 5.5 and 5.6.

Neurosurgical 'causes' account for 128 cases, 51·00 per cent of the total. Data were incomplete in 6 cases.

Table 5.5

Analysis of 249 Cases of Spastic Paraplegia of Spinal Origin: Surgical Causes (128)

Disorder	*No. of Cases*
Adhesive arachnoiditis	24
Pott's paraplegia	15
Neurofibroma	15
Spondylotic myelopathy	14
Meningioma	11
Lymphoma	7
Craniovertebral anomaly	6
Cord compression: type unknown	5
Acute cervical cord contusion	4
Fracture dislocation	3
Intramedullary tuberculoma	3
Intramedullary tumour	3
Fluorosis	3
Extramedullary tumour	2
Intramedullary angioma	2
Severe kyphoscoliosis	1
Spina bifida occulta	1
Extradural tuberculosis	1
Extradural haematoma	1
Haemangio-endothelioma	1
Haemangio-endotheliosarcoma	1
Metastases	1
Intramedullary epidermoid	1
Intramedullary astrocytoma	1
?Spondylotic myelopathy	1
?Adhesive arachnoiditis	1
Total	*128*

Adhesive arachnoiditis was by far the most common single cause of cord compression in this series; it accounted for 9·63 per cent of all paraplegias of spinal origin. The cause is believed to be tuberculous in the majority.

The incidence of *Pott's paraplegia* may be higher than shown since some cases go to orthopaedic surgeons.

Of the 15 cases of *neurofibroma*, one turned out to be a histologically verified malignant schwannoma. All the 11 cases of *meningioma* were verified histologically; six males and five females. There were six cases of craniovertebral anomaly, of which three showed atlanto-axial dislocation. The three cases of *fluorosis* came from three villages in the Anantapur District of Andhra Pradesh, where endemic fluorosis is known to exist.

It is noteworthy that there was only a solitary instance of a possible metastatic lesion in this series of paraplegias. The primary tumour was not detected. Metastatic lesions in the central nervous system or the remote effects of carcinoma on the nervous system are rare in our experience. We have seen only two instances of the latter so far.

Table 5.6

Analysis of 249 Cases of Spastic Paraplegia of Spinal Origin: Medical Causes (117)

Disorder	*No. of Cases*
Tropical spastic paraplegia	45
Paraplegia: type unknown	13
Syphilitic meningomyelitis	10
?Syphilitic meningomyelitis	10
Multiple sclerosis	8
Amyotrophic lateral sclerosis	7
Anterior spinal artery occlusion	6
? Multiple sclerosis	4
Transverse myelopathy	6
Neuromyelitis optica	2
Post-vaccinial myelopathy	2
Syringomyelia	2
Total	*115*

In TABLE 5.6 are listed the various medical diagnostic categories of spastic paraplegia during this 5-year period. There were 115 cases (46·20 per cent). *Tropical spastic paraplegia* was the commonest with 45 cases, and this will be discussed later in this chapter.

A diagnosis of *syphilitic meningomyelitis* was entertained when there was an acute or subacute onset of a transverse segmental lesion of the cord, associated with a positive blood VDRL of 1 in 8 dilution or above, and/or a definite positive serological reaction, irrespective of the dilution, in the spinal fluid. There were only ten such cases in 5 years. Myelography excluded any associated arachnoiditis.

In 10 cases, a diagnosis of *?syphilitic meningomyelitis* has been made provisionally. These were patients with a comparable clinical picture who were said to have had 'bad blood' in the past and had received 'milky-white injections'. The blood VDRL was either negative, or positive but only in very weak dilutions. The spinal fluid was essentially normal and the serology negative. It is difficult to accept these cases as definite instances of luetic meningomyelitis since rapid seroconversion with treatment is very unusual in the South Indian subject (Rajam, 1966). These cases could well be due to other, as yet unknown, causes.

The seven instances of *amyotrophic lateral sclerosis* all conformed to the classical pattern. A diagnosis of *anterior spinal artery occlusion* (six cases) was made when there was a rapid onset—in seconds or minutes—of a transection of the anterior two-thirds of the cord. There was no antecedent trauma nor any evidence of lues. Myelography was invariably carried out to exclude an angioma of the cord.

A diagnosis of *multiple sclerosis* was made in only eight cases. There were 4 further cases in which this disease may have been present. All had evidence of subacute and recurrent lesion at the same level of the cord, with a clear-cut remission in between. In six there was a subacute transverse myelopathy reaching its peak in 48 to 72 hours; recovery was complete in three, incomplete in one, and two had died.

TROPICAL SPASTIC PARAPLEGIA: 45 CASES

The nature and differential diagnosis of the spastic paraplegias pose a particularly difficult problem, because autopsies are rarely obtained. In India in the 40s and even 50s of this century syphilis figured prominently as an aetiological factor. In the late 50s, with the advent

Table 5.7
Rural-Urban Distribution of 249 Paraplegics

District	*TSP*	*Non-TSP*
Rural	15	83
Urban	30	121
Bangalore City	16	85
Total	*45*	*204*

of neurosurgery, the emphasis shifted to the various types of cord compression which were revealed. It also became apparent that primary demyelinating diseases were uncommon.

As the material on paraplegias of unknown type accumulated, a fairly clear-cut pattern began to emerge in certain cases with regard to type of onset, pattern of cord involvement, and the course of the illness. All the available tools of clinical investigation gave negative results, and as far as possible established diagnostic categories are excluded. In this section an analysis of these cases is presented. Formerly designated South Indian paraplegia we now speak of this disease as tropical spastic paraplegia.

During the 5-year period 1963–68, 45 cases of tropical spastic paraplegia (TSP) have been studied in this department [FIG. 5.1] and this represents the largest diagnostic group (18·10 per cent) in the total series of 249 cases of paraplegia. Other forms of paraplegia served as a control group.

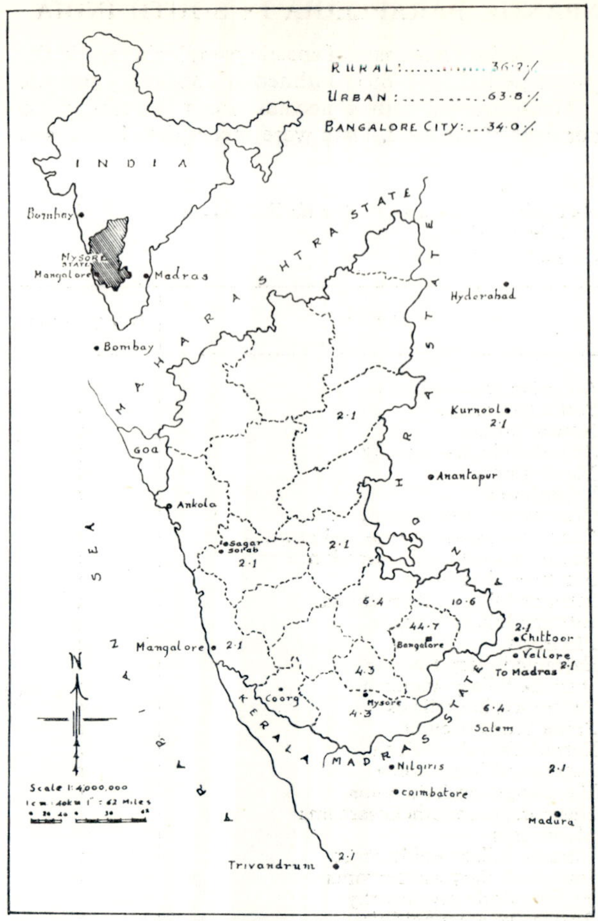

FIG. 5.1. Tropical spastic paraplegia in Mysore state. Note the percentage and distribution by districts of patients with tropical spastic paraplegia, seen during the 5-year prospective study.

Clinical Features

Sex, Age, and Socio-economic Status

There were 29 males and 16 females. The age at onset of symptoms was from 9 to 65 years, with a mean of 34·5 years, and a peak in the third, fourth and fifth decades.

The patients were divided into six economic classes on an arbitrary scale based on total family income, ranging from Class I (rich) to Class VI (destitute). Three-quarters were in Classes IV and V, but none of the top three classes was exempt.

Diet and Habits

The dietary pattern of both groups of paraplegias was no different from the rest of the population. About 60 per cent equally of patients and controls were non-vegetarian, taking small amounts of meat, fish and eggs with a frequency varying from twice a week to once a month. Tapioca (cassava) is eaten rarely in Mysore state. Neither *Lathyrus sativus* nor *Vicia sativa* was knowingly consumed.

Cooking utensils were made of earthenware, aluminium or steel, or of brass coated with a compound of tin and lead known locally as 'Kalai'. Kalai vessels had been used at some time or another by about 60 per cent of patients and of controls.

Antecedent and Family History

A history of exposure to venereal infection was obtained in nine out of 29 TSP patients, of whom six had a local sore or urethral discharge as a sequel, and in 12 out of 31 paraplegic controls. No other unusual features were apparent in the past history. Antecedent febrile illness, inoculation, or history suggestive of multiple sclerosis were conspicuous by their absence. Family histories were negative.

Symptoms

There was insidious development of the disease over a period of several weeks or months in 43 cases. In two the disability reached its peak within 4 weeks, but none suffered sudden severe paralysis. The duration of symptoms at the time of admission varied from 6 weeks to 20 years, being 6 months to 2 years in 53·3 per cent.

The patients presented with difficulty in walking due to weakness and/or stiffness of the lower limbs. In more than half the symptoms were asymmetrical, either in time of onset or in severity. Numbness, and tingling or burning paraesthesiae, particularly of the feet and/or hands, were present in 73 per cent of cases, but they were seldom prominent and usually not voluntarily mentioned. They were mainly distal in distribution. The trunk or face was never involved in these sensory phenomena.

Many of the patients complained of a dragging pain in the lower limbs, and stiffness or pain in the lumbar or lower thoracic regions. Involuntary jerks and flexion movements of the lower limbs, particularly at night, were common. Bladder symptoms were present at the time of first admission in 87 per cent of cases: 69 per cent had precipitancy or urgency, and 40 per cent each hesitancy and frequency of micturition: only five cases required catheterization for retention with overflow. Bladder sensation was obviously not impaired: the majority of men suffered loss of potency.

Fifty-six per cent of patients admitted to weakness of the upper limbs, but this was disabling in only two instances. Three cases had features of an organic psychosis and two had generalized grand mal convulsions. Two patients each complained of disturbance of vision and hearing respectively; four had noted slurring of speech and one difficulty in chewing. These symptoms referable to the cranial nerves were far from impressive, and were not complained of voluntarily.

Neurological Signs

Weakness in the upper limbs was never severe. In no instance was there a persistent asymmetry in the objective weakness of the limbs. Spasticity of varying degrees was seen in all the four limbs, although it tended to be mild in the upper limbs. In general, the disability was due mainly to the spasticity, and in some patients it was the most disabling feature. The deep reflexes in the lower limbs were exaggerated in over 95 per cent of cases and in the upper limbs were pathologically brisk in 80 per cent. The abdominal reflexes were absent in just over three-quarters of the cases. A classical extensor plantar response was elicited in 40 cases.

Objective evidence of sensory deficit was elicited in over 80 per cent of the cases. The diminution of appreciation of touch, pain and temperature was far from impressive. In no case was there a clear-cut segmental level below which sensations were either lost or definitely diminished. Diminution of proprioception or vibration sense was usually present over the toes and fingers and seldom above. Nine patients had a positive Romberg's sign, which, however, was never marked. The gait was predominantly spastic and never primarily high-steppage and ataxic in character. Peripheral neuropathy as evidenced by calf tenderness, weakness and/or wasting of feet and/or hands, was present in 23·4 per cent of cases but was seldom more than mild.

Stray instances of brisk jaw jerk (five cases), mild degree of primary optic atrophy (four cases), and first degree vestibular type of nystagmus (one case) were also encountered.

Other Physical Signs

No classical mucocutaneous signs of vitamin deficiency were present, but unusual dryness of the skin, mosaic dermatoses of the legs, muddy conjunctivae, and Bitot's spots were seen more frequently in patients with TSP than in the paraplegic controls. None of the patients in either group showed the dark pigmentation of the dorsum of the fingers, which is generally considered, when present, to be a useful clinical sign of vitamin B_{12} or folate deficiency in South India (Baker and Mathan, 1971). The general body build in both groups was that of an average South Indian subject.

Investigations

Radiological studies of the chest and cervical spine were non-contributory apart from revealing mild cervical spondylosis in six. Myelography was performed in all the 45 cases and showed mild spondylotic bars in four over the age of 50 years; it was normal in the remainder.

Liver function tests were normal and the mean serum albumin and globulin levels did not differ significantly from the control figures. The erythrocyte sedimentation rate was raised in 12 out of 34 cases, but in most of these there was a possible urinary infection from increased residual urine.

Eosinophilia was present in 22 (48·89 per cent) of the TSP cases and 16 (18·18 per cent) of the paraplegic controls, but this was marked in only three and six cases respectively. Haemoglobin of less than 10·5 g/100 ml was seen in 11 (24·44 per cent) cases of TSP and 12 out of 90 (13·33 per cent) paraplegic controls. The peripheral smears in these 11 cases of TSP were suggestive either of simple iron-deficiency anaemia or anaemia of infection, except for one case with slight macrocytosis. Achlorhydria was no more frequent in this group than in the paraplegic controls. Bone-marrow biopsies were available in 28 TSP cases and four control paraplegics; three of the former and two of the latter showed early megaloblastic changes.

Serum estimations of cyanocobalamin, folate, nicotinic acid and ascorbic acid in TSP patients and control paraplegics showed that only the serum B_{12} levels in both the TSP cases and the paraplegic controls were significantly lower than in normal controls. It is possible that the changes in the marrow and the lower levels of serum B_{12} were a result of loss of employment and impaired nutrition rather than the cause of the malady. These findings, however, are only of limited value as the majority of both the paraplegic groups had previously received vitamin therapy elsewhere.

The plasma thiocyanate levels in 13 patients with TSP were all, with one exception, below the mean normal for seven healthy Nigerian controls and nine Indian non-smokers (Dastur, 1970).

The blood VDRL reaction was negative in all but two, who also showed a positive fluorescent treponema antibody (FTA) test. The incidence of positive blood VDRL in our hospital population is 4 per cent.

The spinal fluid was examined in all cases: normal cell counts in 40; normal protein (<60 mg) in 30; 60 mg to 190 mg in 15.

The spinal fluid sediment was stained with toluidine blue for fungal elements in 33 cases with negative results. The spinal fluid VDRL reaction was negative in all 45 cases; 21 of them also showed a negative reaction with Reiter's protein complement-fixation test and fluorescent treponema antibody (FTA) test. The latter alone was positive in one instance and the patient came to autopsy.

Serum and spinal fluid of nine TSP cases, five paraplegic controls and three normal controls (serum only) were tested for immune reactions using rabbit brain, and liver and calf thymus extracts. The results suggested only non-specific effects of tissue damage.

Biopsies of the peroneus brevis muscle (18 cases) and the first dorsal interosseous nerve of the foot (21 cases) were not informative; two of the former showed denervation atrophy and both had footdrop. In the latter, there was a variable density of myelin, but none was clearly abnormal.

The spinal fluid in nine cases of TSP was cultured for *Mycobacterium tuberculosis*, but with negative findings. In two instances, the spinal fluid was inoculated into Sabouraud's medium for fungi but with negative results. Electroencephalograms in 9 cases of TSP gave normal results in six and mild non-specific abnormalities in three.

Natural History

All patients have been followed up from 6 months to 8½ years, 39 of them for over 2 years and 22 for over 5 years. In no case was there evidence of remissions or relapses with fresh focal signs. In some there were minor fluctuations in disability. During the course of the illness, over a third of the patients could walk unaided, or with a stick, albeit slowly; less than a third could not walk at all, and of these two could not even sit up.

Therapeutic trials with betamethasone, vitamin B_1, B_{12}, B complex, calcium pantothenate and British anti-lewisite dimercaprol have failed to influence the course of the illness.

Follow-up has shown that of the 45 cases, none had improved, 14 showed no change, 20 were worse, and 11 died.

Autopsies have been performed in only two cases, but they were not wholly typical of the majority, and the significance of the pathological findings is questionable. One of these cases died of a subarachnoid haemorrhage, but no aneurysm or angioma was demonstrable. There was post-mortem evidence of luetic aortitis, while the patient had shown a positive FTA test in his serum and spinal fluid during life. Autolytic changes unfortunately precluded a detailed histological study of the brain. The spinal cord, which was better preserved, showed myelin loss evident in the posterior and lateral columns. In the second case cerebral symptoms and signs followed the spastic paraplegia after 5 years, leading to death a year later. At autopsy there was a diffuse chronic meningomyelopathy with perivascular cuffing and remarkable hyalinoid thickening of the vascular adventitia and media, with secondary long-tract degeneration and demyelination, as in the Jamaican neuropathy.

Comment

As we have seen, the commonest form of paraplegia in South India is a spastic disorder with slight sensory impairment, which cannot be identified on the basis of standard classifications of known disorders of the nervous system. In any such series, autopsy studies may eventually reveal that odd cases of a classical kind, such as multiple sclerosis, syphilis, amyotrophic lateral sclerosis or lathyrism, may cause confusion, but it is clearly evident that a majority belong to a group of a different nature. No clues to the aetiology have been discovered. They resemble and may be related to the spastic cord disorders which have now been described in many parts of the tropical world, and for the present may be referred to as tropical spastic paraplegia.

References

BAKER, S. J. (1970) Personal communication.

BAKER, S. J., and MATHAN, V. I. (1966) Megaloblastic anaemia in South India, *Abstr. XI Cong. int. Soc. Haemat.*, Sydney, p. 94.

BAKER, S. J., and MATHAN, V. I. (1971) Tropical sprue in Southern India, in *Tropical Sprue and Megaloblastic Anaemia: A Wellcome Trust Collaborative Study*, London.

CHARAS, THOMNOON, and SILLAWAL (1966) Quoted by Spillane, J. D. (1969).

DASTUR, D. K. (1970) Unpublished observations.

JAGANNATHAN, K., ARJUN DAS, G., and RAMAMURTHI, B. (1965) Symptomatology of subarachnoid haemorrhage, *Neurology (India)*, 13, 44.

KUWABARA, T., and TSUKAMOTO, Y. (1967) Quoted by Pillai, K. M. (1968).

MANI, K. S., GOPALAKRISHNAN, P. N., VYAS, J. N., and PILLAI, M. S. (1968) 'Hot-water epilepsy'—a peculiar type of reflex epilepsy. A preliminary report, *Neurology (India)*, 16, 107.

MANI, K. S., SRIRAMACHARI, S., and KISHORE, B. (1964) Subacute panencephalitis in childhood: report of four cases, *Neurology (India)*, 12, 42.

MATHAI, K. V., and CHANDY, J. (1965) Incidence of subarachnoid haemorrhage, *Neurology (India)*, 13, 40.

PILLAI, K. M. (1968) Pineal gland calcification, *Neurology (India)*, 16, 35.

PRABHAKAR, V. (1968) Personal communication.

RAJAM, R. V. (1966) Personal communication.

RAMAMURTHI, B. (1965) Are subarachnoid haemorrhages uncommon in India?, *Neurology (India)*, 13, 42.

RAO, SRIDHARA RAMA (1970) Unpublished observations.

SPILLANE, J. D. (1969) Tropical neurology, *Proc. roy. Soc. Med.*, 62, 403,

6 Cerebrovascular Disorders in South India

J. ABRAHAM

Two aspects of cerebrovascular disease in South India are discussed in this chapter. One is an epidemiological study assessing the prevalence of hemiplegics in the population and the other is an analysis of stroke in the young adult.

EPIDEMIOLOGY

The incidence of cerebrovascular disease varies in different parts of the world and this group of disorders has become of vital importance in world health with the increasing age of populations. Cerebrovascular disease ranks third as a cause of death in the United States, and every year about half a million people are crippled or killed by stroke.

Data regarding the incidence of cerebrovascular disease in India are not available through any population-based studies, though some information on the hospital incidence of stroke is available from a few centres in India (Bharucha and Umerji, 1962; Dalal, 1965; Misra, Misra, Agarwal, and Sircar, 1967; Padmavati, 1958; Naik, Satyanarayana Rao, and Ramvilas Saboo, 1966). It is generally agreed, however, that hospital incidence of a disease is a fallacious figure by which to judge the prevalence of the disease in a population.

An epidemiological study covering a population of about 200 000 in and around Vellore was undertaken during the years 1968 and 1969 by the Departments of Neurological Sciences and Biostatistics of the Christian Medical College Hospital, Vellore, South India, to assess the prevalence of hemiplegia. All cases of completed stroke[1] with hemiplegia due to cerebrovascular disease or to any other aetiology were included in the study.

The entire town of Vellore and two of the adjacent rural areas of about 10·5 sq km or 39 sq miles in area were included in this study. The total population actually surveyed in both the urban (Vellore town) and the rural areas was 258 576. The age-sex distribution of the sampled population is given in TABLE 6.1.

A total of 1245 persons were identified as suffering from paralysis, paresis, inability to use a limb, bed-ridden, etc. and classified as 'suspects' by the field workers. Of the 1245 'suspects' 174 were identified by the neurologists as cases of genuine stroke with hemiplegia.

The prevalence rate per 100 000 population is 68·5 in males and 44·8 in females.

[1]The word 'stroke' as used here is taken to mean hemiplegia due to any aetiology. Approximately 85 per cent were completed strokes, 13 per cent infantile hemiplegia, and 2 per cent miscellaneous causes.

Table 6.1
Age and Sex Distribution of Population Surveyed

Age Group (in Years)	*Population*		*Total*
	Male	*Female*	
0–9	34 941	37 743	72 684
10–19	26 872	23 856	50 728
20–29	20 932	21 783	42 715
30–39	18 291	16 013	34 304
40–49	13 708	11 978	25 686
50–59	8 679	8 132	16 811
60–69	5 281	5 142	10 423
70 and above	2 705	2 520	5 225

This is not a biased sample as it compares well with the 1961 census figures.

It is evident that the prevalence rate increases with age and that there is a statistically significant male preponderance in the age-groups above 50 years ($p<·01$).

While the female rates are lower in both rural and urban areas the rural rates are lower than urban. It is also observed that 40 of the confirmed hemiplegics among the 147, nearly 25 per cent, were under 40 years of age.

The prevalence rate of 13·1 per 100 000 in the 0–9 year age-group is disconcerting. This large number denotes that birth injuries and early infective lesions leaving hemiplegia as a sequela are still important factors. Unless the aetiology is understood and proper preventive measures are taken, this group of patients with a fairly long life expectancy will increase the demands on an already economically overburdened society.

The surveyed population in Vellore town and in the surrounding rural areas represents quite adequately the conditions of villages and towns in Southern India excluding major cities such as Madras. The southern states in India, which include Andhra Pradesh, Tamil Nadu, Pondicherry, Mysore and Kerala had an estimated population of 131 million in 1969. Thus, we could expect at least 75 000 persons affected with hemiplegia due to stroke. Although other regions of India might differ from the southern areas both in terms of climatic factors and dietary habits, one could reasonably expect similar conditions with regard to environmental and social conditions. We might therefore expect at least 300 000 live hemiplegics in the whole of India. The total number of people who suffer from cerebrovascular disease of all types will naturally be considerably higher. However, as autopsy and morbidity studies have not been done in India, the exact extent of this disease is unknown.

STROKE IN THE YOUNG ADULT

Stroke in the young adult is rare and in children rarer still (Ford, 1960; Fisher, 1951). Wells and Timberger (1961) in a study of patients with cerebral thrombosis under the age of 50 years found 77 cases in a 28-year period: there were 22 patients below the age of 40 years. Less than 2 per cent of strokes in Sweden occur below the age of 40 years (Sjostrom, 1967). In the present series, out of 407 consecutive cases of cerebrovascular disease 127, or 32 per cent, were in the 11 to 40-year age-group. Of all patients with cerebrovascular disease admitted 43·6 per cent were below the age of 45 years. They constitute 24 per cent of all cases of neurological disorders admitted to the neurological wards.

The basic diagnostic categories in cerebrovascular disease applicable to both clinical and mortality data are contained in the international statistical classification of cerebrovascular disease, carrying the rubrics 330 to 334. Unfortunately these categories are not strictly defined; 332, for example, groups together embolism and thrombosis, and various equivalents of cerebral and cerebellar 'softening or necrosis and apoplexy'. Be that as it may, for clinical purposes an exhaustive classification of stroke was drawn up by the *ad hoc* committee of the United States Academy of Neurology in 1958. We have classified our cases modifying the above recommendation in conjunction with the angiographic findings.

Classification of Cases

The diagnosis and distribution by age and sex of 127 cases of stroke in the under-40 year age-group is given in TABLE 6.2.

Much ambiguity and uncertainty in diagnosis still persists; for example some cases without an angiographic study, classified under cerebral infarction in this series, may be due to internal carotid artery thrombosis, embolism or infarction from some other cause such as 'small vessel disease'.

Cerebral Thrombosis (Infarction)

Of all strokes in the younger age-group 44·9 per cent were classified as suffering from cerebral ischaemia as a result of cerebral arterial thrombosis, 42 were men and 15 women. The right side was paralysed in 47·4 per cent and the left in 52·6 per cent The onset of the ictus was acute in 87·5 per cent. A little more than half were engaged in some activity when it occurred. A 'stuttering' onset was found in approximately 9 per cent of cases. Loss of consciousness occurred in less than half the number and did not last more than an hour in most. Seizures at the onset of ictus occurred in approximately 13 per cent. There was no apparent correlation between cerebral infarction and socio-economic status. In 11 per cent of cases the serological test for syphilis was positive. Hypertension was present in 20 per cent, of which this was associated with diabetes in less than half. The serum cholesterol levels were found to be borderline to high in 6·7 per cent.

Approximately a quarter of the patients revealed some abnormality in the ECG. Sixteen per cent had evidence of an ischaemic lesion of the heart not associated with hypertension, diabetes or a high cholesterol.

Electroencephalographic studies revealed abnormalities in the waking record in more than half the number of cases. Focal abnormalities in the appropriate cerebral hemisphere were seen in 84 per cent.

Forty-three out of 57 cases in this group were studied angiographically and 19 were found to have abnormalities. Ten per cent had extracranial, and 90 per cent intracranial, abnormalities, the most common lesion

Table 6.2
Diagnosis and Distribution by Age and Sex of 127 Young Stroke Patients

Diagnosis	*Age in Years*			*Sex*		*No. of Cases*	*Percentage*
	11–20	21–30	31–40	*M*	*F*		
Cerebral (thrombosis) infarction	3	18	36	42	15	57	44·9
Cerebral embolism	3	6	8	7	10	17	13·4
Internal carotid artery thrombosis	1	5	10	14	2	16	12·6
Infantile hemiplegia	9	1	—	6	4	10	7·9
Cortical venous thrombosis (post-partum)	1	5	3	—	9	9	7·1
Subarachnoid haemorrhage (without demonstrable abnormality)	—	—	5	3	2	5	3·9
Aortic arch syndrome	1	—	3	1	3	4	3·1
AV malformations	2	—	2	4	—	4	3·1
Hypertensive encephalopathy	—	—	3	2	1	3	2·4
Intracranial aneurysm	—	2	—	2	—	2	1·6

being middle cerebral artery occlusion which was present in 42 per cent.

Cerebral Embolism

Cerebral embolism was the second commonest cause of stroke in the young adult. The site of origin of the embolus was the heart in all but two of the cases. The most commonly embolized arterial territory was that of the middle cerebral artery. The onset of the embolic phenomenon was acute in nearly all cases, with loss of consciousness in a higher percentage and for a more prolonged period of time than in cerebral infarction. Electroencephalographic abnormalities were found in 50 per cent of the cases.

Internal Carotid Artery Thrombosis

Internal carotid artery thrombosis was the third commonest cause of stroke in the younger age-group. There were 14 males and two females and the right internal carotid artery was thrombosed in ten while the left was thrombosed in six. The site of thrombosis was extracranial in all but one. In three of the cases there was obvious hypertension. The electroencephalographic recordings were abnormal in 64·3 per cent.

Authors from other parts of India (Misra, Misra, Agarwal, and Sircar, 1967; Dalal, Shah, Aiyar, and Kikani, 1968) have also found that between 20 per cent and 25 per cent of all strokes due to thrombo-embolism occur in the below 40-year age-group; 78·1 per cent (Khan and Rao, 1951) and 46·7 per cent (Krishna and Teja, 1965) of stroke patients were under 49 years of age. The high incidence of stroke in the younger age-group, therefore, is not peculiar to the south.

In two other series in India the relative proportion of cerebral thrombo-embolism comprising cerebrovascular disease was 82 per cent (Misra, Misra, Agarwal and Sircar, 1967; Dalal, Shah, Aiyar, and Kikani, 1968) for all age-groups. Osuntokun, Odeku, Dada, and Adeloye (1969) in Nigeria found that thrombo-embolism was the cause of stroke in 73 per cent in all age-groups. It is interesting to compare our figure of 70 per cent to the weighted mean of the population-based studies in America of 62 per cent (Eisenberg *et al.*, 1964; Kurland, Choi, and Sayre 1967; Kannel, 1966; Kannel *et al.*, 1965). In the present series cerebral infarction (cerebral arterial thrombosis 44·9 per cent, cerebral embolism 13·4 per cent, internal carotid artery thrombosis 12·6 per cent) accounted for 70 per cent of all cerebrovascular diseases. The sex ratios (male/female) in thrombosis, embolism and internal carotid artery thrombosis are respectively 2·8, 0·7 and 7. The overall male/female ratio of thrombosis and embolism together is 1·9, compared to 1·72 from the cooperative stroke study in seven centres in the United States for all age-groups (Fisher, 1961). The relative frequency of cerebral thrombosis versus embolism in this series was 0·23 as compared to 0·07 (Groch, McDevitt, and Wright, 1961) and 0·18 (Carter, 1963) for all ages from hospital series in the West.

In discussing the aetiological mechanisms of cerebral atherosclerosis Resch and Baker (1964) found no atherosclerosis in 71·9 per cent of males and 79·2 per cent of females in the 31 to 40-year age-group, while 7·3 per cent of patients had severe atherosclerosis. Baker, Kinnard, Iannone (1961) stated that hypertension and diabetes would produce a definite increase in the appearance and severity of atherosclerosis. It is interesting to note that in Wells and Timberger's series (1961), 32 out of the 77 (42 per cent) patients suffering from cerebral thrombosis below the age of 50 years were hypertensive. In the present series 19·3 per cent with cerebral thrombosis had hypertension; hypertension with diabetes was seen in only 8·8 per cent. The serum cholesterol was borderline to high in 6·7 per cent. A high cholesterol as the only abnormality detected was found in six cases. According to Osuntokun, Odeku, Dada and Adeloye (1969), except in hypertensive and diabetic patients non-embolic ischaemic cerebrovascular disease from atherosclerotic occlusion is uncommon in Nigerians. This observation is borne out by the findings of Resch, Williams, Loewenson, and Wagner (1969) who found that atherosclerosis was less common in Nigeria than in Minnesota and also less common than in ethnologically related American Negroes in Alabama, Maryland, and Tennessee.

No hypertension, diabetes or hypercholesterolaemia was found in 73 per cent of our cases of cerebral infarction. Sixteen per cent had evidence of ischaemic heart disease unrelated to the presence of hypertension or diabetes. The absence of angiographic patterns showing atheroma, and the histological evidence of its absence from internal carotid artery biopsies suggest that there are some systemic and local factors at work in the production of stroke in the younger age-group.

Large vessel arteritis producing pulseless disease has been reported in India (Basu, 1961; Hirsch, Aikat, and Basu, 1964). This, however, was an uncommon aetiological factor in our series of cases. An auto-immune process affecting vessels of smaller calibre is an interesting possibility. The finding of LE cells in the peripheral blood smear, altered albumin-globulin ratios, abnormal serum electrophoretic patterns, coupled with the occasional finding of microfilariae in the blood, tuberculous infection, syphilis and leprosy in some of our patients, cause us to speculate whether the process affecting the cerebral vascular tree is an allergic manifestation of some of the chronic diseases found in the tropics.

In a comparative study of the pattern of vessel involvement in stroke between a Japanese and Minnesota population (Resch *et al.*, 1969) it was pointed out that the Japanese had predominantly small vessel involvement. In the analysis of our angiographic data for stroke in the young we are also impressed by the very much higher incidence of abnormalities of the small vessels.

Katsuki and Omae (1967), writing of stroke profiles in the Japanese, made the following observation:

> Frequency of stenotic lesions in the affected side of the cerebral hemisphere: complete occlusion was more frequently seen at ages below 40, in which cases with occlusion due to arteritis or arteriopathy of unknown aetiology were included. These findings indicate that a definite occlusive arterial disease is responsible for cerebral infarction in a considerable number of cases below age 40 . . . complete occlusion was found in 10 per cent in those above 60 years, compared with 30 per cent in the ages below 40 years.

It seems probable that in some of the Afro-Asian countries and in the Orient arteriopathies of as yet unknown aetiology are responsible for the fairly widespread occurrence of occlusive vascular disorder in the young adult.

Another factor which merits comment is the relative infrequency of intracranial aneurysms in this series. In an analysis of cerebrovascular disease of young adults in Mississippi, Haerer, Smith, and Spencer (1969) found ruptured aneurysms in 27 per cent of cases. Our incidence of subarachnoid haemorrhage was 3·9 per cent and of demonstrable intracranial aneurysm 1·6 per cent. The relative infrequency of aneurysm in India has been commented on by another worker (Ramamurthi, 1965). The reason for the low incidence is not established.

Infantile Hemiplegia

Infantile hemiplegia was the fourth largest entity in this group. Ten out of the 127 patients were diagnosed as infantile hemiplegics of which four were females and six males. Angiographic study was made on six cases: all were found to be normal.

The nature of onset was assessed in eight of these cases, five had acute and three had a gradual onset. Out of the ten cases, six had fever prior to the onset of the hemiplegia. Loss of consciousness was reported in nly one case. In four out of the ten cases, seizures were associated with the onset; two were of a focal nature and two generalized.

All the cases were normotensive. EEG was done in nine: all had focal abnormality originating in the appropriate hemisphere. In addition, four cases had focal abnormality in the opposite hemisphere. Diffuse abnormality on the side of the affected area was seen in four cases, and of these two had diffuse abnormality on the contralateral side as well.

Cortical Venous Thrombosis

Cortical venous thrombosis is the second largest cause of stroke in young females. There were 46 young females with stroke; nine (20 per cent) were diagnosed as cortical venous thrombosis. This constitutes 7·1 per cent of all the young strokes.

The onset was acute in seven, gradual in one and stuttering in another. Prodromes of mild systemic reactions such as fever and headache were present in all the cases. Five had convulsions associated with the onset, and of these two were of a focal and three were of a generalized nature.

Angiograms were performed on six: all were normal. Blood pressure was high in one case. Eight had abnormal EEGs. Focal abnormalities on the infarcted hemisphere were seen in five cases; focal abnormality on the normal side was seen in one case. Diffuse abnormalities on the ipsilateral and contralateral sides of the infarcted area were seen in six and three cases respectively.

Subarachnoid Haemorrhage

This was the presenting feature in eight out of 127 cases; no demonstrable pathology was found in five of these.

Intracerebral Aneurysms. Only one intracerebral aneurysm was visualized on angiography; three others may have been aneurysms which leaked but were not demonstrated angiographically. All four presented as subarachnoid haemorrhage and were in the fourth decade. Three were males and one was female. The aneurysm demonstrated by angiography was a large one involving the left middle cerebral artery. Another had an associated cirsoid aneurysm of the scalp.

Hypertensive Intracerebral Haemorrhage. This condition was diagnosed in two cases. Both were known hypertensives on irregular treatment, both were males in the fourth decade, and both pesented as subarachnoid haemorrhage with evidence of increasing intracranial tension. One died a few hours after admission.

Arteriovenous Malformations

Four patients had arteriovenous malformations. All were males; the ages were 17, 19, 32 and 32 years respectively. The 17-year-old had an arteriovenous malformation of the sylvian area with an associated cirsoid aneurysm of the scalp. The 19-year-old presented as a subarachnoid haemorrhage with focal fits involving the right side. Angiogram showed a small malformation in the ganglionic area. One of the 32-year-old men presented with an acute attack of left-sided hemiparesis. A right brachial angiogram revealed a malformation in the neck involving the subclavian artery with atheromatous changes in the right common carotid artery which was probably the site of embolization. The other 32-year-old man presented as an infantile hemiplegic with a history of 22 years of hemiplegia of the left side following a bout of unconsciousness which lasted for 1 week. Angiogram revealed a fairly large arteriovenous malformation of the right hemisphere.

Hypertensive Encephalopathy

There were three cases diagnosed as hypertensive encephalopathy; all were in the fourth decade, two were males and one female.

Aortic Arch Syndrome

This syndrome was seen in four cases; three were females and one male. The youngest female was 14 years, the other two were in the fourth decade. The one male, in the fourth decade, had all the major vessels supplying the brain occluded except for one vertebral artery.

Survival

From a total of 127 cases included in this study 17 died while in hospital, giving a mortality rate of 13·4 per cent. Some of these died within a few hours after admission. The condition of those discharged was as follows: recovered 11 (8·6 per cent); improved 78 (61·4 per cent); unchanged 19 (15 per cent); worse 2 (1·6 per cent).

Case survival rate showed that there were 11 deaths in the first 6 months, two in the next 6 months, and a total of 17 deaths in 3 years, only six of which occurred after the first 6 months of discharge.

According to Robinson *et al.* (1959) the initial thrombotic episode was fatal in 21 per cent; 15 per cent died in 1 year and 50 per cent died in 4·1 years. Lindgren (1958) found that 34 per cent died in 2 years. A 28 per cent mortality within 3 years has been previously reported in patients not selected according to age who had survived one episode of cerebral thrombosis (Marshall and Shaw, 1969). Berlin, Tumarkin, and Martin (1955) reported only one death in 13 patients under the age of 40 years. We find that the case fatality rate of the under 40-year group differs from the figures of stroke survivals (of all age-groups) given by Western authors.

SUMMARY

An epidemiological study of the prevalence of hemiplegia in South India reveals a rate of 68·5 in males and 44·8 in females per 100 000 population.

Attention is drawn to a 32 per cent incidence of stroke in the under 40-year age-group. It is suggested that atherosclerosis is probably not an important aetiological factor in non-embolic ischaemic lesions. The small intracranial vessels were more involved. Haemorrhagic and possible haemorrhage-producing lesions constituted only 8·6 per cent of all the cases. It is conjectured that arteritis secondary to common tropical diseases may play a role in the causation of stroke in the young adult.

References

BAKER, A. B., KINNARD, J., and IANNONE, A. (1961) Cerebrovascular disease, VIII. Role of nutritional factors, *Neurology (Minneap.)*, 11, 380.

BASU, A. K. (1961) Occlusive disease of the aorta and its main branches, *Brit. J. Surg.*, 49, 148.

BERLIN, L., TUMARKIN, B., and MARTIN, H. L. (1955) Cerebral thrombosis in young adults, *New Engl. J. Med.*, 252, 162.

BHARUCHA, E. P., and UMERJI, R. S. (1962) Cerebrovascular disease in India, *Neurology (India)*, **10**, 137.

CARTER, A. B. (1963) Strokes: natural history and prognosis. *Proc. roy. Soc. Med.*, 56, 483.

DALAL, P. M. (1965) Incidence of cerebral vascular lesions at the Nair Hospital, Bombay, *Neurology (India)*, **13**, 37.

DALAL, P. M., SHAH, P. M., AIYAR, R. R., and KIKANI, B. J. (1968) Cerebrovascular diseases in West Central India. A report on angiographic findings from a prospective study, *Brit. med. J.*, **3**, 769.

EISENBERG, H., MORRISON, J. T., SULLIVAN, P., and FOOTE, F. M. (1964) Cerebrovascular accidents. Incidence and survival rates in a defined population, Middlesex County, Connecticut, *J. Amer. med. Ass.*, **189**, 883.

FISHER, C. M. (1961) Anticoagulant therapy in cerebral thrombosis and cerebral embolism. A national cooperative study, interim report, *Neurology (Minneap.)*, 11, 119.

FISHER, M. (1951) Occlusion of the internal carotid artery, *Arch. Neurol. Psychiat. (Chic.)*, 65, 346.

FORD, F. R. (1960) *Diseases of the Nervous System in Infancy, Childhood and Adolesence*, 4th ed., Springfield, Ill., pp. 882–6.

GROCH, S. N., MCDEVITT, E., and WRIGHT, I. S. (1961) A long-term study of cerebral vascular disease, *Ann. intern. Med.*, 55, 358.

HAERER, A. F., SMITH, R. R., and SPENCER, W. A. (1969) Cerebrovascular disease of young adults in Mississippi, paper presented at the 9th International Congress of Neurology, *Excerpta med. (Amst.), Int. Cong. Ser.*, **193**, 225.

HIRSCH, M. S., AIKAT, B. K., and BASU, A. K. (1964) Takayasu's arteritis. Report of five cases with immunologic studies, *Bull. Johns Hopk. Hosp.*, **115**, 29.

KANNEL, W. B. (1966) An epidemiologic study of cerebrovascular disease, in *Transactions of the Fifth Princeton Conference*, eds. Siekert, R. G., and Whisuant, J. P., New York, pp. 53–66.

KANNEL, W. B., DAWBER, T. R., COHEN, M. E., and MCNAMARA, P. M. (1965) Vascular disease of the brain—epidemiologic aspects. The Framingham Study, *Amer. J. publ. Hlth*, 55, 1355.

KATSUKI, S., and OMAE, T. (1967) Stroke prone profiles in the Japanese, in *Thule International Symposia: Stroke*, eds. Erych, A., and Larsson, T., Stockholm, p. 215.

KHAN, N., and RAO, A. V. N. (1951) Cerebral vascular accidents, *Indian J. med. Sci.*, 5, 632.

KRISHNA, A. G., and TEJA, B. S. (1965) A clinical analysis of 189 cases of cerebrovascular disease, *Neurology (India)*, 13, 126.

KURLAND, L. T., CHOI, N. W., and SAYRE, G. P. (1967) Current status of the epidemiology of cerebrovascular diseases, in *Stroke Rehabilitation. Basic Concepts and Research Trends*, eds. Fields, W. S., and Spencer, W. A., pp.3–22, St. Louis, Mo.

LINDGREN, S. O. (1958) Course and prognosis in spontaneous occlusion of cerebral arteries, *Acta psychiat. scand.*, 33, 343.

MARSHALL, J., and SHAW, D. A. (1959) The natural history of cerebrovascular disease, *Brit. med. J.*, 1, 1614.

MISRA, S. S., MISRA, R. N., AGARWAL, P. S., and SIRCAR, A. R. (1967) Cerebrovascular accidents. A review of 454 consecutive cases, *J. Indian. med. Ass.*, 48, 525.

NAIK, B. K., SATYANARAYANA RAO, P., and RAMVILAS SABOO (1966) Incidence of ischaemic heart disease and cerebrovascular disease in Hyderabad, *Indian Heart J.*, 18, 37.

OSUNTOKUN, B. O., ODEKU, E. L., DADA, T. O., and ADELOYE, R. B. A. (1969) Cerebrovascular accidents in Nigerians. A clinical study, paper presented at the Ninth International Congress of Neurology, *Excerpta med., Int. Cong. Ser.*, 193, 262.

PADMAVATI, S. (1958) A five-year survey of heart disease in Delhi (1951–1955), *Indian Heart J.*, 10, 33.

RAMAMURTHI, B. (1965) Are subarachnoid haemorrhages uncommon in India? *Neurology (India)*, 13, 42.

RESCH, J. A., and BAKER, A. B. (1964) Etiologic mechanisms in cerebral atherosclerosis. Preliminary study of 3839 cases, *Arch. Neurol. (Chic.)*, 10, 617.

RESCH, J. A., OKABE, N., LOEWENSON, R. B., KIMOTO, K., KATSUKI, S., and BAKER, A. B. (1969) Pattern of vessel involvement in cerebral atherosclerosis. A comparative study between a Japanese and Minnesota population, *J. Atheroscler. Res.*, 9, 239.

RESCH, J. A., WILLIAMS, A. O., LOEWENSON, R. B., and WAGNER, J. (1969) Cerebral atherosclerosis. A comparative autopsy between Nigerian Negroes and American Negroes and Caucasians, paper presented at the Ninth International Congress of Neurology, *Excerpta med. (Amst.), Int. Cong. Ser.*, 193, 271.

ROBINSON, R. W., COHEN, W. D., HIGANO, N., MEYER, R., LUKOWSKY, G. H., MCLAUGHLIN, R. B., and MACGILPIN, H. H. (1959) Lifetable analysis of survival after cerebral thrombosis: ten-year experience, *J. Amer. med. Ass.*, 169, 1149.

SJOSTROM, A. (1967) Hospitalized cases of stroke in a Swedish hospital region, in *Thule International Symposia: Stroke*, eds. Engel, A., and Larsson, T., Stockholm, pp. 41–50.

WELLS, C. E., and TIMBERGER, R. J. (1961) Cerebral thrombosis in patients under fifty years of age, *Arch. Neurol. (Chic.)*, 4, 268.

7 The Aortic Arch Syndrome

AN IDIOPATHIC FORM OF NON-INFLAMMATORY OCCLUSIVE VASCULAR DISEASE

P. M. DALAL

This intriguing clinical syndrome is characterized by diminution or absence of the arterial pulsations in the vessels of the arms and the neck, the seat of the disease, irrespective of its aetiology, being located near the origins of the great vessels arising from the aortic arch.

In the recent literature reports on this malady have appeared under various descriptive terms such as 'reversed coarctation' (Giffin, Dry, and Horton, 1939), 'syndrome of obliteration of supra-aortic trunks' (Martorell and Fabre, 1944, 1954; Frövig and Löken, 1951), 'pulseless disease' (Shimizu and Sano, 1951), 'Takayasu's disease' (Caccamise and Whitman, 1952), and 'young female arteritis' (Ross and McKusick, 1953), but excellent clinical descriptions have also appeared in the past (Gull, 1855; Savory, 1856; Broadbent, 1875). It is noteworthy that in Takayasu's original report (1908) on peculiar changes in the central vessels of the retina, he did not stress the diminished or absent vascular pulsations in his patient. Recently, simultaneous involvement of the abdominal aorta and and its branches has also been described (Danaraj and Wong, 1959; Isaacson, 1961; Inada *et al.*, 1962; Schrire and Asherson, 1964).

From a review of the reported cases in the world literature, Ross and McKusick (1953) observed that of many aetiological factors (congenital anomalies, trauma with or without aneurysm, chronic dissecting aneurysm, mediastinal tumours, thrombophilia, etc.) syphilitic aortitis, rather than atheromatosis, appeared to be one of the common causes of this syndrome, and that an arteritis of undetermined origin was responsible for a good number of female cases. Likewise, it has been a prevalent impression that nearly all the cases of aortic arch syndrome reported from India are a form of arteritis of rheumatic, syphilitic or undetermined origin (Misra, Prakash, and Agrawal, 1959; Pahwa, Pandey, and Gupta, 1959; Basu, 1961; Divekar, Deodhare, and Chitale, 1961; Sen *et al.*, 1962; Hirsch, Aikat, and Basu, 1964; Sood, Sachdeva, and Verma, 1970).

It has now been appreciated that the primary lesion in such cases, and particularly in men, may not always be an arteritis (Sen Gupta, and Ghosh, 1957; Ramchandra Rao, Reddy, and Reddy, 1969) and in this chapter an attempt has been made to review the clinical features, laboratory data, angiographic findings, and pathological observations on cases of aortic arch syndrome resulting only from occlusive vascular disease, and where there was no evidence of arteritis.

ILLUSTRATIVE CASE-HISTORY

Case 1. An elderly (?80-year-old) Christian male, on the morning of the day of ictus, was found in an obtunded state and was unable to communicate or move the right-sided limbs. In the evening of the day before the stroke, and after having accidently slipped over a banana skin, he had complained of 'giddiness' and 'dark vision'; subsequent to this fall, however, he ate, spoke and moved the limbs without any noticeable defect. Early in the morning of the day of the stroke, he had also received a milk delivery after which he retired to bed as usual but did not wake up at the expected time. Except for a history of intermittent productive cough without haemoptysis or fever, the family described him as 'very active for his age' and no one was aware of any significant major illness.

Physical examination showed an averagely built man (5 feet 5 inches, 110 pounds) with a temperature of 98.6°F, respirations 16 per minute, and a slow rising pulse of 86 per minute with frequent extrasystoles. Pulsations of the left carotid, left superficial temporal, left subclavian and left radial arteries were feeble, whereas a grade 2/6 systolic bruit was heard over the easily palpable right carotid and right subclavian arteries. The right radial, both femorals and the posterior tibial pulsations were well felt. The cuff pressure readings were 130/60 mm Hg in the right upper limb, 100/60 mm Hg in left upper limb, and 180/60 in the lower limbs. Except for a loud and ringing aortic valve closure sound associated with a grade 2/6 systolic murmur, the remainder of the chest and abdominal examination was unremarkable; no trophic changes were seen in the eyes, face or the limbs.

On neurological examination, 6 hours after the stroke, he was drowsy and unable to communicate even though he did follow some simple commands. The optic fundi were normal. Right homonymous hemianopia was present. There was a conjugate deviation of the gaze to the left, but the reflex eye movements and the pupillary responses were normal. A diminished right corneal reflex was accompanied by a moderate supranuclear type weakness of the right face. There was no paralysis of jaw, palate or tongue. The hypotonic right limbs were motionless even to pinch stimuli, whereas the normotonic left limbs moved spontaneously and in response to pain. Deep tendon reflexes on the right side were exaggerated, and the plantar responses were extensor bilaterally. The rest of the examination was non-contributory.

Except for mild anaemia, routine blood counts and urinalysis were normal. Serum levels for urea nitrogen, sugar and cholesterol were 22.5, 120 and 260 mg per cent respectively. Examination of the cerebrospinal fluid and serological tests for syphilis revealed no abnormality. Electrocardiogram revealed a pattern suggestive of right bundle branch block.

A right carotid angiogram revealed normal outline of the carotid, right middle cerebral, and both anterior cerebral arteries. A retrograde right carotid injection showed normal outline of the right common carotid, right subclavian, and right vertebral arteries, and there was also a good retrograde filling of the entire left vertebral-subclavian circulation ('subclavian steal'). A retrograde thoracic aortogram revealed a normal outline of the innominate and right common carotid arteries, whereas the left carotid and the left subclavian arteries showed complete non-filling near their origin; the origin of the right subclavian artery showed moderate stenosis with a post-stenotic dilatation.

Over the next week there was no significant improvement in the neurological deficit and on the seventh day after the stroke he died from pulmonary complications.

At necropsy, the lungs showed evidence of bronchopneumonia and pulmonary oedema. The heart was normal in size and weighed 290 gm; there was no evidence of endocardial, valvular, or myocardial disease. The left renal artery was thin and vestigial and the renal parenchyma of the atrophic left kidney was mostly replaced by fibrous tissue. The study of other organs was unremarkable from an aetiological or neurovascular point of view.

The ascending aorta was somewhat dilated and the aortic valve leaflets were soft, pliable and revealed no evidence of valvular disease. The intimal surface of the ascending aorta revealed mild tree-bark appearance and contained many pearly-white plaques. The mouth of the right coronary artery was totally occluded by a firm-feeling, pearly-white, fibrous tissue but no evidence of myocardial infarction was seen in its territory. Similar lesions were also seen in the arch of the aorta where firm, pearly-white material had totally occluded the mouths of the left common carotid and left subclavian arteries [Plate 16a]. Pearly-white material had also narrowed the origin of the right subclavian artery. However, the entire descending thoracic and abdominal aorta and all other major extra and intracranial cerebral vessels were remarkably free from atheroma or the pearly-white material. The stem of the left middle cerebral artery as far as its bifurcation, although free from atherosclerosis, was uniformly distended by a reddish-brown ante-mortem blood clot. A similar clot was also seen on the distal side of the fibrous block near the origin of the left common carotid artery. An ischaemic cerebral infarction was present in the central territory of the occluded left middle cerebral artery; the remainder of the serial cerebral cuts were unremarkable.

Microscopic examination of the serial sections of the entire aortic arch showed subintimal proliferation of connective tissue, gradually leading to total occlusion of the ostium of the left subclavian artery. Similar changes were present in the stem of the left common carotid artery, where a fresh as well as an old organized and recanalized thrombus was also found attached to the sclerosed intimal surface [Plate 16b]. Electron-microscopic examination of the thickened intima showed a preponderance of young as well as mature connective tissue (collagen fibres) arranged in a random, non-lamellar, fashion [Plate 16c and d]. Changes suggestive of atheroma were not encountered; but fat-filled macrophages were often seen near the internal elastic lamina. The internal elastic lamina itself was virtually broken up and disintegrated at many places. There was, however, no evidence of coagulation necrosis or granuloma formation. The media, too, showed fragmentation of its elastic fibres, but focal or diffuse productive inflammation with lymphocytes or plasma cells, fibrous scars, and features suggestive of cystic media necrosis or meso-aortitis were absent. In places the adventitial coat appeared somewhat thickened and tiny homogeneous foci made of cells resembling small lymphocytes were occasionally seen around the vasa vasorum; frank evidence of inflammatory change was, however, not found, and fibrous thickening of the intima and media of the vasa vasorum leading to luminal narrowing was also not seen. Furthermore, microscopic lesions suggestive of active, healing, or healed arteritis were not found in the cerebral, pulmonary, renal, and other vessels.

Comments

The patient's recent cerebral infarction resulting from occlusion of the stem of the left middle cerebral artery explains the neurovascular syndrome. It is noteworthy that although the origin of the left common carotid artery was totally occluded by fibrous tissue suggestive of an old process, nevertheless a recent ante-mortem blood clot was found attached to its cranial end. The ante-mortem blood clot in the stem of the left middle cerebral artery could have been a 'washed-out' embolus from the carotid site. Prior to the occurrence of the stroke, the circulation in the occluded carotid territory was presumably maintained through collaterals from across the circle of Willis, but abrupt embolic blockage of the left middle cerebral stem and its penetrating branches possibly resulted in a complete shut-down of the blood flow to this region, resulting in cerebral infarction of its central territory; properly functioning leptomeningeal collaterals probably prevented infarction of its superficial cortical territory.

Connective tissue proliferation had totally occluded the mouths of two arch vessels, and here the degree of atheromatous changes was none to minimal. The histological appearance of subintimal proliferation of connective tissue was also identical with that seen in other cases where the vessels were remarkably free from atherosclerosis. In the segments of the blood vessels showing early stenosis, sudanophilic material was no doubt seen in the deeper zones of the subintimal connective tissue, but histological changes suggestive of atheromatosis were not found. Thus, the morphogenesis of these fibrous lesions, and their exact relationship to early lesions of atheroma, need to be carefully evaluated.

The absence of histological features suggestive of arteritis (active, healing, or healed), fibromuscular hyperplasia, or atheroma, and the lean build of our patient, who had normal levels for serum cholesterol and lipids, are all noteworthy observations.

INCIDENCE

In view of the diverse clinical manifestations, patients with minor symptoms are probably not seen and hence the exact prevalence rate for this disease is so far not known. Reports of the overall incidence for aortic arch syndrome have also varied from one author to another.

For example, during an 11-year random survey for

obliterative vascular disease of the aorta and its peripheral branches at a surgical clinic of a large Indian teaching hospital, in a total of 77 cases Sen *et al.* (1965) recorded only three cases of aortic arch syndrome. On the other hand, Ramchandra Rao, Reddy, and Reddy (1969), working in a medical unit, saw 14 cases in a span of 6 years. Furthermore, during a 7-month prospective study of all the consecutive cases of acute stroke coming to a large teaching hospital, Dalal *et al.* (1968) recorded an incidence of about 4 per cent for aortic arch syndrome, and in the same series about 30 per cent had an occlusive lesion in either the internal carotid or in the vertebral artery. In this series, strokes accounted for 1 per cent of all the hospital admissions and 4 per cent of all the medical admissions.

In Dalal's series (1968) the syndrome was more frequently met with in men, and the disease commonly manifested between 35 to 55 years of age; the youngest patient being 16 and the oldest 80 years of age. There was no significant difference in its incidence in Hindus, Muslims, and Christians.

CLINICAL SYNDROMES

Diminished or absent arterial pulsations in the vessels of the neck, head and arms are characteristic features of this syndrome, and the clinical manifestations are mainly attributable to a decrease in the blood flow to the brachiocephalic circulation. The symptoms and signs are highly variable. Depending upon the degree of the development of the extracranial collateral anastomoses in a particular case, and despite the occlusion of many vessels of the aortic arch, the presenting symptoms may vary from minor to catastrophic; cardiovascular and cerebrovascular syndromes mainly dominate the clinical picture.

Case 2. A 60-year-old Muslim male was seen by aortography to have complete occlusion of the origin of the left subclavian and both common carotid arteries. There was paucity of extracranial collateral anastomoses, and despite this the entire cerebral circulation was effectively maintained through the only patent right vertebral artery via a symmetrical circle of Willis. Although the vertebral artery blood flow was partly obstructed by extensive cervical osteoarthritis, the patient had no cerebral complaints; on direct questioning he denied transitory symptoms such as giddiness, fainting, diminished visual acuity, sensory paraesthesia or focal motor weakness in any limb. A neurological examination was essentially negative. Apart from feeble to impalpable carotid, subclavian and radial artery pulsations on both sides, a general examination revealed no trophic changes in the tissues of the face, eyes, or limbs. The patient suffered from severe exertional dyspnoea and showed signs of congestive cardiac failure with cardiomegaly resulting from an ischaemic heart disease. The cardiac failure proved increasingly resistant to treatment, and 2 years later he died from acute left ventricular failure. Necropsy revealed cardiac dilatation and hypertrophy, old myocardial infarction resulting from occlusion of the circumflex branch of the left coronary artery, pulmonary oedema and chronic passive congestion of various organs, chronic pyelonephritis and nephrosclerosis, and occlusion of various arch vessels. The brain revealed no significant macroscopic or microscopic lesions. The circle of Willis was patent, symmetrical and free from atherosclerosis.

When the cerebral circulation, through various collateral anastomoses, proves to be inadequate, cerebrovascular symptoms manifest either in the form of focal transient symptoms in the carotid or vertebral artery territory, or may present as a persistent focal neurological deficit.

Case 3. An averagely nourished 52-year-old Hindu male was seen by aortography to have complete occlusion of the origins of the innominate and the left subclavian arteries. In addition, the only patent artery, the left common carotid, showed severe stenosis of its ostium. The cerebral circulation was, however, maintained through an extensive network of various cervical collateral anastomoses. Over the subsequent 7 years he suffered from over 100 episodes of transient focal cerebral ischaemia consisting of episodic vertigo with 'helpless feeling' in all the limbs, transient mono-ocular blindness in the right or the left eye, episodic dysarthria with 'twisting' of the face, and transitory but focal weakness of the left-sided limbs (cortical type). Apart from feeble to impalpable pulsations in both arms and in the right side of the neck, associated with an easily palpable vascular thrill over the left carotid pulse, a general and systemic examination and interictal neurological examinations were essentially negative. There were no trophic changes, and the optic fundi revealed no abnormality. Seven years later, he developed intense obstructive jaundice and marked cachexia from an undifferentiated malignancy of the lung with multiple metastases in the liver. Examination of the brain revealed multiple tiny foci of microinfarcts, recent as well as old, resulting from platelet-fibrin embolic plugs. The circle of Willis was free from atherosclerosis, but atheromatous lesions were seen in the region of the occluded arch vessels.

Despite the extension or progression of an occlusive lesion, presumed to be responsible for the cerebral syndrome, some recovery from focal neurological deficit is a common occurrence.

Case 4. A 35-year-old handloom operator, while at work, noticed that his right hand was numb and somewhat clumsy. These symptoms gradually progressed and by the evening of that day there was moderately severe paralysis of the right upper extremity; he experienced no difficulty with speech or gait. By the morning of the next day, however, the face was twisted, the speech was mushy, and the right upper limb was 'lifeless'. On examination, apart from absent to feeble left carotid and radial pulse, he had global aphasia with right homonymous hemianopia accompanied by a severe sensory motor paralysis of the right upper limb; early weakness was also noticed in the right lower limb. Among several other investigations, an arch aortogram showed total occlusion of the origin of the left subclavian artery. The ostium of the left common carotid artery showed a severe degree of tapering stenosis. Other arch vessels were patent. Distal to the severely stenosed segment of the left common carotid artery, the carotid artery was patent and all branches of the middle cerebral artery were well visualized. The remaining intracranial vessels were patent and showed normal calibre. Over the subsequent 6 weeks he made almost complete recovery in speech and in the functions of the right upper limb. Two year later, another arch aortogram showed total occlusion of the left common carotid artery at its origin and a dacron bypass graft was successfully implanted between the patent left internal carotid artery and the aortic arch. A thrombo-endarteriectomy with arterial biopsy at the site of previous occlusion revealed an old organized and recanalized thrombus, and the entire circumference of arterial wall at that site revealed no evidence of active or healed arteritis or atheroma.

When the cerebral circulation is well maintained through various collateral anastomotic channels, a fresh thrombotic episode in a vessel irrigating a large territory of the brain may precipitate a major catastrophic event.

Case 5. A Muslim male aged 35 years was brought to the hospital in an unconscious state. Several months prior to the present stroke, he had suffered a left-sided hemiplegia from which he had made a good recovery. On examination, he was in semicoma with the head and the eyes conjugately deviated to the left. The right carotid and the left subclavian pulses were not felt. Thin non-pulsating 'white' vessels were seen over an atrophic right optic disc. The left pupil was small and reacted well to light but the semi-dilated right pupil reacted only consensually. When the head was tilted vertical eye movements were restricted. In addition to a supranuclear type weakness of the right face, the right limbs were flaccid, areflexic and motionless even to painful stimuli. The hypertonic left limbs showed brisk tendon reflexes and moved both spontaneously and in response to pain. Angiography revealed complete occlusion of the mouth of the left subclavian artery, but a 'subclavian-vertebral steal' phenomenon was present. The right internal carotid artery was totally occluded near its origin; retrograde collateral circulation in the right middle cerebral territory was, however, maintained through well-developed cervical extracranial anastomoses and intracranial leptomeningeal anastomoses. He died from respiratory complications. At necropsy there was no evidence of atherosclerosis anywhere. Pearly-white fibrous tissue had gradually occluded the lumen of the left subclavian artery. Likewise, the right internal carotid lumen was occluded by similar material, and distal to this the vessels appeared thin and 'white' and contained 'stasis thrombi'. A shrivelled area of old cystic infarction was seen in the region of the right external capsule, and this was thought to be responsible for the previous stroke. Pearly-white fibrous tissue had severely narrowed the terminal intracranial segment of the left internal carotid artery, and a fresh thrombus at this site had occluded the rest of the lumen. A massive ischaemic infarction with brain swelling was seen in the entire territory of the left middle cerebral and both the anterior cerebral arteries. Microscopic examination of the vessels failed to reveal evidence of arteritis or atheroma anywhere, and the material occluding the lumen was predominantly subintimal and fibrous in nature.

In general, and despite the severity of circulatory inadequacy, trophic changes such as loss of teeth or hair, ulceration of the tip of the nose or lips, perforation of the nasal septum or the palate, atrophy of the iris or the ciliary muscles, cataracts or facial atrophy, were not present in our cases. Baldness and cataract, when present, appeared to be related more to the advancing age of our patients.

Constitutional symptoms and other findings such as fever, loss of weight, joint pains and arthropathy, cutaneous lesions, leucocytosis, high sedimentation rate, increase of alpha$_2$ and gamma globulins, etc., were not commonly seen, and coincidental tuberculous or syphilitic infection was relatively rare.

Tachycardia, extrasystoles, syncopal episodes, exertional dyspnoea, signs of cardiac failure and cardiomegaly were usually secondary to the underlying ischaemic heart disease. The occurrence of endocardial valvular and pericardial lesions, discovered on investigation or at necropsy, was indeed rare. On the other hand, harsh systolic murmurs over stenosed segments of a vessel, and soft flow murmurs over various anastomotic channels were frequently heard.

Symptoms suggestive of intermittent claudication (easy fatigability, coldness, paraesthesia, cramp-like pains, etc.) were only present when the collateral circulation reaching a limb was found to be inadequate. On the other hand, feeble or absent pedal pulsations suggestive of peripheral vascular disease was a frequent finding in elderly subjects.

LABORATORY DATA

Hypochromic microcytic anaemia or dimorphic anaemia was a common finding and appeared to be related more to the poor nutritional status of our patients. Sickle cells, target cells and other similar abnormalities or haemoglobinopathies were not found. The corrected erythrocytic sedimentation rate, apart from during an intercurrent infection, was observed to be in the normal range. Unless a renal pathology was present, the routine urinalysis revealed no abnormality. Despite several preparations made at random intervals over many years, LE cells were not detected. By and large, the serological tests for syphilis in the blood and the spinal fluid were negative. In the necropsy material, too, *Treponema pallidum* could not be demonstrated in various tissues examined by the Levaditi's method, and lesions suggestive of syphilitic meso-aortitis were also absent. The results of tuberculin tests revealed no significant abnormality when compared with the general population. Except for coincidental occurrence of pulmonary tuberculosis in one case, evidence of tuberculous infection elsewhere in the body, on investigation or at necropsy, was not present in the overall material. Blood levels for urea, sugar, various lipids, and cholesterol were in the normal range. Likewise, serial biochemical and electrophoretic estimations of various fractions of serum proteins revealed no significant abnormality; any unusual rise of $alpha_2$ or gamma globulins was not detected. Most of the liver functions were within the normal range, and an abnormality was only noticed when a coincidental liver disease (e.g. congestive hepatomegaly, carcinoma, etc.) was present.

During an acute ictus, however, the blood levels of fibrinogen were high and the euglobulin clot-lysis time was deranged, but other coagulation factors or parameters showed no significant change.

Electrocardiographic abnormalities, such as ventricular premature beats, bundle-branch block, ventricular hypertrophy, and changes suggestive of myocardial ischaemia or infarction, were frequently seen.

RADIOLOGICAL FINDINGS

Plain X-ray of the chest usually revealed clear lung fields, but in one case an apical scar suggestive of an old tuberculous infection was seen. In patients with signs of cardiac failure, mostly resulting from an ischaemic heart disease, the cardiac silhouette was uniformly enlarged. In some cases the thoracic aorta appeared somewhat elongated or dilated and the lumen often showed irregularities resulting from spotty calcification of its wall; extensive calcification, however, was not seen.

An arch aortogram usually delineated the extent as well as the severity of the vascular damage. Irregular contour of the aortic arch was commonly seen but aneurysm formation or findings suggestive of aortic leak were not present. Likewise, spotty calcification of the descending thoracic and abdominal aorta was not infrequently seen, but radiological features diagnostic of 'atypical coarctation' or 'stenosing aortitis' were not found.

On aortography, gradual constriction of the ostium of various arch vessels, with or without post-stenotic dilatation, leading to almost complete occlusion was a characteristic feature. The arterial segments so occluded, were however, only a few centimetres long, and the lumen of the vessels both proximal and distal to such a block often showed a smooth outline. From serial aortography over many years in several cases it was observed that the disease process resulting in gradual constriction of the vascular lumen evolved slowly, and this probably allowed sufficient time for the development of collateral anastomoses. On sequential films extensive networks of large and tortuous costocervical and thyrocervical collateral anastomotic channels linking the carotid and the vertebral circulation were readily identified. The cerebral circulation in an occluded vascular territory was also maintained by the intracranial leptomeningeal anastomoses. Absence of atheromatous changes in the extra- and intracranial vessels was a significant finding and this was confirmed at necropsy in many cases. It was therefore not surprising to see examples in which many arch vessels were occluded and yet the clinical picture was not alarming.

PATHOLOGY

The characteristic lesions were seen in the arch of the aorta and its major branches and were comprised mainly of irregular or diffuse thickening of the intimal surface by firm-feeling, pearly-white material. These subintimal nodules or plaques often protruded into the ostium of various arch vessels and gradually constricted their lumen, resulting in partial or total occlusion. Since the disease process was segmental or patchy in distribution, it was not uncommon to find areas completely free from this change, while, at the same time fibrous lesions were often found at distant sites such as the sinus region of the internal carotid artery, the intracranial carotid bifurcation, and the origin of the subclavian or vertebral arteries. Not infrequently, mural thrombi in various stages were seen attached to the sclerosed intimal surface, and in elderly subjects atheromatous changes, too, appeared grafted over such lesions. By and large, the descending thoracic and abdominal aorta and their major branches were free from the above changes.

The adventitial coat of the vessel was thickened in places, and foci of lymphocytes showing homogeneity of cell type were occasionally seen around the vasa vasorum; such homogeneous collections of small lymphocytes have consistently been found in the adventitial coat of atheromatous vessels (Schwartz and Mitchell, 1962). Intimal thickening and onion-skin-like cicatrization of the media of the vasa vasorum, or inflammatory changes suggestive of arteritis were not found.

The medial coat was somewhat thin. Patchy but generalized fragmentation of the elastic fibres of the media was a constant finding. However, coagulation necrosis, cystic media necrosis, aneurysm formation, or cicatrization was not found, and bands of inflammatory cells (polymorphs, lymphocytes, plasma cells, giant cells, etc.), or granuloma formation were nowhere seen in the serial sections of the whole of the aortic arch with its main branches.

The intimal layer appeared unusually thick. The zone between the endothelial cells and the internal elastic laminae was mainly composed of connective tissue. Electron-microscopic examination confirmed the preponderance of young as well as mature collagen fibres and these were arranged in a random, non-lamellar, manner. The subintimal proliferation of fibrous tissue had considerably narrowed the lumen of various arch vessels, and, in some cases, sudanophilic material (fat-filled macrophages) was present near the internal elastic laminae. In the overall material, focal fibrinoid necrosis, micro-abscesses, cholesterol clefts, or atheromatous lesions were not seen. In general, the internal elastic lamina was broken up and disintegrated at many places and it was not unusual to see an occasional giant cell nearby; it must, however, be emphasized that the mere presence of giant cells in the vicinity of broken elastic fibres by itself does not constitute evidence in favour of arteritis (Koszewski and Hubbard, 1957).

On the surface of the intimal nodules or plaques, and sometimes on the distal side of a complete occlusion, thrombi were found in various stages of organization. Morphologically, such thrombi, though attached to the sclerosed intima, appeared distinctly separate from the subintimal lesions. Transitional lesions, where an organizing thrombus gradually merged into the subintimal fibrous nodule, were not encountered. The collagen fibres of the subintimal lesion, too, were not oriented in a lamellar fashion to suggest resorption of thrombi.

Multiple microinfarcts or massive ischaemic cerebral infarction, recent as well as old, were often seen in the territory of major vessels showing an occlusive lesion. Except for platelet fibrin embolic plugs or stasis thrombi, the leptomeningeal and smaller cerebral vessels were free from an atheromatous or other intimal change. The coronary vessels, on the other hand, often contained typical intimal and subintimal lesions, and myocardial infarction in the territory of such occluded vessels was not an uncommon finding. Any pathological changes in other organs (e.g. bronchopneumonia, tuberculosis, malignancy, pyelonephritis, etc.) was mainly due to a co-existing disease.

AETIOLOGICAL CONSIDERATIONS

The real nature of the disease process and its pathogenetic aspects remain an enigma, and any views as to its aetiology will be highly speculative.

On the whole, the clinical features, laboratory findings, and histopathological lesions in our material, when compared with other reports (Hirsch, Aikat, and Basu, 1964; Heggtveit, 1964; Ask-Upmark and Fajers, 1956; Frövig and Löken, 1951; Nasu, 1963; Ross and McKusick, 1953), were not suggestive of rheumatic, syphilitic, tuberculous, allergic, Buerger's or Takayasu's type of arteritis or a collagen disease.

From serial angiographic observations in our cases it appeared that the occlusive lesion gradually grew in length and breadth, and histological examination of such partial and uncomplicated lesions showed subintimal fibrous tissue in relation to the damaged elastic fibres. It was difficult to determine if the intimal thickening was primary or secondary to the fragmented elastica. It is, however, noteworthy that Ssolowjew (1932) was able to produce intimal thickening resulting from connective tissue proliferation at the site of experimentally induced tears of elastica, and if the experimental rabbits which he used were fed a cholesterol-rich meal it was also possible to see fatty material in the subintimal lesion of such vessels.

The clinical picture, topographic location of lesions, fibrous plaques in the region of thin media containing damaged elastic fibres, the presence of sudanophilic material in some lesions, the homogeneous collections of small lymphocytes in the adventitial coat without any evidence of arteritis, and the age-groups of our patients, may raise the possibility of juvenile or premature atherosclerosis. The anatomical locations of the lesions may have been governed by factors such as strain hypertrophy, shearing force, intravascular pressure and turbulence or trauma, but these are mere speculations.

The role of any viral agent, endogenous or exogenous toxin, or other similar unidentifiable factor must also be kept in mind. Until this has been done, it would be best to classify this disease as of idiopathic or unknown origin.

COURSE AND PROGNOSIS

We have as yet very little information on the natural history of this disease, and as a result only general observations can be made.

In the neurologically asymptomatic group, in which the cerebral blood flow is probably maintained through various collateral anastomoses, the patient usually lives a relatively normal life unless co-existing illness such as a decompensated heart disease (e.g. Case 2) proves to be fatal.

In the group in which transient cerebral symptoms manifest frequently, the otherwise normal life of the subject is only interrupted by episodes of reversible focal neurological deficit. However, another coincidental disease such as cancer (e.g. Case 3) may prove fatal in outcome.

In the group in which a focal neurological deficit evolves slowly, the chances of recovery after a period of stabilization are usually good (e.g. Case 4). However, another stroke in the same or a different territory usually carries a grave prognosis. If the focal neurological deficit progresses at a faster rate, or if the patient is deeply comatose, the chances of survival from such massive cerebral infarction are poor (e.g. Case 5).

Belonging to an elderly age-group, presence of hypertension, associated heart disease or renal disease, uncontrolled diabetes mellitus, and pulmonary complications are of grave prognostic significance.

TREATMENT

There is no specific treatment. During the acute phase of the illness, general medical and nursing care are most important. The paralysed limb should be maintained in the best possible position to prevent overstretching, contractures and deformities. Frequent passive movements through the full range of motion at all joints is beneficial. Meticulous nursing care of the eyes, mouth, skin, bladder and bowels to prevent xerosis, parotitis, bed sores, and urinary tract infection will prove most rewarding. Every effort should be made to keep the airway patent, and also to prevent pulmonary aspiration of food or vomitus. In the presence of anoxia, oxygen therapy is advisable. Prompt treatment of pulmonary infection with appropriate antibiotics is mandatory.

Correction of anaemia, polycythaemia, fluid and electrolyte balance, and metabolic acidosis are advisable. Incipient cardiac failure or pulmonary oedema should be treated with appropriate decongestive measures, and the blood pressure should be maintained at a near normal level with the judicious use of vasopressor or antihypertensive agents.

Attempts to improve cerebral circulation (e.g. vasodilator therapy), to prevent adhesion of platelets and other blood elements (e.g. infusion of low-molecular-weight dextran), to prevent further extension of thrombus or embolization (e.g. anticoagulant therapy), to decrease brain swelling (e.g. steroid or diuretic therapy), and to prevent convulsions (e.g. *Dilantin Rx*) merit consideration in each and every case.

When a patient shows signs of neurological recovery, with some volitional movements, active physiotherapeutic measures for early rehabilitation should be undertaken at once.

Reconstructive vascular surgery (thrombo-endarteriectomy with or without patch graft angioplasty, or major bypass procedures) to re-establish adequate circulation in an occluded vascular territory, and also to remove a potential source of embolization, may be undertaken during an interictal period in patients who suffer from recurrent focal symptoms, and in those who have recovered from a major deficit. Since the disease process is restricted to a limited segment of the vessel wall near the aortic arch, the success rate of bypass procedures is relatively high.

References

ASK-UPMARK, E., and FAJERS, C. M. (1956) Further observations on Takayasu's syndrome, *Acta med. scand.*, 155, 275.

BASU, A. K. (1961) Occlusive disease of the aorta and its main branches, *Brit. J. Surg.*, 49, 148.

BROADBENT, W. H. (1875) Absence of pulsations in both radial arteries, the vessels being full of blood, *Trans. clin. Soc. Lond.*, 8, 165.

CACCAMISE, W. C., and WHITMAN, J. F. (1952) Pulseless disease. A preliminary case report, *Amer. Heart J.*, 44, 629.

DALAL, P. M., SHAH, P. M., AIYAR, R. R., and KIKANI, B. J. (1968) Cerebrovascular diseases in West Central India. A report on angiographic findings from a prospective study, *Brit. med. J.*, 3, 769.

DANARAJ, T. J., and WONG, H. O. (1959) Primary arteritis of abdominal aorta in children causing bilateral stenosis of renal arteries and hypertension, *Circulation*, 20, 856.

DIVEKAR, M. V., DEODHARE, S. G., and CHITALE, G. K. (1961) Takayasu's or pulseless disease, *J. postgrad. Med.*, 7, 119.

FRÖVIG, A. G., and LÖKEN, A. C. (1951) The syndrome of obliteration of the arterial branches of the aortic arch, due to arteritis, *Acta psychiat. scand.*, 26, 313.

GIFFIN, H. M., DRY, T. J., and HORTON, B. T. (1939) Reversed coarctation and vasomotor gradient; report of a cardiovascular anomaly with symptoms of brain tumor, *Proc. Mayo Clin.*, 14, 561.

GULL, W. (1855) Thickening and dilatation of the arch of the aorta with occlusion of the innominate and left carotid: atrophic softening of the brain, *Guy's Hosp. Rep.*, 16, 12.

HEGGTVEIT, H. A. (1964) Syphilitic aortitis: a clinicopathologic autopsy study of 100 cases, *Circulation*, 29, 346.

HIRSCH, M. S., AIKAT, B. K., and BASU, A. K. (1964) Takayasu's arteritis. Report of five cases with immunologic studies, *Bull. Johns Hopk. Hosp.*, 115, 29.

INADA, K., SHIMIZU, H., KOBAYASHI, I., ISHIAI, S., and KAWAMOTO, S. (1962) Pulseless disease and atypical coarctation, *Arch. Surg.*, 84, 306.

ISAACSON, C. (1961) An idiopathic aortitis in young Africans, *J. Path. Bact.*, 81, 69.

KOSZEWSKI, B. J., and HUBBARD, T. F. (1957) Pulseless disease due to branchial arteritis, *Circulation*, 16, 406.

MARTORELL, F., and FABRE, T. J. (1944) El sindrome de obliteracion de los troncos supraaorticos, *Med. clin. (Barcelona)*, 2, 26.

MARTORELL, F., and FABRE, T. J. (1954) The syndrome of obliteration of the supra-aortic branches, *Angiology*, 5, 39.

MISRA, S. S., PRAKASH, S., and AGRAWAL, P. L. (1959) Pulseless disease (Takayasu's syndrome), *Amer. Heart J.*, 57, 177.

NASU, T. (1963) Pathology of pulseless disease, *Angiology*, 14, 225.

PAHWA, J. M., PANDEY, M. P. N., and GUPTA, D. P. (1959) Pulseless disease or Takayasu's disease, *Brit. med. J.*, 2, 1439.

RAMCHANDRA RAO, N., REDDY, C. R., and REDDY, M. R. (1969) Occlusive disease of the aorta and its main branches, *J. Indian med. Ass.* 53, 425.

ROSS, R. S., and MCKUSICK, V. A. (1953) Aortic arch syndromes; diminished or absent pulses in arteries arising from arch of aorta, *Arch. intern. Med.*, 92, 701.

SAVORY, W. S. (1856) Case of a young woman in whom the main arteries of both upper extremities and of the left side of the neck were throughout completely obliterated, *Med.-chir. Trans.*, 39, 205.

SCHRIRE, V., and ASHERSON, R. A. (1964) Arteritis of the aorta and its major branches, *Quart. J. Med.*, 33, 439.

SCHWARTZ, C. J., and MITCHELL, J. R. A. (1962) Cellular infiltration of the human arterial adventitia associated with atheromatous plaques, *Circulation*, 26, 73.

SEN, P. K., KINARE, S. G., KULKARNI, T. P., and PARULKAR, G. B. (1962) Stenosing aortitis of unknown aetiology, *Surgery*, 51, 317.

SEN, P. K., PARULKAR, G. B., KELKAR, M. D., and DESHMUKH, S. M. (1965) Experiences in vascular reconstructive surgery, *J. Indian med. Ass.*, 45, 660.

SEN GUPTA, S. N., and GHOSH, J. C. (1957) Case of reverse coarctation syndrome, *Brit. med. J.*, 1, 137.

SHIMIZU, K., and SANO, K. (1951) Pulseless disease, *J. Neuropath. exp. Neurol.*, 1, 37.

SOOD, S., SACHDEVA, S., and VERMA, S. N. (1970) Aortic arch syndrome, *J. Ass. Phycns India*, 18, 939.

SSOLOWJEW, A. (1932) Über experimentall Hervogerufene Elasticarisse der Arterien und deren Bedentung für die Lipoidablagerung, *Virchows Arch. path. Anat.*, 283, 213.

TAKAYASU, M. (1908) A case with peculiar changes in central vessels of the retina, *Acta Soc. Ophthal. Japan*, 12, 554.

8 Congenital Atlanto-Axial Dislocation and its Manifestations due to Spinal Cord Compression

N. H. WADIA

The single median and the two lateral joints between the atlas and the axis, which function together as a unit, maintain their stability by the interlocking of the anterior arch of the atlas with the odontoid process of the axis (dens), which in turn is kept firmly in position from behind by the tough, strap-like transverse ligament. The other ligaments, especially the alar, may play an additional role. The principal movement at this joint (for convenience the singular will be used throughout)—rotation of the neck—is facilitated, and dislocation, especially forward dislocation, is thus prevented, unless this arrangement is disturbed by congenital malformation or acquired disease. Acute or chronic compression of the upper cervical cord or medullospinal junction, from dislocation following acquired diseases of the atlas and axis, has been well known since Hilton's first description in 1866 (Pandya, 1970). On the other hand, dislocation and compressive myelopathy, caused by congenital maldevelopment of the articulating bones or ligaments, has not been sufficiently well recognized (Wadia, 1960, 1967). The present writer pointed out its unusually high frequency in India, and this was borne out by subsequent case-reports throughout the country (Bharucha and Dastur, 1964; Srinivasan, Balasubramaniam, and Ramamurthi, 1967; Singh, Dutta, and Gupta, 1969). A similar high incidence has been mentioned by neurologists from Ceylon and Thailand. As opposed to this, Greenberg (1968) was able to collect only 94 cases from the Western literature since Giacomini first described his patient in 1886.

The credit must go to List (1941) for describing the occurrence of 'neurological syndromes accompanying developmental anomalies of the occipital bone, atlas and axis'. He clearly differentiated the neurological syndrome of medullospinal compression, due to dislocation of the atlanto-axial joint accompanying occipitalization of the atlas, from other entities like basilar invagination, the Klippel-Feil anomaly, and Arnold-Chiari malformation. He mentioned valuable radiological and autopsy findings. McRae (1953), and McRae and Barnum (1953) later made important contributions, especially to the radiology of this problem. Spillane, Pallis, and Jones (1957), and Bharucha and Dastur (1964) mentioned the neurological manifestations of a few cases, mostly during the course of an analysis of symptoms caused by craniovertebral anomalies as a group.

The present writer has always felt that the clinical and radiological features of this condition are distinct from the rest of the craniovertebral anomalies; the prognosis and correct surgical treatment depend on this identification. An analysis of 52 cases personally examined and nine autopsies is used throughout this text.

SYMPTOMATOLOGY AND NATURAL HISTORY

There were three main groups of symptoms:

1. Cervical pain and stiffness.
2. Transitory attacks.
3. Progressive neurological disturbance.

These symptoms were seen singly or together in different chronological order.

Cervical Symptoms

In congenital dislocation the cervical symptoms [Table 8·1] rarely predominate as in the acquired ones. When there is pain and neck stiffness a history of a sudden jerk or twist of the neck, or manipulation is usually obtained. Limitation of neck movements, often unnoticed by the patient, was found in 50 per cent of our patients. It was remarkable how often flexion and extension remained free when there was limitation, often severe, of lateral rotation. Torticollis or a slight tilt of the neck was occasionally observed.

A short neck and low hair-line have been mentioned constantly in the literature on craniovertebral anomalies, and are frequently seen in a specific subgroup of dislocation to be mentioned later.

Neurological Manifestations

As will also be shown later, different varieties of atlanto-axial dislocations can be radiologically identified, and which have a different embryological basis. However, their neurological manifestations are common.

There were four main modes of presentation in our patients:

1. Those with attacks of transitory disturbance of the central nervous system only.	4
2. Those with a history of transitory attacks and persistent neurological signs with gradual, but partial, improvement after the last episode.	2
3. Those with a history of transitory attacks followed by a progressive neurological disorder.	15
4. Those with progressive neurological manifestations not preceded by any transitory attack.	31
	52

Table 8.1

Clinical Manifestations of Congenital Dislocation

Group	No. of Cases	Paralysis	Transitory Attacks[1]			Pain in Neck	Restricted Cervical Spine Movements		Short Neck/Low Hairline	Associated Congenital Anomalies[2]
			Paraesthesiae	Unconsciousness	Blindness		Mild	Severe		
I	29	4	1	5	—	9	8	10	19	29
II	15	6	6	7	2	2	4	2	5	7
III	8	3	2	—	—	2	—	2	—	3
Whole Series	*52*	*13*	*9*	*12*	*2*	*13*	*12*	*14*	*24*	*39*

[1]Total 21 cases.
[2]Other than those of the odontoid.

For the sake of clarity and convenience, the transitory attacks observed in Groups 1, 2, and 3 will be described first, and the progressive or residual neurological signs as seen in 2, 3, and 4 will be subsequently mentioned.

Transitory Attacks

Transitory attacks of paralysis of the upper cervical cord or the lowermost part of the medulla form a very characteristic part of the symptomatology of chronic atlanto-axial dislocation, whether congenital or acquired.

Elliot and Sachs (1912) were the first to mention 'a number of attacks of paresis' spread over 30 years in an autopsy-proven case of traumatic atlanto-axial dislocation. Subsequently, these attacks have been mentioned in congenital dislocation by many authors (McRae, 1953; McRae and Barnum, 1953; Illingworth, 1956; Bharucha and Dastur, 1964; Wadia, 1967).

Twenty-one out of 52 patients gave a history of such attacks [TABLE 8.1]. Each episode comprised paralysis of the limbs, paraesthesiae below the neck, unconsciousness and, more rarely, blurring of vision or blindness, singly or together. The paralysis usually affected all four limbs, but occasionally only one side or one limb was involved. The paraesthesiae consisted of intense tingling, and pins and needles; the loss of consciousness was sudden and unaccompanied by any convulsion or incontinence; and the visual symptoms of blurring or blindness were bilateral and symmetrical. These attacks were always precipitated by exaggerated flexion or extension, or even rotation of the neck. The best illustrations of these are given in the words of our patients: 'A light smack on the back of the head playfully given by a friend'; 'Vigorously towelling the back of the head and neck after a bath'; and 'A jump from a moderate height onto my feet'.

Most of the episodes lasted for a few minutes to about half an hour, although some patients continued to feel 'weak' for several weeks. The frequency varied from a single episode recalled only on direct inquiry to a large number over many years. The patients were symptom-free between the attacks but examination revealed a combination of exaggerated deep jerks, absent abdominal reflexes and extensor plantar responses. In some the Lhermitte sign could be elicited.

There were 15 patients, as mentioned in Group 3, in whom progressive neurological disorder followed the transitory attacks. The longest period between the first episode and such neurological disorder was 48 years, interspersed with repeated attacks. In others it was 14 and 16 years, but the majority came within months. The progressive myelopathy often commenced with the last episode.

Group 2 of 2 patients, fell between Groups 1 and 3. These patients came because their recovery from the latest episode was proceeding too slowly.

It must be stressed here that when a patient presents with symptoms suggesting a high cervical cord lesion, a specific direct question about such attacks must be asked, because if they are brief and occasional, then a voluntary account of them is unlikely to be made.

Neurological Symptoms and Signs

The neurological symptoms and signs of Groups 2, 3 and 4 are shown in TABLE 8.2. The predominant affection was of the pyramidal tracts in all limbs. The signs were clearly more marked on one side in many patients, and quite a few of them maintained that the other side was quite normal.

In many of the patients, the legs were more affected than the arms, but in some it was the other way round. Spasticity with clonus was at times a greater handicap than loss of power. The exaggeration of deep reflexes and extensor plantar responses were consistently seen, but the abdominal reflexes were more often preserved than absent. We found no specific order of involvement of the limbs, as mentioned by Symonds and Meadows

Table 8.2
Neurological Manifestations
(48 *Cases*)

Manifestation		*No. of Cases*
1. Motor disability and pyramidal signs:		47
one side more affected than the other	*21*	
2. Paraesthesiae:		13
(a) Spontaneous	*11*	
(b) On neck flexion only	*2*	
3. Posterior column deficit:		34
upper limbs more affected than lower limbs	*8*	
4. Localized wasting (upper limbs)		15
5. Cerebellar signs		10
6. Cutaneous sensory loss:		8
(a) Localized to one limb	*5*	
(b) Sensory level on the trunk	*3*	
7. Urinary symptoms		8
8. Nystagmus		4
9. Horner's syndrome		3

(1937), in spinal cord compression near the foramen magnum. Most patients, though still mobile, were functionally severely handicapped.

Urinary symptoms were uncommon even with severe paralysis. Dyspnoea from intercostal and accessory respiratory muscle weakness was seen only in advanced cases. Paraesthesiae, mostly of tingling, numbness, pins and needles, and 'sand in the palms', usually followed the paralysis affecting all four limbs in most patients, but occasionally remained confined to the upper limbs. Some patients experienced paraesthesiae in the limbs only on flexion of the neck. The paraesthesiae were considered trivial in comparison with the motor disability.

The posterior column signs were less evident than the pyramidal tract signs in all except one patient, who showed only the former. Vibration sense was symmetrically impaired or lost as far as the clavicles in most, although at times it was more evident on the side of greater paralysis. Occasionally, both legs and one of the more paralysed upper limbs showed this impairment only. The vibration and postural loss usually corresponded, but occasionally vibration alone was lost, especially in the lower limbs. As in other craniovertebral anomalies the postural loss in some instances was remarkably greater in the upper than the lower limbs, the more paralysed arm being the worst affected. In the more severe cases, pseudoathetosis and even astereognosis were seen.

Disturbed spinothalamic sensation was noticed only occasionally; in the majority of patients it was confined to the more severely paralysed arm, but in some the loss was evident up to the C2–C4 level, on the side opposite to the more severely paralysed limbs.

Although intention tremor, abnormal gait, and disturbed coordination tests were sometimes found, symptoms of cerebellar disturbance were infrequently volunteered. Nystagmus was infrequent. None had dysarthria.

Localized wasting and weakness of the shoulder or hand muscles, and occasionally fasciculations, were seen in 15 patients. In spite of this evidence of lower motor neurone involvement, the deep reflexes were exaggerated in the upper limbs in all but one of these patients, a sign of diagnostic value distinguishing this condition from syringomyelia and other craniovertebral anomalies, where these reflexes are depressed.

Horner's syndrome was seen unilaterally in 3 patients, on the same side as the more paralysed limbs.

No cranial nerve palsies were seen in our patients.

Other writers on this subject (List, 1941; McRae, 1953; Bharucha and Dastur, 1964) have similarly commented on the frequency of pyramidal tract and posterior column signs, and on the paucity of cervical symptoms. The latter two, however, mentioned a slightly higher frequency of 'bulbar' signs and ataxia, especially in cases where there was associated occipitalization. Bharucha and Dastur (1964) also found a greater percentage of forequarter spinothalamic loss, but as not all their cases of occipitalization had associated dislocation, it is difficult to decide if compression due to a dislocating atlanto-axial joint was the only cause of the signs seen in their cases.

The duration of symptoms can be seen in TABLE 8.3. The course was slowly progressive or somewhat remittent; we saw no cases with sudden onset as mentioned by Bharucha and Dastur (1964).

Table 8.3
Duration of Symptoms

Time-span	*No. of cases*
Within 6 months (3 within a week)	18
6 months to 1 year	8
1 year to 5 years	11
5 years to 10 years	4
10 years to 15 years	4
15 years to 20 years	3
20 years to 25 years	1
40 years	1
48 years	1
Uncertain	1
Total	*52*

A variety of associated congenital anomalies, either clinically or radiologically evident, have been seen in

Table 8.4
Associated Congenital Anomalies

Clinical	*No. of Cases*
Short neck	24
Dysplastic face	11
Dolichocephaly	1
Kyphoscoliosis	7
Sprengel's shoulder	2
Digital anomalies—simian thumb	1
Congenital aqueduct stenosis	1
Holmes-Adie syndrome	1
Congenital athetosis	1
Mirror movements	1
Congenital heart anomaly	1
Anomalous radial artery	1
RADIOLOGICAL	
Occipitalization	29
Cervical vertebrae fusion[1]	30
Hemivertebra	4
Small hypoplastic atlas	2
Cervical spina bifida	6
Cervical rib	2
Flat squamous part of occipital bone	1

[1] 24 of these 30 had fusion of C2 to C3 vertebrae.

our patients [TABLES 8.4 and 8.6]. Greenberg (1968) has mentioned a higher frequency of dislocation with mongolism; we have seen it occur once with von Recklinghausen's disease, though in the presence of a 'cervical spinal neurofibroma', it was uncertain which of the two caused the spinal signs. Similar familial anomalies were seen once; the brother of one of our patients had polydactyly, syndactyly, and craniostenosis.

In our series there were 42 males and 10 females: male preponderance occurs in this disease as in other craniovertebral anomalies. The age factor has been analysed in TABLE 8.5.

Table 8.5
Age Distribution in the Various Groups

Group	*No. of Cases*	*Average Age (in years)*	
		At onset	*At Hospitalization*
I	29	21·8	28·3
II	15	16·9	25·0
III	8	47·7	50·2
Whole series	*52*	*24·0*	*30·7*

INVESTIGATIONS

Radiology

The diagnosis rests almost entirely on good radiology The examination should comprise:

1. Routine skiagrams of the skull and cervical spine (lateral view in flexion and extension), and a through-the-mouth view of the atlanto-axial joint.

2. Lateral cervical tomography in flexion and extension; AP tomography and myelography are undertaken when further elucidation is required. Teleradiological visualization of neck movements is extremely useful.

In a normal individual, the odontoid process lies immediately behind the anterior arch of the atlas and its tip is at the level of, or just above, the superior rim. Its anterior surface is in continuity with that of the axis. Radiological diagnosis is made by visualizing the dislocation, and its degree can be judged by applying certain recommended measurements (McRae, 1953; McRae and Barnum, 1953; Bachs *et al.*, 1955; Hinck and Hopkins, 1960).

There are two main measurements:

1. In the lateral flexion skiagram in an adult, a maximum distance of 3 mm between the odontoid and the anterior arch of the atlas (the *medium joint*) is considered as normal. In a child up to 4·5 mm is permissible. The formula of Hinck and Hopkins (1960) may be applied to judge normality according to age. In all our patients with an intact odontoid the distance was over 5 mm, this was as great as 12 mm in one patient, but in most was between 7 to 9 mm. When the odontoid was separated from the body of axis or was absent, this measurement could not be used. In this case the distance between the inferior rim of the anterior arch of the atlas, and the remaining attached part of the odontoid or the anterior superior edge of the body of the axis (the two closest bony points in the skiagram) was considered; normally no gap exists. In these patients, the dislocation forward of the atlas was clearly visualized, and the distance varied from 7 to 12 mm in flexion.

2. The *spinal canal*, as measured in a lateral (straight) skiagram of the cervical spine at this level, is the distance between the posterior surface of the odontoid and the nearest bony projection on the posterior rim of the foramen magnum or the occipitalized atlas. There is normally no appreciable change on flexion or extension of the neck. It measures 19 to 32 mm. McRae (1953) suggested a safety distance (in flexion) of 19 mm, below which neurological signs were very likely to arise. He maintained that if neurological signs were present, and the spinal canal was less than 19 mm, then these were due to the compressive effect of the narrowed canal on the spinal cord or medullospinal junction, although occasionally patients were seen to be symptom-free with a canal slightly narrower than that.

In those patients in whom the odontoid is absent or separated from the body of the axis, the anterior point of the spinal canal is measured from the posterior superior edge of the body of the axis.

In dislocation, the spinal canal is narrowest in flexion. In none of our cases was it more than 15 mm in flexion, and in 30 of the 52 patients it was less than 10 mm. It was as narrow as 3 to 4 mm in some patients.

If there was no substantial change in the measurements between flexion and extension of the neck, the dislocation was designated as spontaneously irreducible or 'fixed'. The irreducibility was partial or complete. If the dislocation was easily corrected on straightening the neck, it was considered a reducible or 'gliding' dislocation (subluxation).

We also noticed in the lateral cervical spine skiagram that the odontoid was dislocated not only backward [PLATE 17a], but in 13 patients somewhat upwards. Here, it was not uncommon to see the body of the axis or even the fused junction of the C2 to C3 vertebrae behind the anterior arch of the atlas, with the dens raised well within the foramen magnum.

Basilar invagination can be differentiated by using the known measurements and techniques (Chamberlain's line, McGregor's line, Bull's angle, digastric line, AP and lateral tomography), although it is known that there are many fallacies in the measurement of these artificial, eponymously named, lines (Spillane, Pallis, and Jones, 1957). The long and the upward and backwardly dislocated dens, as seen in our cases, are two instances when an impression of basilar invagination may be created when judged by these lines although none actually exists.

We came across only one patient with a co-existent basilar invagination and atlanto-axial dislocation, although we have seen 23 cases of basilar invagination in the same period as when this series was collected.

Table 8.6
Radiological Classification

Group	No. of Cases	Atlas	Axis (Odontoid)								Reducible[3]	Irreducible
		Occipitalization	Normal	Long	Abnormal Odontoid[2] Type I	Type II	Type III	Type IV	Type V	Unclassifiable		
I	29	29[1]	18	4	—	—	—	7	—	—	—	29
II	15	—	—	—	—	8	—	5	1	1	15	—
III	8	—	8	—	—	—	—	—	—	—	6	2
Whole Series	*52*	*29*	*26*	*4*	—	*8*	—	*12*	*1*	*1*	*21*	*31*

[1] C2 and C3 fused in 24 cases
[2] Refers to Greenberg's classification (see text).
[3] Partial or complete.

Classification of the Dislocation

There are various ways in which this can be done (McRae, 1953; Wadia, 1967; Greenberg, 1968). Taking all these points of view, a classification is suggested here [TABLE 8.6] which is a modification of that suggested earlier (Wadia, 1967).

As can be seen from the table, three main groups can be clearly identified.

Group I

This is the largest group, in which the combination of occipitalization of the atlas, frequent fusion of C2 to C3 vertebrae (and occasionally of other cervical vertebrae), dislocation backward of the odontoid process from the median atlanto-axial joint [PLATE 17a], and compression of the adjacent spinal cord were seen. The odontoid was normal in 18, long in 4, and short and peg-like in 7 [PLATE 17a and b]. The long odontoid protruded into the middle of the foramen magnum. The short odontoid represented a congenital anomaly, embryologically representing the basal segment only of the developing odontoid process, and about which more will be said later. This form of dislocation was seen to be partially or completely irreducible.

Group II

In this group of 15 patients there was no occipitalization of the atlas. The basic congenital anomaly was the maldevelopment of the odontoid process. As the odontoid is developed in two parts, the apical and basal segments, Greenberg (1968) has claimed to have radiologically identified five types of odontoid anomalies:

Type I. A normally developed dens which has failed to unite with the body of the axis (OS odontoideum).

Type II. A failure of fusion between the apical and basal segments (ossiculum terminale).

Type III. An apical segment normally developed but whose base has failed to develop (agenesis of the odontoid base or an extreme form of ossiculum terminale).

Type IV. Failure of development of the apical portion of the dens, leaving behind a small peg-like dens or a rounded (round-shouldered) bulge representing the basal segment (agenesis of basal segment).

Type V. Where the whole odontoid has failed to develop, leaving behind a hollow in the superior surface of the body of the axis.

Greenberg mentioned that Types II and IV are much commoner, as can also be seen in TABLE 8.6 [PLATE 17d]. In this group, the dislocation is freely reducible on neck extension in the large majority of patients. It is for this reason that the dislocation may be completely missed in the skiagram of the cervical spine in the straight position. It cannot be too strongly stressed that skiagrams in a flexed position of the neck must be taken.

The congenital nature of this group is evident by its associations, but traumatic fracture or avulsion of the odontoid with an immediate or delayed myelopathy, as mentioned by Corner (1907), Bachs *et al.* (1955), and Blockey and Purser (1956), has to be differentiated, especially in the absence of a history of sufficient trauma or other congenital anomalies. Although McRae (1953) thought that it may be impossible to decide between the two in adults, Harris (1959), Wollin (1963), and Greenberg (1968) have discussed many interesting points of differentiation.

No cases of basilar invagination were encountered in this group either, but in the presence of anomalies of the odontoid the various lines had to be dispensed with and other criteria used.

Group III

This was the smallest group with eight cases only. Here there was no occipitalization, and the odontoid was normal in shape and size and attached to the body of the axis. The dislocation was clearly seen in flexion, and the odontoid was seen to be merely dislocated backwards and not upwards.

It was often difficult to identify these cases from an acquired variety of 'spontaneous atlanto-axial dislocation' (Werne, 1957; Greenberg, 1968). However, three points can be used in favour of congenital malformation:

1. Absence of any recent or past history of paracervical infections, rheumatoid arthritis, or other factors known to cause spontaneous atlanto-axial dislocation.
2. Presence of other congenital anomalies in the cervical spine or elsewhere in the body.
3. Presentation principally with neurological symptoms.

As is known, a majority of patients with spontaneous atlanto-axial dislocation present with neck stiffness and torticollis and few neurological complications, but the reverse is true in this congenital group. There were no cases of basilar invagination in this group either.

The dislocation here was totally or partially spontaneously reducible by neck extension in all but two of these patients [TABLE 8·6].

The main points of differentiation between the three groups [TABLES 8.1, 8.5 and 8.6] are:

1. Groups I and II contained much younger patients than Group III.
2. Short neck and low hair-line predominated in Group I (19 out of 29), was seen occasionally in Group II (5 out of 15), and not at all in Group III.
3. Cervical symptoms were seen most in Group I. The movements of the neck were most free in Group II, where all dislocations were completely or at least partially reducible on neck extension. They were almost equally free in Group III, where spontaneous reducibility was also seen, though not as often complete as in Group II. In Group I, lateral rotation of the neck was limited in quite a few patients, and very little spontaneous change was seen in the dislocation on neck extension.
4. Associated dysplastic facies and congenital anomalies were most frequent in Group I and least so in Group III.
5. Transitory attacks were found to be more or less equally frequent in all groups.

Myelography

Lumbar myelography should essentially be performed when:

1. The clinical diagnosis is uncertain.
2. More than one congenital anomaly exists in the cervical spine; when one has to make sure that the compression is at the site of the atlanto-axial dislocation and not elsewhere.
3. Differentiation from syringomyelia or basilar invagination has to be made.

The CSF examination is usually normal, although occasionally the protein may be as high as 80 to 90 mg; in one of our cases, it was 190 mg.

PATHOLOGY AND PATHOGENESIS

These will be dicussed under two headings:

1. The mechanism of the dislocation.
2. Pathological changes in the underlying spinal cord or medullospinal junction.

The Mechanism of the Dislocation

The probable reasons for dislocation at the atlanto-axial joint are enumerated below.

Maldevelopment or Malfunctioning of the Transverse Ligament

This is the primary defect in causing dislocations in cases belonging to Groups I and III, although the role of the alar ligaments and the joint capsules is perhaps insufficiently stressed. It appears that the basic congenital defect is an absence of proper formation of well-defined strong ligaments from the original amorphous fibrous mass around the dens during early life, rather than a clear laxity of well-developed ligaments; 'laxity' or 'incompetence' of the transverse ligament has often been mentioned, but has nowhere been demonstrated by any writer.

In six out of our seven autopsied cases of Groups I and III, no transverse ligament could be found, and in its place ill-defined fibrous tissue was seen on careful dissection. List (1941) expressed the same view when he said that 'a large amount of dense fibrous tissue firmly fixed the odontoid process to the base of the skull, but no transverse ligament existed'.

Maldevelopment of the Odontoid Process

Much has been written on the embryological development and the various maldevelopments of the odontoid process and their role in congenital atlanto-axial dislocation (Harris, 1959; Wollin, 1963; Greenberg, 1968). Greenberg described five different maldevelopments of the odontoid, and he claimed to have separately identified each of them in all the recorded cases in the world literature; although such retrospective analysis of printed skiagrams leaves much to be desired. The fact that in 22 out of our 52 cases (7 in Group I and 15 in Group II) a maldeveloped odontoid was the sole or major cause for the dislocation further stresses its role in maintaining stability at this joint. In cases like those belonging to our Group I a short peg-like odontoid process representing the basal segment only can easily slip below a poorly developed transverse ligament. In Group II a similar situation arises, or an intact but separate apical segment allows a free dislocation of the atlas, while the apical segment is itself carried with it.

Maldevelopment of the Lateral Articulating Facets Between the Atlas and the Axis

PLATE 17b illustrates not only the asymmetry in the level of the superior articular facets of the axis, but also the different directions in which they face. When the articular facets of the axis slope sharply downward and forward instead of being 'square-shouldered', the atlas dislocates forward and downward, giving rise to the apparently upward and backward dislocation of the odontoid seen radiologically and mentioned earlier in Group I.

Occipitalization of the Atlas

This, especially with fusion of C2 to C3 into a block vertebra, throws an undue strain on the atlanto-axial joint, because according to List (1941), the nodding (flexion) movements which normally take place at the atlanto-occipital joint, now occur instead at other cervical joints including the atlanto-axial.

The Underlying Spinal Cord (Medullospinal Junction)

Macroscopic

The maximum compression is usually at C1 but List (1941) and Wadia (1967) reported cases in which it was seen at C2 and even C2–C3 levels (PLATE 17c), and McRae and Barnum (1953) and Dastur *et al.* (1965) found a pit in the anterior surface of the lower end of the medulla oblongata where the dislocated dens fitted. The latter is reported with a congenitally long dens but we would also expect it to occur in those cases of our Group I in which the dislocation was not only backward but upward. The spinal cord is often distorted and thinned over 2 cm or more of its length [PLATE 17c].

A dural band at the site of compression arising as a result of constant abnormal movements has been seen by surgeons and pathologists (Bharucha and Dastur, 1964; Dastur *et al.*, 1965) [PLATE 17c], and may play some role in the advanced case.

No cavitation of the cord was seen resulting from the compression, but in our last case a smooth-lined, non-communicating cavity (syrinx) was found in the region of one posterior horn from C3 to C6 segments. This was considered as an associated anomaly of the neuraxis, which did not contribute to the symptoms.

No basilar invagination or Arnold-Chiari malformation were found.

Microscopic

These changes are not very different from those seen with any chronic compression and have been thoroughly discussed by Dastur *et al.* (1965).

DIFFERENTIAL DIAGNOSIS

When the full flow of the natural history is evident from the transitory attacks precipitated by exaggerated neck movements, the subsequent progressive high cervical cord lesion, the dysplastic face, the short neck, the associated congenital anomalies, and the absence of cranial nerve palsies, the diagnosis is straightforward. Radiology often merely confirms the clinical diagnosis.

With a slightly variant picture, however, the diagnosis may not be so straightforward, even after radiology, from the acquired dislocations. Tuberculous and non-tuberculous infections, and malignant deposits of the atlas and axis cause a dislocation and progressive myelopathy of much shorter span; the transitory attacks are absent; neck pain and stiffness are more remarkable and the general health of these patients is poorer. The differences between our Group II and traumatic dislocation, and between our Group III and spontaneous atlanto-axial dislocation from paracervical infections, rheumatoid arthritis, etc., have already been pointed out earlier in this chapter.

The clinical distinction between early spinal cord compression from tumour, high cervical spondylosis and atlanto-axial dislocation may be wellnigh impossible when no history of transitory attacks is forthcoming. The CSF may be normal or show slightly raised protein in all these conditions; only careful radiology and myelography will settle the matter.

Differentiation from amyotrophic lateral sclerosis, posterolateral sclerosis, syringomyelia and spastic diplegia in children (cerebral palsy) has to be made under certain circumstances. A clinical picture of syringomyelia and pathological changes of intramedullary cavitation are familiar in cases of basilar invagination and the Arnold-Chiari malformation; syringomyelia may either co-exist as a separate anomaly or, as is now believed, result from the effects of the disorder around the foramen magnum. On the other hand, syringomyelia as a diagnosis has occasionally been suggested by the referring physicians, but a significant cavitation within the cord has not been seen in our autopsies. Yet, when a forequarter spinothalamic sensory loss in an upper limb is detected as a sign of the myelopathy of atlanto-axial dislocation, a co-existing independent syringomyelia has to be carefully excluded. Unlike classical syringomyelia, where the deep reflexes of the upper limbs are usually absent, in dislocation the spinothalamic loss is accompanied by exaggerated deep reflexes. Trophic ulcers of the hands have not been reported with this myelopathy, while they constantly occur in syringomyelia. The presence of cerebellar ataxia and marked pyramidal tract signs in all the limbs makes the differentiation easier.

Basilar invagination, occipitalization of the atlas, Klippel-Feil anomaly, and the Arnold-Chiari malformation are very often considered together with congenital atlanto-axial dislocation under the single heading of craniovertebral anomalies, but it should be possible to make clinical and radiological differentiation between them.

In basilar invagination, the transitory attacks have rarely been described; on the other hand, lower cranial nerve palsies, cerebellar signs, the spinothalamic variety of sensory loss over the arms, and signs of raised intracranial pressure are seen more often with it. Basilar invagination essentially presents a picture of a posterior fossa lesion, while atlanto-axial dislocation largely causes a cervical myelopathy.

Occipitalization, or fusion of other cervical vertebrae (Klippel-Feil anomaly), is asymptomatic; neurological signs seen with this arise from other associated anomalies.

Finally, the Arnold-Chiari malformation usually presents with cerebellar signs and a syringomyelia or syringobulbia-like picture in contrast to the largely pyramidal tract disturbance of atlanto-axial disease. Supine myelography and vertebral angiography should clear up one's doubts.

Diagnosis of hysteria, peripheral neuritis, multiple sclerosis and even cerebrovascular (vertebrobasilar) insufficiency have been suggested by the referring physicians for those of our patients in whom the history of intermittent episodes was predominant. A careful history and assessment should clearly indicate the nature of such episodes.

PROGNOSIS AND TREATMENT

The prognosis is intimately connected with surgical treatment. We advise surgical treatment for all patients with neurological signs, however slight, except those over 60 years who are in poor general health and have little neurological disturbance.

The prognosis will depend on how effective the surgical procedure is in decompressing the spinal cord, and at what stage the operation is undertaken. If the operation is performed as a prophylactic measure, as was done in some of our patients with intermittent attacks and little neurological disturbance, the result will be excellent, barring the immediate postoperative complications. Even at a well-developed stage of the disease, a successful operation arrests the deterioration and may even provide some improvement; advanced cases are doomed to lead a paraplegic life or die from complications of decubitus.

The details and the merits and demerits of the various surgical techniques will not be discussed here; it may be said, however, that the standard operation of removal of the posterior arch of the atlas and posterior margin of the foramen magnum performed for basilar invagination or Arnold-Chiari malformation, without previous traction of the neck or attempt at reduction, can result in a disastrous postoperative haematomyelia (Dastur *et al.*, 1965). It is therefore important to differentiate, pre-operatively, atlanto-axial dislocation from other craniovertebral anomalies. Today, our practice is to reduce the dislocation spontaneously by neck extension, or if this is not possible, by skull traction. The lateral atlanto-axial joints are then fused by an anterior approach. A majority of the patients improve with this procedure and postoperative haematomyelia is avoided. For those in whom no substantial improvement is seen a later posterior decompression and sectioning of dural bands, if found, is recommended.

References

BACHS, A., BARRAQUER-BORDAS, L., BARRAQUER-FERRE, L., CANANDELL, J. M., and MODOLELL, A. (1955) Delayed myelopathy following atlanto-axial dislocation by separated odontoid process, *Brain*, 78, 537.

BHARUCHA, E. P., and DASTUR, H. M. (1964) Craniovertebral anomalies, *Brain*, 87, 469.

BLOCKEY, N. J., and PURSER, D. W. (1956) Fractures of the odontoid process of the axis, *J. Bone Jt Surg.*, 38B, 794.

CORNER, E. M. (1907) Quoted by Blockey, N. J., and Purser, D. W. (1956).

DASTUR, D. K., WADIA, N. H., DESAI, A. D., and SINH, G. (1965) Medullospinal compression due to atlanto-axial dislocation and sudden haematomyelia during decompression, *Brain*, 88, 897.

ELLIOTT, G. R., and SACHS, E. (1912) Observations on

fracture of the odontoid process of the axis with intermittent pressure paralysis, *Ann. Surg.*, **56**, 876.

GREENBERG, A. D. (1968) Atlanto-axial dislocations, *Brain*, **91**, 655.

HARRIS, R. I. (1959) in *Modern Trends in Diseases of the Vertebral Column*, eds. Nassim, R., and Burrows, H. J., London, p. 29.

HINCK, V. C., and HOPKINS, C. E. (1960) Measurement of the atlantodental interval in the adult, *Amer. J. Roentgenol.*, **84**, 945.

ILLINGWORTH, R. S. (1956) Attacks of unconsciousness in association with fused cervical vertebrae, *Arch. Dis. Childh.*, **31**, 8.

LIST, C. F. (1941) Neurologic syndromes accompanying developmental anomalies of occipital bone, atlas and axis, *Arch. Neurol. Psychiat. (Chic.)*, **45**, 577.

MCRAE, D. L. (1953) Bony abnormalities in the region of the foramen magnum, *Acta radiol. (Stockh.)*, **40**, 335.

MCRAE, D. L., and BARNUM, A. S. (1953) Occipitalization of the atlas, *Amer. J. Roentgenol.*, **70**, 23.

PANDYA, S. K. (1970) John Hilton's contributions on atlanto-axial disease, *Neurology (India)*, **18**, 147.

SINGH, S., DUTTA, A. K., and GUPTA, S. (1969) Craniovertebral anomalies with neurological deficit, *J. Ass. Phycns India*, **17**, 469.

SPILLANE, J. D., PALLIS, C. A., and JONES, A. M. (1957) Developmental abnormalities in the region of the foramen magnum, *Brain*, **80**, 11.

SRINIVASAN, K., BALASUBRAMANIAM, V., and RAMAMURTHI, B. (1967) Craniovertebral anomalies, *Neurology (India)*, **15**, 42.

SYMONDS, C. P., and MEADOWS, S. P. (1937) Compression of the spinal cord in the neighbourhood of the foramen magnum, *Brain*, **60**, 52.

WADIA, N. H. (1960) Chronic progressive myelopathy complicating atlanto-axial dislocation due to congenital abnormality, *Neurology (Bombay)*, **8**, 81.

WADIA, N. H. (1967) Myelopathy complicating congenital atlanto-axial dislocation, *Brain*, **90**, 449.

WERNE, S. (1957) Studies in spontaneous atlas dislocation, *Acta orthop. scand.*, Suppl. 23.

WOLLIN, D. G. (1963) The os odontoideum, *J. Bone Jt Surg.*, **45A**, 1459.

9 Anterior Encephaloceles

P. N. TANDON

INCIDENCE

Of the major congenital malformations those of the central nervous system are by far the commonest in most countries. There are, however, well-recognized geographical variations. Penrose (1957) pointed out that although there is great variation in frequency of occurrence of these malformations in different parts of Europe, the incidence is on the whole greater among Europeans than among Asians and Africans.

The incidence of three major malformations of the central nervous system reported from different countries is summarized in TABLE 9.1. It is apparent that the highest incidence of these malformations is reported from India; the United Kingdom comes next. In the United Kingdom the incidence is much higher in Birmingham (McKeown and Record, 1960; Leck, 1966) than in Northamptonshire (Pleydell, 1960). Giroud (1960) reported a west to east diminution in frequency in France. The figures from Sweden and the United States are generally comparable (Böök, 1951; Alter, 1962; Wacker, 1963), while those from Japan (Neel, 1958) show a significantly lower incidence of spina bifida and hydrocephalus; anencephaly is equally as frequent as that in the United States. Alter (1962), from South Carolina, reported that anencephaly and spina bifida appeared to be less common in Negroes than in whites, while hydrocephalus was somewhat more frequent in Negroes. In contrast to these figures, Simpkiss and Lowe (1961), from Kampala, Uganda, reported a negligible incidence of anencephaly and spina bifida, and quoted Kahn (1956) as having observed a low incidence of these lesions among native Africans in Johannesburg and Pretoria. That this may not be true of all African countries is apparent from the report by Odeku (1967) from Western Nigeria who between 1957 and 1966 collected 97 patients with congenital malformations of the spine and spinal cord, and 36 cases of cranium bifidum.

Table 9.2

Incidence of Encephaloceles at Various Sites (Dekaban, 1959)

Collected figures from three large series reported from the United States

Site	*No.*	*Percentage*
Occipital	203	72·2
Parietal	34	12·1
Frontal	26	9·3
Nasal	17	6·0
Nasopharyngeal	1	0·4
Total	*281*	*100·0*

Apart from variations in the overall frequency of malformations of the central nervous system, there is evidence to suggest a difference in the relative incidence of various lesions. The relative frequency of encephalocele to spina bifida aperta seems to vary from centre to centre. Reports from the United States generally suggest a ratio of 1:6 (Ingraham and Matson, 1954; Dekaban, 1959), while it is reported as 1:5 from the United Kingdom (Lorber, 1961; Norman, 1963). Odeku (1967), in Nigeria, found a relative incidence of 1:3. Even among the encephaloceles there appears to be some geographical predilection for a particular site. Anterior encephaloceles are reported as uncommon lesions in the United States (Kahn and Lemmen 1952;

Table 9.1

Incidence of Congenital Malformations of the Central Nervous System per 1000 Births Reported from Various Parts of the World

Authors	*India* Khanna and Prasad 1967	Saifullah *et al.* 1967	Ghosh and Bali 1963	Mittal and Grewal 1969	*Uganda* Simkiss and Lowe 1961	*USA* Alter 1962	Wacker 1963	*Sweden* Böök 1951	*Japan* Neel 1958	*UK* McKeown and Record 1960	Pleydell 1960	Leck 1966
Total births analysed	5 376	1 000	4 353	4 150	2 068	55 156	19 615	44 109	64 570	56 760	62 224	524 274
Overall incidence of malformations	36·0	?	34	22·41	54	?	?	11·18	12·22	17·30	?	?
Anencephaly	4·0	4	2·9	2·17	0	0·53	0·71	0·54	0·63	1·96	1·0	2·16
Spinal bifida	5·0	4	2·06	0·72	0	0·71	0·45	1·09–1·45	0·26	2·80	1·9	2·14
Hydrocephalus	3·0	3	1·8	1·21	1·5	0·96	1·06	1·00	0·32	1·76	0·6	
Encephalocele	?	1	?	0·48	0	?	?	?	?	?	?	0·37

Davis and Alexander, 1959; Ingraham and Swan, 1943; Fisher, Uihlein, and Keith, 1952). Most reports from Western countries would suggest a relative incidence of basal to sincipital and occipital encephaloceles to be 1:1·5:6. Blumenfeld and Skolnik (1965) reported the relative incidence of various encephaloceles as basal 10 per cent, sincipital 15 per cent, occipital 75 per cent. Collected figures from three large series reported from the United States are summarized in TABLE 9.2 (Dekaban, 1959).

However, Odeku (1967), in Ibadan, Western Nigeria, reported a proportionately higher incidence of encephaloceles located anteriorly and basally as compared with reports from the West: occipital 25; nasofrontal 6; parieto-occipital 3; parietal 1; tempero-orbital 1. Acquaviva *et al.* (1965), from Casablanca, Morocco, found 39 out of 98 meningo-encephaloceles situated anteriorly. Tandon (1970), in a series of 40 cases of cranium bifidum, reported 11 situated anteriorly. We have since operated on six more cases of fronto-ethmoidal encephaloceles. It may, however, be mentioned that this apparently higher incidence of anterior encephaloceles seen by us at Lucknow and Delhi, has not been reported from other centres in India. Ramamurthi (1970) from Madras, South India, has seen only three cases in the last 20 years. The highest incidence of fronto-ethmoidal encephaloceles has been reported from Bangkok, Thailand, by Suwanwela *et al.* (1969), who have collected 82 cases in 7 years. They have calculated the incidence of this disease in the Thai population to be 1 in 5000. In their experience the sincipital encephalocele is more frequent than the occipital variety. They also referred to a high incidence of this lesion in Malaysia and Indonesia and a lower incidence in Japan and Hong Kong. A low incidence is also reported from Ceylon (Weinman, 1970).

CLASSIFICATION

Between the two extremes of cranium bifidum occultum and anencephaly, there is a variety of lesions grouped under the common term of 'encephaloceles'. An encephalocele may present through a defect anywhere in the skull but the common sites are the occipital, sincipital, or basal regions. The sincipital variety with which we are concerned here is further subdivided into: frontal, frontonasal, fronto-ethmoidal, and naso-orbital.

1. *Frontal:* the cranial defect is in the frontal bone, nearly always in the midline.
2. *Frontonasal:* the hernia is through a defect in the skull at the junction of the frontal bone with the nasal bone.
3. *Fronto-ethmoidal:* the protrusion of the intracranial contents is through the foramen caecum, i.e. the junction of the frontal and ethmoid bones. It extends beneath the nasal bone to present on the surface at the junction of the nasal bone and the cartilage.
4. *Naso-orbital:* the encephalocele protrudes through the medial wall of the orbit, involving the frontal, ethmoid, and lacrimal bones.

Depending upon the contents of the sac these lesions have been further classified as cranial meningocele, encephalomeningocele, encephalocystocele and encephalo-cystomeningocele. There is no particular merit in this subdivision.

AETIOPATHOGENESIS

The aetiology of meningoencephalocele is not known. Experimental teratology has, however, helped greatly in the understanding of some of these malformations. Encephaloceles and meningoceles, as well as anencephaly, are produced at the same stage of embryonic development and in the same conditions, indicating that these processes are minor alterations in the closure of the encephalic tube (Giroud, 1960). According to Blumenfeld and Skolnik (1965), the most acceptable theory of aetiology is that of St. Hilaire who postulated that the encephaloceles arise in the embryo through adhesions of the brain anlage to the germinal membranes. The adhesions disappear and leave scars which interfere with normal development. Several other theories have been postulated. Failure of the ethmoidal plate to close around the olfactory nerves may result in an osseous defect, the herniation of the brain occurring later in embryonic development. In contrast to this, others believe that the hernia is caused by localized increase in intraventricular pressure during embryonic development forcing the brain through the as yet unformed osseous structures.

The sensitive period at which the anomaly is produced is the end of the gastrulation stage, i.e. 8 to 10 days in mice and rats or about the sixteenth day in humans. If one accepts the hypothesis that encephaloceles are a minor variant of anencephaly, in experimental animals these defects can be produced by a variety of factors, e.g. X-rays, anoxia, some vitamin deficiencies or hypervitaminosis A, a variety of chemicals including prochlorperazine and actinomycin, acting at critical periods of development.

Data obtained in humans indicate some genetic influence. The frequency of the O blood group among mothers of anencephalics has suggested an influence of genetic constitution (Coffey and Jessop, 1957).

The incidence of anencephaly or other gross neural defects in the family of an anencephalic is 3 per cent, compared with an average figure of 0·1 per cent in the general population (Penrose, 1957; Lamy and Frezal, 1959); consanguinity increases the frequency. Thus Penrose (1957, 1960) proposed a genetic hypothesis involving either a recessive gene, or chromosome translocation, or fresh mutation; at the same time he could not rule out the influence of external factors.

Coffey and Jessop (1957) noticed that the state of nutrition was often a little lower in mothers of anencephalics. The haemoglobin and plasma-protein levels of these mothers were lower than in controls. According to Penrose (1957) the geographical variations may be influenced by the presence or absence of trace elements in water.

A relatively high incidence of anterior encephaloceles has only been reported from Thailand, Nigeria, Casablanca, and Delhi. All our patients belonged to the lower socio-economic group. The possible role of malnutrition in the aetiology of this condition must therefore be considered. No two patients in our series or in that of Suwanwela *et al.* (1969) belonged to the same family.

PATHOLOGICAL ANATOMY

An appreciation of the site of the defect in the skull is important in planning the management of encephaloceles. In frontal encephaloceles the defect is in the frontal bone, while in the frontonasal variety it is at the junction of the frontal bone with the nasal bone. The neck of the sac in these two groups is therefore at the external surface of the cranium. In the fronto-ethmoidal variety the herniation takes place through an enlarged foramen caecum, i.e. the junction of the frontal and ethmoid bones. The neck of the sac is therefore situated intracranially just in front of the crista galli (Tandon, 1966). Usually, both frontal poles herniate through the defect but we have encountered unilateral cases. In the latter, the midline defect tends to appear more towards one side. In some cases the defect may be very large, and it then encroaches upon the roof of the orbits.

The herniated brain, as in all encephaloceles, is gliosed and usually adherent to the overlying skin in the region of the apex of the sac. This is particularly so in the fronto-ethmoidal variety, in which case it may be difficult to deliver it into the cranial cavity during an intracranial operation.

The foramen of Munro may be partially or completely obliterated as a result of the deformity produced by traction and herniation of the brain. This may result in unilateral or bilateral hydrocephalus.

As in other encephaloceles, there is a higher incidence of associated anomalies of the brain. Localized cortical atrophy, subarachnoid cyst, agenesis of corpus·callosum etc., have been encountered.

CLINICAL FEATURES

Anterior encephaloceles, unlike the basal variety, are obvious at birth, presenting as a mass at any site ranging from the middle of the forehead, the root of the nose, the bridge of the nose, or its side. The exact location of this mass is of practical significance as it indicates the type of defect. Frontal and naso-orbital varieties are easily recognized. There seems to be some confusion, however, regarding the frontonasal and fronto-ethmoidal groups. Many authors have used these terms as synonymous. This differentiation is, however, of practical importance for planning a correct surgical approach (Tandon, 1970). The frontonasal encephalocele presents at the root of the nose over the bregma, through a defect at the frontonasal junction; the nasal bone is thus below the mass. It is usually globular, the contents being mostly fluid. In contrast to this, the fronto-ethmoidal encephalocele presents below the root of the nose, at the junction of the bone and the cartilage. The nasal bone is above the mass. It overrides the bridge of the nose and if unilateral it may be on one side rather than in the midline. It presents a lobulated appearance, usually with a depression or groove in the midline. It is always sessile and the contents are mostly solid, though cystic lesions are infrequently seen [PLATE 18a].

The size of the encephalocele varies a great deal. At birth the lesion is usually small but it tends to enlarge as the child grows.

Most anterior encephaloceles are covered with full-thickness skin and only rarely have cases been reported with exposed brain tissue without any covering. The thickness of the skin covering is variable; it is thick and even puckered in smaller lesions, and thin, shiny and stretched in larger ones.

Depending upon the contents of the encephalocele, the mass may be compressible though usually not completely reducible. It may be possible to elicit cross-fluctuations with the anterior fontanelle. It generally enlarges and becomes tense when the child cries. Transillumination in a dark room may be helpful in estimating the contents of the sac but small portions of neural tissue may not cast sufficient shadow to be detected.

These malformations are usually associated with deformity of the face which tends to worsen with progressive enlargement of the encephalocele. A broad bridge and elongation of the nose, and hypertelorism are constant findings in cases of the fronto-ethmoidal lesion. Associated microcephaly has been reported, but overt hydrocephalus is uncommon.

The naso-orbital encephalocele, also called anterior orbital, protrudes forwards from the inner canthus on to the face and displaces the eyeball laterally. It is frequently associated with anomalies of the eyes, such as coloboma, microcornea, microphthalmos, hydrophthalmos, and apparent anophthalmos. We have encountered no examples of this particular variety, although a number have been reported from other centres in India (Pahwa and Patney, 1963; Consul and Kulshresthra, 1965). Posterior orbital encephaloceles present as axial exophthalmos, their true nature being disclosed only after surgical exploration (Mortada and El-Toraci, 1960). An excellent review of this subject is available with a case report by Strandberg (1949). We have seen only one such case in Delhi (Tandon, 1970).

Neurological Examination

Owing to their location there is seldom any associated neurological deficit. The possibility of mental retardation must, however, be seriously considered, especially in a case with a sizable hernia of both frontal poles.

A search should be made for other anomalies of the nervous system and also elsewhere in the body.

INVESTIGATIONS

Plain skull X-rays with anteroposterior and lateral views will show a defect in the frontal bone or at the junction of the frontal bone with the nasal bone, in the frontal and the frontonasal encephaloceles respectively. In the fronto-ethmoidal variety no bony defect is seen from such views, but the presence of a soft tissue mass over the bridge of the nose with a normal frontonasal junction should point to the correct diagnosis. Postero-anterior projections at various angles and frontal tomograms may reveal the opening anterior to the crista galli (Suwanwela and Hongsaprabhas, 1966).

A careful evaluation of the cerebrospinal fluid pathways is an essential pre-operative investigation. In contrast to occipital encephaloceles, the anteriorly situated lesions are only infrequently associated with hydrocephalus. However, now and again one encounters dilatation of one or both lateral ventricles [PLATES 18c and d]. It may be mentioned that the size of the head or the state of the fontanelle often fails to provide an indication of a co-existent hydrocephalus (Lorber, 1961; Tandon, 1970).

DIFFERENTIAL DIAGNOSIS

Generally the diagnosis is obvious on inspection alone. Infrequently the encephalocele may have to be differentiated from a congenital tumour, e.g. a dermoid or

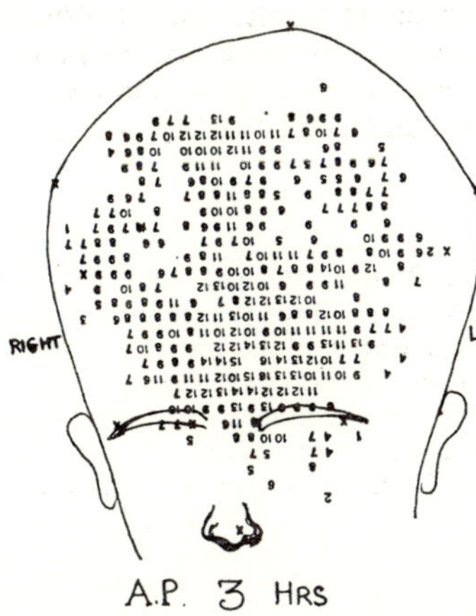

FIG. 9.1. RHISA cisternogram 3 hours after injection of the isotope into the lumbar theca: evidence of communication between the subarachnoid space and the swelling on the nose.

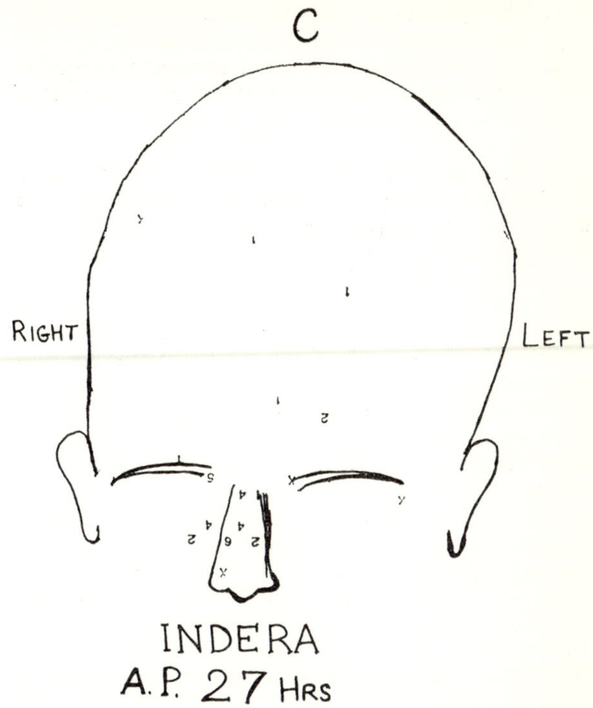

FIG. 9.2. Same patient as in FIGURE 9.1. RHISA cisternogram 27 hours after injection of the isotope.

nasal glioma. Aspiration of the mass, if cystic, and determination of the sugar content of the fluid may be helpful. Roentgenographic demonstration of the underlying bone defect or a communication between the swelling and the cranial cavity will establish the diagnosis. RHISA cisternography may demonstrate this communication where routine radiological investigations have failed (Tandon *et al.*, 1970). PLATE 18b is a clinical photograph of a 10-year-old girl who presented with a small cystic swelling on the left side of the nose. A similar swelling was reported to have been excised in early childhood; a full history and operative findings were not available. A RHISA cisternogram unequivocally demonstrated a communication between this swelling and the CSF pathways [FIGS. 9.1. and 9.2].

TREATMENT

The guiding principles for treatment of an encephalocele are the same irrespective of its location. For planning the management of an encephalocele, the following factors need consideration (Tandon, 1970):

1. Pathological anatomy:
   (a) The site of the bone defect.
   (b) The size of the encephalocele.
   (c) The contents of the sac.

2. The state of the cerebrospinal fluid pathway.
3. The neurological status of the patient.
4. The presence or absence of associated anomalies of the central nervous sytem and other regions of the body.

While a gross neurological deficit or an associated malformation incompatible with useful survival would contra-indicate surgery the evaluation of the first two factors helps to plan the correct surgical procedure.

The aim of surgery in these cases is to excise the sac at its neck and provide a water-tight closure of the dural defect. Precise knowledge of the site of the bone defect, where the neck of the sac is situated, is thus essential for planning the correct approach. An extra-cranial approach would provide an adequate exposure of the neck of a frontal or a frontonasal encephalocele. An elliptical incision is made around the base of the herniated mass, preserving enough skin to provide closure of the wound without tension. The incision is deepened to dissect the neck of the sac. The sac is then opened. Adhesions are released between the herniated brain and the sac, especially in the region of the apex and neck. The gliosed brain is excised and the amputated frontal lobe is allowed to retract into the cranial cavity. The sac is excised at the level of the skull defect. A piece of periosteum is then sutured to the dura with interrupted silk sutures at 1–2 mm intervals. The skull defect, if large, is covered with a stainless steel wire mesh and the scalp stitched in layers.

An intracranial approach is essential in dealing with fronto-ethmoidal and naso-orbital encephaloceles. Through a coronal incision a bilateral frontal craniotomy is performed. By means of a combined intra- and extradural approach the defect in the dura and the bone is outlined. An attempt is made to deliver the herniated frontal poles intracranially. Except with small encephaloceles this may not be possible, in which case it may be amputated at the cranial end of the orifice. As much as possible of the herniated portion is then removed by suction and sharp dissection. The remaining portion, in the case of large encephaloceles, may have to be removed at a second-stage, extracranial operation. It is important to outline the defect in the dura completely. It is then closed with a piece of periosteum, fascia or synthetic 'dura'. The graft, which should always be much bigger than the defect, is properly anchored in place by interrupted stitches all round. Some difficulty may be encountered near the posterior rim of the defect. It may be enough, however, to spread out the graft beyond the defect in this region, if it is adequately anchored elsewhere. A piece of gelfoam is placed over the graft and the brain is allowed to fall over it. The dura is then closed. In cases in which the bone defect is larger than a centimetre it is advisable to cover it extradurally with a stainless steel mesh or a bone graft. Rusonova (1967) advocated closure of the cranial defect with plexiglass. We have no experience with this material though we have successfully used a silastic button, fashioned to the size of the defect, in one of our recent cases. Even after a successful intra-cranial operation, a number of cases of fronto-ethmoidal encephalocele are left with an unsightly nose. They require a second-stage plastic operation to remove the remaining contents of the sac, excise the redundant skin, and reconstruct the nose.

Co-existing hydrocephalus, though uncommon in anterior encephaloceles, should be searched for and treated before any attempt is made to excise the latter. Failure to do so would result in either a postoperative cerebrospinal fluid leak or a recurrence of the swelling. The large encephalocele shown in PLATE 19a was repaired intracranially. Immediately postoperative the swelling had markedly reduced [PLATE 19b]. Four weeks later, however, it started to enlarge again [PLATE 19c]. An associated communicating hydrocephalus was treated by means of a thecoperitoneal shunt. The encephalocele regressed completely following this procedure [PLATE 19d].

PROGNOSIS

The majority of anterior encephaloceles are isolated malformations and do not preclude normal mental and physical development. The prognosis depends upon the size of the defect, the amount of neural tissue in the sac, and the presence or absence of associated anomalies, especially of microcephaly and hydrocephalus. It is advisable to correct the defect early in life, to prevent increasing hernia of the brain. We prefer to operate upon these infants when they are 6 to 8 weeks old. Smaller lesions are easier to repair, require sacrifice of only a small amount of neural tissue and leave minimal deformity. In contrast, the larger lesions, even after successful repair, require several operations to achieve a reasonable cosmetic result. Hypertelorism and some residual deformity of the nose may be inevitable. This has also been emphasized by Suwanwela *et al.* (1969) and Mealey, Dzenitis, and Hockey (1970).

References

ACQUAVIVA, R., TAMIC, P. M., BRU, P., LEBASCLE, J., and KERDOUDI, H. (1965) Anterior-basal meningo-encephaloceles: observations on 39 personal cases. *Excerpta Med. (Aust.), Int. Cong. Ser.*, 93, 165.

ALTER, M. (1962) Anencephalus, hydrocephalus and spina bifida epidemiology with special reference to a survey in Charleston S.C., *Arch. Neurol. (Chic.)*, 7, 411.

BLUMENFELD, R., and SKOLNIK, E. M. (1965) Intranasal encephaloceles, *Arch. Otolaryng.*, 82, 527.

BÖÖK, J. A. (1951) Quoted by Mckeown, T., and Record, R. G. (1960).

COFFEY, V. P., and JESSOP, W. J. E. (1957) Quoted by Giroud, A. (1960).

CONSUL, B. N., and KULSHRESTHA, O. P. (1965) Orbital meningocele, *Brit. J. Ophthal.*, 49, 374.

DAVIS, C. H., JR., and ALEXANDER, E., JR. (1959) Congenital naso-frontal encephalomeningoceles and teratoma. Review of seven cases, *J. Neurosurg.*, **16**, 365.

DEKABAN, A. (1959) *Neurology of Infancy*, Baltimore, Md., p. 181.

FISHER, R. G., UIHLEIN, A., and KEITH, H. M. (1952) Spina bifida and cranium bifidum. Study of 530 cases, *Proc. Mayo Clin.*, 27, 33.

GHOSH, S., and BALI, L. (1963) Congenital malformations in the newborn, *Indian J. Child Hlth*, Vol. 12, No. 2 448–452.

GIROUD, A. (1960) Causes and morphogenesis of anencephaly, in *Congenital Malformation: A Ciba Foundation Symposium*, London, pp. 199–212.

INGRAHAM, F. D., and MATSON, D. D. (1954) *Neurosurgery of Infancy and Childhood*, Springfield, Ill., p. 456.

INGRAHAM, F. D., and SWAN, H. (1943) Spina bifida and cranium bifidum—a survey of 546 cases, *New Engl. J. Med.*, 228, 559.

KAHN, E. A. (1956) Quoted as a personal communication by Simpkiss and Lowe (1961) *Arch. Dis. Childh.*, **36**, 404–6.

KAHN, E. A., and LEMMEN, L. J. (1952) Unusual congenital anomalies of neurosurgical interest in infants and children, *J. Neurosurg.*, **9**, 59.

KHANNA, K. K., and PRASAD, L. S. N. (1967) Congenital malformations in the new-born, *Indian J. Pediat.*, 34, 63.

LAMY, M., and FREZAL, J. (1959) Quoted by Giroud, A. (1960).

LECK, I. (1966) Changes in the incidence of neural-tube defect, *Lancet*, ii, 791.

LORBER, J. (1961) Systematic ventriculographic studies in infants born with meningomyelocele and encephalocele. The incidence and development of hydrocephalus, *Arch. Dis. Childh.*, **36**, 381.

MCKEOWN, T., and RECORD, R. G. (1960) Malformations in a population observed for five years after birth, in *Congenital Malformation: A Ciba Foundation Symposium*, London, pp. 2–16.

MEALEY, J., DZENITIS, A. J., and HOCKEY, A. A. (1970) The prognosis of encephaloceles, *J. Neurosurg.*, 32, 209.

MITTAL, V. K., and GREWAL, R. S. (1969) Congenital anomalies in neonates, *Indian J. Pediat.*, 36, 356.

MORTADA, A., and EL-TORACI, I. (1960) Orbital meningo-encephalocele and exophthalmos, *Brit. J. Ophthal.*, 44, 309.

NEEL, J. V. (1958) Quoted by McKeown, T., and Record, R. G. (1960).

NORMAN, A. P. (1963) *Congenital Abnormalities in Infancy*, Oxford, p. 21.

ODEKU, E. L. (1967) Congenital malformations of the cerebrospinal axis seen in Western Nigeria: the African child with 'encephalocele', *Int. Surg.*, 48, 52.

PAHWA, J. M., and PATNEY, H. L. (1963) Anterior meningo-encephalocele with a report of three cases, *J. All-India ophthal. Soc.*, 11, 100.

PENROSE, L. S. (1957) Quoted by Giroud, A. (1960).

PENROSE, L. S. (1960) Genetical cause of malformations and the search for their origins, in *Congenital Malformations: A Ciba Foundation Symposium*, London, p. 22.

PLEYDELL, M. J. (1960) Anencephaly and other congenital abnormalities. An epidemiological study in Northamptonshire, *Brit. med. J.*, 1, 309.

RAMAMURTHI, B. (1970) Personal communication.

RUSONOVA, A. A. (1967) Surgical treatment of anterior encephalocele, *Khirurgiya* (*Mosk.*), 6, 67.

SAIFULLAH, S., CHANDRA, R. K., PATHAK, I. C., and DHALL, G. I. (1967) Congenital malformations in new-born. A prospective longitudinal study. A preliminary report on 1 000 consecutive births, *Indian Pediat.*, 4, 251.

SCHWIDDE, J. T. (1952) Spina bifida: survey of 225 encephaloceles and myelomeningoceles, *Amer. J. Dis. Child.*, 84, 35.

SIMPKISS, M., and LOWE, A., (1961) Congenital abnormalities in the African new-born, *Arch. Dis. Childh.*, **36**, 404–6.

STRANDBERG, B. (1949) Cephalocele of posterior part of orbit, *Arch. Ophthal.*, 42, 254.

SUWANWELA, C., and HONGSAPRABHAS, C. (1966) Fronto-ethmoidal encephalomeningocele, *J. Neurosurg.*, 25, 172.

SUWANWELA, C., HONGSPRABHAS, C., SRIKASIDUL, S., SUKABOTE, C., SUWANWELA, N., and CHIENPRADIT, K. (1969) Frontoethmoidal encephalomeningocoele, *Chula. med. J.*, 14, 179.

TANDON, P. N. (1966) Meningoencephalocele, *Neurology* (*India*), 14, 161.

TANDON, P. N. (1970) Meningoencephaloceles, *Acta neurol. scand.*, 46, 369.

TANDON, P. N., RAO, M. A. P., PATHAK, S. N., and DAS, B. S. (1970) *Use of I^{131}-labelled Human Serum Albumin in the Scanning of CSF Pathways*, paper presented at the Second Annual Conference of the Society of Nuclear Medicine, 23 October, New Delhi.

WACKER, M. N. (1963) Congenital abnormalities. A survey of 296 cases occurring in a 10-year period, *Amer. J. Obstet. Gynec.*, 86, 310.

WEINMAN, D. (1970) Personal communication.

10 The Infantile Tremor Syndrome

P. N. TANDON and P. C. BAJPAI

A clinical syndrome affecting infants between the ages of 6 to 24 months and characterized by a sudden onset of moderately coarse tremors, with a frequency of 6 to 12 cycles per second, associated with a preceding developmental retardation, apathy and hypokinesia, has been described under different names by a number of workers in India during the past decade (Pohowalla *et al.*, 1960; Bajpai *et al.*, 1965, 1968 *a* and *b*; Kaul, Prasan, and Chowdhry, 1963; Sachdeva, Manchanda, and Lal, 1965; Garg and Srivastav 1969; Mathur *et al.*, 1969). In spite of some minor differences in the various reports, it is generally agreed that the salient clinical features are sufficiently characteristic to merit its acceptance as a clinical syndrome seen in all parts of India. These cases cannot be classified with any of the commonly accepted clinical states characterized by tremors, and they have not been reported from outside India. They do not much resemble the encephalitis tremens of Wright and Morley (1958), the new tremor syndrome of Wilson, Zigas, and Gajdusek (1959), kuru (Gajdusek and Zigas, 1957; Klatzo, Gajdusek and Zigas, 1959), or the kwashiorkor recovery state described by Kahn (1954), and Kahn and Falcke (1956).

In the absence of any precise knowledge of the aetiology we have preferred to label this condition as the 'infantile tremor syndrome' taking into consideration the two constant features—the age of the patients and the tremors.

CLINICAL FEATURES

The clinical features described are based upon a personal study of 212 cases of this syndrome seen over the past 10 years.

Age Incidence

The average age of these patients was 13 months with a minimum of 5 months and a maximum of 30 months. This is in agreement with all other reported series.

Sex

Males were affected almost twice as frequently as females.

Family History

All these patients belonged to the lower socio-economic group. No history of significant neurological disease was available in the families. Familial incidence was not observed, with one solitary exception; no two cases were reported from the same family.

Birth History

Most of these children had a full-term, normal delivery. Only occasionally was prematurity recorded. History of birth trauma or its suggestive features was not elicited in any of the patients.

Post-natal History

Failure to attain the expected milestones of psychomotor development prior to the onset of disease was a common finding in these patients. On the basis of a modified Gesell's scale for mental assessment, a little over half the patients (54·1 per cent) were considered grossly retarded, while only 47 could be regarded as normal. The remaining 46 were adjudged as being borderline. The failure of psychomotor development was an insidious process and it was difficult to ascertain the time of its onset. Onset of retardation preceded the development tremors by 6 to 16 weeks.

Past Illness

Besides common ailments of infancy, such as gastro-intestinal and/or respiratory infections, no significant past illness was recorded in these infants.

Seasonal Incidence

The maximum number of patients were admitted in the hot summer months of April, May and June. Isolated cases were seen throughout the year. FIGURE 10.1 shows the seasonal incidence of this disease.

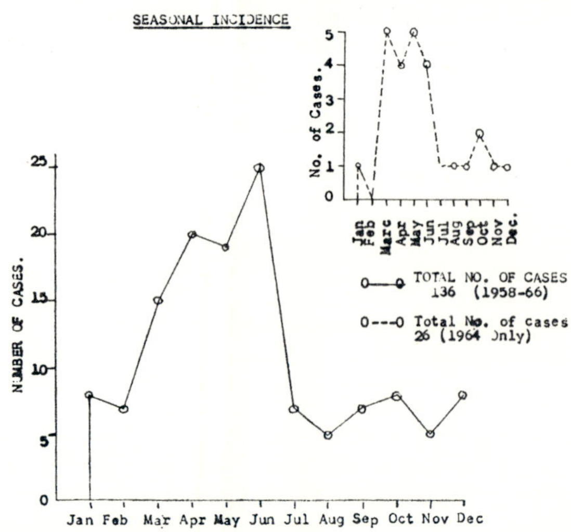

FIG. 10.1. Graph showing seasonal incidence of infantile tremor syndrome.

Presenting Symptoms

The presenting symptoms of 212 patients are summarized in TABLE 10.1. The most constant symptom was tremors. The onset of the tremors was invariably abrupt, a dramatic event in the illness. The parents would date the onset of the illness to appearance of the tremors even though it was apparent on careful interrogation that they had observed an insidious and progressive developmental regression over a few weeks prior to the onset of the tremors. Fever, simultaneous with the development of tremors or in some instances preceding it, was reported in a little over one-half (52·3 per cent) of the patients. Some other children developed fever during the course of the hospital stay, usually associated with an intercurrent respiratory tract infection. Other presenting symptoms were infrequent and inconstant.

Table 10.1

Presenting Symptoms

(Total number of cases 212)

Presenting Symptoms	*No. of Cases*	*Percentage*
1. Tremors on admission	198	93·4
2. Fever	107	50·4
3. Cough	54	25·4
4. Listlessness and lethargy	70	33·0
5. Diarrhoea	26	12·2
6. Pallor	53	25·0
7. Pigmentation	33	15·5
8. Rolling up of eyeballs	11	5·2
9. Oedema	8	3·8
10. Dyspnoea	15	7·1
11. Excessive sleep	14	6·6

Physical Examination

The majority of these children looked apparently well-built for their age. In spite of the fact that these children belonged to a low socio-economic group, significant malnutrition was infrequent. The incidence of overt malnutrition was between 9·5 per cent and 10·8 per cent in the various reported series. Only 31 of our 212 patients (14·6 per cent) were noted to have clinical evidence of some vitamin deficiency, while eight had nutritional oedema.

Characteristically, the children were plump and well-covered [PLATE 20a]. The majority were, however, pale and anaemic. An open mouth, vacant expressionless look, light-coloured sparse silky hair, pallor and plumpness of the face constitute the characteristic facies of the syndrome [PLATE 20b]. So typical is this physiognomy that on a number of occasions it has been possible to predict the impending onset of the tremors on the basis of these features. Hyperpigmentation of the skin, chiefly in the peripheral parts of the limbs, was observed in approximately one-fifth of these patients. Dark patches in the oral mucous membrane were seen in three instances. Sometimes a venocapillary dilatation, giving a honeycomb reticulation of the skin, was seen on the thighs and lower abdomen.

The patients maintained full consciousness throughout the illness but listlessness and apathy were dominant and constant features especially in the early stages of the disease. Paucity of spontaneous movements, lack of interest in their surroundings and poor response to colourful objects were the manifestations of a psychomotor regression so characteristic of the disease. As mentioned earlier this often preceded the onset of tremors, and a reversal of this to normality heralded the remission of tremors.

The tremors were generalized in 80 per cent of the children. In the rest one or more parts of the body were involved in various combinations [TABLE 10.2]. The upper limbs were almost always involved. In the face, they were most marked in the perioral region and around the eyes. Tremulousness of the voice was noted when the child cried.

Table 10.2

Distribution of Tremors

S. No.	*Distribution of Tremors*	*No. of Cases*	
1.	*Generalized* (face + four limbs and four limbs without face involvement)	169	
2.	*Localized*	43	
	(a) Half of the body		*13*
	(b) One limb		*2*
	(c) Both upper limbs		*20*
	(d) Both lower limbs		*1*
	(e) Face alone or face + no limb		*7*
	Total	*212*	

The tremors varied in intensity but were generally fast and of high amplitude. Their rate varied from 6 to 12 cycles per second [PLATE 20c]. In the same child the rate and the amplitude may vary from one limb to another. At rest they were present nearly constantly but were absent during sleep. Focal or generalized myoclonic jerks or choreiform movements were observed in a few instances along with the tremors.

Focal neurological deficit was rarely seen either during the acute illness or in the follow-up period. One patient had hemiparesis. In a few infants (29 out of 212) a posture like a 'bird with wings spread out' was observed. This consisted of abduction of the arms to approximately 90 degrees at the shoulders, full flexion at the elbows and wrists and pronation of the forearms. The hand showed ulnar deviation while the fingers were flexed at all joints. This attitude remained unchanged despite the change in the position of the child. It persisted throughout the illness for a variable time after the complete disappearance of tremors.

Muscle power, nutrition and tone were normal in the majority of infants. Forty-seven children, including 29 with the peculiar posture described above, had a plastic rigidity of the upper limbs. Hypotonia has also been described in some cases. Superficial and deep tendon reflexes were generally normal and no sensory loss was detected.

During the acute stage of the disease it was not possible to test for coordination owing to the paucity of spontaneous or induced motor activity. However, in some cases, during recovery, incoordination on attempted movements was observed.

THE COURSE OF THE DISEASE

On the basis of the history, physical examination and follow-up, the course of the illness can be divided into three stages: the 'pretremor' phase, 'tremor' phase, and the 'post-tremor' phase.

The pretremor phase is characterized by a psychomotor regression, pallor and sometimes a tremulous voice. In some cases there may be a pyrexial illness though the fever is seldom high. It was possible to recognize some of the potential cases of infantile tremor syndrome from the facies and a combination of the above signs.

The tremor phase usually starts in an acute manner. There is rapid evolution of the disease at this stage, the full-blown picture being established within a few days. The condition then remains stationary for a varying length of time, when the child starts to manifest spontaneous recovery. In the patients who were followed fully until there was complete remission of tremors, the average duration of this phase was 43·4 days with a minimum of 3 days and a maximum of 400 days. The disappearance of tremors is not as abrupt as their onset. The tremors subside gradually in amplitude and severity and then become intermittent, persisting for a longer period in one or two extremities than in the rest of the body.

The post-tremor phase often overlaps with the tremor-phase, in which the child becomes more active and mentally alert. The patient starts to take interest in his surroundings, attempts to play with toys, turns in bed and takes feeds better, even while the tremors persist. The mental state shows evidence of progressive improvement and the disease appears to have a self-limiting course. We have so far seen no case in which the tremors persisted indefinitely. The other features of the disease also regress and the physical growth of the child continues unaffected.

LABORATORY INVESTIGATIONS

Anaemia has been one of the most constant abnormalities. Eighty per cent of the children were found to be anaemic; in nearly half the patients the haemoglobin was below 8 g per cent and in only 20 per cent was it above 10 g per cent. Bone-marrow examination in 104 patients revealed a normoblastic hyperplasia in all except 11 who had a megaloblastic reaction. Serum vitamin B_{12} level was estimated in 20 cases of typical tremor syndrome. None of the infants had a serum vitamin B_{12} level below 100 μg per ml, which is regarded as significant of a vitamin B_{12} deficiency state (Bajpai *et al.*, 1968 *b*).

Routine examination of blood, urine, stool, serum protein, serum albumin and blood sugar failed to reveal any abnormality. Only 8 patients had hypo-albuminaemia. VDRL was negative in all. Tuberculin test was positive in twenty infants. In none of our patients did we find any abnormality of CSF. Tests for phenylpyruvic acid in urine, liver functions, and liver biopsy were carried out in a number of cases and were consistently normal.

Electroencephalography (EEG) could be done only in a small number of cases. Nearly half of these had an abnormal EEG; generally the abnormality was diffuse but frequently it was more marked on one side. Most of the abnormal records showed multifocal or diffuse epileptiform activity [PLATE 20d].

Roentgen examination of the skull revealed no abnormality. However, pneumoencephalography performed in 43 patients revealed significant abnormality in the majority. This consisted of central, cortical or global atrophy of varying degree [TABLE 10.3]. Evan's ratio estimated to evaluate the central atrophy suggested severe atrophy in 5 cases, moderate in 13 and mild in 15. Excessive subarachnoid air in the sulci indicative of cortical atrophy was observed in 33 out of the 43 cases. The abnormality was diffuse in eight, and seen only in the frontal or frontoparietal region in the remaining. An interesting observation was the occurrence of unilateral central and/or cortical atrophy in three cases with typical tremors restricted to the contralateral side of the body [PLATE 21a].

Table 10.3
Analysis of Pneumoencephalograms
(Total number of cases 43)

Evan's Ratio	*No. of Cases*	*Remark*
Below 0·25	7	Normal
0·25–0·29	15	Mild central atrophy
0·30–0·35	13	Moderate central atrophy
Above 0·35	5	Severe central atrophy
Difficult to assess	3	Unsatisfactory for measurement

Brain Biopsy

In spite of the limitations inherent in a small brain biopsy, obtained through a trephine opening from the frontal region it is significant to note that 70 per cent of cases showed evidence of inflammation involving the meninges, brain or both [TABLE 10.4]. Parenchymatous inflammatory response was very sparse and restricted to small foci of perivascular infiltration. The inflammation was never very acute or intense. Another frequent finding in brain biopsies was a significant degree of astrogliosis, with hypertrophy of astrocytes and increased subpial, perivascular and pericellular glial fibres [PLATE 21b].

Table 10.4
Analysis of Biopsies
(Total number of cases 34)

Finding	*No. of Cases*
Meningeal infiltration with inflammatory cells	9
Meningeal and perivascular parenchymatous infiltration	5
Parenchymatous perivascular infiltration alone	5
Astrocytosis or gliosis	11
1. In association with evidence of inflammation	*6*
2. In association with myelin loss	*3*
3. Without any associated abnormality	*2*
Myelin loss or reduction	6
No abnormality seen	10

TREATMENT

There is no specific treatment for this condition. Oral or parenteral iron is administered to correct anaemia. Blood transfusion may be required for a severely anaemic child. Intercurrent infection is treated with appropriate antibiotics. Nutritional requirements are assessed and supplemented, if found deficient. Administration of vitamins B_{12} or B_6 has not proved to be helpful in altering the course of illness. Phenobarbitone and *Dilantin Sodium* are administered to children manifesting focal seizures.

PROGNOSIS

The disease tends to run a self-limiting course, seldom resulting in any physical disability. Only one child had residual hemiparesis, while some developed focal or generalized seizures in the follow-up period. The incidence of mental retardation was, however, very high. In a small series of cases followed up for an average of 4 years, a comparative evaluation of pre-illness and follow-up developmental quotient (DQ) and/or intelligence quotient (IQ) revealed that 81·5 per cent were found to have deteriorated. Undoubtedly, occasional children escape unaffected and some are capable of normal intellectual attainments.

The disease is only rarely fatal, and mortality is mainly due to some intercurrent infection.

DISCUSSION

An analysis of our 212 cases and an additional 267 cases reported by others leaves little doubt about the existence of a well-defined clinical syndrome which has so far been reported only from India. The syndrome is characterized by a sudden onset of high amplitude, fast tremors, usually generalized but often restricted to some part of the body, affecting infants mostly between the ages of 6 and 24 months. The majority of these infants appear well-covered, often plump, only a few manifesting overt malnutrition. Light-coloured, sparse and fine hair and mental retardation antedate the onset of tremors in many instances. A varying period of developmental regression, apathy and hypokinesia preceded and accompanied the tremors. Fever preceding and/or accompanying the tremors, skin pigmentation, respiratory tract infection, or gastro-intestinal upsets are frequent features. Except for a moderate degree of anaemia, routine laboratory investigations failed to reveal any abnormality in blood, urine, stool or CSF. Pneumoencephalography demonstrated significant cerebral atrophy in most of the cases thus investigated. Brain biopsy suggested an inflammatory pathology in nearly two-thirds of the cases submitted to this procedure (Bajpai *et al.*, 1971). Visiting colleagues from abroad who had seen these patients in India, and discussions at International Congress (Tandon, Bajpai, and Misra, 1967, 1969), where we presented our experience, would confirm our suspicion that identical cases have not been observed elsewhere.

In spite of a general awareness of this condition among paediatricians and neurologists in India, the aetiopathogenesis of the syndrome remains uncertain. There has been no post-mortem study on any of the fatal cases. Until recently there has been a paucity of objective evidence in favour of or against any of the postulated aetiological factors, i.e. malnutrition or infection. A history of administration of drugs or indigenous herbal medicines was not available in any of the patients.

Considering the wide prevalence of malnutrition in children of this age-group in India, it is natural that a number of workers tend to implicate it in most disease states of unknown aetiology. Practically all reported cases have been confined to children from the lower socio-economic group. The disease is also restricted to the nutritionally vulnerable age. The dietetic history of these infants frequently revealed inadequacy, with a large number still breast-fed at the time of onset of the disease even though they were well past the age of weaning. The frequent findings of mild to moderate anaemia, light-coloured hair and skin pigmentation added to the suspicion that a single or polyvalent nutrient deficiency, or imbalanced nutrition was responsible for this syndrome. Jadhav *et al.* (1962) ascribed it to primary deficiency of vitamin B_{12}. Our studies (Bajpai *et al.*, 1968 *a* and *b*) as well as those of Kaul, Prasan, and Chowdhry (1963) and Sachdev, Manchanda, and Lal (1965) failed to substantiate this. A therapeutic trial with vitamin B_{12} did not alter the course and duration of the tremors. Furthermore, administration of vitamin B_{12} in the pretremor phase has been shown to be ineffective in preventing the progression of these cases to the fully-fledged tremor syndrome.

Mathur *et al.* (1969) have attributed this condition to protein-calorie malnutrition. They reported normal or low total plasma proteins and consistently lower serum albumin in all the 30 cases studied by them. We have found this abnormality in only eight out of the 108 cases thus investigated. It may be mentioned that in some of the cases reported by Mathur *et al.* (1969), the clinical picture remained unaltered even after reversal of the serum chemistry to normal.

Probably influenced by the publication of Kahn (1954), from Johannesburg, an imbalanced nutritional state leading to a biochemical derangement was held responsible for this condition by Sachdev, Manchanda and Lal (1965). Kahn (1954) reported a neurological syndrome in infants recovering from severe malnutrition 1 to 8 weeks after being put on an adequate diet. The syndrome was characterized by irritability, coarse parkinsonian tremors, cogwheel rigidity of the affected limbs, disturbance in posture and grossly exaggerated deep tendon reflexes. The clinical picture of these cases does have some superficial similarity to that of our patients. Kahn (1954) originally suggested that an imbalanced repair process produced by a diet rich in protein but deficient in vitamins was responsible for the condition of his patients. However, 2 years later, Kahn and Falcke (1956) could no longer consider this hypothesis as tenable.

Pohowalla *et al.* (1960), from Indore, described this condition under the title of 'infantile meningo-encephalitic syndrome', assuming an infective aetiology. However, no objective evidence of infection was provided by them and they could not rule out the possibility of an undetermined metabolic disorder.

A frequent history of pyrexia preceding or accompanying the onset of tremors, the suggestion of a seasonal incidence (the maximum number of cases are seen in the months of April, May and June when other infective illnesses are very frequent in our country), the age of the patients, the restriction of the disease to a lower socio-economic group, and the self-limiting course suggest the possibility of an infective illness. Consistently normal CSF findings tended to detract from such an aetiology. However, the results of our study of brain biopsy (Bajpai *et al.*, 1971) point strongly in this direction. Unequivocal, though variable, evidence of meningeal and/or parenchymatous inflammatory lesion was observed in 70 per cent of cases. The absence of findings in the remaining cases may be due to the limitations imposed by a small biopsy, or else the disease may have burnt out by the time the biopsy was performed. Undoubtedly, the abnormalities seen in a limited biopsy specimen are only a pointer to the more widespread pathology which will only be elucidated when a complete autopsy is achieved.

The striking association of astrocytic proliferation and hypertrophy, with or without non-specific meningeal or parenchymatous leucocytic infiltration, suggests a possible viral aetiology. Greenfield and Meyer (1963), and Zlotnic (1968) have pointed out that in some encephalitides of viral aetiology the degree of astrocytic reaction may be out of proportion to the amount of neuronal damage. In slow virus infections like kuru and scrapie (Hadlow, 1961), astrocytic hyperplasia may be the only abnormality in the absence of any leucocytic infiltration. Even though the clinical course of the disease is unlike that of the accepted slow virus infections, on the basis of a brief review of our material, neither Gajdusek (1969) nor Field (1969) could rule out such a possibility. Detailed virus studies would be necessary to prove or disprove it.

The possibility of the co-existence of malnutrition and infection, either preceding the other, also needs to be considered. Failure to thrive leading to overt malnutrition has been reported to occur in primary brain atrophies in infants.

References

BAJPAI, P. C., MISRA, P. K., TANDON, P. N., NIGAM, G. J., VORA, V. C., and MALAVIYA, A. (1968 *a*) Serum vitamin B_{12} in 'infantile tremor syndrome', *Indian J. med. Res.*, 56, 1398–1405.

BAJPAI, P. C., MISRA, P. K., and TANDON, P. N. (1968 *b*) Further observations on 'infantile tremor syndrome' *Indian Pediat.*, 5, 297–307.

BAJPAI, P. C., MISRA, P. K., TANDON, P. N., WAHAL, K. M., and NEWTON, G. (1971) Brain biopsy in 'infantile tremor syndrome', *Indian J. med. Res.*, 59, 413–18.

BAJPAI, P. C., TANDON, P. N., SHARMA, N. L., and MISRA, P. K. (1965) Infantile tremor syndrome, *Acta neurol. scand.*, 41, 473–86.

FIELD, E. G. (1969) Personal communication.

GAJDUSEK, D. C. (1969) Personal communication.

GAJDUSEK, D. C., and ZIGAS, V. (1957) Degenerative disease of the central nervous system in New Guinea. The endemic occurrence of 'Kuru' in the native population, *New Engl. J. Med.*, 257, 974–8.

GARG, B. K., and SRIVASTAV, J. R. (1969) 'Infantile tremor syndrome', *Indian J. Pediat.*, 36, 213–18.

GREENFIELD, J. G., and MEYER, A. (1963) in *Greenfield's Neuropathology* 2nd ed., London.

JADHAV, M., WEBB, J. K. G., VAISHNAVA, S., and BAKER, S. J. (1962) Vitamin B_{12} deficiency in Indian infants—a clinical syndrome, *Lancet*, ii, 903–8.

KAHN, E. A. (1954) A neurological syndrome in infants recovering from malnutrition, *Arch Dis. Childh.*, 29, 256–61.

KAHN, E. A., and FALCKE, H. C. (1956) A syndrome simulating encephalitis affecting children recovering from malnutrition (kwashiorkor), *Pediatrics*, 49, 37–45.

KAUL, K. K., PRASAN, N., and CHOWDHRY, R. M. (1963) Some clinical observations and impressions on a syndrome of tremors in infants from India, *J. Pediat.*, 63, 1158–160.

KLATZO, I., GAJDUSEK, D. C., and ZIGAS, V. (1959) Pathology of kuru, *Lab. Invest.*, 8, 799–847.

MATHUR, G. P., DAYAL, R. S., PRASAD, R., and MATHUR, S. (1969) Tremors, mental and physical retardation, light coloured hair and anaemia in malnourished children, *Indian Pediat.*, 6, 483–7.

POHOWALLA, J. N., KAUL, K. K., BHANDARI, N. R., and SINGH, S. D. (1960) Infantile meningoencephalitic syndrome, *Indian J. Pediat.*, 27, 49–54.

SACHDEV, K. K., MANCHANDA, S. S., and LAL, H. (1965) The syndrome of tremors, mental regression and anaemia in infants and young children, *Indian Pediat.*, 2, 239–51.

TANDON, P. N., BAJPAI, P. C., and MISRA, P. K. (1967) *Infantile Tremor Syndrome*, paper presented at the Joint Conference of the Neurological Society of India and the Middle East Neurosurgical Society, December 1967, New Delhi.

TANDON, P. N., BAJPAI, P. C., MISRA, P. K. (1969) *Infantile Tremor Syndrome. A Review of Ten Years Study*, paper presented at the World Congress of Neurological Sciences, September 1969, New York.

WILSON, K., ZIGAS, V., and GAJDUSEK, D. C. (1959) New tremor syndrome, *Lancet* ii, 699–702.

WRIGHT, I., and MORLEY, D. C. (1958) Encephalitis tremens, *Lancet*, ii, 871–3.

ZLOTNIK, I. (1968) The reaction of astrocytes to acute virus infections of the central venous system. *Brit. J. exp. Path.*, 555–564.

11 Painful Ophthalmoplegia

N. T. MATHEW

'Painful ophthalmoplegia' is a self-limiting ophthalmoplegic syndrome, characterized by acute or subacute onset associated with pain, spontaneous remissions, recurrences, and a dramatic response to corticosteroid therapy in the acute stage of the disease. Its synonyms are superior orbital fissure syndrome; superior orbital fissuritis; sphenoidal syndrome; indolent inflammation of the cavernous sinus; Tolosa-Hunt syndrome; and Collier's syndrome. Collier (1921) was probably the first to point out the occurrence of such an entity. Hunt *et al.* (1961) and Smith and Taxdal (1966) reported a few cases of this disease and stressed the importance of recognizing and differentiating it from diabetic ophthalmoplegia, intracavernous carotid aneurysm, and nasopharyngeal tumour infiltrating the base of the skull. They also pointed out the beneficial effect of corticosteroids in this condition. Mathew and Chandy (1970) have given a comprehensive account of this disease from their experience in India. This syndrome of painful ophthalmoplegia is the commonest type of acute ophthalmoplegia in South India, where the incidence of intracranial berry aneurysms is low (Ramamurthi, 1969) and diabetic ophthalmoplegia is rare. Statistics from the Department of Neurological Sciences, Christian Medical College Hospital, Vellore, for a 5-year period between 1965–70 are given in TABLE 11.1

Table 11.1
Christian Medical College Hospital, Vellore: Cases Presenting with Oculomotor Palsy 1965–1970

Disease	*No. of Patients*
Intracranial aneurysms	4
Diabetes	3
Nasopharyngeal carcinoma	3
Tuberculous basal meningitis	12
Painful ophthalmoplegia	30
Uncertain	4
Total	*56*

CLINICAL FEATURES

Sex and Age Incidence

Painful ophthalmoplegia affects both males and females, the sex ratio being roughly 3:1. It has been found to affect both young and old with a range from 8 years to 65 years. Maximum incidence is found in young adults and the middle-aged. Occupation, economic status and nutrition of the patient appear to bear no relationship to the occurrence of painful ophthalmoplegia. Moreover, heredofamilial factors seem to play no part in this disease, unlike the cases reported by Currie (1970).

Onset of Symptoms

Symptoms usually begin with pain unilaterally around the eye, in the retro-orbital region or in a hemicranial distribution. Pain is of a continuous and boring type. It may last for days or weeks before opththalmoplegia appears. Movements of the eyeball become painful at the beginning of the illness in some cases. Diplopia ensues and the majority develop ptosis of varying degree. General constitutional symptoms, malaise and mild fever are noted in occasional cases.

Physical Signs

By the time a patient consults an ophthalmologist, neurologist or neurosurgeon, he has developed diplopia and ocular palsy. This is predominantly a unilateral condition, although the other eye may be affected during a subsequent attack. It is extremely rare to have both eyes affected simultaneously.

Various combinations of involvement of the third, fourth, sixth, ophthalmie division of the fifth nerve, second, and oculosympathetic nerves are seen. Partial or complete paralysis of the extra-ocular muscles supplied by the third nerve is the commonest finding. Ptosis varies in degree from case to case. In some it is total. It is interesting to note that there is no iridoplegia in most cases in spite of the paralysis of the extra-ocular muscles supplied by the third nerve. Of 30 cases with third nerve involvement studied by the author, 23 had a normal-sized pupil which reacted fairly well to light though not as briskly as on the unaffected side. A cocaine test performed in a few of them by instilling two drops of 10 per cent cocaine solution into both eyes showed poor mydriasis on the affected side, suggesting a lesion of the oculosympathetic nerve.

Paresis of the lateral rectus and superior rectus are also seen, although less frequently than paresis of muscles supplied by the third nerve.

Hypaesthesia and hypalgesia in the distribution of the ophthalmic division of the fifth nerve are seen in about 40 per cent of cases. Corneal sensation may be diminished in these cases. The maxillary division of the fifth nerve is not usually affected. Involvement of the optic nerve is an occasional feature. In the author's experience with 34 cases, nine patients complained of diminished acuity of vision and three patients developed pallor of the disc with attenuation of the arteries suggesting a primary optic atrophy. One patient had an attack of optic neuritis in the opposite eye, 1 month prior to the onset of ophthalmoplegia.

In the acute stage minimal prominence of the eyeball is a frequent finding. Occasionally, the proptosis may be moderate in degree. Usually there is no displacement of the eyeball. Slight periorbital oedema and minimal congestion of the conjunctiva are other less frequent findings. TABLE 11.2 summarizes the physical findings in 34 cases.

Table 11.2

Painful Ophthalmoplegia: Neurological Findings in 34 Cases

Positive Findings	*No. of Patients*
Third nerve lesion (partial or complete)	30
Fourth nerve lesion	15
Sixth nerve lesion	22
Ophthalmic division of fifth nerve (hypoaesthesia or hyperaesthesia)	15
Second nerve including primary optic atrophy	9
Size of the pupil (normal or slightly dilated pupil in the presence of third nerve palsy)	23
Slight periorbital oedema, slight congestion of the conjunctiva	9
Slight proptosis	17

The remaining cranial nerves and the central and peripheral nervous systems are not involved. Moreover, systemic examination reveals nothing specifically abnormal. Five patients out of 34 gave a history of past tuberculosis, and two of these had evidence of a healed lesion in the lungs.

INVESTIGATIONS

Haemoglobin and packed cell volume are within normal limits. White blood corpuscles (WBC) total count shows values usually between 7000/c mm and 11 000/c mm. Moderate eosinophilia (absolute eosinophil count between 1000 and 2400/c mm) may be seen in some cases. There are no abnormal cells in the blood smear. Raised ESR in the range of 20 mm/hr to 60 mm/hr is observed in the acute stage in certain cases. Blood examination for microfilariae was done in 14 cases, of which five were positive for *Microfilaria bancrofti*. No other blood parasite was found.

LE cell test was positive in seven out of 14 cases in which it was performed. Tests for rheumatoid arthritis factor (the Rose-Waaler test) and antinuclear factor were carried out in four patients, and the rheumatoid arthritis factor was found to be significantly positive in two cases, and the antinuclear factor in one case.

The serum protein estimations, serum albumin-globulin ratio, serum protein electrophoresis, serum cholesterol, blood urea, blood sugar, and glucose tolerance tests are all normal. The cerebrospinal fluid (CSF) cell count, biochemistry, CSF protein electrophoresis and colloid mastic reactions are within normal limits. CSF cultures, including those for tuberculous bacilli and fungi, are negative. There is no serological evidence of syphilitic infection. Routine urine examination is normal.

Otorhinolaryngological examination was carried out in all cases and none of them showed evidence of sinusitis or nasopharyngeal growth. Nasopharyngeal biopsy in eight cases showed no evidence of any malignant growth. Temporal artery biopsies performed in seven cases were normal.

X-rays of the skull, including anteroposterior, lateral, and special views for superior orbital fissure and sinuses, showed no abnormality. X-ray of the chest showed evidence of healed pulmonary tuberculosis in two cases, but in others it was normal.

Pneumoencephalogram reveals nothing abnormal in such cases. Carotid angiogram is essentially normal except occasional irregular narrowing of the intracavernous portion of the internal carotid artery, as observed in one of the cases by the author. A similar observation was made by Tolosa (1954) in one case.

COURSE AND TREATMENT

In untreated cases the pain lasts for about 2–4 weeks and then gradually subsides. Pain and concern about the condition of the eye make victims anxious and depressed. The neurological symptoms and signs persist longer, usually up to 3–4 months. The majority of untreated patients show gradual improvement with either complete or partial recovery. An occasional patient may be left with permanent ophthalmoplegia or primary optic atrophy.

Corticosteroid Therapy

Eighteen patients were put on prednisolone, 60 mg daily in divided doses; this was later tapered off and the drug withdrawn after 4 weeks. The effect of steroids is dramatic, and evident in 24–72 hours. In almost all patients pain diminishes in intensity in 24–48 hours and subsides completely within 4–5 days. Ptosis and eye movements show improvement by the third or the fourth day and in most cases movements of the lid and eyeball return to normal within a fortnight. The response to corticosteroids is quick and convincing; it can be used as a therapeutic test before other elaborate and expensive investigations are contemplated (Smith, 1967).

In an occasional case, if prednisolone is not fully effective, other immunosuppressive agents may be tried. In one of my patients who did not respond well to corticosteroid therapy, a 3-week course of oral cyclophosphamide (*Endoxan*), 200 mg daily was tried. The response was adequate and the patient's eye returned to normal by the end of the course.

Table 11.3
Number of Episodes of Ophthalmoplegia

No. of Episodes	*No. of Patients*
Single episode	21
Two episodes	9
Three episodes	4
Total	*34*

Recurrence is a feature of this disease; one-third of the patients had a recurrence. TABLE 11.3 shows the number of episodes of ophthalmoplegia in 34 patients. Recurrence may take place within a few months, or a number of years may elapse before a second attack. Recurrence is usually on the same side but in this series there were instances of contralateral involvement during the subsequent episode. Response to steroid therapy during the second or third episode is as good as in the first attack. No specific factor appeared to be responsible for the recurrences.

DIFFERENTIAL DIAGNOSIS

Clinical examination and investigations on the lines mentioned above rule out conditions which produce ophthalmoplegia such as meningitis, syphilis, intracavernous aneurysm, space-occupying lesions, nasopharyngeal tumours, temporal arteritis, and periostitis of the superior orbital fissure.

Third nerve palsy in painful ophthalmoplegia resembles diabetic ophthalmoplegia which is typically that of a third nerve palsy without iridoplegia. Absence of iridoplegia may be taken as the most useful single feature which distinguishes diabetic ophthalmoplegia and painful ophthalmoplegia from ophthalmoplegia due to aneurysm. Moreover, the presence of overt or latent diabetes helps to distinguish diabetic ophthalmoplegia from the syndrome of painful ophthalmoplegia. It is not certain why the pupils are spared in these conditions. In a case of diabetic ophthalmoplegia Dreyfus, Hakim, and Adam (1957) found focal changes mostly in the central regions of the intracavernous portion of the third nerve, and the sparing of the subepineural fibres was held to explain the absence of iridoplegia.

Ophthalmoplegic migraine can be excluded by the negative history. None of my patients with painful ophthalmoplegia had a history of migraine.

Pseudo-tumour of the orbit must be considered in the differential diagnosis but it is unlikely because in painful ophthalmoplegia the paralysis is neurogenic rather than myogenic. In orbital pseudo-tumours the paralysis is more a myogenic process. The observation by Jellinek (1969) that vertical movement of the eyeball is more frequently affected in pseudo-tumour justifies the above statement. Florid features of chemosis, marked proptosis and displacement of the eyeball, so characteristic of pseudo-tumour, are not found. Ptosis is not a feature of pseudo-tumour oculi. However, it is possible that pseudo-tumour oculi and painful ophthalmoplegia are related disorders.

Endocrine ophthalmopathy also enters into the differential diagnosis but none of the patients showed any symptom or sign of endocrine disturbance either at the time of the disease or on follow-up.

Recurrent cranial nerve palsies described by Symonds (1958) and the polyneuritis cranialis of the Guillain-Barré syndrome (Brain, 1962) are different syndromes. There, the cranial nerve involvement is more widespread; it is not confined to the nerves passing through the superior orbital fissure. CSF protein may be elevated in some cases of polyneuritis cranialis whereas it is normal in painful ophthalmoplegia.

The syndrome of ophthalmoplegia, ataxia and areflexia described by Miller Fisher (1956) need not be considered further because the ophthalmoplegia is the only lesion.

It is evident from TABLE 11.1 that tuberculous basal meningitis is an important cause of cranial nerve palsies in India. Involvement of cranial nerves other than those passing through the superior orbital fissure, the bilateral nature of the involvement, the CSF cellular reaction and raised protein, and culture for tubercle bacilli help in differentiating these cases from painful ophthalmoplegia.

SITE AND PATHOLOGY OF THE LESION

A combination of third nerve, fourth nerve, sixth nerve, oculosympathetic, and the ophthalmic division of the fifth nerve would place the lesion in the posterior part of the orbit or in the superior orbital fissure or anterior part of the cavernous sinus. Occasional involvement of the optic nerve would mean that the lesion is not wholly confined to the cavernous sinus or superior orbital fissure. A frank intra-orbital lesion such as pseudo-tumour oculi, abscess or orbital myositis is unlikely for reasons already stated. A classical cavernous sinus thrombosis is also unlikely because of the absence of chemosis, marked proptosis and venous congestion or papilloedema, and the strictly unilateral nature of the condition even in the acute state. But a different type of lesion is possible in the cavernous sinus or superior orbital fissure, as shown by Tolosa (1954). He demonstrated a granulomatous inflammatory lesion around the carotid artery in the cavernous sinus. The carotid angiogram of his patient showed an irregular narrowing of the intracavernous portion of the carotid artery, similar to one of my cases which I presumed to be due to a similar periarteritic inflammatory lesion. Extensive studies, including carotid angiography and pneumoencephalography, and exploratory surgery in one case, failed to reveal any lesion outside the cavernous sinus. Hunt *et al.* (1961) also had a similar experience with one of their cases which was explored. Until pathological confirmation is obtained we can only assume that our cases are similar pathologically to those described by Tolosa.

AETIOLOGICAL CONSIDERATIONS

In the 34 cases studied, no direct aetiological factor was identified but there were some findings of possible significance:

1. Five patients showed evidence of past tuberculous infection.
2. Five patients out of 14 showed microfilariae in their blood. One patient among them later turned up with filarial fever.
3. Seven out of 14 patients showed positive LE cell phenomenon.
4. Two out of four patients showed a positive Rose-Waaler test.
5. Eosinophilia was noted in 10 patients out of 24.
6. ESR was raised in 13 patients who were seen in the acute states.

There was no evidence of systemic collagen disease in any of the cases. Temporal artery biopsies were negative. These patients therefore cannot be said to suffer from any known collagen disease. The LE cell phenomenon is not specific for systemic lupus erythematosus and it may be positive in conditions with an altered immune mechanism. Tait (1934) described a case in which he considered rheumatoid periostitis of the superior orbital fissure a possibility.

From the clinical history, high ESR, eosinophilia, LE cell phenomenon, positive Rose-Waaler Test in two cases, and dramatic response to steroids, it may be inferred that the pathological process is a result of some immuno-allergic lesion. This may be related to infection or infestation. Whether tuberculosis or filarial infection could be indirectly responsible for the altered immune mechanism is a matter for consideration. Immunological studies using modern techniques may be rewarding.

But certain questions would still have to be answered. Why should a process like this confine itself to the superior orbital fissure or cavernous sinus? Is it some anatomical peculiarity of that region or some other factor which is responsible for this localization? In this context there is a similarity between this syndrome and Bell's palsy, as suggested by Collier (1921).

References

BRAIN, R. (1962) Polyneuritis cranialis, in *Diseases of the Nervous System*, London, p. 731.

COLLIER, J. (1921) Discussion on ocular palsies, *Proc. roy. Soc. Med.*, 14, 10–11.

CURRIE, S., (1970) Familial oculomotor palsy with Bell's palsy, *Brain*, 93, 193–8.

DREYFUS, P. M., HAKIM, S., and ADAM, R. D. (1957) Diabetic ophthalmoplegia, report of a case with post-mortem study and comments on the vascular supply of human oculomotor nerve, *Arch. Neurol. Psychiat.* (*Chic.*), 77, 337–49.

FISHER, C. M. (1956) An unusual variant of acute idiopathic polyneuritis (syndrome of ophthalmoplegia, ataxia, areflexia), *New Engl. J. Med.*, 255, 57.

HUNT, W. E., MEAGHER, J. N., LEFEVER, H. E., and ZEMAN, W. (1961) Painful ophthalmoplegia. Its relation to indolent inflammation of cavernous sinus, *Neurology* (*Minneap.*), 11, 56–62.

JELLINEK, E. H. (1969) The orbital pseudo-tumour syndrome, *Brain*, 92, 35–58.

MATHEW, N. T., and CHANDY, J. (1970) Painful ophthalmoplegia, *J. neurol. Sci.*, 11, 243–56.

RAMAMURTHI, B. (1969) The rarity of bleeding aneurysms in India, *Excerpta med.* (*Aust.*), *Int. Cong. Ser.*, 193, 149.

SMITH, J. L. (1967) *Neuro-ophthalmology*, Vol. III, Symposium of the University of Miami and Bascon Palmer Eye Institute, Saint Louis, p. 10.

SMITH, J. L., and TADAL, D. S. R. (1966) Painful ophthalmoplegia. The Tolosa-Hunt syndrome, *Amer. J. Ophthal.*, 61, 1466–72.

SYMONDS, C. P. (1958) Recurrent multiple cranial nerve palsies, *J. Neurol. Neurosurg. Psychiat.*, 21, 95–101.

TAIT, C. B. V. (1934) Ophthalmoplegia associated with bony changes in the region of sphenoid fissure, *Brit. J. Ophthal.*, 18, 532–5.

TOLOSA, E., (1954) Periateritic lesion of carotid syphon with clinical features of carotid infraclinoidal aneurysm, *J. Neurol. Neurosurg. Psychiat.*, 17, 300–2.

12 Endemic Fluorosis in India

A. H. SIDDIQUI

Fluorine is a non-metallic element of the halogen group and is present in teeth and bone. It is also found in foodstuffs and in drinking-water in areas of endemic fluorosis.

Fluorides, containing fluorine, are widely used in the manufacture of glass and enamel, and the conversion of phosphate into superphosphate, a common fertilizer. Industrial exposure to fluorides and ingestion of water containing them are known to produce a form of osteosclerosis to which the name fluorosis has been given by its Danish discoverers Möller and Gudjonsson (1932). Consumption of inexpensive wines to which sodium fluoride has been added as a preservative produces 'wine fluorosis' (Soriano and Manchon, 1966).

Roholm (1937) described in detail the various aspects of fluorine intoxication. Endemic fluorosis was first reported from India (Shortt *et al.*, 1937), and areas with a high natural content of fluorides in drinking-water have been described by various workers (Pandit *et al.*, 1940 *a* and *b*; Raghavachari and Venkataramanan, 1940; Daver, 1945; Khan and Wig, 1945; Venkateshwarlu, Rao, and Rao, 1952; Murti, Rao, and Venkateshwarlu, 1953; Siddiqui, 1955; Singh *et al.*, 1962 *a* and *b*). Jolly *et al.* (1969) recorded 25 ppm fluoride (25 mg/L) in water, the highest figure reported from India. The disease occurs with varying intensity in Andhra Pradesh, Tamilnadu, Mysore, Punjab and Kerala. Singh *et al.* (1962 *a* and *b*) have calculated that at least one-fourth of the Punjab contains a belt in which the fluoride content of drinking-water is high. This exposes roughly 5 million people to the toxic potentialities of this ion. A larger population is exposed to the risk of fluorine intoxication in Andhra Pradesh and Tamilnadu.

PATHOGENESIS

Fluorine has a marked affinity for the hard tissues and is deposited in the teeth and bones. It combines readily with mineralized tissue in children, being deposited in the permanent teeth during the calcification of the crowns. In adults it is deposited in the skeleton, producing osteosclerosis and the formation of exostoses and osteophytes. Bones subjected to the greatest stress are most affected.

The pathogenesis of the spinal cord lesion in fluorosis is complex and a number of factors are concerned, the most important being compression of the spinal nerves and spinal cord by osteophytes, fluorotic bars or protrusions (Lyth, 1945; Singh *et al.*, 1962 *a* and *b*), and interference with the blood supply which may be temporary or permanent.

Cervical cord compression is likely to occur when the sagittal diameter of the spinal canal is 11 mm or less; the average diameter of the cord in the cervical enlargement is 10 mm. The diameter of the spinal canal is variable; neurological complications are liable to occur when the spinal canal is narrow.

The blood supply of the spinal cord in the cervical region is derived from the anterior spinal and radicular arteries. The radicular arteries running along the cervical roots may be compressed if there is gross narrowing of the intervertebral foramina due to osteophytic outgrowths, or if there is marked root-sleeve fibrosis.

Tetraplegia resulting from sudden compression of the spinal cord in severe flexion or hyperextension of the neck has been described in fluorosis (Singh *et al.*, 1962 *a* and *b*; Siddiqui, 1970). Minor falls may exacerbate the disability.

CLINICAL MANIFESTATIONS

Mottled tooth enamel is one of the earliest, most sensitive and easily distinguishable signs of excessive intake of fluorine in childhood. The condition is largely confined to the permanent teeth, although in areas of high incidence of the disease the deciduous teeth may occasionally be affected. The enamel is abnormally opaque and chalky white. White blotchy areas are usually interspersed with areas of more or less normal enamel—the so-called 'mottling'. In the later years of childhood there are patches or bands of brown or black pigment deposited in the defective enamel. These changes are permanent [PLATE 22b].

Prolonged ingestion of water with a high fluoride content causes skeletal fluorosis in adults. The initial symptom is a recurrent general tingling sensation in the limbs or all over the body. Pain and stiffness next appear in the lumbar region, and later also involve the thoracic and cervical spine. Extension is more painful than flexion. The stiffness increases until the entire spine appears to be one column of bone and the patient develops a 'poker-back' [PLATE 21c]. Later the joints of the limbs become stiff and painful. Bony exostoses can be seen or felt [PLATE 21d]. By this time the individual is between 20 and 40 years of age.

In advanced stages, the patient is wasted and there are usually signs of spinal cord compression with impotence and loss of sphincter control [PLATE 22a]. In the final bed-ridden state mental powers remain unimpaired.

NEUROLOGICAL COMPLICATIONS

Involvement of the nervous system has been reported mostly from India. The earliest description was that of Shortt *et al.* in 1937. Detailed studies were subsequently made by Siddiqui (1955, 1970), Singh *et al.* (1961, 1962 *a* and *b*) Singh and Jolly (1961), Singh, Jolly, and Bansal (1961), Rao and Siddiqui, 1962. Only two cases of neural involvement in fluorosis have been reported from outside India; from the United States (Sauerbrunn, Ryan, and Shaw, 1965) and England (Webb-Peploe and Bradley, 1966).

The severity of the disease is related to the concentration of fluorine in water, to the period of ingestion, to meteorological factors (e.g. temperature) and to the physical strains to which the patients are subjected (Siddiqui, 1955). The lowest concentration of the fluorine in water causing skeletal fluorosis with tetraplegia was 1·35 ppm (Siddiqui 1970); with paraplegia it was 1·2 ppm (Singh *et al.* 1962 *b*).

The cardinal clinical manifestations are paraesthesiae and patchy sensory loss, weakness of the limbs, wasting of the small muscles of the hands, fibrillary twitchings of muscles, and spasticity of the lower limbs with loss of sphincter control.

The physical signs depend on the anatomical factors of maximum narrowing of the spinal canal and the vertebral foramina, and on whether the compression is chiefly at one site or several. The cervical vertebrae are relatively less affected than those of the dorsal and lumbar regions, so that neurological cervical syndromes are less severe. Inversion of the radial reflex is not uncommon. The clinical picture then resembles that of cervical spondylosis. The pathogenic mechanisms of root and cord compression are similar, although cord compression is more characteristic of fluorosis and root compression of cervical spondylosis.

When the skull is involved there may be some perceptive deafness. This probably results from pressure on the eighth nerve in the sclerosed and narrowed auditory canal (Rao and Siddiqui, 1962). Hearing loss is for higher frequencies [FIG. 12.1]. It commences at 3000 cps and is marked (up to 60 decibels) at 8000 cps. Bone conduction is affected more than air conduction.

RADIOGRAPHY

Radiological changes in skeletal fluorosis are quite characteristic and diagnostic. Osteosclerosis is observed throughout the skeleton with the most pronounced changes in the spine and pelvis. Osteosclerosis and irregular osteophyte formation involve the body of the vertebra, its transverse and spinous processes, pedicles and lamina [PLATE 23a]. The beak-like lipping and chalky-white, ground-glass appearance of the entire vertebral column provide a characteristic appearance. There is calcification of the intervertebral ligaments [PLATE 22c].

In the pelvis there is calcification of the sacrotuberous and sacrospinous ligaments.

In the limbs irregular periosteal bone formation occurs involving the tendons, fasciae, and muscular attachments including the interosseous membranes of the forearms and legs and the deltoid tuberosity. Calcification of the interosseous membrane of the forearm is a very helpful radiological sign, especially when osteosclerosis is slight [PLATE 22c].

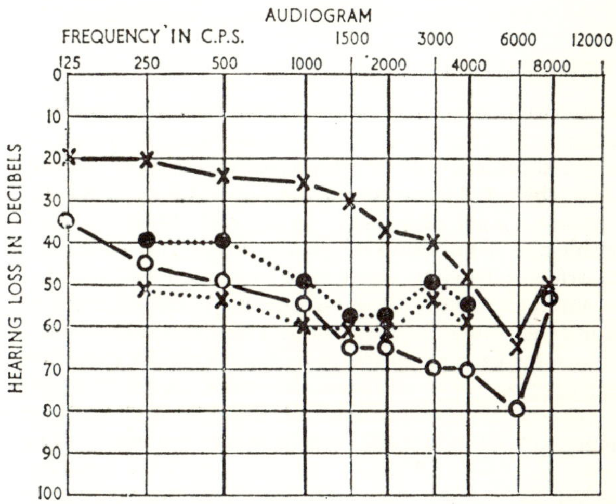

FIG. 12.1. Endemic fluorosis. Audiogram in a patient with bilateral perceptive deafness.

BIOCHEMISTRY

In skeletal fluorosis the serum calcium and inorganic phosphorus levels are normal, the alkaline phosphatase is elevated, and the calcium balance is markedly positive (Srikantia and Siddiqui 1965; Rao, Siddiqui, and Srikantia, 1968).

Fluorine estimation in drinking-water, blood, urine and bone ash are diagnostic laboratory procedures adopted for the confirmation of diagnosis. Urinary fluorine estimation is one of the most important investigations because it bears a linear relationship with intake.

Osteophytosis of the spine and calcification of the spinal ligaments make a lumbar puncture difficult [PLATE 22d]. There are no special changes in the composition of the spinal fluid, but in advanced cases with cord compression, the manometric and chemical abnormalities are similar to those observed in other causes of spinal cord compression.

PROGNOSIS

The dental and skeletal changes are permanent but they may be arrested when the individual leaves an endemic area, although he may continue to excrete fluorine in his urine at high levels for many years (Siddiqui, 1955).

DIAGNOSIS

If a patient comes from an endemic area or has left such an area and complains of pain and stiffness of the spine and the joints, fluorosis should be suspected. Mottling of the teeth, bony exostoses, osteosclerosis, osteophytosis, and calcification of the ligaments of the spine, tendon insertions, and interosseous membrane of the forearm are the principal features of fluorosis. Elevated blood and urinary fluorine levels are diagnostic.

TREATMENT

Preventive aspects of endemic fluorisis are very important as there is no specific treatment. A supply of water containing sub-mottling concentration of fluoride (less than 0·8 ppm to 0·8 mg/L) is ideal. Venkateshwarlu, Rao, and Rao (1952) and Siddiqui (unpublished data) found 0·9 to 1 pmm (0·9 to 1·0 mg/L) fluoride in drinking-water to be associated with mottled enamel; almost the same amount that is incorporated in domestic water supplies in Europe and the United States for the prevention of dental caries. In India hot weather not only increases the water intake but also increases the concentration of fluoride, and leads to ingestion of abnormal amounts of sediment. The optimal concentration of fluoride could be achieved either by drilling tube-wells or by defluoridation of water.

In cases of spinal compression laminectomy has been tried with favourable results, although there is a high mortality (Agarwal and Singh, 1964; Siddiqui, 1970).

References

AGARWAL, H. D., and SINGH, H. (1964) Management of fluorotic myelopathy, *Singapore med. J.*, 5, 208.

DAVER, M. B. (1945) Occurrence of fluorosis in endemic form in Hyderabad state, *Indian med. Gaz.*, 30, 332.

JOLLY, S. S., SINGH, I. D., PRASED, S., SHARMA, R., SINGH, B. M., and MATHUR, O. C. (1969) An epidemiological study of endemic fluorosis in Punjab, *Indian J. med. Res.*, 57, 1333.

KHAN, Y. M., and WIG, K. L. (1945) Chronic endemic fluorosis (with bone affections) in the Punjab, *Indian med. Gaz.*, 80, 429

LYTH, O. (1946) Endemic fluorosis in Kweichow, China, *Lancet*, i, 233.

MÖLLER, P. F., and GUDJONSSON, S. V. (1932) Massive fluorosis of bones and ligaments, *Acta radiol.* (*Stockh.*), 13, 269.

MURTI, G. V. S., RAO, D. N., and VENKATESHWARLU, P. (1953) Spinal compression due to skeletal fluorosis, *J. Indian med. Ass.*, 22, 396.

PANDIT, C. G., RAGHVACHARI, T. N. S., RAO, D. S., and KRISHANA MURTI, V. (1940 *a*) Endemic fluorosis in South India, *Indian J. med. Res.*, 28, 533.

PANDIT, C. G., and NARAYAN RAO, D. (1940 *b*) Endemic fluorosis in South India, *Indian J. med. Res.*, 28, 559.

RAGHAVACHARI, T. N. S., and VENKATARAMANAN, K. (1940) Endemic fluorosis in South India, *Indian J. med. Res.*, 28, 517.

RAO, B. S. N., SIDDIQUI, A. H., and SRIKANTIA, S. G. (1968) A study of calcium 45 turnover in skeletal fluorosis, *Metabolism*, 17, 366.

RAO, A. B. N., and SIDDIQUI, A. H. (1962) Some observations on eighth nerve functions in fluorosis, *J. Laryng.*, 74, 94.

ROHOLM, K. (1937) *Fluorine Intoxication*, London.

SAUERBRUNN, B. J., RYAN, C. M., and SHAW, J. F. (1965) Chronic fluoride intoxication with fluorotic radiculomyelopathy, *Ann. intern. Med.*, 63, 1074.

SHORTT, H. E., MCROBERT, G. R., BERNARD, T. W., and NAYYAR, A. S. M. (1937) Endemic fluorosis in Madras Presidency, *Indian J. med. Res.*, 25, 553.

SIDDIQUI, A. H. (1955) Fluorosis in Nalgonda District, Hyerabad-Deccan, *Brit. med. J.*, 2, 1408.

SIDDIQUI, A. H. (1970) Neurological complications of skeletal fluorosis with special reference to lesions in the cervical region, *Fluoride*, 3, 91.

SINGH, A., and JOLLY, S. S. (1961) Endemic fluorosis with particular reference to fluorotic radiculomyelopathy, *Quart. J. Med.*, 30, 357.

SINGH, A., JOLLY, S. S., and BANSAL, B. C. (1961) Skeletal fluorosis and its neurological complications, *Lancet*, i, 197.

SINGH, A., DASS, R., HAYARAH, S. S., and JOLLY, S. S. (1962 *a*) Skeletal changes in endemic fluorosis, *J. Bone Jt Surg.*, 44, 806.

SINGH, A., DEVI, P., BANASAL, B. C., and SINGH, S. S. (1962 *b*) Endemic fluorosis, *Indian J. med. Res.*, 50, 387.

SRIKANTIA, S. G., and SIDDIQUI, A. H. (1965) Metabolic studies in endemic fluorosis, *Clin. Sci.*, 28, 477.

SORIANO, M., and MANCHON, F. (1966) Radiological aspects of a new type of bone fluorosis, periostitis deformans, *Radiology*, 87, 1089.

VENKATESHWARLU, P., RAO, D. H., and RAO, K. R. (1952) Studies in endemic fluorosis: Vishakapatanam and suburban areas, *Indian J. med. Res.*, 44, 535.

WEBB-PEPLOE, M. M., and BRADLEY, W. G. (1966) Endemic fluorosis with neurological complications in a Hampshire man, *J. Neurol. Neurosurg. Psychiat.*, 29, 577.

13 Juvenile Motor Neurone Disease

K. JAGANNATHAN

INTRODUCTION

The pattern of neurological disorders witnessed in the area of Madras is similar to that seen elsewhere in India, characterized by a high incidence of infections such as tuberculous meningitis, particularly in children, and the classical neurological disorders. Although nutritional standards are generally poor, primary nutritional neurological disorders are not common in the area. A large number of obscure spastic paraplegias, primary optic atrophy and polyneuropathy are encountered but their relationship to nutritional deficiencies has not been established. Degenerative diseases of the central nervous system, such as spino-cerebellar degeneration, are seen in about the same frequency as elsewhere. Although consanguinity in marriage is common in South India, familial neurological disorders are not seen in any great number. However, juvenile motor neurone disease is one of the unusual forms of disease seen in South India, and an account of it is presented here.

Motor neurone disease is a progressive disorder of unknown aetiology chiefly affecting the motor neurones of the spinal cord, brain stem and cerebral cortex, resulting in weakness and atrophy of muscles, usually associated with exaggeration of tendon reflexes. The disease is mainly encountered in middle life, from the fourth to the sixth decades. It includes amyotrophic lateral sclerosis, progressive muscular atrophy, and progressive bulbar palsy. Some workers tend to include a clinical state dominated by spasticity and hyper-reflexia, without wasting of the muscles, called 'primary lateral sclerosis'. The concept that these variations in the clinical pattern of the disease are underlined by a common aetiological agent has yet to be substantiated.

EPIDEMIOLOGY

Motor neurone disease is worldwide in its incidence. The 'classical' motor neurone disease occurring in the older age-groups and documented in all temperate regions is not uncommon in the tropics. In its age of onset, progression of symptoms, termination within 3 to 5 years, and modes of clinical presentation, it does not differ from that described in the West. In recent years attention has been focused on the increased occurrence of the disease in certain geographical areas such as Guam (Kurland, 1954) and New Guinea (Gajdusek, 1963). Although the exact pattern of the disease does not greatly vary in these pockets of high incidence, its curious association with dementia, and/or the parkinsonian syndrome in such closed communities has raised the possibility of an underlying genetic factor. Cases are on record of the familial nature of amyotrophic lateral sclerosis (Serci, 1963; Poser, 1965), but the classical variety is usually sporadic. Aetiological theories are many: cell abiotrophy (Gowers); a viral infection (Buniha, 1962; Zilber, 1963), ischaemia of the motor neurone cells (van Gehuchten, 1963) and manganese deficiency (Kimura, 1963). McMenemy (1962) has referred to toxins like mercury and lead, exposure to triorthocresyl phosphate and benzol, and to trauma, including electrical injuries, as occasional aetiological agents. A chronic form of infection from the poliovirus has also been suggested (Amici, 1959). The basic error may be at the biochemical enzymatic level, contributed to or precipitated by an unknown exogenous factor (Mathai, 1969).

In South India, the disease is not uncommon and occurs with much the same frequency as elsewhere. The clinical picture conforms to classical accounts, although progress may be slower. We see 35 to 40 cases each year; total annual admissions to hospital are over 3000. But in addition to the classical type of the disease, we see it in younger age-groups and the course of the disease is then much slower (Meenakashi Sundaram, Jagannathan, and Ramamurthi, 1970) [TABLE 13.1].

This group of patients usually present as follows:

1. Weakness and wasting of the extremities.
2. Twitching of muscles.
3. Nasal regurgitation and nasal twang.
4. Difficulty in swallowing and articulation.
5. Defective hearing.
6. Difficulty in walking.

The diagnosis of motor neurone disease is arrived at by a process of exclusion of other similar clinical conditions such as craniovertebral anomalies and cervical cord disease. The clinical diagnosis is confirmed by electromyographic studies and muscle biopsies. No autopsies have been performed since all patients are still living.

The disorder usually appears before the end of the third decade. One patient even developed wasting and fasciculation at the age of 8 years. In a series of 14 patients observed during the 4 years 1966–70, the average age was 15 years. In this part of India this juvenile form of the disease comprises nearly 10 per cent of all types of motor neurone disease.

Table 13.1

'Juvenile' Motor Neurone Disease: 14 Cases

Case No.	Age at investigation	Sex	Age at onset	Family history	Mode of onset	Distribution and symmetry	Cranial nerve involvement	Deafness	Fasciculation	Reflexes TR; PR	Myelogram	Sensation	Electromyography	Biopsy	Serology
1	16	M	10	Nil	Insidious	UL > LL R > L	Normal	—	+	++ ↑ ↑	N	N	Fibrillation + Denervation + Motor conduction normal	Not done	—
2	19	M	18	Nil	„	LL = UL R > L	10, 12	—	+	++ ↑ ↓	Not done	N	„	Not done	—
3	14	M	13	Nil	„	UL > LL R > L	7, 8, 10, 12	+	+	+ ↑ ↑	N	N	„	+	—
4	20	M	14	Nil	„	LL ⩾ UL L ⩾ R	Normal	—	+	++ ↑ ↑	Not done	N	„	+	—
5	18	F	17	Nil	„	LL = UL L = R	7, 8, 10, 12	+	+	++ ↑ ↑	Not done	N	„	Not done	—
6	19	M	18	Nil	„	LL = UL R = L	7, 8, 10, 12	+	+	+ ↑ ↑	Not done	N	„	Not done	—
7	13	F	12	Nil	„	LL = UL L > R	7, 8, 10, 12	+	+	++ ⇂ ↑	Not done	N	„	Not done	—
8	19	M	12	Nil	„	LL > UL R > L	N	—	+	++ ↑ ↓	N	N	„	Not done	—
9	20	M	15	Nil	„	LL > UL R > L	12	—	+	++ ↑ ↑	N	N	„	+	—
10	16	F	11	Nil	„	LL = UL R = L	7, 8, 11, 12	+	+	+— ↑ ↑	Not done	N	„	+	—
11	20	M	17	Nil	„	LL > UL L > R	7, 10, 12	—	+	++ ↓ ↑	N	N	„	+	—
12	24	M	8	Nil	„	LL > UL L > R	N	—	+	++ ↓ ↑	N	N	„	+	—
13	16	F	15	Nil	„	UL > LL R > L	7, 12	—	+	++ ↑ ↑	Not done	N	„	+	—
14	18	M	17	Nil	„	UL > LL R > L	10, 12	—	+	++ ⇂ ↑	Not done	N	„	+	—

Males are twice as often affected as females, and the ratio is comparable to that of classical motor neurone disease (Spillane, 1962).

FAMILY HISTORY

When chronic spinal amyotrophy occurs in the young, there is often a family history as in the cases of Kugelberg and Welander (1956). In these Madras cases, however, the family history is negative and, with signs of pyramidal involvement, this group may be distinguished from the spinal atrophy of Kugelberg and Welander. In Japan, spinal atrophy with preserved tendon reflexes and a dominant mode of inheritance has been described (Tsukagoshi and Tsubaki, 1965). The Madras cases thus differ from both other variants of spinal amyotrophy.

CLINICAL FEATURES

The patient usually belongs to a low socio-economic group but no nutritional or calorie deficiency can be traced on general examination. Higher functions are well preserved unlike the juvenile spinal atrophy described by Ford (1966) and that by Münch-Peterson (1931). The cranial nerves show a high incidence of involvement of up to 60 per cent. The muscles most often affected are those innervated by the lower cranial nerves with resultant wasting of the tongue [PLATE 23c), defective palatal movement, nasal regurgitation, hoarseness of voice, and facial paralysis. Facial muscles are often affected asymmetrically [PLATE 23b]. Involvement of the trapezius and sternomastoid muscles is less frequent. Limb muscles are usually affected in an asymmetrical fashion. Although such asymmetrical involvement, at least in the early phase of the disease, does occur in classical cases of motor neurone disease (Spillane, 1962; Nishigaki, 1964), continued asymmetry is unusual and is more typical of the juvenile form. All muscles affected show characteristic fasciculation. The muscular wasting is more distal than proximal: bilateral footdrop is common. Pelvic girdle weakness gives the patient a waddling gait. The hands show typical clawing in varying degrees, although the patient continues to work and is able to use his hands in many ways.

Tendon reflexes are usually hyperactive in all limbs, although sometimes the upper limb reflexes are impaired when wasting of muscles is profound. Asymmetry of reflex activity and wasting is often marked. Generalized reflex impairment is unusual. The plantar reflex is always extensor. All modalities of sensation are normal. Bilateral perceptive deafness occurs in a third of the patients, and is possibly due to degeneration of the cells of the auditory nerve nuclei. The sphincters are not affected.

LABORATORY DATA

The haemogram, blood chemistry, and ESR are normal. The glucose tolerance test and the exocrine function of the pancreas are within normal limits. The fractional test-meal is normal. Serum GOT, and GPT levels are normal. Radiographs of the cervical spine are normal; there are no signs of any craniovertebral anomaly. The cerebrospinal fluid is normal, and both the blood and cerebrospinal fluid are serologically non-reactive for syphilis. High cervical cord compression has always been excluded by opaque myelography.

The electromyographic pattern is typical of denervation, and the characteristic features of fibrillation potentials on the oscilloscope and amplifier are distinctive. The interference pattern and the amplitude of the action potentials are reduced. Giant polyphasic potentials are seen. Conduction velocities are essentially normal. These electromyographic investigations thus exclude polyneuritis and primary muscle disease.

Muscle biopsy helps in establishing the diagnosis of neurogenic atrophy. Degenerating fibres are seen side by side with normal ones with marked shrinkage of the affected fibres. There are no cellular infiltrations. The vessels appear normal in all their aspects.

SUMMARY

The incidence of classical motor neurone disease in South India is comparable to that in other areas. A special subgroup of motor neurone disease is recognized by its frequent occurrence in younger age-groups before the third decade. The clinical features are characterized by a high incidence of involvement of the bulbar nuclei and facial nerve nuclei, the prolonged asymmetrical distribution of the wasting of the extremities, the presence of pyramidal signs and the high incidence of bilateral nerve deafness. The condition is not familial and the diagnosis of anterior horn cell disease is supported by electrical and muscle biopsy studies. The disease is a very chronic one which may last for many years, but higher cerebral functions remain intact.

There is no clue to the aetiology of this disorder nor to the explanation for its onset at an earlier age than in the classical form of motor neurone disease. It is not known why its course is longer, enabling patients to continue to work for years. There are no significant antecedent illnesses and none of the cases had suffered from poliomyelitis.

It remains to be seen whether post-morten studies will throw light on the nature of the illness and whether other foci of early-onset motor neurone disease will come to light.

References

AMICI, R. (1959) Late sequelae of poliomyelitis in childhood, *Reg. Neuro-biol.*, 5, 617.

BUNIHA, A. (1962) Cell inclusions in familial ALS, *Tr. Akad. Nauk USSR*, 4, 62, 1293.

FORD, F. R. (1906) *Diseases of the Nervous System in*

Infancy, Childhood and Adolescence, 5th ed., ed. Chandy, E., Springfield, Ill., p. 276.

GAJDUSEK, D. C. (1963) Motor neurone disease in natives of New Guinea, *New. Engl. J. Med.*, **266**, 9.

GEHUCHTEN, VAN (1963) Amyotrophic lateral sclerosis, *Acta neurol. Belg.*, **63**, 821.

KIMURA, K. (1963) Study of amyotrophic lateral sclerosis, *Psychiat. Neurol. jap.*, **65**, 31.

KUGELBERG, I., and WELANDER, M. (1956) Heredofamilial juvenile muscular dystrophy, *Arch. Neurol. Psychiat. (Chic.)*, 75, 500.

KURLAND, L. T., and MULDER, D. W. (1954) Epidemiologic investigations of amyotrophic lateral sclerosis, 1. Preliminary report on geographic distribution, with special reference to the Mariana Islands, including clinical and pathological observations, *Neurology (Minneap.)*, **4**, 355–78, 438–48.

MATHAI, N. (1969) *Amyotrophic Lateral Sclerosis and Parkinsonism Dementia in the Mariana Islands*, paper presented at the Ninth International Congress of Tropical Medicine and Malaria, Teheran.

MCMENEMY, W. H. (1962) in discussion on motor neurone disease, *Proc. roy. Soc. Med.*, 55, 1019.

MEENAKASHI SUNDARAM, E., JAGANNATHAN, K., and RAMAMURTHI, B. (1970) Clinical pattern of motor neurone disease in younger age groups, *Neurology (India)*, 8, Suppl. 1, 104.

MÜNCH-PETERSON, F. J. (1931) Studien über erbliche Erkrankungen des Zentrenervunsystems, II. Die familare amyotrophische Lateralsclerose, *Acta psychiat. (Kbh.)*, **6**, 55.

NISHIGAKI, N. (1964) Amyotrophic lateral sclerosis. Report of 48 cases, *Clin. Neurol. jap.*, **4**, 499.

POSER, C. M. (1965) Familial amyotrophic lateral sclerosis, *Dis. nerv. Syst.*, **26**, 697.

SERCI, M. (1963) On familial incidence of amyotrophic lateral sclerosis, *Acta neurol. scand.*, **39**, 169.

SPILLANE, J. D. (1962) in discussion on motor neurone disease, *Proc. roy. Soc. Med.*, 55, 1019.

TSUKAGOSHI, F., and TSUBAKI, T. (1965) Hereditary proximal neurogenic muscular atrophy in adults, *Arch. Neurol. (Chic.)*, **12**, 597.

ZILBER, F. (1963) Study of etiology of amyotrophic lateral sclerosis, *Bull. Wld Hlth Org.*, **29**, 449.

ZILKHA, K. J. (1962) in discussion on motor neurone disease, *Proc. roy. Soc. Med.*, 55, 1019.

Part Two

AFRICA

See PLATES 24–25

14 Neurological Disorders in Senegal

H. COLLOMB, M. DUMAS, and P. L. GIRARD

INTRODUCTION

The Republic of Senegal is situated on the west coast of Africa, covers an area of 196 722 sq km or 78 000 sq miles and has a population of about four million inhabitants. In northern and eastern districts the climate and vegetation is Saharan, and is therefore hot and dry. The rearing of cattle and the growing of millet are its principal resources. In the west, along the coast, the climate is damper and in the south, in the Casamancia region, it is hot and humid. This region is mainly forested and rice is cultivated here. Senegal became independent in 1960 after having been under French rule for 300 years.

Seventy per cent of the population are under the age of 30 years; there are slightly more women than men. It is a mainly rural population (75 per cent); 90 per cent follow the Islamic faith. The country's main activity is agriculture (especially groundnuts) and fishing.

The Wolofs are ethnically predominant, followed by the Serer tribe, the Tukulor tribe, the Peula, and the Diolas—marriages are very often 'endogamic', especially in the north.

The traditional diet consists of rice, fish, millet, and groundnuts. The average caloric intake per head of population is sufficient and often excessive. The diet is not a balanced one, however; fats exceed proteins, a fact, which is due to the large consumption of groundnuts. Greens are as yet rarely eaten.

For purposes of medical administration the country is divided into seven large regions which themselves are divided into districts (prefectures). Each region is governed by a chief medical officer who has at his disposal a hospital with departments of medicine, surgery, obstetrics, radiology, and bacteriology. Each district has a medical officer in charge of a centre with hospital beds, a maternity ward, and a laboratory. Medical practice is poorly developed in the hinterland where technical facilities are lacking as well as medicaments and medical personnel.

On the other hand, in Dakar (450 000 inhabitants) the position is reversed. There one finds three-quarters of the medical practitioners, half the hospital beds, all the research units of the country, and the Faculty of Medicine. The Dakar School of Medicine was founded in 1918. The medical course lasted 4 years and graduates then served in different parts of Black Africa under French control. Since 1949 the medical curriculum has been identical to that of French faculties. Dakar University was founded in 1957, and remained French until 1960 when it then became Senegalese. It is the oldest university founded by the French in Black Africa, and is also one of the best equipped. In addition to the mixed Faculty of Medicine and Pharmacology, there are faculties of law, economics, arts, science and the humanities. There are also numerous research units and institutes.

In the Faculty of Medicine in 1970 there were 720 students. The doctorate of medicine is equivalent to a French diploma or degree.

NEUROLOGICAL PRACTICE

The neurological clinic was founded 10 year ago and is part of the University Hospital Centre of Dakar. It forms part of a neuropsychiatric group which consists of:

Hospital beds: 65 allocated to neurology, 130 to psychiatry, and 30 to neurosurgery.

Laboratories: clinical psychology, clinical electroencephalography, neuroradiology and neuropathology.

An outpatient consultation service.

A mobile re-education service.

This group is situated in a general hospital (Fann Hospital Centre) which also has general and specialized services and beds for infectious diseases, tuberculosis and leprosy.

The neurology department receives patients from Dakar's other two hospitals and from the various medical centres of the Republic (some come from other Black African countries). Some patients are admitted after neuropsychiatric consultations.

As the hospital is situated in Dakar, most of the sick suffering from acute affections (comas, cerebrovascular accidents and epileptic disorders) come from the city; this is not so in the case of chronic affections: these are more representative of the population as a whole.

In the hinterland, the sick are first taken to their local healer following the traditional procedure. This means that proper treatment is delayed, especially in cases of syphilis of the nervous system, tuberculous meningitis, and cord compressions.

Hospital beds are inadequate especially as there are so many patients requiring long-term stay, as in tuberculous meningitis, Pott's disease, nutritional neuropathy, trypanosomiasis and syphilis of the nervous system.

There are three neurologists, and for the past 10 years systematic studies of all diseases of the nervous system encountered have been pursued. In our neuropathological laboratory 95 per cent of the fatal cases are autopsied.

Analysis of Neurological Admissions

In the 10-year period from January 1961 to December 1970 there were 4519 admissions. The diagnostic categories which they comprised are shown in Table 14.1.

Table 14.1

Analysis of Neurological Admissions
January 1961–December 1970

Etiologies	*Nombre de Cas*			
	Total	*Hommes*	*Femmes*	*Frequence*
A. V. C. Ischémique	1 144	626	518	25·31
A. V. C. Hémorragique	560	303	257	12·39
Epilepsie	447	261	186	9·86
Neuropathie nutrionnelle	172	69	103	3·80
Tumeur cérébrale	155	107	48	3·42
Trauma—cranien	133	108	25	2·94
Mal de Pott	116	75	41	2·56
Encéphalite	108	63	45	2·38
Tuberculose nerveuse	96	67	29	2·12
Encéphalopathie infantile	84	55	29	1·85
Hydrocéphalie	71	45	26	1·57
Polynévrite	69	46	23	1·52
P.A.A. & P.A.C.	63	48	15	1·39
Syphilis nerveuse	61	52	9	1·34
Tumeur rachis	59	47	12	1·08
Neuropaludisme	55	41	14	1·21
Méningite purulente	55	44	11	1·21
Sciatique	54	39	15	1·19
Nerfs craniens	52	42	10	1·15
Nerfs periphériques	52	34	18	1·15
Parkinson	50	39	11	1·10
Céphalées	50	21	29	1·10
S.L.A. & syndrome S.L.A.	47	39	8	1·04
Hérédo—degénérescence	44	35	9	0·97
Méningo—encéphalite	42	31	11	0·92
Myélite	39	26	13	0·86
Abcès cerveau	38	31	7	0·84
Encéphalopathie	34	18	16	0·75
Trypanosomiase	34	19	15	0·75
Méningiome	33	12	21	0·73
Arachnoidite	30	20	10	0·66
Polyradiculonévrite	30	21	9	0·66
Méningo-encéph.-mylo.-rad.	29	16	13	0·64
Myopathie	27	23	4	0·59
Chorée	19	7	12	0·42
Thrombophlébite cérébrale	17	7	10	0·37
Tumeur médul. & Q. de chev.	17	11	6	0·37
Malformations S.N.C.	15	10	5	0·33
Phacomatose	14	10	4	0·30
Parasitose & S.N.	1	5	6	0·24
Affection demyélinisante	11	8	3	0·24
Spondilodiscite non tuberc.	9	7	2	0·19
Intoxication & S.N.	7	4	3	0·15
Myasthénie	6	2	4	0·13
Epidurite	5	3	2	0·11
Divers	255	146	109	5·64
total	*4 519*	*2 743*	*1 776*	*100%*

These figures underline the importance of vascular pathology, infectious pathology, and epilepsy. They are, however, not very accurate with regard to tumour pathology as a number of patients with cerebral tumours are admitted direct to the neurosurgical clinic.

Spinal cord compression is very often due to tuberculous lesions of the spine (Pott's disease). Nutritional neuropathies are a particular group found in many African reports. Multiple sclerosis is conspicuous by its virtual absence (Collomb, 1961).

The remaining affections are no different from those of Europe.

INFECTIONS AND INFESTATIONS

The role of infectious, parasitic and mycotic agents in the pathology of the nervous system is of great importance in the African environment.

Bacterial Purulent Meningitis

The problem of the epidemics of meningococcal meningitis which occur during the dry season in subtropical regions will not be discussed here. Purulent meningitis in infancy and early childhood has been carefully studied in Dakar (Charpentier, 1956; Sénécal, Dupin, and Charpentier, 1957). Pfeiffer's bacillus (*Haemophilus influenzae*) is responsible for 39 per cent of cases, the illness occurring mainly during the wet season, while the pneumococcus (19 per cent) and the meningococcus (16 per cent) follow in the dry season. In meningitis caused by Pfeiffer's bacillus, the most dangerous of these organisms, disorders of muscular tonus and of the respiratory rhythm are encountered, and tetaniform features occur. There is a high mortality rate and this seems to be due to delay in diagnosis. If an early diagnosis is made, however, the mortality rate drops from 39 to 5 per cent.

Acute Meningitis with Clear Fluid

This appears to be the outcome of viral aetiology in a great number of cases (Armengaud and Baylet, 1962). In fact, according to certain workers (Baylet, 1967; Baylet *et al.*, 1962) it is responsible for 93 per cent of the cases. The poliomyelitis virus is responsible for more than a quarter of the cases and is prevalent in Type II; Type III is rare. The Coxsackie virus is found in 12·5 per cent, and echoviruses in 7·5 per cent. The influenzal virus is sometimes isolated. One notes the absence of the mumps virus (less than 1 per cent). On the other hand, the frequency of positive reactions to adenoviruses (10 per cent) must be mentioned, although, of course, its significance in the aetiology of acute lymphocytic meningitis is not known.

Non-viral aetiologies seem much rarer by comparison; 7 per cent are related to infections such as typhoid, malaria, syphilis and, most important of all, tuberculosis. Leptospiral meningitis (caused by *Leptospira icterohaemorrhagiae*) is rarely seen.

Encephalitis and Meningo-encephalitis

These are very numerous and of various aetiology—bacterial, viral, parasitic or mycotic. There are two clinical forms:

1. Acute or fulminating cases which present with disorders of consciousness, as in malignant malaria, viral encephalitis and tuberculous meningitis.

2. Subacute or chronic cases with mental deterioration as the salient feature. Trypanosomiasis and syphilis are the commonest causes. Helminthiasis is rarely responsible. One must add rare aetiologies such as subacute sclerosing encephalitis. Chronic forms of

encephalitis have also been observed; it has not been possible to be precise about their aetiology (Martino, Bartoli, and Giordano, 1965).

Encephalopathies of Bacterial Origin

Tuberculous Meningitis

According to hospital statistics this seems to be relatively rare (100 cases in 5 years), but tuberculosis is nevertheless very important in Senegal. In the neuropsychiatric department the practice of routine autopsy has, however, revealed that tuberculous meningitis is widespread in Dakar's urban area (Collomb *et al.*, 1965 *b*). The difficulties of diagnosis have been studied by many workers (Collomb *et al.*, 1967 *b*; Collomb, Courson, and Dumas, 1968; Diop Mar *et al.*, 1969). Patients are usually from 1 to 35 years of age with maximum vulnerability between the ages of 1 to 4. In the infant, the symptoms are classic, with a meningeal onset in 70 per cent and convulsions in 25 per cent. Forty per cent of the patients are admitted in a state of deep coma.

In the adult, symptomatology is polymorphic; onset is accompanied by a meningitic syndrome in 50 per cent, with psychic disorders in 30 per cent of the cases. Sphincter disorders are common. There may be ocular paralyses, abnormal movements, or hemiplegia. Some cases present as a problem of intracranial hypertension, others as a spinal paraplegia. The EEG remains normal in 10 per cent.

Early diagnosis presents many problems. Pulmonary or glandular tuberculosis is present in 80 per cent of cases, but bacteriological proof is not obtained in more than 50 per cent; laboratory standards are inadequate. The CSF is opalescent in half of the cases: usually there is a lymphocytosis of 50 to 300/100 ml; protein is raised above 100 mg/100 ml in 50 per cent. About 17 per cent of our patients have had BCG vaccination. The mortality rate is 54 per cent, and 21 per cent of survivors are disabled.

Neurological Manifestations of Whooping Cough

These appear more frequently in subtropical Africa (Ancelle, 1968; Lafaix *et al.*, 1968 *a*) than in the temperate regions of the Northern Hemisphere. They arise mainly during the third week of the illness. In one-fifth of cases there are simple convulsions which carry a good prognosis but in the remainder acute toxic-anoxic encephalopathies occur. World mortality appears to be about 66 per cent.

Encephalitic Forms of Typhoid Fever

These are particularly common in Senegal (Lafaix *et al.*, 1968 *b*). Ten per cent of our patients with typhoid present in this way; children are particularly susceptible. Antibiotic therapy seems to be an aggravating factor in some cases; corticosteroids seem to be of little use.

Acute Chorea

This is sometimes seen. Its relationship with streptoccocal infection here is not apparent (Giordano *et al.*, 1965).

Viral Infections

Enteroviruses

In Senegal poliomyelitis is a disease of infancy and childhood; 90 per cent of our patients are less than 3 years of age and the disease is rarely seen after 7 years of age. Type I virus is the most frequent (Chignara, 1965; Diop Mar, Rey, and Baylet, 1967). Encephalitic forms of poliomyelitis are not uncommon (11 out of 186 cases in one series). Convulsive phenomena may be the presenting feature (Collomb *et al.*, 1962 *b*).

Coxsackie, echo- and adenovirus encephalitis are seen in infants and children, often in small epidemics. Headache, fever and convulsions are common but there may be pyramidal, striatal or cerebellar signs as well. There is usually a moderate CSF pleocytosis (Vanel, 1965; Baylet, 1967; Collomb *et al.*, 1962 *a*).

Arboviruses

Infection with Type B arboviruses has been demonstrated. Meningeal and psychiatric syndromes occur; insomnia, visual hallucinations, and behavioural disorders have been witnessed.

An epidemic of yellow fever occurred in Senegal in 1965 and numerous cases of postvaccinial encephalitis were observed. It followed the use of both the Dakar and the Rockefeller vaccines; 1 in 30 000 were affected, and 90 per cent of our patients were children from 2 to 11 years of age. About the twelfth day after inoculation there was an onset of fever and headache, the development of a lymphocytic meningitis, convulsions (in two-thirds), confusion and delirium (in one-half), involuntary movements, and the development of coma in at least one-third of the cases. There was a mortality of 10 per cent. The electroencephalogram was usually very abnormal with widespread delta activity. The illness was usually acute, but subacute and chronic forms were described in which personality change, disorders of stance and gait, and involuntary movements were noted. Some patients bore residual signs of cerebral damage (Baylet, Collomb, and Grelier, 1963; Diop Mar *et al.*, 1967; Bert and Collomb, 1966).

Myxoviruses

Cerebral complications during the course of measles are usually due to an encephalopathy rather than a true virus encephalitis. High rates of incidence have been reported; 7 per cent, 18 per cent, and 23 per cent respectively by Armengaud, Louvain, and Frament (1961), Frament (1962) and Rey *et al.* (1970). The risk of this complication increases with age, and malaria, whooping cough, and herpetic infections are not uncommonly present. In 50 per cent of cases the onset of cerebral symptoms occurs on the third to the fifth day of the eruption. Convulsions and stupor are prominent; mortality does not exceed 30 per cent. In two-thirds of the fatal cases death occurs within 48 hours. The cerebrospinal fluid remains normal in two-thirds of all cases. In those that recover there appear to be no residual disorders.

Subacute sclerosing panencephalitis is seen in Senegal and it does not appear to differ in any way from the European variety. We have seen nine cases in 7 years (Collomb *et al.*, 1970*b*). Antimeasles antibodies in serum and cerebrospinal fluid have always been present in abundance when looked for. The EEG has always shown the characteristic rhythmical disorder. Only one patient recovered, a child of 5 years.

Other Viruses

Animal rabies is endemic in rural Senegal. Thirty examples of infection in domestic animals have been reported in the past 5 years; there have been six fatal human cases.

In children infection with herpes viruses can be generalized; this is a primary infection, and encephalitis is rare.

Cerebral complications during the course of varicella, hepatitis and cytomegalovirus infections have all been observed.

Syphilis

Syphilis of the nervous system is relatively frequent in Senegal, and is essentially an urban disease. It is responsible for some 2 per cent of cases attending a neuropsychiatric clinic (Collomb *et al.*, 1965*a*; Collomb, Ayats, and Diop, 1966). General paresis is the commonest neurological manifestation (80 per cent of cases) and the onset is often acute. Pupillary abnormalities are rare (12 per cent), CSF changes are characteristic and constant, and there is a mortality rate of 25 per cent.

Cerebrovascular syphilis is responsible for 3·5 per cent of all cases of cerebrovascular disorder.

Tabes dorsalis is exceptionally rare.

Trypanosomiasis

This is not a major problem in Senegal although there are small endemic foci. There were less than 50 cases in the country in 1968. This is the chronic form of infection of the nervous system by *Trypanosoma gambiense* which is seen in the neurological clinic (Collomb and Diop, 1967). Indifference and apathy are the cardinal features. Intellectual deterioration occurs but it may be more apparent than real. At times there are acute symptoms, hallucinations, delirium and mania, and in children coma may be the presenting feature. Inversion of sleep rhythms (Collomb, Ayats, and Martino, 1962), speech difficulties, aggressive tendencies and various forms of psychomotor retardation are common.

Electroencephalographic signs are very characteristic. In the early stages there is slowing of the alpha rhythm, a general instability and fluctuating theta activity. Later, there is conspicuous delta activity with striking variations from one day to the next and bisynchronous outbursts. Tracings during night sleep become very abnormal, continuously interrupted by waking rhythms. During recovery from the disease abnormal sleep rhythms are the last to subside.

Diagnosis normally depends on the discovery of trypanosomes in the blood, lymph glands and spinal fluid. CSF inoculation into the Gambian rat may reveal the presence of the parasite. There is a striking increase of gamma globulin in the blood and CSF. Immunoelectrophoresis shows a significant increase of IgM globulins in serum and a high level in the CSF (Mattern, 1967).

Drugs used in the generalized phase of the illness, such as suramin (urea derivative) or pentamidine (aromatic diamidine), are not effective when the nervous system is involved as they do not penetrate the blood-brain barrier. Arsenical compounds are then necessary. *Arsobal* (Mel B), a preparation of melarsen oxide and dimercaprol (BAL), is given intravenously in 3·6 per cent solution in propylene glycol. We usually give one to three courses of treatment, each of three injections.

The mortality rate remains high at about 20 per cent. Neuroleptics and tranquillizers seem to be dangerous; they carry a risk of cardiovascular collapse, itself a complication of the untreated disease (Collomb and Bartoli, 1967; Collomb *et al.*, 1968).

Cerebral Malaria

Malaria ranks third after measles and tetanus among patients admitted to the department of infectious diseases in Dakar. Sixty-three per cent of these malarial patients have some cerebral involvement. The mortality rate is about 30 per cent. Infants and young children suffer most, and cerebral malaria is rare over the age of 20 years. The clinical picture is well known. In 20 per cent the onset is catastrophic, and convulsions occur in two-thirds. The EEG shows major changes in two-thirds. At autopsy the perivascular and vascular lesions involve particularly the white matter, there are the usual anoxic signs, but whether 'vascular silting-up' is the basis for all the cerebral lesions is doubtful; the parasite may have some direct toxic effect on cell mitochondria (Collomb and Rey, 1967; Rey *et al.*, 1968; Lemercier *et al.*, 1969).

Helminthiasis

Invasion of the nervous system is rare in the majority of human worm infestations. Cerebral cysticercosis was not recognized in Senegal until 1961 (Collomb, Lariviere, and Philippe, 1961). Bilharziasis of the nervous system has not yet been observed here. There are many forms of filarial infection but although meningeal syndromes have been described in Senegal there is no clear link between the parasite and the cerebral lesion.

Mycoses

Parasitic fungal infections of the nervous system are rare here. *Cryptococcus neoformans* strains have been isolated and the clinical similarity to tuberculous meningitis has been observed.

CEREBRAL LESIONS

Cerebrovascular Disorders

Cerebrovascular accidents are a serious problem in Senegal. They comprise more than 20 per cent of our neurological admissions. On the other hand coronary atherosclerosis is rare: the importance of atherosclerosis in relation to cerebrovascular accidents is much the same in Senegal as in white races, but we have gained the impression that in Senegal involvement of the vertebrobasilar system is much less common.

Non-embolic ischaemic episodes comprise about two-thirds of our cases; men and women are affected in the same proportions; the mortality rate is low (19 per cent of the total cases of cerebrovascular accidents). Arteriographic and pathological studies show that the main lesions are situated in the middle cerebral artery in 41 per cent, in the internal carotid artery in 40 per cent, while they affect the vertebrobasilar system in only 6 per cent. Hypertension is rarely found in cerebral infarction of this type.

Cerebral haemorrhage is responsible for one-third of cerebrovascular accidents; it is commoner in women and mainly affects those over 50 years of age. The mortality rate is 90 per cent. Hypertension and atherosclerosis are responsible for 50 per cent of our cases of intracranial haemorrhage; 32 per cent result from rupture of a vascular anomaly (aneurysm or angioma); 12 per cent are meningeal and 6 per cent subdural.

We see many young patients with acute cerebrovascular accidents of an occlusive nature. Cases under 30 years of age comprise 10 per cent of our series. If we compare the thrombotic and non-thrombotic cases over a 10-year period, we find that where there is no thrombosis only 1 per cent are under the age of 30 years; when thrombosis is present this rate rises to 21·5 per cent. Such a high thrombosis rate does not occur in the young white population. These occlusive episodes are not the result of atherosclerosis but are probably infective in nature. They usually involve an internal carotid artery or the root of a middle cerebral artery. These young patients rarely die and arterial obstruction is usually an arteriographic observation. Some form of arteritis exists. Few of these cases prove to be due to haemoglobinopathy or the result of embolism in cardiomyopathy.

The reader is referred to the following papers for further information on our studies of cerebrovascular disorders in Senegal: Dumas, 1961, 1968; Fernex, 1961; Payet *et al.*, 1961; Sankale, 1961; Pene, Sankale, and Ancelle, 1961; Lemercier *et al.*, 1970 *a*.

Intracranial Tumours

For a long time considered to be rare in the African, we find an increasing incidence of intracranial tumour as the years pass. In Dakar, from 1960 to 1969, we have seen 120 cerebral tumours: 50 gliomas, 23 meningiomas, 6 pituitary tumours, 3 auditory neurinomas and the remainder a miscellaneous group including 17 metastatic tumours. In the latter group the primary cancer was in the liver in three, and in the lung in four cases. In the same period we saw 20 tuberculomas and 28 cerebral abscesses.

In their clinical and pathological features these intracranial masses do not differ from those seen in the West. Parasitic lesions have not been encountered. Mycotic lesions are infrequent (*Nocardia asteroides* and *Cladosporium trichinoides*).

Hydrocephalus

We have investigated 110 cases, 58 per cent of which were under 1 year of age (Courson *et al.*, 1970 *a*). Seventy per cent were postinfective by nature; 17 per cent were congenital; 13 per cent undetermined.

Epilepsy

The incidence of epilepsy in Senegal is probably about seven or eight per thousand inhabitants. The clinical manifestations and EEG findings do not differ from those described elsewhere, but petit mal is rarely encountered and the symptomatic variety is probably commoner than in Europe as a consequence of meningitis, encephalitis and trauma. Childhood infectious diseases are more severe and carry a higher mortality; survivors often suffer from epilepsy. In medical centres epilepsy occurs in 55 per cent of malaria cases, 23 per cent of pertussis, 21 per cent of meningitis, and 17 per cent of measles cases (Collomb *et al.*, 1970 *a*).

Our experience does not differ significantly from that of Billinghurst in Uganda [p. 199], Haddock in Ghana [p. 148] and Osuntokun and Dada in Nigeria [p. 166].

SPINAL CORD LESIONS

Infective lesions of the spinal cord, such as acute poliomyelitis and acute myelitis, are commonly seen and present no unusual features. The main poliomyelitis virus is Type I; epidemics of Type II also occur. In the majority of cases of acute myelitis the cause is unknown, although antirabies vaccination is responsible for a few. There may or may not be an associated encephalitis. Syphilis is not often the cause of acute myelitis (only four of the last 20 cases seen).

Acute paraplegias are usually due to injury or tuberculosis of the spine. Many of the latter are not admitted to the Department of Neurology, where only 13 per cent of paraplegias are due to Pott's disease. Paraplegia during the course of typhoid or brucellosis is encountered but is rare. Parasitic infestation of the spinal cord is also very rare.

Primary tumours of the spine are responsible for 35 per cent of compressive lesions of the spinal cord; plasmacytomas are particularly frequent (6 per cent of all compression lesions); metastatic lesions are responsible for 25 per cent of cases (Courson *et al.*, 1970 *b*; Carayon *et al.*, 1968). Carcinoma of the liver and prostrate is responsible for approximately two-thirds of the metastatic lesions. Next in frequency is carcinoma of the breast; carcinoma of the lung is still rare among the black African population. Some 14 per cent of compressive lesions of the cord are the result of infection of the epidural space (excluding Pott's disease). Subacute and chronic forms of spinal arachnoiditis comprise 25 per cent of all the compressive lesions of the spinal cord. In a third of these cases tuberculosis seems to be the cause; the aetiology of the remainder is not known. Myelography is essential in diagnosis.

In summary, we can say that carcinoma of the liver, spinal arachnoiditis, and spinal epidural infections play a larger role in the aetiology of paraplegias in Senegal than they do in Europe. Subacute combined degeneration (vitamin B_{12} neuropathy) is practically unknown in Senegal. The rarity of multiple sclerosis and the frequency of nutritional lesions of the spinal cord will be discussed later.

PERIPHERAL NERVE LESIONS

Polyradiculoneuritis (Guillain-Barré syndrome) is sometimes encountered (4 per cent of paraplegias). Sensorimotor neuropathy is responsible for some 23 per cent of our paraplegias, but the aetiology is known in only about a quarter of the cases (vitamin B_1 neuropathy 15 per cent; alcoholism 10 per cent; diabetes 3 per cent). Vitamin B; neuropathy following isoniazid therapy for tuberculosis is exceptional. Chronic polyneuropathy is seen in the alcoholic male, and subacute forms in females during and after pregnancy; cardiac beriberi is a frequent associated feature of the latter cases.

Symptoms and signs of peripheral neuropathy are frequently encountered in the nutritional neuropathies considered below.

Sciatica is rare; lumbar disc lesions are much less frequently encountered than in the European, and of upper situation.

DISORDERS OF MUSCLE

There have been few reports from Senegal (Collomb *et al.*, 1962 *c*). Dermatomyositis in childhood, polymyositis in adults and occasional cases of muscular dystrophy are encountered. The majority of the latter are of the characteristic Duchenne type; limb-girdle types and facioscapulo-humeral types have yet to be described in Senegal. Myasthenia has been identified but it is rare.

DEGENERATIVE AND HEREDITARY DISORDERS

Parkinson's disease is common in the African in Senegal and conforms to classical descriptions. Amyotrophic lateral sclerosis is also common, presenting with the usual symptoms and signs, but in some 25 per cent of cases deterioration is slower and patients may survive for years. It is not always easy to differentiate the latter from chronic spinal arachnoiditis or chronic cervical myelopathy.

The African environment makes the study of hereditary disorders exceptionally difficult and few observations have been reported. We have recognized peroneal muscular atrophy and various forms of hereditary spinocerebellar degeneration.

DEMYELINATING DISORDERS

Multiple sclerosis is virtually absent in Senegal, but three cases with autopsy confirmation have been described (Collomb, Lemercier, and Dumas, 1968; Collomb *et al.*, 1970 *c*; Lemercier *et al.*, 1970 *b*). In each case the onset was very acute and the progress of the disease rapid. We have published an account of five cases of neuromyelitis optica (Collomb and Virieu, 1967).

NEUROLOGICAL DISORDERS IN KWASHIORKOR

Convulsions and hemiplegia during the course of kwashiorkor have been described in Senegal and are usually due to subdural haematoma, cortical thrombophlebitis, or cerebral atrophy (Satgé *et al.*, 1964). Striatal symptoms and signs have also been described during the period of recovery from the illness (Satgé *et al.*, 1970). Ten to 20 days after the beginning of treatment, when the weight is rising, the oedema subsiding, and serum proteins are improving, a fairly characteristic neurological syndrome makes its appearance. There is a general state of tremor with akinesia, striatal rigidity and brisk pouting reflexes. These appearances usually subside in a few days, without sequelae and without affecting the general progress of the patient. The precise cerebral disturbance responsible for these manifestations is not known; the role of magnesium deficiency or excess of amino acids have been considered.

The long-term sequelae of kwashiorkor and of protein malnutrition in infancy in general are of considerable importance. The cranial circumference is usually less than normal up to the age of 5 or 6 years and may not reach normal proportions until puberty. Clinical and electroencephalographic studies on infants with protein malnutrition must clearly be followed by accurate psychometric assessment of the ultimate consequences of this widespread disorder (Collomb, Diop, and Valantin, 1970).

NUTRITIONAL NEUROPATHY

One of the most interesting and perplexing problems for the neurologist in Senegal is the group of paraplegias of unknown causation which occur in poor communities living on a grossly inadequate diet. We believe they are nutritional in origin but perhaps it would be more accurate to use the term 'obscure neuropathy' as suggested by Cruickshank, Montgomery, and Spillane (1961). Gastric achlorhydria, altered hepatic histology, the satisfactory nature of the therapeutic response to a nourishing diet and vitamin B complex preparations, if used in the early stages of the disorder, nevertheless suggest that a nutritional disturbance is certainly present.

It is difficult to determine the precise incidence of these disorders throughout Senegal, but in Dakar they comprise 6 per cent of admissions to the Department of Neurology and some 27 per cent of paraplegias. Children are rarely affected; 68 per cent of the patients are female; this is significant because, in general, male admissions are far greater than female. Seventy per cent of cases are between the ages of 20 and 40 years; only 6 per cent are less than 20 years (Collomb *et al.*, 1967 *a*).

Clinical Features

There are three main forms of clinical presentation but with some general admixture between them:

1. Polyneuritic type; 62·5 per cent
2. Pyramidal type; 21·5 per cent
3. Combined sclerosis type; 16 per cent

The first type is characterized by the onset of paraesthesiae in the distal portions of the extremities and by weakness and clumsiness in the hands and feet. The paraesthesiae are frequently burning and usually painful. Gait soon becomes affected. In half the cases the onset is fairly rapid and in 32 per cent there is a recent history of gastrointestinal troubles or diarrhoea. General fatigue is another preliminary complaint in a further 17 per cent.

In women the onset of these symptoms is frequently during pregnancy or just before or after confinement. Indeed, the disease affects women three times more commonly than men. It is most often diagnosed in natives of Dakar or Central Senegal (the Wolof ethnic group) and in Casamancias in the south of the country. The two other forms of the disease are also seen in the Wolofs but only the polyneuritic form is seen in the Casamancias. The diet of the latter includes rice and fresh fish but fat consumption is lower than elsewhere in Senegal and consists essentially of palm oil, which is rich in vitamin A. In this Casamancia region the diet is markedly deficient in thiamine but, although it is also lacking in vitamin B_2, ascorbic acid and calcium, it does not differ in these respects from other regions of Senegal.

Characteristic signs of a sensorimotor neuropathy are found in the limbs especially the lower limbs. Intense discomfort and pains are felt in the feet and legs and there may be quite striking muscular atrophy.

In the second type the onset is usually slower and much more insidious. Women are twice as commonly affected as men and the majority are in their late thirties. They do not present any general features suggestive of nutritional deficiency, as do the first group, but pregnancy or an intercurrent illness may accelerate the disability and determine admission to hospital. The disorder is usually considerable by this time and therapy is not very effective. Weakness and spasticity of the lower limbs are the oustanding signs and hyper-reflexia is marked; clonus is common. The plantar reflexes may be extensor. Although pains and limb discomfort are complained of there is usually no objective sensory loss of note. On the other hand, impairment of sight and hearing is frequently encountered. This pyramidal affliction is found among the Wolofs and in patients from the north of the country.

In the third type the symptoms and signs indicate involvement of the posterior columns of the spinal cord in addition to the pyramidal pathways. There are subjective sensory complaints, largely taking the form of paraesthesiae and pains in the distal portion of the extremities, together with weakness and spasticity of the lower limbs, ataxia and progressive gait disorder. The onset is insidious; ataxia is the main feature when patients are examined 18 months after onset. Pyramidal involvement varies in intensity; loss of posture and vibration also varies in degree and extent. Males are twice as commonly affected as women; most of our patients are in their late thirities. In about 25 per cent there is complaint of impairment of vision and/or hearing. Gastrointestinal symptoms occur in about one-third. This third type of presentation is also encountered mainly in the Wolofs and in patients from the north.

We therefore see that all three forms of the disorder are to be found among the Wolofs who are distributed throughout Senegal in a wider fashion than other ethnic groups. In the forested regions of the south, where the Casamancias live, it is the polyneuritic form that is mainly found. In the dry regions of the north we see only the pyramidal or combined forms of the disorder. Although rice is the staple diet in all these regions of Senegal, in the north millet, maize and tubers (sweet potato and cassava) are also eaten. So far as we know the cassava-producing neuropathies of Nigeria are not seen in Senegal.

Investigations

Routine investigations of blood (sugar, urea, proteins, cellular content, etc.) and cerebrospinal fluid are normal. Serological tests of both are negative.

We have also carried out the following tests and the majority gave normal results: marrow biopsy; serum protein electrophoresis, serum iron, serum amylase, serum transaminase, tryptophan tests for vitamin B_6 deficiency, bisulphite binding tests for vitamin B_1 deficiency, the Schilling test, stool examination for parasites, liver flocculation tests, gastric acidity, and liver biopsy.

In 60 per cent of cases we have found complete or subtotal achlorhydria or a negative response to histamine injection. In a further 24 per cent there is hypochlorhydria. In all these cases there are no changes in the blood or bone marrow.

Liver puncture biopsy has been carried out almost routinely and histological examinations have been made by Professor Camain. The staining methods he has used are the haematoxylin-eosin, Masson, Hotchkiss-MacManus, Ziehl, and Tierman-Schmeltzer. No evidence of infiltrates or fibrosis has been detected. On the other hand, changes in the cytoplasm and nuclei of the hepatic cells have been constant and characteristic. The nuclei are divided and deformed, they vary in size, shape and colour and there is excess lipofuscin in the cytoplasm. These changes vary in intensity from one case to the next but there is no relation between the degree or amount of hepatic cell alteration and the severity or type of clinical disability.

In 13 patients a Schilling test indicated defective absorption of vitamin B_{12} (Bresson *et al.*, 1968).

Pathology

Although four of our patients have died we have been able to study the nervous system at autopsy in only one case (Lemercier, Jacquin-Cotton, and Collomb, 1971). The patient was a man of 22 years with a year's history of difficulty in walking and some impairment in hearing. He had a pyramidal syndrome and although he complained of paraesthesiae and cramps we could not detect any objective sensory loss. He showed the characteristic hepatic cellular changes. He died suddenly but autopsy did not reveal the cause of death. There was obvious demyelination of the pyramidal pathways from the cervical to the lumbar regions but there were also less marked changes in the sensory pathways and in the anterior spinal nerve roots. There were no signs suggestive of inflammatory infiltrates as in some of the cases of Jamaican neuropathy, but the lesions were similar to those described by Grieve, Jacobson, and Proctor (1967) in nutritional neuropathies among the Bantu. It is of interest that death was also sudden in our three other fatal cases.

We feel that there are several factors which point to the nutritional nature of these neuropathies in Senegal: the common story of preceding gastrointestinal symptoms, aggravation by pregnancy, the poor social origins of the patients, the unbalanced diet, the reduced gastric acidity, and the hepatic cell changes which are not those seen in hepatitis or cirrhosis. In addition there is the suggestive evidence of defective absorption of vitamin B_{12}.

The precise nature of this nutritional fault is unknown. Several mechanisms have to be considered. We may be seeing the result of the operation of some toxic substance acting as an antivitamin, or in some other way. But in Senegal the role of cassava does not appear to be important. On the other hand defective absorption and/or assimilation may be responsible. The issue is clearly a very complex one and its resolution necessitates intensive studies in the future. We hope that in carrying out such studies we may also discover clues to the aetiology of neurological disorders in other climates.

References

ANCELLE, G. (1968) Complications neurologiques de la coqueluche, *Thèse Dakar*, No. 11, 141.

ARMENGAUD, M., and BAYLET, R. J. (1962) Intérêt et limites des recherches virologiques en médecine africaine. Considérations à propos d'une étude portant sur 449 malades hospitalisés à Dakar, *Presse méd.*, 70, 925.

ARMENGAUD, M., LOUVAIN, M., and FRAMENT, V. (1961) La mort dans la rougeole en pays tropical (à propos de 125 observations), *Bull. Fac. mixte Méd. Pharm. Dakar*, 9, 262.

BAYLET, E. J. (1967) Les entérovirus au Sénégal, *Gaz. méd. Fr.*, 74, 1627.

BAYLET, R. J., COLLOMB, H., and GRELIER, L. (1963) L'étiologie de l'encéphalite vaccinale (à propos de 4 observations), *Rev. neurol.*, 108, 790.

BAYLET, R. J., DUBOIS, P., ARDOUIN, C., GRELIER, L., and KHOURY, B. (1962) Syndromes méningés à liquide clair (recherches virologiques), *Bull. Soc. Path. exot.*, 55, 275.

BERT, J., and COLLOMB, H. (1966) L'E.E.G. dans l'encéphalite vaccinale (vaccination anti-amarile), *Bull. Soc. méd. Afr. noire Langue franc.*, 11, 591.

BRESSON, Y., COLLOMB, H., BALLON, G., DUMAS, M., and PETIT, M. (1968) Le test de Schilling dans les neuropathies nutritionnelles, *Bull. Soc. méd. Afr. noire Langue franç.*, 13, 632.

CARAYON, A., COURSON, B., VIRIEU, R., and PIQUARD, R. (1968) Compression médullaire par métastase d'un cancer du foie cliniquement inapparent (à propos de 10) observations), *Bull. Soc. méd. Afr. noire Langue franç.*, 13, 586.

CHARPENTIER (1955). Les méningites suppurées du nourrisson africain. Etude critique de 202 cas observés à l'Hôpital A. le Dantec. Thése Paris, No. 1704, p. 42.

CHIGNARA, P. A. (1965) La poliomyélite au Sénégal, *Thèse Dakar*, No. 6, p. 129.

COLLOMB, H., LARIVIERE, M., and PHILIPPE, Y. (1961) Cysticercose cérébrale (premier cas au Sénégal), *Bull. Soc. méd. Afr. noire Langue franç.*, 6, 695.

COLLOMB, H., AYATS, H., and MARTINO, P. (1962) Les troubles du sommeil dans la trypanosomiase, *Journées méd. France Commun. Nancy*, 217.

COLLOMB, H., DUBOIS, P., BAYLET, R., GRELIER, L., and BERT, J. (1962 *a*) Méningoencéphalites aiguës de l'enfance à entéro-virus non poliomyélitique, *Bull. Soc. méd. Afr. noire Langue franç.*, 7, 716.

COLLOMB, H., GUERINEAU, P., BAYLET, R., and GRELIER, L. (1962 *b*) La poliomyélite à Dakar chez l'enfant (Importance des formes encéphalitiques convulsivantes), *Bull. Soc. méd. Afr. noire Langue franç.*, 7, 703.

COLLOMB, H., PHILIPPE, Y., BERT, J., and DIOP, B. (1962 *c*

Atrophies musculaires progressives chez l'Africain, *Bull. Soc. méd. Afr. noire Langue franç.*, 7, 326.

Collomb, H., Ayats, H., Mattern, P., and Bonnardot, R. (1965 *a*) La syphilis nerveuse en milieu africain. Journées Nationales de Dermatologie et Syphiligraphie, Marseille 2–4 octobre 1964, *Bull. Soc. franç. Derm. Syph.*, 72, 583.

Collomb, H., Plassart, H., Lemercier, G., Bourgeade, A., Bartoli, D., and Giordano, C. (1965 *b*) Les méningites tuberculeuses en milieu africain à Dakar. A propos de 40 observations, *Bull. Soc. méd. Afr. noire Langue franç.*, 10, 357.

Collomb, H., Ayats, H., and Diop, M. (1966) La paralysie générale en milieu africain, *Afr. méd.* 5, 13.

Collomb, H., Lemercier, G., and Dumas, M. (1966) Encéphalomyelite disséminée aiguë ou sclérose en plaques? (à propos d'un cas chez un noir Africain; étude anatomique), *Bull. Soc. méd. Afr. noire Langue franç.*, 11, 184.

Collomb, H., and Bartoli, D. (1967) Le coeur dans la trypanosomiase humaine africaine à *Trypanosoma gambiense, Bull. Soc. Path. exot.*, 60, 142.

Collomb, H., and Diop, M. (1967) Diagnostic de la trypanosomiase humaine africaine à *Trypanosoma gambiense, Afr. méd.*, 6, 159.

Collomb, H., and Rey, M. (1967) Accès pernicieux palustre en zone d'endémie, *Méd. Afr. noire*, 16, 219.

Collomb, H., and Virieu, R. (1967) Neuromyélite optique aiguë au Sénégal (à propos de 5 observations), *Bull. Soc. méd. Afr. noire Langue franç.*, 12, 92.

Collomb, H., Quere, M. A., Cros, J., and Giordano, C. (1967 *a*) Les neuropathies dites nutritionnelles au Sénégal, *J. neurol. Sci.*, 5, 159.

Collomb, H., Virieu, R., Lemercier, G., and Dumas, M. (1967 *b*) Thromboses vasculaires cérébrales multiples par artérite au cours d'une méningite tuberculeuse, *Bull. Soc. med. Afr. noire Langue franç.*, 12, 813.

Collomb, H., Bartoli, D., Ayats, H., and Koate, P. (1968) Les atteintes cardiaques dans la trypanosomiase humaine africaine à *Trypanosoma gambiense, Bull. Soc. méd. Afr. noire Langue franç.*, 12, 337.

Collomb, H., Courson, B., and Dumas, M. (1968) Les sténoses de l'aqueduc de Sylvius d'origine tuberculeuse. Discussion étiopathogénique à propos d'un cas, *Bull. Soc. méd. Afr. noire Langue franç.*, 13, 204.

Collomb, H., Diop, B., and Valantin, S. (1970) La malnutrition protidique chez l'enfant (références sénégalaises) in *Proceedings of the Second Panafrican Psychiatric Workshop*, Ile Maurice, p. 91.

Collomb, H., Dumas, M., Ayats, H., Virieu, R., Simon, M., and Roger, J. (1970 *a*) Epidémiologie de l'épilepsie au Sénégal, *Afr. J. med. Sci.*, 1, 125.

Collomb, H., Dumas, M., Baylet, R., Girard, P. L., and Jacquin-Cotton, L. (1970 *b*) Panencéphalites sclérosantes subaigués au Sénëgal. Etude clinique et biologique, *Bull. Soc. méd. Afr. noire Langue franç.*, 15, 442.

Collomb, H., Dumas, M., Lemercier, G., and Girard, P. L. (1970 *c*) Sclérose en plaques au Sénégal, *Afr. J. med. Sci.*, 1, 253.

Courson, B., Toure, P., Izarn, R., and Collomb, H. (1970 *a*) Aspects étiologiques et anatomiques des hydrocéphalies non tumorales du nourrisson et de l'enfant, *Afr. méd.*, 9, 515.

Courson, B., Jacquin-Cotton, L., Toure, P., and Collomb, H. (1970 *b*) Paraplégies chirurgicales non traumatiques, mal de Pott exclu, *Afr. méd.*, 9, 503.

Cruickshank, E. K., Montgomery, R. D., and Spillane, J. D. (1961) Obscure neurologic disorders in Jamaica, *Wld Neurol.*, 2, 199.

Diop Mar, I., Niang, I., Guicheney, A., Berne, C., Collomb, H., Rey, M., and Satgé, P. (1967) Encéphalites consécutives à la vaccination anti-amarile (d'après 248 cas observés à Dakar en 1965), *Ann. Pédiat.*, 43, 181.

Diop Mar, I., Rey, M., and Baylet, R. (1967) Place de la paralysie infantile dans la pathologie infectieuse en milieu hospitalier dakarois, *Bull. Soc. méd. Afr. noire Langue franç.*, 12, 326.

Diop Mar, I., Guerin, M., Lafaix, C., and Rey, M. (1969) Les méningites tuberculeuses à Dakar (difficultés du diagnostic, gravité), *Méd. Afr. noire*, 16, 411.

Dumas, M. (1961) Accidents vasculaires cérébraux chez l'Africain. A propos de 142 observations, *Thése Dakar*, No. 3, p. 182.

Dumas, M. (1968) La pathologie vasculaire cérébrale au Sénégal. Considérations générales, *Afr. méd.*, 7, 517.

Fernex, M. (1961) Observations sur l'état anatomohistologique des artères des malades africains, *Méd. Afr. noire*, 8, 66.

Frament, V. (1962) Contribution à l'étude de la rougeole en pays tropical, *Thèse Dakar*, No. 1, p. 131.

Giordano, C., Bartoli, D., Ayats, H., and Collomb, H. (1965) Chorées aiguës de l'enfant, à Dakar, *Bull. Soc. méd. Afr. noire Langue franç.*, 10, 504.

Grieve, S., Jacobson, S., and Proctor, N. S. F. (1967) A nutritional myelopathy occurring in the Bantu on the Witwatersrand, *Neurology (Minneap.)*, 17, 1205.

Lafaix, C. Lemercier, G., Dumas, M., Diop Mar, I., Ancelle, G., and Rey, M. (1968 *a*) Manifestations nerveuses de la coqueluche d'après 84 observations, *Bull. Soc. méd. Afr. noire Langue franç.*, 13, 746.

Lafaix, C., Rey, M., Diop Mar, I., and Alihonou, E. (1968 *b*) Manifestations encéphalitiques de la fièvre typhoide (17 observations), *Bull. Soc. méd. Afr. noire Langue franç.*, 13, 517.

Lemercier, G., Bert, H., Nouhouayi, A., Rey, M., and Collomb, H. (1969) Le neuropaludisme: aspects électroencéphalographiques, neuropathologiques. Problèmes physiopathologiques, *Path. et Biol.*, 17, 459.

Lemercier, G., Quenum, C., Richir, C., and Collomb, H. (1970 *a*) Athérosclérose cérébrale au Sénégal. Etude anatomopathologique, *Atherosclerosis*, 12, 107.

Lemercier, G., Virieu, R., Dumas, M., and Collomb, H. (1970 *b*) Sclérose en plaques au Sénégal, *Acta neurol. belg.*, 70, 309.

Lemercier, G., Jacquin-Cotton, L., and Collomb, H. (1971) Myelopathy of obscure aetiology—nutritional syndrome, *Neurology (Minneap.)*, 21, 185.

Martino, P., Bartoli, D., and Giordano, C. (1965) Méningoencéphalites chroniques d'origine indéterminée, *Bull. Soc. méd. Afr. noire Langue franç.*, 10, 201.

Mattern, P. (1967) Les globulins du sérum et du LCR dans la trypanosomiase humaine à *Trypanosoma gambiense, Afr. méd.* 6, 1963.

Payet, M., Sankale, M., Pene, P., and Fernex, M. (1961) Les aspects anatomo-cliniques de l'athérosclérose chez le noir africain (à propos de 200 cas), *Rev. Athérosclér.*, 3, 67.

PENE, P., SANKALE, M., and ANCELLE, J. P. (1961) L'hypertension artérielle chez l'Africain à Dakar. Rapport IIèmes Journées Médicales de Dakar, 13–21 décembre 1960, *Méd. Afr. noire*, special July No., 57–64.

REY, M., CAMERLYNCK, P., DIOP MAR, I., LAFAIX, C., and SOW, A. (1968) Le paludisme dans l'agglomération dakaroise en 1966–1967 (d'après une expérience hospitalière), *Bull. Soc. méd. Afr. noire Langue franç.*, 13, 353.

REY, M., LEMERCIER, G., GIRARD, P. L., LAFAIX, C., and SOW, A. (1970) Encéphalites et encéphalopathies de la rougeole, *Bull. Soc. méd. Afr. noire Langue franç.*, 15, 3.

SANKALE, M. (1961) L'athérosclérose chez le noir africain. Rapport IIèmes Journées Médicales de Dakar, 1960, *Méd. Afr. noire*, Special July No., 49–56.

SATGÉ, P., LAFFONT, M., BERT, J., CARAYON, A., and GIORDANO, C. (1964) Troubles neurologiques d'origine vasculaire dans la convalescence d'un Kwashiokor, *Bull. Soc. méd. Afr. noire Langue franç.*, 9, 305.

SATGÉ, P., ZOHOUN, I., COLLOMB, H., and DUMAS, M. (1970) Syndrome Extrapyramidal au Cours de la Période de Récupération du Kwashiorkor, paper presented at the Second Pan-African Congress of Neurological Sciences, 13–17 January, Ibadan.

SÉNÉCAL, J., DUPIN, H., and CHARPENTIER, P. (1957) A propos de 302 cas de méningites aiguës du nourrisson. Considérations épidémiologiques cliniques et thérapeutiques, *Bull. méd. A.O.F.*, 2, 241.

VANEL, J. (1965) Les infections à virus Coxackie à Dakar. (Considérations cliniques et épidémiologiques), *Thèse Dakar*, No. 4, p.139.

15 Neurological Disorders in Ghana

D. R. W. HADDOCK

INTRODUCTION

Ghana is placed more or less centrally among the countries strung along the Guinea Coast of West Africa bounded by the sea on the south. The Ivory Coast lies to the west; Togoland, Dahomey and Nigeria lie to the east. To the north lies the Upper Volta. The area of the country is 92 100 sq miles which is roughly the size of the United Kingdom. In shape Ghana is rectangular with a long axis north to south (some 420 miles) and its short axis east to west (about 334 miles). The Ghanaian coast is 4 deg. N of the equator and the Greenwich Meridian runs through Eastern Ghana.

There is a flat coastal plain extending for up to 30 miles inland but there are many mountain ridges beyond (up to 2 000 feet). In the centre of the country is a plain and the great man-created Volta Lake. The land becomes higher in the north (about 1–2 000 feet).

Climate

The chief characteristics of Ghana's climate are the relatively high temperatures (mean annual temperatures of 79 deg. to 84 deg.F), the great variation in the rainfall from north to south, and the tendency of the dry seasons to grow longer and more intense with distance from the sea. The climate is strongly influenced by the dry hot north-east trade winds from the Sahara (the Harmattan) and opposing them the cooler, moister south-west winds (the monsoon) blowing from the sea. The rainfall around coastal Accra is only about 25 to 30 inches a year but this is exceptionally low, as most of the country has a rainfall of 40 to 60 inches per annum—the north being drier and the west wetter. The rain is concentrated into a single or double rainy season depending upon the region. Relative humidity is very high at the coast but diminishes inland. Humidity drops sharply with the Harmattan in January.

Vegetation

The distribution of the vegetation depends on the rainfall and length of the dry season. Savannah woodland is the most extensive vegetation covering about 65 000 sq miles in the northern and south-eastern areas of the country. There is a large area of high forest in the south-west with a canopy in places at about 130 feet. Some trees are up to 200 feet high. A coastal plain stretches up to 20 miles inland consisting of scrub and grasslands. In the immediate coastal area there is often a mangrove strip.

Economy

The economy is largely dependent on the cocoa crop (cocoa makes up about 65 per cent of the value of exports). Gold, diamonds, bauxite and timber are also exported. Maize, cassava, rice, yams, millet and sugar are grown as food-crops. The Volta dam is an important source of hydro-electric power. Local industries are not very highly developed as yet but clothes, plastic goods, household utensils, alcoholic beverages, canned and bottled foods are produced in some quantity. Cattle rearing is important in the north.

Population

The estimated population of Ghana in 1969 was 8 400 000, of whom about 80 per cent lived in rural areas. The estimated crude birth rate is 47–55 per thousand population, and the infant mortality rate 90–160 per thousand live births. The population may be increasing at a rate of 2·5 per cent per annum. The life expectancy at birth is 48 years and about 43 per cent of the population are under 15.

The Medical Services

In 1969 there were 581 doctors in Ghana of whom 307 were Ghanaian and 274 expatriates giving a ratio of one doctor to 14 440 people in Ghana. This ratio is, of course, very low by European standards. There were about 600 Ghanaian medical students in training in 1968. Most of the doctors work in government hospitals, polyclinics or dispensaries; some are missionaries and relatively few are in private practice. Patients who attend government hospitals and polyclinics pay no fees, except for X-rays and a small lodging fee as inpatients.

There are about 7 750 beds in government hospitals and 2 950 in mission hospitals. The Medical School o the University of Ghana is based on Korle Bu Hospital, Accra, a large hospital of 1 500 beds with modern blocks for the main departments. The first 39 graduates qualified in 1969 and are doing their preregistration appointments. Soon there will be 50–60 graduates a year.

Disease in Ghana

The disease picture of Ghana is that which one finds in most developing, tropical countries; it is strongly influenced by poverty, low-protein diets, poor sanitation, and an abundance of insect vectors of disease. There is a large childhood mortality due to malaria, protein-calorie malnutrition, respiratory infections, measles and gastroenteritis. Malaria, schistosomiasis, onchocerciasis, leprosy, typhoid, amoebiasis, bacillary dysentery, virus hepatitis, meningitis, tetanus, and guinea-worm infections are common endemic diseases. Trypanosomiasis is now less common. Hypertension and strokes are very prevalent, cardiomyopathies of various types are common, but coronary artery disease is very rare. Neoplasia is less prevalent than in the West but primary carcinoma of the liver, carcinoma of the breast and cervix are common. Burkitt's tumour is the commonest tumour of childhood. Carcinoma of the bronchus is very rare. Duodenal ulcer, cirrhosis of the liver, and diabetes are frequently found. There is still widespread ignorance of the causation of disease and the germ theory. Many people consider witchcraft and juju to be responsible for disease. Thus, people often consult the traditional healer or prophet before seeking proper medical advice. Such delay is frequently disastrous.

Neurological Practice in Ghana

There are general physicians in regional hospitals in the country but the only two physicians specializing in neurology are at the Korle Bu teaching hospital where there is now also a neurosurgeon. Investigative facilities are limited, but electroencephalography, cerebral angiography and ventriculography are available in Accra. Weekly neurological, epilepsy and neurosurgical clinics are held at Korle Bu Hospital. Table 15.1 gives the incidence of neurological disease in Ghana.

The following account is based on practice in the teaching hospital with cases referred from many areas and may therefore not be typical of the whole country.

NEUROLOGICAL DISEASE IN ACCRA

Most of the neurological diseases seen in Europe and the United States (with the striking exceptions of multiple sclerosis and subacute combined degeneration) are seen in Ghana. The proportions of the different types of disease are rather different, and this fact may be seen in Table 15.2 which records the patients seen at the neurological clinic in a 2-year period, and neurological inpatients admitted to a 42-bed general medical unit with a neurological bias.

The following comments will deal with each disease group in Table 15.2 in turn and may serve as a *general commentary* on neurological disease in Ghana. Neurological complications of other endemic diseases will be briefly described later.

Table 15.1

Incidence of Neurological Disease in Ghana

Incidence probably similar to European	*Deviations from European Incidence*			*Peculiar to local Peoples*
	More common	*Less Common*	*Not met*	
Cerebral abscess	Pyogenic meningitis	Cerebrovascular disease	Multiple sclerosis	
	TB meningitis	Secondary cerebral tumour	Ménière's syndrome	Haemoglobinopathic vascular disease of the CNS
Primary cerebral tumour	Cerebral malaria	Cervical and lumbar spondylosis	Subacute combined degeneration	
Brain injuries	Arbovirus encephalitis			Trypanosomiasis
Subdural haematoma	Tetanus	Neurological syndromes associated with malignancy	Friedreich's ataxia	
Acute infective polyneuritis	Rabies		Periodic paralysis	Amoebic brain abscess
	Febrile convulsions	Motor neurone disease		Onchocercal optic atrophy
Bell's palsy	Snake-bite (neurotoxicity)	Parkinsonism		
Radial pressure palsies				
Idiopathic epilepsy	Obscure paraplegias	Chorea (Sydenham's and Huntington's)		
	Leprosy neuritis			
Neurosis	Ataxic neuropathy			
Hysteria	Burning feet syndrome	Carpal tunnel syndrome		
	Nutritional neuropathy	Trigeminal neuralgia		
	Hepatic encephalopathy	Herpes zoster		
		Narcotic poisoning		

Infections of the CNS

Infections of the central nervous system are common in Ghana and they have a high morbidity and mortality rate. From the point of view of therapy and prevention they are of the greatest importance among diseases of the nervous system. The unholy tetrad of ignorance, poverty, inability to reach hospital, and unwillingness to go to hospital plays an important part in the high mortality found in these diseases.

Meningitis

Pyogenic meningitis is a significant cause of death (the sixth highest cause of death in childhood). The case mortality rate is high. In 1965 among 79 cases of pyogenic meningitis in Accra 30 were pneumococcal, 7 meningococcal, 5 due to *Haemophilus influenzae*, 2 due to *Escherichia coli* and 1 due to *Streptococcus faecalis* (Sodhi and Djorjevic, 1966). In the remaining 34 no pathogens were isolated, possibly because of prior antibiotic administration. Pneumococci are the most common identified organisms in children and adults. The high mortality rate is distressing and is probably related to the high prevalence of pneumococcal infections and the frequent late clinical presentation. In Northern Ghana epidemic meningococcal meningitis is the commonest variety. Tuberculous meningitis is perhaps less common than anticipated in view of the abundance of pulmonary tuberculosis. Christian (1967) found four cases of TBM in 373 consecutive autopsies in children aged 0 to 14 years.

Encephalitis

Encephalitis is often misdiagnosed and confused with cerebral malaria, and sometimes with massive intracerebral sickling. Antibodies to arboviruses are widespread in Ghana. Five cases of probable virus encephalitis and one case of measles encephalitis were found in Christian's series of 373 post-mortems on children. Rabies is not uncommon and not infrequently follows incomplete vaccination. Paralytic poliomyelitis is seen and is almost exclusively a childhood disease.

Tetanus

Tetanus is very prevalent among adults and children in the tropics (Ogbeide, 1969; Fendall and Grounds, 1965; Haddock, 1965). Neonatal tetanus caused 15·4 per cent of neonatal deaths at Korle Bu in 1968, with a case mortality rate of over 80 per cent (Ofosu-Amaah and Brookman-Amissah, 1970). This neonatal killer is preventable and is due to improper management of the umbilical cord, for the cord is often cut with bamboo knives, broken bottles, razors, etc., and dressed with herbal concoctions and black powder (Asirifi, 1966). About half as many children had tetanus from the ages of 1 month to 14 years in 1965 as in the neonatal period, the mortality rate being 44 per cent. In the tetanus unit in 1968 and 1969, 192 cases of tetanus were admitted and 76 died.

Tetanus after criminal abortion is common and carries a high mortality rate. Many of the cases had wounds so small as hardly to merit hospital attention initially, and thus prophylactic wound treatment can only prevent a proportion of cases. The valuable therapeutic procedures of tracheostomy and assisted ventilation require skilled staff who are not yet generally available in Ghana.

Prevention by widespread active immunization, and measures to prevent criminal abortion appear to be the most fruitful way to deal with this important tropical disease.

Cerebral Abscess

This is not uncommon, often following neglected sinusitis as well as otitis media and septicaemia.

Neurosyphilis

On the whole this appears uncommon, particularly tabes dorsalis. The fact that malaria and fever have therapeutic benefit in neurosyphilis may be relevant. Possible protection by previous infection with yaws is now becoming less common as the latter diminishes.

Tumours of the CNS

No special studies of tumours of the CNS have been made in Ghana. Hitherto there has been little interest in them as only recently has neurosurgery become available. Secondary tumours in adults appear to be less common than in the United Kingdom, probably because of the almost complete absence of bronchial carcinoma. Hepatocarcinoma is common but rarely metastasizes to the brain. In children, however, Burkitt's tumour of the spine is probably the commonest cause of paraplegia (Wosornu, Nkrumah, and Perkins, 1971) and cerebral metastases are also seen. Among primary tumours, meningiomas, astrocytomas, glioblastomas and pituitary tumours have all been seen. Spinal meningiomas and Schwannomas have also been described (Addae and Mitra (1970).

Disorders of the Cerebral Circulation (Haddock, 1970)

These are very common and rank sixth as a cause of death in adults. A full description is given later [p. 152].

Injuries of the Brain

Head injuries are important in African countries but are usually tended by the surgeons. Motor vehicles, falls and brawls are usually the villains of the piece. Subdural haematomas, however, sometimes reach medical wards in Ghana (Archampong, 1968) and the diagnosis can be very difficult in the absence of a history of trauma, particularly in the elderly. A high index of suspicion is the most important safeguard. Postconcussion syndromes appear to be relatively uncommon. This

Table 15.2

Outpatient Attendance at the Neurology Clinic and Neurological Admissions to Medical Unit with Interest in Neurology, Korle Bu Teaching Hospital, Accra, 1968 and 1969

Disease	*Outpatient*	*Admissions*	*Deaths*
Infections of the CNS			
Pyogenic meningitis	2	19	11
TB meningitis		2	
Encephalitis		6	2
Tetanus		2	
Subdural abscess		1	
Tabes dorsalis	1		
Tumours of the CNS			
Primary cerebral	7	14	1
Secondary cerebral	1		
Primary spinal		2	
Secondary spinal		2	
Retinoblastoma		2	
Disorders of the Cerebral Circulation			
Cerebrovascular accidents	16	116	47
Hypertensive encephalopathy		1	
Temporal arteritis	1		
Intracranial aneurysm	1		
Cavernous sinus thrombosis		2	2
Infantile hemiplegia	5	1	
Injuries of the Brain			
Postconcussion syndromes	6		
Subdural haematomata	2	3	2
Extrapyramidal Syndromes			
Parkinsonism	9	2	
Spasmodic torticollis	1		
Disorders of the Spinal Cord			
Paraplegia of uncertain origin	3	14	1
Transverse myelitis	2	1	
Traumatic tetraplegia		1	
Spinal cord injury		1	
Cervical spondylosis	10	1	
Lumbar spondylosis	4	2	
Cervical cord lesion (cause?)		2	
Probable spinal vascular occlusion	2		
?Demyelinating spinal lesion	2		
Motor neurone disease	1		
Cauda equina lesion (traumatic)		1	
Disorders of the Cranial Nerves			
Bell's palsy	17	1	
Oculomotor paralysis (1 diabetic)	2	3	
Abducent paralysis (cause?)	1	1	
Polyneuritis cranialis		1	
Retrobulbar neuritis	3		
Optic atrophy (primary, cause?)		2	
Unexplained bulbar lesions	1		
Disorders of the Peripheral Nerves			
Peripheral neuropathy (cause uncertain)	5	5	
Infective polyneuritis	1	3	
Tropical ataxic neuropathy	1		

Table 15.2 (continued)

Disease	*Outpatient*	*Admissions*	*Deaths*
Burning feet syndrome	1		
Sarcoid neuropathy	1		
Pressure palsies (5 radial, 1 ext. popliteal)	6		
Carpal tunnel syndrome	2		
Herpes zoster	2		
Disorders of Muscle			
Muscular dystrophy	3		
Myokymia	1		
Myasthenia gravis	1	1	
Paroxysmal and Convulsive Disorders			
Epilepsy (*Note:* 260 *patients* with epilepsy were seen at a separate clinic 1968–69)	See note	37	
Migraine	12		
Syncopal attacks	4	1	
Ménière's syndrome (a European)	1		
Benign paroxysmal vertigo	2		
Psychogenic and Psychiatric			
Tension headaches	11	2	
Anxiety states	5	3	
Hysteria	11	6	
Depressive states	6	2	
Schizophrenia	2	4	
Post-partum psychosis		1	
Neurosis	8	1	
Writer's cramp	4	1	
Miscellaneous			
Hyperhydrosis	2		
Magnesium sulphate poisoning		2	
Barbiturate poisoning		1	
Hereditary cerebellar ataxia		1	
Organic dementia (cause ?)		1	
Total	*192*	*280*	*67*

Notes:

1. All but 15 patients were of African descent.
2. Epileptics attended a separate clinic.
3. Most cases of tetanus and many cases of meningitis were admitted to the Infectious Fevers Unit.
4. Some outpatients were subsequently admitted.

may be related to a lesser public awareness of litigation possibilities than exists in the West.

Extrapyramidal Syndromes

Parkinsonism is probably less evident than in Europe and seems to be occasionally postencephalitic but usually occurs in the elderly. Chorea (Huntington's and Sydenham's), athetosis and torsion spasm have been seen but are rare.

Disorders of the Spinal Cord

Paraplegia

Paraplegia is a significant tropical neurological problem. Common causes of paraplegia in Ghana include trauma, spinal tuberculosis, and Burkitt's tumour in childhood. Other less common causes of paraplegia seen in Accra include central disc protrusions, vertebral neoplasms including Hodgkin's disease and other secondaries, meningovascular syphilis, transverse myelitis, infective polyneuritis and extradural abscess due to guinea-worm infestation (Mitra and Haddock, 1970). However, in approximately 40 per cent of paraplegias seen in the medical wards in Accra no definite cause can be found. This is in accordance with experience in other African countries. Various possible causes of obscure paraplegia in the tropics include arachnoiditis, schistosomal granulomas in the cord (Bird, 1965; Faust, 1948), spinal cysticercosis (Powell *et al.*, 1966), atypical neurosyphilis, paragonimiasis of the cord (Adams and Macgraith, 1964), lathyrism, and tropical neuropathy. Definite diagnosis is difficult in these patients with obscure paraplegias as they rarely come to autopsy. Many present late, when any CSF evidence of transverse myelitis or infective polyneuritis may have disappeared.

Myelography is often essential if surgically remediable conditions are to be excluded. In such obscure cases the myelogram may appear normal, while in a few there is evidence of arachnoiditis and occasionally a block is shown. In two such cases laminectomy revealed a swollen segment of cord (apparently not tumerous), and in one laminectomy was followed by marked clinical improvement. Schistosomiasis is widespread in Ghana and schistosomiasis of the cord has occasionally been found elsewhere in Africa although it can only be indubitably proven at post-mortem. Although success has been claimed for treatment of the schistosomiasis it is difficult to see how such chemotherapy can influence a granuloma produced as a reaction to dying ova. We have found the prognosis for improvement in these obscure paraplegias to be rather poor, but the patients are sometimes able to walk and often have bladder control.

Spinal Cord Injury

This is quite common and usually the result of motor vehicle accidents. Falling from palm trees and fracturing vertebrae L1 or L2 while harvesting the nuts is a particular African hazard. Some fall while carrying a heavy load on their head and injure the lower cervical cord.

Cervical and Lumbar Spondylosis

Intervertebral disc degeneration with protrusion and root and cord pressure is probably less common than in the United Kingdom although about 15 cases were seen in 2 years and an appreciable number of lumbar disc cases attended the general medical and orthopaedic clinics. Clinical and radiological osteoarthrosis of the spine and knees are very common in the elderly Ghanaian.

Other Spinal Cord Diseases

The rarity of multiple sclerosis in the tropics is well known. We have never seen a convincing example in Accra although a case of neuromyelitis optica has been found. Motor neurone disease is rare. Some patients with amyotrophic lateral sclerosis may fall into the obscure paraplegia group. Addisonian anaemia is rare in Africa, and subacute combined degeneration has not been identified in Ghana.

Disorders of the Cranial Nerves

Two comments may be made about cranial nerve disorders:

1. There are many cases of unexplained isolated optic atrophy in which investigations are unrevealing. The possibility of local toxins cannot be ignored.
2. Trigeminal neuralgia appears to be rare.

Disorders of the Peripheral Nerves

In the urban environment of Accra peripheral neuropathy appears to be much less prevalent than in rural Nigeria. This may be due to differences in cassava preparation and consumption, and in general nutrition. Alcoholism is common and so is alcoholic hypoglycaemic coma, but alcoholic neuropathy is only occasionally seen. It should be remembered that not all cases of peripheral neuropathy in the African are associated with cassava consumption. Some appear to be neuritic beriberi and some are associated with pellagra (Ebrahim and Haddock, 1964).

Disorders of Muscle

Muscular rheumatism is not included in TABLE 15.2 but is frequently diagnosed. Muscular dystrophy is rare. I have now seen four cases of myasthenia gravis in Accra.

Epilepsy

As can be seen from TABLE 15.2 over 250 patients attended the Epilepsy Clinic (established in 1966) in Accra during 1968 and 1969. After clinical, EEG and other investigations, we considered that just over half our epileptics had symptomatic epilepsy although the cause was not usually clear (Edoo and Haddock, 1970). The commonest identified causes of epilepsy were trauma and cerebrovascular disease. Possession of the sickle-cell gene did not appear to predispose to epilepsy. Grand mal epilepsy was the variety of fit in over 80 per cent of the patients. Petit mal is not often recognized and may be considered not worthy of medical attention by the parents of a victim. In a small survey the approximate prevalence of epilepsy in Accra was considered to be 4·1 per thousand (Haddock, 1967).

As in the rest of Africa, epilepsy is predominantly a social problem. Owing to belief in supernatural causation and fear of acquiring the disease by contagion, the unfortunate sufferers are often shunned, deprived of schooling and occupation, and sometimes deserted by their spouses. The social prognosis in Accra is fair if fits are few and begin after school age and if there is no physical or mental handicap (Haddock and Edoo, 1970). Attendance at the clinic has been irregular and disappointing despite attempts at education. This is due to the local conception that medicine should be permanently effective after a short-term course, to difficulty in travel to the clinic, and to lack of cooperation on the part of employers and school teachers. In those who have attended regularly results of drug treatment have usually been satisfactory.

Migraine

Migraine is fairly prevalent but often unrecognized. One severe case has been seen with unilateral optic atrophy following occlusion of the central artery of the retina. Classical Ménière's syndrome has not been seen in an African.

Psychogenic and Psychiatric Disorders in Ghana (Foster, 1966)

These cannot be reviewed comprehensively but certain features worthy of note by the physician will be commented upon.

Aetiology

Society and the way of life are changing very rapidly for many Africans. There is a rapid drift towards towns often resulting in isolation from the family, poverty, poor living conditions, loneliness, and unemployment. There are considerable pressures on the young to reach high and sometimes unattainable scholastic levels. The man who achieves financial success will be expected to help and support many relatives. Despite sophistication, education, and a widespread belief in Christianity, many people still believe in and fear supernatural influences (e.g. ghosts and juju). Polygamy and childlessness are other common worries. These stresses and conflicts are important in producing mental breakdowns. Foster (1966), in a study of mental disease in Accra, emphasized poverty and low academic attainment as important factors.

Children of Muslims seemed to him less liable to mental illness than children of Christians. He also rightly stressed the importance of eliminating organic disease (e.g. typhoid, malaria, trypanosomiasis) as the cause of mental illness. Indian hemp consumption is quite prevalent in Accra and is responsible for many acute but usually transient psychoses.

Types of Mental Disturbance

Neurosis. Anxiety states are the commonest neurosis and often take the form of a cardiac neurosis. To many Ghanaians any frontal chest pain or palpitation implies heart trouble and danger of death. In the sterile woman who fears divorce, desertion or ridicule, abdominal pains without organic basis are common. Hysterical paralyses and comas are not uncommon. Depression (often combined with anxiety) is frequently seen and may be associated with impotence which is regarded very seriously.

The Psychoses. Schizophrenia and manic-depressive psychoses are usually seen by the psychiatrists after preliminary visits to traditional healers, witch doctors or 'prophets'. Acute short-term confusional episodes without obvious organic causes are not uncommon, as in other parts of Africa.

Miscellaneous and Poisoning

Suicidal poisoning is fortunately still uncommon in Accra—barbiturates are rarely taken in dangerous quantities. A few cases of magnesium sulphate poisoning have been seen due to the almost universal habit of swallowing large quantities of mist alba to move the bowels at the onset of any sickness and for real or imaginary constipation. Sometimes significant systemic absorption takes place (possibly due to overdosage and overdilution without purgation), giving rise to acute toxic effects. The patient, often a child, is semi-comatose; more or less paralysed, areflexic and hypotensive. Several serious cases have been seen. The toxicity of local herbal preparations is uncertain. Cow's urine for epileptic revival does not seem to be widely used as in Nigeria.

Neurological Complications of Endemic Diseases

Many neurological problems are encountered as presentations or complications of endemic diseases. An attempt to summarize the problem in Ghana is made in TABLE 15.3.

Neurological Complications of the Haemoglobinopathies

Two to 3 per cent of children born in Southern Ghana have a serious haemoglobinopathy (SS, SC or S thalassaemia). Persons with haemoglobinopathy are liable to neurological complications—estimates of the frequency of these complications vary considerably but in Adeloye and Odeku's recent series from Nigeria (1970) it was 12·8 per cent in SS disease admissions. SS and SC disease patients dying in sickle-cell crises may show pathological changes in the nervous system including diffuse microcirculatory stasis and congestion with secondary neural anoxic changes and pericapillary haemorrhages (Baird *et al.*, 1964; Diggs, 1959). Sometimes cerebral or subarachnoid haemorrhages, subdural haematoma, or cerebral thrombosis are found.

In our experience febrile convulsions and hysterical behaviour are quite common in sickle-cell crisis. True psychotic incidents during crisis are sometimes seen. Focal signs due to vascular occlusion seem much less common. Electroencephalographic changes in crisis, usually diffuse and resembling those of diffuse encephalopathy produced by anoxia, are very common (Haddock, Edoo, and Konotey-Ahulu, 1970; Lemmi and Ang, 1965). These EEG changes are not usually accompanied by clear-cut neurological signs. Ocular complications such as retinopathy and monocular blindness with optic atrophy (Konotey-Ahulu, 1968) are seen. Serious cerebrovascular occlusion may be readily precipitated by hypoxia during anaesthesia in people with SS and SC disease and even in those with the sickle-cell trait (AS). Pneumococcal meningitis is a not-infrequent complication of sickle-cell disease, and

Table 15.3

Epidemic and Endemic Diseases in Ghana with Neurological Complications

Disease	*Neurological Complications*	*Comments with relevance to Ghana*
Viral Measles	Convulsions, encephalitis, SSLE	Common illness. Fourth ranking cause of death in children but encephalitis uncommon
Smallpox	Convulsions, encephalitis	Now uncommon in Ghana
Virus hepatitis (Morrow *et al.*, 1968)	Liver failure with neuropsychiatric manifestations	Distressingly prevalent with considerable mortality. A common cause of coma
Arbovirus infections	Encephalitis	Infection with arboviruses widespread—occasional encephalitis seen
Bacterial Typhoid	1. Toxic psychosis 2. Meningitis 3. Peripheral neuritis	Typhoid is prevalent. Complications (1) often seen; (2) and (3) rare
Bacillary dysentry	Peripheral neuropathy	Neuropathy is occasionally seen
Leprosy	Peripheral neuropathy	Neuropathy is common and crippling
Relapsing fever	1. Optic Atropy 2. Meningitis 3. Paraplegia and hemiplegia 4. Cranial nerve palsies	A serious disease but now rare in Ghana
Protozoal Falciparum malaria	Febrile convulsions, cerebral malaria	Malaria universal in children. Cerebral malaria common and often fatal
Amoebiasis	Cerebral abscess, peripheral neuropathy and neuromuscular block due to emetine (Salako, 1970)	Amoebiasis rife. Cerebral abscess rare. Emetine now falling out of use
Trypanosomiasis (Scott, 1965)	Chronic meningo-encephalitis	Trypanosomiasis (Gambiense) still found in Northern Ghana
Toxoplasmosis	Encephalomyelitis, granulomata in CNS	Cerebral toxoplasmosis reported in Ghana (Christian, 1970)

Table 15.3 (continued)

Disease	*Neurological Complications*	*Comments with relevance to Ghana*
Metazoal Onchocerciasis	Optic atrophy	Very common in parts of Ghana—a leading cause of blindness
Guinea-worm infection	Spinal extradural abscess causing paraplegia	Guinea-worm infection common. Cases of paraplegia reported
Schistosoma haematobium and *mansoni*	Cerebral and spinal granulomata	*S. haematobium* widespread in Ghana, *S. mansoni* less common. Neurological complications probably rare and unreported in Ghana
Toxocariasis	Epilepsy and increased liability to poliomyelitis (Woodruff, Bisseru, and Bowe, 1966)	High incidence of positive skin tests in Accra but significance uncertain
Cysticercosis	Epilepsy	One case reported in Ghana but probably rare (Odamtten and Laing, 1967)
Miscellaneous Haemoglobinopathy SS, SC, S thalassaemia	Cerebral and cord vascular occlusion and haemorrhage, optic atrophy, acute encephalopathy and EEG changes. Liability to pneumococcal meningitis (Greer and Schotland, 1962)	High incidence of haemoglobinopathy; neurological complications fairly common
Snake-bite	Motor paralysis, respiratory failure, ptosis an early sign	Snake-bite common. Envenomation in perhaps 10 per cent of victims

in this connexion it is interesting to note that a specific immunological deficiency of polymorphs against pneumococci has been described in sickle-cell disease (Winkelstein and Drachman, 1968).

References

ADAMS, A. R. D., and MAEGRAITH, B. G. (1964) *Clinical Tropical Diseases*, 3rd ed., Oxford, p. 77, 510–512.

ADDAE, R. O., and MITRA, A. K. (1970) Recovery from paraplegia following timely removal of cord tumours, *Ghana med. J.*, 9, 125.

ADELOYE, A., and ODEKU, E. L. (1970) The nervous system in sickle cell disease, *Afr. J. med. Sci.*, **1**, 33.

ARCHAMPONG, E. Q. (1968) Diagnosis of subdural haematoma, *Ghana med. J.*, 7, 124.

ASIRIFI, Y. (1966) Patterns of disease as seen in hospital, *Ghana med. J.*, 5, 137.

BAIRD, R. L., WEISS, D. L., FERGUSON, A. D., FRENCH, J. H., and SCOTT, R. B. (1964) Studies on sickle cell anaemia: XXI. Clinicopathological aspects of neurological manifestations, *Pediatrics*, 34, 92.

BIRD, A. V. (1965) Spinal cord complications of bilharziasis, *S. Afr. med. J.*, 39, 158.

CHRISTIAN, E. C. (1967) Why do our children die ?, *Ghana med. J.*, 6, 111.

CHRISTIAN, E. C. (1970) Human toxoplasmosis in Ghana, *Ghana med. J.*, 9, 80.

DIGGS, L. W. (1959) Studies on sickle cell anaemia: XXI. Clinicopathological aspects of neurological manifestations, *Proc. VIth int. Cong. trop. Med. Malar.*, 6, 442.

EBRAHIM, G. J., and HADDOCK, D. R. W. (1964) Polyneuropathy of probable nutritional origin in Dar-es-Salaam, Tanganyika, *Trans. roy. Soc. trop. Med. Hyg.*, 58, 246.

EDOO, B. B., and HADDOCK, D. R. W. (1970) Epilepsy in Accra, Ghana: a report on classification and etiology, *Afr. J. med. Sci.*, 1, 207.

FAUST, E. C. (1948) Inquiry into ectopic lesions in schistosomiasis, *Amer. J. trop. Med.*, 28, 175.

FENDALL, N. R. E., and GROUNDS, J. G. (1965) The incidence and epidemiology of disease in Kenya: I. Some diseases of social significance, *J. trop. Med. Hyg.*, **68**, 77.

FOSTER, E. B. (1966) A longitudinal ecological study of one hundred consecutive admissions to the Accra mental hospital, *Ghana med. J.*, **5**, 123.

GREER, M., and SCHOTLAND, D. (1962) Abnormal haemoglobin as a cause of neurologic disease, *Neurology (Minneap.)*, **12**, 114.

HADDOCK, D. R. W. (1965) Neurological disorders in Tanzania, *J. trop. Med. Hyg.*, **68**, 161.

HADDOCK, D. R. W. (1967) An attempt to assess the prevalence of epilepsy in Accra, *Ghana med. J.*, **6**, 140.

HADDOCK, D. R. W. (1970) Cerebrovascular accidents in Ghana, *Trans. roy. Soc. trop. Med. Hyg.*, **64**, 300.

HADDOCK, D. R. W., and EDOO, B. B. (1970) The social aspects of epilepsy in Accra, Ghana, *Epilepsia (Amst.)*, **11**, 217–22.

HADDOCK, D. R. W., EDOO, B. B., and KONOTEY-AHULU, F. I. D. (1970) *Electroencephalographic Changes in Sickle Cell Disease*, paper presented at the Second Pan-African Congress of Neurological Sciences, 13–17 January, Ibadan.

KONOTEY-AHULU, F. I. D. (1968) Sickle-cell disease and monocular blindness in Africans, *Lancet*, **ii**, 222.

LEMMI, H., and ANG, R. (1965) Electroencephalographic studies in sickle-cell crises in adults in *Proceedings of the Eighth International Congress of Neurology, Vienna, 1965*.

MITRA, A. K., and HADDOCK, D. R. W. (1970) Paraplegia due to guinea-worm infection, *Trans. roy. Soc. trop. Med. Hyg.*, **64**, 102–6.

MORROW, R. H., SMETANA, H. F., SIA, F. T., and EDGCOMB, J. H. (1968) Unusual features of viral hepatitis in Accra, Ghana, *Ann. intern. Med.*, **68**, 1250.

ODAMTTEN, S. E., and LAING, W. N. (1967) Cysticercosis of the brain, *Ghana med. J.*, **6**, 97–105.

OFOSU-AMAAH, S., and BROOKMAN-AMISSAH, E. (1970) Analysis of deaths in the department of child health, Korle Bu Hospital, 1968, *Ghana med. J.*, **9**, 12–22.

OGBEIDE, M. I. (1969) Prednisolone in the treatment of tetanus in infants and children, *W. Afr. med. J.*, **18**, 7.

POWELL, S. J., PROCTOR, E. M., WILMOT, A. J., and BARNETT, A. M. (1966) Neurological complications of cysticercosis in Africans: a clinical and serological study, *Ann. trop. Med. Parasit.*, **60**, 159.

SALAKO, L. A. (1970) Emetine-induced muscular paralysis, *Ghana med. J.*, **9**, 137.

SCOTT, D. (1965) *Epidemic Disease in Ghana, 1901–1960*, London, pp. 138–83.

SODHI, H. S., and DJORJEVIC, L. (1966) Pyogenic meningitis, *Ghana med. J.*, **5**, 115.

WINKELSTEIN, J. A., and DRACHMAN, R. H. (1968) Deficiency of pneumococcal serum opsonizing activity in sickle-cell disease, *New Engl. J. Med.*, **279**, 459.

WOODRUFF, A. W., BISSERU, B., BOWE, J. C. (1966) Infection with animal helminths as a factor in causing poliomyelitis and epilepsy, *Brit. med. J.*, **1**, 1576.

WOSORNU, J. L., NKRUMAH, F. K., and PERKINS, I. V. (1971) Survival of Burkitt's lymphoma patients in Ghana, *Brit. J. Cancer*, **25**, 479–86.

CEREBROVASCULAR DISEASE

Increasing interest is being taken in cerebrovascular disease in the Western world for the following reasons:

1. Cerebrovascular accidents are a leading cause of death and disability. The high incidence and mortality are partly due to an ageing population and also to a diminishing death rate from infection.

2. Cerebral angiography has improved topographical diagnosis and led to the possibility of prophylactic surgical treatment of diseased extracranial vessels.

3. Epidemiological studies have defined some risk factors.

It is only comparatively recently however that cerebrovascular disease in the tropics has been studied (Collomb, Dumas, and Lemercier, 1966; Dalal *et al.*, 1968; Osuntokun, Odeku, and Adeloye, 1969; Dada, Johnson, and Araba, 1969; Gwee *et al.*, 1970; Haddock, 1970 *a*). The following review is based on personal experience in Tanzania and Ghana and on a study of the relevant literature. Differences in cerebrovascular disease in tropical and non-tropical countries and possible aetiological and epidemiological factors will be emphasized, but the general clinical manifestations, the methods of investigation and the principles of management will not be stressed, because they are universal.

Cerebrovascular disease is primarily a disease of arteries; atherosclerosis and hypertension are of predominant importance, while cerebral disturbances are secondary. The key to prevention therefore lies in exploring the causation and prevention of vascular disease. It seems likely that cerebral atherosclerosis is largely environmental rather than racial in origin, although it appears to be more severe and occurs at a younger age in American Negroes than in Whites (Takahashi, 1962; Stallones, 1965). There is a general impression that vascular disease is uncommon in the tropics. This certainly appears to be true of coronary artery disease and limb vessel occlusion (Reef and Isaacson, 1962; Virieu and Collomb, 1968), but hypertension is probably as common in many parts of the tropics as in the West (Stuart, 1968). In some parts of the tropics, such as Tanzania (Haddock, 1965 *b*; Forsyth, 1969) and among the Samburu in Kenya (Shaper, Williams, and Spencer, 1961), hypertension appears less prevalent and this emphasizes the need that the tropics should not be regarded as one homogeneous area with identical medical problems and conditions.

However, factors which may affect the prevalence of atherosclerosis can be noted:

1. The majority of tropical people live in rural areas and engage in agriculture, usually at a subsistence level. They are thinner, more physically active, and much poorer than their Western counterparts.

2. The tropical diet is higher in unrefined carbohydrates and lower in proteins, animal fats, and often in calories.

3. In the tropics there is a high childhood mortality and continuing exposure to severe infectious disease, so there is a smaller proportion of people over 50 years of age than in the West.

4. Cigarette smoking is less prevalent and much less heavy.

These factors may lessen the incidence of atherosclerosis. Circumstances are changing in the tropics, however, with increasing urbanization, a drift from agricultural activity, and consumption of more sophisticated foodstuffs including large amounts of sugar in some areas. Hypertension and diabetes may be increasing, physical activity is lessening, and populations are becoming older. These changing circumstances will probably cause a gradual increase in atherosclerotic disease. Although haemorrhagic and occlusive pathologies are often found in the same brain and haemorrhagic and occlusive strokes show many similarities, the epidemiology, aetiology, management and mortality show differences, and it is desirable to consider them separately.

Prevalence of Cerebrovascular Disease in Ghana

Mortality Statistics

These are not comprehensive. In the 29 compulsory registration areas of Ghana in 1967 cerebrovacular disease was the tenth commonest cause of death (3·5 per cent of deaths). In Lagos, Nigeria, in 1963, CVD was the eleventh commonest cause of death (2·8 per cent of deaths) (Humponu-Wusa, 1969). These percentages may be compared with the 14½ per cent of all deaths caused by strokes in the United Kingdom (Acheson and Fairbairn, 1970).

Epidemiology

Vital statistics are neither complete nor accurate in most parts of the tropics. Much dependence has to be placed on hospital statistics, which are not reliable in estimating the full extent of cerebrovascular disease in the community.

In Table 15·4 some indication of hospital prevalence of cerebrovascular disease in the tropics is given. Haemorrhagic and ischaemic strokes are not differentiated.

Hospital admissions may depend on the clinicians' interests, availability of beds for chronic cases, relatives' willingness to allow admission of patients with certain diseases, and ease of access to the hospital for patients. The hospital burden of cerebrovascular disease is probably less in the tropics but is very variable from area to area and is probably smaller in country areas than in towns.

The varieties of cerebrovascular accidents are difficult to differentiate on purely clinical grounds. The simplest and most commonly used differential method is examination of the CSF, but even this is liable to fallacy as in 20 per cent of cases of cerebral haemorrhage the CSF may not be blood-stained. The figures often given for the different varieties of stroke are therefore liable to considerable error depending on the criteria of diagnosis. Autopsy diagnoses are heavily biased towards cerebral haemorrhage as haemorrhagic strokes are much more often fatal than ischaemic. Some statistics on differing varieties of stroke are given in Table 15.5.

Comments

On the whole these figures are remarkably consistent for the tropics, the United States and London; ischaemic strokes predominate. Intracranial haemorrhage comprises 13 per cent to 23 per cent of the cases and subarachnoid haemorrhage 5 per cent to 13 per cent. Cerebral embolism is less common except in Bombay and Uganda, where 20 per cent of strokes were embolic.

Table 15.4
Cerebrovascular Accidents as Proportion of Hospital Admissions

Country	*Author*	*CVA*	
		Percentage of Admissions	*Percentage of Neurological Admissions*
Uganda	Hutton (1956)	—	9·2
Uganda (Kampala)	Billinghurst (1966)	—	34·0
Tanzania	Haddock (1965*a*)	0·86	6·5
Nigeria (Lagos)	Dada, Johnson, and Araba (1969)	—	16·8
Kenya (Nairobi)	Ojiambo (1966)	—	20·0
Nigeria (Ibadan)	Kaushik (1961)	0·15	7·0
Nigeria (Ibadan)	Osuntokun, Odeku, and Adeloye (1969)	—	12·7
Ghana (Accra)	Haddock (1970*a*)	4·00	41·0
India (Bombay)	Dalal *et al.* (1968)	1·00	—
United Kingdom (London)	Glynn (1956)	6·00	—
S. Africa (Natal)	Cosnett (1969)	—	33·0

Table 15.5

Varieties of CVA in the Tropics and the West

Country	Author	Diagnostic Method	No. of Cases	Ischaemic (Non-Embolic)	Haemorrhagic		Embolic	Unclassified
					* IC	† SAH		CVA
				%	%	%	%	%
Nigeria (Ibadan)	Osuntokun, Odeku, and Adeloye (1969)	LP autopsy	472	49·8	19·5	12·1	4·4	—
Nigeria (Lagos)	Dada, Johnson, and Araba (1969)	Clinical autopsy	205	57·6	22·3	13·6	4·9	1·5
Ghana (Accra)	Haddock (1970*a*)	LP clinical autopsy	280	23·0	19·0	—	2·0	54·0[1]
Senegal (Dakar)	Dumas (1968)	LP angiogram autopsy	600	68·0	13·0	11·0	—	—
Uganda (Makerere)	Shaper and Shaper (1958)	LP clinical	—	63·0	12·5	—	23·0	—
India (Bombay)	Dalal *et al.* (1968)	LP angiogram autopsy	127	52·0	13·0	4·0	20·0	10·0
Malaysia (Singapore)	Gwee *et al.* (1970)	LP autopsy	241	69·0	22·0	9·0	1·0	—
London (United Kingdom)	Glynn (1956)[2]	LP clinical autopsy	315	52·0	23·0	10·0	2·0	7·0
New York (United States)	Groch, McDevitt, and Wright (1961)	LP angiogram autopsy	688	70·0	7·0	5·0	5·0	9·0
United States	Merritt (1967)	LP clinical	604	66·0	21·0	8·0	5·0	—

[1] Mainly ischaemic in fact but no LP.
[2] Also 6 per cent transient ischaemic included.
* IC Intracerebral.
† SAH Subarachnoid haemorrhage.
All percentages do not total 100 per cent as some included subdural haematoma and tumour haemorrhage.

Non-Embolic Ischaemic Cerebrovascular Disease

Ischaemic cerebrovascular disease is commoner than haemorrhagic disease in the tropics but we lack statisics.

Pathology

There have been several reviews of the pathophysiology of cerebral ischaemic vascular disease recently (Crawford and Crompton, 1968; Yates, 1964). Some recent concepts may be emphasized:

1. The frequency of extracranial stenosis of carotid and vertebral arteries as a cause of cerebral ischaemia.

2. The importance of anastomoses in the circle of Willis and between extracranial (e.g. ophthalmic) and intracranial arteries in maintaining imperilled cerebral circulation.

3. The abandonment of the concept of cerebral vasospasm except after subarachnoid haemorrhage and possibly hypertensive encephalopathy. Transient attacks are more likely to be embolic in origin, arising from carotid plaques.

4. A large cerebral infarct may swell and act as an acute expanding intracranial lesion (Adams, 1966).

5. The recognition of two topographical types of cerebral infarcts—those occurring within particular arterial areas and those occurring in the boundary zones or 'watersheds' (Adams, 1967).

6. After unilateral cerebral infarction there may be bilateral reduction of regional blood flow for up to 3 weeks, possibly accounting for early stupor, coma and obtundity after a stroke (Meyer, 1970).

Literature on cerebrovascular pathology in Africa is sparse, but accounts have come from Nigeria (Williams, Resch, and Loewenson, 1969; Edington and Gilles, 1969 *a*); Ghana (Edington, 1954; Laing, 1969); Senegal (Collomb *et al.*, 1966; Collomb, Dumas, and Lemercier, 1966); Uganda (Davies, 1948; Hutt and Coles, 1969) and South Africa (Laurie and Woods, 1968; Reef and Isaacson, 1962). The findings of these authors have much in common and may be summarized as follows.

Cerebral atherosclerosis is fairly common but much less marked than in developed countries. The most severe atherosclerosis is seen in association with hypertension; diabetes is important but syphilis is not. Severe cerebral atherosclerosis without hypertension is less common than in the West thus emphasizing the possibly greater significance, aetiologically, of hypertension in ischaemic strokes in the tropics. In Senegal, Collomb does not think that hypertension and diabetes play such a predominant role and he believes that cerebral atherosclerosis is little different from that in the West. All agree, however, that coronary and limb atherosclerosis are much less intense and common in Africa. Stallones (1965) says, 'The pattern of geographic distribution of cerebrovascular ischaemic deaths does not resemble that attributed to atherosclerotic heart disease'. In South Africa considerable chemical differences in composition were found between the aortas and coronary arteries of adult whites and blacks, but no marked differences in the cerebral arteries.

Pathological and angiographic studies have shown that extracranial arterial stenosis is common in tropical patients, although the incidence is less than the 50 per cent cited by Hutchinson and Yates (1957). When the figures of the earlier publications are compared with those of the later ones, the impression is that CVD is increasing in autopsy findings in the tropics.

Incidence

The authors' findings in TABLE 15.4 from Ibadan, Lagos, Ghana, India and Senegal record a hospital male preponderance in ischaemic vascular diseases, the male to female ratios in these areas being 1·8:1; 1·4:1; 1·5:1; 2·2:1, and 1·4:1 respectively. In Singapore the sex ratio was equal. In tropical hospitals there are almost always considerably more male than female admissions and this may mean that the recorded male preponderance in Africa is not genuine.

Age is difficult to assess in the tropics as many people do not know their date of birth. There are relatively fewer old people than young and therefore fewer at risk of stroke. Hypertension is relatively common in young people in parts of the tropics (Akinkugbe, 1969).

In the series of cases from Lagos, Accra and Bombay the peak age incidence was 51–60 years for males and females; In Ibadan 51–60 years for males and 41–50 years for females; in Singapore the figures were 51–60 years for males and 61–70 years for females. In Senegal 55 per cent of cases occurred before the age of 50.

In the West the average age for ischaemic stroke is probably at least a decade higher (Glynn, 1956; Chapman *et al.*, 1966; Merritt, 1967). This difference may be related to the differing population structures.

The Completed Non-embolic Stroke

One would not expect any marked differences in clinical manifestations but presentation may be modified, as those with less severe disabilities such as isolated dysphasia, dementia or brachial monoplegia may not be seen. Over 90 per cent of the patients in Osuntokun's and Haddock's series had hemiplegia; 60 per cent to 70 per cent of those with right hemiplegia had dysphasia, and 10 per cent to 15 per cent of left hemiplegics were dysphasic. There was an unexplained and quite marked excess of right as opposed to left hemiplegics in the Ibadan and Lagos series but the incidence was equal in Accra. Carotid strokes were very much commoner than vertebral strokes. The modes of onset did not differ from standard accounts.

Transient Ischaemic Attacks (TIA)

Transient ischaemic attacks are variously defined according to the maximal allowed duration, from 1 hour to 1 week (Jennett, 1967; Gwee *et al.*, 1970). The subject has been well reviewed by Marshall (1968 *a*) who believes that they may be due to disturbance of blood flow, to small infarcts or to small haemorrhages, and that it may be impossible to differentiate these causes clinically. They are an important aspect of cerebrovascular disease as they offer an opportunity to prevent completed strokes by anticoagulant therapy, vascular surgery, treatment of anaemia or hypotensive drugs where appropriate. Osuntokun, Odeku, and Adeloye (1969), Dada (1970) and Gwee *et al.* (1970) found that about 10 per cent of their cases of stroke (ischaemic cases only in Osuntokun's series) presented with TIA. Transient ischaemic attacks are uncommon presenting features of strokes in Accra, with less than 2 per cent of cases presenting thus. However, if patients with ischaemic strokes are questioned, about 5 per cent give stories of previous attacks (Haddock, 1970 *b*). Many patients with transient ischaemic attacks in the tropics probably do not seek medical attention; the prevalence may be as high as elsewhere.

Epilepsy

This is a not uncommon sequel of cerebrovascular diseases; Osuntokum, Odeku, and Adeloye (1969) found it in nine of their 235 cases (3·8 per cent), and CVD ranks high in the list of known causes of symptomatic epilepsy in Ibadan, Accra and Dakar. Osuntokun and Odeku (1970) found it responsible for 2·7 per cent of their epileptics; Haddock (1970 *a*), for 3·4 per cent and Collomb *et al.* (1966) for 10 per cent (these authors included acute stroke in their series).

Hypertension

In the series from Ibadan, Lagos, Accra, Senegal, Bombay and Singapore 63 per cent, 57 per cent, 62 per cent, 53 per cent, 51 per cent and 46 per cent respectively of the patients with ischaemic stroke were hypertensive. On the basis of unexplained ECG left ventricular hypertrophy in 28 per cent of his 'normotensive' patients at Accra, Haddock (1970 *b*) believes that the true prevalence of hypertension may be even higher than 62 per cent. The prevalence of hypertension in these series does not greatly differ from American and European series.

In over 60 per cent of cases in the Ibadan series and in over 80 per cent of the Accra series hypertension was not known to be present before the stroke. As treatment with hypotensives can prevent CVA this situation shows one method of stroke prevention by detecting and treating hypertension.

Diabetes Mellitus

Diabetes is not uncommon in the tropics although its prevalence varies widely from place to place and the disease is almost certainly increasing in many areas (Tulloch, 1962). The association of diabetes with ischaemic CVD has long been recognized. In Accra and Ibadan glucose tolerance tests were done where possible and diabetes was found in 24 per cent and 20 per cent respectively in cases of ischaemic CVD. In Bombay and Singapore diabetes was found in 21 per cent and 14 per cent but in Lagos and Senegal diabetes was diagnosed in only 2 per cent and 3 per cent. These differences may, however, be related to the intensity of search. Diabetes is probably a factor of major importance in the tropics as in the West.

Obesity

In the tropics obesity, high socio-economic status and serum lipids are probably interrelated to varying extents. Obesity tends to be associated with relative material prosperity in the tropics, in contrast to the situation in the United States where it is less common in the higher socio-economic groups. In the tropics obesity may be viewed as a sign of good health, high social status and in the female even of physical beauty.

There has been little study of obesity in the tropics but it is probably a fairly common problem in middle-aged urban West African women (Virieu and Collomb, 1968; Haddock, 1969). Tulloch (1962) found a variable prevalence; it is low in nomadic groups. Johnson (1970) found Nigerian men and women in Lagos to be heavier (at equivalent heights) than English people. Parry (1969) believes obesity is associated with hypertension as does Haddock (1969); Shaper *et al.* (1969) found no evidence of the association in 'nomadic warriors in the Kenyan army'. Virieu and Collomb (1968), Dalal *et al.* (1968), Haddock (1970 *a*) and Dada (1970) have all shown an abnormally high prevalence of obesity in ischaemic CVD.

In the Accra series obesity was particularly common in middle-aged females and was correlated with hypertension; in males it showed some correlation with diabetes.

Serum Lipids

In the West there is some association between elevation of serum lipids and cerebrovascular disease but it is much less strong than the association of hyperlipaemia with ischaemic heart disease. Dada (1970) found nearly 50 per cent of his cases to have hypercholesterolaemia; Osuntokun, Odeku, and Adeloye (1969) found the mean cholesterol levels in ischaemic stroke to be higher than normal but believed that the serum cholesterol level was a reflection of socio-economic status; Haddock (1970 *a*) found elevated serum cholesterol and beta lipoprotein levels in ischaemic and haemorrhagic CVD. Dalal *et al.* (1968) found relatively little hypercholesterolaemia. In general, in the tropics the serum lipid levels were raised above the local mean levels but were not high by Western standards.

Socio-economic Status

Chapman *et al.* (1966) found a positive correlation in the United States between upper socio-economic status and occlusive CVD. In Ibadan and Accra there is evidence of a similar relationship; Dada, Johnson and Araba (1969) found 27·8 per cent of their patients in Lagos to be in the middle and upper income groups.

Urbanism

Urbanism may predipose to CVD (Howe, 1963). In tropical countries urbanism is often associated with lessened physical activity, higher intake of refined carbohydrates, and obesity. Although conclusive evidence is lacking, stroke in the tropics is probably more common in urban than rural areas.

Sickle-cell Disease

Cerebral infarction in sickle-cell diseases in childhood and adolescence occasionally occurs, but it appears to be rare in adult life (Adeloye and Odeku, 1970). The prevalence of the sickle-cell gene was normal in ischaemic CVD at Ibadan and Accra but in Lagos there was a suspicion of increased sickle-cell dsease. Haemoglobinopathy is probably not an important factor in adult CVD. Dada, Johnson, and Araba (1969) found an increased blood viscosity in their cases. In controls the viscosity was highest in genotypes CC and SC and increased above normal in AS and SS. This finding needs investigation.

Prognosis

In the tropical series the early mortalities for non-embolic ischaemic CVD recorded by Osuntokun, Odeku, and Adeloye (1969), Haddock (1970 *a*), Dalal *et al.* (1968), Collomb, Dumas, and Lemercier (1966), and Gwee *et al.* (1970) were 15·3 per cent, 15 per cent, 30 per cent, 19·2 per cent and 15 per cent respectively. Apart from the Bombay series these mortalities are lower than in most Western series. This may be due to the fact that the average age was considerably lower than in the West and may also imply selection of cases that reach hospital. One suspects that in the tropics the very old and the very ill are less often sent to hospital. Figures for long-term prognosis are not available. Impressions gained at Accra suggest that about 50 per cent of survivors become fairly independent, that men do better than women, and that the gross obesity often seen in the latter is a bad omen for eventual mobility, independence, and indeed survival.

Prevention

Hypertension is a considerable problem in many parts of the tropics. Abrahams and Alele (1960), Smith (1966), and Akinkugbe (1969), working in Nigeria, consider most cases of hypertension to be essential in origin although a significant percentage may be renal (over 40 per cent in Smith's series). Hutt and Coles (1969), describing an autopsy series on Ugandan hypertensives, found more renal than essential hypertension. In Smith's series, 55 of 207 hypertensive patients presented with stroke which caused 47 per cent of the deaths. Aetiological factors are obscure. Salt intake and balance (Dahl and Love, 1954; Shaper *et al.*, 1969), low protein and high-carbohydrate diets (Kaneta *et al.*, 1964), schistosomiasis (Akinkugbe, 1969) and malarial renal lesions (Edington and Gilles, 1969 *b*), are possibilities worthy of further investigation. Much early renal disease in the tropics is unrecognized and untreated.

Detection and treatment of hypertension is the most obvious way of preventing ischaemic and haemorrhagic CVD. Any such comprehensive programme involves important considerations of priorities, lack of medical staff and cost. Many of our hypertensive patients are well controlled with thiazides with or without reserpine, and in view of its relative cheapness this combination is suitable as a first approach in mild or moderate hypertension.

In Accra a year's treatment with reserpine, 0·25 mg, and polythiazide, 2 mg daily, costs about £10; methyldopa, 250 mg t.i.d. for 1 year, costs about £32. Clearly, long-term hypotensive treatment of large numbers can be extremely expensive.

Cerebral Embolism

The diagnosis of cerebral embolism is usually made when a stroke occurs in a person with an obvious source of embolism. It is now thought that TIA or so-called cerebral thrombosis may sometimes be due to emboli from sclerotic plaques in major cervical arteries. In the tropical series described, embolism occurred in about 5 per cent of CVA cases, except in Bombay and Uganda where the proportion was about 20 per cent. Information on sources of cerebral emboli in the tropics is scanty and is summarized in TABLE 15.6.

The following comments may be made:

1. Mitral regurgitation is common in many parts of the tropics and is often due to endomyocardial fibrosis although many cases are of obscure origin. Embolic phenomena are not common in endomyocardial fibrosis but do occur. Emboli are probably commoner in other obscure tropical cardiomyopathies such as heart muscle disease and annular subvalvular left ventricular aneurysm (Edington and Gilles, 1969 *c*).

2. True rheumatic heart disease is fairly common in Africa and India and subacute bacterial endocarditis is often seen.

3. Secondary cerebral emboli from chorionepithelioma and cerebral abscesses may both present as strokes.

4. Pulmonary thromboses are common in sickle-cell disease and are a conceivable source of cerebral emboli.

5. Coronary thrombosis and embolism after cardiac operations are rare causes in Africa.

6. High mortality rates are usually due to underlying cardiac disease.

Cerebral Haemorrhage

Cerebral haemorrhage, although less common than ischaemic vascular disease, kills more people because of its considerably higher mortality rate. A distinction should be made between primary intracerebral haemorrhage and subarachnoid haemorrhage as the aetiology, clinical manifestations and management are different. In intracerebral haemorrhage blood commonly leaks into the subarachnoid space. In perhaps 20 per cent of cases of subarachnoid haemorrhage there may be focal signs of cerebral damage due to bleeding into brain tissue or to postictal vasospasm. Clinical distinction may be difficult. There is a very close connexion between intracerebral haemorrhage and hypertension and a fairly close one between subarachnoid haemorrhage and hypertension.

Intracerebral Haemorrhage (ICH)

Prevalence. As described in the section on ischaemic strokes, intracerebral haemorrhage is believed to account for 15 per cent to 30 per cent of CVA. In Japan cerebral haemorrhage is apparently more common than ischaemic disease (Kaneta *et al.*, 1964) although

Table 15.6

Sources of Embolism and Mortality in Cerebral Embolic Disease

	Osuntokun, Odeku and Adeloye, Ibadan (1969)	*Haddock, Accra* (1970 *b*)	*Carter, United Kingdom* (1957)
Number of Cases	21	14	60
Mortality rate	42·9%	50%	42%
Sources of Embolism			
Mitral disease	9	3	5
Mitral disease and AF[1]	3	0	31
Bacterial endocarditis	6	3	3
Aortic aneurysm	0	1	—
Hypertension and AF	0	6	—
Coronary thrombosis	0	1	11
Endomyocardial fibrosis	2	0	—
Heart muscle disease	1	0	—
AF (cause ?)	—	—	6
Thyrotoxicosis AF	—	—	4

[1]AF = atrial fibrillation.

accuracy of diagnosis has been questioned. Freytag (1968) in the United States found fatal intracerebral haematomas commoner in Negroes than Caucasians, particularly in the younger age-groups where the rate was approximately six times higher in Negroes.

This may be due to the higher prevalence of hypertension in younger Negroes (Merrill, 1964). Stallones (1965), commenting on this, says the difference between the races may be diminishing, and may be environmental (perhaps associated with poverty and poor medical attention) rather than racial in origin. In autopsy series of strokes, haemorrhage predominates owing to its higher mortality (Merritt, 1967; Edington, 1954). Some investigators (Yates, 1964; Stallones, 1965) believe that in the Western world cerebral haemorrhage is decreasing while ischaemic CVD is increasing. Anderson and McKay (1968), basing their findings on early death within 24 hours of onset as being strongly suggestive of haemorrhagic stroke, believe that the relative incidence of intracerebral haemorrhage and ischaemic stroke has really remained fairly constant during this century.

Accounts of the pathology of cerebrovascular disease in the tropics recorded in the section on ischaemic CVD include descriptions of cerebral haemorrhage. The pathological accounts appear to show no clear difference from those in Europe and America, although one suspects that cerebral haemorrhage may occur in younger subjects in Africa with less severe arterial pathology than in Europe.

Age Incidence. In Lagos, Accra and Bombay the peak age incidence of intracerebral haemorrhage was found to be between 51 and 60 years. In Ibadan and Dakar it appeared to be lower, between 40 and 60 years. In Singapore it was between 61 and 70 years (in Singapore the age of people with CVA was higher than in the other areas). In each case the mean age was a few years younger than in the case of non-embolic ischaemic stroke. An appreciable proportion of victims were under 40. In Glynn's United Kingdom series (1956) the mean age for ICH was 56·6 years, some 5 years younger than for cerebral thrombosis. Merritt's American series (1967) of intracerebral haemorrhage was slightly younger. There were very few in these Western series under 40.

Thus, in the tropics cerebral haemorrhage appears to occur in younger people than in the West and in a slightly younger age-group than occlusive strokes.

Sex Incidence. We have already said that more males utilize hospitals in the tropics than females, so that hospital statistics of relative sex incidences are not reliable. In the tropical series males outnumber females but the male preponderance is rather less marked than in the case of ischaemic CVA. The exception is Singapore, where cerebral haemorrhage appears relatively commoner in men than women when compared with ischaemic CVD.

Experience in Lagos, Ibadan and Accra shows that the clinical presentation resembles that described in the West, with coma present at an early stage in over half the patients and the onset being nearly always abrupt. Although the mortality is high, some of the survivors of ICH make a surprisingly good functional recovery. Severe residual hemiplegia, epilepsy and recurrent strokes are complications seen in the tropics as well as the West.

The prevalence of hypertension, often severe, in cerebral haemorrhage in Ibadan, Accra, Dakar and Bombay was 81·5 per cent, 77 per cent, 71 per cent, and 54 per cent respectively.

Features which are associated with hypertension such as albuminuria and obesity are as common in cerebral haemorrhage in the tropics as elsewhere. Other features such as hypercholesterolaemia and diabetes, more fundamentally associated with atherosclerosis, are common in ICH but perhaps not so important as in ischaemic CVD.

Bleeding disease such as leukaemia and aplastic anaemia are present in a proportion of cases of ICH. These were found in 4 per cent of Osuntokun's series and in 3 per cent of Dalal's series.

Prognosis. Marshall (1968 *b*) believes that the mortality of ICH is 60 per cent to 70 per cent and is much worse than that of cerebral infarction. McKissock, Richardson, and Taylor (1961) and others have found that the level of consciousness 24 hours after onset was crucial in deciding the prognosis; if the patient is in coma at this time the outlook is almost hopeless. Experience in the tropics is similar—the recorded mortalities from intracerebral haemorrhage in Ibadan, Accra, Dakar, Singapore and Bombay were 77 per cent, 67 per cent, 66 per cent, 77 per cent, and 82 per cent. The evil significance of coma after 24 hours was confirmed in Lagos and Accra. The ultimate fate of those discharged from hospital is not known in the tropics but probably half are severely incapacitated.

Subarachnoid Haemorrhage (SAH)

Primary subarachnoid haemorrhage occurs when there is rupture of a vessel in the subarachnoid space; secondary subarachnoid haemorrhage is a consequence of intracerebral haemorrhage. Common causes are trauma, intracranial aneurysm, and angioma. Less common causes included bleeding diseases, anticoagulants, cerebral tumours, spinal tumours, acute hypertensive reactions, meningitis and encephalitis.

Although constituting only about 10 per cent of strokes subarachnoid haemorrhage is of great importance, as the victims are often younger, with less generalized vascular disease and with surgery offering a hopeful prospect.

In Senegal, Dumas (1968) found internal carotid aneurysms to be the commonest, with anterior cerebral and anterior communicating, aneurysms next in frequency. Subarachnoid haemorrhage accounted for 12.1 per cent, 13·6 per cent, 11 per cent, 9 per cent and 9 per cent of strokes in Ibadan, Lagos, Senegal, Bombay and Singapore respectively. In Accra it appears to cause about 10 per cent of CVA. At autopsy in Accra, Edington (1954) found subarachnoid haemorrhage in 13 and intracerebral haemorrhage in 53 out of 3645 subjects. The difficulties in differentiating primary subarachnoid and intracerebral haemorrhage without autopsy or angiography are well known.

In Dakar and Lagos females predominate (68 per cent and 57 per cent respectively) while in Ibadan, Accra and Singapore women made up 30 per cent to 40 per cent of the total. The average age of patients with subarachnoid haemorrhage is lower than in ischaemic stroke or ICH and is usually in the fifth and sixth decades in the West. This rather late age peak incidence is due to the fact that hypertension and arteriosclerosis play a part in determining rupture. Bleeding from angiomas tends to occur earlier. In the tropical series the peak age incidences were earlier than in the other types of stroke; the median ages of patients with SAH were 21–30 years; 31–40 years, 41–50 years and 51–60 years in Ibadan, Accra, Lagos and Singapore. The low age of the Ibadan series was partly contributed to by a few cases due to sickle-cell diseases.

Hypertensive Encephalopathy

Hypertensive encephalopathy is a relatively uncommon form of cerebrovascular disease. In the tropics it is most commonly seen as a result of acute glomerulonephritis or eclampsia. Hypertensive encephalopathy was present in 5·9 per cent of patients in the Ibadan series.

Conclusions

Cerebrovascular disease is a significant problem in the tropics and probably a growing one. This increase may be related to ageing of the population due to survival from infectious disease and to more atherosclerosis and hypertension. Cerebral atherosclerosis and hypertension are common in Africa, ischaemic heart disease is rare. The African with hypertension is liable to cerebral haemorrhage and infarction at a comparatively early age as well as hypertensive cardiac failure and uraemia. Urbanization, less physical exertion, and larger caloric intakes are on the increase in many areas and will probably cause more atherosclerosis.

A leader in *The Lancet* (1969) states: 'As Africa overcomes its problems with infections and parasitic diseases hypertension seems likely to grow in importance and it will then be interesting to see whether its incidence and characteristics resemble those in the American Negro'. The prevalence of hypertension and strokes in the latter is greater than in American whites.

It is suggested that the picture of vascular disease in certain parts of South-East Asia is intermediate between those seen in Africa and in the West.

Prevention is potentially the most fruitful approach to CVD. More investigation into the causation of hypertension is needed with particular reference to salt intake, pyelonephritis, malarial nephrosis, and bilharzia. It is of interest that in one area of Japan long-term limitation of salt intake has reduced blood pressure levels in the population.

Detection and prolonged drug treatment of hypertension is desirable but it is expensive in money and medical manpower; resources are limited in the tropics. So-called diseases of civilization such as atherosclerosis and diabetes are probably becoming more prevalent in the tropics. Yet this changing pattern should not be considered inevitable; halting it will require fundamental changes in fields other than that of medicine.

References

ABRAHAMS, D. G., and ALELE, C. A. (1960) Clinical study of hypertensive disease in West Africa, *W. Afr. med. J.*, 9, 183.

ACHESON, R. M., and FAIRBAIRN, A. S. (1970) Burden of cerebrovascular disorders in the Oxford area in 1963 and 1964, *Brit. med. J.*, 2, 621.

ADAMS, J. H. (1966) Echoencephalography, *Lancet*, 1, 487.

ADAMS, J. H. (1967) Patterns of cerebral infarction: some comments on their topography and pathogenesis, *Scot. med. J.*, 12, 339.

ADELOYE, A., and ODEKU, E. L. (1970) The nervous system in sickle cell disease, *Afr. J. med. Sci.*, 1, 33.

ANDERSON, T. W., and MCKAY, J. S. (1968) A critical re-appraisal of the epidemiology of cerebrovascular disease, *Lancet*, 1, 1137.

AKINKUGBE, O. O. (1969) School survey of arterial pressure and proteinuria in Ibadan, Nigeria, *E. Afr. med. J.*, 46, 257.

BILLINGHURST, J. R. (1966) Analysis of neurological admissions to Mulago Hospital, Kampala 1965–66, *E. Afr. med. J.*, 42, 566.

CARTER, A. B. (1957) The immediate treatment of cerebral embolism, *Quart. J. Med.*, 26, 335–48.

CHAPMAN, J. M., REEDER, L. E., BORUN, E. R., CLARK, V. A., and COULSON, A. H. (1966) Epidemiology of vascular lesions affecting the central nervous system, the occurrence of strokes in a sample population under observation for cardiovascular disease, *Amer. J. publ. Hlth*, 56, 191.

COLLOMB, H, COURSON, B., DUMAS, M., LEMERCIER, G., and TAP., D. (1966) La part des malformations vasculaires dans les accidents hémorragiques cérébraux, *Bull. Soc. méd. Afr. noire Langue franç.*, 11, 243.

COLLOMB, H., DUMAS, M., and LEMERCIER, G. (1966) La pathologie vasculaire cerebrale chez l'African (a propos de 600 cas), *Bull. Soc. méd. Afr. noire Langue franc.*, 11, 54.

COSNETT, J. E. (1969) Strokes in young people: experience in a Bantu hospital, *S. Afr. med. J.*, 43, 501.

CRAWFORD, T., and CROMPTON, M. R. (1968) The pathology of strokes, in *The Management of Cerebrovascular Disease*, 2nd ed., Marshall, J., London, p. 26.

DADA, T. O. (1970) Clinical syndromes of cerebral atherosclerosis in Nigerians, *Ghana med. J.*, 9, 167.

DADA, T. O., JOHNSON, F. A., and ARABA, A. B. (1969) Cerebrovascular accidents in Nigerians; a review of 205 cases, *W. Afr. med. J.*, 18, 95.

DAHL, L. K., and LOVE, R. A. (1954) Evidence for relationship between sodium chloride intake and human essential hypertension, *Arch. intern. Med.*, 94, 525.

DALAL, P. M., SHAH, P. M., AIYAR, R. P., and KIKANI, B. J. (1968) Cerebrovascular diseases in West Central India. A report on angiographic findings from a prospective study, *Brit. med. J.*, 3, 769.

DAVIES, J. N. P. (1948) Pathology of central African natives, Mulago Hospital. P.M. studies IX, *E. Afr. med. J.*, 25, 454.

DUMAS, M. (1968) La pathologie vasculaire cérébrale au Senegal, considérations générales, *Afr. Med.*, 7, 517.

EDINGTON, G. M. (1954) Cardiovascular disease as a cause of death in the Gold Coast African, *Trans. roy. Soc. trop. Med. Hyg.*, 48, 419.

EDINGTON, G. M., and GILLES, H. M. (1969 *a*) *Pathology in the Tropics*, London p. 519.

EDINGTON, G. M., and GILLES, H. M. (1969 *b*) *Pathology in the Tropics*, *London*, pp. 26, 27, 534.

EDINGTON, G. M., and GILLES, H. M. (1969 *c*) *Pathology in the Tropics*, London, p. 301.

FORSYTH, D. M. (1969) Hypertension in Tanzania, *E. Afr. med. J.*, 46, 309.

FREYTAG, E. (1968) Fatal intracerebral haematomas. A survey of the pathological anatomy of 393 cases, *J. Neurol. Neurosurg. Psychiat.*, 31, 616.

GLYNN, A. A. (1956) Vascular diseases of the nervous system, *Brit. med. J.*, 1, 1216.

GROCH, S. N., MCDEVITT, E., and WRIGHT, I. S. (1961) A long-term study of cerebral vascular disease, *Ann. intern. Med.*, 55, 358.

GWEE, A. L., THAM, N. B., CHEE, E. K. H., and CHEW, L. S. (1970) Cerebrovascular disease—epidemiological and clinical considerations, *Singapore med. J.*, 11, 2.

HADDOCK, D. R. W. (1965 *a*) Neurological disorders in Tanzania, *J. trop. Med. Hyg.*, 68, 161.

HADDOCK, D. R. W. (1965 *b*) Blood pressure levels in inpatients in Dar-es-Salaam, *E. Afr. med. J.*, 42, 42.

HADDOCK, D. R. W. (1969) Obesity in medical outpatients in Accra, *Ghana med. J.*, 8, 251.

HADDOCK, D. R. W. (1970 *a*) Cerebrovascular accidents in Ghana, *Trans. roy. Soc. trop. Med. Hyg.*, 64, 300.

HADDOCK, D. R. W. (1970 *b*) Unpublished observations.

HOWE, G. M. (1963) *National Atlas of Disease Mortality in the United Kingdom*, London.

HUMPONU-WUSA, O. O. (1969) A look at some health problems in Nigeria, *W. Afr. med. J.*, 18, 181.

HUTCHINSON, E. C., and YATES, P. O. (1957) Carotico-vertebral stenosis, *Lancet*, i, 2.

HUTT, M. S. R., and COLES, R. (1969) Post-mortem findings in hypertensive subjects in Kampala, Uganda, *E. Afr. med. J.*, 46, 342.

HUTTON, P. W. (1956) Neurological disorders in Uganda, *E. Afr. med. J.*, 33, 209.

JENNETT, W. B. (1967) Ischaemic carotid strokes, *Scot. med. J.*, 12, 368.

JOHNSON, T. O. (1970) Height and weight patterns of an urban African population sample in Nigeria, *Trop. geogr. Med.*, 22, 65.

KANETA, S. ISHIGURO, K., KOBAYASHI, S., and TAKASHI, E. (1964) An experimental study on nutrition and cerebrovascular disease in Tohoku area of Japan, *Tohoku J. exp. Med.* 83, 398.

KAUSHIK, S. C. (1961) The pattern of neurological disease in Ibadan, in *First Pan-African Psychiatric Conference, 12–18 November* 1961, *Abeokuta*, ed. Lambo, T. A., Ibadan p. 78.

LAING, W. N. (1969) The pattern of cardiovascular and renal causes of obscure deaths in Ghana, *Ghana med. J.*, 8, 254.

LAURIE, W., and WOODS, J. D. (1958) Atherosclerosis and its cerebral complications in the South African Bantu, *Lancet*, i, 231.

MCKISSOCK, W., RICHARDSON, A., and TAYLOR, J. C. (1961) Primary intracerebral haemorrhage. A controlled trial of surgical and conservative treatment in 180 unselected cases, *Lancet*, ii, 221.

MARSHALL, J. (1968 *a*) *The Management of Cerebrovascular Disease*, 2nd ed., London, p. 122.

MARSHALL, J. (1968 *b*) *The Management of Cerebrovascular Disease*, 2nd ed., London, p. 92.

MERRILL, J. P. (1964) in *Principles of Internal Medicine*, ed. Harrison, T. R., *et al.*, New York.

MERRITT, A. H. (1967) *A Textbook of Neurology*, 4th ed., Philadelphia, p. 159.

MEYER, J. S. (1970) Newer concepts of cerebral vascular disease, *Med. Clin. N. Amer.*, 54, 349.

OJIAMBO, H. O. (1966) Neurological disease at Kenyatta National Hospital, Nairobi. A retrospective study of 75 cases, *E. Afr. med. J.*, 43, 366.

OSUNTOKUN, B. O., and ODEKU, E. L. (1970) Epilepsy in Nigerians, *Trop. geogr. Med.*, 22, 1.

OSUNTOKUN, B. O., ODEKU, E. L., and ADELOYE, R. B. A. (1969) Non-embolic ischaemic cerebrovascular disease in Nigerians, *J. neurol. Sci.*, 9, 361.

PARRY, E. H. O. (1969) The casual blood pressure in Ethiopian highlanders in Addis Ababa, *E. Afr. med. J.*, 46, 247.

REEF, H., and ISAACSON, C. (1962) Atherosclerosis in the Bantu; distribution of atheromatous lesions in Africans over 50 years of age, *Circulation*, 28, 25.

SHAPER, A. G., LEONARD, P. J., JONES, K. W., and JONES, M. (1969) Environmental effects on the body build, blood pressure and blood chemistry of nomadic warriors serving in the army in Kenya, *E. Afr. med. J.*, 46, 282.

SHAPER, A. G., WILLIAMS, A. W., and SPENCER, P. E. (1961) Blood pressure and body build in an African tribe living on a diet of milk and meat, *E. Afr. med. J.*, 38, 569.

SHAPER, A. G., and SHAPER, L. (1958) Analysis of medical admissions to Mulago Hospital, 1957, *E. Afr. med. J.*, 35, 647.

SMITH, A. J. (1966) Arterial hypertension in Lagos Teaching Hospital, *W. Afr. med. J.*, 15, 97.

STALLONES, R. A. (1965) Epidemiology of cerebrovascular disease; a review, *J. chron. Dis.*, 18, 859.

STUART, K. L. (1968) Hypertension in the tropics, *Brit. med. J.*, 1, 103.

TAKAHASHI, E. (1962) On the geographic distribution of death rates from vascular lesions affecting the central nervous system in the United States of America, *Tohoku J. exp. Med.*, 76, 224.

TULLOCH, J. A. (1962) *Diabetes Mellitus in the Tropics*, Edinburgh.

VIRIEU, R., and COLLOMB, H. (1968) Les aspects épidémiologiques de l'athérosclérose, *Afr. med.*, 7, 499.

WILLIAMS, A. O., RESCH, J. A., and LOEWENSON, R. B. (1969) Cerebral atherosclerosis: a comparative study between Nigerian Negroes and American Negroes and Caucasians, *Neurology* (*Minneap.*), 19, 205.

YATES, P. O. (1964). A change in the pattern of cerebrovascular disease, *Lancet*, i, 65.

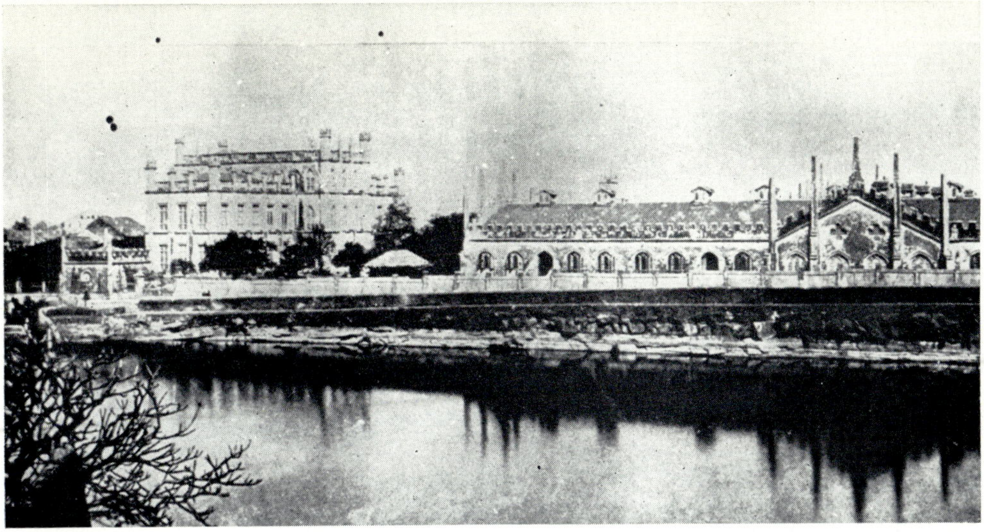

a. *India.* The Sir J. J. Hospital, Bombay. The original Babula tank is in the foreground, with the medical college (*left*) and the hospital (*right*) behind it.

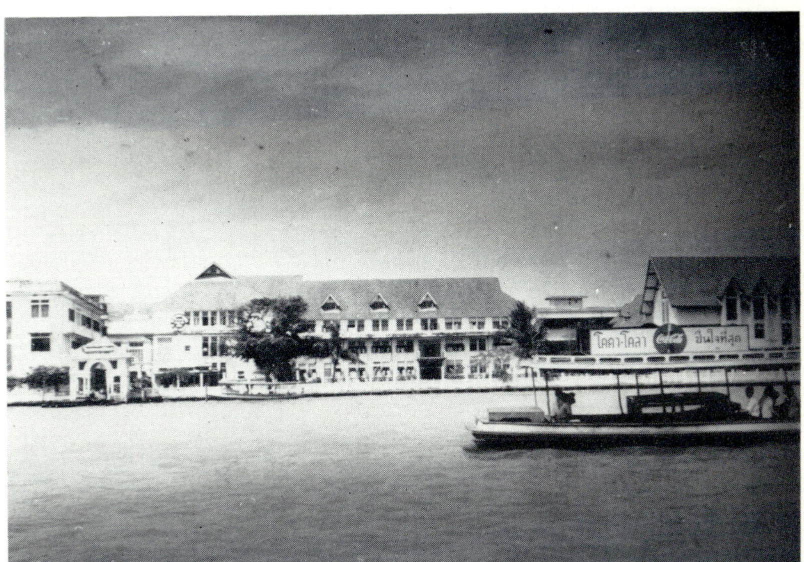

b. *Thailand.* Siriraj Teaching Hospital, Bangkok. (Photograph by J. D. Spillane.)

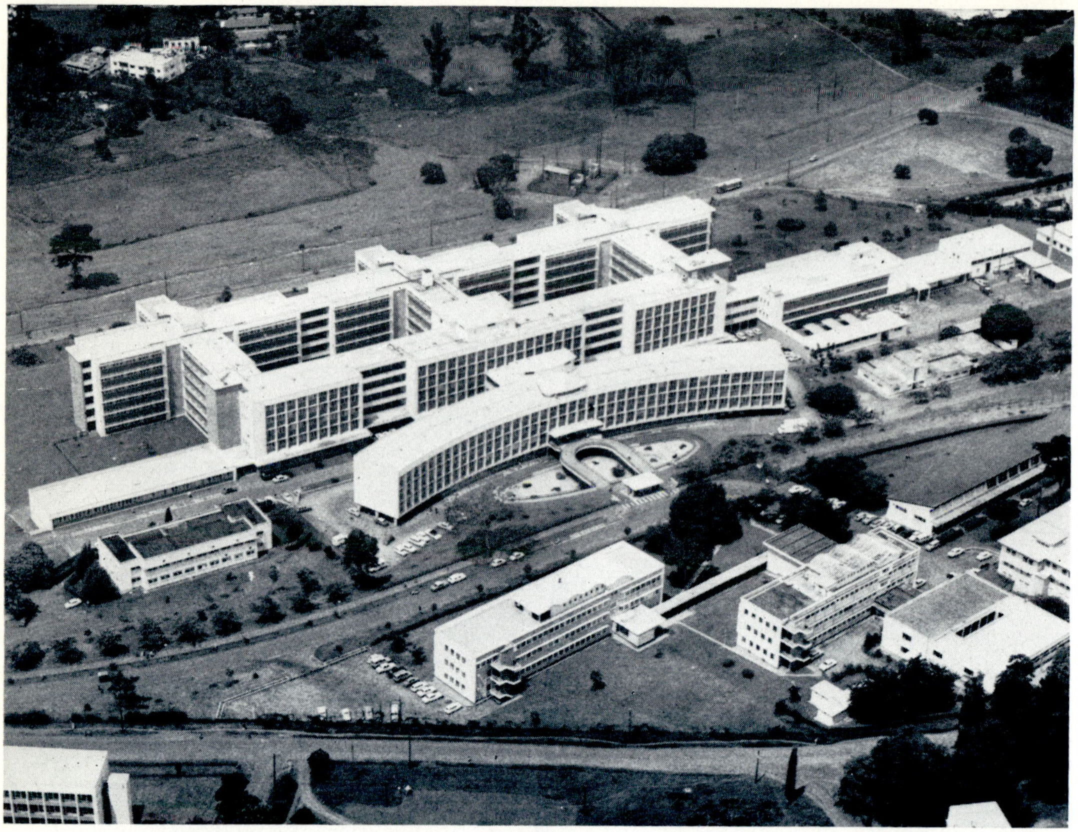

a. *Uganda*. Mulago Hospital and Makerere Medical School, Kampala. (By courtesy of the Department of Medical Illustration, Makerere Medical School.)

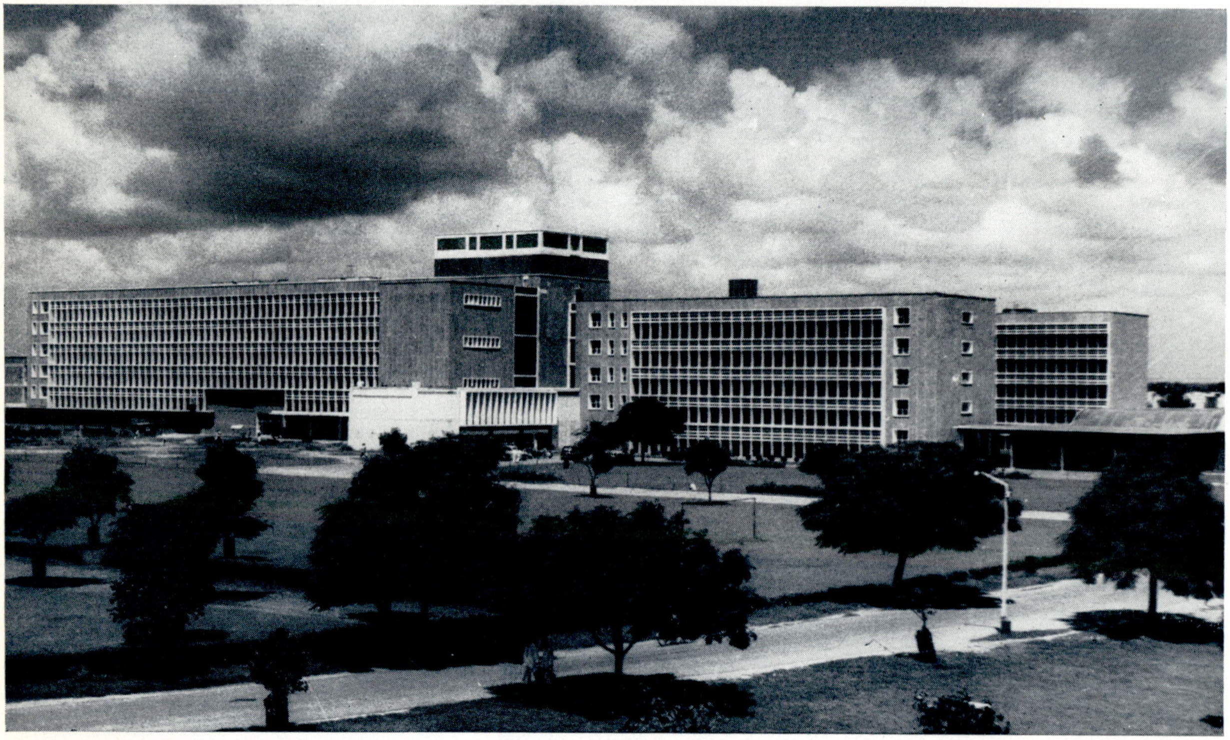

b. *India*. The All India Institute of Medical Sciences, New Delhi.

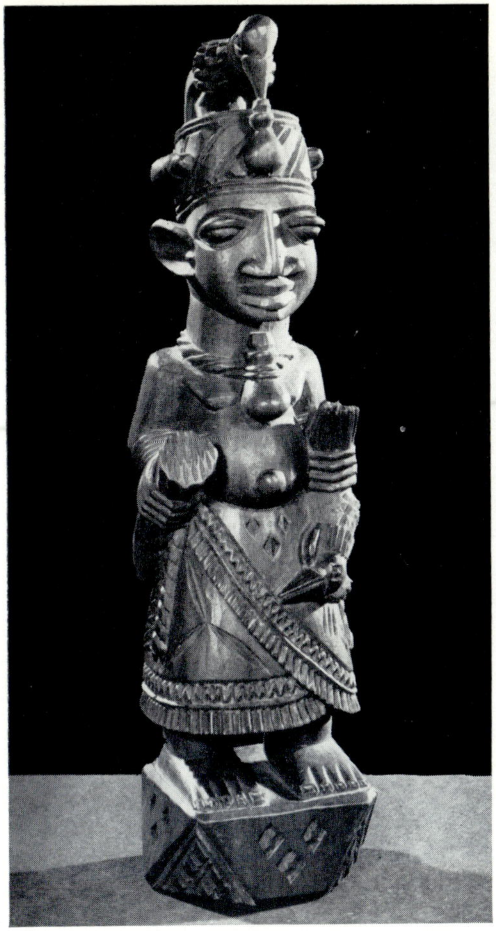

a. *Nigeria*. Woodcarving of a native doctor, or *Babalawo*. Sacrificial bird in one hand and staff of power in the other. Pear-shaped gourds contain his potent remedies. (Photograph by J. D. Spillane.)

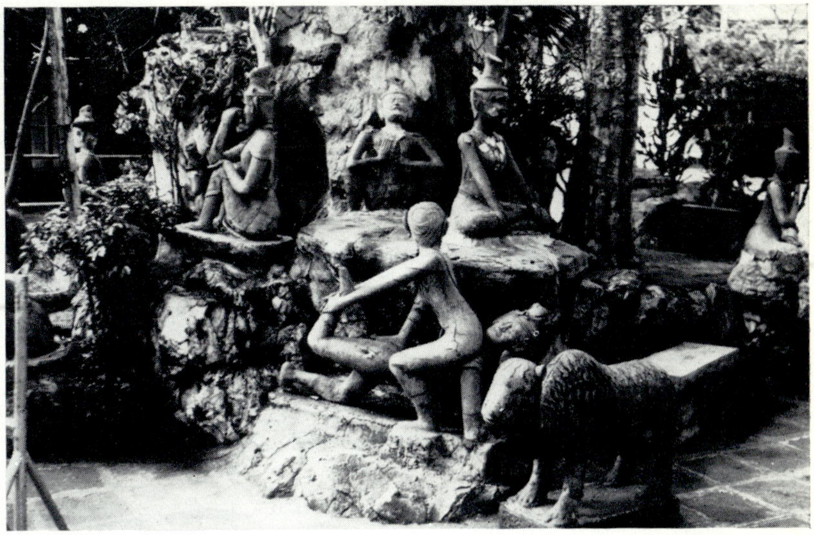

b. *Thailand*. Ancient physiotherapy, in a Bangkok wat. (Photograph by J. D. Spillane.)

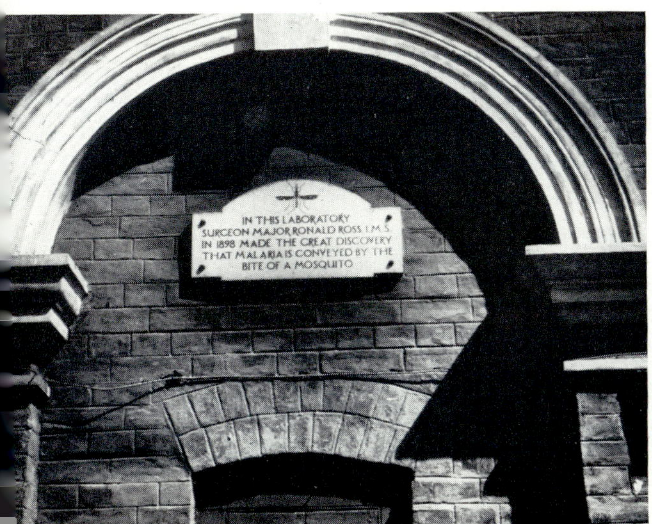
IN THIS LABORATORY
SURGEON MAJOR RONALD ROSS I.M.S.
IN 1898 MADE THE GREAT DISCOVERY
THAT MALARIA IS CONVEYED BY THE
BITE OF A MOSQUITO

c. *India*. The Ross commemoration tablet on the wall of the old laboratory in Calcutta Medical School. (Photograph by J. D. Spillane.)

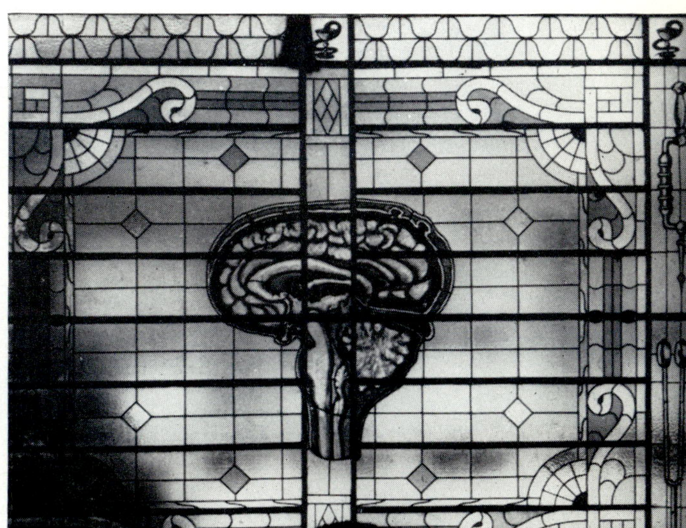

d. *Brazil*. Latin American artistic temperament showing itself in the stained-glass windows of the Neurological Institute of Rio de Janeiro. (Photograph by J. D. Spillane.)

PLATE 4
Introduction

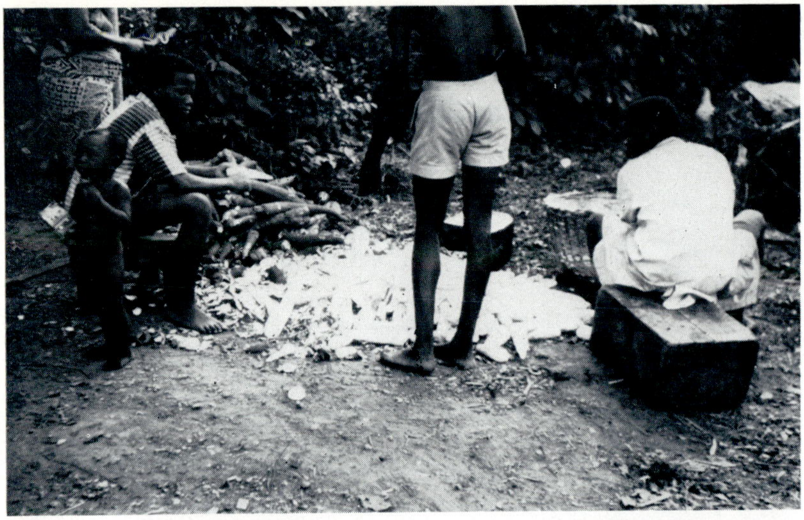

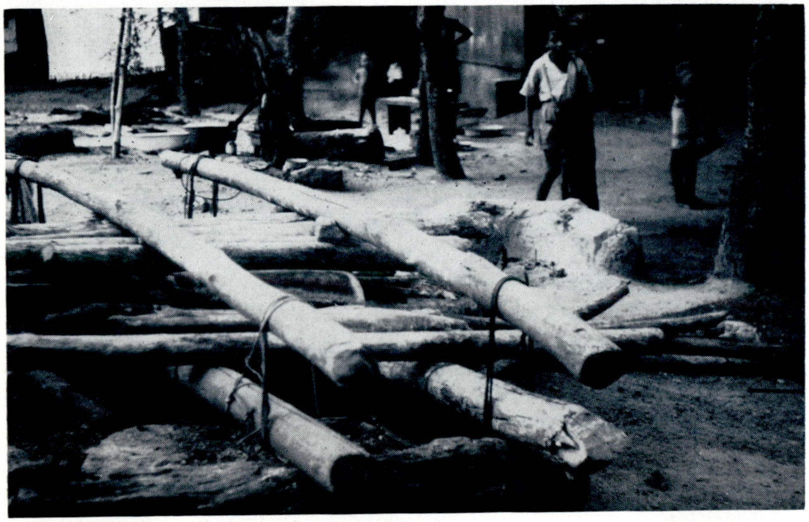

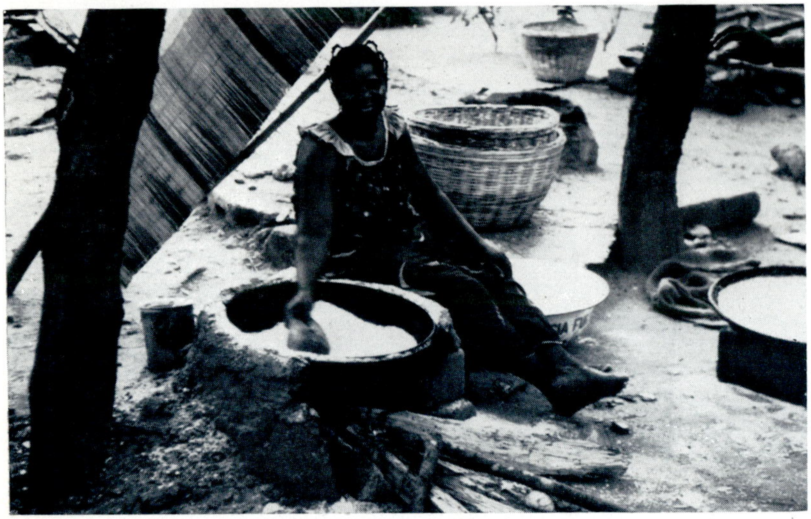

Cassava preparation in Nigeria. *Above:* the tubers are peeled and sliced; *centre:* pressed in sacks between logs; *below:* pounded into a flour. The ataxic neuropathy of Nigeria tends to occur in districts where there is a high consumption of cassava. Cassava contains cyanide-producing glycosides. (Photographs by J. D. Spillane.)

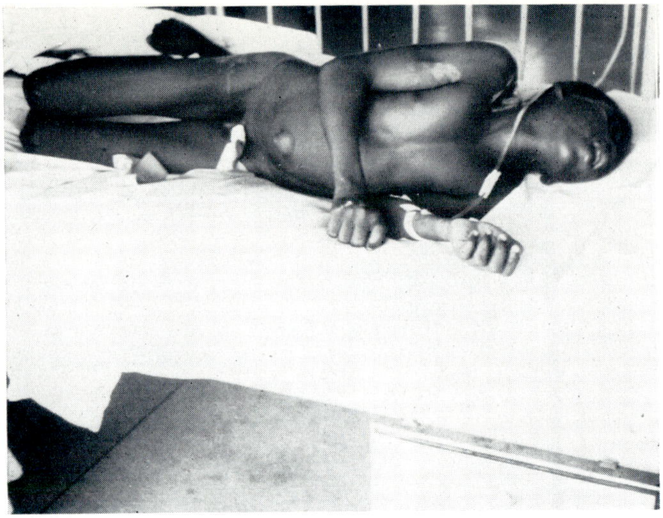

a. Tetanus in a Nigerian. (Photograph by J. D. Spillane.)

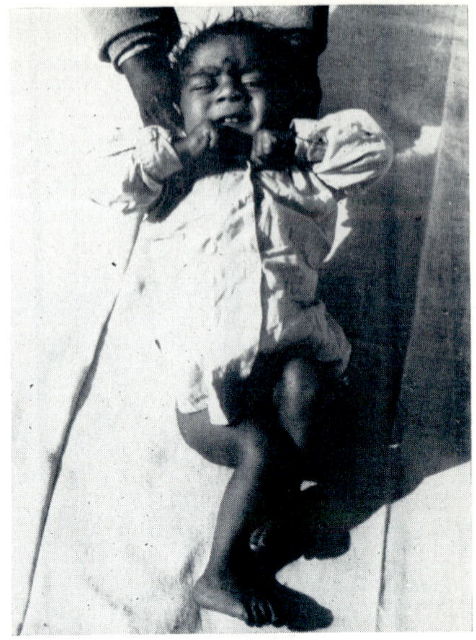

b. Infantile tremor syndrome (India; see p. 114). The infant is conscious, the upper limbs are abducted at the shoulders and flexed at the elbows; fists are clenched; fluttering tremors affect mainly the face and the limbs. (Photograph by J. D. Spillane.)

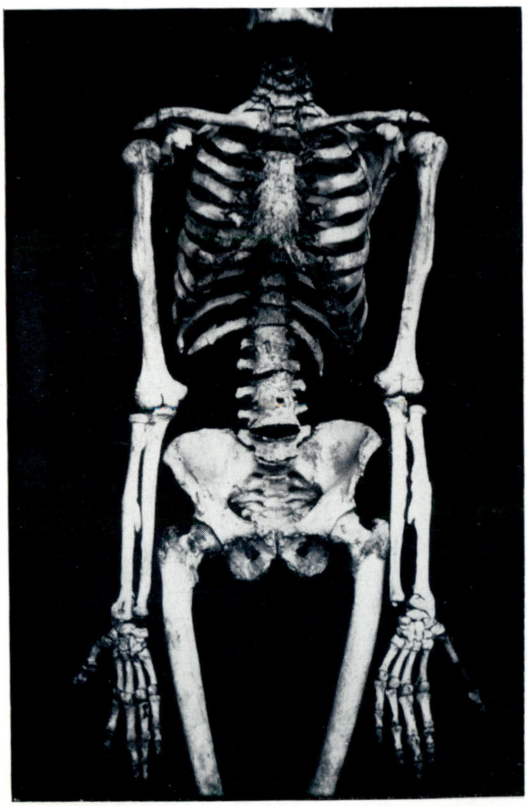

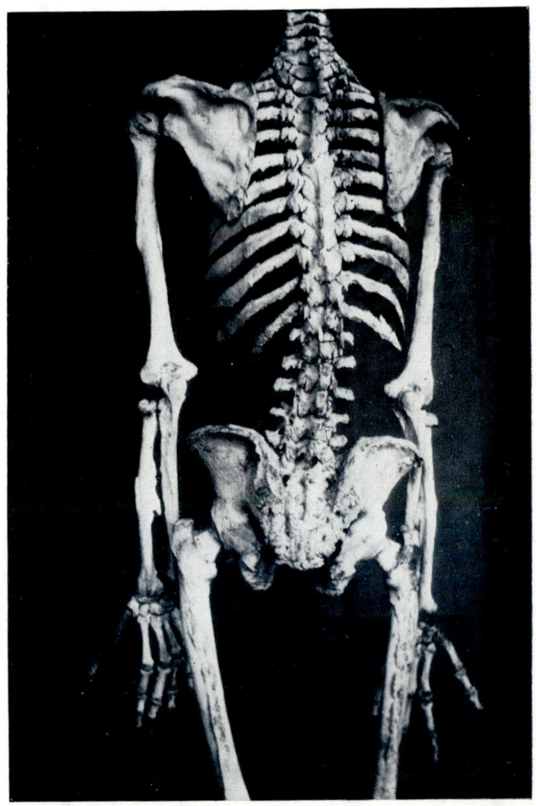

c. and d. Endemic fluorosis (India). A skeleton in the museum of the Department of Anatomy in Madras University Medical College. Diffuse osteosclerosis, irregular periosteal bone formation, calcification of vertebral and pelvic ligaments and the interosseous membranes of the forearms. Deafness and paraplegia are common consequences. (Photographs by J. D. Spillane.)

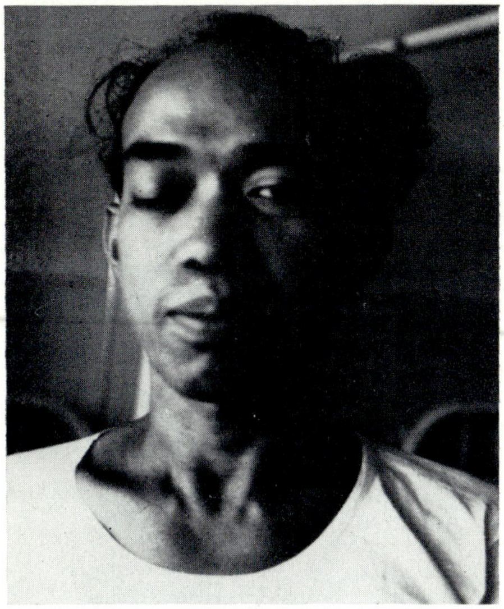

a. *Bangkok*. A right third nerve palsy in a patient recovering from encephalomyelitis due to antirabic vaccine. (Photograph by J. D. Spillane.)

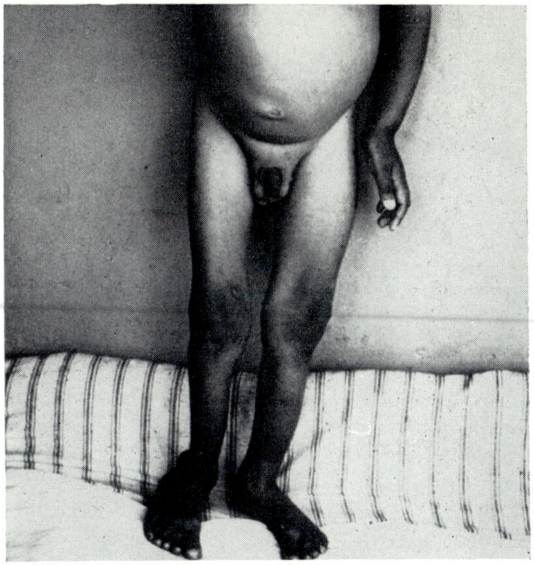

b. Rickets in an Indian child. (Photograph by J. D. Spillane.)

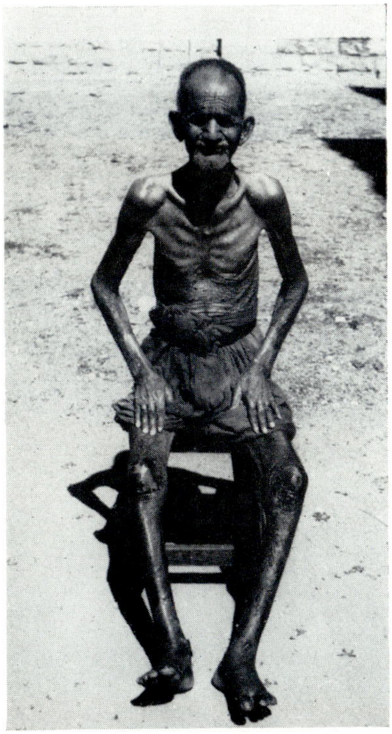

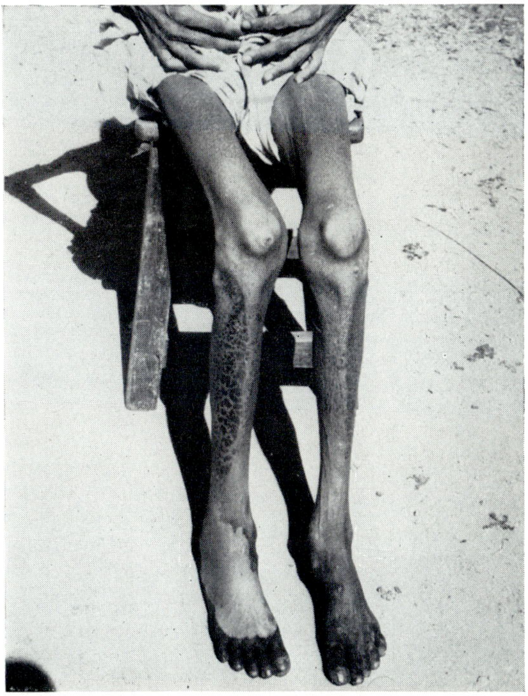

c. and d. Pellagra in Hyderabad, India. Note the general evidence of gross malnutrition and the mosaic dermatitis of the limbs. (Photographs by J. D. Spillane.)

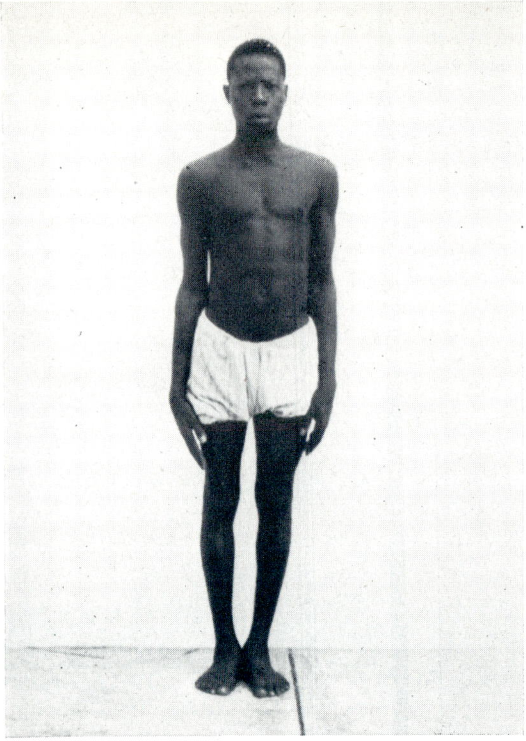

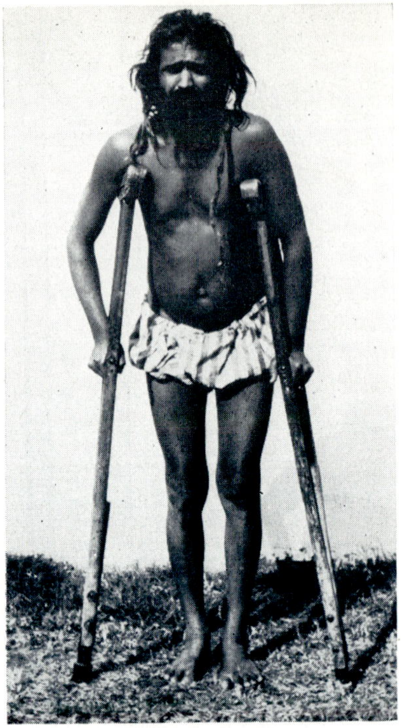

b. Lathyrism: epidemic spastic paraplegia in Central India. (Photograph by J. D. Spillane.)

a. and c. Ataxic neuropathy of Nigeria. Two young men with a sensory ataxia, powerful upper limbs and a slight weakness of the lower limbs; note the difference between the musculature of the upper and lower limbs. (Photographs by J. D. Spillane.)

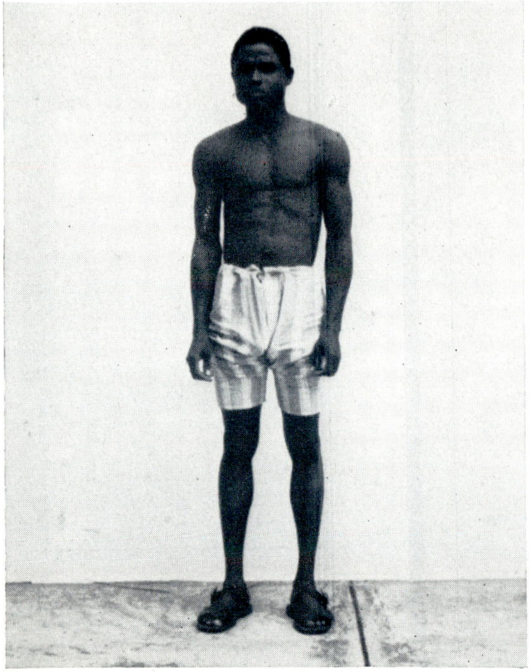

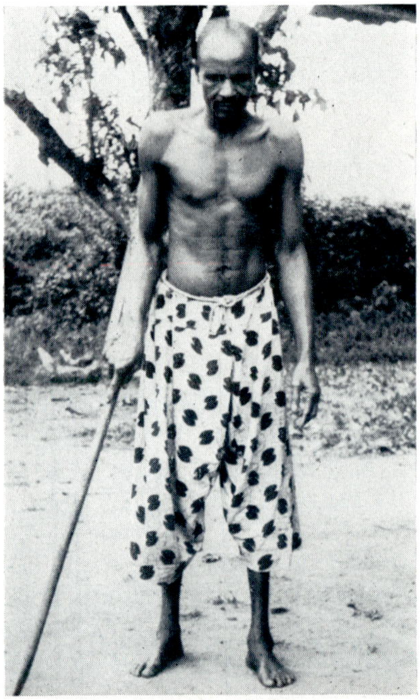

d. Middle-aged man, husband of woman in PLATE 8a. Bilateral foot-drop and gross ataxia in ataxic neuropathy of Nigeria. (Photograph by J. D. Spillane.)

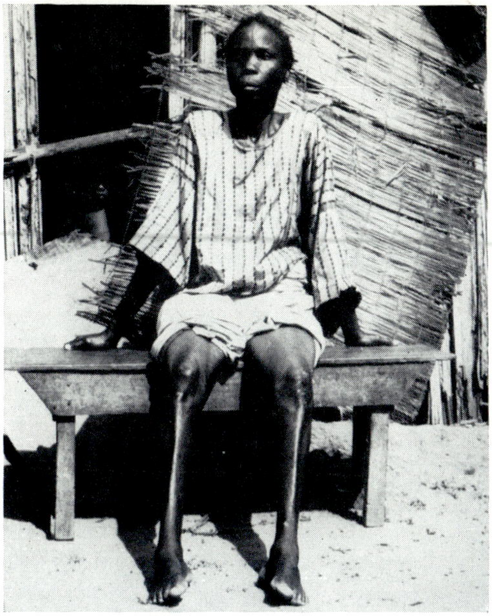

a. Middle-aged woman, wife of man in PLATE 7d. Bilateral foot-drop and gross ataxia in ataxic neuropathy of Nigeria. (Photograph by J. D. Spillane.)

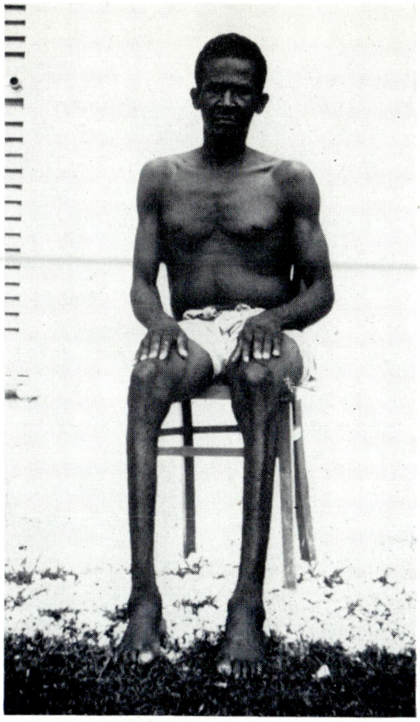

b.

b. and c. Jamaican neuropathy. The great majority of cases are spastic; a smaller group are ataxic. The majority do not show the gross degree of muscular atrophy of the legs as seen in these illustrations. (Photographs by J. D. Spillane.)

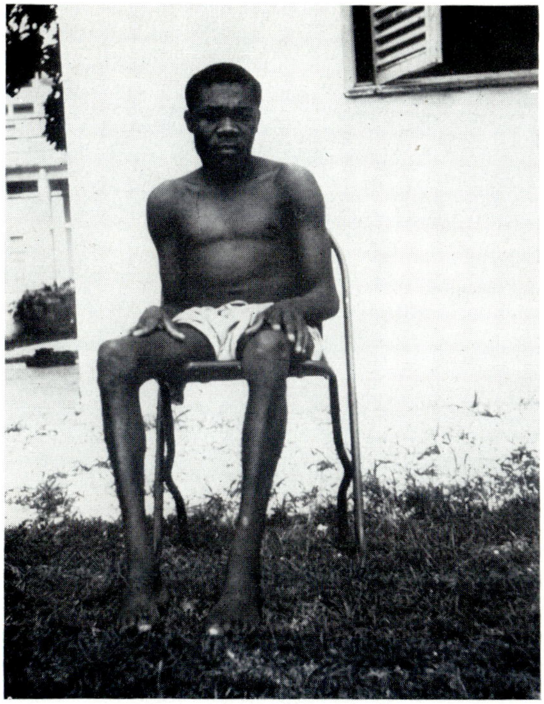

c.

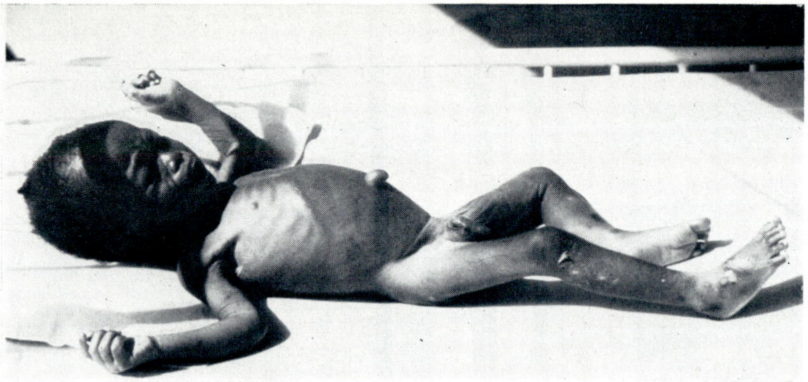

a. Kwashiorkor: protein-calorie malnutrition in a Jamaican infant. (Photograph by J. D. Spillane.)

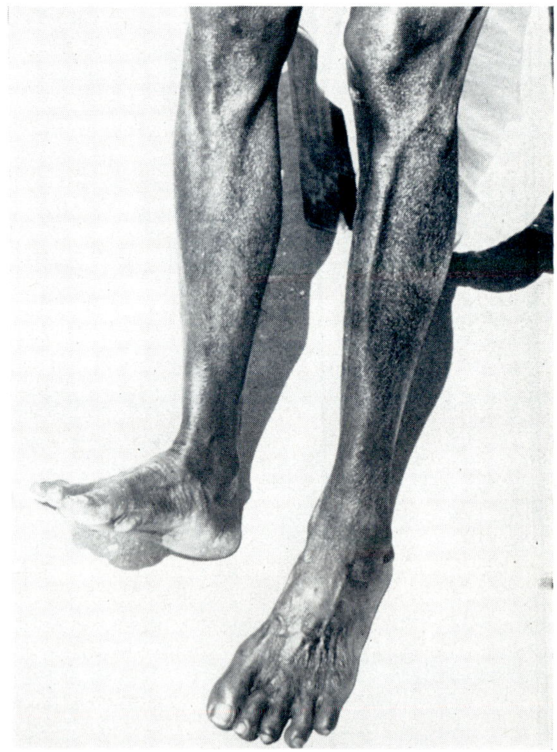

b. Leprosy: left foot-drop; note wasting of anterior tibial muscle group. (Photograph by J. D. Spillane.)

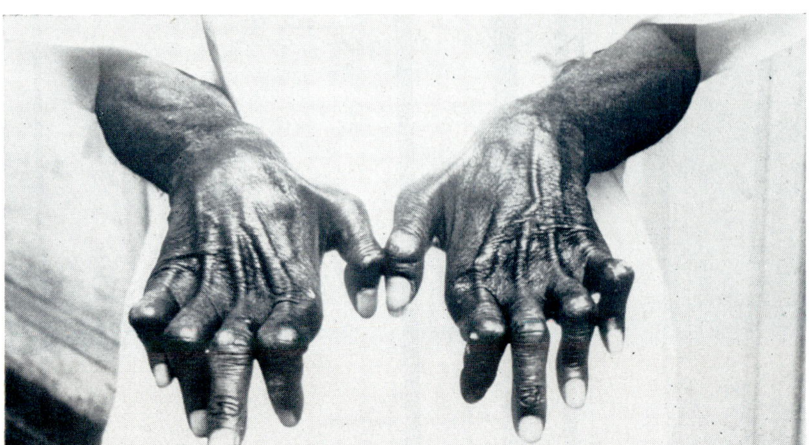

c. The consequences of leprosy: claw hands. (Photograph by J. D. Spillane.)

PLATE 10
India

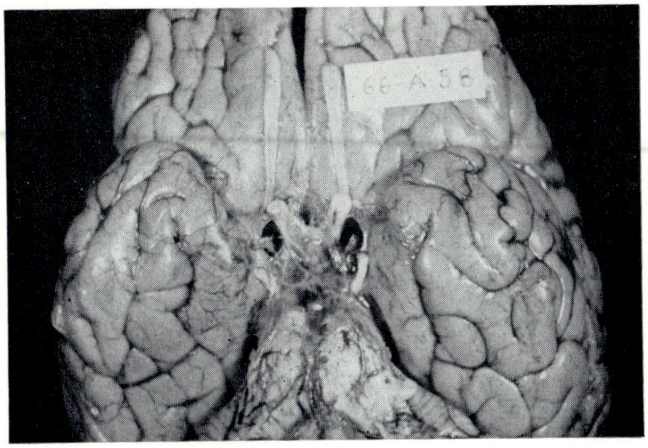

a. and b. Tuberculous meningitis with the brunt of the lesion in the basal region.

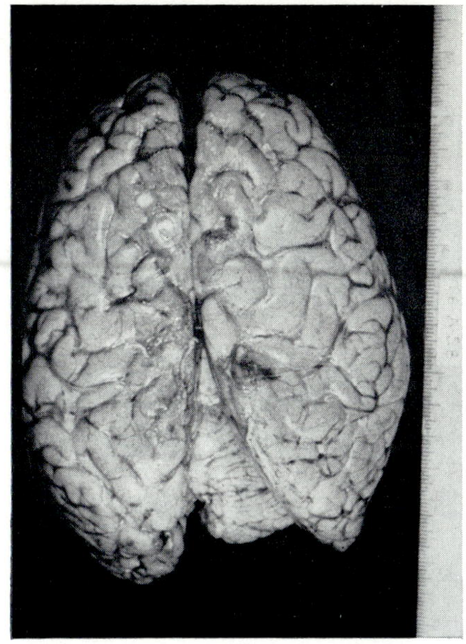

b.

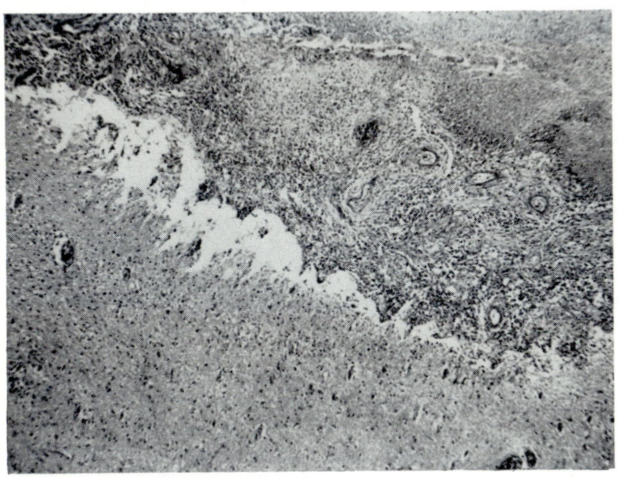

c. Microphotograph showing characteristic tuberculous inflammation of the meninges and involvement of the underlying brain (H & E × 36).

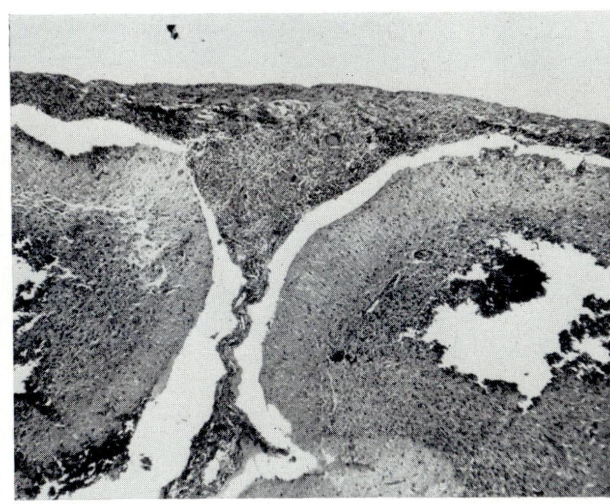

d. Microphotograph showing characteristic tuberculous meningitis with infarction of the underlying brain.

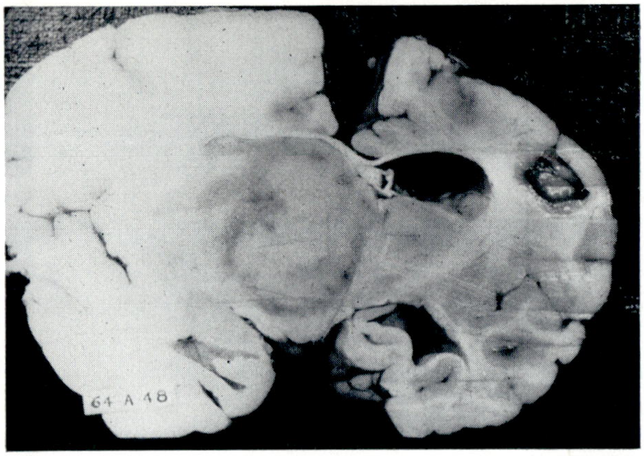

a. Thalamic tuberculoma.

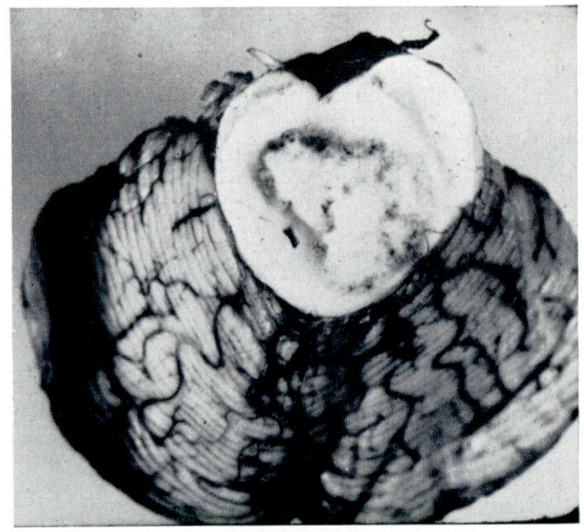

b. Brain stem tuberculoma.

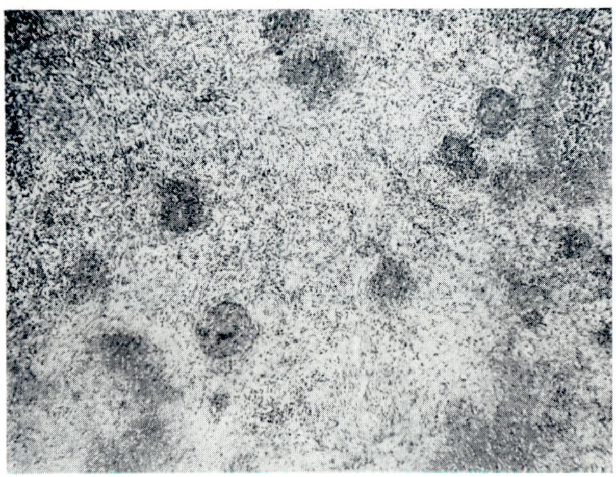

c. Tuberculoma of the brain with surrounding satellite granulomas (H & E × 46).

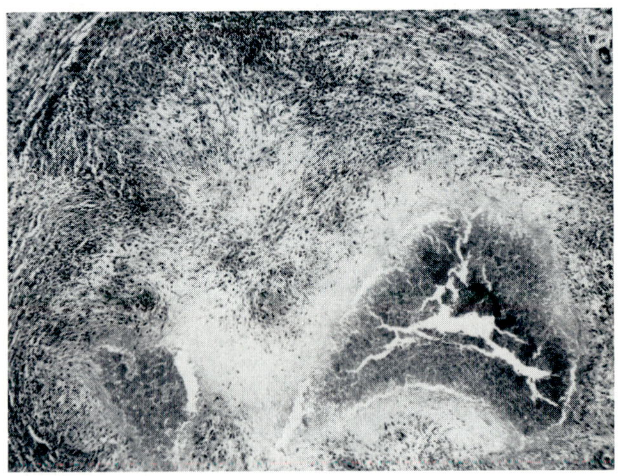

d. Tuberculoma of the brain showing coalescence of three enlarging caseating granulomas (H & C × 36).

PLATE 12
India

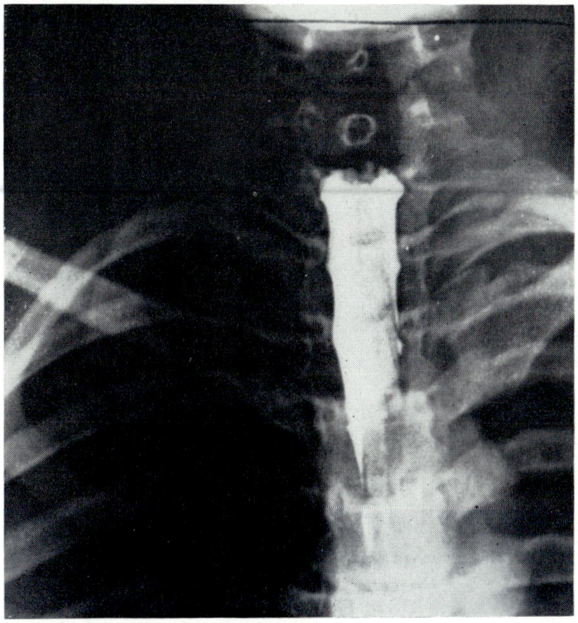

a. Cisternal myelogram in a case of Pott's paraplegia showing an extradural type of block starting at T.3 level.

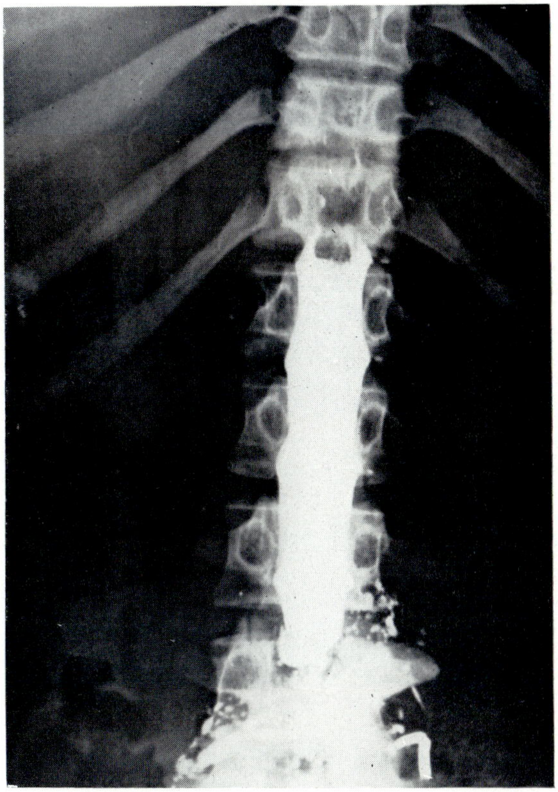

b. Lumbar myelogram of the same patient revealing a block at the lower border of T.12. Note the fuzzy outline and narrowing of the T.11–T.12 intervertebral space.

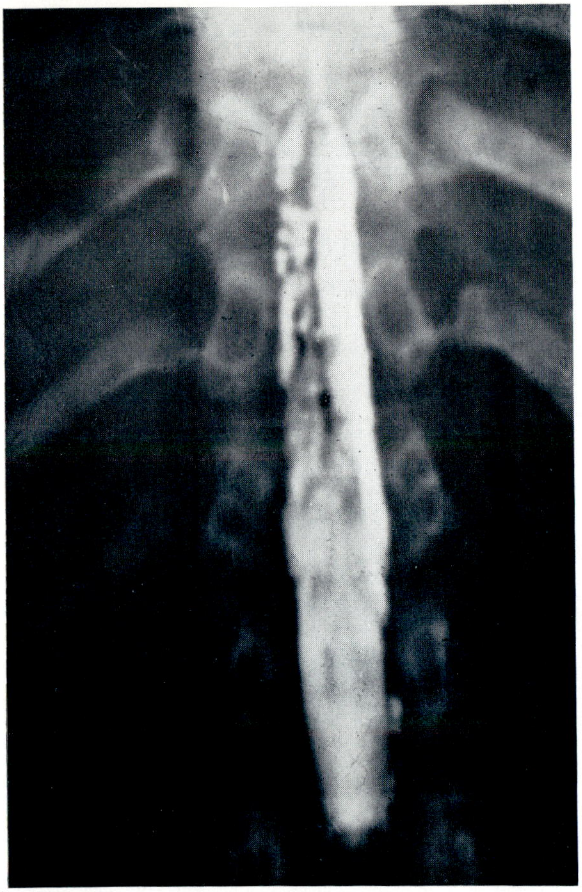

a. Radiculomyelopathy; lumbar myelogram: complete block at T.9–T.10 level with an irregular myodil column over T.10–T.11 vertebrae. Note its similarity to an angioma. (By courtesy of the Editor, *Journal of Neurological Sciences.*)

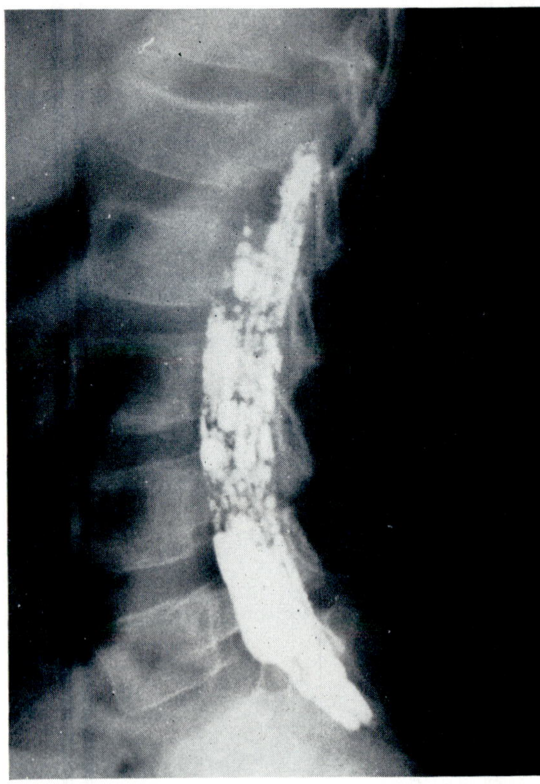

b. Lumbar myelogram, lateral view: a 'spotty' myodil column with a complete block at L.I (By courtesy of the Editor, *Journal of Neurological Sciences.*)

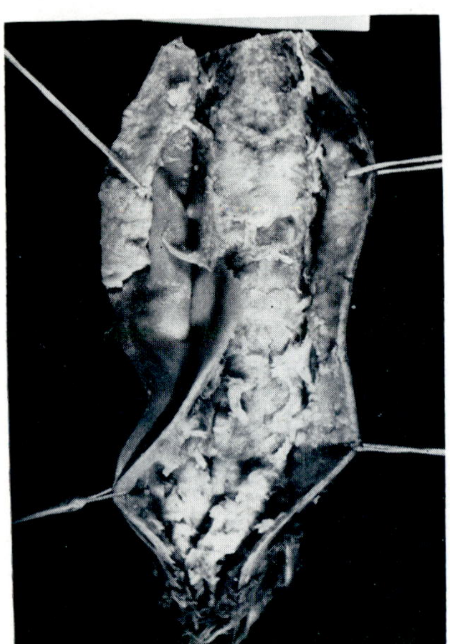

c. Lower end of the spinal cord where dense adhesive exudate is being torn as the dura is reflected. (By courtesy of the Editor, *Journal of Neurological Sciences.*)

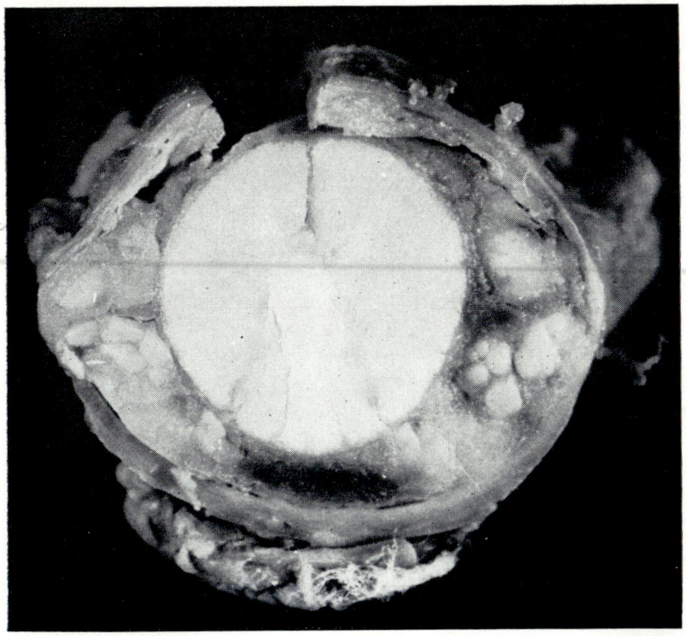

a. Radiculomyelopathy: a transverse section of the cord showing dense granulomatous exudate with tuberculoid nodules on one side. (By courtesy of the Editor, *Journal of Neurological Sciences.*)

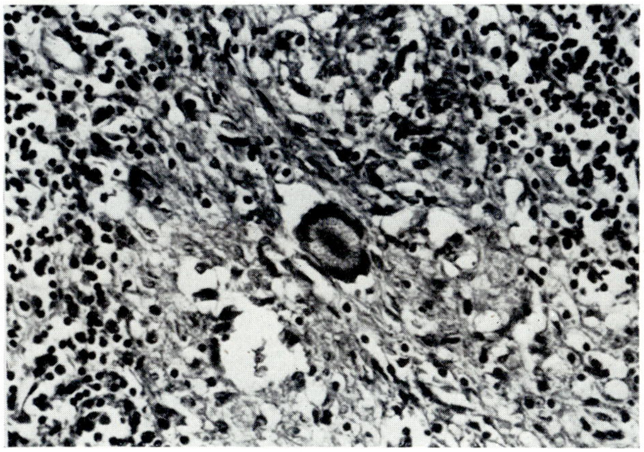

b. Spinal exudate showing a typical 'tubercle' with central giant cells surrounded by epithelioid cells and then by small mononuclear cells (H & E × 275). (By courtesy of the Editor, *Journal of Neurological Sciences.*)

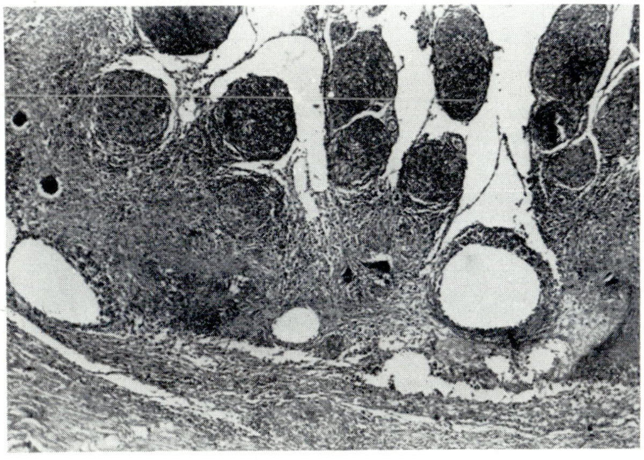

c. Exudate showing microcysts and multiple giant cell systems and infiltration of some of the roots (H & E × 40). (By courtesy of the Editor, *Journal of Neurological Sciences.*)

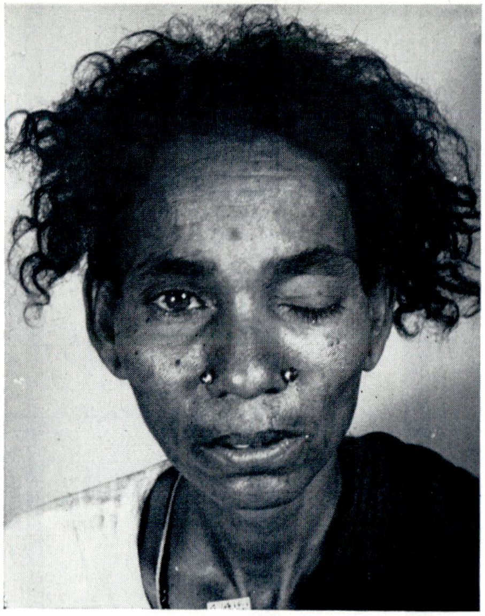

a. 45-year old woman with painful ophthalmoplegia on the left side. Note the complete ptosis. (By courtesy of the Editor, *Journal of Neurological Sciences.*)

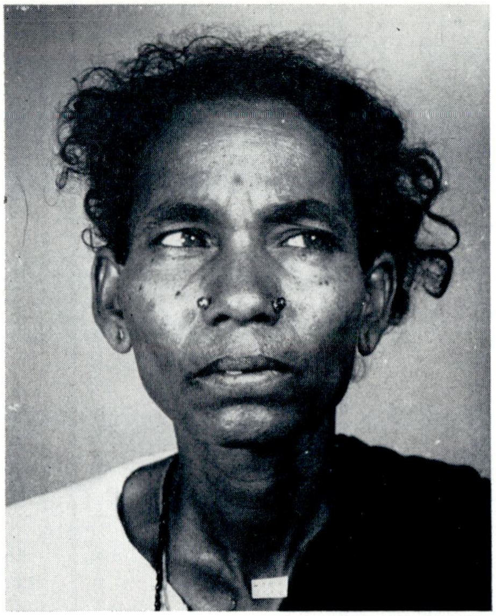

b. Same patient as in PLATE 15a, on the tenth day of corticosteroid therapy, with complete disappearance of her symptoms and signs. (By courtesy of the Ed1ior, *Journal of Neurological Sciences.*)

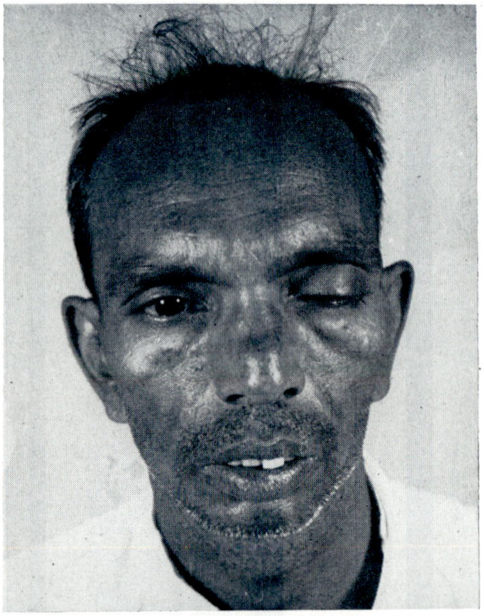

c. 48-year-old man in the acute stage of painful ophthalmoplegia. Note the ptosis, slight prominence of the eye and minimal periorbital oedema on the left side. (By courtesy of the Editor, *Journal of Neurological Sciences.*)

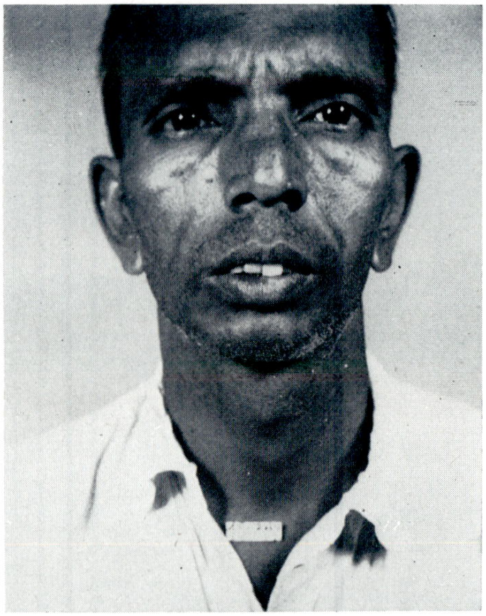

d. Same patient after a week of treatment with prednisolone. (By courtesy of the Editor, *Journal of Neurological Sciences.*)

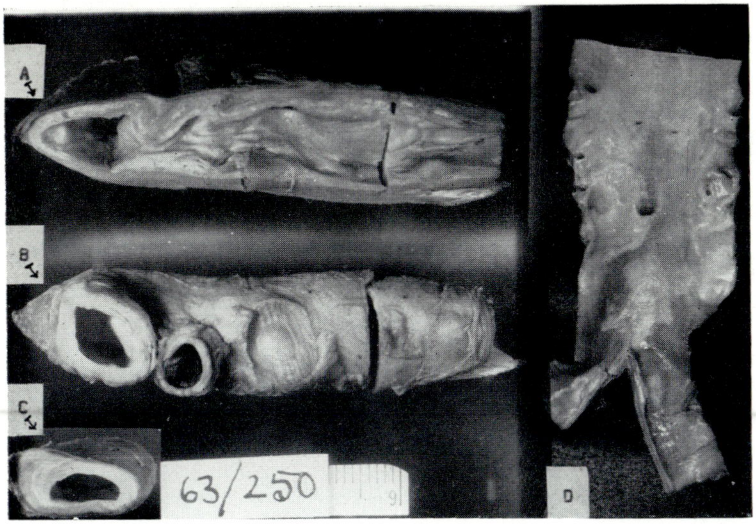

a. Aortic arch syndrome: (*a*) The intimal surface of the aortic arch showing pearly-white subintimal nodular lesions; a mild bark-like appearance is also present.
(*b*) The superior surface of the aortic arch showing complete occlusion of the ostium of the left subclavian artery by pearly-white material. The lumen of the left common carotid artery contains an ante-mortem blood clot. The innominate artery shows irregular stenosis of its lumen.
(*c*) A partial stenotic lesion at the origin of the right subclavian artery.
(*d*) The abdominal aorta, until its bifurcation, is relatively free from atherosclerosis.

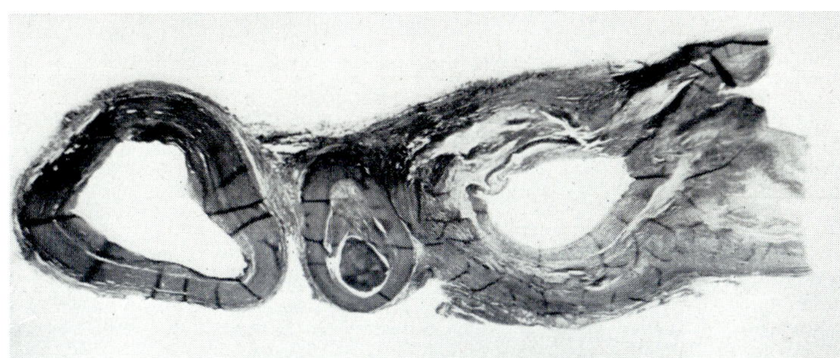

b. Cross-section of the main vessels of the aortic arch showing intimal and adventitial thickening. The lumen of the left common carotid artery contains an ante-mortem blood clot. The medial coat is somewhat thin but appears well preserved (Verhoeff–van Gieson stain × 3.5).

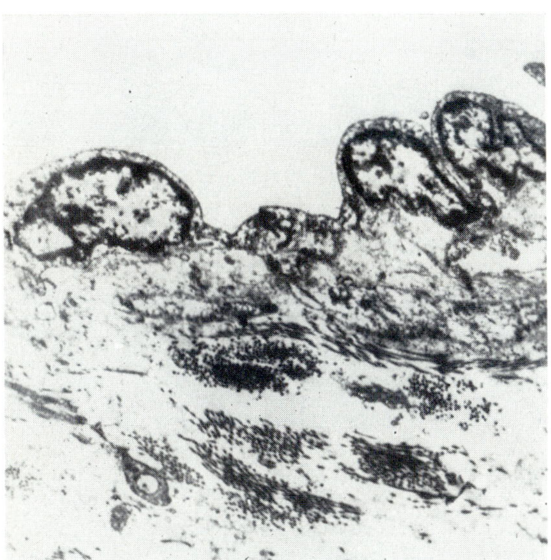

c. Electronmicrograph of a section through the intimal and subintimal region of the material as seen in PLATE 16a, showing bundles of collagen fibres in whorls together with cells resembling fibrocytes (× 1400, reduced).

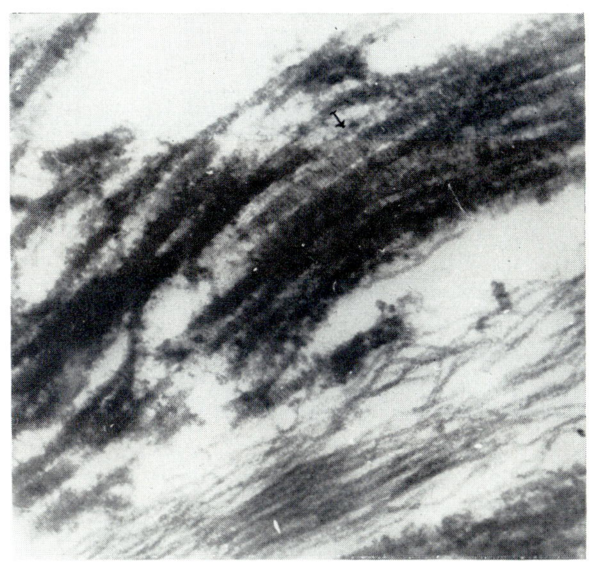

d. High-power view of the collagen fibres showing (see arrow) characteristic banded appearance (× 42,700, reduced). (Tissues treated with 1 per cent phosphotungstic acid before embedding in araldite.)

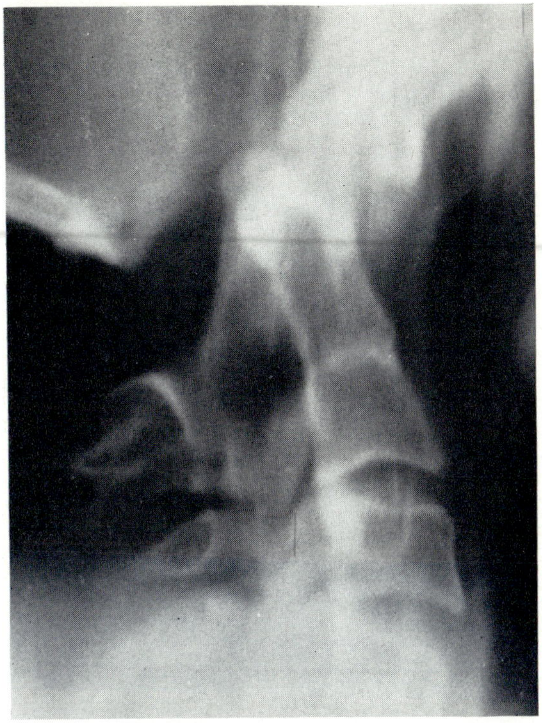

a. Lateral tomogram of craniovertebral junction in a case of congenital atlanto-axial dislocation. The fused C.2–C.3 form a block vertebra. There is a large gap between the occipitalized anterior arch and the odontoid. The odontoid is peg-like.

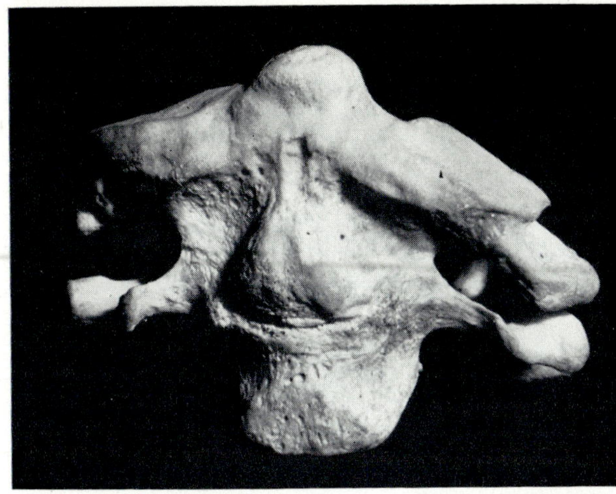

b. A macerated specimen of Group I cases of atlanto-axial dislocation seen from the front. *Note:* (*a*) the short odontoid; (*b*) the asymmetrical superior articular facets, especially the acutely sloping left one; (*c*) the fused C.2 and C.3 vertebrae.

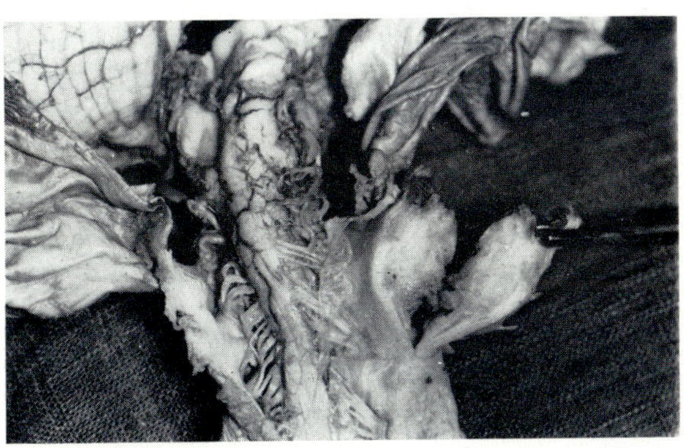

c. Attenuated upper cervical cord from prolonged compression. The forceps is holding a thick dural band at the same site.

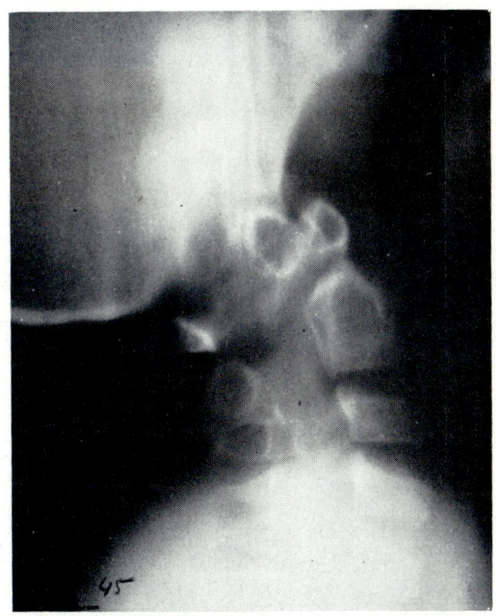

d. Tomogram of the lateral view of the cervical spine, illustrating Group II (Type II) cases. The separate apical segment of the odontoid is clearly seen behind the anterior arch of the atlas (ossiculum terminale). The basal segment is represented by a small bulge upwards from the body of the axis. *Note:* No dislocation in extension; and value of tomography.

PLATE 18
India

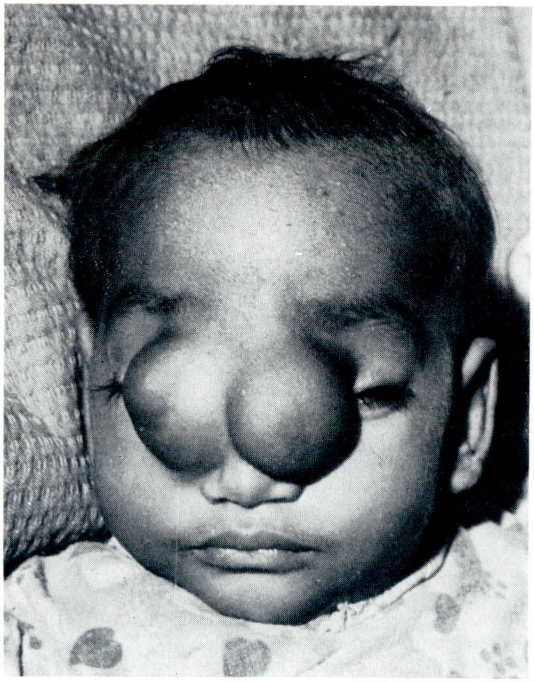

a. Anterior encephaloceles: typical fronto-ethmoidal-encephaloceles.

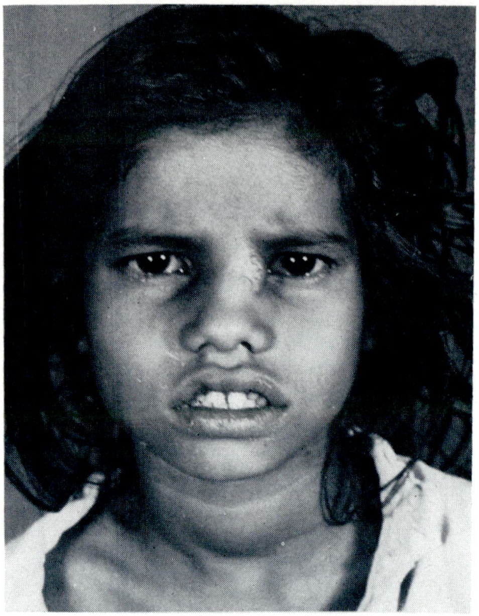

b. Cystic swelling on the left side of the nose.

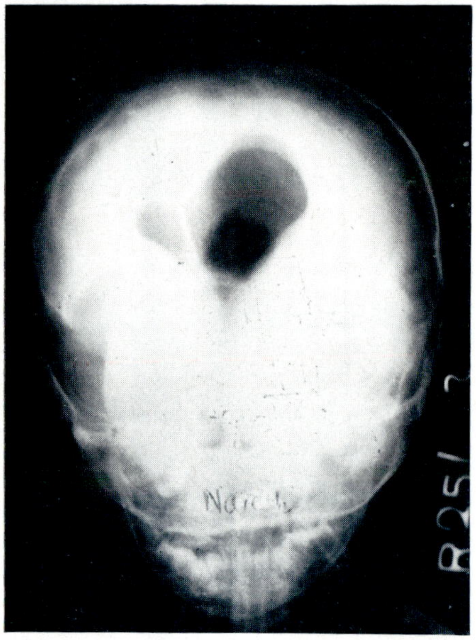

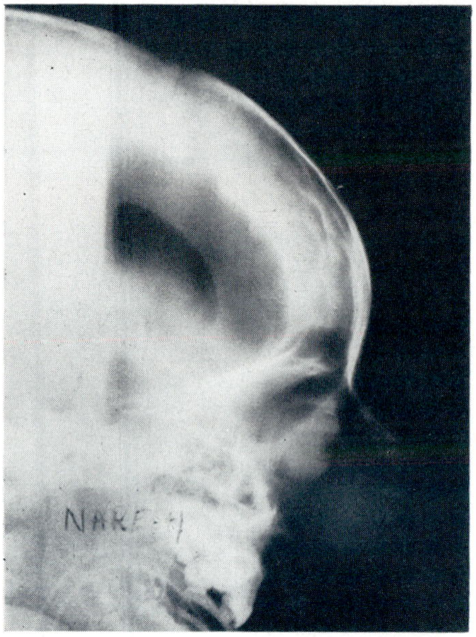

c. and d. Ventriculogram: brow-up AP and lateral views. Note the unilateral dilatation of the lateral ventricle.

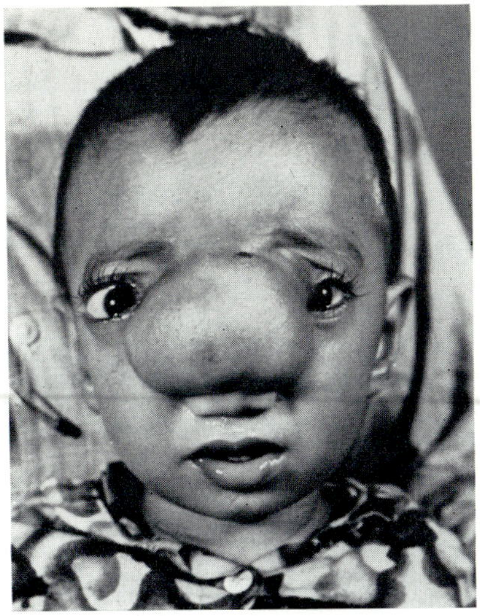

a. Pre-operative photograph: fronto-ethmoidal encephalocele.

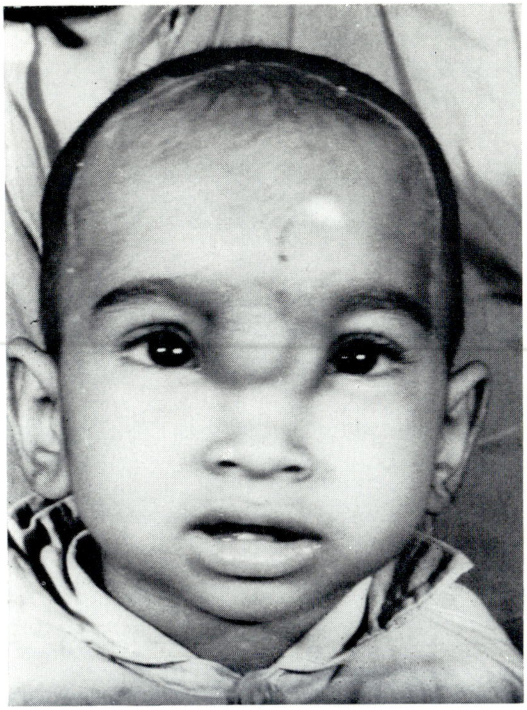

b. Post-operative photograph: 10 days post-operative with small residual swellings.

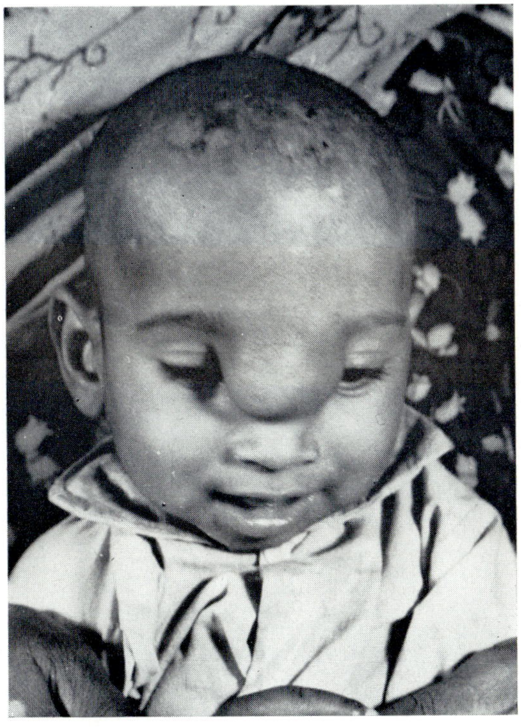

c. Three weeks post-operative, with enlarging swelling.

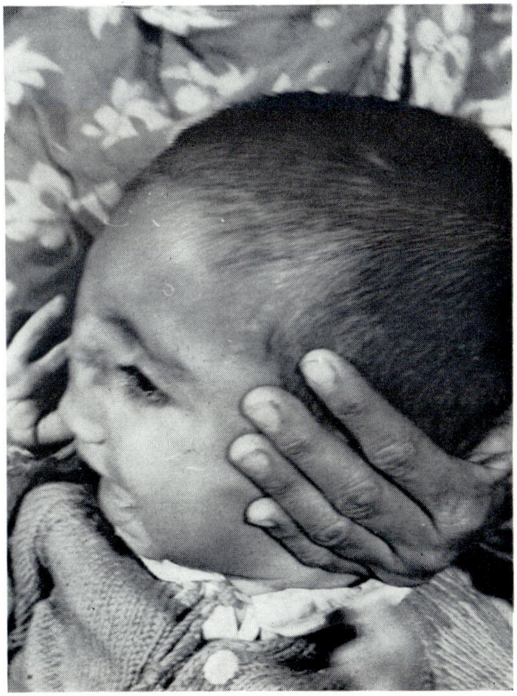

d. Following the co-peritoneal shunt: complete regression of the encephalocele.

PLATE 20
India

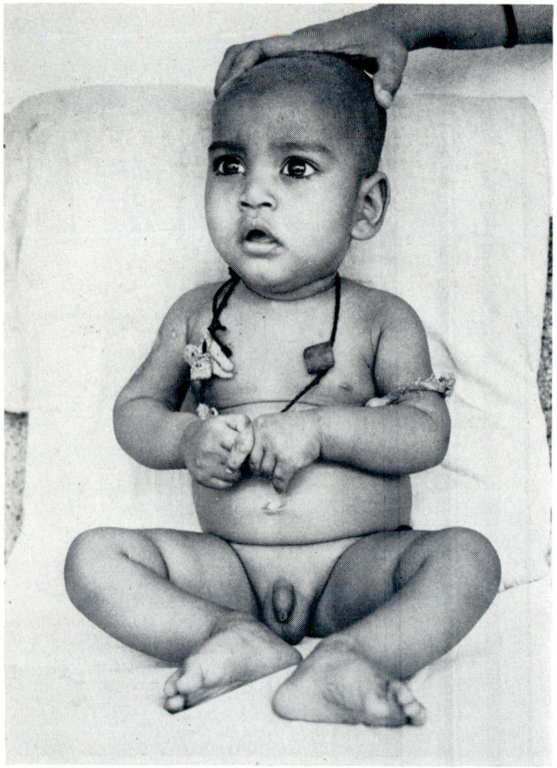

a. Infantile tremor syndrome: infant recovering from the 'tremor phase'. (See PLATE 5b for tremor phase.)

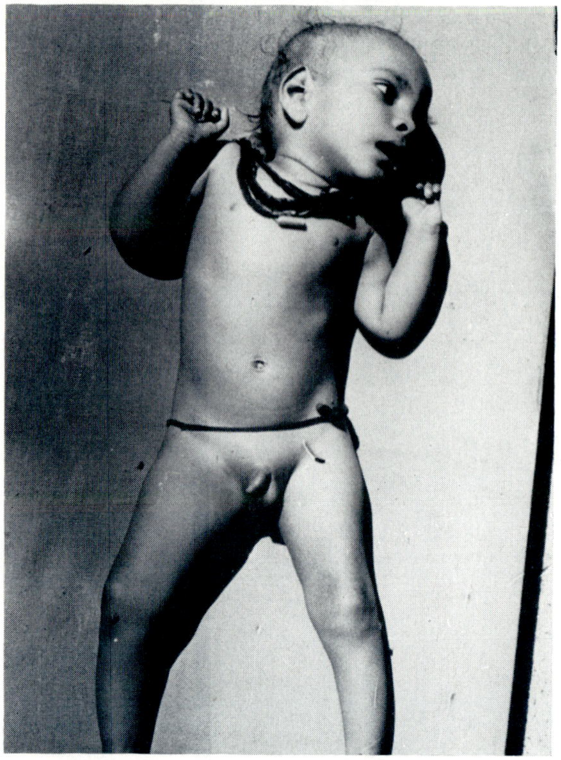

b. Infant showing postural abnormality.

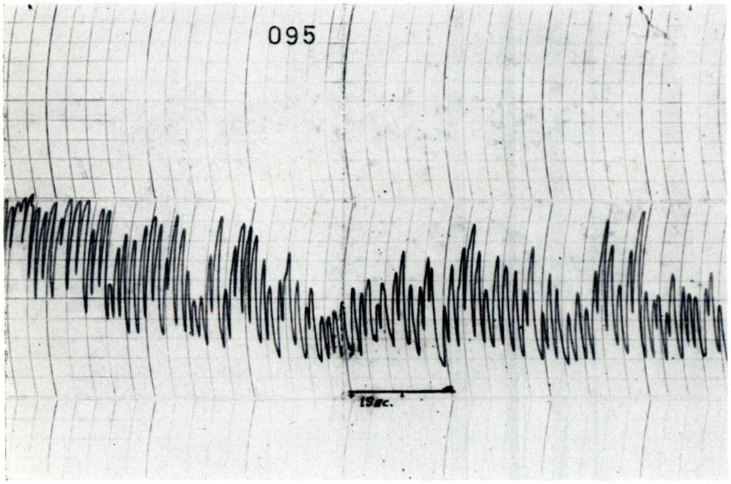

c. Polygraphic record of tremors.

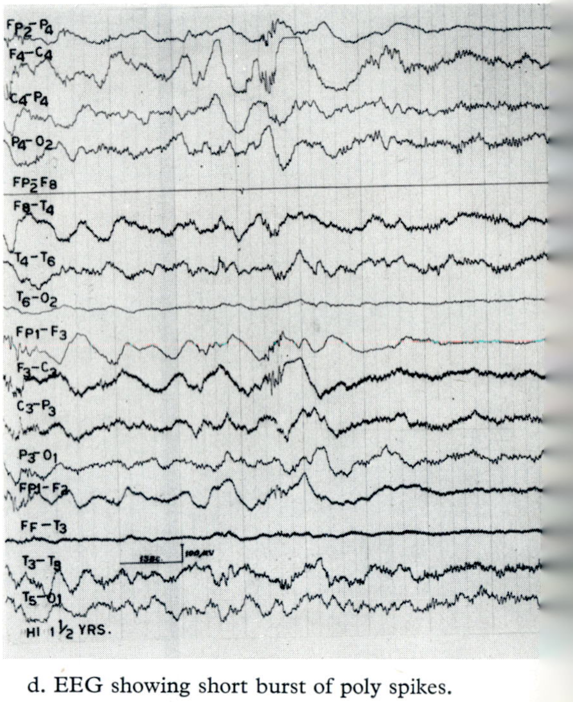

d. EEG showing short burst of poly spikes.

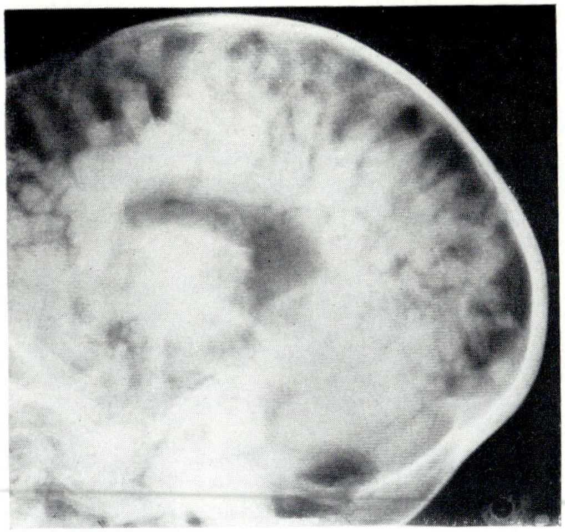

a. Infantile tremor syndrome: typical pneumo-encephalographic findings: cerebral atrophy.

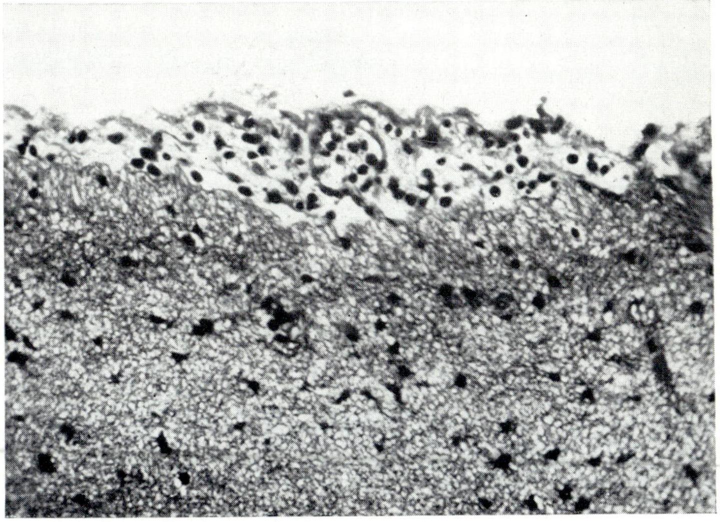

b. Microphotograph: mild meningeal infiltrate with well-defined subpial gliosis (H & E × 330).

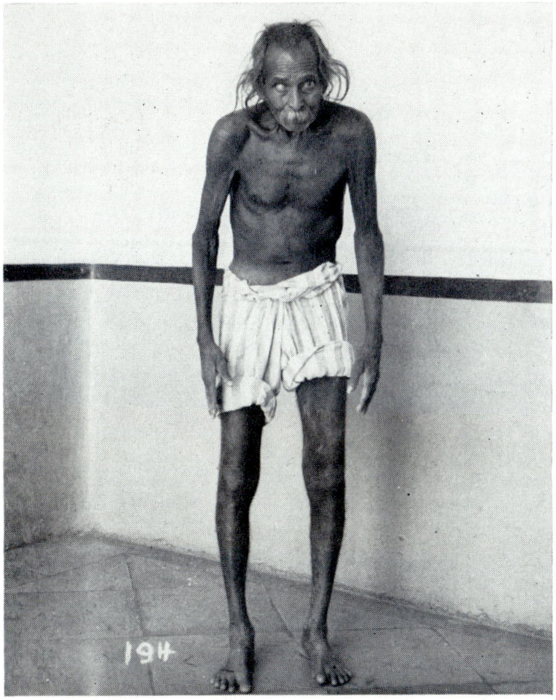

c. Endemic fluorosis: progressive rigidity and kyphosis. Spinal stiffness usually precedes limb joint stiffness.

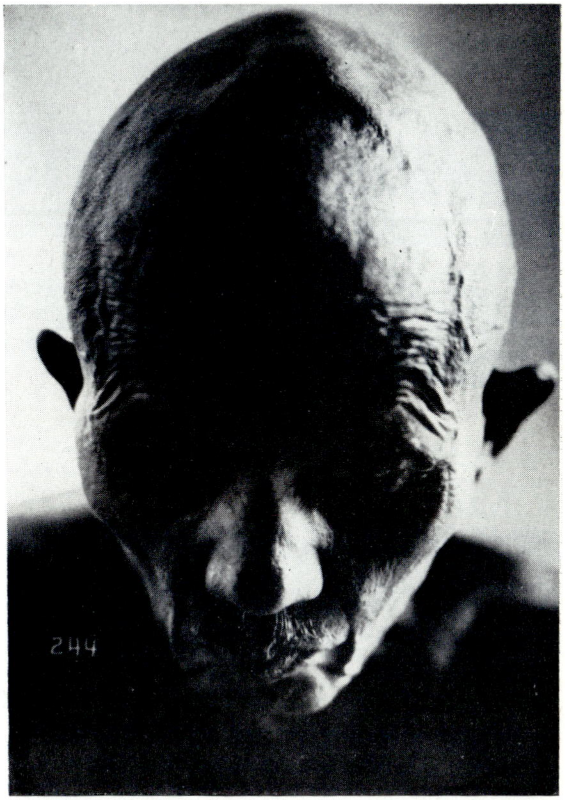

d. Endemic fluorosis: cranial exostosis at junction of coronal and sagittal sutures.

PLATE 22
India

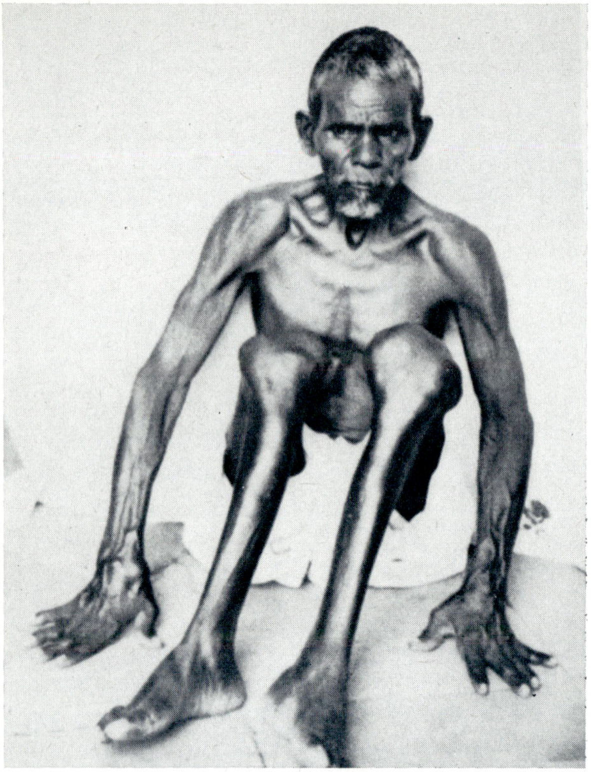

a. Endemic fluorosis: end stage of the disease in an old man. Tetraplegia with incontinence and contractures of lower limbs. Mental faculties retained.

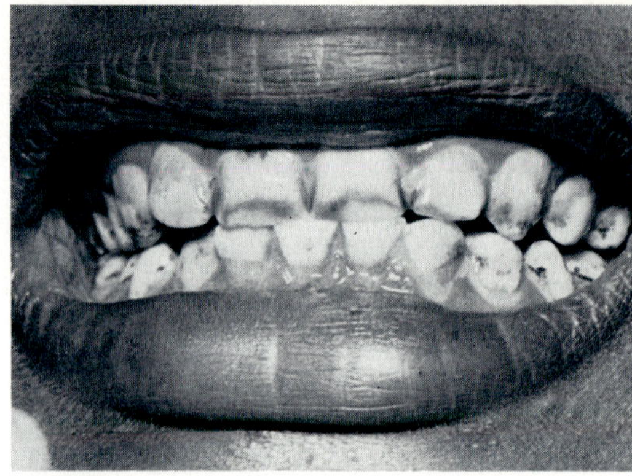

b. The tooth enamel is abnormally opaque and chalky white; white blotchy areas give appearance of mottling; later stages are characterized by deposits of dark pigment in the defective enamel.

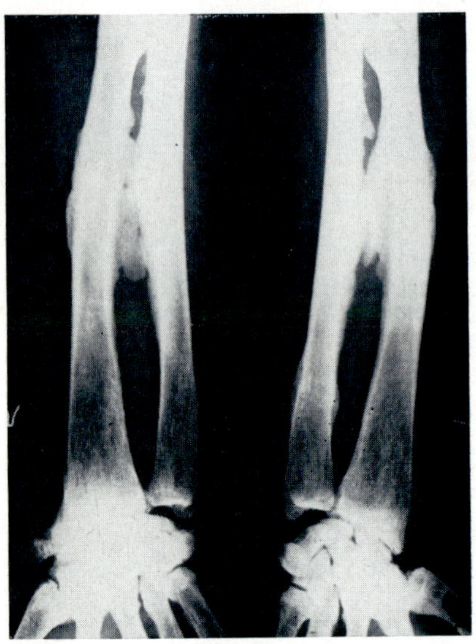

c. Radiograph of forearms to show calcification in the interosseous ligaments.

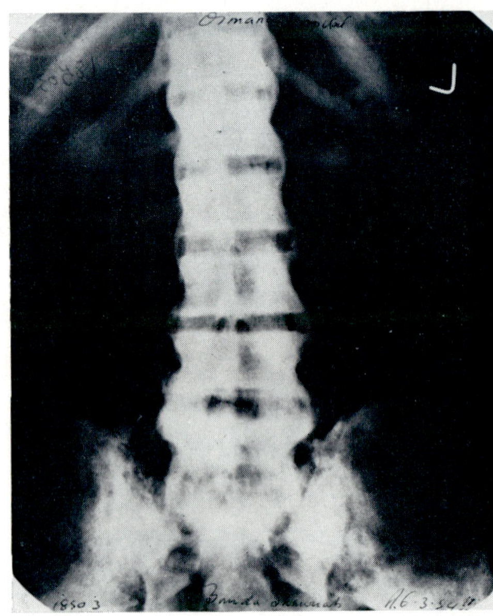

d. Radiograph of lumbar spine showing dense osteosclerosis involving the bodies and pedicles of the vertebrae and their spinous processes, together with calcification of spinous ligaments and osteophytosis.

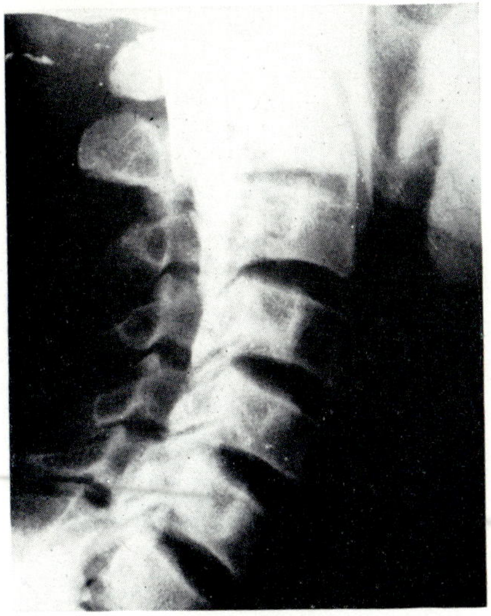

a. Endemic fluorosis: myelogram showing partial block at C.2–C.3 in a patient with tetraparesis; note osteosclerosis of pedicles. Good degree of recovery following decompressive laminectomy.

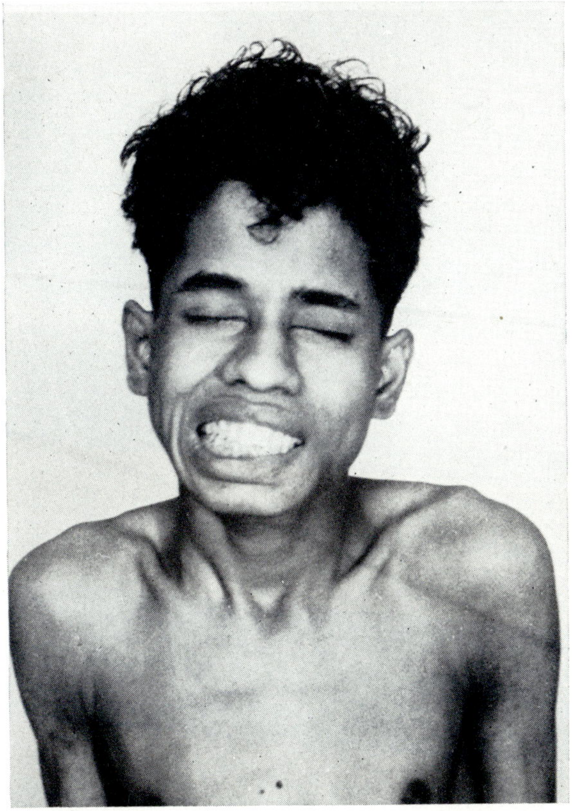

b. Juvenile motor neurone disease: left lower facial weakness and bilateral paresis of orbicularis oculi, in patient aged 18 years, with onset at 15. General muscular atrophy, hyperactive reflexes, bilateral extensor plantar responses. Patient showed asymmetrical wasting of thoracic musculature.

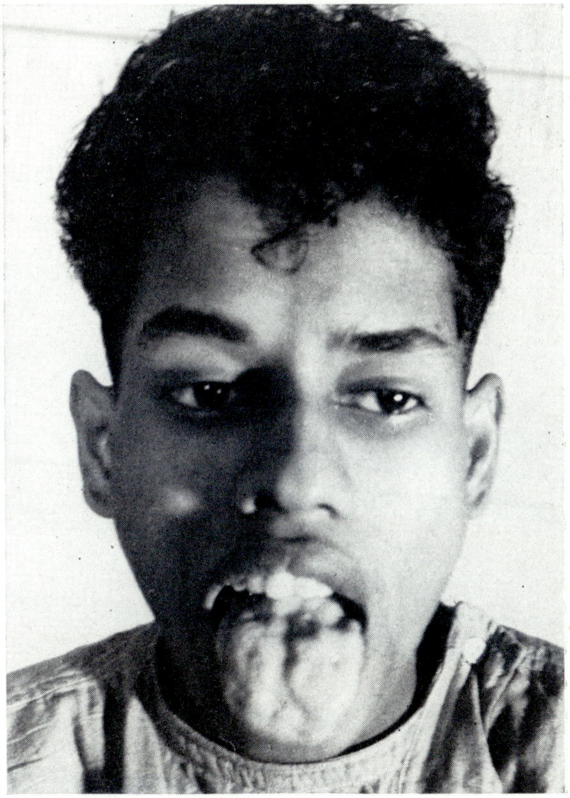

c. Wasting of the tongue in the same patient.

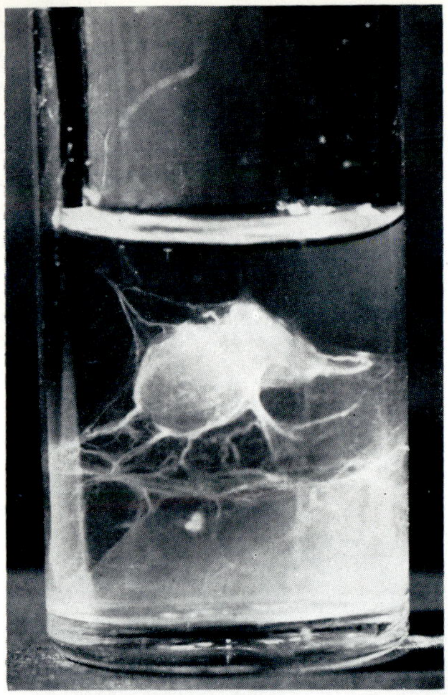

a. Spontaneous 'spider-web' clot in cerebrospinal fluid from a Nigerian patient suffering from tuberculous meningitis.

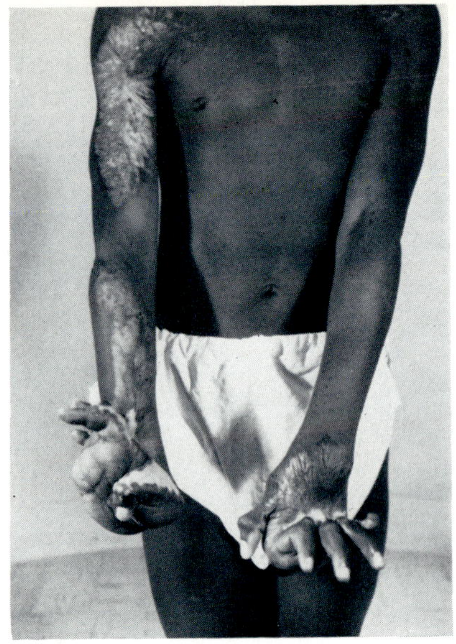

b. Severe contractures of the hands as a result of burns applied as a 'resuscitative' measure by a Nigerian parent to a son in epileptic coma.

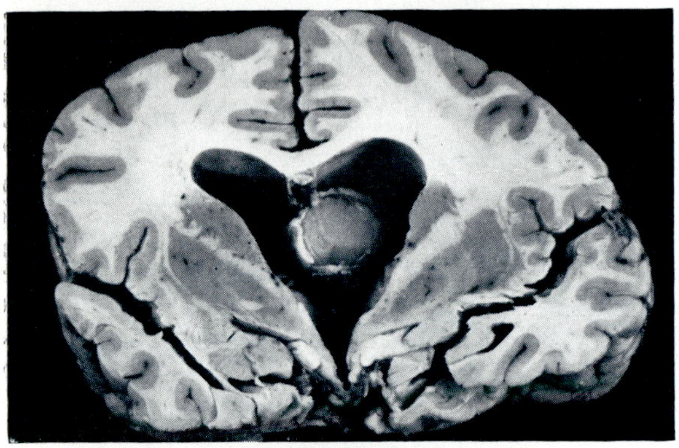

c. Colloid cyst of third ventricle from a Nigerian patient. (By courtesy of the Editor, *Tropical and Geographical Medicine*.)

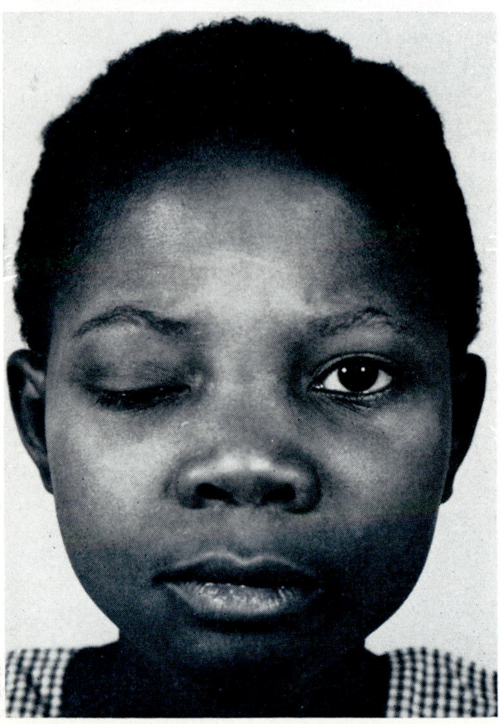

d. Ocular presentation of Burkitt's neoplasm in a Nigerian girl before treatment.

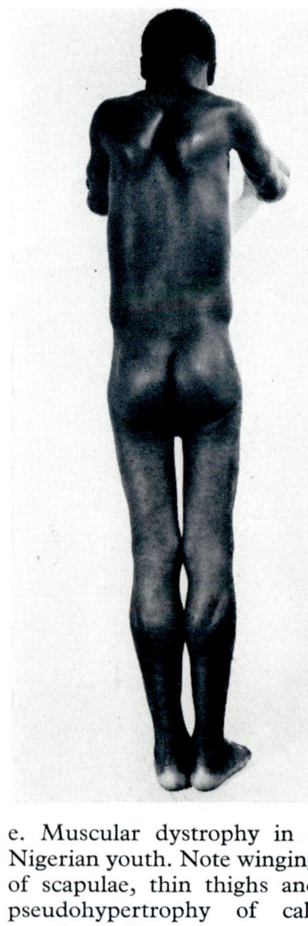

e. Muscular dystrophy in a Nigerian youth. Note winging of scapulae, thin thighs and pseudohypertrophy of calf muscles. (By courtesy of Professor A. O. Williams.)

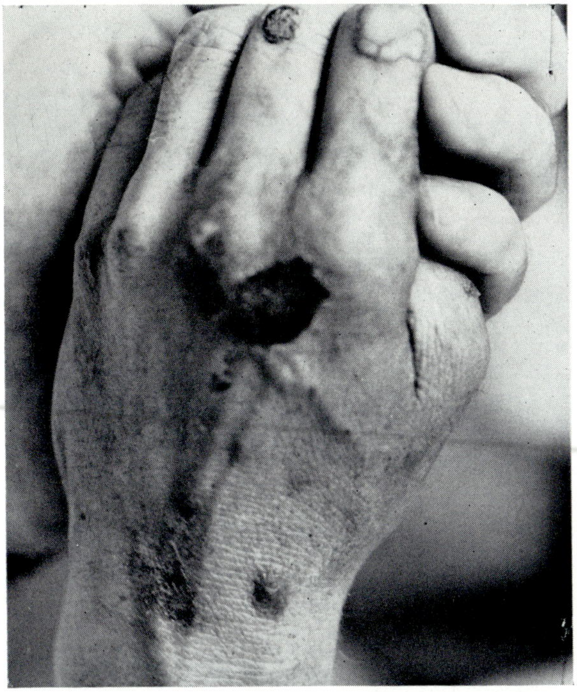

a. *South Africa:* the hand of a man with porphyria variegata, showing blisters, sores and scarring. His sister, who did not have skin sensitivity, had an attack of acute porphyria.

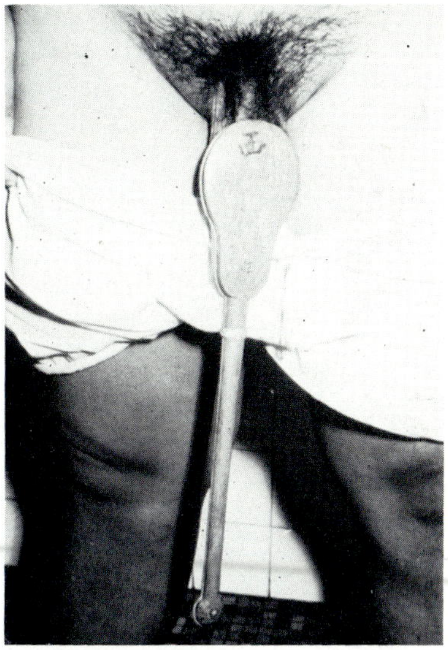

b. *Singapore:* Koro: a clamp used by a Singapore Chinese to fasten on his penis which he feared would retract into his abdomen with a fatal outcome. Koro is a form of epidemic hysteria.

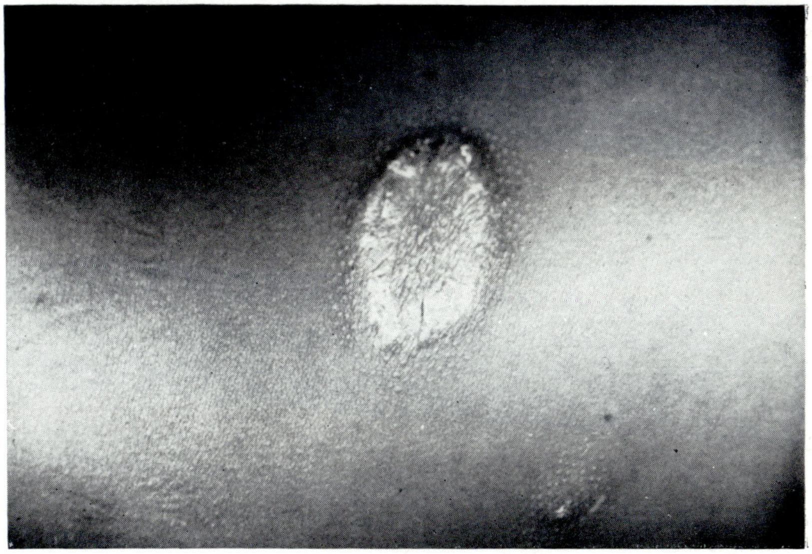

c. *Kuala Lumpur:* tuberculoid lesion in a case of leprosy. Erythematous, scaly and well demarcated.

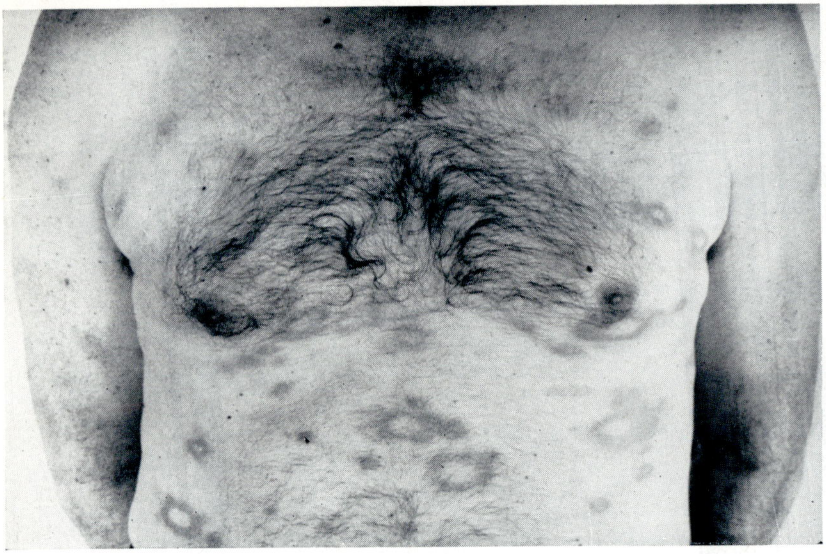

a. *Kuala Lumpur:* classical borderline leprosy in a Caucasian. Numerous well-defined lesions with a central clearing, giving an annular appearance.

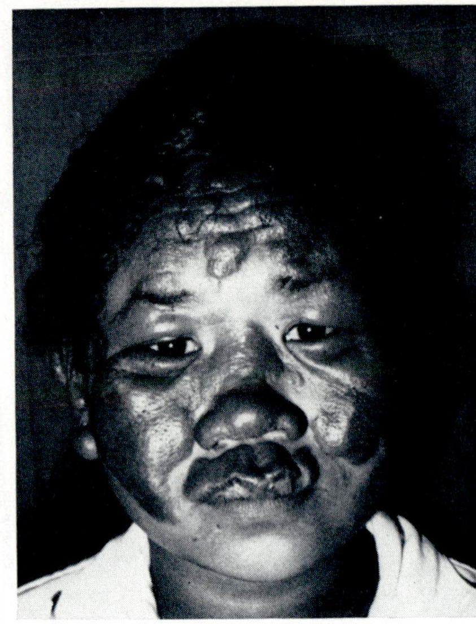

b. Borderline leprosy: severe Type I reaction.

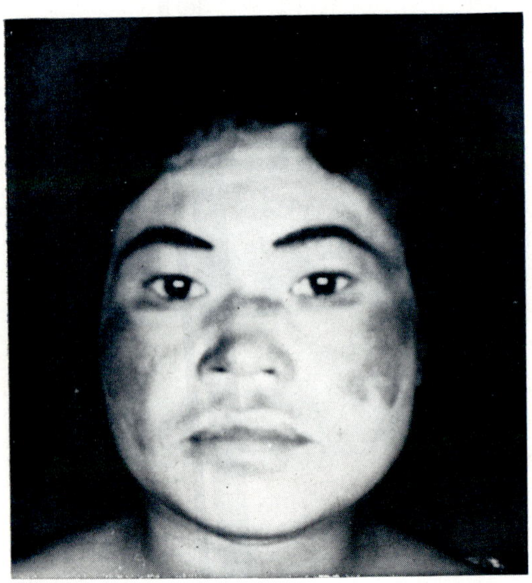

c. Borderline leprosy, same patient as in PLATE 26b. Reaction has subsided, leaving hyperpigmentation; histology showed that the reaction was of the 'reversal' type.

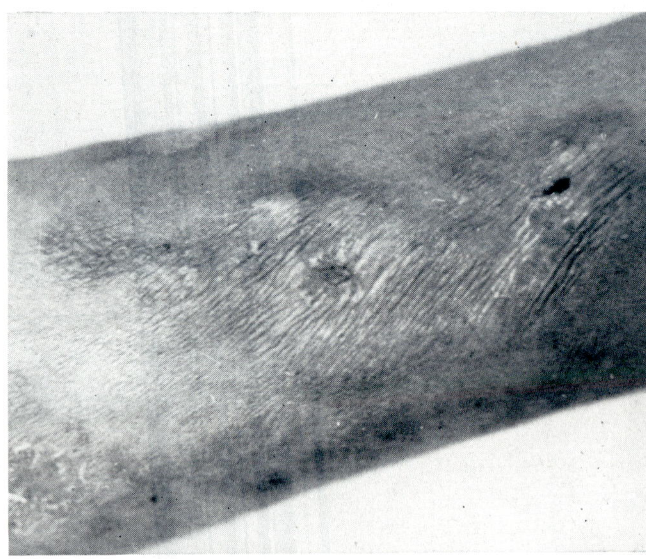

d. Erythema nodosum leprosy with a tendency towards necrosis in the centre of some of the lesions.

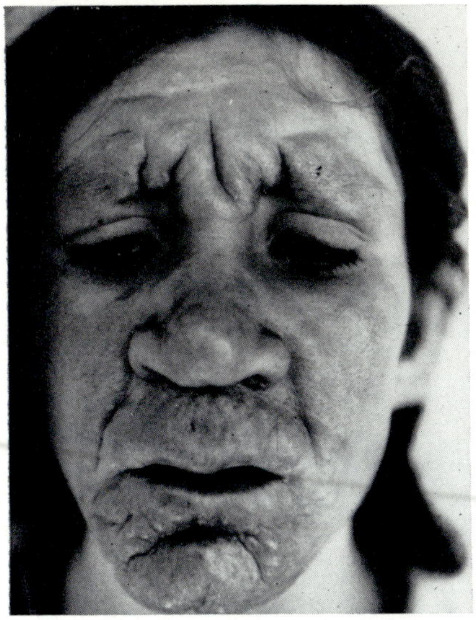

a. *Kuala Lumpur:* severe nodular lepromatous leprosy in an Iranian woman.

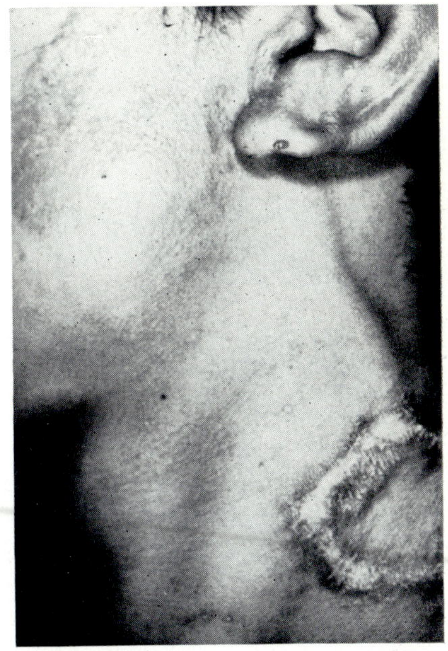

b. Tuberculoid (BT) leprosy of the ear and neck, with an enlarged pre-auricular nerve, in a Chinese patient.

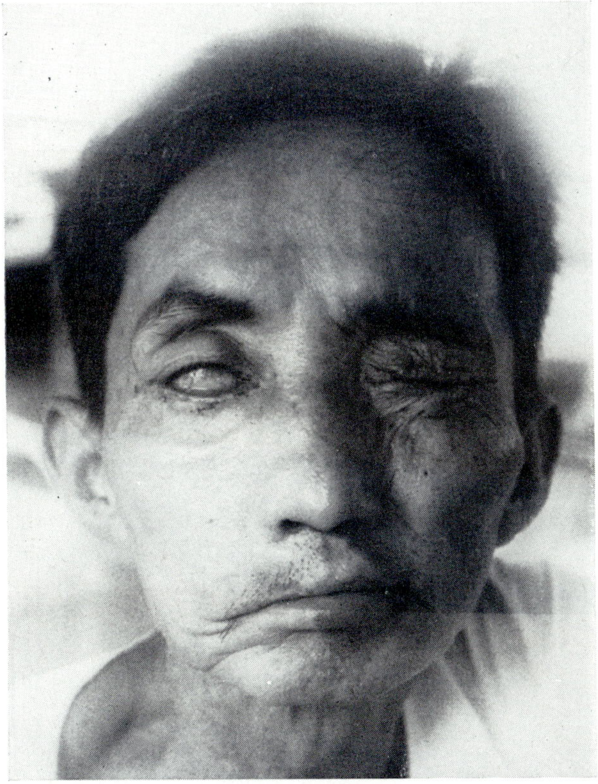

c. Leprosy. Facial paralysis following Type I reaction. Corneal exposure will cause trouble unless there is surgical help.

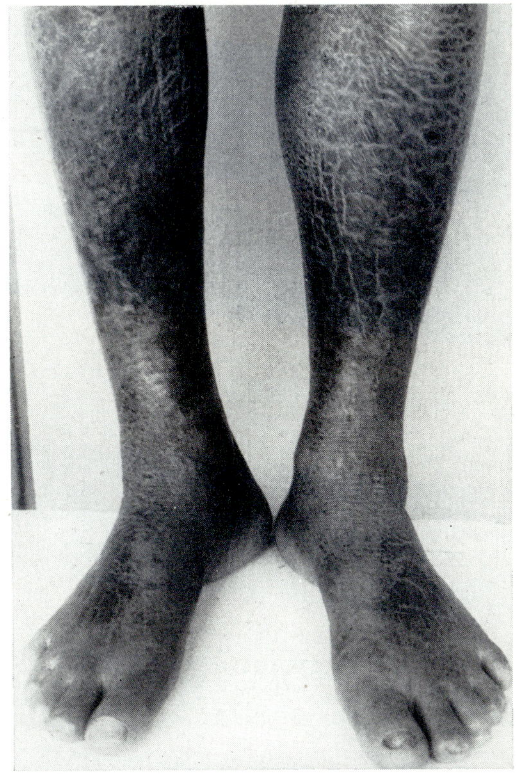

d. Secondary xeroderma associated with diffuse anaesthesia in a lepromatous case of long standing.

PLATE 28
South-East Asia

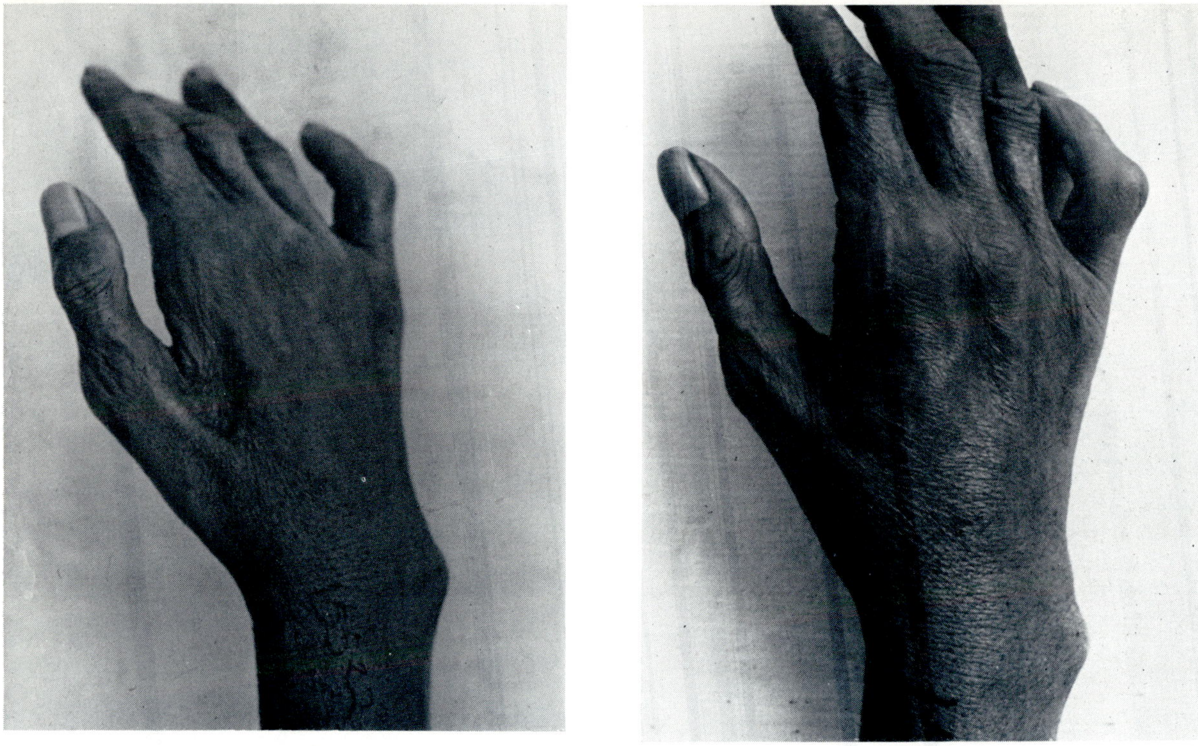

a. and b. *Kuala Lumpur:* surgical obliteration of the hollow between thumb and index finger, formed by interosseal wasting in tuberculoid leprosy. This sign is well known to the Chinese, and patients like to have a fat graft or a plastic repair to fill out the hollow between thumb and index.

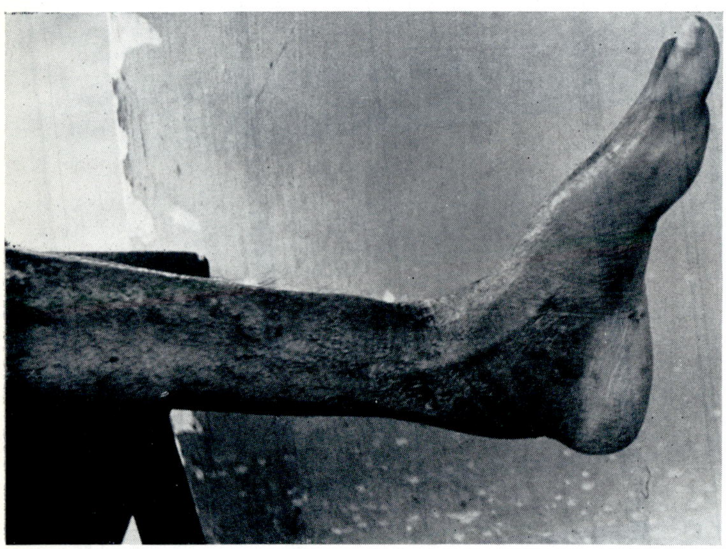

c. Leprosy. Charcot arthropathy of ankle joint. (Photograph by J. D. Spillane.)

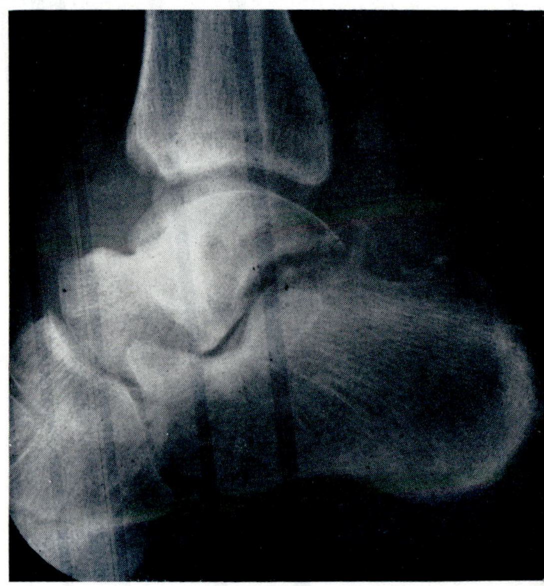

d. Charcot arthropathy of ankle joint. Note the parrot' beak deformity of the talus.

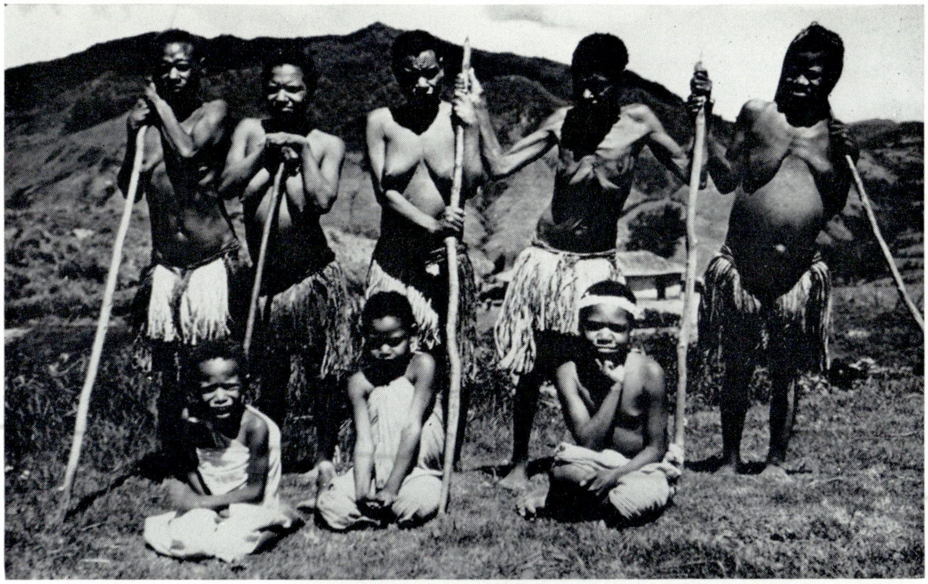

New Guinea: groups of kuru patients in 1957 at the Kuru Research Hospital. All died within a year of photography. The pictures show many pre-adolescent child victims of kuru, of an age-group in which kuru has not occurred in recent years.

a. Eight kuru patients in the first, or ambulatory, stage of the disease. Five adult women are holding sticks to maintain their balance. Three girls, who are still able to walk without the aid of a stick but with severe ataxia, sit in front of the women.

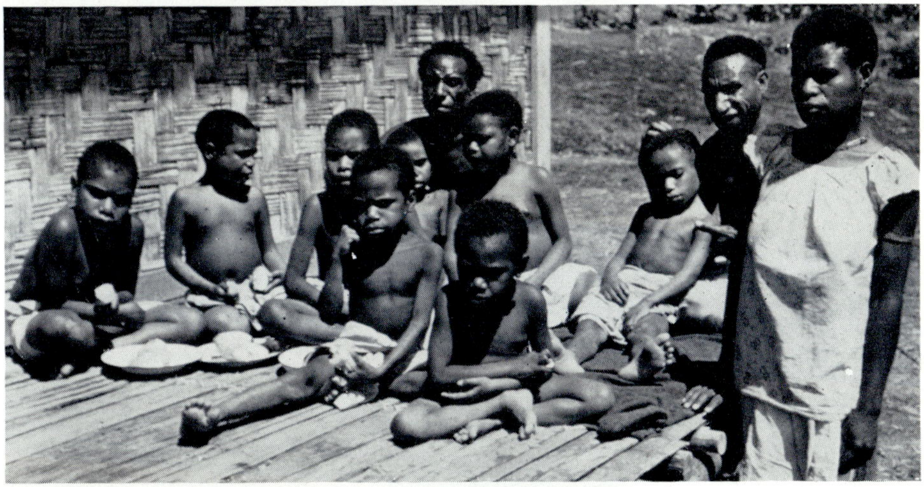

b. Eight pre-adolescent children, four boys and four girls, with kuru. The girl at the far right in her father's lap is the same child as that on the left in a, now 2 months later and in the secondary, sedentary, stage of kuru.

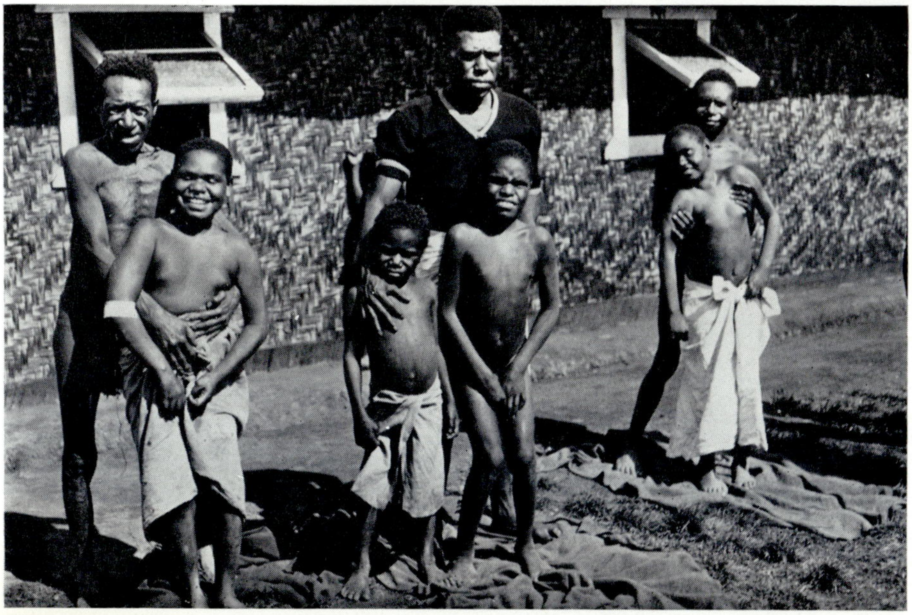

c. Four children with kuru; two boys in the centre; a girl on each side. All are just passing from the first, or ambulatory, to the second, sedentary, stage of the disease.

New Guinea: three child victims of kuru late in stages 1, 2, and 3, respectively.

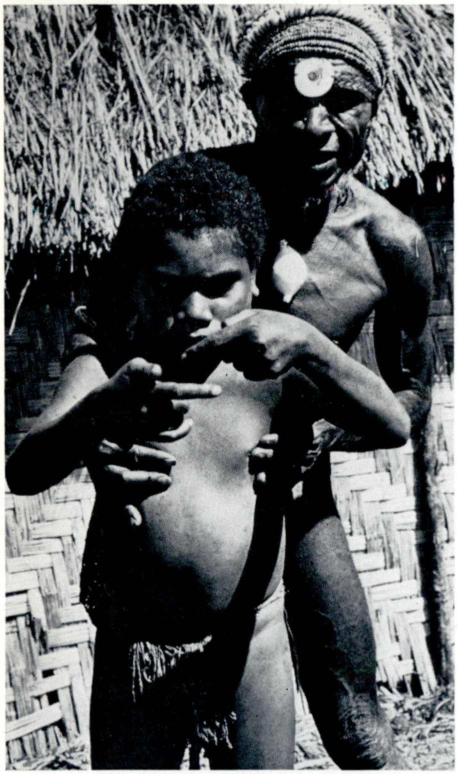

a. A Gimi boy in late stage 1, or the ambulatory stage, of kuru attempts to execute the finger-to-finger test while supported by his father so that he will not fall. He could still walk alone with the aid of a stick. He showed marked internal strabismus.

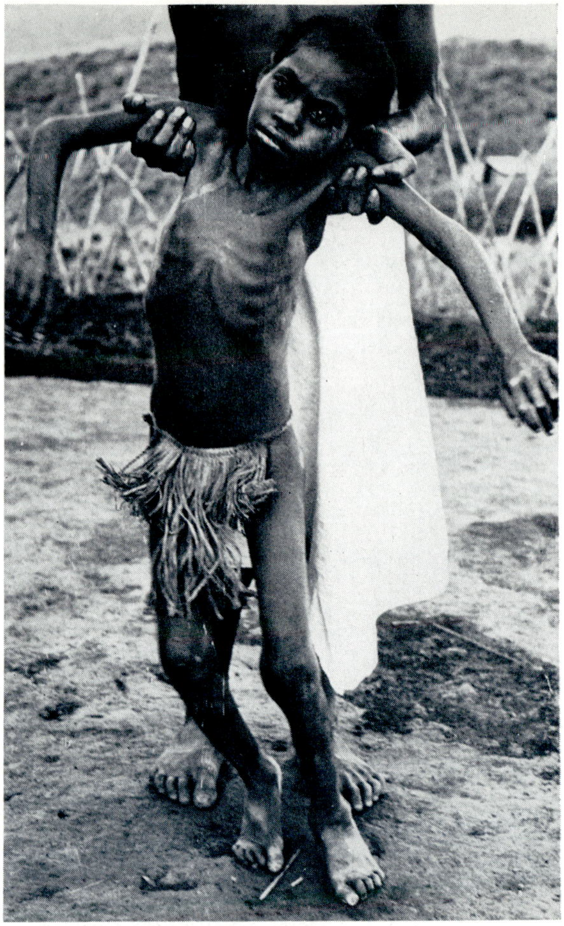

b. A South Fore girl late in stage 2, or the sedentary stage, of kuru. She could no longer sit up unsupported and was remarkably dysarthric.

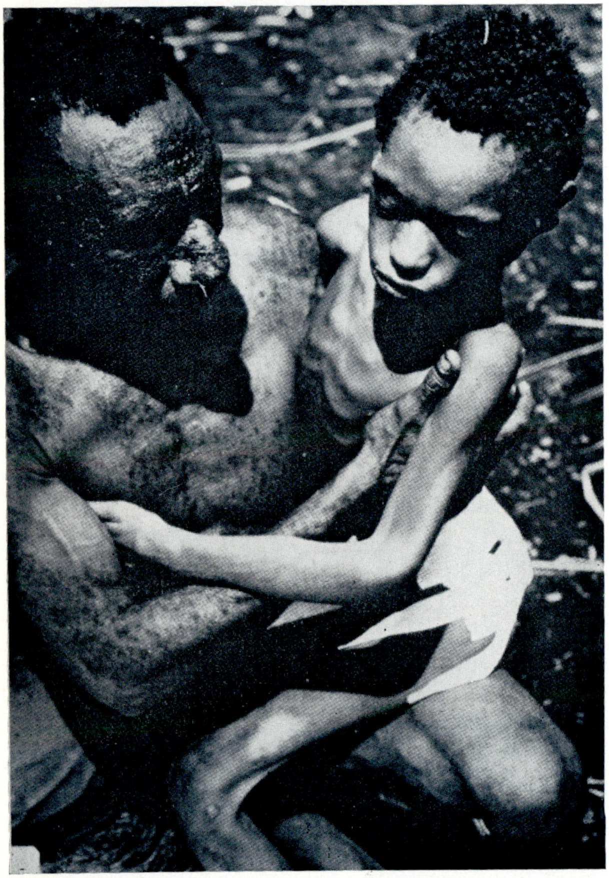

c. A South Fore girl in the third or terminal stage of kuru, already suffering from deep decubitus ulcers and emaciation as a result of dysphagia. She was totally aphonic yet remained alert and conscious, though unable to direct her gaze or reply to questions without setting off jerky startle responses.

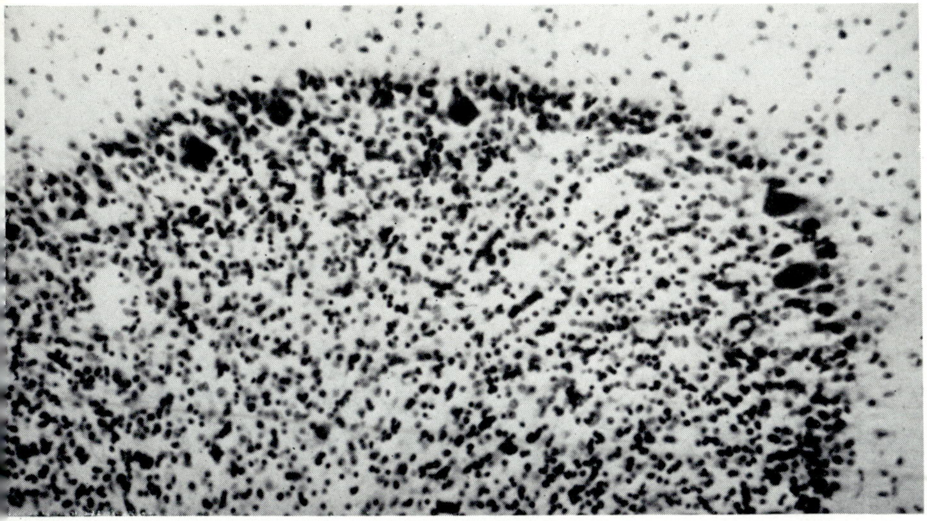

a. *New Guinea:* Kuru. The extensive loss of Purkinje cells and neurones of the granular layer of the cerebellum in a kuru victim. The sparsity of intact neurones is readily appreciated when one contrasts the section with a normal cerebellum. Silver impregnation techniques permit the demonstration of empty fibrous baskets where Purkinje cells have disappeared.

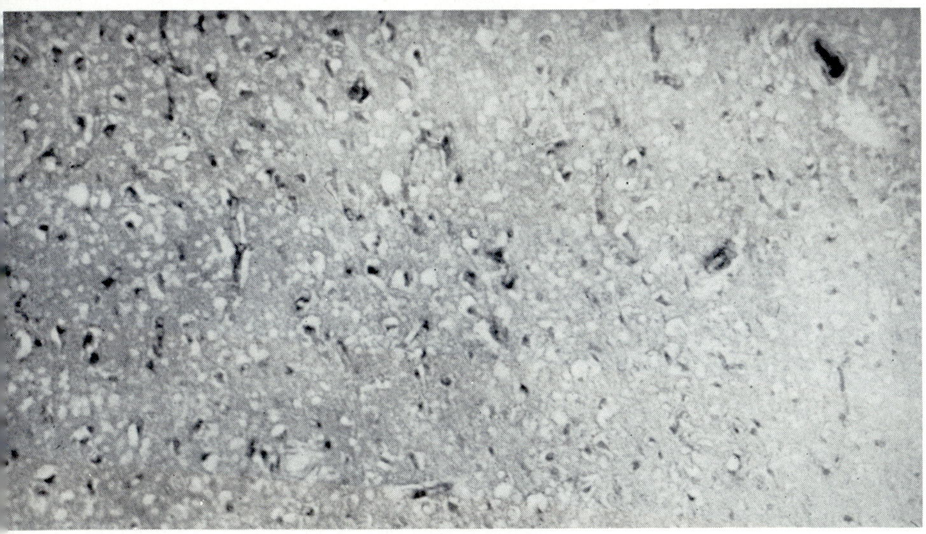

b. Status spongiosus of grey matter in the cerebral cortex of a kuru patient. The holes are intracellular vacuolation caused by coalescing vacuoles in the axonal and dendritic processes of the neurones, and also in some of the glial cells.

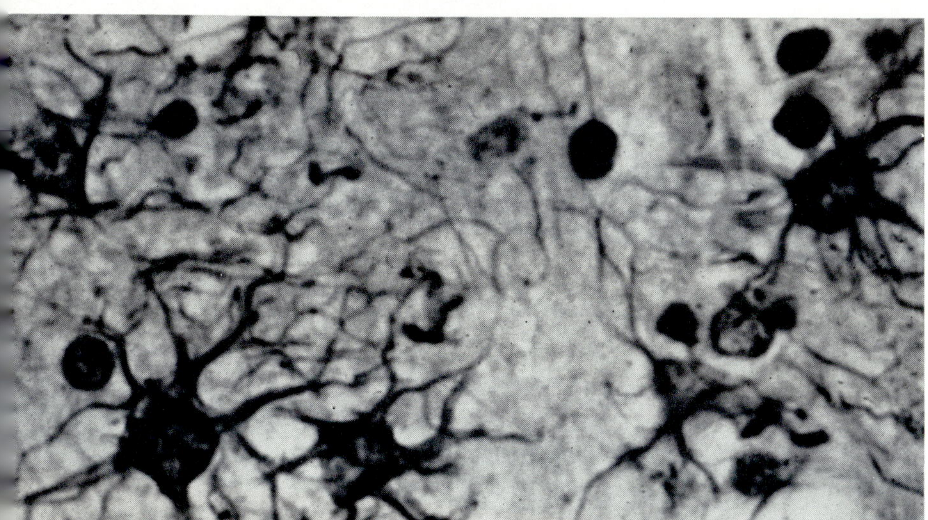

c. Extensive astroglial hypertrophy and proliferation in the cerebral cortex of a kuru victim.

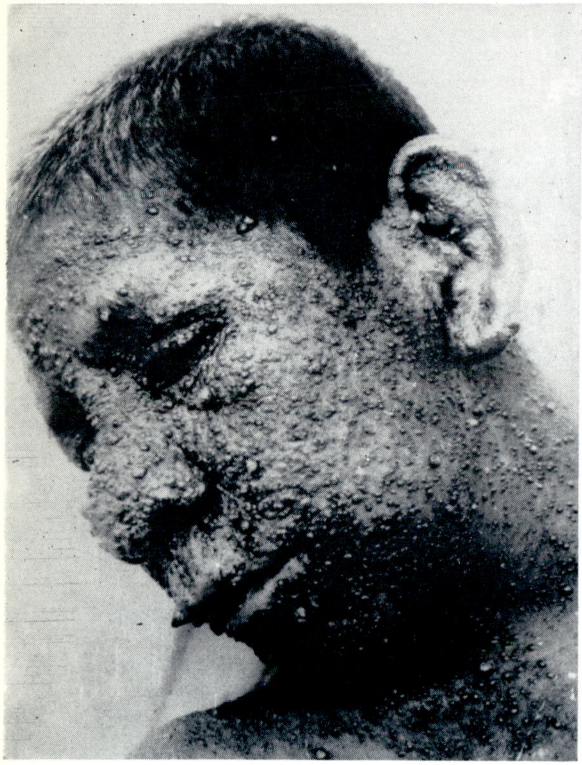

a. and b. *Peru:* verruga peruana. The eruptive phase of the illness showing the warty nature of the cutaneous lesions.

a. b.

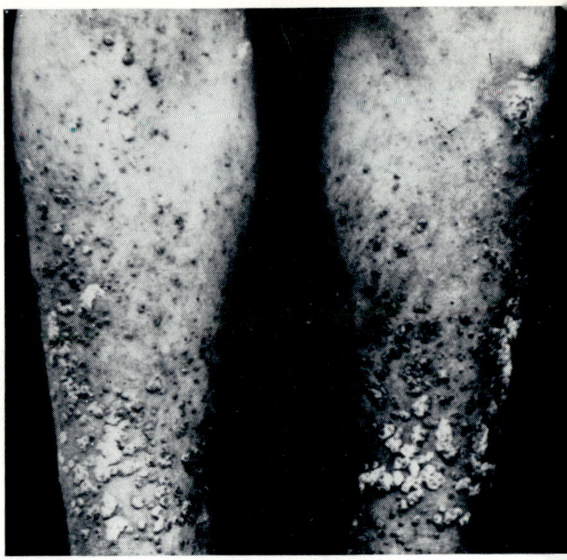

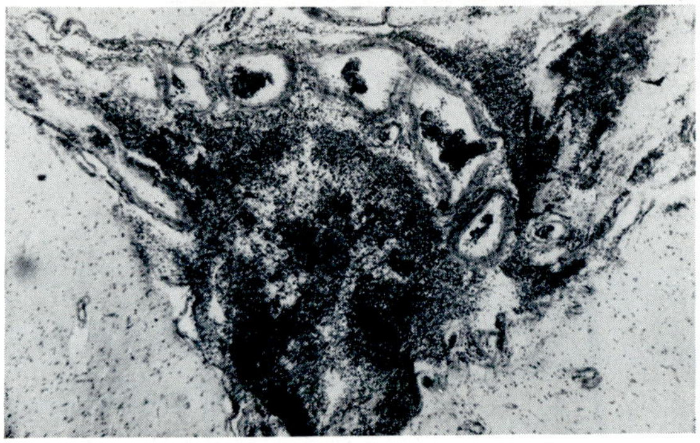

c. Meningeal and vascular cortical reactions in verruga peruana.

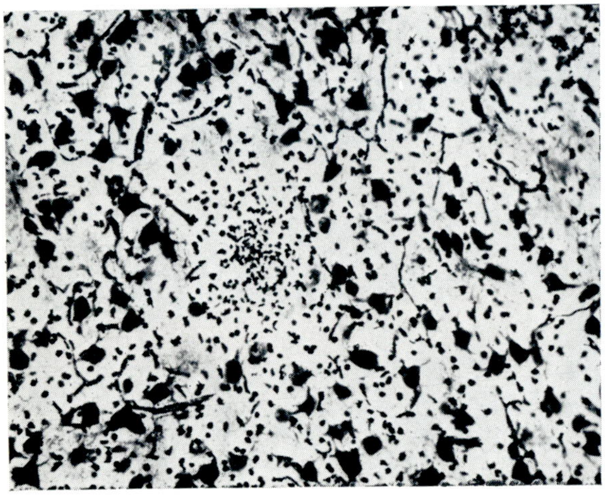

d. Neuronal and glial alterations; glial nodule formation in the pontine nuclei.

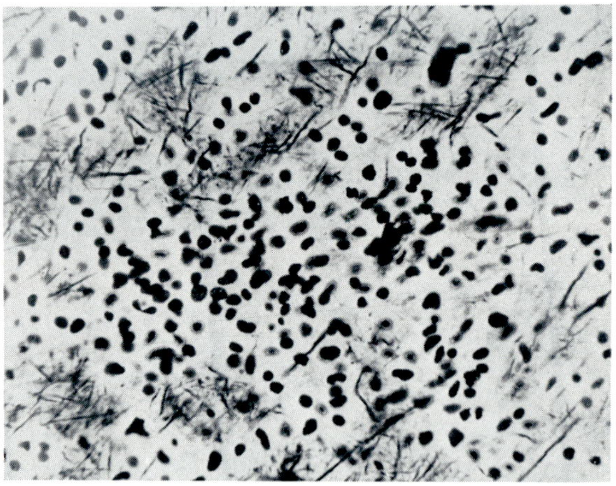

e. Frontal cortex; glial infiltration and axonal alterations.

PLATE 33
Latin America

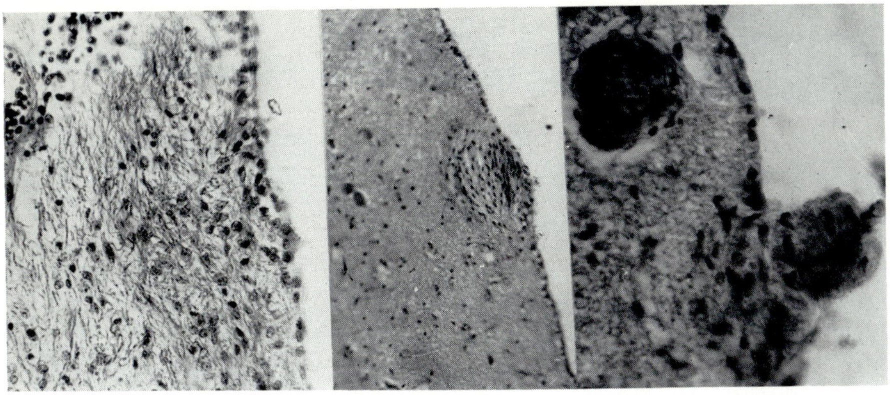

a. *Peru:* verruga peruana. Three phases of verruca formation in the brain.

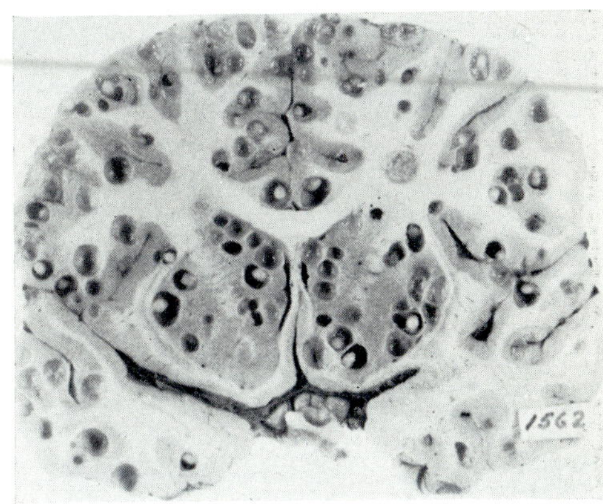

b. Cystic cysticercosis: there were 1200 cysts in this brain, 129 in this section. No calcification.

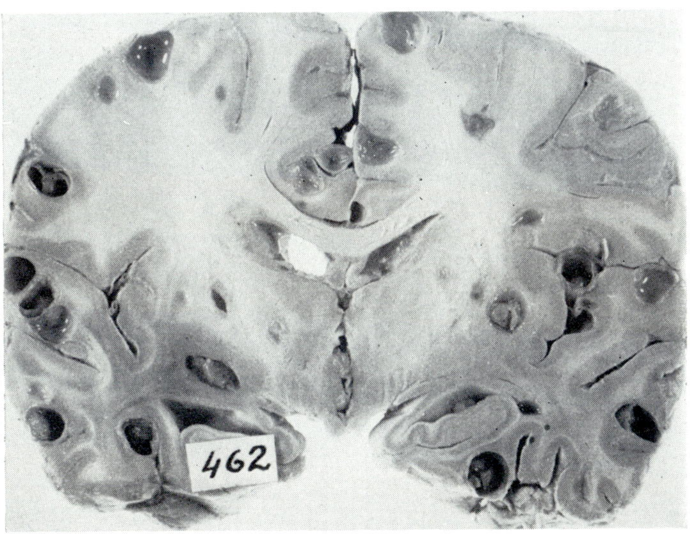

c. Cystic cysticercosis: note invasion of the ventricles.

PLATE 34
Latin America

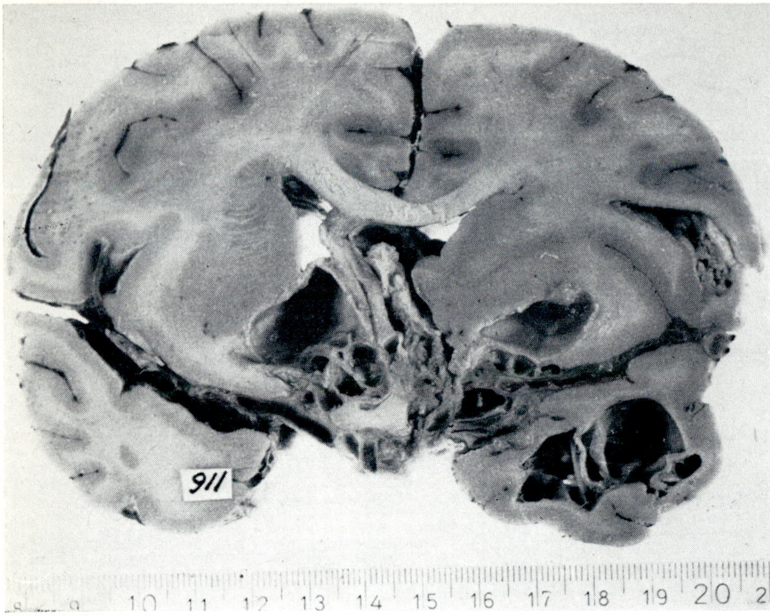

a. *Peru:* racemose form of cysticercosis with massive basal involvement

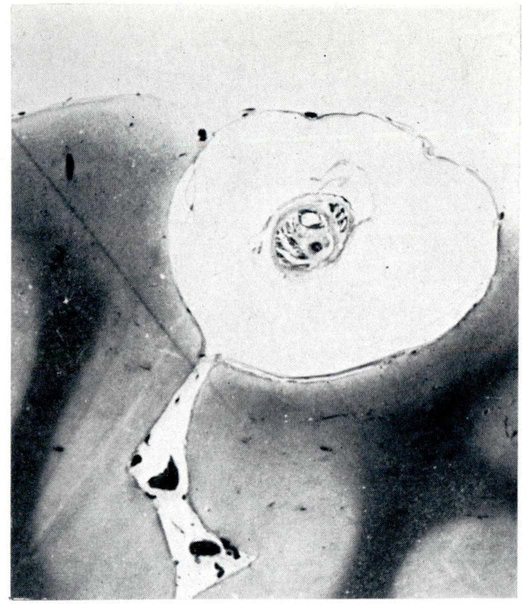

b. Subpial vesicle with scolex; note compression of underlying cortex.

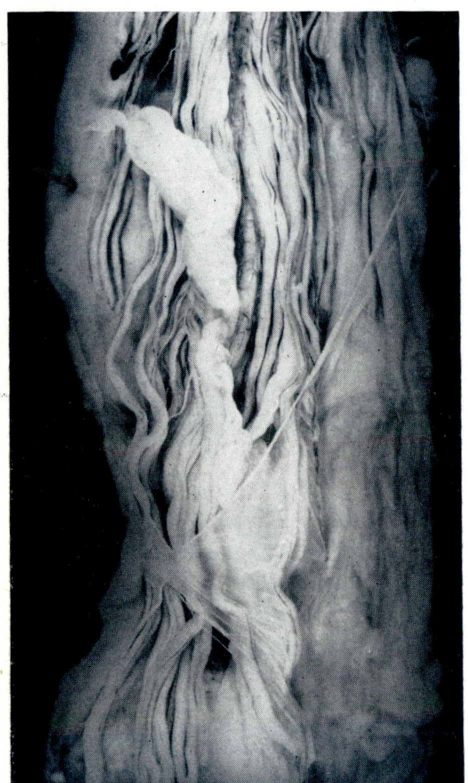

c. Racemose vesicle in the cauda equina.

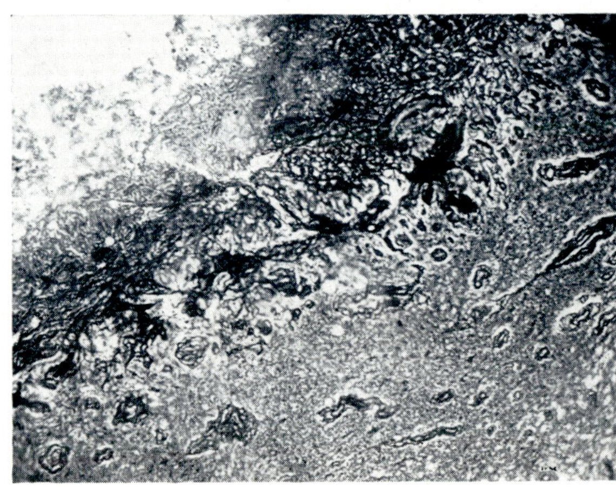

d. Fibrovascular connective tissue reaction surrounding a disintegrating parasite.

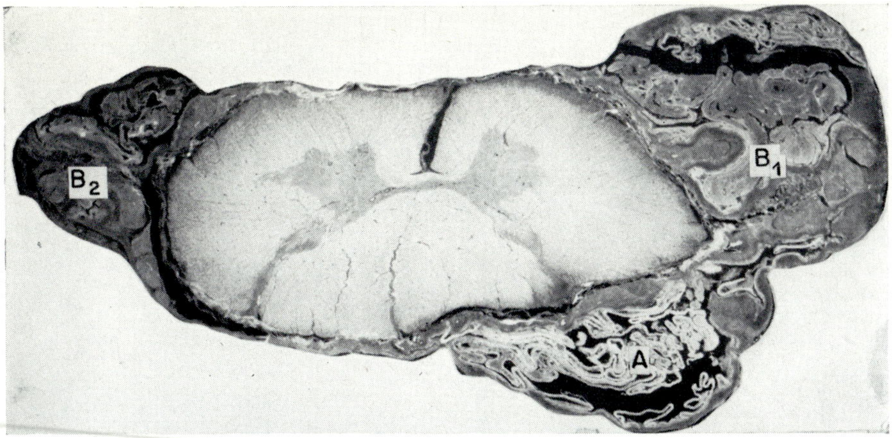

a. *Peru:* cystic cysticercosis. Spinal cord: meningeal involvement; vesicle membranes in stage of disintegration (A, B_1, B_2).

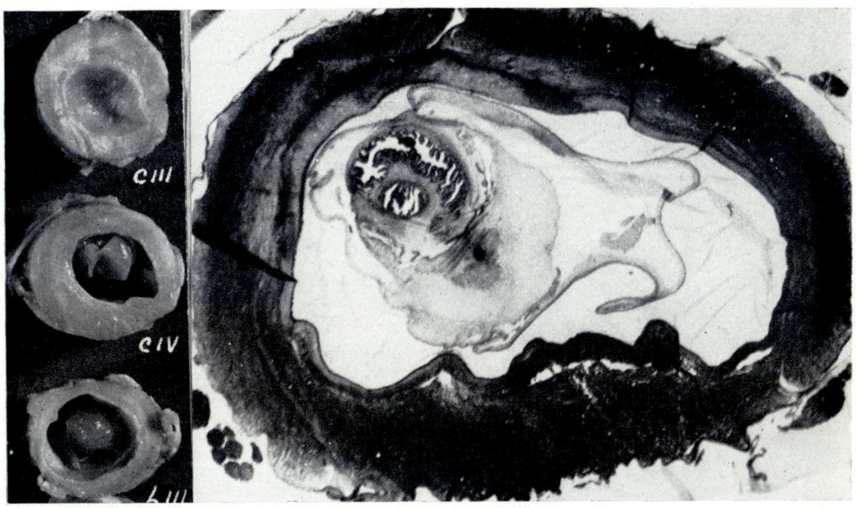

b. Spinal cord. *Left:* intraspinal vesicles at cervical and lumbar levels. *Right:* parasite within vesicle displacing cord tissues.

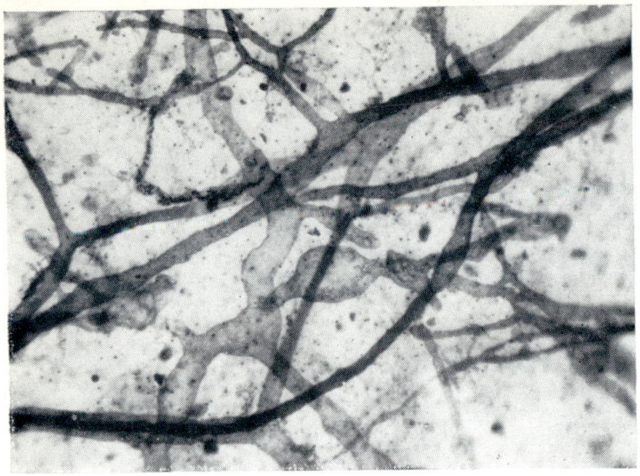

a. *Peru:* cystic cysticercosis. Deep fibrocanalicular layer of the vesicular membrane.

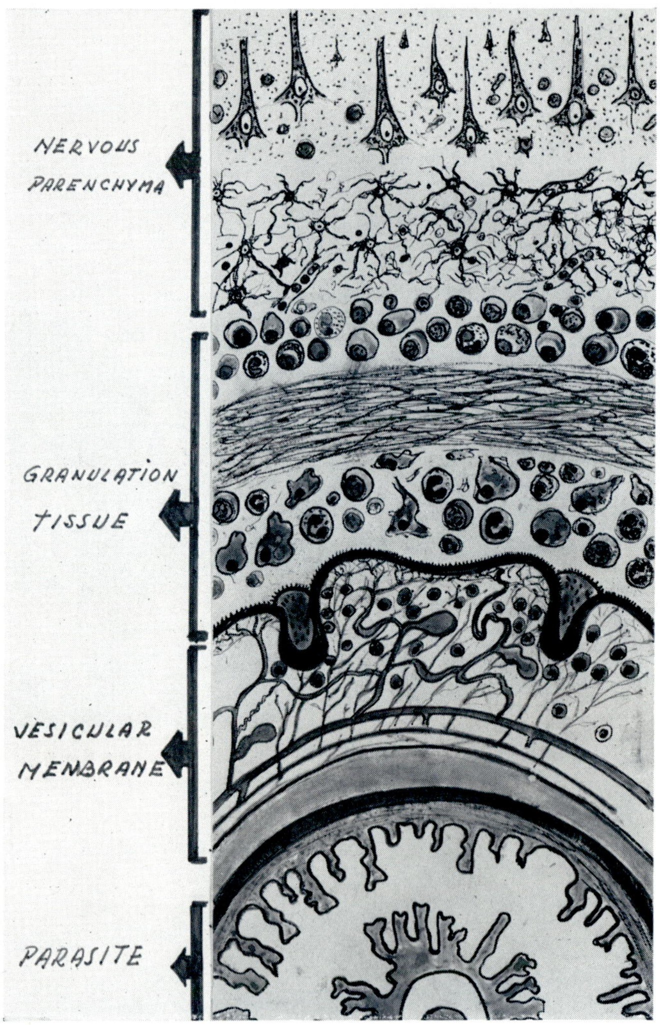

b. Schematic representation of the reaction produced by the cysticercus in brain tissues. Superposition of the parasite, the vesicular membrane, the reactional tissue and the nervous parenchyma, showing different structural layers.

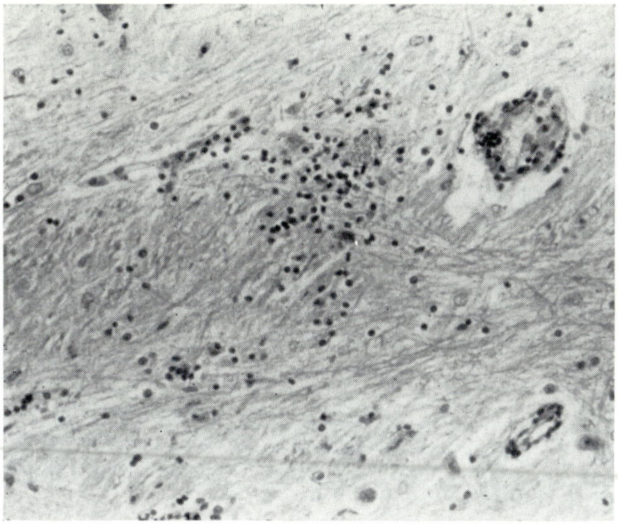

a. *Brazil:* human Chagas' acute encephalitis. Microglial granuloma (H & E × 20).

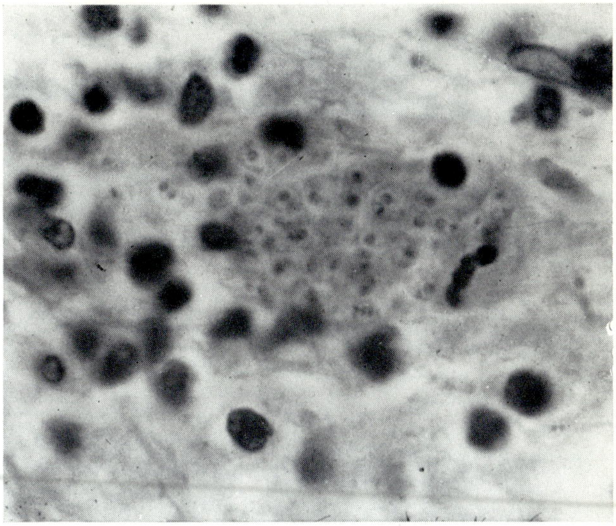

b. Parasitic pseudocyst in cerebral white matter in human Chagas' acute encephalitis (H & E × 320).

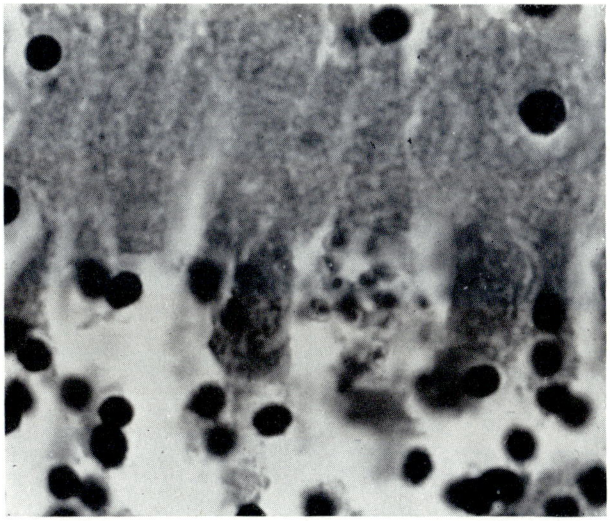

c. Experimental Chagas' infection in mouse. Parasitic pseudocyst in Purkinje layer of cerebellum (H & E × 320).

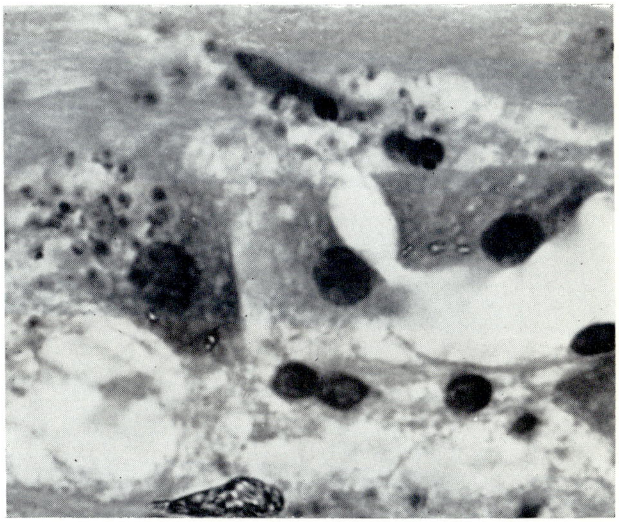

d. Experimental Chagas' infection in mouse. Parasitic pseudocyst in intestinal myoenteric plexus (H & E × 320).

PLATE 38
Latin America

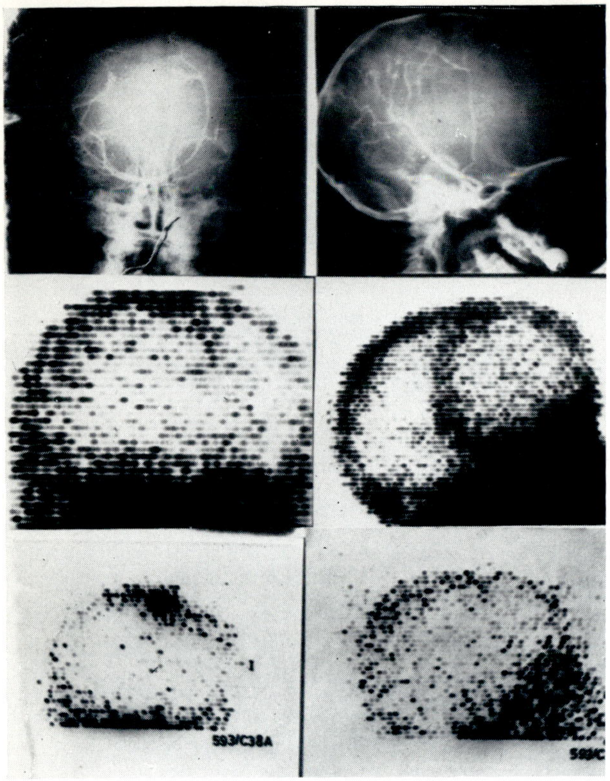

a. *Uruguay:* hydatid disease of the nervous system. *Upper row:* angiogram in a case of frontal cyst showing the circumferential disposition of ACA (anterior cerebral artery) and MCA (middle cerebral artery). *Middle row:* scintillography of the same patient showing hyporadioactive area surrounded by a more intensive radioactive band. *Lower row:* another case showing the more usually encountered hyper-radioactive area.

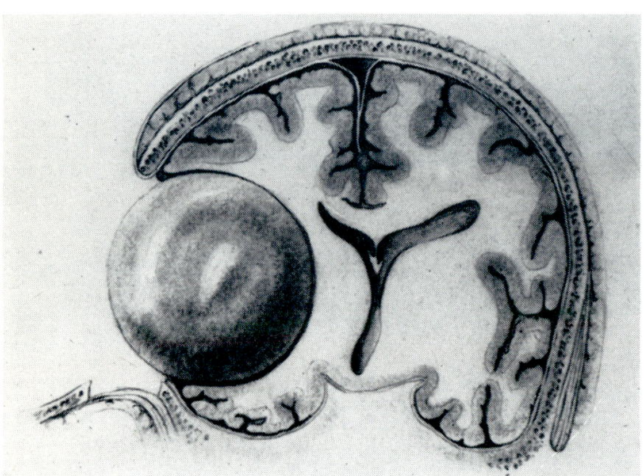

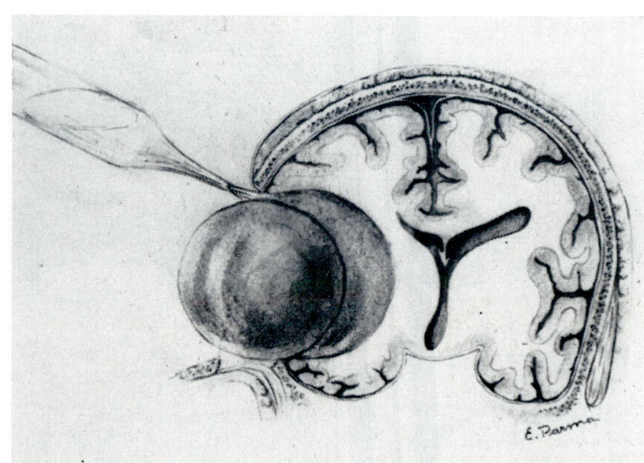

b. and c. Schematic explanation of San Julián and Arana-Iñiguez's procedure.

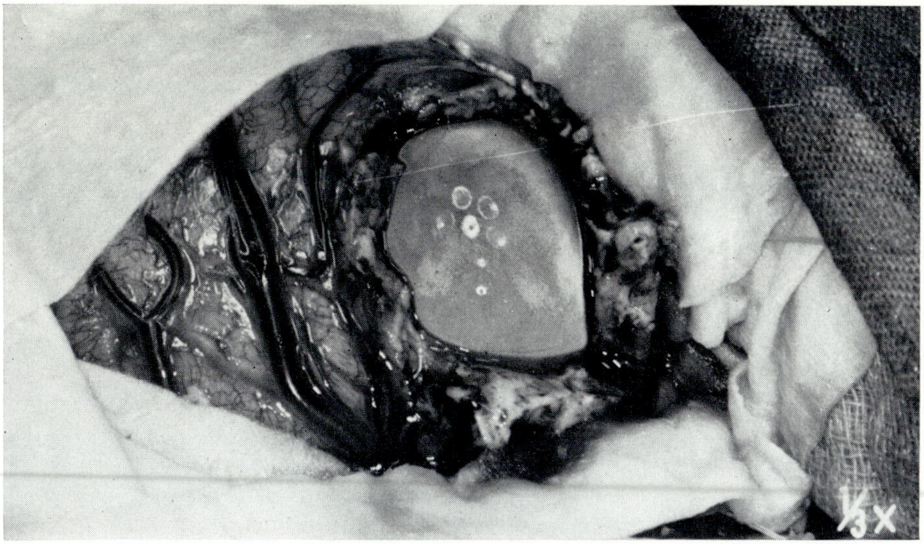

Uruguay: hydatid disease of the nervous system. Three stages in the surgical procedure of evacuating a hydatid cyst of the brain.

a. Note the whitish colour of the brain at the site of the hydatid cyst.

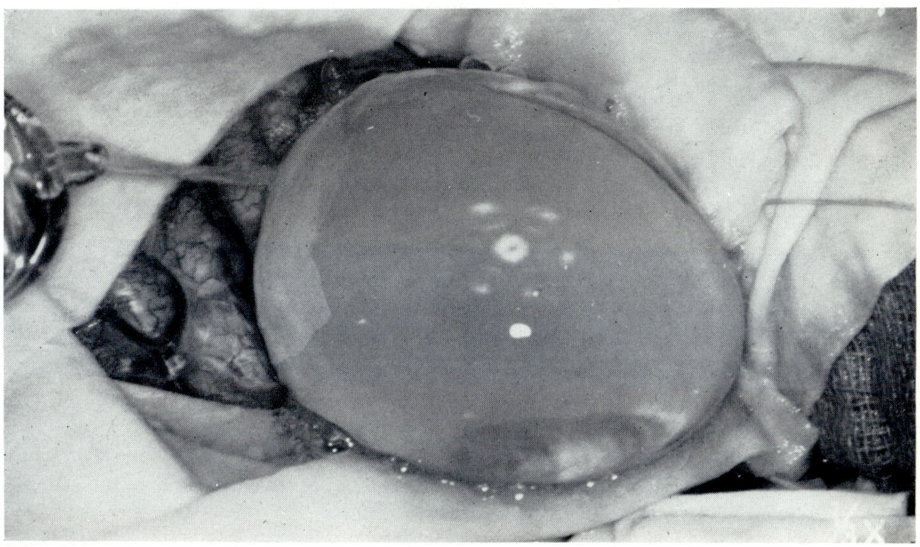

b. Satisfactory exposure of the cyst.

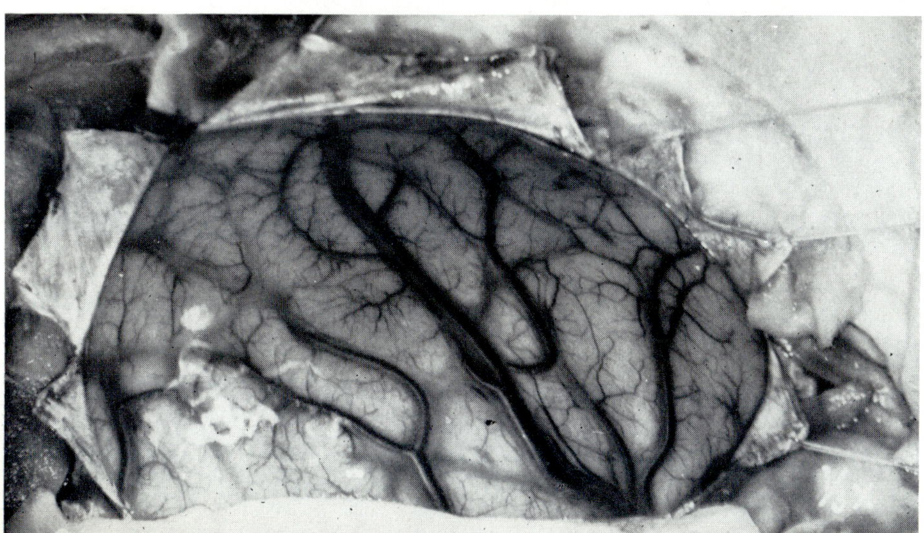

c. Saline is injected between the cyst and the brain.

PLATE 40
Latin America

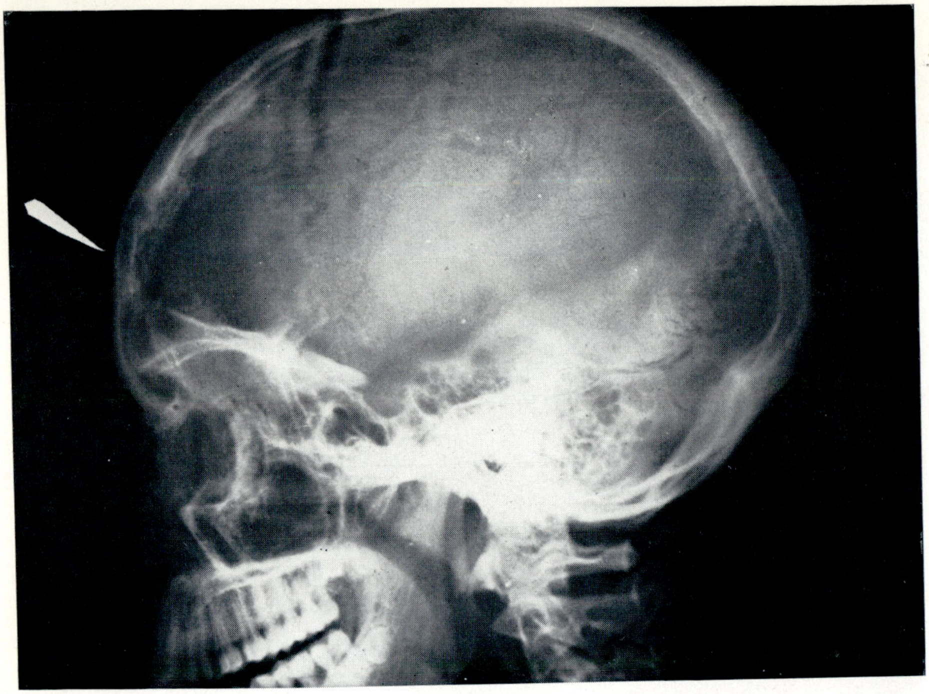

a. *Uruguay:* hydatid disease of the nervous system. Cranial hydatidosis: prominent geodes in the frontal bone overlying frontal hydatid cyst.

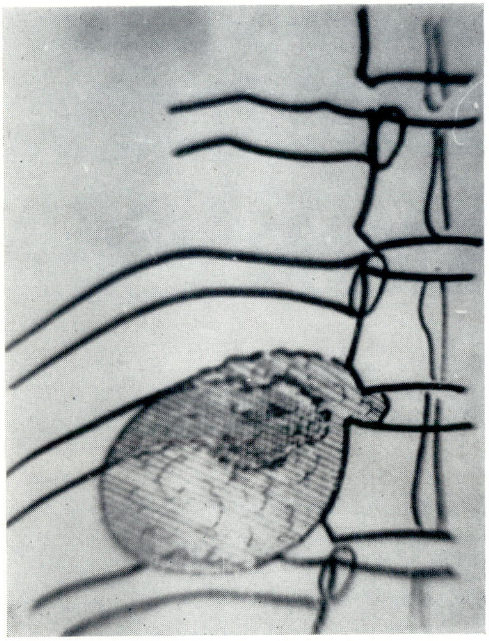

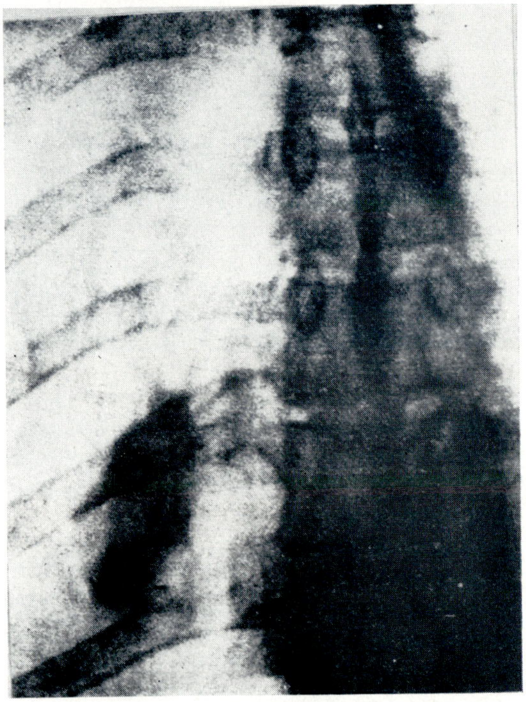

b. and c. Vertebral hydatidosis. Note the costal geode, the missing 'coffee bean' (pedicle), the paravertebral ossifluent abscess, and the intact intervertebral disc.

16 Neurological Disorders in Nigeria

B. O. OSUNTOKUN

INTRODUCTION

Nigeria, the most populous African country with an estimated population of 64 million, i.e. a quarter of the population in Africa, and occupying a land area of 356 000 sq miles, is situated entirely in the tropics, between latitudes 4 deg. N and 13 deg. N. Nigeria comprises a conglomeration of peoples, first welded into 'one nation' by British colonial administrators. National unity, a precarious thing for the 6 years after Independence in 1960, has now apparently been firmly consolidated, though not without the thunder and fire of a 3-year civil war, producing over two million deaths, the first war between African peoples fought with sophisticated weapons of the twentieth century. Peoples such as the Hausas and Fulanis in the North, the Benins and the Yorubas in the South, can boast of age-long history, social and political civilization and culture or arts dating back several centuries, and proudly reminisce in their history of extensive empires that were well known and held in awe and respect in most parts of West Africa. Nigeria is largely peopled by what have been termed the 'West African Negroes' [FIG. 16.1] (Akinkugbe, 1969)—usually over five and a half feet tall, with dark-brown to black spiralled hair and a broad flat nose, and by and large farmers or traders, and in the savannah country, itinerant herdsmen with few cattle.

The climate of Nigeria varies from the warm humid weather in the south to the drier, but still warm, weather in the north. This is also reflected in the vegetation of the country, for the mangrove forests of the coastal areas give way to evergreen forest belts as one moves away from the coast, then to rolling savannah, and finally in the far north of the country to the sand-dunes of the Sahara desert. The annual rainfall varies from over 150 inches in Lagos, the capital of Nigeria, to 20 inches in Maiduguri in the North-Eastern State.

Nigeria is mainly an agricultural country, although in recent times huge deposits of petroleum have been discovered and the country is now the tenth largest oil-producing country in the world. However, most of the people are still poor with a *per capita* income of £30 per annum and live in villages or in slum areas in the cities. In contrast there is an *élite* section, probably constituting about 1 per cent of the population, who are disproportionately affluent, and who live in modern houses often in specially reserved areas of the towns and cities. This latter group is mainly comprised of civil servants, business executives, university teachers, officers of the armed forces, clergymen and graduate teachers. The diet of most of the population comprises carbohydrate, mainly derived from yam and cassava (manihot or manioc), and supplemented by beans, rice, vegetables and occasionally meat. The poorer peasants often go without meat or fish for months. The diet of the *élite*, even when predominantly Nigerian in its composition of carbohydrate, is usually adequately supplemented by meat and fish, and sometimes approximates to a European diet.

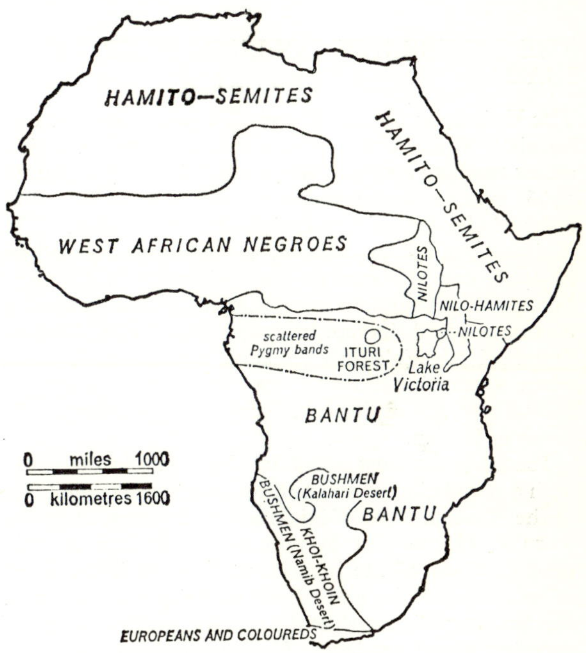

FIG. 16.1. The major racial groups in Africa. *Source:* Greenberg, A. (1955) *Studies in African Linguistic Classification:* revised as *The Languages of Africa*, 1963, The Hague. (By courtesy of Professor O. O. Akinkugbe.)

GENERAL MEDICAL SERVICES IN NIGERIA

Nigeria's medical services are provided mainly by a chain of general and specialist hospitals (about 300), maintained and run either by the Government or by voluntary agencies, such as the various missionary societies; there are also a number of private hospitals (mainly situated in the big towns and cities) and rural health centres. In addition, there are three university teaching hospitals at Ibadan, Lagos, and Zaria. (The Medical School of the University of Nigeria, Nsukka, which ceased to function during the Nigerian civil war is now being reactivated, and new medical schools are to be started in Benin City and in Ife.) By and large, the curative health services in Nigeria are grossly inadequate, especially in rural areas, where a Western-trained doctor is rarely if ever seen or where he attends only once a month, when he runs a mobile clinic, or holds consultative clinics in the numerous dispensaries and maternity centres scattered over the country side and generally poorly equipped and staffed. The doctor to population ratio in Nigeria is 1:30 000, but three-fifths of the doctors available live in the cities of Ibadan, Lagos, Kaduna, Zaria and Kano (with a total population of about three million). In the rural areas, therefore, the traditional native healers have extensive practice.

THE UNIVERSITY COLLEGE HOSPITAL, IBADAN

The University College Hospital, Ibadan, the teaching hospital of the University of Ibadan, and Nigeria's oldest teaching hospital, was opened in 1957 and until 1966 trained undergraduates for the M.B., B.S. external degrees of the University of London. (The University of Ibadan, founded as the University College in 1948, and affiliated to the University of London, became an autonomous institution in 1962 and awarded its first medical degrees in 1967.) The UCH, Ibadan, remained Nigeria's only teaching hospital until 1963, when a teaching hospital was founded in Lagos, a coastal city, the capital of Nigeria, and 90 miles to the south of Ibadan.

Ibadan is the most populous Negro city in the world with a population of one million, and is the capital city of the Western State of Nigeria, largely peopled by the Yorubas (13 million in population) a pure negroid people. Many of the inhabitants live on farms a few miles from the city and return only for the weekends. Ibadan lies 7 deg. north of the equator, and at a height of 750 feet above sea-level. A Neurosurgical Unit, the first in Nigeria, was established in 1962, followed by a Neurological Unit in 1964. The UCH, Ibadan, has remained the centre of excellence in Nigeria for curative medicine, and patients are referred from all parts of Nigeria and not infrequently from other West African countries. Most of the patients seen are of Yoruba origin, but at least 2 per cent come from all parts of Nigeria. An average of 60 000 patients (male to female ratio being 3:2) are seen annually in the general medical outpatient clinics and half of these are further investigated in the various specialist clinics. The hospital has a consultant staff of 80, and 110 other doctors in its service.

This account of neurology in Nigeria is based largely on experience at Ibadan during the last 5 years and on a review of the hospital records of the past 13 years (1957–1970), during which about 10 000 patients with neurological diseases (excluding head injury, traumatic paraplegia and febrile convulsions) were seen. A modern neurological service is available only at Ibadan and Lagos, each with a neurologist and two neurosurgeons.

GENERAL PATTERN OF NEUROLOGICAL PRACTICE AND ILLNESS IN NIGERIA

> A [Yoruba] patient consulting a Babalawo (native doctor) is not even required to tell the doctor what his problem is—he merely whispers it inaudibily into the divining apparatus. The Babalawo rendered omniscient through his dealings with the spirit would know the problem and the treatment without recourse to the patient. The Yoruba patient approaches the 'European' doctor with the same expectations and the discussion of his problem with the doctor is culturally irrelevant.
>
> (Prince, 1961.)
>
> The diviner (the native doctor) is consulted and has to find out himself whether the complaint is an illness, lost stock, an unfaithful wife or other difficulties. If it is an illness, the diviner has to describe all the symptoms to the patient. Most patients refuse to give a history. When persuaded, they grudgingly give a few symptoms, reserving the major complaint for discovery by the doctor.
>
> (Ntsekhe, 1961.)

The above quotations illustrate some of the difficulties encountered in the practice of neurology in most African countries. The history, considered essential elsewhere, especially among Caucasians, is often unhelpful and grossly distorted by cultural taboos and idiosyncrasies, and by disregard and contempt for details and temporal sequence on the part of the patient. The physical examination is not infrequently regarded as an ordeal by the illiterate Nigerian patient, who finds it difficult to appreciate the cooperation required from him to enable an examiner to elicit physical signs. His attitude is usually that the doctor should and ought to know what is wrong with him without bothering him so much. Sometimes, his enthusiasm to please confuses the doctor by the absurdity of his responses to questions.

There are other difficulties, and one that is outstanding is the unreliability of the sign of Babinski—the most important physical sign in clinical neurology. It is not infrequently absent or replaced by a flexor response when it ought to be present, a phenomenon that prompted the editor of this book on a visit to Ibadan, to remark, 'The great Babinski would never have discovered his famous sign if he had lived and practised neurology in Africa'. There are, of course, plausible explanations for the frequent absence of this sign in Africans, the most likely being the fact that they wear no shoes (Osuntokun, 1968; Osuntokun, Odeku, and Adeloye, 1969 *a*). Subclinical dietary deficiencies may also be important and may account for the high frequency of absent tendon reflexes in apparently neurologically normal samples. For example, among 154 apparently well-nourished Nigerian civil servants in the upper and middle socio-economic groups, 25 per cent had absent knee and ankle jerks (Osuntokun, 1969). Among Tanzanians, Haddock (1963) found that one or more tendon reflexes were absent in 17 per cent.

PREVALENCE OF NEUROLOGICAL DISEASE IN HOSPITAL POPULATION

The data presented below represent only the minimum figures for prevalence. The prevalence of neurological diseases in the hospital population is 4·2 per cent (Osuntokun, 1971*a*).

nfections of the Nervous System

In Nigeria, infections of the nervous system constitute the commonest neurological problems and account for over 40 per cent of all neurological diseases seen in Ibadan. The frequency in the hospital population is 19 per thousand [Table 16.1].

The Meningitides

Apart from aseptic meningitis, tuberculous, pneumococcal and *Haemophilus influenzae* meningitis are the commonest forms of this disease.

Tuberculous Meningitis. Sixty-five per cent of patients with tuberculous meningitis (TBM) were under 10 years of age and only 4 per cent were above the age of 40 (Osuntokun, 1971 *a*). In a review of 194 patients seen in the UCH, Ibadan, between 1965 and 1969 (Osuntokun, Adeuja, and Familusi, 1971), the male to female ration was 6:5; the highest incidence occurred in the first and second years of life, with 18 and 24 per cent of cases. These Nigerian patients often presented late in hospital. Signs of meningeal irritation were found in four-fifths and impaired consciousness in three-fifths. Mantoux or Heaf test was negative in 15 per cent of the patients. Over 50 per cent developed focal neurological deficit on admission or soon afterwards. Signs of meningeal irritation were occasionally absent in children, and TBM should therefore be considered in the differential diagnosis of any fever in a Nigerian child. Characteristic changes in the cerebrospinal fluid were sometimes absent [Plate 24a] although in the majority the concentration of protein was usually raised. Polymorphonuclear leucocytosis was found in 13 patients—an unusual finding recently emphasized by others (Taylor, Smith, and Vollum, 1955; Kocen and Parsons, 1970). The mortality of tuberculous meningitis was 50 per cent. Elevated concentration of protein in CSF, the presence of miliary tuberculosis, a rising temperature on admission, impaired consciousness, and associated diseases such as haemoglobinopathy and measles, adversely influenced the morbidity rate. Fifty-two per cent of survivors developed neurological deficit [Table 16.2]. Long

Table 16.1

Infections of the Nervous System: UCH, Ibadan, 1957–1970

Disorder	*No. of Cases*	*Frequency per 1 000 in Hospital Population*
Meningitides	1 310	6·00
Tuberculous	315	
Pneumococcal	315	
H. influenzae	171	
Meningococcal	42	
Other organisms	41	
Aseptic	427	
Intracranial abscess	78	0·35
Encephalitis	335	1·50
Obscure encephalopathy	21	
Poliomyelitis	248	1·10
Herpes zoster	10	
Tetanus	1 881	8·30
Neurosyphilis	46	0·20
Cerebral malaria	121	0·53

Table 16.2

Neurological Complications of Tuberculous Meningitis in 194 Nigerians
(Osuntokun, Adeuja, and Familusi, 1971)

Disorder	*No. of Cases*
Cranial nerve palsies	
Facial nerve	25
Oculomotor nerve	14
Abducens	6
Optic atrophy	4
Sensorineural deafness	5
Polyneuritis cranialis	1
Others	
Hemiplegia/hemiparesis	22
Diffuse brain damage	23
Hydrocephalus	20
Tetraplegia	16
Paraplegia	7
Cortical blindness	6
Epilepsy	5
Aphasia	3
Personality changes	1
Athetosis	1
Diabetes insipidus	1
Horner's syndrome	1

duration of symptoms before treatment, impaired consciousness on admission, and miliary tuberculosis also adversely influenced the mortality rate. I believe that because of the high morbidity and mortality of TBM in Nigerians treatment should include intrathecal administration of isonicotinic acid anhydride (10–50 mg per dose according to age), streptomycin (10–50 mg per dose according to age) and hydrocortisone (10 mg) on alternate days until the CSF returns to normal, or for a minimum of 10 doses, in addition to the usual oral and systemic administration of INH, PAS, and streptomycin. The best results in the treatment of TBM have been obtained when intrathecal therapy was given as a routine (Lorber, 1960; Fitzsimmons and Smith, 1963; *British Medical Journal*, 1971). In those not responding to treatment, the new antituberculous drugs should be considered, especially rifampicin.

Pneumococcal Meningitis. In pneumococcal meningitis, 43 per cent of the Nigerian patients were under the age of 10, and 10 per cent were over 40 years. Pneumococcal meningitis is common in Southern Nigeria (Lucas, 1964 *a*). Pregnancy and sickle-cell disease increase the susceptibility to the disease (Lucas, 1964 *a*; Adeloye and Odeku, 1970). In the two last named conditions, there may be an interference with the production of antibody to pneumococcal antigen (Lucas, 1964 *a*; Robinson and Watson, 1966). In the Nigerian environment, pneumoccoccal menginitis is frequently complicated by hyperpyrexia and fatal heat stroke (Lucas, 1964 *b*). As reported in other parts of Africa (Trowell, 1960), cases of pneumococcal meningeal infection in the absence of an obvious primary focus are rather frequent in Nigerians. In a series of 77 cases from Ibadan, reported by Lucas (1964 *a*), 55 per cent of the patients had no obvious focus of infection: this has also been noted by other workers in Africa (Hutton, 1956; Gelfand, 1957), who have also pointed out that the African Negro is peculiarly susceptible to pneumococcal infections. With treatment by massive dosage (24–36 mega units) of penicillin and soluble sulphonamides, with or without systemic corticosteroids, the mortality rate of pneumococcal meningitis in Nigerians is rather high at 47 per cent (Lucas, 1964 *a*), and the morbidity rate is high, at 30 per cent of survivors. Intramuscular administration of penicillin is preferable to addition of penicillin to intravenous fluids, as there is considerable evidence that most of the penicillin added to intravenous fluids is inactivated. Not infrequently, however, pneumococcal meningitis may present in some bizarre ways: among Nigerians these include psychotic maniacal states (Lucas, 1964 *b*).

Other Meningitides. Meningococcal meningitis was found to be evenly distributed throughout all age-groups, but is commoner in the drier parts of Northern Nigeria, and in these and in other areas of the dry savannah zone of Africa, epidemic outbreaks are frequent. They are virtually unknown in Southern Nigeria.

Meningitis due to *Haemophilus influenzae* predominantly afflicted children, as out of the 171 cases in the period under review, only four patients were older than 9 years. Meningitis due to *Escherichia coli* is not uncommon among Nigerian children.

Most of the cases (74 per cent) of aseptic meningitis occurred in children and were usually associated with lymphocytic pleocytosis with normal CSF sugar content; they may have been due to virus infections. Four per cent of aseptic meningitis occurred in adults over 40 years old. However, some may have been cases of tuberculous meningitis in which *Mycobacterium tuberculosis* was not isolated.

Other organisms found to cause meningitis in Nigerians are *Salmonella*, *Pseudomonas*, *Proteus*, *Candida albicans* and *Torula* (*Cryptococcus neoformans*). A meningitic syndrome has been seen as a primary presentation of Burkitt's lymphoma and Burkitt's cells were readily identified by phase-contrast microscopy and tissue-culture techniques.

The Viral Encephalitides

In Southern Nigeria, the most frequently isolated viruses in patients with encephalitis are the arboviruses, herpes group of viruses, and the enteroviruses (Boorman and Draper, 1968; Causey, Kemp, Madbouly, and Lee, 1969). Sixty-five per cent of the patients seen in UCH, Ibadan, were in the first decade of life. Although the prevalence of measles infection is high in Nigerians (Gans *et al.*, 1961; Morley, Woodland, and Martin, 1963) and encephalitis complicating measles within the first week is not uncommon (Kaushik, 1961), subacute inclusion encephalitis (subacute sclerosing panencephalitis) is uncommon among Nigerians, with only two cases recognized in Ibadan in the last 10 years. The rarity of subacute inclusion encephalitis may be related to its aetiological link with a persisting tolerated infection and altered thymic-mediated immunological reaction to the measles virus (Burnet, 1968). In general, auto-immune diseases are rare in Nigerians (Greenwood, 1968).

Other Viral Infections

Rabies is not uncommon in Nigeria. In Ibadan, in the last 10 years, 13 patients suffered and died from rabies.

The dreadfully virulent Lassa virus, causing an almost invariably fatal disease with encephalitis, haemorrhagic diathesis, myositis, myocarditis, hepatitis and nephritis (White, 1970) seems to be confined to a small area of the Northern region of Nigeria.

In paralytic poliomyelitis, 90 per cent of the patients were in the first decade, 35 per cent were less than a year old, and 65 per cent were under 4 years of age. No indigenous Nigerian who had lived in Nigeria throughout childhood contracted paralytic poliomyelitis after the age of 10 years. Three Nigerians who had grown up abroad and returned to Nigeria as adults, subsequently developed paralytic poliomyelitis. Epidemics of poliomyelitis are rare in the tropics—although occasional ones have occurred in Tanzania (Laufer, 1958) and in Kenya (Fendall and Lake, 1958). That nearly 100 per cent of African patients who suffer from paralytic poliomyelitis are under the age of 10 years is probably due to the fact that acquired immunity occurs early in a population with a low standard of hygiene and reaches nearly 100 per cent by the age of 10 years (Trowell, 1960).

Other Infectious Diseases

Thirty-two per cent of cases of cerebral abscess occurred in the first decade of life, 76 per cent of the patients were under the age of 30 years. There were 42 males and 36 females. Eighty per cent of the cases were complications of infections of the paranasal (especially frontal) sinuses and middle ear.

Tetanus is by far the commonest neurological disease seen in Ibadan, and accounts for 20 per cent of all neurological diseases. Forty-two per cent of the patients were under the age of 10, and this included a large number of cases of neonatal tetanus. Otherwise, the disease was fairly uniformly distributed throughout the second to fifth decades. Six per cent of the patients were above the age of 50 years. Males predominate, the ratio of male to female being 3:2. There was no apparent site of entry in 23 per cent of the patients. The standard treatment at Ibadan consists of the administration of 20 000 units of antitetanus serum, intravenous fluids, sedation with chlorpromazine, sodium amytal, diazepam and paraldehyde. Severe cases and those with laryngeal spasm had tracheostomy with or without intermittent positive pressure respiration. The mortality rate was 45 per cent. A short period of onset, the severity of the disease on admission (as determined by frequency of spasms), excessive sweating, hyperpyrexia, laryngeal spasms, and tachycardia were of grave prognostic significance. Of those who had tracheostomy, 80 per cent died, a reflection of the severity of the disease rather than a result of the tracheostomy. It should be pointed out however, that tracheostomy, except in well-equipped hospitals and when its aftercare is handled by well-trained nursing staff, carries its own enormous risks.

Neurosyphilis, common in Northern Nigeria, is uncommon in the south probably due to the protective effect of infection with *Treponema pertennue* (the causative agent of yaws), which confers cross-immunity. Yaws occurred in high prevalence in Southern Nigeria a decade or two ago, but seems to have been successfully wiped out by elaborate public health measures. In the future, the incidence of neurosyphilis in Southern Nigerians may increase. Clinical presentations of neurosyphilis as seen in Ibadan, include dementia, myelopathy, deafness, vertigo, epilepsy, tabes dorsalis and occlusive cerebrovascular disease.

Cerebral malaria in the indigenous Nigerian is a disease of very young children. Ninety-eight per cent of our cases occurred in the first decade, and 90 per cent occurred in patients less than 2 years old. Cerebral malaria was not encountered within the first 3 months of life nor in patients who were homozygous for haemoglobin S gene.

Vascular Diseases of the Nervous System

Cerebral atherosclerosis is not rare in Nigerians especially among the middle and upper socio-economic groups, the diabetics and hypertensives (Osuntokun, Odeku, and Adelyoye, 1969*a* and *b*; Dada, Johnson, and Araba, 1969), but is less common than among American Negroes and American Caucasians (Williams, Resch, and Loewenson, 1969).

Among Nigerians [Table 16.3], non-embolic ischaemic cerebrovascular disease constitutes two-thirds of all

Table 16.3

Vascular Disease of the Nervous System in Nigerians as seen in UCH, Ibadan, 1957–1960

Disorder	*No. of Cases*	*Frequency per 1000 in Hospital Population*
Non-embolic ischaemic cerebrovascular disease	263	1·20
Cerebral haemorrhage	105	0·48
Primary subarachnoid haemorrhage	63	0·30
Subdural haematoma	41	0·18
Embolic ischaemic cerebrovascular disease	36	0·16
Hypertensive encephalopathy	34	0·15
Intracranial venous thrombosis	43	0·19
Vascular myelopathy	4	
Intermittent claudication of the spinal cord	2	
Haematomyelia	1	

cerebrovascular accidents (i.e. ischaemic infarction and haemorrhage but excluding spontaneous subarachnoid haemorrhage). Cerebral haemorrhage accounts for one-quarter of cerebrovascular accidents. There is a male preponderance in all three categories. The peak frequency of non-embolic disease and cerebral haemorrhage is in the sixth decade.

The most important predisposing factors to non-embolic infarction and cerebral haemorrhage are hypertension and diabetes mellitus. The former is commoner in cerebral haemorrhage than in infarction, and the latter is commoner in cerebral infarction than in cerebral haemorrhage. Rheumatic heart disease and subacute bacterial endocarditis are the major predisposing conditions to embolic infarction. A third of the patients with non-embolic infarction and cerebral haemorrhage come from the upper and middle socio-economic groups.

The prognosis in transient ischaemic attacks in Nigerians is worse than in Caucasians. In Nigerians, the prognosis with regard to completed strokes is better in intermittent ischaemia of the vertebrobasilar territory than in intermittent ischaemia of the internal carotid territory.

Although the frequency of haemoglobin S in the Nigerian population is 24 per cent, haemoglobinopathy is not a factor in the aetiopathogenesis of stroke in the adult, but may be in children. The serum levels of cholesterol, phospholipids and non-esterified fatty acids in Nigerian patients with cerebral haemorrhage and non-embolic infarction merely reflect the high socio-economic groups of these patients; the levels are no different from those of normal Nigerians in the same socio-economic groups.

The mortality of cerebral haemorrhage (77 per cent) is the highest, compared with a 16 per cent mortality in non-embolic ischaemic infarction and 43 per cent in embolic infarction. Cerebral haemorrhage is more commonly seen at autopsy than cerebral infarction. Epilepsy is a more frequent sequel of cerebral infarction, whether non-embolic or embolic, than of cerebral haemorrhage.

Berry aneurysm is a more common cause of primary subarachnoid haemorrhage than arteriovenous malformation. Angioma, Sturge-Weber disease and aneurysmal dilatation of the vein of Galen as a cause of subarachnoid bleeding have all been encountered. Multiple aneurysms were demonstrated in 22 per cent of patients with primary subarachnoid haemorrhage. Sickle-cell anaemia is now recognized as a cause of subarachnoid haemorrhage in young Nigerians (Adeloye and Odeku, 1970). Other neurological manifestations of sickle-cell disease, as encountered in Nigerians, include mental changes, disturbance of consciousness, convulsions, meningism, cranial nerve palsies, cerebrovascular accidents, dural sinus thrombosis and increased susceptibility to pneumococcal meningitis.

Epilepsy and Other Paroxysmal Disorders of the Nervous System [Table 16.4]

After tetanus and meningitis, epilepsy is the next commonest disease of the nervous system in Nigerians. The incidence in the hospital population is 3·2 per thousand. In 70 per cent of the patients no cause was found. Other causes encountered were infections (9·4 per cent), vascular lesions (6·5 per cent), trauma (6 per cent), neoplasms (3·6 per cent), metabolic causes (1·5 per cent), and birth injury (1·3 per cent). Males predominated in symptomatic epilepsy by 3 to 1. The sex incidence in idiopathic epilepsy is equal. Megaloblastic anaemia following anticonvulsant therapy was very rare.

The prevalence of epilepsy in Nigerians and in other Africans shows no difference as compared with the prevalence in Caucasians (Dada and Odeku, 1966; Osuntokun and Odeku, 1970), except that there is an apparent rarity of petit mal, probably due to parents' difficulty in recognizing the transient symptoms of the disease in a child. Febrile convulsion in Nigerian children, however, is not the benign illness that it may be elsewhere. The mortality and morbidity rates in Nigerian children are high, being largely due to administration at home of a concoction whose main ingredient is cow's urine, to burns [Plate 24b], and to other resuscitative measures such as rubbing alligator pepper into the eyes thereby causing severe conjunctivitis (Osuntokun, Odeku, and Sinnette, 1969). These measures are taken in an attempt by anxious, frightened, and illiterate parents to 'wake up' children in the stage of post-ictal coma or stupor. Cow's urine apparently possesses a hypoglycaemic action and often causes irreversible neuronal damage including cortical blindness.

Migraine and polymyositis constitute the only two non-gynaecological diseases in Nigerians in which there is an outstanding predominance of females (Osuntokun, 1971 *a*). The male to female ratio among Nigerians who suffer from migraine is 2:5. Response to ergotamine tartrate has been very good, and most patients have benefited from tranquillosedatives. The four patients in Table 16.4 with periodic migrainous neuralgia (Horton's syndrome) were all females. In 95 per cent of the patients, the onset of migrainous headaches began before the age of 20, in 85 per cent of them in the

Table 16.4

Epilepsy and Other Paroxysmal Disturbances in Nigerians, UCH, Ibadan, 1957–1970

Disorder	*No. of Cases*	*Frequency per 1000 in Hospital Population*
Epilepsy	702	3·20
Grand mal without aura	*389*	
Petit mal	*15*	
Akinetic attack	*1*	
Myoclonic epilepsy	*8*	
Grand mal with aura	*135*	
Temporal lobe epilepsy	*50*	
Jacksonian epilepsy	*52*	
Epilepsia partialis continua	*8*	
Adversive attacks	*5*	
Spinal epilepsy	*1*	
Status epilepticus	*18*	
Migraine	74	0·32
Periodic migrainous neuralgia	4	—
Ménière's syndrome	12	0·05
Narcolepsy and related syndromes	14	—
Hypersensitive carotid sinus	2	—
Vasomotor syncope	10	—

second decade. One of the patients also had idiopathic epilepsy.

Ménière's syndrome is rare in Nigerians.

Of the 14 patients with narcolepsy and related disorder, 11 were males, and three females. The ages of the patients ranged from 10 to 55. Irresistible attacks of normal sleep was the only constant feature. Two of the patients were obese, but there was no clinical and biochemical evidence of chronic hypoventilation. Sleep paralysis and nightmares were present in 50 per cent of the patients. None had cataplexy. Two male patients aged 12 and 22 respectively exhibited megaphagia and bulimia (Kleine-Levin syndrome). Investigations including urinary steroids, insulin sensitivity, cerebrospinal fluid examination, plain radiographs of the skull, and in four patients pneumoencephalography, were normal. In most patients there has been excellent response to medication with amphetamine, which had been given in a dose as large as 60 mg daily before maximal therapeutic effect was obtained. The patients tolerated the drug very well.

Intracranial Tumours

Primary intracranial tumours are not uncommon. More than 80 have now been recorded at Ibadan, of which 45 per cent were gliomas and 25 per cent were meningiomas (Odeku, Osuntokun, Adeloye, and Williams, 1970). The rest include craniopharyngioma, pituitary adenoma, pinealoma, teratoma, colloid cysts of the third ventricle [PLATE 24c], and primary intracranial Burkitt's neoplasm. The nervous system is frequently involved in Burkitt's neoplasm and manifestations encountered among Nigerians include those of solitary solid brain tumour, polyneuritis cranialis with bilateral or unilateral proptosis, spinal cord compression due to epidural deposits, and polyradiculopathy. Not infrequently, the involvement of the nervous system is the first manifestation of Burkitt's neoplasm (Odeku and Osuntokun, 1968). The response of Burkitt's neoplasm involving the nervous system to cytotoxic drug therapy (*Endoxan*) is often dramatically impressive [PLATE 24d] although relapse is quite common.

All of the 14 intracranial tuberculomas seen were supratentorial: all these patients showed a positive Heaf or Mantoux test and only five had either treated pulmonary tuberculosis or evidence of tuberculous infection elsewhere (Adeloye and Odeku, 1969).

In Nigerian patients with metastatic tumour deposits in the brain, choriocarcinoma was the commonest primary, accounting for 70 per cent (Adeloye and Odeku, 1969). The breast and kidney were the other main sites, each accounting for 12 per cent of cases. Carcinoma of the lung is uncommon in Nigerians. Only one patient was encountered with adenocarcinoma of the lung and brain metastasis. Although primary carcinoma of the liver is very common in Nigerians, it does not metastasize to the brain; it may, however, present with skeletal metastases and hence with neurological deficit such as paraplegia.

Head Injury

In Nigeria, which has the highest rate in the world of automobile accidents per million vehicle miles (Schram, 1969), head injury is quite common, over 1500 cases having been treated in Ibadan in the last 10 years. The postconcussion syndrome characterized by postural dizziness, lack of concentration, impaired memory and insomnia is not uncommon in Nigerians, having been encountered in over 150 cases in the last 5 years. Persistence of these symptoms in association with clear-cut evidence of anxiety neurosis and unwillingness to return to work or self-declaration of being unfit to work (Miller, 1961 *a* and *b*) has been seen in Nigerian peasants who had never heard of insurance companies or compensation, as well as among Nigerian soldiers during the civil war after trivial head injury. Accident neurosis was not encountered among soldiers with penetrating missile injuries of the head and other forms of severe head injuries. It appears that in *some* Nigerians, as in Caucasians, some form of motivation—conscious or subconscious—may be pre-eminent in the aetiology of accident neurosis.

Congenital Malformations [TABLE 16.5]

In Nigerians, spina bifida cystica and encephaloceles are not uncommon; in the former tetanus neonatorum is a common cause of death (Odeku, Grant, and Ekop, 1967; Odeku, 1967; Odeku, 1971). In addition to 260 cases of congenital hydrocephalus, over 60 cases of acquired hydrocephalus (postmeningitic, posthaemorrhagic, neoplastic) have been seen. More than half of these patients have been operated on or treated by ventriculoperitoneal and ventriculojugular shunts with considerable success.

Table 16.5
Congenital Malformations in UCH, Ibadan

Disorder	*No. of Cases*	*Frequency per 1000 in Hospital Population*
Spina bifida occulta	95	0·43
Spina bifida manifesta	106	0·48
Arnold-Chiari malformation	6	—
Platybasia	2	—
Congenital hydrocephalus	260	1·20

Heredofamilial and Other Degenerative Diseases [TABLE 16.6]

The heredofamilial spinocerebellar degenerations are rare in Nigerians. Of the 12 patients with neurofibromatosis, two had severe diastolic hypertension; associated phaeochromocytoma was suspected but not confirmed by detailed investigation: one had bilateral acoustic neuromas.

Table 16.6
Other Congenital and Degenerative Diseases

Disorder	*No. of Cases*	*Frequency per 1000 in Hospital Population*
Cerebral palsy	444	2·00
Tuberous sclerosis	4	—
Sturge-Weber disease	4	—
Heredofamilial spinocerebellar degeneration	2	—
Idiopathic cerebellar degeneration	16	—
Non-metastatic neoplastic cerebellar degeneration	2	—
Ataxia telangiectasia	2	—
Neurofibromatosis	12	—
Motor neurone disease	79	0·35

Motor neurone disease is not uncommon; the incidence in the hospital population is 3·5 per 10 000. The disease was found in all age-groups, the peak incidence being in the fifth decade, when the onset of the disease occurred in 30 per cent of the patients. However, at onset, 55 per cent of the patients were below the age of 40. Males predominated, and the ratio of male to female was 3:1. Only in one patient was the disease familial. The clinical syndromes encountered are as follows: progressive muscular atrophy, 5; amyotrophic lateral sclerosis, 60; chronic spinal muscular atrophy (mimicking muscular dystrophy), 5; pure lateral sclerosis, 5; and infantile neurogenic spinal muscular atrophy, 4. Two of the patients with the clinical picture of amyotrophic lateral sclerosis had suffered as infants from paralytic poliomyelitis. There were two middle-aged patients who showed the clinical picture of chronic progressive bulbar palsy alone, probably motor neurone disease. Thirteen other patients also excluded from this series, who suffered from the Nigerian nutritional ataxic neuropathy (Money, 1959; Osuntokun, 1968), showed clinical and electrophysiological evidence of widespread motor neurone disease, and clinical evidence of parkinsonism, cerebellar degeneration, and dementia. In Nigerians, motor neurone disease does not appear to carry the same inexorably poor prognosis as has been described for Caucasian patients; in several patients the disease has remained static over the past 7 to 10 years. Motor neurone disease is common in relatively young Nigerians, an observation previously noted by Brown (1961). The absence of a family history of the disease in most of the Nigerian patients makes it unlikely that these patients suffered from Kugelberg-Welander-Wohlfart disease or variants of it, although it is possible that non-familial, benign, chronic spinal muscular atrophy of young people may occur sporadically.

Peroneal muscular atrophy and other hereditary or genetically determined peripheral neuropathic syndromes have not been seen in Nigerians.

Diseases of the Extrapyramidal System [TABLE 16.7]

Of the patients with the parkinsonian syndrome, the male to female ratio was 4:1. The peak incidence occurred in the sixth decade, and 35 per cent of patients in this series showed the earliest manifestation in this decade. At onset of the disease, 72 per cent of the patients were over the age of 50 and 90 per cent were over the age of 40. Severe diastolic hypertension, without other evidence of cerebrovascular disease, was present in 25 per cent of the patients. In 10 patients there had been previous episodes of cerebrovascular accidents. Diabetes mellitus was present in 10, and in four of them was associated with severe hypertension. In a male patient aged 12, parkinsonism followed an encephalitic-like illness, after an interval of 1 month. Therapy with phenothiazine was the cause of parkinsonism in seven patients. In one patient it was due to direct infiltration of the basal ganglia by carcinoma of the ethmoid, and in another patient, aged 32 at onset, there was a family history of Parkinson's disease and essential tremor. Glucose-tolerance test with and without steroid priming, and serum cholesterol levels

Table 16.7
Extrapyramidal Syndromes seen in UCH, Ibadan, 1957–1970

Syndrome	*No. of Cases*	*Frequency per 1000 in Hospital Population*
The parkinsonian syndrome	107	0·47
Choreo-athetosis	52	0·23
Sydenham's chorea	3	—
Huntington's chorea	3	—
Spasmodic torticollis	2	—
Torsion dystonia	2	—
Creutzfeldt-Jakob disease	1	—
Hepatolenticular disease	6	—
Familial essential tremor	3	—
Multiple tics	2	—

were normal in the non-diabetic patients. In six patients there was co-existent liver disease; in three of them—all under 50 years of age—histology of liver biopsy showed eosinophilic inclusion bodies; in two other patients aged 18 and 50 respectively Laënnec's cirrhosis of the liver was found. There was no evidence of abnormal copper transport and deposition and no amino-aciduria. In another male patient aged 55, in addition to hepatomegaly, idiopathic tropical splenomegaly was also present; liver biopsy was not done because of thrombocytopenia. One of the patients who suffered from cirrhosis of the liver died, and autopsy showed lenticular cavitation and confirmed cirrhosis of the liver. In one 8-year-old female patient, whose haemoglobin electrophoretic fractionation showed a genotype *Hb* SS, Kayser-Fleischer ring was present in the cornea, and liver biopsy showed cirrhosis at histology; there was no neurological evidence of disease of the basal ganglia and no family history of liver disease or neurological illness.

The main causes of choreo-athetosis as found in this series are birth injury, postexanthemata syndrome, and cerebrovascular disease. In about 50 per cent of the patients no cause was obvious.

Demyelinating Diseases [Table 16.8]

Multiple sclerosis is rare among African Negroes. There were two Nigerian patients who may have been cases of multiple sclerosis; however, without autopsy confirmation, the diagnosis will remain speculative. These two patients had never lived outside Nigeria. One, a female patient aged 22 in 1964, presented with vertigo, diplopia, and tetraparesis, and was found to have evidence of multiple neuronal lesions, but these subsequently cleared up apparently completely. In 1969, however, she again presented with fairly acute onset neurological disease with tetraparesis, asymmetrical pyramidal tract involvement, and posterior column sensory loss; cerebrospinal fluid examination, pneumoencephalogram, and carotid and vertebral angiography were normal. Over a period of 4 weeks, she recovered almost completely being left with exaggerated tendon reflexes and sustained bilateral ankle clonus. The other patient, a male aged 24, had an episode of ataxic nystagmus in association with bilateral extensor plantar responses, absent abdominal reflexes, and posterior column sensory loss, which eventually cleared up completely. Contrast neuroradiological investigations showed no abnormality.

Table 16.8

Demyelinating Disease, UCH, Ibadan, 1957–1970

Disorder	*No. of Cases*	*Frequency per 1000 in Hospital Population*
Multiple sclerosis	2	—
Postinfectious encephalomyelitis	12	—
Neuromyelitis optica	95	0·43
Acute bilateral retrobulbar neuritis	11	—
Acute transverse myelitis	22	—

Of the patients with neuromyelitis optica (Devic's disease), most of them (85 per cent) were under the age of 40. The onset was sudden with bilateral retrobulbar neuritis and transverse myelitis, one preceding the other usually by a few days. Corticosteroid therapy produced more striking improvement in the visual defect than in the spinal cord lesions. Eleven patients who presented with acute retrobulbar neuritis only responded very well to treatment with prednisolone. Twenty-two patients with isolated transverse myelitis showed poor response to treatment with prednisolone.

Table 16.9

Spinal Cord Syndromes as seen in UCH, Ibadan

Disorder	*No. of Cases*	*Frequency per 1000 in Hospital Population*
Tuberculosis of the spine with spinal cord compression	406	2·10
Intraspinal canal neoplasms	54	0·24
Other causes of spinal cord compression	76	0·34
Obscure myelopathy	90	0·41
Tropical ataxic neuropathy	395	1·80
Arachnoiditis	6	—
Myelopathy secondary to portacaval shunt	1	—
Spondylotic myelopathy	65	0·30
Syringomyelia	3	—

Spinal Cord Syndromes [Table 16.9]

Tuberculosis of the spine with spinal cord compression, tropical ataxic neuropathy [p. 173], and spinal cord compression constitute the commonest spinal cord syndromes.

Of the intraspinal canal masses, epidural tumours were by far the commonest (75 per cent), and most of them were either Burkitt's neoplasm or metastatic tumour deposits. There were three patients with non-tuberculous chronic epidural granuloma. The primary cord tumours include meningioma, 4; neurofibroma, 3; schwannoma, 3; melanoma, 1. Unusual causes of spinal cord compression encountered include paravertebral abscess, due to brucellosis, and intramedullary schistosomal granuloma.

There was a group of patients with isolated spinal cord disease of insidious onset presenting primarily as spastic paraparesis, normal sphincteric function, normal cerebrospinal fluid, absence of radiological evidence of spondylosis, normal myelographic examination, and liver function tests. This group has been labelled obscure myelopathy. In a few of them, at laminectomy, no definitive lesion apart from slight softening of the spinal cord was found.

Diseases of Peripheral Nerves [Table 16.10]

Excluding diabetic neuropathy, symmetrical peripheral neuropathy (without involvement of the cranial nerves) is common; aetiological diagnoses are as follows:

Table 16.10
Diseases of the Peripheral Nerves

Disorder	*No. of Cases*	*Frequency per 1000 in Hospital Population*
Peripheral polyneuropathy (not tropical ataxia)	466	2·10
Guillain-Barré syndrome	26	—
Porphyria	4	—
Polyneuritis cranialis	75	0·34
Isolated oculomotor palsy	36	—
Sarcoidosis of the nervous system	2	—
Sciatica	21	—
Neuralgic amyotrophy	15	—
Trigeminal neuralgia	5	—
Facial palsy (lower motor neurone type)	105	0·48
Obstetric neuropraxia	24	—
Mononeuritis simplex		
Carpal tunnel syndrome	9	—
Others (common peroneal, ulnar, radial, lateral cutaneous nerve of thigh)	14	—

	%
Nutritional	40·0
Idiopathic	33·0
Primary presentation of diabetes mellitus	4·0
Guillain-Barré syndrome	5·0
Alcoholic	4·0
Malignant disease	3·0
Drug-induced (nitrofurantoin, phenytoin, isoniazid)	3·0
Miscellaneous	8·0

In the nutritional peripheral neuropathies, there was usually other evidence of malnutrition, such as mucocutaneous lesions and malabsorption. This group of pure peripheral neuropathies showed no clinical evidence of disease of the spinal cord or the cranial nerves, and this readily distinguished them from the tropical ataxic neuropathy as found in Nigerians [p. 173]. In many patients the onset of the disease occurred during pregnancy or lactation. The miscellaneous group of peripheral neuropathies includes leprosy and those aetiologically linked to uraemia or renal failure, porphyria, enteritis, polyarteritis nodosa, myelomatosis, and amyloidosis. Most Nigerian patients who suffer from leprosy are usually seen at leprosaria in various parts of Nigeria. Peripheral neuropathy is a common complication of diabetes mellitus and was found in 48 per cent of 830 Nigerian diabetics seen at Ibadan. In 21 of these patients sensory peripheral neuropathy was the primary presentation of diabetes mellitus (Osuntokun, 1971 *b*).

The commonest causes of polyneuritis cranialis were malignant disease of the paranasal sinuses and Burkitt's tumour. In most cases of involvement of the nervous system by Burkitt's neoplasm, the diagnosis was obvious at phase-contrast microscopy of cells in the cerebrospinal fluid, as characteristic cells of Burkitt's tumour are readily recognized. Other causes of polyneuritis cranialis in Nigerians included haemoglobin SS disease, bacterial and carcinomatous meningitides, and very rarely sarcoidosis.

Isolated optic atrophy (non-glaucomatous), a not uncommon finding, was generally due to retrobulbar neuritis, choroidoretinitis (possibly due to toxoplasmosis), and occasionally pituitary and medial sphenoidal ridge tumours. In more than 50 per cent of the patients seen at Ibadan no cause was found.

Sciatica was relatively uncommon, for ruptured intervertebral disc was rarely encountered, as found among other African Negroes (Hutton, 1956; Trowell, 1960). Pelvic malignant disease, especially in the female, was found to be a common cause of this symptom complex in Nigerians. In Nigerians, cervical spondylosis does occur, but over the age of 50 it is only half as common as in Caucasians (Spillane, 1969).

Neuralgic amyotrophy or brachial neuritis was found as a complication of serotherapy and vaccinations. Trigeminal neuralgia is rare in Nigerians and this again is probably due to the low percentage of elderly Nigerians in the population.

The commonest cause of infranuclear facial paralysis was Bell's palsy (idiopathic facial palsy) in 95 per cent of cases. In Bell's palsy in Nigerians response to treatment with prednisolone or adrenocorticotrophic hormone has been so good that steroid therapy is now offered to most patients, although this therapeutic observation is uncontrolled. Other causes of infranuclear facial palsy encountered are the Guillain-Barré syndrome (usually bilateral), the Ramsay Hunt syndrome (herpes infection), trauma and metastases (in one patient, from carcinoma of the cervix).

Obstetric neuropraxia usually presented as dropped

foot, often unilateral, but occasionally bilateral. It was found in short women with contracted pelvis, and usually but not always the result of prolonged labour. The prognosis was usually good, except when associated with fistula formation in the genito-urinary tract—evidence of prolonged obstruction. From clinical and electrophysiological studies carried out on these patients, it appears that it is essentially a neuropraxia of the lumbosacral cord of the sacral plexus. Some patients, however, did have clinical evidence of a transient lesion of the femoral nerve.

The carpal tunnel syndrome was associated with gross obesity, 2; acromegaly, 1; rheumatoid arthritis, 2; pregnancy, 2; there was no evidence of a predisposing factor in two patients. Of the 14 patients who presented with other forms of mononeuritis simplex, leprosy was present in six, while four others suffered from diabetes mellitus, and the rest from pressure palsies.

Diseases of the Muscles [TABLE 16.11]

Muscular dystrophy is not a particularly rare disease in Nigerians. In the last 4 years I have seen on an average four patients per year. The clinical presentations are in no way different from those described for Caucasian patients [PLATE 24e]. Four of the five patients who suffered from dystrophia myotonica were all first-degree relatives from the same family, in conformity with transmission by the autosomal dominant gene, probably with incomplete penetrance.

Table 16.11

Primary Diseases of Muscles in Nigerians, UCH, Ibadan 1957–1970

Disorder	*No. of Cases*		*Prevalence per 1000 in Hospital Population*
Muscular dystrophies	34		0·14
Duchenne type		*14*	
Limb-girdle		*12*	
Facioscapulohumeral		*3*	
Dystrophia myotonica		*5*	
Polymyositis	42		0·17
Pyomyositis	269		1·10
Myasthenia gravis	14		0·07
Thyrotoxic myopathy	1		
Hypocalcaemic myopathy	2		
McArdle's syndrome	1		

Although muscular dystrophy is not uncommon in Nigerians, it is possible that many patients, especially the younger ones, may be kept away from hospital. Dada and Elliott (1967) have commented on the failure of early recognition of symptoms of the disease by Nigerian parents and relatives, as in many instances such children are initially considered to be lazy.

Of the 42 patients with polymyositis, three had malignant neoplasm, one multiple myeloma, three suffered from rheumatoid arthritis, in three patients there were cutaneous changes of dermatomyositis, and in the others no predisposing disease was found. The male to female ratio was 1:2. Only seven of the patients were above the age of 40 years at the onset of the disease.

The first report of polymyositis in Nigerians was by Barnard and Robertson (1960), who reported three patients at the UCH, Ibadan. The female preponderance among Nigerians is similar to that described among Caucasians (Pearson, 1962; Walton and Gardner-Medwin, 1969). However, other collagen diseases and auto-immune diseases are rare in Nigerians (Greenwood, 1968) and probably in other African races (Trowell, 1960). For example, only three cases of polyarteritis nodosa and one patient with disseminated lupus erythematosus were seen in Ibadan in the period 1957 to 1969, during which time at least 240 000 patients were seen in the various clinics of the hospital. Discoid lupus erythematosus, however, is not rare (Shrank, 1968). Pernicious anaemia and Hashimoto's disease are virtually unknown in Nigerians.

Of the 14 patients with myasthenia gravis, there were five males and nine females. None of the patients appeared to have a thymoma.

Myopathy was associated with hypocalcaemia and osteomalacia in two elderly patients aged 65 and 68. There was considerable symptomatic improvement following treatment with calcium gluconate and vitamin D. One patient with thyrotoxicosis showed clinical and electromyographic evidence of proximal myopathy. Thyrotoxicosis is not uncommon in Nigerians—75 cases have been seen in the last 13 years at Ibadan. Evidence of myopathy was, however, not routinely looked for in these patients.

The one patient who showed the clinical and biochemical features of McArdle's syndrome was of Lebanese parentage, her parents having become naturalized Nigerians.

Pyomyositis, a suppurative disease of the muscles, occurring in the tropics and confined largely to the indigenous population, is by far the commonest primary disease of the muscles in Nigerians. It was mostly found in those under 30 years of age, the highest incidence being in the third decade. FIGURE 16.2 shows the age and sex distribution of cases seen at Ibadan. The abscess may be intramuscular or intermuscular, the former being common in young people. Usually, the lower limbs are involved and sometimes the abscess may be multiple. Fever, pain, tenderness and leucocytosis were usually present in patients with the intramuscular abscess and often absent in those with intermuscular lesions. The commonest muscle involved was the quadriceps femoris, in two-thirds of patients, but other muscles such as the trapezius, latissimus dorsi, biceps, brachialis, sacrospinalis, the glutei, hamstrings, gastrocnemius, and soleus were not infrequently involved. *Staphylococcus pyogenes* was usually isolated from the pus and rarely from the blood. Treatment consists of surgical drainage and administration of antibiotics. It is not quite clear why pyomyositis is such a common suppurative disease in the tropics. It is predominantly a disease of poor people, and malnutrition or undernutrition may be relevant to its high prevalance among the indigenous populations of developing countries in Africa. It is possible that trauma with secondary infection of muscle haematoma accounts for most cases of intramuscular pyomyositis.

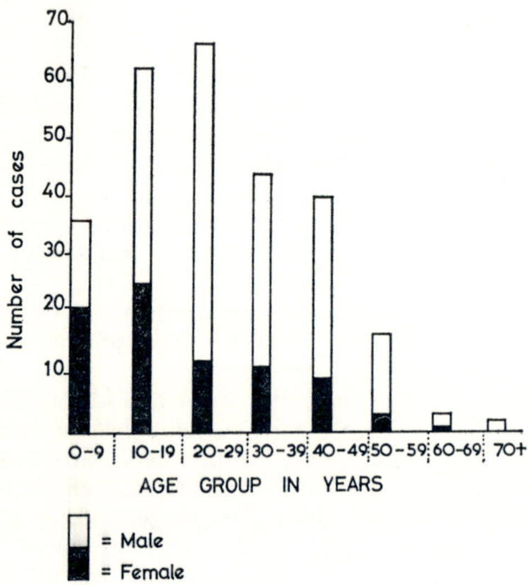

FIG. 16.2. Age and sex distribution of Nigerian patients with pyomyositis.

It is also possible that infection of tracts of wandering parasites such as the guinea-worm is important in the aetiology of intermuscular pyomyositis (Anand and Evans, 1964). It has been suggested that muscle necrosis induced by an unknown factor, possibly a virus, may precede local bacterial invasion (Horn and Master, 1968).

Some classical muscle diseases, especially the metabolic myopathies such as periodic paralysis, have not been encountered in Nigerians, nor have they been described in other Africans. The apparent rarity of any disease may be due to failure of recognition or to shortage of medical personnel. It seems likely that with time and improved medical services, the list of diseases said not to occur in the developing countries is bound to shorten (Shrank, 1968).

Neurology of Non-Viral Infectious Disease

Trypanosomiasis is common in the northern parts of Nigeria where it may account for 60 per cent of Nigerian asylum population (Lambo, 1961). In the southern area, where Ibadan is situated, it is not seen. We have not encountered cysticercosis at Ibadan, probably due to the predominance of Muslims in the population. The neuropsychiatric syndromes which may be caused by trypanosomiasis and cerebral cysticercosis are well known, and include schizophrenic-like psychosis, fluctuating yet persistent disturbances of consciousness, slowly progressive personality changes, progressive dementia, and sometimes affective withdrawal (Lambo, 1965). In the terminal phase, stupor and coma supervene.

In typhoid in a third of the 920 patients seen at Ibadan (1957–68), symptoms of impaired mentation and consciousness were present, most commonly as a confusional state. In three patients the initial diagnosis was schizophrenia. Six patients had a transient reversible parkinsonian syndrome, and in seven other patients, a mild peripheral symmetrical neuropathy was present following recovery from typhoid. Typhoid fever should be considered in the differential diagnosis of confusional and psychotic states in the Nigerian, for the associated pyrexia may be mild initially and hence easily missed.

Occasionally, pneumococcal meningitis may present primarily as a psychiatric illness (Lucas, 1964 *b*).

Miscellaneous

Tension headache is a common form of headache in Nigerians and most patients respond to tranquillo-sedatives, especially chlordiazepoxide. In the more elderly patients, the good response to antidepressant drug therapy suggests that this may also be a form of monosymptomatic depression (Osuntokun, 1971 *a*).

Vestibular neuronitis was encountered as a cause of vertigo in 23 patients. It was self-limiting.

Writer's tremor or writer's cramp was found in those whose occupation involved a lot of writing. Of the 20 patients seen over a period of 4 years (1966–70) by the author, there were six females and 14 males. The ages range from 16 years to 54 years with the peak incidence in the fourth and fifth decades. Eleven of the patients were teachers, and one was a university lecturer. The occupations of the others were nursing, 3; sales clerk, 2; dispensary attendant, 1; student, 2. Fourteen of the patients showed other features of anxiety neurosis, such as palpitations, persistent fear of an impending catastrophe, excessive sweating and insomnia.

In two families two siblings each were encountered with congenital auditory imperception. In one pair of siblings pain asymbolia was also present (Osuntokun, Odeku, and Luzzatto, 1968). In the other pair one sibling was mentally subnormal.

Anxiety neurosis is common in Nigerians. Apart

from the classical presentation, a common symptomatology is somatization of their symptoms, hence bizarre stories of 'worms crawling from the foot to the head and back again' may mislead the newcomer to tropical Africa.

In the years 1966–69, hysterical conversion syndromes were seen in 14 males (including eight soldiers) and nine females. All the females were in the second decade. All the patients except one were under 30 years old; only two of the civilian patients were older than 19. The youngest was 9 years old and the eldest 34. The soldiers developed their symptoms following a battle and were apparently initially shell-shocked. The presentations in the soldiers were as follows, hemiplegia and mutism, 1; deafness and dumbness, 7. Of the others, eight were students, and the rest were self-employed. Other presentations included paralysis, 3; bizarre involuntary movements, 7; hyperventilation tetany, 1; abnormal gait, 1; blindness, 1; dysphonia, 2. The response to treatment was very satisfactory in all the patients, although in three it required prolonged stay in hospital, several episodes of sodium amytal narcosis and suggestive psychotherapy to achieve a cure. One of the patients, a soldier who when first seen had a right hemiplegia, mutism, and deafness, subsequently recovered without any neurological deficit, but eventually went into hypomaniacal states and had to be institutionalized at a mental hospital. Our experience at Ibadan of the hysterical conversion syndromes in Nigerians does not support Elliot Slater's (1965) statement that 'the diagnosis of hysteria is a disguise for ignorance and a fertile source of clinical error'.

NIGERIAN TROPICAL ATAXIC NEUROPATHY

Over the last eight decades it has been established that some forms of neurological degenerative disease (tropical neuropathies) in communities with a low standard of nutrition, and largely from the indigenous population of tropical countries or from prisoner-of-war camps [TABLE 16.12[1] and FIG. 16.3], are due to malnutrition and/or dietary toxins (Spillane, 1947; Money, 1959; Montgomery *et al.*, 1964; Osuntokun, 1968). In their details these tropical neuropathies vary from one part of the world to another, but they have certain features in common. They comprise in varying combinations, lesions of the skin, mucous membranes, and the nervous system. In Nigerians the essential neurological components of the disease are myelopathy, bilateral optic atrophy, bilateral sensorinueral deafness, and usually symmetrical peripheral neuropathy. The diagnosis is made when at least any two of these four main neurological components are present (Osuntokun, 1968), with or without lesions of the skin and mucous membranes suggestive of avitaminosis and malnutrition. In Nigerians, because of the marked sensory ataxia, the disease is often referred to as ataxic neuropathy.

Moore (1934 *a* and *b*, 1937), Clark (1935, 1936) and Oluwole (1935) produced some fragmentary evidence to suggest that the disease as found in Nigerians was aetiologically related to consumption of a cassava diet and chronic cyanide intoxication. Cassava (manihot), a root-crop, contains a high concentration of cyanogenetic glycoside, linamarin, which on hydrolysis yields hydrocyanic acid. However, until recently research on the aetiology of the disease in Nigerians (Money, 1959; Monekosso and Annan, 1964 *a* and *b*; Monekosso, Annan, and Ashby, 1964) belaboured the hypothesis that deficiency of thiamine and riboflavine was the most important factor. Monekosso and Wilson (1966) described raised plasma thiocyanate—a detoxication product of cyanide—and changes in fractions of serum vitamin B_{12} (suggestive of chronic cyanide intoxication) in Nigerian patients with ataxic neuropathy.

Between 1966 and 1970, I carried out clinical, electrophysiological, metabolic and epidemiological studies of the disease. The aims of these studies were to determine if there was any significant correlation of the prevalence of the disease to consumption of cassava diet, and to seek biochemical evidence of chronic exposure to cyanide of dietary origin; to delineate further the clinical neurology and neuropathology of the disease, and to determine the role of protein-calorie and vitamin malnutrition in the aetiology of the disease.

Three hundred and seventy-five Nigerian patients who suffered from ataxic neuropathy have been studied and subjected to detailed neurological, ophthalmological and biochemical investigations. Field surveys were done to assess the prevalence of the disease in the adult populations of three villages, comprising Yorubas, a distinctly anthropologically homogeneous people. Two of the villages are in a district of high cassava consumption and the other village is in a district of low cassava consumption. Biochemical investigations were directed towards determining the nutritional status of the patients with regard to protein-calorie deficiency, vitamin and mineral nutrition, assessment of renal and hepatic function and exclusion of diabetes mellitus, achlorhydria, malabsorption, hypo- or hyperthyroidism, and assessment of chronic cyanide intoxication of dietary origin. Serological tests for syphilis and infections such as typhoid and typhus were done, and appropriately stained blood films examined for malaria parasites. Electromyography and motor nerve conduction tests were carried out on patients admitted to hospital. Percutaneous biopsy of the liver was done in 26 patients, and specimens were subjected to histological examination and also used for determination

[1] References to TABLE 16. 12 may be found in Osuntokun (1969).

Table 16.12

Tropical Nutritional Neuropathy: Review of Literature (1888–1969) *and Neuropathy of Prisoners of War*

Author(s)	Country	Mucocutaneous lesions (Cheilosis stomatoglossitis, Orogenital syndrome, Follicular hyperkeratosis)	Visual defects (optic atrophy; retro-bulbar neuritis)	Sensorineural deafness	Myelopathy: Pyramidal tract	Myelopathy: Posterior columns	Polyneuropathy	Hypotonic ataxic Types mainly = ++	Spastic ataxic Types mainly = ++	Dementia	Others	Presumed Aetiology	Neuropathology
Strachan, 1888, 1897	Jamaica	+	+	+	+	+	+	++	+	+		Malaria	Pigmentation of brain and spinal cord
Van dyne, 1909	Jamaica	+	+	+	+	+	+	++	+	+		Pellagra	
Stannus, 1912, 1913	Nyasaland	+	+	+	+	+	+	++	+	+		Pellagra	
1936	British Guiana	+	+	+	−	+	+	++	−	−	Orogenital syndrome	Malnutrition	
	Sierra Leone	+	+	+	−	+	−	++	−	−		Riboflavine deficiency	
	Barbados	+	+	+	−	+	−	++	−	−			
Scott, 1918	Jamaica	+	+	+	+	+	+	++	+	+		Nutritional deficiency Pellagra	Degeneration of CN I, 2 and 8, peripheral nerves and posterior root ganglia, posterior columns and anterolateral columns of spinal cord
Wright, 1928, 1930, 1934, 1936	Sierra Leone	+	+	+	+	+	+	++	−	−		Vitamin A and B deficiency	
Bradley, 1928	Seychelles	+	+	+	+	+	+	+	+	−		Nutritional deficiency	
Moore, 1930, 1932, 1934, 1937, 1939, 1940, 1943	Nigeria	+	+	+	+	+	+	++	+	−		HCN from capair cassava	
Clarke, 1935, 1936												Nutritional deficiency, e.g. Vitamin B	
Sharples, 1929	British Guiana	+	+	−	−	+	−	++	−	−		Nutritional deficiency	
Dychitan, 1930	Philippine Islands	+	+	+	+	+	+	++	−	−			
St. John, 1930, 1936	Barbados	+	+	−	−	−	−	−	−	−		Vitamin B deficiency	
Browne, 1932, 1939	British Guiana	+	+	+	+ (Mild)	+	+	+	−	−		Toxins from black pepper, and ginger teas especially during puerperium	
Nicholls, 1933, 1934, 1935, 1946	Ceylon	+	+	+	+	+	+	++	−	−	Phrynoderma and keratomalacia were common in this series Diarrhoea††	Vitamin A deficiency	Myelin degeneration in posterior spinal nerve roots, posterior columns and to a lesser extent in anterolateral columns of spinal cord
Landor and Pallister, 1935	Malaya	+	+	−	+	+	+	++	+	+		Pellagra	
Pallister, 1940		+	+	−	+	+	+	++	+	−	Diarrhoea††	Pellagra	Degeneration in biopsy of terminal branch peroneal nerve
Clark, 1937	Jamaica	+	+	−	−	−	+	−	−	−		Vitamin B deficiency	
Ellinger *et al.*, 1937	Egypt	−	−	−	+	+	−	−	++	−		Obscure	
Minchin, 1940	Southern India	−	−	−	++	+	−	−	++	−		Lathyrism	

Table 16.12 (continued)

Raman and Abbu, 1940	India	+	+	−	−	−	−	+	++	−		Pellagra	
Verma, 1942	India	+	+	−	−	−	+	++	−	−		Vitamin A and B deficiencies	
Metevier, 1941	Trinidad	+	+	−	−	−	+	−	−	−		Vitamin B deficiency	
Peraita, 1942, 1946	Spain	+	+	+	+	+	+	−	++	+	Diarrhoea†† achlorhydria	Malnutrition Vitamin B deficiency	
Grande and Jiminez	Spain	+	+	+	+	+	+	+	+	+	Diarrhoea††	Malnutrition Vitamin B deficiency	
White, 1943	Tanganyika	−	−	−	+	−	−	++	−	−		Obscure	
Ransome, 1944	Singapore	+	+	−	−	+	+	++	−	−	Cerebellar ataxia	Vitamin B deficiency	Degeneration of optic nerves, column of Goll, cells in Clarke's column, and posterior root ganglia
Lucasse, 1943, 1950, 1952	Congo (Kinshasha)	+	−	−	+	−	−	−	++	−		Obscure	
Gopalan, 1950	S. India	−	−	−	+	−	−	−	++	−		Obscure No ingestion of lathyrus	
Al witry *et al.*, 1950	Iraq	−	−	−	+	−	−	−	++	−		Obscure	
Knuttgen, 1955	Liberia	+	+	+	+	+	+	++	+	−		Nutritional deficiency	
Rizzotti, 1952	Ethiopia	−	−	−	+	−	−	−	++	−		Lathyrism	
Hutton, 1950, 1956; Shaper and Shaper, 1958	Uganda	+	−	+	+	−	−	+	+	−			
Harries, 1956	Kenya	−	−	−	+	−	−	−	++	−		Obscure	
Degazon, 1956	Jamaica	+	+	−	−	−	−	−	−	−		Vitamin deficiency	
Cruickshank, 1956, 1961; Cruickshank *et al.*, 1961; Montgomery *et al.*, 1964	Jamaica	−	+	+	+	+	+	+	++	−	ii Frequent dysfunction of bladder ii Laryngeal nerve palsy	?Syphilitic (of a queer variant) ?Toxins from plant foodstuffs e.g. HCN	Leptomeningeal thickening with cellular infiltration (perivascular) and reactive gliosis in CNS substance. Demyelination of posterior columns, and anterolateral of spinal cord, tracts, nerve roots, optic and auditory nerves. Degeneration of cells in grey matter of cord, and Clarke's column
Ferroluzzi, 1958	Eritrea	−	−	−	+	−	−	−	++	−		Obscure	
Rowland, H. A. K., 1963	Sierra Leone	−	+	+	+	+	+	+	++	+		Vitamin B deficiency Partial recovery on hospital diet and vitamin B supplement	
Money and Smith, 1955; Money, 1958, 1959, 1960	Nigeria	+	+	+	+	+	+	++	+	−	Endemic focus in S. Nigeria	Vitamin B deficiency	
Money, 1961	Uganda	+	+	+	+	+	+	+	+	−		Vitamin B deficiency	

Table 16.12 (continued)

Author(s)	*Country*	*Mucocutaneous lesions (Cheilosis, Stomatoglossitis, Orogenital syndrome, Follicular hyperkeratosis)*	*Visual defects (optic atrophy; retro-bulbar neuritis)*	*Sensorineural deafness*	*Myelopathy*		*Polyneuropathy*	*Hypotonic ataxic Types mainly = ++*	*Spastic ataxic Types mainly = ++*	*Dementia*	*Others*	*Presumed Aetiology*	*Neuropathology*
					Pyramidal tract	*Posterior columns*							
Haddock *et al.*, 1962	Tanzania (Tanganyika)	+	+	+	+	+	+	++	+	–		Malnutrition	
Ebrahim *et al.*, 1964		–	–	–	+	+	+	++	+	–		Vitamin B deficiency	
Haddock, 1965	Tanzania	–	–	–	+	+	+	+	++	–	Bladder dysfunction	Malnutrition	
Rodgers, 1965	Jamaica	–	+	+	+	+	+	+	++	–		?Treponemal infection ?Neurotoxins of dierary origin	
Osuntokun, 1966, 1968	Nigeria	+	+	+	+	+	+	++	+	+	Occasional bladder dysfunction and laryngeal palsy	HCN from cassava. Deficiency of sulphur containing amino acids. Ariboflavinosis	Segmental demyelination of peripheral nerves
Monekosso and Wilson, 1966	Nigeria	+	+	+	+	+	+	++	+			HCN from cassava	
Ojiambo, 1966	Kenya	–	+	–	+	+	–	++	+	+	Cerebellar ataxia		
Grieve *et al.*, 1967	Witwaters-rand; S. African Bantus	+	–	–	+	+	–	+	++	+	Evidence of liver damage. History of chronic alcoholism usually	Malnutrition Vitamin B deficiency. Liver disease Alcoholism	Degeneration of anterolateral tracts of cord
Collomb *et al.*, 1967	Senegal	–	+	+	+	+	+	++	+	–		Nutritional deficiency of riboflavin and nicotinamide Liver disease	
Osuntokun and Williams, 1969	Nigeria	+	+	+	+	+	+	++	+	+		HCN and malnutrition	Light and electron-microscopic study of peripheral nerves confirm segmental demyelination
Ashcroft *et al.*, 1967 (Suburban survey)	Jamaica	+	+	+	+	+	+	+	++	–		Nutritional deficiency	
		PRISONERS OF WAR											
Spillane and Scott, 1945	N. Africa	+	+	+	–	+	+	+	+	–		Vitamin B deficiency and malnutrition	
Clarke and Sneddon, 1946	Hong Kong	+	+	+	–	+	+	+	+	–		Vitamin B deficiency and malnutrition	
Butler *et al.*, 1945	Philippines	+	+	–	–	+	+	+	+	–	Diarrhoea††	Beriberi, pellagra (and other Vitamin B deficiencies)	

Table 16.12 (continued)

Graves, 1947	Malaya	−	+		+	−	+	+	++	−		Beriberi, pellagra (and other Vitamin B deficiencies)	
Cruickshank, 1946	Malaya	+	+	+	+	−	+	+	+	−		Beriberi Vitamin B deficiency	
Denny-Brown, 1947	Burma, Malaya, Thailand	+	+	+	+	+	+	+	++	−		Vitamin B deficiency	
Smith, 1946	Hong Kong	+	+	−	−	+	+	++	−	−		Vitamin B deficiency	
O'Donnell, 1947	Java	+	+	+	−	−	+	+	+	−		Vitamin B deficiency	
Smitskamp, 1947	Java	+	+	+	−	−	+	+	+	−			
Hobbs and Forbes, 1946	Java	+	+	+	−	−	+	+	+	−		Vitamin B deficiency	
Zimmer *et al.*, 1944	Nimes (Europe)	+	−	−	−	−	+	−	−	+	Oedema Ascites, Diarrhoea +	Beriberi Pellagra Vitamin B deficiency	
Bloom, 1944	N. Africa (British prisoners of war)	+	−	−	−	−	+	−	×	+	Oedema Diarrhoea +	Beriberi Pellagra Vitamin B deficiency	
Spillane 1947	i Europe, Polish refugees	−	−	−	−	−	+	−	−	+	Wernicke's Encephalopathy	Vitamin B deficiency	
	ii German Prisoners from Middle East	+	+	+	−	+	+	++	+	+	Oedema Diarrhoea + Laryngeal palsy Ageusia Anosmia Trigeminal hypo-aesthesiae	Malnutrition Vitamin B deficiency	Atrophy and disappearance of pyramidal cells from Sommer's section in Cornu ammonis; central chromatolysis and degeneration of a few Betz cells Localized disintegration of Corti's organ in the basal coil of cochlea with localized distension of Reissner's membrane with albuminoid coagulum in perilymph
Spillane, 1947	British Prisoners of war from Far East	+	+	+	+	+	+	++	+	−	Laryngeal palsy Diarrhoea +	Malnutrition Vitamin B deficiency	

Source: Osuntokun, B. O. (1969) *Chronic Cyanide Intoxication and a Degeneraive Neuropatthy in Nigerians*, Ph.D. thesis, University of Ibadan.

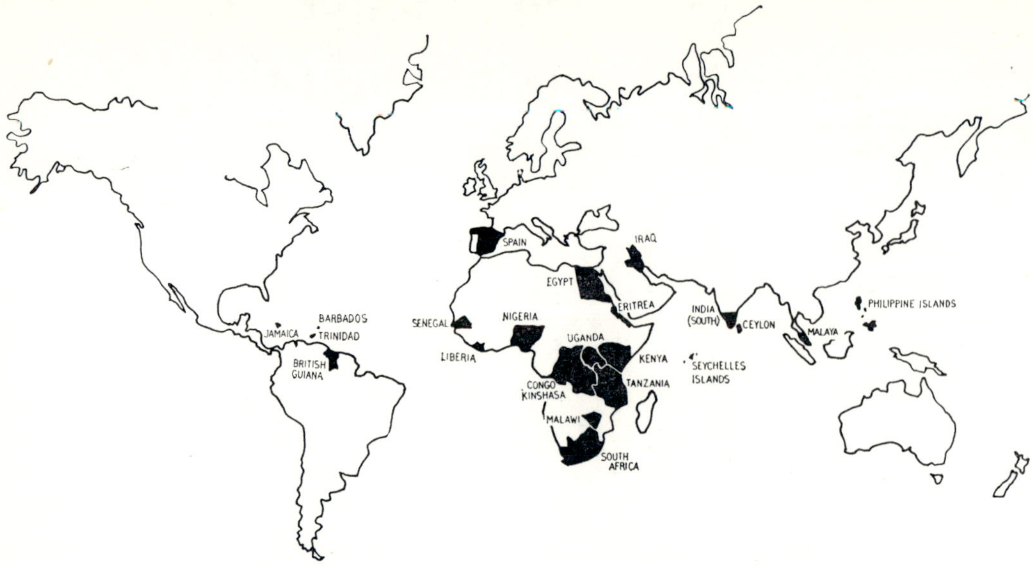

FIG. 16.3. World map showing distribution of the so-called tropical neuropathies.

of rhodanese[2] activity. Biopsy of muscle and of anterior tibial nerve in 23 patients was carried out and the specimens subjected to histological examination including single nerve fibre preparations and electron-microscopy. Details of the methodology employed in these studies have been described elsewhere (Osuntokun, 1968, 1969; Osuntokun, Monekosso, and Wilson, 1969 *a* and *b*; Osuntokun, Aladetoyinbo, and Adeuja, 1970; Osuntokun, Singh, and Martinson, 1970; Osuntokun and Aladetoyinbo, 1971; Aladetoyinbo, Osuntokun, and Adeuja, 1971).

Clinical Features

Age and Sex Distribution [TABLE 16.13]

The youngest at onset was 6 years old, and the oldest was 73. The sex ratio is 1:1. In the child-bearing age for the female, females outnumber males by 13 to 10. The apparent fall in the number of cases in the later years of life in both sexes is probably due to the low expectation of life in a developing country such as Nigeria.

Socio-economic Status

All the patients came from the low socio-economic classes.

[2] Rhodanese or thiosulphate-cyanide: sulphur transferase is the enzyme which catalyses the conversion of cyanide to thiocyanate—this pathway accounts for a variable (60–100 per cent) but major portion of detoxication of cyanide in human beings (Smith and Malcolm, 1930; Baumann, Springson, and Metzger, 1933).

Dietetic History

A history of almost total dependence on a monotonous diet of cassava derivatives was constant in all the patients. Occasional dietary supplements include yam, maize, rice, vegetables and occasional animal protein. Many of the patients, however, ate no other major item of food.

Family History

In 40 per cent of the patients, at least one other person in the family was similarly affected. Not infrequently, a history that several members of the family has 'similar trouble' was obtained. In many cases the afflicted members of the family were seen and further investigated by the author. In all cases the afflicted members of the family had lived in the same environment and had a similar dietetic history. Analysis of the relationship in the affected members showed no evidence of a genetically determined predisposition. The families were poor and members lived communally. Multiple conjugal cases in which husbands, wives and co-wives (in polygamous homes) were affected accounted for 65 per cent of the familial cases. Daughters and sons were affected in only about 10 per cent of these familial cases. Wives were more frequently afflicted than husbands.

Preceding or Predisposing Factors

Thirty patients gave a history of preceding febrile illness, 1 to 8 weeks before the onset of symptoms. In 20 female patients the illness began during the last two trimesters of pregnancy. In 14 other female patients onset of symptoms coincided with lactation.

Table 16.13
Age and Sex Distribution of 375 Nigerian Patients who Suffered from Ataxic Neuropathy

Year	0–9	10–19	20–29	30–39	40–49	50–59	60–69	70+	*Total*
Males	0	13	20	34	43	48	26	4	*188*
Females	4	18	30	54	50	21	8	2	*187*
Total	4	31	50	88	93	69	34	6	*375*

Mode of Onset

This was usually insidious as far as ataxia and weakness were concerned. A history of sudden onset of blurring of vision was obtained in 2 per cent, mostly young patients under 30 years of age who eventually developed other features of the disease; in one patient seen during the acute episode, there were signs of bilateral retrobulbar neuritis.

Intermittency

A history of intermittency in severity of symptoms was obtained in 7·8 per cent. Symptoms were usually worse during the rainy season, during pregnancy, lactation, and during febrile episodes. In two patients true transient remission occurred, confirmed clinically by almost total regression of neurological deficit: both, however, subsequently developed permanent neurological deficit. In the rest of the patients, the illness was initially progressive and subsequently become static. Three patients suffered from periodic attacks of vertigo accompanied by diplopia—both lasting a few days: they were not seen during these episodes. Four other patients suffered from intermittent psychotic episodes.

Symptoms and Signs [TABLES 16.14, 16.15, 16.16, 16.17]

The initial and commonest symptoms consist of various forms of paraesthesiae and dysaesthesiae starting in the distal parts of the lower limbs. The next commonest was blurring or loss of vision: this was then followed by ataxia of gait, tinnitus, deafness, weakness and thinning of legs. Seven per cent of the patients complained of girdle pains, usually in the lumbar region. In 4 per cent of the patients, sphincteric symptoms were present; all had normal myelographic examination.

Recurrent angular sores and painful tongue were complained of in 40 per cent of the patients.

Other rare symptoms include vertigo, diplopia, hoarseness of voice, rest tremor of hands, spontaneous twitching of muscles, and colicky abdominal pain.

The commonest signs were posterior column sensory loss in the lower limbs in four-fifths of the patients, and in the upper limbs in only 4 per cent of the patients.

Table 16.14
Symptomatology in 375 Patients

Symptoms	*Present in percentage of Cases*
Neurological	
Sensory symptoms (paraesthesiae, dysaesthesiae, often or initially confined to the lower limbs)	85
Visual symptoms	81
Abnormal gait	52
Tinnitus	48
Deafness	36
Weakness (usually or initially in lower limbs)	35
Sphincteric disturbance	4
Hoarseness/altered voice	2
Symptoms of mental or psychotic illness	9
Recurrent mucocutaneous lesions	40
Colicky abdominal pain	4

Bilateral optic atrophy with loss in visual acuity was found almost as frequently as posterior column sensory loss. Remarkably, the typical visual field loss was concentric diminution of the visual field proceeding to tubular vision, and central or paracentral scotomata were demonstrable in less than 5 per cent of the patients. Bilateral temporal pallor and advanced optic atrophy were commonly seen at fundoscopy.

Deafness of the sensorineural type was present in 41 per cent and was usually bilaterally symmetrical. Audiometric examination usually showed severe loss in the low and high frequencies with almost normal hearing in the middle range of 1000–3000 cps [FIG. 16.4 *a* and *b*]. In severe cases there was loss of hearing at

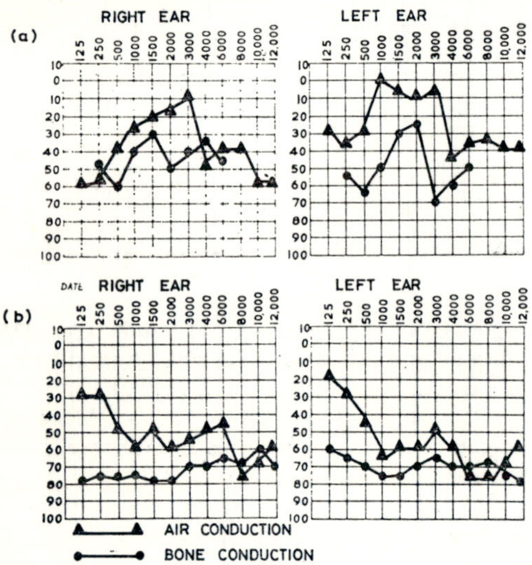

FIG. 16.4. (*a*) Hearing loss in a moderately severe case of Nigerian ataxic neuropathy. (*b*) Hearing loss in a severe case of Nigerian ataxic neuropathy.

all frequencies. Temporary threshold shift, or the phenomenon whereby a subject demonstrates a decline in his auditory threshold for a sustained tone as a function of time, was found in patients with less advanced deafness. This was usually found at low frequencies (250–1000 cps). Caloric tests usually showed no abnormality.

Weakness was found in the lower limbs in a third of the patients—more often in the distal musculature, and was uncommon in the upper limbs except in a few cases. In advanced cases, the lower limbs assumed the 'inverted champagne bottle' appearance.

Other findings include symmetrical superficial sensory loss (to light touch and pain) of stocking, and less commonly glove, distribution in 16 per cent, calf tenderness in 11 per cent, and laryngeal palsy in 2 per cent.

Ataxia of gait was demonstrable in 60 per cent. Seventeen per cent of the patients showed hypertonia of muscles of the lower limbs. The rest were hypotonic. Absent tendon reflexes were common, especially in the lower limbs (58 per cent). In 7 per cent of the patients, extensor plantar responses were obtained, and 3 per cent showed sustained ankle clonus.

Various combinations of cerebellar degeneration, motor neurone disease, Parkinson's disease, and dementia, were present in 4 per cent.

Table 16.15
Physical Findings in 375 Patients

Physical findings	*Present in percentage of Cases*	
Posterior column sensory loss (usually confined to or initially in lower limbs)	83	
Bilateral optic atrophy	81	
Alteration in tone in limb muscles	70	
Hypotonia		*53*
Hypertonia		*17*
Demonstrable ataxia of gait	60	
Impaired coordination (sensory ataxia in lower limbs usually)	43	
Bilateral perceptive deafness	41	
Weakness in limbs (usually lower limbs)	30	
Proximal musculature only		*13*
Distal and proximal musculature		*17*
Wasting of muscles	12	
Superficial stocking (and less commonly glove) sensory loss	16	
Calf tenderness	11	
Laryngeal palsy	2	
Cortico-extrapyramidal-cerebellar-motor neurone degeneration	4	

Neuropsychiatric findings in this series include dementia, in 7 per cent, schizophrenic-like psychosis in 2 per cent and euphoria in 1 per cent.

Mucocutaneous evidence of malnutrition was Present in two-fifths of the patients. Three per cent of the patients were overweight; 10 per cent were underweight. In 2 per cent non-toxic goitre was present [Table 16.18].

Natural History

So far, no patient has died from the disease. Predominantly posterior column myelopathy was the commonest and earliest feature, closely followed by optic atrophy. The peripheral nerves appear to be the last to be involved.

Investigations

Cerebrospinal fluid (CSF) examination was usually normal; only six patients had CSF protein concentration greater than 50 mg per cent. All had normal myelographic examination.

Kahn or VDRL test was positive in blood in nine patients and in two of them in the CSF as well. All gave a history of yaws in childhood.

Plain radiographs of chest, vertebral column, sacro-iliac joints, long bones of lower limbs, and of hands revealed occasional abnormalities such as fuzzy margins of the sacro-iliac joints, sclerosis of the shafts of long bones and vertebrae, and very rarely osteoporosis.

Table 16.16

A Comparison of Tendon Reflex Status in 375 Nigerian Patients with Tropical Ataxic Neuropathy and 375 Nigerian Normals, Mainly Civil Servants (Matched for Age and Sex)

Reflex	Patients: Absent in %	Patients: Exaggerated in %	Normals: Absent in %	Normals: Exaggerated in %
Biceps jerk	5	14	0	5
Triceps jerk	14	14	0	5
Supinator jerk	16	14	0	5
Knee jerk	44	19	24	5
Ankle jerk	60	19	25	4

Table 16.17

Neuropsychiatric Findings in 375 Nigerian Patients with Ataxic Neuropathy

Findings	Present in percentage of cases
Dementia	7
Schizophrenic-like psychosis	2
Euphoria	1
Phobic-anxiety state	1
Drowsiness/confusional state	1

Only six patients showed achlorhydria; this was histamine-fast in two patients.

Transient albuminuria was present in one patient. None had porphyrinuria, or schistosomal ova in urine. Amino-aciduria was absent.

Liver-function tests, glucose-tolerance tests, serum calcium and phosphate, alkaline phosphatase, and plasma-bound iodine, I^{125} tri-iodothyronine red blood cell uptake and I^{131}-uptake of thyroid on scanning were usually normal. No patient had biochemical evidence of malabsorption.

Table 16.18

Other Findings

Findings	Present in percentage of cases
Mucocutaneous evidence of malnutrition (angular stomatitis glossitis gingivitis and gum hyperplasia caries non-haemorrhagic follicular hyperkeratosis)	40
Underweight	11
Obesity or overweight	3
Non-toxic goitre	2

Scanty trophozoites of *Plasmodium falciparum* were found in 17 patients.

Liver biopsy in 26 patients showed only occasional non-specific periportal lymphocytic infiltration.

Electromyographic evidence of denervation was present in patients with clinical evidence of symmetrical peripheral polyneuropathy. Profuse fasciculation even in clinically normal muscles was seen in patients who suffered from motor neurone disease as well. Motor nerve conduction velocity was significantly reduced in the peripheral nerves compared with the normals, and this was often so even in patients with no clinical evidence of peripheral neuropathy (Osuntokun, 1970 *a*). The slowing was greatest in the common peroneal nerve [Fig. 16.5] and was most marked in patients with clinical evidence of sensorimotor polyneuropathy (usually) in the lower limbs.

Histological examination of a single nerve fibre preparation of biopsy specimens of anterior tibial nerves showed segmental demyelination and marked variation in internodal lengths; demyelination was confirmed by electron-microscopy of nerves from four patients (Osuntokun, 1969; Williams and Osuntokun, 1969). In five patients with wasting of the distal musculature of the lower limbs, histological examination of the extensor digitorum brevis showed neurogenic atrophy.

Electrocardiographic (ECG) abnormalities were uncommon. Sinus tachycardia was present in six patients without other ECG evidence of cardiomyopathy. Low voltage tracings and non-specific T wave changes were found in 16 other patients. In none was these sufficiently widespread to suggest diffuse myocardial disease.

Assessment of Nutritional Status

Protein Nutrition. Haemoglobin concentration, serum albumin and transferrin fall in protein malnutrition. Serum transferrin is said to be a sensitive

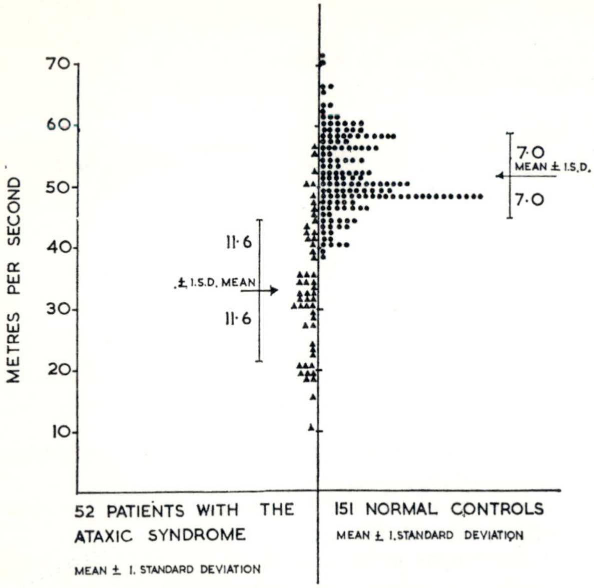

FIG. 16.5. Scattergram showing motor nerve conduction velocities in m/sec in Nigerian patients suffering from tropical ataxic neuropathy, and in normal controls (Nigerian).

index of protein nutrition (MacFarlane *et al.*, 1969). Haemoglobin levels, serum albumin and transferrin concentrations were normal in the patients. Anaemia was rare. Haemoglobin concentration greater than 16 g/100 ml was not uncommon in patients in this series. In two patients haemoglobin concentration exceeded 19 g/100 ml, but white cell counts were normal.

Calorie Nutrition. Using serum cholesterol as an index of calorie consumption in relation to requirement (Mann *et al.*, 1955; Edozien, 1965), no significant difference was found in the concentration of serum cholesterol in the patients compared with unaffected peasants from areas known to be free of the disease.

Vitamin Nutrition. There was diminished excretion of riboflavine as found in 29 patients, and serum riboflavine was significantly reduced compared with normals (Osuntokun, 1969; Aladetoyinbo, Osuntokun, and Adeuja, 1971). Intake of nicotinic acid and thiamine seemed to be adequate judging from urinary excretion values of *N*-methylnicotinamide and thiamine. Transketolase activity of red blood cells, a sensitive index of thiamine intake, was found to be normal compared with that of normal Nigerians (Osuntokun, 1971 *c*). Serum levels of folic acid were normal.

Serum caeruloplasmin was significantly lower in patients compared with normals (Osuntokun and Williams, 1970).

There was no evidence of increased frequency of urinary infections in patients. Widal and Felix tests showed normal results.

Investigation of Cyanide Metabolism and Assessment of Exposure to Cyanide of Dietary Origin in Patients

Cyanide is detoxicated in the body [FIG. 16.6] largely by conversion to thiocyanate, catalysed mainly by rhodanese present in most tissues (and in the highest concentration in the liver) in man, and to a lesser extent by mercaptopyruvate: cyanide sulphur transferase. The major substrates for this conversion are thiosulphate and 3-mercaptopyruvate, derived mainly from cysteine. Cyanide in body fluids is in dynamic equilibrium with thiocyanate, the equimolar concentration of cyanide varying between 0·25 and 0·5 per cent of that of thiocyanate (Boxer and Rickards, 1952). The enzyme thiocyanate oxidase present in blood cells (Goldstein and Rieders, 1953) helps to maintain the equilibrium by oxidizing thiocyanate to cyanide. Cyanide may also react spontaneously *in vitro* with cystine to form 2-aminothiazoline-4-carboxylic acid or its stochiometric isomer, 2-imino-4-thiazolidine carboxylic acid (Schoberl and Hamm, 1948; Schoberl, Kawohl, and Hamm, 1951; Aldridge, 1951; Behringer and Zillikens, 1951; Wood and Cooley, 1956). Cyanide by interaction with hydroxocobalamin is incorporated into the 1-carbon metabolic pool, and cyanide is thereby converted into cyanocobalamin and probably to thiocyanate as well (Wokes, Badenoch, and Sinclair, 1955; Wokes and Picard, 1955). Chronic cyanide intoxication may therefore be assessed biochemically by estimation of:

1. Thiocyanate, and cyanide in body fluids.
2. Changes in amino acid pattern in the plasma especially with regard to sulphur-containing amino acids (cysteine, cystine, and methionine).
3. Quantitative changes in fractions of vitamin B_{12} (especially hydroxocobalamin and cyanocobalamin).

TABLE 16.19 shows the plasma thiocyanate and cyanide levels and urinary thiocyanate excretion in Nigerian patients with ataxic neuropathy compared with levels in normal Nigerians. The latter comprised hospital workers, most of whom belong to the upper and middle socio-economic groups; many of them did not eat cassava at all, or no more than once or twice a week. In addition, the level of free cyanide as distinct from bound cyanide in the blood of patients is significantly raised compared with that of normals (Osuntokun, Aladetoyinbo, and Adeuja, 1970). Plasma thiocyanate and cyanide levels in other Nigerian patients suffering from diseases unrelated or dissimilar to tropical ataxic neuropathy are normal (Osuntokun, 1968). In the patients with tropical ataxic neuropathy, the concentration of plasma thiocyanate and cyanide and urinary thiocyanate fell when they were fed on a hospital diet which contained cassava meals only twice a week [TABLE 16.20]. The patients not infrequently showed definite clinical improvement with hospitalization. When the patients were discharged and returned to their usual diet of cassava, the plasma cyanide and

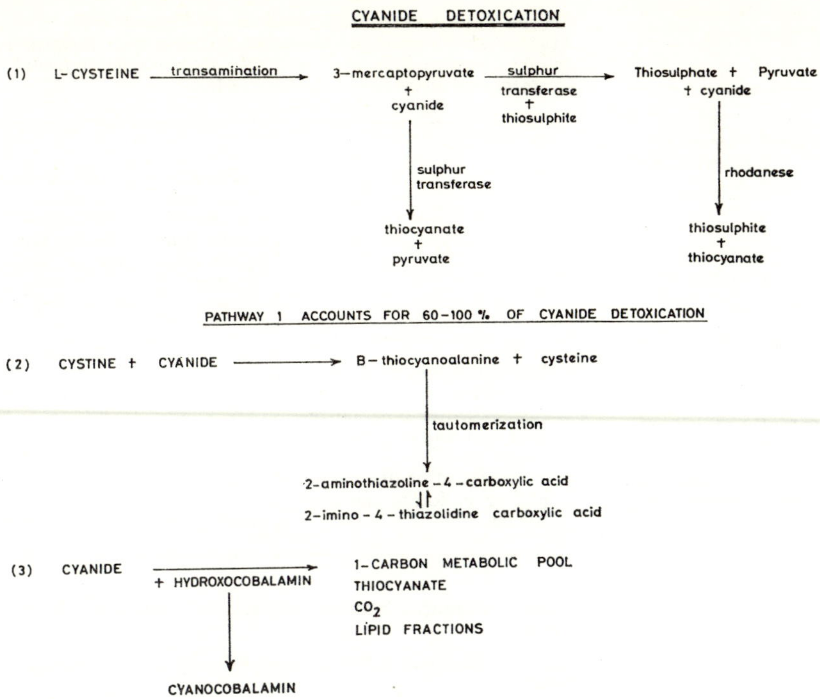

FIG. 16.6. Detoxication of cyanide in man.

thiocyanate levels rose again [TABLE 16.21]. This was usually associated with clinical deterioration.

Rhodanese activity in liver biopsy specimens in patients was found to be within normal limits.

TABLE 16.22 shows the serum levels of vitamin B_{12} in patients and controls. Total serum B_{12} level was normal or high. Serum cyanocobalamin, an intermediary in the detoxication of cyanide involving hydroxocobalamin, was higher in patients than in controls. The level of serum hydroxocobalamin was lower in patients compared with normals. There was a significant positive correlation between cyanocobalamin and plasma thiocyanate ($r = +0{\cdot}14$, $p < 0{\cdot}01$), and a significant negative correlation between plasma thiocyanate and hydroxocobalamin ($r = -0{\cdot}33$, $p < 0{\cdot}001$).

Preliminary results of analysis of various fractions of B_{12} in serum, using chromatography and bio-autographic technique (Lindstrand and Stahlberg, 1963) showed that cyanocobalamin, a detoxication product of cyanide was present in excess in the patients with ataxic neuropathy (Osuntokun, 1969).

Sulphur-containing amino-acids were absent in 60 per cent of patients with ataxic neuropathy and greatly reduced in the others. The essential amino acids were reduced, but the pattern was unlike that found in

Table 16.19

Urinary Thiocyanate, Plasma Thiocyanate and Cyanide (Determined Within 48 Hours of Admission) in Nigerian Patients with Tropical Ataxic Neuropathy and Normal Nigerians

	Urinary thiocyanate in micromoles per kg. body weight per 24 hours (mean + standard error)	*Plasma thiocyanate in micromoles per 100 ml (mean + standard error)*	*Plasma cyanide in micromoles per 100 ml (mean + standard error)*
Patients with tropical amblyopia	2·4 + 0·1 ($n = 67$)	11·4 + 0·2 ($n = 375$)	0·1 + 0·004 ($n = 108$)
Normal Nigerians	0·6 + 0·05 ($n = 40$)	2·9 + 0·02 ($n = 106$)	0·03 + 0·002 ($n = 106$)
	$p < 0{\cdot}001$	$p < 0{\cdot}001$	$p < 0{\cdot}001$

Table 16.20

Fall in Plasma Thiocyanate and Cyanide and Urinary Thiocyanate in 67 Patients with Tropical Amblyopia after 6 Weeks on Hospital Diet

	On admission	After 6 weeks on hospital diet
Plasma thiocyanate in micromoles per 100 ml (mean + standard error)	11·1 + 0·4	2·8 + 0·1
Plasma cyanide in micromoles per 100 ml (mean + standard error)	0·09 + 0·004	0·03 + 0·001
Urinary thiocyanate in micromoles per kg body weight, per 24 hours (mean + standard error)	2·4 + 0·1	0·7 + 0·03

Note: The differences between the concentration on admission and after 6 weeks on hospital diet are statistically significant ($p < 0·001$ for each variant).

Table 16.21

Plasma Thiocyanate and Cyanide in 35 Patients with Tropical Amblyopia, on Admission, 6 Weeks after Admission, and on Hospital Diet, and 12 Weeks after Discharge from Hospital and Reversion to Cassava Meals

	A Plasma thiocyanate in micromoles per 100 ml (mean + standard error)	B Plasma cyanide in micromoles per 100 ml (mean + standard error)
1. Within 48 hours of admission	11·9 + 0·8	0·1 + 0·006
2. 6 weeks after hospitalization and on hospital diet	2·8 + 0·3	0·025 + 0·002
3. 12 weeks after discharge and reversion to cassava meals	12·8 + 0·9	0·110 + 0·07

For differences between 1A and 2A, 2A and 3A, $p < 0·0001$.

For differences between 1B and 2B, 2B and 3B, $p < 0·0001$.

No significant differences between 1A and 3A, 1B and 3B.

Table 16.22

Serum Vitamin B_{12} in pg/ml and Plasma Thiocyanate in Nigerian Patients with Ataxic Neuropathy and Normal Controls (Nigerians)

Groups	No.	A Serum B_{12} with cyanide extraction[1] in pg/ml (≡Total B_{12}) Mean ± SEM	B Serum B_{12} without cyanide extraction[1] (≡cyanocobalamin) Mean ± SEM	A–B ≡hydroxocobalamin Mean ± SEM	C Plasma SCN^- in mole/100 ml Mean ± SEM
1. Patients with ataxic neuropathy	320	1764 ± 76	1141 ± 57	587 ± 31	11·3 ± 0·24
2. Normal Nigerians	114	1430 ± 94	575 ± 44	864 ± 68	2·7 ± 0·17

For difference between 1A and 2A, $p < 0·01$.
For difference between 1B and 2B, $p < 0·002$.
For difference between 1A–B, and 2A–B, $p < 0·002$.
For difference between 1C and 2C, $p < 0·0001$.
SEM = Standard Error of Mean.

[1] On Smith's (1961) hypothesis, the concentration obtained in the lactobacillus assay of B_{12} represents total B_{12} when cyanide was added to the buffer used to extract serum B_{12}; the concentration obtained without cyanide added to the buffer represents cyanocobalamin, and the difference which is normally substantial represents hydroxocobalamin. Estimation of vitamin B_{12} microbiologically, with and without added cyanide to the extracting buffer, may possibly therefore, in view of the experience of other workers (Matthews, Wilson, and Zilkha, 1965; Wilson and Matthews, 1966) be used in assessing the amounts of hydroxocobalamin and cyanocobalamin. Smith's hypothesis may not necessarily be true, however. Vitamin B_{12} is known to consist of at least six components of which four—hydroxocobalamin, cyanocobalamin, methylcobalamin and deoxyadenosyl B_{12} (DNB Co-enzyme B_{12})—are found in human sera. Chromatographic with bio-autographic techniques appear to be more reliable in assessing the quantitative changes in B_{12} fractions.

kwashiorkor, the classical disease of protein-calorie deficiency (Osuntokun, Durowoju, MacFarlane, and Wilson, 1968; Osuntokun, 1969).

The raised plasma thiocyanate in Nigerian patients was not of dietary origin as the thiocyanate concentrations of cassava derivatives are very low (Osuntokun, 1969). Nigerians do not consume large amounts of food, such as cabbage and milk, known to contain a high concentration of thiocyanate. We have shown that cyanide was released in considerable amounts from cassava derivatives during dilute acid hydrolysis *in vitro* and during intragastric hydrolysis of cassava meals (Osuntokun, 1969; Osuntokun and Aladetoyinbo, 1971).

Epidemiological Studies

Most of the patients (95 per cent) come from areas in Nigeria where cassava is intensely cultivated (Oke, 1968; Osuntokun, 1969).

There is biochemical evidence of increased exposure to cyanide in families in endemic areas where multiple or conjugal cases were found, compared with members of normal families from the same endemic area [TABLE 16.23]. The ataxic families consumed more cassava meals (Osuntokun, 1969). In families in endemic areas there is a statistically significant positive correlation between age and plasma thiocyanate, suggesting that prolonged exposure to cyanide may be important in determining the onset of the disease (Osuntokun, 1969).

The biochemical evidence of cyanide exposure in families in endemic areas showed a remarkable trend towards equal values in many members of the same family, except in those who were very young (Osuntokun, 1969). A common cooking pot, and what is cooked, appear to be more important than heredity in determining concentrations of plasma thiocyanate.

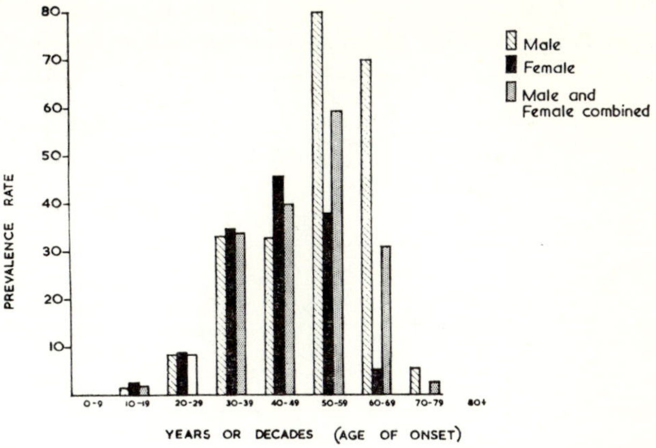

FIG. 16.7. Prevalence of tropical ataxic neuropathy per 1000 per decade of life, as found during a neurological survey of Epe carried out in 1967. (By courtesy of the Editor, *West African Medical Journal*.)

Employing haemoglobin electrophoretic genotypes, colour blindness and ability to taste phenylthiocarbamide (PTC) in members of afflicted and normal families in endemic areas, no evidence was found of a genetically determined predisposition in these endemic areas (Osuntokun, 1969).

The results of field surveys of three villages show marked differences in the prevalence of ataxic neuropathy, and in the neurological profiles [TABLE 16.24]. Details of prevalence rates for each decade for Epe are shown in FIGURE 16.7. It is worthy of note that the highest prevalence—as high as 80 per 1000 [FIG. 16.7]—occurs in the same decade in which the maximum incidence was found among cases studied in hospital. There is biochemical evidence of increased exposure to cyanide in the high cassava-eating areas (Osuntokun,

Table 16.23
Metabolic Studies in Families in Endemic Areas of Epe and Ososa

	No. of families	*No. of individuals*	*Plasma SCN^- in μ moles/100 ml* Mean ± SEM	*Serum B_{12} in pg/ml with CN^- extraction = 1* Mean ± SEM	*Serum B_{12} in pg/ml without CN^- extraction = 2* Mean ± SEM	*1–2 = hydroxocobalamin* Mean ± SEM	*Age in years* Mean + SEM
Families with ataxic neuropathy	43	139					
Patients with ataxic neuropathy		79	12·7 ± 0·5	1716 ± 147	1140 ± 100	593 ± 57	49·6 ± 1·5
Patients with isolated myelopathy or optic atrophy		9	9·2 ± 0·8	1115 ± 304	887 ± 303	253 ± 58	41·0 + 4·4
Normals from families with ataxic neuropathy		55	6·5 ± 0·4	2031 ±203	925 ± 78	1070 ± 147	25·5 + 2·3
Normals from normal families in endemic area	25	93	5·8 ± 0·2	1671 ± 109	801 ± 59	867 ± 71	37·0 + 1·7
Normals from staff of UCH Ibadan		114	2·7 ± 0·17	1430 ± 94	575 ± 44	864 ± 68	25·0 + 1·8

Table 16.24

Neurological Syndromes Found in Ososa, Epe and Akinmorin

	High cassava-eating villages				*Low cassava-eating village*	
	Ososa		*Epe*		*Akinmorin*	
Neurological Syndromes	*No. of patients*	*Prevalence per 1 000 adult population > 10 years*	*No. of patients*	*Prevalence per 1000 adult population > 10 years*	*No. of patients*	*Prevalence per 1000 adult population > 10 years*
Ataxic neuropathy	55	24·1	162	21·6	1	Less than 0·1
Ataxic neuropathy + motor neurone disease + Parkinson's disease + cerebellar degeneration + dementia	3		3		0	
Ataxic neuropathy + motor neurone disease	1		1		0	
Ataxic neuropathy + Parkinson's disease	1		0		0	
Ataxic neuropathy + cerebellar degeneration + motor neurone disease	0		3		0	
Parkinson's disease	2		4		1	
Motor neurone disease	0		2		0	
Tuberous sclerosis	0		1		0	
Peripheral neuropathy	2		4		0	
Epilepsy	0		2		0	

Monekosso, and Wilson, 1969*a* and *b*; Osuntokun, 1969). There is also some evidence that cassava farmers and processers may be at risk of developing the disease (Osuntokun, Monekosso, and Wilson, 1969*a*; Osuntokun, 1969).

Goitre is common in the areas endemic for Nigerian tropical ataxic neuropathy (Oluwasanmi and Alli, 1968) and is not uncommon in Nigerian patients suffering from ataxic neuropathy (Osuntokun, 1969). In experimental animals cassava is goitrogenic (Ekpechi, 1967).

Comments

It is possible that the neurological syndromes resembling Nigerian ataxic neuropathy, described from many tropical and a few subtropical countries, and from prisoner-of-war camps, may have a *nutritional* basis in common. It is unlikely, however, that the specific aetiological factor involved—whether a deficiency, such as lack of a specific vitamin or inadequate protein intake, or a dietary toxin—is the same in *all* countries or places where the cases have been described. The geographical zones where these syndromes occur cover wide areas and include a conglomeration of peoples who differ in most cases in culture, feeding habits and common dietary items usually consumed. Signs such as glossitis, cheilosis and angular stomatitis, common in ataxic neuropathy and classically attributed to vitamin B deficiency, are probably non-specific and merely represent clinical evidence of impaired oxidative metabolism in rapidly regenerating epithelium. Thiamine deficiency causes impaired oxidative decarboxylation of the keto-acids, deficiency of nicotinic acid and riboflavine with impaired function of nicotinamide-adenine-dinucleotide (NAD), nicotinamide-adenine-dinucleotide phosphate (NADP), flavin-mononucleotide (FMN) and flavin-adenine-dinucleotide (FAD); iron deficiency, with impaired function of cytochrome system or cyanide-induced inhibition of cytochrome oxidase, will produce more or less the same biochemical end-result, by impairing transfer of electron to molecular oxygen and retarding oxidative metabolism. Hence, the mucocutaneous signs mentioned above may occur in clinical states associated with deficiency of most components of vitamin B complex and in chronic cyanide intoxication. Of course, if multiple defects occur in oxidative metabolism it is likely that the effects will summate. One substance may also be important for the normal function of another. For example, the decyanation of cyanocobalamin to the physiologically active vitamin B_{12} (hydroxocobalamin and co-enzyme B_{12}) requires NADP, FMN and FAD (Cima, Levorato, and Mantovan, 1967).

The neuropathological effects of chronic cyanide intoxication in experimental animals and man have been extensively studied, and predominantly include demyelination and focal necrosis of neurones (Hirano, Levine, and Zimmerman, 1967; Bass, 1968). In recent times there has been some considerable evidence that chronic cyanide intoxication is the major factor in the pathogenesis of tobacco ambylopia (Heaton, McCormick, and Freeman, 1958; Freeman and Heaton, 1961), subacute combined degeneration of pernicious anaemia (Wilson and Langman, 1966), Leber's hereditary optic atrophy (Wilson, 1965), and lathyrism (Ressler, Redstone, and Erenberg, 1961; Dastur, 1962; Ressler, 1962), and these diseases bear some clinical similarity to Nigerian tropical ataxic neuropathy. Although precise neuropathological demonstration of the lesions in the nervous system in Nigerian tropical ataxic neuropathy is lacking, for there has been no post-mortem study as no patient has died in hospital, segmental demyelination has been demonstrated in biopsy specimens of peripheral nerves (Osuntokun, 1969; Williams and Osuntokun, 1969). This is confirmed by the finding of reduced motor nerve conduction velocity in the Nigerian patients. Conceivably, chronic cyanide intoxication is a cause of segmental demyelinating neuropathy. A segmental neuropathy has been produced in Wistar rats fed for 12–18 months on a diet of which 80 per cent was made up of cassava derivatives. In these rats, the plasma level of thiocyanate was significantly raised (Osuntokun, 1969, 1970 *b*).

The impression or conclusion at the moment is that although there are similarities between ataxic neuropathy in Nigerians and some nutritional neuropathies seen in other tropical and subtropical countries, it is not justifiable to assume that these represent clinical variants of the same disease, and hence, in the context of the Nigerian experience, that they are all related aetiologically to chronic cyanide intoxication. It has been pointed out above how the same biochemical end-result, and probably the same neuropathic effects, may be caused by deficiencies of various vitamins or by the presence of a cellular poison such as cyanide. When a diet is poor, multiple nutritional deficiencies often occur together, and hence may summate to produce the final clinical picture. However, at least in the Nigerians who suffer from tropical ataxic neuropathy, chronic cyanide intoxication appears to be the most important factor in the causation and pathogenesis of the disease. Deficiency of riboflavine also occurs in the Nigerian patients.

In the treatment of the disease, a double-blind controlled trial of hydroxocobalamin and riboflavine has shown no beneficial effect in favour of the drugs (Osuntokun, Wilson, Langman, and Aladetoyinbo, 1970). Another trial employing hydroxocobalamin injections, riboflavine and cysteine tablets is at the moment in progress.

References

ADELOYE, A., and ODEKU, E. L. (1969) Metastatic neoplasms of the brain in Nigeria, *Brit. J. Cancer*, 23, 340–8.

ADELOYE, A., and ODEKU, E. L. (1970) The nervous system in sickle cell disease, *Afr. J. med. Sci.*, 1, 33–48.

AKINKUGBE, O. O. (1969) *Observations on High Blood Pressure in the West African*, M.D. thesis, University of London.

ALADETOYINBO, A., OSUNTOKUN, B. O., and ADEUJA, A. O. G. (1971) Serum riboflavin in nutritional neuropathy in Nigerians, *W. Afr. J. biol. Chem.*, 14, 3–5.

ALDRIDGE, W. N. (1951) The conversion of cyanogen chloride to cyanide in the presence of blood protein and sulphydryl compounds, *Biochem. J.*, 48, 271–6.

ANAND, S. V., and EVANS, K. J. (1964) Polymyositis, *Brit. J. Surg.*, 51, 917–20.

BARNARD, B. G., and ROBERTSON, J. H. (1960) Polymyositis: report on 3 cases from West Africa, *Brit. med. J.*, 1, 1473–6.

BASS, N. H. (1968) Pathogenesis of myelin lesions in experimental cyanide poisoning: a microchemical study, *Neurology (Minneap.)*, 18, 167–77.

BAUMANN, E. J., SPRINGSON, D. B., and METZGER, N. (1933) Thyroid and cyanide metabolism, *J. biol. Chem.*, 100, 13.

BEHRINGER, H., and ZILLIKENS, P. (1951) *Ann. Chem.*, 574, 140, quoted by Wood and Cooley (1956).

BOORMAN, J. P. T., and DRAPER, C. C. (1968) Isolation of arboviruses in the Lagos area of Nigeria, and a survey of antibodies to them in man and animals, *Trans. roy. Soc. trop. Med. Hyg.*, 62, 269–77.

BOXER, G. E., and RICKARDS, J. C. (1952) Studies on metabolism of carbon of cyanide and thiocyanate *Arch. Biochem.*, 39, 7–14.

BRITISH MEDICAL JOURNAL (1971) Tuberculous meningitis in children, [leading article], *Brit. med. J.*, 1, 1.

BROWN, A. (1961) The pattern of disease in Nigeria, in *First Pan-African Psychiatric Conference, 12–18 November*, 1961, *Abeokuta*, ed. Lambo, T. A., Ibadan, pp. 134–8.

BURNET, F. M. (1968) Measles as an index of immunological function, *Lancet*, ii, 610–13.

CAUSEY, P. O. R., KEMP, G. E., MADBOULY, M. H., and LEE, V. H. (1969) Arbovirus surveillance in Nigeria; 1964–1967, *Bull. Soc. Path. exot.*, 62, 249–53.

CIMA, L., LEVORATO, C., and MANTOVAN, R. (1967) Enzymatic decyanation of cyanocobalamin in rat tissues, *J. Pharm. Pharmacol.*, 19, 32–40.

CLARK, A. (1935) On the aetiology of pellagra and allied nutritional diseases, *W. Afr. med. J.*, 8, 7–9.

CLARK, A. (1936) Report on effects of certain poisons contained in food plants of West Africa upon health of certain native races, *J. trop. Med. Hyg.*, 39, 69, 285.

DADA, T. O., and ELLIOTT, B. A. (1967) Muscular dystrophy of Duchenne type in Nigerians, *J. neurol. Sci.*, 4, 435–44.

DADA, T. O., JOHNSON, F. A., and ARABA, A. B. (1969) Cerebrovascular accidents in Nigerians: a review of 205 cases, *W. Afr. med. J.*, 18, 95–108.

DADA, T. O., and ODEKU, E. L. (1966) Epilepsy in Nigerian patients: a review of 234 cases, *W. Afr. med. J.*, 15, 153–63.

DASTUR, D. K. (1962) Lathyrism. Some aspects of the disease in man and animals, *Wld Neurol.*, 3, 721–30.

EDOZIEN, J. C. (1965) Establishment of a biochemical norm for evaluation of nutritional status in West Africa, *J. W. Afr. Sci. Ass.*, 10, 3–21.

EKPECHI, O. L. (1967) Pathogenesis of endemic goitre in Eastern Nigeria, *Brit. J. Nutr.*, 21, 537–45.

FENDALL, N. R. E., and LAKE, B. M. (1958) Poliomyelitis in Kenya, *J. trop. Med. Hyg.*, 61, 135–44.

FITZSIMMONS, J. M., and SMITH, H. M. V. (1963) Tuberculous meningitis: special features of treatment, *Tubercle*, 44, 103–11.

FREEMAN, A. G., and HEATON, J. M. (1961) The aetiology of rectrobulbar neuritis in Addisonian pernicious anaemia, *Lancet*, ii, 908–11.

GANS, B., MACNAMARA, F. N., MORLEY, D. C., THOMSON, S. W., and WATT, A. (1961) Some observations on the epidemiology of measles in West Africa, *W. Afr. med. J.*, 10, 253–62.

GELFAND, M (1957) *The Sick African: A Clinical Study*, 3rd ed., Cape Town, p. 26.

GOLDSTEIN, F., and RIEDERS, F. (1953) Conversion of thiocyanate to cyanide by an erythrocytic enzyme, *Amer. J. Physiol.*, 173, 287–90.

GREENBERG, A. (1955) *Studies in African Linguistic Classification;* revised as *The Languages of Africa*, 1963, The Hague.

GREENWOOD, B. M. (1968) Autoimmune disease and parasitic infections in Nigerians, *Lancet*, ii, 380–2.

HADDOCK, D. R. W. (1963) Neurological signs in African patients without overt neurological disease, *E. Afr. med. J.*, 40, 601–8.

HEATON, J. M., MCCORMICK, A. J. A., and FREEMAN, A. G. (1958) Tobacco amblyopia: a clinical manifestation of vitamin B_{12} deficiency, *Lancet*, ii, 286–90.

HIRANO, A., LEVINE, S., and ZIMMERMAN, A. (1967) Experimental cyanide encephalopathy: electron microscopic observations of early lesions in white matter, *J. Neuropath. exp. Neurol.*, 26, 200–13.

HORN, C. V., and MASTER, S. (1968) Polymyositis tropicans in Uganda, *E. Afr. med. J.*, 45, 463–71.

HUTTON, P. W. (1956) Neurological disorders in Uganda, *E. Afr. med. J.*, 33, 209–33.

KAUSHIK, S. C. (1961) The pattern of neurological disease in Ibadan, in *First Pan-African Psychiatric Conference*, 12–18 *November* 1961, *Abeokuta*, ed., Lambo, T. A., Ibadan, pp. 78–87.

KOCEN, R. S., and PARSONS, M. (1970) Neurological complications of tuberculosis: some unusual manifestations, *Quart. J. Med.*, 39, 17–30.

LAMBO, T. A. (1961) Important areas of research in tropical neurology, in *First Pan-African Psychiatric Conference*, 12–18 *November* 1961, *Abeokuta*, ed. Lambo, T. A., Ibadan, pp. 91–4.

LAMBO, T. A. (1965) Psychiatry in tropics, *Lancet*, ii, 1119–21.

LAUFER, I. (1958) A severe epidemic of paralytic poliomyelitis in Western Province of Tanganyika, 1956, *J. trop. med. Hyg.*, 61, 4–11.

LINDSTRAND, K., and STAHLBERG, K. G. (1963) On vitamin B_{12} forms in human plasma, *Acta med. scand.*, 174, 665–9.

LORBER, J. (1960) Treatment of tuberculous meningitis, *Brit. med. J.*, 1, 1309–12.

LUCAS, A. O. (1964*a*) Pneumococcal meningitis in pregnancy and the puerperium, *Brit. med. J.*, 1, 92–5.

LUCAS, A. O. (1964*b*) *Pneumococcal Meningitis in Nigerian Adults*, M.D. thesis, University of Newcastle upon Tyne.

MACFARLANE, H., *et al.* (1969) Biochemical assessment of protein-calorie malnutrition, *Lancet*, i, 392–5.

MANN, G. V., TEEL, K., HAYES, O., MCNALLY, A., and BRUNO, D. (1955) Exercise in the diposition of dietary calories. Regulation of serum lipoprotein and cholesterol levels in human subjects, *New Engl. J. Med.*, 253, 349–55.

MATTHEWS, D. M., WILSON, J., and ZILKHA, K. J. (1965) Cyanide metabolism and vitamin B_{12} in multiple sclerosis, *J. Neurol. Neurosurg. Psychiat.*, 28, 426–8.

MILLER, H. G. (1961*a*) Accident neurosis, *Brit. med. J.*, i, 919–25.

MILLER, H. G. (1961*b*) Accident neurosis, *Brit. med. J.*, i, 992–8.

MONEKOSSO, G. L., and ANNAN, W. G. T. (1964*a*) Clinical epidemiological observations on an ataxic syndrome in Western Nigeria, *Trop. geogr. Med.*, 4, 316–23.

MONEKOSSO, G. L., and ANNAN, W. G. T. (1964*b*) Pyruvate metabolism in an ataxic syndrome in Western Nigeria, *W. Afr. J. biol. Chem.*, 7, 43–6.

MONEKOSSO, G. L., ANNAN, W. G. T., and ASHBY, P. H. (1964) Therapeutic effect of vitamin B complex on an ataxic syndrome in Western Nigeria, *Trans. roy. Soc. trop. Med. Hyg.*, 58, 432–6.

MONEKOSSO, G. L., and WILSON, J. (1966) Plasma thiocyanate and vitamin B_{12} in Nigerian patients with degenerative neurological diseases, *Lancet*, i, 1062–4.

MONEY, G. L. (1959) Clinical aspects of tropical ataxic neuropathies related to malnutrition, *W. Afr. med. J.*, 8, 3–17.

MONTGOMERY, R. D. CRUICKSHANK, E. K., ROBERTSON, W. B., and MCMENEMEY, W. H. (1964) Clinical and pathological observations on Jamaican neuropathy: a report on 206 cases, *Brain*, 87, 425–62.

MOORE, D. G. F. (1934*a*) Retrobulbar neuritis and partial optic atrophy as sequelae of avitaminosis, *Ann. trop. Med. Parasit.*, 28, 295–303.

MOORE, D. G. F. (1934*b*) Retrobulbar neuritis cum avitaminosis, *W. Afr. med. J.*, 7, 119–20.

MOORE, D. G. F. (1937) Retrobulbar neuritis cum avitaminosis followed by post-partial optic atrophy—now shown to be of pellagrinous nature. Its serious incidence and its need for general investigation, *W. Afr. med. J.*, 9, 35–40.

MORLEY, D. C., WOODLAND, M., and MARTIN, N. J. (1963) Measles in Nigerian children: a study of the disease in West Africa and its manifestations in England and other countries during different epochs, *J. Hyg. (Lond.)*, 61, 135–41.

NTSEKHE, V. (1963) Observations on psychiatric problems in Basutoland, in *First Pan-African Psychiatric Conference*, 12–18 *November*, 1961, *Abeokuta*, ed. Lambo, T. A., Ibadan, pp. 234–6.

ODEKU, E. L. (1967) Congenital malformations of the cerebrospinal axis seen in Western Nigeria: the African child with 'encephalocele', *Int. Surg.*, 48, 52–62.

ODEKU, E. L. (1971) Personal communication.

ODEKU, E. L., GRANT, I. H., and EKOP, A. C. (1967) Congenital malformations of the cerebrospinal axis seen in Western Nigeria: the spinal meningoceles, *Int. Surg.*, 47, 580–96.

ODEKU, E. L., and OSUNTOKUN, B. O. (1968) The clinical neurology of Burkitt's neoplasm, a preliminary evaluation based on 105 cases, *W. Afr. med. J.*, 17, 263–7.

ODEKU, E. L., OSUNTOKUN, B. O., ADELOYE, A., and WILLIAMS, A. O. (1970) Intracranial tumours: an African series, in *Abstracts of the Second Pan-African Congress on Neurologial Sciences, 13–17 January 1970, Ibadan*, Ibadan.

OKE, O. L. (1968) Cassava as food in Nigeria, *Wld Rev. Nutr. Diet.*, 9, 227–50.

OLUWASANMI, J. O., and ALLI, A. F. (1968) Goitre in Western Nigeria, *Trop. geogr. Med.*, 20, 357–66.

OLUWOLE, I. L. (1935) On the aetiology of pellagra and allied nutritional diseases, *W. Afr. med. J.*, 8, 7–9, quoted by Clark (1935).

OSUNTOKUN, B. O. (1968) An ataxic neuropathy in Nigeria: a clinical, biochemical and electrophysiological study, *Brain*, 91, 275–48.

OSUNTOKUN, B. O. (1969) *Chronic Cyanide Intoxication and a Degenerative Neuropathy in Nigerians*. Ph.D. thesis, University of Ibadan.

OSUNTOKUN, B. O. (1970 *a*) Electrophysiological study of neuromuscular function in tropical ataxic neuropathy, *W. Afr. med. J.*, 19, 126–9.

OSUNTOKUN, B. O. (1970 *b*) Cassava diet and cyanide metabolism in Wistar rats, *Brit. J. Nutr.*, 24, 377–80.

OSUNTOKUN, B. O. (1971 *a*) The pattern of neurology in the tropics: experience at Ibadan, Nigeria, *J. neurol. Sci.*, 12, 417–42.

OSUNTOKUN, B. O. (1971 *b*) *The Neurology of Diabetes Mellitus in Nigerians*, M.D. thesis, University of London.

OSUNTOKUN, B. O. (1971 *c*) Unpublished data.

OSUNTOKUN, B. O., ADEUJA, A. O. G., and FAMILUSI, J. B. (1971) Tuberculous meningitis in Nigerians: a review of 194 patients, *Trop. geogr. Med.*, 23, 225–31.

OSUNTOKUN, B. O., and ALADETOYINBO, A. (1971) Plasma cyanide and hepatic thiosulphate: cyanide sulphur transferase activity in the tropical ataxic neuropathy, *Nig. J. Sci.*, 4, 209–30.

OSUNTOKUN, B. O., ALADETOYINBO, A., and ADEUJA, A. O. G. (1970) Free cyanide levels in tropical ataxic neuropathy, *Lancet*, ii, 372–3.

OSUNTOKUN, B. O., DUROWOJU, M. E. O., MACFARLANE, H., and WILSON, J. (1968) Plasma amino-acids in the Nigerian nutritional ataxic neuropathy, *Brit. med. J.*, 3, 647–9.

OSUNTOKUN, B. O., MONEKOSSO, G. L., and WILSON, J. (1969*a*) Relationship of a degenerative tropical neuropathy to diet: report of a field survey, *Brit. med. J.*, 1, 547–9.

OSUNTOKUN, B. O., MONEKOSSO, G. L., and WILSON, J. (1969*b*) Cassava diet and a chronic degenerative neuropathy: an epidemiology study, *Nig. J. Sci.*, 3, 3–15.

OSUNTOKUN, B. O., and ODEKU, E. L. (1970) Convulsive disorders in Nigerians: the adult epilepsies, *Afr. J. med. Sci.*, 1, 185–200.

OSUNTOKUN, B. O., ODEKU, E. L., and ADELOYE, R. B. A. (1969 *a*) Non-embolic ischaemic cerebrovascular disease in Nigerians, *J. neurol. Sci.*, 9, 361–88.

OSUNTOKUN, B. O., ODEKU, E. L., and ADELOYE, R. B. A. (1969 *b*) Cerebrovascular accidents in Nigerians: a study of 348 patients, *W. Afr. med. J.*, 18, 160–73.

OSUNTOKUN, B. O., ODEKU, E. L., and LUZZATTO, L. (1968) Pain asymbolia and congenital auditory imperception, *J. Neurol. Neurosurg. Psychiat.*, 31, 291–6.

OSUNTOKUN, B. O., ODEKU, E. L., and SINNETTE, C. H. (1969) Convulsive disorders in Nigerians: febrile convulsions, *E. Afr. med. J.*, 46, 385–94.

OSUNTOKUN, B. O., SINGH, S. P., and MARTINSON, F. D. (1970) Deafness in tropical nutritional ataxic neuropathy, *Trop. geogr. Med.*, 22, 281–8.

OSUNTOKUN, B. O., and WILLIAMS, A. O. (1970) Metal-containing proteins in Nigerian nutritional ataxic neuropathy, *Ghana med. J.*, 9, 184–6.

OSUNTOKUN, B. O., WILSON, J., LANGMAN, M. J. S., and ALADETOYINBO, A. (1970) Report of a controlled trial of hydroxocobalamin and riboflavin in Nigerian ataxic neuropathy, *J. Neurol. Neurosurg. Psychiat.*, 33, 663–6.

PEARSON, G. M. (1962) Polymyositis: clinical forms, diagnosis and therapy, *Postgrad. med. J.*, 31, 450–8.

PRINCE, R. (1961) Some notes on Yoruba native doctors and their management of mental illness, in *First Pan-African Psychiatric Conference, 12–18 November 1961, Abeokuta*, ed. Lambo, T. A., Ibadan, pp. 279–288.

RESSLER, C. (1962) Isolation and identification from common vetch of the neurotoxin B-cyano-L-alanine, a possible factor in neurolathyrism, *J. biol. Chem.*, 237, 733–5.

RESSLER, C., REDSTONE, P. A., and ERENBERG, R. H. (1961) Isolation and identification of a neuro-active factor from *Lathyrus latifolius*, *Science*, 134, 188–90.

ROBINSON, M. G., and WATSON, R. J. (1966) Pneumococcal meningitis in sickle cell anaemia, *New Engl. J. Med.*, 274, 1006–8.

SCHOBERL, A., and HAMM, R. (1948) Über der Alpha-amino-beta-Rhodanpropionsaure und über die Umsetzung zwischen Cystin und Kalium Cyanid, *Chem. Berl.*, 81, 210–14.

SCHOBERL, A., KAWOHL, M., and HAMM, R. (1951) Die Umsetzung von Cystin und Cystamin mit Kalium Cyanid ein neuer Weg in die Thiazolinchemie, *Chem. Berl.*, 84, 571–6.

SCHRAM, R. (1969) Accident services and protection in Africa, with special reference to Uganda road accidents, in *Integrating Rehabilitation in Africa*, ed. Barry, B. O., National Fund for Research into Crippling Diseases, London.

SHRANK, A. B. (1968) Autoimmune disease in Nigerians, *Lancet*, ii, 513.

SLATER, E. (1965) Diagnosis of hysteria, *Brit. med. J.*, 1, 1395–9.

SMITH, A. D. M. (1961) Retrobulbar neuritis in Addisonian pernicious anaemia, *Lancet*, 1, 1001.

SMITH, R. G., and MALCOLM, R. L. (1930) Urinary sulphur and thiocyanate excretion in cyanide poisoning, *J. Pharmacol. exp. Ther.*, 40, 457–71.

SPILLANE, J. D. (1947) *Nutritional Disorders of the Nervous System*, Edinburgh.

SPILLANE, J. D. (1969). Tropical neurology, *Proc. roy. Soc. Med.*, 62, 403–10.

TAYLOR, K. B., SMITH, H. V., and VOLLUM, R. L. (1955) Tuberculous meningitis of acute onset, *J. Neurol. Neurosurg. Psychiat.*, 18, 165–73.

TROWELL, H. C. (1960) *Non-infective Disease in Africa*, London.

WALTON, J. N., and GARDNER-MEDWIN, D. (1969) Progressive muscular dystrophy and the myotonic disorders, in *Disorders of Voluntary Muscle*. ed. Walton, J. N., London, p. 483.

WHITE, H. (1970) Lassa fever: an account of 26 cases, in *Proceedings of the Annual Scientific Conference of the Association of Physicians of Nigeria*, University of Ibadan, p. 5.

WILLIAMS, A. O., and OSUNTOKUN, B.O. (1969) Light and electron microscopy of peripheral nerves in tropical ataxic neuropathy, *Arch. Neurol.* (*Chic.*), 21, 475–92.

WILLIAMS, A. O., RESCH, J. A., and LOEWENSON, R. B. (1969) Cerebral atherosclerosis: a comparative study between Nigerian Negroes and American Negroes and Caucasians, *Neurology* (*Minneap.*), 19, 205–10.

WILSON, J. (1965) Leber's hereditary optic atrophy: a possible defect of cyanide metabolism, *Clin. Sci.*, 29, 505–15.

WILSON, J., and LANGMAN, M. J. S. (1966) Relation of subacute combined degeneration of the cord to vitamin B_{12} deficiency, *Nature* (*Lond.*), 212, 787–9.

WILSON, J., and MATTHEWS, D. M. (1966) Metabolic inter-relationships between cyanide, thiocyanate, and vitamin B_{12} in smokers and non-smokers, *Clin. Sci.*, 31, 1–7.

WOKES, F., BADENOCH, J., and SINCLAIR, H. M. (1955) Human dietary deficiency of vitamin B_{12}, *Amer. J. clin. Nutr.*, 3, 375–82.

WOKES, F., and PICARD, C. W. (1955) The role of vitamin B_{12} in human nutrition, *Amer. J. clin. Nutr.*, 3, 383–90.

WOOD, J. L., and COOLEY, S. L. (1956) Detoxication of cyanide by cystine, *J. biol. Chem.*, 218, 449–57.

17 Neurological Disorders in Uganda

J. R. BILLINGHURST

INTRODUCTION

Uganda, aptly described by the great explorer and journalist Henry Stanley as the 'pearl of Africa', lies at the heart of the continent. Though far from the sea its southern boundary is marked by the shores of Lake Victoria, the source of the River Nile, discovered by Speke in 1862.

En route Speke and his party had passed through the lush territory of Buganda, inhabited by a highly evolved tribe who impressed not only Speke but also their next white visitor, Henry Stanley. Arriving in 1875, he wrote his famous letter to the *Daily Telegraph* in London urging that missionaries should be sent out from England, a step which led to the opening up of the whole region. What is now Uganda became in 1902 a British protectorate. Subsequent constitutional developments led to the declaration of full independence within the Commonwealth in 1962 and the adoption of a republican constitution in 1967. Buganda lies at the heart of Uganda and the site of its ancient capital is now the capital city of Kampala.

The early history of the region is incomparably described by Moorehead in his book *The White Nile*.

Uganda is almost rectangular is shape and covers an area of 91 000 sq miles. The long western border with the Congo follows roughly the line of the great Western Rift system of lakes and mountains. The uplift caused by the Western Rift reversed the flow in many rivers, causing the sluggishly moving water in wide valleys to become choked with extensive papyrus swamps. It is estimated that one-fifth of Uganda is covered by water, a feature which imparts to most of the country a relatively humid and equable climate. A further moderating factor is the elevation of the land, as 84 per cent of the surface lies between 3000 and 5000 feet above sea-level.

The dry north-eastern corner is very sparsely populated by nomadic cattle people akin to those in the Northern Frontier District of Kenya. The very fertile areas around Mount Elgon in the east, along the lakeside, and in the mountainous south-west are heavily cultivated by settled tribes belonging to the great Bantu-speaking ethnic group which occupies most of the continent south to the Cape and west across the Congo basin to Cameroun. The tribes in the centre and north have some affinities with those in Sudan, and cultivate land, herd goats, or catch fish according to local circumstances. Cattle are widely distributed except in pockets in the south-east and north-west where tsetse flies abound. The local cattle are noted more for their relative resistance to certain infections (and in some breeds for their long horns) than for the volume of their milk yield.

The population is about 9½ million, almost all being of African race. The people tend to live in individual homesteads or in scattered hamlets rather than in towns, thus making it difficult to gather epidemiological data on a large scale. There are no valid vital statistics.

Although tribal and local preferences have some influence on diet, the main determining factor is climate. For the Bantu-speaking tribes living in the wetter areas the chief food item is the cooking banana or plantain, a staple containing virtually no first-class protein. The main meal would be likely to include sweet potato, brown beans and a sauce made from groundnuts. In other parts of the country millet or sorghum may be the chief item. Maize is widely cultivated. Cassava (manioc) is also widely grown as a 'famine crop' as it can stand poor soil, drought and insect attacks, but it is not regularly used as the main dietary item. Substantial amounts of animal protein are consumed by few; beef, chicken and goat's flesh are the commonest sources, whereas fish is only available to a limited group. Eggs and milk are not widely consumed. Tribal taboos limit the use of some sources of animal protein, and protein derived from vegetable sources thus assumes a heightened importance.

While severe undernutrition is seldom seen, protein-calorie malnutrition (kwashiorkor) is deplorably common in weanling infants, and not infrequent in children around the age of 6 years; when found occasionally in adults it is likely to be due to extreme poverty, alcoholism, or malabsorption.

Subsistence farming or rearing of livestock occupies the life of most Ugandans. The two great cash-crops are cotton and coffee. Tea and sugar tend to be grown on estates. Copper is the only metal mined in any considerable quantity and industrialization is still in its infancy. Wild animals survive in considerable numbers and abound in the magnificent game parks.

In the old pattern of life the individual was very much part of an extended family group and of a local community, but migratory labour, higher education, and urbanization are now breaking up these patterns. Uganda suffers less than some countries but drunkenness, sexual promiscuity, and a rising toll of neurotic illnesses are symptoms of the malaise of a society adapting itself to the world at large.

The first hospital was opened in 1897 by a missionary doctor, Sir Albert Cook. Syphilis was thought (probably incorrectly) to be a major menace at the time. Attention was soon focused on the appalling outbreak of trypanosomiasis (sleeping sickness). Both diseases, however, have shown a sharp decline in frequency since then. Malaria is hyperendemic in central Uganda, rare or unknown in the uplands. Accidents, anaemias, worms, gastroenteritis, pneumonia, tuberculosis, and gonorrhoea are all major causes of morbidity. The Government, which provides free medical services, is building an increasing number of hospitals and dispensaries, and mission or church-related hospitals still make a substantial contribution. These developments in a moderately heavily populated land with good communications are leading to a standard of patient care which compares favourably with other parts of Africa.

A vital factor in the improvement of standards has been the Makerere Medical School, an integral part of Makerere University, Kampala. Currently, 90 students are admitted each year. Clinical training actually began at Mulago Hospital, Kampala, in 1923; the new hospital, a well-equipped institution with 900 beds, was completed in 1962.

NEUROLOGICAL PRACTICE

The Neurological Clinic at Mulago Hospital was established in 1968: some 200 new patients are seen annually. Neurosurgical facilities became available in 1969, with neuroradiology evolving concurrently, although not electroencephalography. In the mid-1960s most admissions to all wards were of the acute or emergency variety, in contrast to special centres and even to other teaching hospitals in Africa, where selection affects statistics. Chronic neurological cases were usually only admitted when specific diagnostic or therapeutic procedures were necessary.

Adult neurological admissions were analysed over a 2-year period, 1966–68 (Billinghurst, 1970*b*), as part of an analysis of admissions to adult medical wards (Patel and Lwanga, 1971). A similar analysis, including children, was carried out for a 1-year period in 1965–66. The pattern of adult disorders in the two series was compared and it was found that, apart from a rise in total numbers per year from 283 to 324, the proportionate distribution between diagnoses was almost identical. Either series can therefore be compared with previously reported series from Mulago and other African centres [TABLES 17.1 and 17.2].

The patients included in the analyses were almost entirely of African race; there were no Europeans and only a handful of Asians. It is important to note this point when consideration is taken of the epidemiological significance of the odd and the rare. Furthermore, all were patients admitted into general wards or attending general outpatient clinics, and the great majority were from the lower socio-economic groups. The analyses did not include private patients who tend to come from the higher socio-economic groups; their case-notes are filed elsewhere in the hospital. Among such private patients, though few in number, there would be a disproportionately large number with diseases such as diabetes mellitus.

Table 17.1

The Changing Pattern of Neurological Admissions at Mulago Hospital

Adults and Children				*Adults only*	
1940–42[1] 2 yrs	1947–52[2] 6 yrs	1965–66 1 yr		1957[3] 1 yr	1966–68 2 yrs
104	46	—	Cases excluded	12	—
165	681	594	Total number (included)	256	648
83	114	594	Annual average	256	324
Annual Rates			*Disorder*	*Annual Rates*	
1 (1·2%)	11 (10%)	105 (18%)	All vascular disorders (except syphilis)	30 (12%)	101 (31%)
33 (40%)	29 (26%)	9 (1·5%)	Neurosyphilis	21 (8%)	13 (3·9%)
17 (21%)	33 (29%)	160 (27%)	Meningitis	118 (46%)	53 (16%)
8 (9%)	5 (4·1%)	44 (7%)	Encephalitis	12 (4·7%)	22 (7%)
6 (7%)	*4 (3·8%)	95 (16%)	Cerebral malaria	NR	28 (8%)
3 (3·6%)	8 (7%)	34 (6%)	Epilepsy	17 (7%)	32 (10%)
—	2 (1·5%)	14 (2·4%)	Intracranial tumour	2 (0·8%)	13 (3·9%)
—	1 (1·0%)	4 (0·7%)	Motor neurone disease	3 (1·2%)	7 (2·2%)
3 (3·0%)	2 (1·9%)	3 (0·5%)	Polyneuropathy	7 (2·7%)	11 (3·4%)

* *Note:* Autopsy cases only. Muwazi and Trowell (1944),[1] Hutton (1956),[2] and Shaper and Shaper (1958).[3]

For various reasons the following conditions were excluded from the published analyses before TABLES 17.1 and 17.2 were drawn up:

- 'Encephalopathy', 'poisoning', 'toxic coma', etc.
- Psychiatric and functional disturbances
- Polymyositis and pyomyositis
- Trauma and birth injury
- Tuberculosis of spine
- Tetanus
- Cerebral palsy
- Indefinite and undiagnosed disorders

Annual rates are quoted in TABLE 17.1 but the percentages are worked out from total numbers.

In order to assist in making comparisons, percentages are stated and quoted to the nearest whole number if this was 5 or more, since the figures do not have the exact accuracy of scientific measurements. Annual patient rates are also quoted to the nearest whole number.

Neurological cases accounted for approximately 10 per cent of all adult and all paediatric medical admissions in the 1965–66 analysis and for the same proportion of all adult medical admissions in the 1966–68 and 1957 analyses [TABLES 17.1 and 17·2].

The Interpretation of Symptoms and Signs

Formidable barriers of language and comprehension make difficult the evaluation of neurological symptoms and the elicitation of certain physical signs. Visits to local herbalists are likely to have preceded hospital consultation, which may be delayed until the disease process reaches an advanced stage with astonishingly florid signs. The time-scale becomes hazy as events are traced into the past, and the grossest underestimates may be given for the duration of insidiously progressive conditions. Cultural attitudes among the Bantu-speaking tribes of the south and west lead to the utmost politeness, an intense desire to please, and a submissive attitude towards pain, death, and the strange complexities of hospital life. The Nilotic and other ethnic groups of the north tend to be more abrupt, and at the same time more direct in their communications. History taking does not seem to be regarded by Ugandans as irrelevant or unwarranted; they do not expect doctors to be diviners, as do the Yorubas in Nigeria [CHAPTER 16 p. 162]. The balance of symptoms, however, may seem to the interrogator to be curiously distorted. Shame may lead to the deliberate concealment of a past or family history of tuberculosis,

Table 17.2a

Distribution of Neurological Disorders in some Centres in Sub-Saharan Africa: Geographical Comparisons Adults and Children

	Kampala Uganda 1965–66 *1 yr*	*Ibadan*[1] *Nigeria* 1957–68 *12 yrs*	*Johannesburg*[2] *S. Africa* 1957 *1 yr*
Cases excluded	—	3338	283
Total number (included)	594	6231	1101
Annual average	594	519	1101
All vascular disorders	105 (18%)	586 (9%)	287 (26%)
All infections	331 (56%)	2169 (35%)	272 (25%)
Total meningitis	160 (27%)	1310 (21%)	NR
Purulent meningitis	124 (21%)	568 (9%)	not included
Tuberculous meningitis	19 (3·2%)	315 (5%)	133 (12%)
Encephalitis	44 (7%)	335 (5%)	?24 (2·2%)
Cerebral malaria	95 (16%)	121 (1·9%)	1 (<0·1%)
Brain abscess	4 (0·7%)	78 (1·3%)	19 (1·7%)
Neurosyphilis	9 (1·5%)	46 (0·7%)	13 (1·2%)
Epilepsy	34 (6%)	702 (11%)	296 (27%)
Intracranial tumour	14 (2·4%)	—	17 (1·5%)
Motor neurone disease	4 (0·7%)	76 (1·2%)	5 (0·5%)
Spinal cord disorders (excluding tropical ataxic neuropathy)	34 (6%)	294 (4·7%)	NR
Polyneuropathy	3 (0·5%)	596 (10%)	75 (7%)
Myasthenia and muscle disorders	4 (0·7%)	47 (0·8%)	7 (0·6%)

[1] Osuntokun (1971).
[2] Reef, Lipschitz, and Block (1958).

epilepsy and madness; these diseases together with leprosy are greatly feared, far more than cancer.

The newly-arrived practitioner, most of whose patients are likely to be Baganda if he is working in Kampala, is struck by the extraordinary prevalence of such symptoms as giddiness, palpitations, and chest pains. Orley (1970 *b*) gives an excellent account of the image of the body and its functions held by Baganda. Of the symptoms which could indicate neurological disease giddiness is the commonest. It is thought to be a precursor of epilepsy. It is also recognized as a feature of anaemia, which is very common and is often associated with generalized weakness. Such generalized weakness may lead, *inter alia*, to impairment of potency in the male and since great store is set on the satisfaction of the female in sexual intercourse any degree of impotence or fear of it is a major source of anxiety. Giddiness is, therefore, a symptom with potentially disastrous consequences. Yet, although so often mentioned, it rarely has a detectable cause.

Similarly, fear that pain on the top of the head (typical of tension headache) may be an early symptom of 'spoiling' of the brain creates more anxiety and depression in an individual already afflicted with either 'Masanyalaze' (literally electricity), a useful term for paraesthesiae, is too often mentioned to be really helpfull in diagnosis. Undue sleepiness, though common, is hardly ever due to narcolepsy.

When the complainant appears to be robustly healthy and has no abnormal signs, anxiety neurosis or hypochondriacal personality is commonly inferred. (For a dynamic review of the picture of psychiatry in Uganda, see German, 1972.)

In the course of physical examination, sensory testing can be agonisingly time-consuming and inconclusive. Worse still for the neurologist is the absence of the plantar response in those (the majority) who do not wear shoes most of the time. Unlike Haddock (1963) in Tanzania, the author would not expect to find knee or ankle jerks absent in a significant proportion of casual examinations.

Table 17.2b

Distribution of Neurological Disorders in Some Centres in Sub-Saharan Africa: Geographical Comparisons Adults Only

	Kampala *Uganda* 1966–68 *2 yrs*	*Nairobi*[1] *Kenya* 1965 *0·6 yr*	*Lagos*[2] *Nigeria* 1962–67 *6 yrs*	*Natal*[3] *S. Africa* 1959–62 *3·8 yrs*
Cases excluded	—	5	450	87
Total number (included)	648	70	750	1215
Annual average	324	120	125	320
All vascular disorders	202 (31%)	19 (27%)	205 (27%)	378 (31%)
All infections	249 (38%)	32 (46%)	140 (19%)	328 (27%)
Total meningitis	106 (16%)	24 (34%)	102 (14%)	134 (11%)
Purulent meningitis	80 (12%)	19 (27%)	NR	?
Tuberculous meningitis	18 (2·8%)	5 (7%)	NR	50 (4·1%)
Encephalitis	44 (7%)	2 (2·9%)	?15 (2·0%)	23 (1·9%)
Cerebral malaria	55 (8%)	NR	NR	NR
Brain abscess	10 (1·5%)	1	NR	27 (2·2%)
Neurosyphilis	25 (3·9%)	2 (2·9%)	15 (2·0%)	106 (9%)
Epilepsy	64 (10%)	1	124 (17%)	207 (17%)
Intracranial tumour	25 (3·9%)	1	NR	9 (0·7%)
Motor neurone disease	14 (2·2%)	2 (2·9%)	—	6 (0·5%)
Spinal cord disorders (excluding tropical ataxic neuropathy)	36 (5%)	4 (6%)	109 (15%)	41 (3·4%)
Polyneuropathy	22 (3·4%)	6 (9%)	51 (7%)	6 (0·5%)
Myasthenia and muscle disorders	4 (0·6%)	NR	NR	2 (0·2%)

[1] Ojiambo (1966).
[2] Dada *et al.* (1969).
[3] Cosnett (1964).

Modes of Presentation of Illness

Of the various abnormalities of function of the nervous system the commonest are disturbed consciousness and behaviour. They are present in nearly a quarter of the adult medical admissions at Mulago Hospital.

'Acute brain syndrome' is a useful term for disturbed

behaviour or consciousness where the disturbance is of relatively acute onset and short duration. It is, of course, only a descriptive term, and corresponds roughly to 'toxic confusional state'. It nearly always has an organic basis and more often than not the primary cause lies outside the nervous system. Diagnosis and management of these cases are some of the most exacting responsibilities of a doctor in the tropics.

'Chronic brain syndrome', where the onset is more gradual and the duration longer, is also a diagnostic challenge but the urgency of the situation is less harassing.

German (1972) has drawn attention to the high frequency in Uganda of acute and chronic brain syndromes. They accounted for 46 per cent of all admissions to Butabika Mental Hospital, Kampala, and more than three-quarters of the patients were aged less than 40 years. He comments on 'the ease with which apparently trivial systemic disturbances can trigger off the typical clinical picture', and wonders whether this is the result of pre-existent subclinical brain damage from trauma, alcohol, malnutrition, or syphilis. He mentions the interesting but as yet unproved hypothesis of Cravioto and de Licardie (1968) that infantile protein-calorie malnutrition (kwashiorkor) may render the adult brain more susceptible to insult.

Acute Brain Syndrome

In adults the commonest causes of acute brain syndrome are as follows:

1. *Systemic disorders:*
   - Alcohol
   - Hypoglycaemia (often associated with alcohol)
   - Lobar pneumonia
   - Haemorrhage; shock; peripheral circulatory failure
   - Typhoid fever
   - Cholaemia
   - Uraemia
   - Hypovitaminoses.
2. *Intracranial disorders*
   - Purulent meningitis
   - Head injury and post-traumatic states
   - Cerebral malaria
   - Encephalitis
   - Subdural haematoma
   - Primary intracerebral haemorrhage and infarction
   - Epilepsy.

So commonly is hypoglycaemia suspected that intravenous hypertonic glucose is routinely administered to such patients. Dramatic, complete and sustained response is often the diagnostic and gratifying response. Unfortunately, poor response does not exclude the diagnosis; it may simply indicate irremediable delay. Such brain-damaged adults succumb speedily or survive for an unpredictable period. Prolonged alcoholic debauch is by far the commonest recognizable precipitating factor. There is widespread ignorance about the effects and dangers of alcohol, especially of illicitly distilled spirits, and acute excessive intake may prove to be rapidly fatal. Insulin overdosage is only occasionally encountered.

The signs of lobar pneumonia are only too readily missed in the early stages, especially in an uncooperative patient. At autopsy it proves to be the commonest undiagnosed cause of coma.

Typhoid fever, cirrhosis, and chronic renal disease are all commonly met with at Mulago, so hepatic and renal failure have to be considered. Pellagra is rather infrequently seen; the patient is far more likely to be an alcoholic than an exclusive maize-eater.

Intracranial causes are considered later [p. 199]. The nosological entities of cerebral malaria and encephalitis in survivors (the majority) are imprecise to a degree; it may be more accurate to speak of a febrile encephalopathy associated with malaria or an undiagnosed infection.

Chronic Brain Syndrome

Many of the conditions causing acute brain syndrome may leave residual persisting brain damage, notably alcohol, hypoglycaemia, and head injury. Chronic alcoholism, dementia paralytica (GPI), and arteriosclerotic brain disease must also be considered here. Presenile dementias are seldom diagnosed.

Historical Trends at Mulago Hospital, Kampala

TABLE 17.1, which covers a span of almost 30 years, is arranged in such a way that figures for adults and children and those for adults alone can be compared. Approximate annual rates are quoted for easy comparability. The proportion of patients with 'encephalitis' has remained fairly constant at between 4 per cent and 10 per cent. No consistent trend is discernible for meningitis or cerebral malaria. There is a gradual increase in the proportion of intracranial tumours but the numbers involved are very small. On the other hand, trends in neurosyphilis and vascular disorders are striking. Even if syphilis was overdiagnosed in the past this alone could not explain such a marked decline over the years. Vascular disorders on the other hand have shown an equally striking upward trend.

Geographical Comparisons in Sub-Saharan Africa

TABLES 17.2a and 17.2b enable comparisons to be drawn regarding the geographical distribution of neurological disorders in certain parts of sub-Saharan Africa over the past decade or so. In many respects exact comparability is not possible. For instance, the series from Ibadan and Lagos do not include intracranial tumours, which are dealt with by separate neurosurgical units. Tetanus and pyomyositis are not included in most published analyses and were therefore excluded from the table. Cerebral malaria, on the other hand, often finds a place and when it does its incidence shows striking variations. It was one of the commonest diagnoses in children at Mulago, in the year 1965–66, where it accounted for 16 per cent of all adult and childhood admissions, whereas at Ibadan the proportion was about 2 per cent and at Johannesburg there was only one case in a total of 1384. Polyneuropathies are commoner in Nigeria than elsewhere, and Nigerian ataxic neuropathy is conspicuous by its absence in reports from Kenya and Uganda. Motor neurone disease accounts for between 1 per cent and 2 per cent of all cases in many series, and myasthenia gravis and muscle disorders (other than pyomyositis) for 1 per cent or less. Everywhere neurosyphilis is seen to be infrequent, whereas vascular disorders are common; even the distribution of individual vascular conditions is similar. In these respects Uganda may be seen to be taking part in historical and geographical trends that are of continent-wide distribution.

Geographical Variations within Uganda

Meningococcal Meningitis

The far north of Uganda is just within that great belt of savannah which, lying south of the Sahara, stretches across the continent from west to east and is characterized by a long intense dry season. Geographers may sometimes apply to this region the term 'Sudan'; epidemiologists refer to it as the 'meningitis belt'. There meningococcal meningitis is endemic, and sometimes disastrously epidemic. Kampala, like most of Uganda, lies outside this belt and *Neisseria meningitidis* is only sporadically isolated at Mulago. When it is, the patient is likely to have travelled recently from the north or is in contact with someone from the endemic area.

Leprosy

Numerically, this well-known infection must rank as one of the most important of all neurological disorders in Uganda. There are about 10 000 new cases every year, 30 000 cases under treatment, and 70 000 disabled. Tuberculoid leprosy is the commonest clinical type (90 per cent of all cases), a fact which may be of great importance in view of the claim by Kinnear Brown, Stone, and Sutherland (1968) that BCG inoculation affords protection against this variety of leprosy.

Prevalence rates vary from one per thousand in the south-west to 43 per thousand in the east-central area. The prevalence is low around Kampala but the diagnosis must be constantly borne in mind in view of the number of immigrants in the city's environs.

Trypanosomiasis (*Sleeping Sickness*)

Trypanosomiasis is included because it presents as a low-grade meningo-encephalitis, fatal if not treated in its early stages. The course of the disease in *Trypanosoma gambiense* infection is relatively slow. The organism was probably introduced from the Congo around 1900 and over the next two decades caused the death of up to one-third of a million people. Compulsory evacuation of the affected areas, bush clearance, and spraying directed against the vector tsetse fly brought about the abatement of the epidemic. From the historical point of view it put Uganda 'on the map', attracting distinguished investigators to the country. The organism was first identified near Kampala in 1902 (Foster, 1970). A more acute form of the disease, due to *T. rhodesiense*, appeared in 1940 in South Busoga (on the shoreline of Lake Victoria), possibly introduced by immigrant labourers. A focus of human *T. rhodesiense* persists there, and one of *T. gambiense* in West Nile (the north-west corner of Uganda). Between 1961 and 1967, 20 to 70 cases from infected districts were confirmed each year and treated at the East African Trypanosomiasis Research Organization's centre at Tororo.

Barnley (1968), however, stated that 'over 200 new cases per year' are occurring in the South Busoga area and that 'unless effective measures are taken there is every danger of a most serious epidemic'. Resettlement of the area originally evacuated had become haphazard and bush clearance was irregular, both circumstances predisposing to the increased hazard of contact between man and infected vector.

Occasional cases are seen at Mulago Hospital. The north shore of the Kavirondo Gulf of Lake Victoria is an important focus.

Rabies

The whole of western and north-western Uganda can be regarded as an endemic area for rabies. In 1964–65 four human fatalities were reported in south-western Uganda. At that time quarantine regulations were being strictly enforced by Uganda but not by Congo or Rwanda. Immunization of dogs is strongly encouraged but probably not widely practised outside Kampala.

TABLE 17.3 shows the broad diagnostic groups in 648 patients admitted to Mulago Hospital, Kampala, during the 2 years 1966–68. Reasons have already been given for regarding the patients as fairly unselected, and representative of Uganda as a whole. There is nevertheless an inevitable lopsidedness to these figures as they deal only with admissions.

A general commentary follows.

PNEUMOCOCCAL MENINGITIS

Streptoccus pneumoniae was by far the commonest organism isolated in meningitis at Mulago (54 cases out of 80 with purulent meningitis in the 1966–68 analysis). In almost one-third more of cases no organism was identified. Possible explanations included technical

Table 17.3
Adult Neurological Admissions, Mulago Hospital, 1966–68

Main diagnostic categories	*Male*	*Female*	*Total*
Infections (including cerebral malaria)	198	51	249 (38·4%)
Vascular disorders	136	66	202 (31·2%)
Epilepsy	43	21	64 (9·9%)
Intracranial tumour	19	6	25 (3·9%)
Extrapyramidal disorders	14	3	17 (2·6%)
Motor neurone disease	11	3	14 (2·2%)
Spinal cord disorders	26	9	35 (5·4%)
Polyneuropathy	15	7	22 (3·4%)
Disorders of roots or individual nerves	8	2	10 (1·5%)
Myasthenia and muscle disorders	3	1	4 (0·6%)
Miscellaneous	4		6 (0·9%)
Total:	*477*	*171*	*648*
All medical cases	3928	2216	6144

problems and in some cases the presumed administration of an antibiotic prior to admission. The 'no organism' group differed in no important clinical or prognostic respect from the pneumococcal group.

The majority of sufferers from pneumococcal meningitis were young adults; males outnumbered females by 7 to 2. Overall mortality was 57 per cent. Kaushik (1961) noted a mortality rate of 51 per cent at Ibadan.

Unfavourable prognostic factors at Mulago were: age exceeding 60 years (all died); admission in coma (all died); the presence of concomitant pneumonia or endocarditis; delay in diagnosis after admission; and 'inadequate' initial doses of penicillin. Duration of symptoms prior to admission did not have any predictable influence on prognosis; healthy young adults may die within 2 days, while others could struggle for a week before receiving massive therapy, and yet recover. The level of CSF sugar bore no relation to prognosis.

Favourable prognostic factors were: the absence of any focus of pneumococcal infection other than the meningitis; the presence of otitis or mastoiditis; a normal CSF pressure; and normal mental state on admission. 'Adequate' penicillin dosage was a total of 12 to 24 million units daily given intramuscularly in divided doses at 2-hourly intervals. The intravenous route was not used. Chloramphenicol was only given (with the penicillin) in eight cases, five of whom perished. Intrathecal penicillin was given to one (fatal) case. Recovery when it occurred was usually gratifyingly complete.

The pattern described is very similar to that seen in the 23 cases reviewed by Hutton, Shaper, and Wilson (1962). They estimated the CSF level of penicillin between 7 and 24 hours after the initiation of therapy and established that a 2-hourly intramuscular injection of 1 million units gave a mean CSF concentration of 1 unit per ml which was well above the minimal inhibitory concentration required for most organisms tested. So a daily parenteral dose of 12 to 24 million units can be considered 'adequate' therapy without the necessity to resort to intrathecal administration, an opinion shared by most authors.

At Mulago there are insufficient data to indicate whether or not the addition of corticosteroids improves prognosis, but experience outside Africa has not been encouraging on this point. Although it is not possible to confirm the suggestion of Hutton and his colleagues that prognosis is critically influenced by mechanical factors deforming the midbrain and the vessels at the tentorial hiatus, the overwhelmingly sinister prognosis of coma is a strong pointer in that direction.

Experience in Nigeria is similar to that in Uganda (Kaushik, 1961) [Chapter 16, p. 164], even in the frequency of pneumococcal meningitis in the humid south and meningococcal meningitis in the dry north. Pneumococcal lobar pneumonia is a very common disease at Mulago. The peculiar susceptibility of the African to pneumococcal infection is well established.

Other Forms of Meningitis

Haemophilus influenzae was the commonest organism recognized in children with meningitis aged 3 years or less. It was scarcely ever seen in a child over the age of 6 years. The prognosis is rather better than that of pneumococcal meningitis (16 per cent of 37 cases died).

Tuberculous Meningitis

This occurred in approximately equal numbers in children (9 cases) and adults (10 cases) in 1965–66, and there were 18 adult cases in 1966–68. Overall mortality for adults over the 3 years was 54 per cent; childhood mortality was 33 per cent.

Amoebic Meningitis

A unique case of chronic meningitis due to an unidentified amoeba has been reported by Grundy and Blowers (1970). The clinical picture resembled that of a very low-grade tuberculous meningitis. Apart from a residual mild facial nerve palsy (lower motor neurone type) the young man made a complete recovery on prolonged chloroquine therapy and was well when last seen at the Neurological Clinic 18 months later. As the clinical picture was totally different from that of the very acute and usually fatal meningo-encephalitis reported in *Hartmanella* infections, the organism was presumed to be different. Efforts to identify it fully were not successful.

Other Organisms

These are listed by Foster and Hawgood (1966) and Mpairwe (1968). Mpairwe and Patel (1970) have described cases of cryptococcal meningitis.

POLIOMYELITIS

Acute anterior *poliomyelitis* does not figure prominently in hospital statistics. Exposure to the virus is almost certain to occur early in life and most clinically detected cases are children. The effectiveness of oral vaccine is sometimes vitiated by interference from other commonly occurring enteroviruses. In paralytic cases Huckstep (1966) found that 58 per cent were not seen by a doctor until more than 3 months after the onset of paralysis; in 36 per cent the delay was more than a year, by which time deformities were often severe. There are estimated to be 30 000 cripples with untreated paralytic poliomyelitis in Uganda. TABLE 17.4 shows how this number compares with other physically disabling conditions with a neurological basis.

Table 17.4

Main Causes of Disablement in Uganda
(after Huckstep, 1970)

Disorder	*Estimated number in Uganda*
Leprosy	70 000
Residual paralytic poliomyelitis	90 000
Cerebral palsy	20 000
Tuberculosis of bone and joint	10 000
Congenital deformities	5 000
Surviving paraplegic patients	2 000
Residual disabilities following injuries, burns, osteomyelitis, septic arthritis, amputations, etc.	
Total number of disabled patients	250 000[1]

[1] Official figure of International Labour Organization Survey.

NEUROSYPHILIS

The appalling outbreak of trypanosomiasis at the beginning of the century first put Uganda 'on the map', but a few years later it was the turn of syphilis, which Sir Albert Cook described as 'rampant everywhere'. Colonel Lambton, sent out by the Colonial Office in 1907, reported an incidence of 14 per cent and opined that there was a large epidemic of syphilis in Uganda. Foster (1970) has reviewed this historical problem and considers that those views were incorrect and that a great deal of the treponemal infection detected at that time was non-venereally transmitted syphilis or yaws.

TABLE 17.5 reveals the marked decline in the incidence of neurosyphilis over a 26-year period, from

Table 17.5

Manifestations of Neurosyphilis

Manifestation	1937–41 *5 yrs*	1960–64 *5 yrs*	1966–68 *2 yrs*
Cerebral vascular accidents	34 (31%)	6 (32%)	11 (44%)
Dementia paralytica (GPI)	18 (16%)	4 (21%)	8 (32%)
Meningitis	35 (32%)	2 (10%)	1 (4%)
Myelopathy	15 (13%)	5 (27%)	5 (20%)
Tabes dorsalis	—	1	—
All other cases	9 (8%)	1	—
Total:	*111*	*19*	*25*
Total admissions (excluding obstetric cases)	34,859	51,643	
Cases of neurosyphilis (expressed as a percentage of all admissions)	0·3%	0·036%	

40 per cent of all adult and childhood neurological admissions in 1940–42 to 1·5 per cent in 1965–66.

The manifestations of neurosyphilis recorded by Billington (1966) and by the author are summarized in TABLE 17.5. 'Syphilitic amyotrophy' is a clinical type not encountered by the author. The problem of isolated syphilitic optic atrophy is considered on page 202. No account of neurosyphilis in Africa can be complete without mention of the extreme rarity of both tabes dorsalis and the Argyll Robertson pupil.

The Mental Hospital at Kampala contains a number of chronic dements presumed to be suffering from arrested dementia paralytica (GPI). Every now and then the diagnosis is disproved at autopsy, a reminder of the probable tendency in the past to overdiagnose neurosyphilis. Maybe there is a current tendency to err in the opposite direction. In retrospective analyses occasional cases are discovered where diagnostic tests were omitted; conversely, the presence of negative tests does not exclude the diagnosis with absolute certainty.

EPILEPSY

Based on a careful study of a defined population in rural Uganda, where he lived for several months, Orly (1970*a*) estimated the prevalence of epilepsy to be between 2·1 and 3·7 per thousand. This is probably an underestimate; even so there must be at least 20 000 epileptics in Uganda.

All reports from Africa comment on the infrequency of petit mal. At Mulago temporal lobe seizures are particularly likely to be diagnosed in the psychiatric clinics. Grand mal is the commonest type encountered. There is a special risk of scalds and burns. Because of the indigenous attitudes, witnesses of a fit, far from assisting the victim, are likely to run away.

About half of the epileptics seen at the Neurological Clinic have had fits for 5 years or more. The main challenge is not the aetiology (83 per cent of cases were cryptogenic, 8 per cent post-traumatic and 8 per cent post-encephalopathic) but the management of the epilepsy. Phenobarbitone has proved to be the drug of choice in most cases; it need only be taken twice a day, and to 'stabilized' patients it can safely be prescribed in considerable quantities, up to 2000 of the 30 mg tablets at a time, thus reducing congestion in the Clinic and time and cost of travel (Billinghurst, 1970*a*). An initial follow-up rate of 83 per cent is being maintained and most patients who can be convinced of the vital importance of regular, unbroken, long-term therapy have had marked reduction or cessation of fits.

In the long term we need a change in the indigenous attitudes towards epilepsy which, associating it with bewitchment, contagiousness, dementia and incurability, currently make it one of the most feared and psychosocially disabling of all common diseases.

INTRACRANIAL TUMOURS

At Mulago facilities for the pathological examination of tumours preceded neurosurgery by many years.

During the 13-year period 1953–65 (Billinghurst, 1966) there were 52 histologically proved intracranial tumours; 28 were primary tumours, four were metastases, and 20 were direct extensions from extracranial sites. Over the same period primary tumours were found at autopsy in four patients from the Kampala Mental Hospitals. Fifty-four per cent of all these primary tumours were gliomas; 16 per cent were meningiomas [TABLE 17.6]. As predicted there has been a sharp rise in numbers since then. In the period 1965–70 Bailey (1971) found 85 primary tumours of which 72 were histologically verified and the remainder presumed on good clinical grounds. Numbers are too

Table 17.6

Intracranial Tumours at Mulago Hospital 1935–1965

Primary Intracranial Tumours	*No. of Cases*
Glioma, all types	17 (54%)
Meningioma	5 (16%)
Craniopharyngioma	3
Pituitary adenoma: chromophobe 1, eosinophil 1	2
Acoustic neuroma	2
Medulloblastoma	2
Malignant tumour of fourth ventricle, type undetermined	1
Total:	*32*
Intracranial Metastases Sources:	
Carcinoma of bronchus	2
Primary hepatoma	1
Pleural mesothelioma	1
Embryonal sarcoma	1
Total:	*5*
Direct Extensions	
Burkitt's lymphoma	9
Carcinoma or sarcoma of nasopharynx	3
Retinoblastoma	3
Adult malignant lymphoma involving skull	2
Carcinoma of ethmoid	1
Sarcoma of eye	1
Metastasis in skull from carcinoma of bronchus	1
Total:	*20*

small to point up any differences in the less common tumours.

In the period 1954–60 primary tumours of the 'brain and other parts of the nervous system' accounted for 1·3 per cent (23 cases) of all tumours in males and 0·8 per cent (9 cases) of all tumours in females recorded in the Kampala Cancer Registry (Davies, Knowelden, and Wilson, 1965). This could be compared with a London series (Davies, 1961) where the brain was the primary site in 1·9 per cent of all tumours in males and 1·1 per cent of all tumours in females. This would suggest that in relation to other neoplasms brain tumours occur almost as frequently in Kampala as in London.

Over the 5-year period 1957–61 Jackson and Okubadejo (1963) noted 13 primary brain tumours in 3489 autopsies at University College Hospital, Ibadan, a rate of 0·37 per cent which is close to the Mulago figure of 0·43 per cent. If primary cerebral tumours are uncommon at Kampala, confirmed metastases are positively rare. From 1953 to 1965 there were only four from Mulago and one from the Mental Hospitals. The primary site in two was the bronchus, a tumour seldom seen in Uganda: only one came from the liver, a very common primary site. Since many patients with advanced malignant disease are either not admitted or not autopsied, the true incidence of metastases may be higher.

In the 5-year period 1961–65 there were 29 intracranial abscesses, and fracture of the skull was the commonest cause; 76 per cent of the patients died (Billinghurst, 1966). Between 1953 and 1965 there were no histologically verified cases of cerebral gumma, tuberculoma or parasitic cysts.

THE NERVOUS SYSTEM IN BURKITT'S LYMPHOMA

Burkitt's lymphoma, of which the characteristic cell is a poorly differentiated lymphoid cell, was first described by Burkitt in Uganda (Burkitt, 1958). It was subsequently found to be of worldwide distribution, but it is predominantly a neoplasm of the African continent; only in Papua and New Guinea is it as common as in Africa. Burkitt's lymphoma has several unique features: it is the commonest childhood tumour in Uganda, Nigeria, Papua, and New Guinea; in Africa it is practically confined to areas where the mean temperature of the coolest month does not fall below 15°C or 59°F or where the annual rainfall is not less than 500 mm or about 20 inches (Haddow, 1963); it commonly presents with easily detectable multicentric swellings in one or more quadrants of the jaws or in the orbits or ovaries; in its earlier stages it responds dramatically to treatment with cytotoxic drugs. Its immune mechanisms, its possible relationship to a virus infection, with or without an insect vector, and the role of reticulo-endothelial system response to tropical infections, notably malaria—these are current topics of intense international research and interest (Burkitt, 1969; Kafuko and Burkitt, 1970).

The involvement of the jaws, orbits and ovaries confers upon it in Africa its clinically distinctive features. Most of the victims are of African race but the condition is not confined to them. Nor is involvement of the organs confined to the sites mentioned; many others are liable to attack, such as deep lymph nodes, bones, abdominal viscera, thyroid and even breasts. There is a curious tendency for superficial lymph nodes to escape (Wright, 1964).

Involvement of the nervous system is a serious prognostic feature. In Uganda surveillance is organized at the Lymphoma Treatment Centre, an 18-bed research ward which was set up at Kampala in 1967 in affiliation with the Makerere Medical School. Prospective studies at the Centre are delineating more exactly the neurological features of the tumour and especially the frequency and significance of tumour cells in the CSF (Ziegler *et al.*, 1970). The pattern in Uganda is similar to that reported in Nigeria (Janota, 1966; Odeku and Osuntokun, 1968) and Kenya (Clifford *et al.*, 1967; Frank, 1968). At least one-third of all patients can be expected to present with, or to develop, some neurological abnormality, usually one or more of the following: myelopathy; cranial neuropathy; disturbance of consciousness or mental state. The presence of Burkitt tumour cells in the CSF (malignant pleocytosis) has a profound effect on prognosis and choice of chemotherapy.

Myelopathy

This may vary from a mild paraparesis with absent or minimal sensory involvement to a complete flaccid paraplegia, with a sensory level and sphincter paralysis. The thoracic cord is most commonly affected, but no part is exempt. The clinical picture is not distinctively different from other examples of cord compression, and if there are no evident tumour masses diagnosis may be delayed. Preceding back pain or root pain is not often described.

Multiple Cranial Neuropathy

The nerves most commonly affected are the oculomotor (third, fourth, and sixth) and the facial; less frequent are lesions of the second, fifth, ninth and twelfth nerves. In the majority there is an obvious tumour in the jaws or orbits but this is not invariable.

Disturbance of Consciousness and Mental State

Mental dullness, apathy and drowsiness, or alternatively and less commonly undue restlessness and irritability, are mentioned in all reports. They form, in fact, the most frequent symptom group in the series from Kenya. These features, together with headache, are well recognized in meningeal leukaemia, and they led Frank to infer that a similar process is occurring in Burkitt's lymphoma.

Convulsions, neck stiffness and focal cerebral symptoms may also occur.

Meticulous examination of the CSF for tumour cells was carried out by Ziegler and his colleagues (1970) in a prospective study. It is the critical investigation which demonstrates whether or not the neoplasm has crossed the blood–brain barrier—information which is essential when assessing the necessity for intrathecal therapy and the long-term therapeutic response. Their paper should be consulted for the technical details.

Malignant pleocytosis may occur in patients in any of the above clinical groups or it may be asymptomatic. Its prognostic import is so sinister that patients with it are placed in the most advanced staging of the disease, whether or not other neurological abnormalities are present. Ziegler and his colleagues find, however, that the majority of patients presenting with paraplegia or cranial neuropathy in the absence of malignant pleocytosis subsequently develop malignant cells in the CSF. It is now their policy to place all such patients in the most advanced staging group.

The floor of the middle or posterior fossa of the skull may be eroded directly or tumour cells may spread along cranial nerves or blood vessel coverings to reach the intracranial space. Janota (1966) has drawn attention to the frequent involvement of the trigeminal ganglion and pituitary gland. The CSF is reached by direct spread across dura and arachnoid. Ziegler and Bluming (1971) have put forward the concept of tumour cells finding in extradural sites a sanctuary from the effects of systemic cytotoxic drugs and immune cytolytic processes, and subsequently seeding the CSF to cause relapses. Discrete intracranial masses are unusual; they are known or presumed to be associated with dural involvement. Microscopic invasion of the brain from the subarachnoid space along the Virchow-Robin spaces is noted (Wright, 1964) and accounted for the nine cases in the author's series (1966). It is presumed that meningeal involvement explains the alterations of consciousness and mental state. Tumour cells are only sometimes present in the CSF in such cases.

Myelographic and pathological evidence indicates that in some patients the myelopathic process is an extradural compression of the cord by direct spread from an osseous focus or from a paravertebral deposit through neural foramina (Cockshott and Evans, 1963). In others it is cord ischaemia due to obstruction of radicular arteries by retroperitoneal or retropleural tumour (Wright, 1964).

Treatment

The treatment of choice is chemotherapy rather than surgery unless it is a question of removing a large accessible tumour mass. Surgical decompression of the cord is not recommended. Current views on the best chemotherapy are undergoing rapid change. Experience at the Lymphoma Treatment Centre indicates that the best regime evolved so far is to give a systemic course of cyclophosphamide with or without sequential courses of vincristine, methotrexate and cytosine arabinoside, and at the same time to administer intrathecally a 4-day course of methotrexate or cytosine arabinoside. Striking remissions are achieved but delayed relapse occurs in the majority and it remains to be seen whether true cure has been achieved in the majority of 'long-term' survivors (Ziegler and Bluming, 1971).

SPINAL CORD DISORDERS

Most of the recognized disorders have been seen in Uganda but there are certain peculiarities to note.

Tuberculous disease of the spine is an important cause of paraplegia, although it is not nearly so common as at Ibadan; the outlook in most cases is hopeful. *Spinal syphilis*, seldom recognized, presents as a vascular episode or as slowly progressive paraplegia; *tabes dorsalis* is of the utmost rarity.

Subacute combined degeneration is rarely seen; this is a reflection of the rarity of vitamin B_{12} deficiency which, when it does occur, is unlikely to be due to Addisonian pernicious anaemia.

Burkitt's lymphoma is the commonest cause of paraplegia in children.

While *syringomyelia* and *syringobulbia* are extremely rare, *various anomalies of the foramen magnum region* have recently been recognized.

Cervical spondylosis is one of the commonest causes of cervical myelopathy but purely radicular syndromes are oddly uncommon. Lumbar disc protrusion is quite frequently diagnosed by surgical colleagues and severe cauda equina involvement by multiple disc protrusions has been confirmed by laminectomy.

Spinal arachnoiditis (arachnoid adhesions) is one of the commoner recognized causes of myelopathy although its aetiology is obscure. The clinical, CSF and radiological features are often so strongly suggestive of a tumour that diagnosis is only made at laminectomy. Suspicious clinical features include a comparatively rapid onset followed by non-progression of symptoms, the absence of back pain, and asymmetrical distribution of signs. Myelography rarely shows the allegedly diagnostic pattern. Histological examination of tissue removed yields no clue as to aetiology. Surgery seldom helps the patient. There is no evidence that the condition is due to tuberculosis, trauma, subarachnoid haemorrhage or meningitis. Past syphilis cannot be excluded.

The tropical ataxic neuropathy of Nigeria is not seen at Mulago and probably nowhere else in Uganda, where cassava, although widely grown as a 'famine crop', is not regularly consumed in great quantities.

Obscure myelopathies of acute or chronic development are seen. The chronic variety, in which the pyramidal tract is predominantly involved, resembles the spastic type described in Jamaica but is completely unlike the ataxic neuropathy of Nigeria. Affected patients in Uganda do not show stigmata of nutritional deficiency or systemic disease. The acute variety ('acute transverse myelitis') often presents as a disastrously severe episode and the spinal cord, if obtainable, shows central necrosis identical to that described by Hughes (1966). The aetiology of both types of myelopathy is bafflingly obscure.

Schistosomiasis involving the cord, although unlikely, cannot be completely excluded. The only fluke likely to be present in the indigenous people is *Schistosoma mansoni*, apart from a pocket of *S. haematobium* in Lango District. Infection rates and degree of parasitization are low in the environs of Kampala. In the 1966–68 analysis none of the 10 patients with obscure myelopathy came from an area of high endemicity. Eosinophilia occurred in the blood of a few but in the CSF of none. Stool examinations were negative. Whether *S. mansoni* is ever a cause of myelopathy in an area of high endemicity, such as the West Nile District, is not known but the possibility has been suggested (Williams and Williams, 1968).

POLYNEUROPATHIES

Compared with other parts of Africa, polyneuropathies constitute a rather small proportion of patients with neurological diseases at Mulago. This may be due to the infrequency of nutritional deficiency as compared with Tanzania (Ebrahim and Haddock, 1964) and Nigeria [CHAPTER 16, p. 186].

The commonest identified type is *acute 'infective' polyneuritis* (Guillain-Barré syndrome) both in the author's series and in those of Hutton for 1947–52 and the Shapers for 1957. It merges with subacute obscure polyneuropathies which constitute the next largest group.

Alcoholic neuropathy is surprisingly uncommon. Muwazi and Trowell (1944) ascribed this to the fact that local beers were consumed with yeast but this explanation would not fit the drinkers of (locally) distilled spirits. Since thiamine deficiency, in the absence of alcoholism, is also an uncommon cause of neuropathy here, one can only conclude that the average local diet is adequate in this respect. Pellagra, alcohol-induced rather than dietary, is not uncommon.

INH-induced neuropathy is rarely seen. This is ascribed both to avoidance of excessive dosage (the optimum daily dose being 300 mg) and to the presence in the majority of the population of genetically determined rapid INH-inactivators (Patel, 1970).

Diabetic neuropathy is usually mild and relatively symptomless. In an outpatient series of 79 diabetics seen by the author there was absence or impairment of ankle jerks in 68 per cent, knee jerks in 62 per cent, vibration sense in 47 per cent, and superficial pain in 23 per cent. Weakness was rare and mononeuritis and autonomic involvement absent (apart from impotence in males.) Chronic pancreatic disease accounts for about 10 per cent of diabetes but the neuropathy is similar.

OPTIC NEURITIS AND OPTIC ATROPHY

Acute optic neuritis is seldom seen in the Department of Ophthalmology at Mulago and its aetiology [TABLE 17.7] is usually not determined (Emiru, 1970). A recognized occasional cause is poisoning by methyl alcohol, an accidental adulterant in local brews (*enguli*). The onset of blindness is sudden, or blindness is noticed on emergence from stupor or coma. At this stage there is often some degree of papilloedema, followed later by optic atrophy. Recovery of sight is variable. Acute retrobulbar neuritis as a manifestation of either multiple sclerosis or neuromyelitis optica (Devic's disease) has not been reported in Uganda. Recently, however, the author saw a woman with retrobulbar neuritis and other neurological features compatible with an acute and partially reversible demyelinating disorder affecting the optic nerves and cerebral hemispheres.

Table 17.7
Causes of Simple Optic Atrophy

Cause	No.
Suspected methyl alcohol (from history)	8
Pituitary tumours (mainly chromophobe adenoma)	6
Suspected syphilis (positive serological test but without other neurological signs)	6
Orbital space-occupying lesion	2
Onchocerciasis	2
Encephalitis	1
Cerebral berry aneurysm	1
Trauma	1
Foster-Kennedy syndrome	1
Undetermined	9
Total:	37

In a personal series of 37 cases of optic atrophy Emiru has noted a variety of causes similar to those seen elsewhere. It is gross visual, rather than endocrine, disturbance which brings a patient with a pituitary tumour to hospital and by then the tumour may be massive. The role of syphilis is uncertain and the occurrence of isolated optic neuritis must be presumed since other neurological features are invariably absent. Onchocerciasis can affect all parts of the eye including the optic nerve. The vector fly, *Simulium*, lives near fast-flowing streams and rivers and is found mainly around Mount Elgon on the Kenya border, by the banks of the Nile just below its source, and all along the western border of the country where up to 100 per cent of the population at risk are infected.

In almost one-quarter of Emiru's 37 cases no cause for the optic atrophy could be determined. Thus, Uganda shares with other countries the problem of 'tropical amblyopia'. The absence of other neurological symptoms or signs in such cases in Uganda precludes the likelihood of tropical ataxic neuropathy.

MISCELLANEOUS DISORDERS

Parkinsonism is often seen: it is not possible to give a valid estimate of its prevalence. Contrary to Hutton's experience in 1947–52, *rheumatic (Sydenham's) chorea* is quite commonly seen in children and occasionally in adults, especially young pregnant women (chorea gravidarum). Sharing the same aetiological basis, chronic carditis is one of the commonest forms of heart disease encountered. On the other hand *Huntington's chorea*, noted by Hutton (1956), has not subsequently been identified in Africans.

Motor neurone disease is in all respects 'classical', with onset in middle life, a spectrum of cord and bulbar involvement and a natural history similar to that seen elsewhere. Abnormally young age at onset is not noted.

Myasthenia gravis presents a clinical profile similar to that noted elsewhere; the purely ocular form is seen (Singh, 1964) as well as the more generalized form.

Of the *muscular dystrophies* seen the most frequent is the pseudohypertrophic type of Duchenne, the clinical picture of which in Uganda is not unusual. Between one and four new cases are seen annually. Limb-girdle muscular dystrophy is occasionally seen but the facioscapulohumeral type has not been recognized by the author. *Dystrophia myotonica* and *myotonia congenita* have not been noted.

Peroneal muscular atrophy (Charcot-Marie-Tooth) and *Friedreich's and other hereditary ataxias* have not been recognized in Uganda in typical form. The missing disease which arouses the greatest degree of interest, however, is *multiple sclerosis*. It has not been seen in a person of African race in Uganda. Yet the author has seen five Europeans and two Asians who have developed a first or subsequent episode of this disease in Uganda, proof that it is not the tropical environment itself which provides absolute protection.

Trigeminal neuralgia and *Ménière's disease* are rare. *Bell's palsy* is common, as are *neuralgic amyotrophy*, and *compression syndromes of radial, median and ulnar nerves*.

NEUROLOGICAL DISORDERS IN CHILDREN

Children constitute about 40 per cent of the patients attending Mulago Hospital (and probably most hospitals in the tropics).

The pattern of childhood neurological admissions (307 cases) at Mulago over the course of a year (1965–66) has been analysed by the author. As with adults, the distortion which is inevitable when attention is directed only towards inpatients can to some extent be rectified by drawing on experience gained by the analysis of 138 children seen over the course of a year 1968–69) at the Paediatric Neurology Clinic at Mulago (Egdell and Stanfield, 1972). Three-quarters of the children attending this clinic were aged less than 5 years and the commonest reason for attendance was failure to achieve expected physical or mental development for age.

TABLE 17.8 shows the distribution of disorders seen in hospital inpatients. Infections (79 per cent) play an overwhelming role and fall mainly within three groups: meningitis (120 cases), cerebral malaria (82), and encephalitis (24).

Table 17.8
Childhood Neurological Admissions, Mulago Hospital, 1965–66

Disorder	*No. of cases*	
All infections	243 (79%)	
Meningitis		*120*
Encephalitis		*24*
Cerebral malaria		*82*
Brain abscess		*1*
Cavernous sinus thrombosis		*1*
Poliomyelitis (new)		*11*
(old)		*4*
Vascular disorders	17	
Epilepsy	8	
Intracranial tumour	1	
Extrapyramidal disorders (rheumatic chorea)	2	
Infantile cerebral palsy	3	
Congenital disorders	27	
Hydrocephalus		*20*
Spina bifida manifesta		*7*
Acute transverse myelitis	1	
Miscellaneous	5	
Total:	*307*	

Detailed information concerning meningitis is given in TABLE 17.9. Of the 37 cases of *Haemophilus influenzae* meningitis 22 (60 per cent) were aged less than 1 year and a further 8 were between 1 and 2 years; one was aged 6 and another 8 years. As with adults, the poor prognosis of pneumococcal infection is evident. Tuberculosis does not figure as prominently as in some centres in Africa.

Cerebral malaria was the diagnosis made in a child with high fever, cerebral disturbance, malarial parasitaemia, normal CSF, and either a rapid and complete response to antimalarial therapy or a rapid progress to death. Of 82 children with this diagnosis 18 died (22 per cent). From birth to the age of 5 years children living in a hyperendemic area (such as the environs of Mulago) are susceptible to this virulent complication. Susceptibility then decreases, due to acquired immunity, until by adult life the victims are almost all immigrants from non-malarious areas.

Table 17.9

Meningitis in Children

Organism	*No. of cases*		*Mortality*
Haemophilus influenzae	37		6 (16%)
Streptococcus pneumoniae	18		12 (67%)
Other specified organisms:	7		2
Esch. coli		*2*	
Non-haemolytic streptococcus		*2*	
Klebsiella		*1*	
Micrococcus		*1*	
Citrobacter		*1*	
Purulent CSF, no organism identified	37		13 (35%)
Mycobacterium tuberculosis	9		3 (33%)
Lymphocytic CSF (? viral)	9		1

Encephalitis was diagnosed when a child had moderate fever, diffuse cerebral disturbance (with or without fits) and a tendency to survive; malarial parasites were absent and the CSF was either normal or showed a slight excess of lymphocytes. It was associated with measles in 7 cases and with pertussis in 3. Recorded residual defects included mental retardation (4 cases), hemiplegia (2), and choreo-athetosis (1).

The diagnostic problems posed in encephalitis in adults are well known. The problem is even greater in children in whom convulsions and mental disturbance may be due to high fever alone without primary brain disease; virus isolation is so infrequently achieved as to make no useful contribution in the majority of cases. The problem is greatest in cerebral malaria, the specific pathology of which can only be proved at autopsy; in a child the presence of malarial parasitaemia does not prove the existence of this pathological process within the brain and *per contra* the absence of parasitaemia does not disprove its existence if the child has very recently received antimalarial therapy.

Stanfield (1969), recently reviewing this entire problem, has quoted the analysis of Patel (1971) who looked into a series of 117 children at Mulago Hospital with fever, convulsions and altered consciousness observed over a 9-month period in 1967–68. Eight children had a recognizable condition, e.g. meningitis. The remainder were divided into two groups; 80 cases with normal CSF cell counts (less than 5 per c mm), and 29 with CSF pleocytosis. Although age distribution and mortality rates were the same in the two groups, the children with normal CSF cell counts had a short-lived fever, convulsions only while febrile, a brief stay in hospital, no neurological signs, and in a few who died no evidence of primary brain disease, whereas the children with CSF pleocytosis had a longer illness, persisting neurological signs and liability to fits after defervescence of fever, and autopsy evidence of cerebral malaria in two and of encephalitis in two.

It would be rash to conclude that a normal CSF cell count excludes encephalitis or cerebral malaria in a child, but it does emphasize the difficulties of attaching precise diagnostic labels. Stanfield suggests the term 'febrile encephalopathy' to cover the whole spectrum of these disorders. Whereas there is no specific drug for encephalitis, it is vital to give chloroquine to all children who are febrile in an endemic or sporadic malarious area and particularly to those who are convulsing or whose consciousness is disturbed.

Retrospective perusal of the clinical notes gave little indication as to the amount and degree of residual damage from 'febrile encephalopathy'. Egdell and Stanfield found that of 132 brain-damaged children seen in their Paediatric Neurology Clinic 21 (16 per cent) were apparently normally developed until they were struck by a catastrophic illness of the type described above.

A form of encephalitis mainly localized to the cerebellum ('acute cerebellitis') has been seen by the author and others in children and young adults. The clinical picture is one of dysarthria and ataxia of limbs and trunk, with acute onset and moderate to complete recovery. The local people recognize the natural history and prognosis and their accounts suggest an infective aetiology.

Vascular disorders (17) constitute less than 6 per cent of the inpatient group. Of the 14 children with non-embolic cerebral infarction 5 had homozygous sickle-cell disease, 4 were associated with high fever (cause undiagnosed), 2 followed meningitis, 1 followed vaccination, 1 was associated with severe dehydration, and in 1 no cause could be found.

Cerebral palsy, mental subnormality and behaviour disorders were common problems in the Clinic. Malnutrition was evident in 12 patients. In only three was kernicterus believed to be an aetiological factor, in marked contrast to experience at Lagos, where the cause of cerebral palsy in 97 (50 per cent) of 196 children was ascribed to kernicterus (Animashaun, 1971).

Of the developmental defects of the nervous system encountered in children, congenital hydrocephalus and spina bifida manifesta were the ones noted in the inpatient analysis. There has been no systematic survey of the various other defects.

CONCLUDING REMARKS

Among the most striking features which emerge from a review of the picture of neurology as seen in Uganda are the frequency of 'organic' causes of disturbed behaviour and consciousness, the rising tide of cerebral vascular disorders, the decline of neurosyphilis, the appalling prognosis of pneumococcal meningitis, the therapeutic and psychosocial deprivations of epileptics, the absence of multiple sclerosis, and the problem of the aetiology of obscure myelopathies.

References

ANIMASHAUN, A. (1971) Aetiology of cerebral palsy in African children, *Afr. J. med. Sci.*, 2, 165.

BAILEY, I. C. (1971) The pattern and presentation of intracranial tumours in Uganda, *E. Afr. med. J.*, 48, 565.

BARNLEY, G. R. (1968) Resettlement in the South Busoga sleeping sickness area, *E. Afr. med. J.*, 45, 263.

BILLINGHURST, J. R. (1966) Intracranial space-occupying lesions in African patients at Mulago Hospital, Kampala, *E. Afr. med. J.*, 43, 385.

BILLINGHURST, J. R. (1970*a*) Epilepsy challenged: 15 months' experience in the Neurological Clinic, Mulago Hospital, *E. Afr. med. J.*, 47, 288.

BILLINGHURST, J. R. (1970*b*) The pattern of adult neurological admissions to Mulago Hospital, Kampala, *E. Afr. med. J.*, 47, 653.

BILLINGTON, W. R. (1966) Neurosyphilis in Uganda: a comparison of two five-year periods, *E. Afr. med. J.*, 43, 469.

BROWN, J. A. K., STONE, M. M., and SUTHERLAND, I. (1968) BCG vaccination of children against leprosy in Uganda: results at end of second follow-up, *Brit. med. J.*, 1, 24.

BURKITT, D. P. (1958) A sarcoma involving the jaws in African children, *Brit. J. Surg.*, 46, 218.

BURKITT, D. P. (1969) Etiology of Burkitt's lymphoma—an alternative hypothesis to a vectored virus, *J. nat. Cancer Inst.*, 42, 19.

CLIFFORD, P., SINGH, S., STJERNSWÄRD, J., and KLEIN, G. (1967) Long-term survival of patients with Burkitt's lymphoma: an assessment of treatment and other factors which may relate to survival, *Cancer Res.*, 27, 2578.

COCKSHOTT, W. P., and EVANS, K. T. (1963) Childhood paraplegia in lymphosarcoma (Burkitt's tumour), *Brit. J. Radiol.*, 36, 914.

COSNETT, J. E. (1964) Neurological disorders in the Zulu, *Neurology (Minneap.)*, 14, 443.

CRAVIOTO, J., and DE LICARDIE, E. R. (1968) in *Malnutrition, Learning and Behaviour*, ed. Scrimshaw, N. S., and Gordon, J. E., Cambridge, Mass.

DADA, T. O., JOHNSON, F. A., ARRABA, A. B., and ADEGBITE, S. A. (1969) Cerebrovascular accidents in Nigerians: a review of 205 cases, *W. Afr. med. J.*, 18, 95.

DAVIES, J. N. P. (1961) The pattern of African cancer in Uganda, *E. Afr. med. J.*, 38, 486.

DAVIES, J. N. P., KNOWELDEN, J., and WILSON, B. A. (1965) Incidence rates of cancer in Kyadondo County, Uganda, 1954–1960, *J. nat. Cancer Inst.*, 35, 789.

EBRAHIM, G. J., and HADDOCK, D. R. W. (1964) Polyneuropathy of probable nutritional origin in Dar-es-Salaam, Tanganyika, *Trans. roy. Soc. Med. Hyg.*, 58, 246.

EGDELL, H. G., and STANFIELD, J. P. (1972) Paediatric neurology in Africa: a Ugandan report, *Brit. med. J.*, 1, 548.

EMIRU, V. P. (1970) Causes of simple optic atrophy at Mulago Hospital, personal communication.

FOSTER, W. D. (1970) *The Early History of Scientific Medicine in Uganda*, East African Literature Bureau, Kampala.

FOSTER, W. D., and HAWGOOD, B. C. (1966) The aetiology and laboratory diagnosis of meningitis in Kampala, Uganda, *E. Afr. med. J.*, 43, 309.

FRANK, G. L. (1968) Involvement of the nervous system in Burkitt's tumour, in *Cancer in Africa*, eds. Clifford, P., Linsell, C. A., and Timms, G. L., Nairobi.

GERMAN, G. A. (1972) Psychiatric syndromes, in *A Companion to Medical Studies in East Africa*, eds. Shaper, A. G., Hutt, M. S. R., and Kibukamusoke, J. W., London.

GRUNDY, R., and BLOWERS, R. (1970) A case of primary amoebic meningoencephalitis treated with chloroquine, *E. Afr. med. J.*, 47, 153.

HADDOCK, D. R. W. (1963) Neurological signs in African patients without overt neurological disease, *E. Afr. med. J.*, 40, 601.

HADDOW, A. J. (1963) An improved map for the study of Burkitt's lymphoma syndrome in Africa, *E. Afr. med. J.*, 40, 429.

HUCKSTEP, R. L. (1966) Orthopaedic problems in East Africa, *J. roy. Coll. Surg. Edinb.*, 11, 206.

HUCKSTEP, R. L. (1970) The cripple in Africa, *Makerere med. J.* 14, 9.

HUGHES, J. T. (1966) *Pathology of the Spinal Cord*, London.

HUTTON, P. W. (1956) Neurological disorders in Uganda, *E. Afr. med. J.*, 33, 209.

HUTTON, P. W., SHAPTER, A. G., and WILSON, A. M. M. (1962) Acute pneumococcal meningitis: the significance of mechanical factors in influencing mortality, *Trans. roy. Soc. trop. Med. Hyg.*, 56, 149.

JACKSON, J. G., and OKUBADEJO, O. A. (1963) A review of intracranial tumours seen in necropsies at the University College Hospital, Ibadan, Nigeria, between 1957 and 1961, *W. Afr. med. J.*, 12, 251.

JANOTA, I. (1966) Involvement of the nervous system in malignant lymphoma in Nigeria, *Brit. J. Cancer*, 20, 47.

KAFUKO, G. W., and BURKITT, D. P. (1970) Burkitt's lymphoma and malaria, *Int. J. Cancer*, 6, 1.

KAUSHIK, S. C. (1961) The pattern of neurological disease in Ibadan, in *First Pan-African Psychiatric Conference, 12–18 November, 1961, Abeokuta*, ed. Lambo, T. A., Ibadan, p. 78.

MONEKOSSO, G. L., and ASHBY, P. H. (1963) The natural history of an amblyopia syndrome in Western Nigeria, *W. Afr. med. J.*, 12, 226.

MPAIRWE, Y. (1968) Salmonella meningitis in Kampala, *E. Afr. med. J.*, 45, 581.

MPAIRWE, Y., and PATEL, K. M. (1970) Cryptococcal meningitis in Mulago Hospital, Kampala, *E. Afr. med. J.*, 47, 445.

MUWAZI, E. M. K., and TROWELL, H. C. (1944) Neurological disease among African natives of Uganda, a review of 269 cases, *E. Afr. med. J.*, 21, 2.

ODEKU, E. L., and OSUNTOKUN, B. O. (1968) The clinical neurology of Burkitt's neoplasm: a preliminary evaluation based on 105 cases, *W. Afr. med. J.*, 17, 263.

OJIAMBO, H. P. (1966) Neurological disease at Kenyatta National Hospital, Nairobi: a retrospective study of 75 cases, *E. Afr. med. J.*, 43, 366.

ORLEY, J. H. (1970*a*) Epilepsy in Uganda (rural): a study of 83 cases, *Afr. J. med. Sci.*, 1, 155.

ORLEY, J. H. (1970*b*) *Culture and Mental Illness: A Study from Uganda*, Nairobi.

OSUNTOKUN, B. O. (1971) The pattern of neurological illness in tropical Africa: experience at Ibadan, Nigeria, *J. neurol. Sci.*, 12, 417.

PATEL, A. M. (1970) Personal communication.

PATEL, C. C. (1971) Acute febre encephalopathy in Ugandan children, *Afr. J. med. Sci.*, 2, 135.

PATEL, K. M., and LWANGA, S. K. (1971) A study of medical admissions to Mulago Hospital, Kampala (June 1966 to May 1968), *E. Afr. med. J.*, 48, 76.

REEF, H., LIPSCHITZ, R., and BLOCK, J. (1958) Neurological disorders at Baragwanath Hospital: a survey, *Med. Proc.*, 4, 292.

SHAPER, A. G., and SHAPER, L. (1958) Analysis of medica, admissions to Mulago Hospital, 1957, *E. Afr. med. J.* 35, 647.

SINGH, J. S. (1964) Myasthenia gravis in a Musoga girl (case report), *E. Afr. med. J.*, 41, 535.

STANFIELD, J. P. (1969) Fever in children in the tropics, *Brit. med. J.*, 1, 761.

WILLIAMS, E. H., and WILLIAMS, P. H. (1968) Bilharzia in the West Nile District, *Uganda Practit.*, 1, 110.

WRIGHT, D. H. (1964) Burkitt's tumour: a post-mortem study of 50 cases, *Brit. J. Surg.*, 51, 245.

ZIEGLER, J. L., BLUMING, A. Z., MORROW, R., FASS, L., and CARBONE, P. (1970) Central nervous system involvement in Burkitt's lymphoma, *Blood*, 36, 718.

ZIEGLER, J. L., and BLUMING, A. Z. (1971) Intrathecal chemotherapy in Burkitt's lymphoma, *Brit. med. J.*, 2, 508.

18 Neurological Disorders in Kenya

J. R. HARRIES

INTRODUCTION

Kenya is part of a vast tract of the African continent known as East Africa, with Somalia, Ethiopia and the Sudan lying to the north and Tanzania, Malawi and Zambia to the south. Kenya has an area of 247 000 sq miles with an eastern coastline on the shores of the Indian Ocean and Uganda on the western boundary.

The country has very varied scenic and climatic conditions due to the altitude, which rises from sea-level to the snow-capped peak of Mount Kenya at 17 058 feet. From the lush and fertile coastal strip, the terrain changes to rather arid scrub-bush and grass-lands that are renowned as the home of vast concentrations of wild animals.

Then comes the Central Plateau where the capital Nairobi with a population of about 500 000 is situated at an altitude of 5400 feet. Climbing steadily onwards the Escarpment is reached, descending into the Great Rift Valley that cuts across Kenya from north to south. This is one of the most impressive and notable geological features of the country and is studded with both fresh-water and soda lakes, all with wonderful bird life. Lakes Nakuru and Elementeita are world famous for the hundreds of thousands of flamingoes whose massive density paints the lake shores a deep pink clearly visible from several miles away. As in so many regions of Kenya, the hills are of volcanic origin, with many craters, extinct volcanoes, and hot springs.

From the wall of the Western Rift the country continues to rise and the change in climate and crops is most noticeable. There are lovely green pastures in an intensively farmed area, and sometimes newborn lambs, trout streams and similar such glimpses bring to mind the English countryside rather than an equatorial country. Kenya has no really big rivers. Those east of the Rift flow into the Indian Ocean and rivers rising on the western side feed the lakes, many of them flowing into Lake Victoria, which is the largest lake in Africa and equal in size to Ireland. Kisumu is the hub of the Western Province, having a busy and colourful port with the lake boats and railway ferry steamers constantly arriving and departing with their assorted cargoes of indigenous produce. In order to reach Kisumu one has to drop from the Highlands, from the high-rainfall tea-growing areas of Kericho, to the warmer climate of the sugar-growing areas, until finally reaching the vast flat expanse of the Kano plains so often devastated by floods. Much work is being done here in cutting ditches and drainage channels. Finally, there is the little-known Northern Province.

The equator bisects Kenya and accounts for the small variation between the times of sunrise and sunset. Twilight as known in European countries is almost non-existent. At midday the sun's rays are practically vertical. Kenya is poor in mineral wealth—explorations for oil continue but, to date, no strike has been made. Apart from soda ash from Lake Magadi in the Rift Valley, the country has little mineral export. However, Kenya is compensated with what many consider to be the world's best climate. This varies with the terrain and the time of year. The Highlands are dry and warm with refreshingly cool evenings most of the year round, when even a log fire may be desirable. The coastal region is very hot and humid in January, February and March but otherwise pleasant. The climate round Lake Victoria is similar to that of the coast and, in the north, the semidesert has great heat by day and cold at night without variation. There are two seasons of rain—the long rains occurring in April and May sometimes through to June and July, and the short rains from October to November. The annual rainfall for the coast is 50 to 60 inches. In the Highlands it varies from 30 inches to 70 inches in the tea-growing areas of Kericho. In the desert areas, rain can be unknown for a long time. Drought and floods go hand in hand and can unexpectedly alternate, causing great hardship and difficulties for the farming communities. However, temperatures rarely drop below 40°F and do not rise to more than the mid-eighties except at the coast and Lake Victoria in the hot season. In the desert they rise to well over 100°F. Many people consider Kenya's agricultural potential to be unrivalled in the continent of Africa.

The tribes of Kenya fall into five ethnic groups. There is a small remnant of the aboriginal inhabitants, the Wanderobo, who live in the forest areas in Central Kenya. At the time of the Bantu migration southwards, the coastal strip and the bush country bordering the Highland Plateau were occupied, but they were split in two during the subsequent migrations of the Nilohamites, leaving a pocket near Lake Victoria, the Abaluhya. The Nilohamitic tribes comprise the Masai, Kipsigis, and Nandi. The migrating Nilotic tribes from the southern Sudan inhabited the eastern shores of Lake Victoria and an area southwards, mainly consisting of the Luo, Maragoli and Kisii tribes. In the north, pushing all these tribes southwards were the Hamitic groups of Somali, Gabbra and Galla, and Boran. The majority tribe in Kenya is the Bantu Kikuyu—followed closely by the Nilotic Luo with, perhaps, the Bantu Kamba as the third largest tribe.

The diet of these tribes varies—maize being the staple foodstuff of the Bantu. The Nilohamitic tribes which include the Masai have a basic diet of blood and milk, provided by their roving herds of cattle. The jugular vein of the animals is punctured by a reed to obtain the blood. The Nilotic tribes are traditionally fish-eaters.

Kenya is essentially an agricultural country and it is claimed that almost anything will grow—given the right circumstances; but there are many natural hazards with which the farmer has to contend, droughts, floods, army-worm and locusts, to mention a few. The main agricultural activities are in ranching, dairy produce, pigs and sheep. A great deal of excellent quality coffee and tea is grown and exported, as are pyrethrum, maize, cotton, sugar-cane and wattle bark. Sisal exports once had considerable value but in today's markets prices have diminished. Kenya's first-class fruit including pineapples, strawberries and avocado are in good demand from overseas and earn considerable revenue. The flora of both temperate and tropical zones, which flourishes, is also finding markets overseas, thanks to the jet-age, when rare orchids, superb roses and carnations can be transported within 12 hours to European capitals.

Education for the African has been of paramount importance since Independence and much has been done in that way of building primary and secondary schools. Nairobi can boast a modern well-equipped university with most faculties represented. An underlying problem of considerable magnitude lies in finding employment for those whose education has been completed at secondary school level; some 150 000 youths a year are leaving school with only 20–30 per cent having any chance of higher education. The way of life for the masses has not changed very much—women still till the land and are used as 'carriers' in rural areas, while many tribes lead an unfettered, nomadic existence, especially in the northern areas. In the urban areas, a middle-class society is emerging enjoying the so-called fruits of civilization—modern homes, cars, sophisticated national and European dress and the luxuries to which the Western Hemisphere has been accustomed.

Medical Services and Teaching

The organization of the medical services in Kenya follows the pattern which was started under the colonial administration. There are five provinces in the country and each has a central hospital which is usually staffed by a specialist in medicine and surgery together with ancillary staff. There are a varying number of district hospitals throughout these regions, which can refer cases to the regional hospital. Feeding the district hospitals are networks of health centres and dispensaries which are usually staffed by people of hospital assistant qualifications.

The King George VI Hospital of colonial times in Nairobi became known in 1965 as the Kenyatta National Hospital and is the referral hospital for all the regional hospitals, as well as catering for the half-million inhabitants of Nairobi. It is a well-staffed teaching hospital, undergoing expansion. The new hospital is expected to be completed by the end of 1973, with a total bed strength—combining the old and the new—of approximately 2000. The hospital is served by the Medical Research Laboratory, which is also the reference laboratory for the whole country. In addition to the government hospital organization, there are various mission hospitals scattered around. Recently, in the Nyanza Province, a hospital was opened which was built by Russian aid.

The first medical teaching in Nairobi at the King George VI Hospital was carried out by a group of staff members in about 1957. This was at a postgraduate level to encourage doctors to study for higher degrees and it met with considerable success. At one time, there were proposals to set up a postgraduate institute in Nairobi to complement the undergraduate teaching at Makerere University College in Kampala; McGill University, Canada, showed considerable interest in this. However, with the advent of Independence it was decided to set up a full-scale medical school in Kenya, which was done with assistance from Glasgow University, McGill University, and Padua University in addition to the full-time staff employed by the Kenya Government, and part-time consultants working in private practice. The Department of Anatomy and Physiology was established in 1967, although clinical teaching had commenced before this, and the later clinical students from Makerere University Medical School, Uganda, came down for part of their clinical experience at the Kenyatta National Hospital. The first students from the pre-clinical faculties have now begun their clinical work at the Kenyatta National Hospital and the Medical School which is part of Nairobi University.

There is no Department of Neurology, as such, in the hospital but the author has 12 beds and holds an outpatient clinic once a week, comprised solely of neurological patients. Neurological patients are also admitted under the neurosurgeon, and by the various medical firms which often refer to the author for opinions. A part-time neurosurgeon was appointed for the first time to the Kenyatta National Hospital in 1967, and neurosurgery has now been established as a part-time speciality in the hospital.

NEUROLOGICAL PRACTICE IN KENYA

This section is based on 750 personally observed cases of neurological disorders in Kenya. They were seen over a period of 5 years and should provide a general picture of neurological practice here.

Diseases of the Cranial Nerves: 70 Cases

Optic Atrophy

Five cases—four males, one female. In two adult males this was associated with syphilis and in two others with the drinking of methyl alcohol. The other case was a child of $3\frac{1}{2}$ years in association with large haemangioma involving the upper eyelid.

Epidemics of methyl alcohol poisoning occur from time to time from illicit distillations—recently 35 cases were admitted to the Kenyatta National Hospital with 17 deaths. Two of the survivors had optic atrophy with blindness.

Trigeminal Neuralgia

One case.

Third Nerve Palsies

Two cases—both women due to aneurysms of the internal carotid artery.

Facial Palsy

Fifty-four cases—29 males, 25 females; 51 of these cases were classified as Bell's palsy. In one female patient the palsy was bilateral. There were too few patients seen early enough to evaluate the role of ACTH in treatment. It is difficult to be certain of the outcome of such cases as they often do not return for follow-up. However, 14 were noted to have made a good recovery. Of the three other cases, two were due to fractures of the base of the skull and one to chronic otitis media.

Eighth Nerve Deafness

Two cases in males with positive serology for syphilis.

Multiple Cranial Nerve Palsies

Six cases involving the occulomotor nerves and also the vagal, glossopharyngeal and hypoglossal nerves. These were all due to postnasal carcinoma, and usually accompanied by facial pain. Postnasal carcinoma is one of the more common forms of cancer seen in Kenya (Clifford *et al.*, 1963).

The Epilepsies: 260 Cases

Grand Mal Epilepsy

Two hundred and thirty-four cases—164 males, 70 females.

Post-traumatic: 14—13 males, 1 female.
With focal onset: 2 cases.
Mental deficiency: 6 cases.
Due to metabolic disturbances: hypocalcaemia, 2 cases; insulinoma, 1 case.

Petit Mal

With typical 3 per sec spike and wave: 6 cases.
Minor attacks without typical EEG: 2 cases.
Jacksonian motor seizures; 4 cases.
Narcolepsy; 14—all males.

Age-groups in Grand Mal Epilepsy

Age-group in years	*Male*	*Female*
0–10	18	6
11–20	71	38
21–30	38	16
31–40	8	2
41–50	6	2
51–60	2	
Total:	*143*	*64*

The discrepancy in numbers is due to the well-known difficulty we have with many Africans who do not know their ages. Results of treatment are difficult to assess in epilepsy because many patients make only a single attendance at a clinic. But we are able to say that of those in which an adequate follow-up was possible there was good control in 56, i.e. no fits for at least 1 year. Electroencephalography in our patients revealed the characteristic features of epilepsy, in all their varieties, but there is a high incidence of focal discharges.

Pain in the Head: 28 Cases

Migraine: 26 Cases

Common migraine: 16—11 males, 5 females.
Classical migraine: 1 male.
Migrainous neuralgia: 7 males.
Post-traumatic: 2 males.

The frequency of migrainous headaches is, I believe, on the increase in Africans. The patients who suffered from migrainous neuralgias were largely African businessmen.

Congenital and Neonatal Diseases of the Nervous System: 37 Cases

Infantile hemiplegia:	6—5 males, 1 female
Cerebral diplegia:	3—2 males, 1 female
Hydrocephalus:	14
with paraplegia	4—3 males, 1 female
without paraplegia	10—3 males, 7 females
Meningocele and meningomyelocele:	9
with paraplegia	2—1 male, 1 female
without paraplegia	7—3 males, 4 females
Platybasia and Arnold-Chiari malformation:	5—3 males, 2 females
Athetosis:	5—5 females.

These were all female children suffering from varying degrees of mental deficiency.

Five patients with abnormalities of the cervical spine associated with platybasia and the Arnold-Chiari malformation have been seen in the past 2 years presenting with a mixed cord syndrome with long tract pressure and spinocerebellar ataxia. Three of these patients have been submitted to laminectomy and suboccipital decompression without significant improvement.

Heredofamilial Diseases of Nervous Origin and Other Cerebellar Ataxias: 34 Cases

Congenital spastic paraplegia:	1
Friedreich's ataxia:	4
Sanger Brown's ataxia:	1
Olivopontocerebellar ataxia:	4

Cerebellar Ataxias Probably Due to Viral Infections: 6 Cases

Unclassified Cerebellar Ataxias

Eighteen cases—13 males, 5 females.

In Kenya cerebellar ataxias form a significant group of chronic disabling neurological diseases. The heredofamilial ataxias were fairly common in our series but in no instance were other members of the family involved. This is in contradistinction to the situation among Asian patients where three families have been seen with two members affected in each.

Although no viral isolations have been made, the onset of a mild febrile illness with abnormalities in the spinal fluid associated with a cerebellar ataxia makes a viral aetiology probable. In two of the patients, however, the diagnosis was made in retrospect, as the initial episode had occurred many years previously but the ataxia had persisted.

The largest group of unclassified ataxias remains a mystery. In one of these patients *Schistosoma mansoni* eggs were found in the stool and the CSF protein was raised to 89 mg per cent. Of the 18 patients, eight had a pure cerebellar ataxia of moderate to severe degree with no other signs. Investigations included spinal fluid examination with serology and, in some of the patients, studies for brain antibodies, haemograms, skull and chest X-rays, hunts for parasites and serum B_{12} levels and, in other patients, myelography and vertebral angiography, all with completely negative results. In the remaining 10 patients, other physical signs were observed such as extensor plantar responses on one or both sides in five, slight impairment of vibration sense in four, and nystagmus in four, but again all ancillary investigations proved negative. There appears to be neither a nutritional nor an infective factor responsible. Vitamin therapy has not influenced the course of the disease. There has been no evidence of hypothyoidism or underlying malignancy. Although there is no direct evidence for this, plant poisoning may be a possible aetiological factor. A demyelinating condition is also a possibility; could this be the Bantu form of multiple sclerosis?

Infections of the Nervous System: 47

Meningitis: 9 Cases

Pyogenic: 4—2 males, 2 females (all pneumonococcal).
Tuberculous: 3—2 males, 1 female.
Benign lymphocytic: 2—1 male, 1 female.

Encephalitis: 7 Cases

Postpertussis: 3—2 males, 1 female.
Unknown: 4—1 male, 3 females.

Anterior Poliomyelitis

Eight cases—6 males, 2 females.

Two apparently following an injection into the leg.

Trypanosomiasis: 1 Case

This incidence does not, of course, give a true picture of the frequency of meningitis or poliomyelitis which will be dealt with separately.

Chorea

Sydenham's chorea: 15—3 males, 12 females (ages 7–16 years).

Chorea gravidarum: 1.

Chorea is often a prolonged disease in African children and, in cases of undoubted rheumatic chorea, choreic movements may continue for up to 2 years. These movements are often well controlled with diazepam but in three patients α-methyldopa has been used with excellent results. In one child in whom severe movements had lasted for a year or so, complete cessation occurred after 1 week on a dosage of 250 mg daily.

Vascular Disease of the Brain and Spinal Cord: 69 Cases

Hemiplegia

Sixty-one cases—37 males, 24 females (age-range: 10–80 years).

Associated with moderate to severe hypertension—8 males, 4 females, (age-range: 40–80 years).

Probably due to embolism—6:

Aortic regurgitation:	4
Mitral stenosis and auricular fibrillation:	1
Bacterial endocarditis:	1

Associated with carotid artery obstruction—2. One of each sex.

Due to trauma (depressed fracture of the skull):	8 males
Following encephalitis:	2
Probably due to an arteritis:	1
Post-parturient:	1
Associated with ST malaria:	1
Probably syphilitic:	2
Due to sickle-cell anaemia:	1
No cause ascertained:	29—19 males, 10 females

In 29 patients in whom no obvious cause was found the age-groupings were as follows:

Age-groups in years	*No. of cases*
0–10	3
11–20	3
21–30	8
31–40	4
41–50	4
51–60	6
61–70	1

Subdural Haematoma. 4 cases—1 male, 3 females.
Subarachnoid Haemorrhage. 3 cases.
Hemiballismus. 1 case.

The majority of the hemiplegic patients do not fall into the age-group in which arteriosclerosis usually occurs, i.e. 50 plus. No aetiological factor has been discovered, and in those in whom angiography has been carried out no lesions have been found. It has not been possible to study oestrogen levels in these patients but there is evidence to suggest that in African males at least they may be high. This is shown clinically by the relative absence of body hair, the frequency of gynaecomastia, primary carcinoma of the liver, and carcinoma of the male breast, and has been suggested to be related to impairment of liver function in metabolizing oestrogens. This aetiological possibility could be considered in view of the number of cerebrovascular incidents which have occurred as a result of women taking an oestrogen-containing contraceptive pill.

Tumours of the Nervous System: 43 Cases

Cerebral Tumours

Thirty-four cases—19 males, 15 females.

Pituitary Tumours

Four cases: with acromegaly: 3; without acromegaly: 1.

Craniopharyngioma

Three cases.

Hemisphere Tumours

Eleven cases:

Parietal lobe:	7
Frontal lobe:	1
Occipital lobe:	1
Temporal lobe:	2

Of the tumours where histology was available four were glioblastomas, two astrocytomas, and one an oligodendroglioma.

Unclassified probable tumours:	2
Tuberculoma:	2
Meningioma:	3
Hydatid cycsts:	3
Posterior fossa tumours:	6
Eighth nerve tumours:	2
Brain stem ? glioma:	3
Cerebellar ? glioma:	1
Spinal cord lesions:	10
Von Recklinghausen's disease:	1 cervical
Neurofibromata:	1 cervical
Neurinoma:	5; dorsal, 4; cervical, 1
Ependymoma:	1 cervical
Solitary cysts in cord:	2 cervical

Miscellaneous Spinal Cord Conditions: 17 Cases

Cord Compression

Twelve cases:

Cervical spondylosis:	3
Arachnoiditis—all in the dorsal region, one tuberculous:	3
Pott's paraplegia:	3
Odontoid subluxation:	1
Traumatic:	2

Transverse Myelitis

Four cases—all in the dorsal region.

? Schistosoma granuloma

One case.

Diseases of the Peripheral Nerves: 26 Cases

Polyneuritis

Twenty-six cases.

Leprosy

Ten cases—9 males, 1 female (ages 22–50 years).

Hypertrophic Polyneuropathy

Two cases. One probably Refsum's disease. Both male.

Infective Polyneuritis (Landry's Paralysis)

Two cases.

Polyneuropathy of Uncertain Origin

Eleven cases: Associated with raised CSF protein: 4. Normal protein: 7.

Acute Intermittent Porphyria

One case.

Extensive investigations in the obscure polyneuropathies failed to give any evidence of a causative factor. It is of interest to note that one woman with a high CSF protein slowly developed papilloedema during the course of the disease, which subsequently resolved when the CSF protein had fallen. She was in hospital for over 2 years but eventually was able to walk with the aid of crutches. The single patient with porphyria was pregnant and had been given a barbiturate as a hypnotic and then developed a severe widespread paresis, with porphyrins in the urine. She eventually made a good recovery but relapsed during a subsequent pregnancy.

Nutritional Disorders: 13 Cases

Nutritional spastic cord syndromes: 6.
Nutritional ataxic cord syndrome: 3.
Vitamin B_{12} neuropathy: 2.
Subacute combined degeneration of the cord: 1.
Pellagrous cord syndromes: 2.

Peripheral Nerve Injuries or Compressions: 43 Cases

Cervical spondylosis with cord pressure:	5 males (ages 32–62)
Brachial plexus avulsion (birth injury):	1
Erb's palsy (birth injury):	1
Cervical rib:	2
Carpal tunnel syndrome:	1
Radial nerve palsy:	29 males
Ulnar palsy:	3 males
Root pressure on sacral I (disc lesion):	1

Apart from one case in a child due to a stab-wound the remaining 28 cases of radial nerve palsy occurred in men between the ages of 23 and 50 years, all of whom admitted to an excessive consumption of alcohol the previous evening.

Ulnar palsies appeared to be due to pressure at the internal condyle.

Diseases of Muscle: 18 Cases

Muscular Dystrophies

Eight cases: Pseudohypertrophic muscular dystrophy (Duchenne): 6 males. Facioscapulohumeral dystrophy: 2 female.

Myasthenia Gravis

Five cases—4 males, 1 female.

Polymyositis

Four cases—2 males, 2 females.

Thyrotoxic Myopathy

One case.

Myasthenia gravis is rare in Africans. (Harries, 1956; Greenwood and Francis, 1967; Idowu, 1967; Harries, 1969). Four examples were seen among the much smaller European and Asian population over the same period.

In one patient a thymoma was removed. Three patients died of respiratory failure and in two positive pressure respiration was used unsuccessfully. All gave histories of difficulty in swallowing, fatigue on chewing and generalized weakness made worse on exercise, The orbicularis oculi and oris were always affected and two had external ophthalmoplegia. One patient aged 51 had evidence of thyrotoxicosis with tachycardia and proptosis. All responded to edrophonium given intravenously. Large doses of pyridostigmine together with ephedrine were needed to control symptoms in the survivors.

Three of the patients with polymyositis had skin lesions. In two these resembled dermatomyositis, and in the other considerable oedema of the skin was present. The response to steroids was satisfactory.

The patient with thyrotoxic myopathy was a woman with considerable weakness and loss of muscle sense in the limb girdles.

Diseases of Uncertain Origin: 46 Cases

Demyelinating Conditions

Four cases. Only two patients with multiple sclerosis have been seen. There were two other patients with optic atrophy; one patient had associated pyramidal signs; in the other there was retrobulbar neuritis, pyramidal signs, and a paretic Lange curve with a negative CSF Kahn.

Motor Neurone Disease

Eight cases:

Werdnig-Hoffman disease:	1—female of 2½ years
Progressive muscular atrophy:	2—1 male of 22 years; 1 female of 59 years
Amyotrophic lateral sclerosis:	3—2 males, 1 female
Progressive bulbar palsy:	1—male of 35 years
Peroneal muscular atrophy:	1—female of 25 years

Neuralgic Amyotrophy

Three cases—males.

Parkinson's Disease

Twenty-seven cases—17 males, 10 females.

Ages varied from 45 to more than 60 years. Only one patient had hypertension. There was no history of encephalitis. The onset was often unilateral. Outpatient follow-up was very poor. However, Parkinson's disease makes a significant contribution to chronic disabling neurological diseases in Africans.

Choreo-athetosis

One male of 50 years.

Familial Tremor

One male.

Huntington's Chorea

Two cases—1 male, 1 female.

The male patient was a policeman aged about 30, who had violent choreiform movements for 3 years but at the time of examination had no mental changes.

The female was a school-teacher in her late twenties who had noticed choreiform movements for several months and had evidence of intellectual deterioration. Her brother had had similar movements and had committed suicide.

Hysteria: 30 *Cases*

Aphonia:	4—3 males, 1 female
Limb paralysis:	13—6 males, 7 females
Anaesthesias:	5—2 males, 3 females
Abnormal gaits:	2—1 male, 1 female
Tremors:	3—males
Fits:	2—1 male, 1 female
Writer's cramp:	3—males

Hysterical neurological manifestations are quite common in Africans and generally take the form of limb paresis which may be monoplegic, hemiplegic or paraplegic; it is with these forms that the best therapeutic results are obtained with encouragement, physiotherapy and galvanic stimulation. Hysterical aphonia seems particularly difficult to treat.

Benign Intracranial Hypertension: 6 Cases

In areas where medical facilities in country districts are inadequate or where neurological diagnostic facilities are not available, benign intracranial hypertension may go unrecognized and untreated with tragic results. Six cases have been seen in the past 4 years (Mehta *et al.*, 1970). Two became totally blind and one partially so. In these three symptoms had been present for several months before treatment was initiated, and in two the intracranial pressure remained elevated at least intermittently for 2 years. Particulars of these six African cases are given in TABLE 18.1.

Multiple Sclerosis: 2 Cases

Only two cases of this disease have been encountered in the years 1952–69 (Foster and Harries, 1970). Both patients were young Africans with the characteristic features of the illness including paretic Lange curves and negative serology.

ACUTE POLIOMYELITIS

Poliomyelitis continues to be a problem in tropical countries; thus the changing patterns of admission and the forms of treatment evolved over a period of a decade or so, with special reference to young children, are pertinent to this chapter.

In 1955 a polio unit was set up in Nairobi which accepted cases from all parts of East Africa. The cases admitted from other hospitals were primarily life-threatening. Many were transported by air, a flying team being sent out from the unit for this purpose. The unit possessed four Radcliffe and one Engström intermittent positive pressure respiration (IPPR) pumps (Engström, 1954), four tanks, one cuirass respirator, and two rocking beds. During epidemics one Beaver IPPR pump and seven additional tanks were borrowed. At the height of an epidemic in 1956–57, five IPPR machines, six tanks and two oxygen tents were in use at the same time.

Two hundred and twenty-four cases were admitted to the unit during the period November 1956 to September 1957. Only one of these cases was non-paralytic. Of this total 52 were Europeans, 18 Asians, and 154 Africans. The age and sex incidences of each racial groups are presented in TABLES 18.2 and 18.3, showing considerable differences between the age distribution in the different races. In the African group 146 of the 154 admissions (94·8 per cent) were under the age of 5 years; of these 146 cases, 115 were under 2 years of age. In the European group 28 of the 52 admissions (53·8 per cent) were over 20 years of age. All but one of the 18 Asians admitted were under 15 years of age. Among the 154 Africans, 39 could be classified as life-threatening cases; the respective figures for Europeans and Asians were 19 out of 52, and 6 out of 18. This contrasts with the admissions of respiratory cases from 1959 to 1963 when there were 90 African cases compared with two in other races [TABLE 18.4].

In 1960 a large-scale vaccination campaign, using the Sabin attenuated virus, was launched in Kenya. This was begun during the 1959–60 epidemic and appeared to cut short the spread of the disease, as only 15 respiratory cases were admitted in the 3 months following the start of the campaign as against 53 cases in the previous 3 months.

The majority of Europeans and Asians took advantage of polio inoculation after the introduction of the Salk vaccine, and many Africans may have done so. Forty African children with respiratory poliomyelitis, of an average age of 2 years and 2 months were admitted during the 3 years following the advent of vaccination. It would appear from this that vaccination campaigns on a large scale should be undertaken every 2 years to inoculate the newly born.

The main problem now facing those who deal with life-threatening poliomyelitis in tropical Africa is that of the young African child.

Life-threatening Poliomyelitis

This may be classified as follows:

1. Paralysis of the respiratory centre.

2. Bulbar paralysis: pharyngeal paralysis with inability to swallow.

3. Bulbospinal paralysis: pharyngeal paralysis plus involvement of the muscles of respiration.

4. Spinal paralysis: paralysis of intercostals and/or diaphragm.

5. Abdominal paralysis.

Table 18.1

Six African Cases of Benign Intracranial Hypertension

Case	Age	Sex	Race	Prior history	Duration of symptoms	Symptoms on admission			Physical signs			Investigations							Treatment	Follow-up
						Headache	Vomiting	Diplopia	Papilloedema	VI N Palsy	Other CNS	CSF pressure	Protein	Cells	Skull X-Ray	Ventric	Angio	EEG		
1	2	F	Af.	URI Gastro-enteritis Chlortetra-cycline 2 days	2 dys		+		+	+		>300	50	O	N	N			L + S Tetracyclines discontinued	Well after 1 month
2	13	F	Af.	Nil	2 mo.	+			+		L VII nerve weak-ness	>300	32	O	N	N	N Bilat-eral		L + S + D Spitz Holter Valve	Died 21 months after first admission. No post-mortem Acute glaucoma developed 1 year
3	21	F	Af.	Probably 7 months prior	4 mo.	+	+	+	+	+		>300	15	O	N	N	N	A	L + S + D	Optic atrophy was developing on admission
4	16	F	Af.	Nil	2 mo.	+			+			>300	30	O	N	N			L	Well after 2 years
5	24	M	Af.	Nil	6 wks	+	+		+			>300	20	O	N	N			L + S + D	
6	26	F	Af.	Mitral stenosis	4 wks	+	+	+	+	+		>300	30	2	N	N			L + S + D Spitz Holter Valve	Early optic atrophy 3 years later

L — Repeated lumbar punctures
S — Steroids
D — Diuretics
A — Abnormal
N — Normal

Source: Mehta, S., Patel, K. C., Jindani, A., and Harries, J. R. (1970) Benign intracranial hypertension, *E. Afr. med. J.*, **47**, 333.

Table 18.2
Poliomyelitis. Total Admissions[1] by Race, Sex and Age

Age	African			Asian			European		
	M	*F*	*Total*	*M*	*F*	*Total*	*M*	*F*	*Total*
0–1	32	23	55	1	0	1	1	0	1
1–2	37	23	60	4	1	5	3	0	3
2–5	17	14	31	2	5	7	2	4	6
5–15	2	2	4	3	1	4	8	1	9
15–20	1	1	2	0	1	1	3	2	5
20–30	0	2	2	0	0	0	3	14	17
30–50	0	0	0	0	0	0	7	4	11
Total:	*89*	*65*	*154*	*10*	*8*	*18*	*27*	*25*	*52*

(By courtesy of the Editor, *South African Medical Journal.*) [1] 11 months ending September 1957.

Table 18.3
Poliomyelitis. Life-Threatening Cases and Deaths, etc. by Race and Age

	0–5 years			5–20 years			20–50 years		
	Afr	*As*	*Eur*	*Afr*	*As*	*Eur*	*Afr*	*As*	*Eur*
Total	146	13	10	6	5	14	2	0	28
Resp. cases[1]	36	4	1	3	2	1	0		17
Resp. cases as % of total	24·6%	30·7%	10%	50%	40%	7·7%	0		60·7%
Deaths	7	1	0	1	0	0	0		2
Mortality rate	19·5%	25%	0	33·3%	0	0	0		11·7%
Age group as % of all ages	94·8%	72·2%	19·2%	4%	28·8%	27%	1·2%		53·8%

[1] Life-threatening poliomyelitis. (By courtesy of the Editor, *South African Medical Journal.*)

Table 18.4
Poliomyelitis. Respiratory Cases (All Age-Groups)

Race	1957	1959 to March 1960	March 1960 to 1963	Total
African	39	50	40	129
Asian	6	0	1	7
European	19	0	1	20
Total:	*64*	*50*	*42*	*156*

(By courtesy of the Editor, *East African Medical Journal.*)

Diagnosis

Central Paralysis of Respiration

The diagnosis of central paralysis is difficult, but fortunately this condition is rare. It is usually accompanied by other evidence of brain stem involvement such as cranial nerve palsies and sometimes including pharyngeal palsy. Central paralysis of respiration is characterized by an irregular pattern of breathing, accompanied by apnoeic phases associated with changes in blood gas tensions. However, the pattern of breathing in normal children is often very irregular and may mimic that of central paralysis, the distinguishing feature being periods of apnoea in the latter. It should be mentioned in passing that there is an unusual type of central paralysis in which the respiratory centre can be made to function by command. This has been called the 'lazy respiratory centre'. Irregular breathing due to central paralysis may also be confused with that due to obstruction of the upper air passages by the accumulated secretions of bulbar paralysis—the irregularity of the latter case being corrected by adequate suction of the pharynx.

Bulbar Paralysis

Bulbar paralysis may mimic paralysis of the spinal respiratory muscles especially when secretions have been inhaled causing diminished movement of a portion of the chest wall. Children affected with bulbar paralysis will refuse to take food or drink and will cough and splutter if they are made to swallow. Crackling will be heard on auscultation of the pharynx as the air bubbles through the secretions. Examination of the pharynx will reveal bubbly mucus and there may be palatal palsy and/or loss of the gag reflex. The normally obtuse angle between the soft tissues of the floor of the mouth and the larynx becomes acute.

Spinal Respiratory Paralysis

Paralysis of the intercostal muscles with or without paralysis of the diaphragm may be suspected from an increase in the respiratory rate, the pulse rate, and from the use of the alae nasi. In more severe cases the accessory muscles of respiration may be brought into use. It is usually not difficult to observe inequalities of movement of the intercostal muscles and frequently paradoxical movement may be observed. If the diaphragm is intact, the chest wall will fall in as the abdomen expands with diaphragmatic descent. A feeble cry and cough is often noticeable although the feeble cough is more usually due to paralysis of the abdominal muscles.

With diaphragmatic paralysis again paradoxical movement is noticeable—as the chest expands the abdomen retracts. It is not possible to feel the diaphragm descend on inspiration. Litten's sign may be useful in thin patients.

Abdominal Paralysis

Paralysis of the abdominal muscles is a cause of life-threatening disease in children. The child is unable to cough and whereas, by itself, this may not be too serious, if it catches a cold or develops some more severe respiratory infection such as measles, a life-threatening situation may ensue with accumulation of secretions in the lungs.

Distinctive Features

African Cases

Half of the African patients had severe diarrhoea on admission and some were considerably dehydrated. Many were anaemic; one had a haemoglobin level of 35 per cent (Sahli's method) in spite of profound dehydration. A feature among the Africans which was not seen in the other groups was the high proportion of 'wet lungs' (20 out of the 39 life-threatening cases). This condition was mainly due to paralysis of the abdominal muscles with or without diaphragmatic or intercostal paralysis, leading to an inability to cough. Measles or an upper respiratory tract infection superimposed upon this condition, or nursing in the supine position led to a state of 'wet lung' with generalized râles and, in some cases, consolidation and/or atelectasis. Some of these cases gave a history of a febrile illness with paralysis of the limbs some weeks before and had been admitted to a general hospital as cases of bronchitis or bronchopneumonia before being sent to the unit.

Asian Cases

Of the six life-threatening cases, encephalitis predominated in two; one other had bulbospinal poliomyelitis and the remaining three had involvement of the spinal muscles of respiration.

European Cases

In this group there was a high incidence of bulbar and bulbospinal involvement (12 out of 19 life-threatening cases).

The total admissions included 14 married European women of whom six were pregnant. One miscarried at 3 months, one had a stillbirth at 36 weeks and three live babies were delivered at term, one by Caesarean section. The remaining patient was 6 months pregnant and had been an inpatient for 3 months. The Caesarean baby was delivered during the period of infectivity and the virus was isolated from the meconium and cord blood. The virus isolations were carried out by Dr. J. Gear in Johannesburg and both proved to be Type I.

Of the 10 adult European males admitted, eight showed respiratory involvement, six requiring respiratory aids.

Treatment

Statistical details of treatment are shown in TABLES 18.5, 18.6 and 18.7. Very gentle handling by the nursing staff is essential in all patient suffering from life-threatening disease.

Central Paralysis of Respiration

The following description of one of the patients illustrates the problems of treatment of paralysis of the respiratory centre.

In this child the disorder of respiration was accompanied by a bulbar paralysis, paralysis of the fifth and seventh nerves on the left, and loss of consciousness lasting 3 days. The pharynx was kept clear by posture and suction. The respirations were very irregular, often falling to about 10 per minute with several prolonged periods of complete apnoea. Slowing of the respirations was often corrected by intravenous aminophylline and the apnoeic phases were controlled by positive pressure respiration through a face mask. The involvement of the respiratory centre lasted as long as the period of coma. The bulbar paralysis disappeared after 3 weeks and the child made a complete recovery with the exception of a mild residual facial palsy. A tank respirator may be used in such patients but it may be necessary to use high pressures at the beginning of treatment to ensure that the patient's breathing co-ordinates with the tank.

Bulbar Paralysis

Bulbar paralysis is treated by nursing in the prone or semiprone position with the foot of the bed elevated about 9 inches. These patients are usually fed intravenously for the first 2 or 3 days and then by means of a narrow polythene tube introduced into the stomach. If it is not possible to keep a clear airway, pharyngeal suction through the nose and mouth is performed as frequently as necessary.

Table 18.5

Poliomyelitis. Respiratory Cases (Average Age Two Years—1957–1963)

Type and treatment	*Total*	*Deaths*	*Mortality Percentage*
All cases	109	35	32·0
Bulbar	4	0	0·0
Spinal (tank)	80	23	29·0
Bulbospinal (tank)	18	3	16·6
Bulbospinal (tank and tracheostomy)	3	3	100·0
Bulbospinal (IPPR)	4	4	100·0
All bulbospinal cases	25	10	40·0

(By courtesy of the Editor, *East African Medical Journal.*)

Eighteen consecutive patients (all age-groups) have been treated in this manner without a death and without performing a tracheostomy, although this may be necessary if the airway cannot be kept clear.

Spinal Paralysis, i.e. Paralysis of the Intercostals and/or Diaphragm

Adults. Of the 17 cases who needed respiratory aids, 16 were treated in tanks and one by IPPR as he was admitted with total atelectasis of one lung which it was not possible to clear in a tank. Adult cases were put into tank respirators when their vital capacities fell to 30 per cent of the expected normal.

Of the 11 treated in tanks none died. The moment to use tank respirators in infants is judged by a falling or increasing respiratory rate, and any other indications of respiratory distress such as the use of accessory muscles and alae nasi.

Children. The treatment of choice in all children with paralysis of the intercostal muscles and diaphragm is also the tank respirator.

The Alligator type of respirator with a high frequency of respiration and a shorter inspiratory phase is more convenient. The tank should be easy to tilt for the purpose of postural drainage. The indications for using the respirator are the raised respiratory rate and pulse rate, usage of the alae nasi or accessory muscles of respiration with evidence of intercostal or diaphragmatic paralysis or paradoxical respirations. A good case may be made out for its use if there is any evidence of respiratory muscle involvement in an attempt to rest the muscles. Children tolerate the face-down position well and frequent turning into this position is advisable. Children need moderately high pressures, around 12 cm water at a rate of 30/min. Measurement of ventilation in these very small children is difficult and it is usually convenient to use the above arbitrary pressures and frequencies without measuring the minute volume. To avoid the possibility of overventilation, weaning should be early, within 3 days of the temperature reverting to normal. The tank is opened every 4 hours for a few minutes at a time while the pulse and respirations are carefully observed. The time that the tank is opened each day is slowly increased if no untoward effects are observed. The children are given fluid feeds for the first 3 to 4 days. Nine children have been treated in this way with no fatalities. Their average stay in the respirator was 37 days and the average age 2½ years.

Bulbospinal Paralysis

Adults. Seven adult cases were treated with tracheostomy and IPPR machines in the manner described previously by many writers (Lassen, 1953; Smith, Spalding, and Russell, 1954; Macrae *et al.*, 1954; Harries and Lawes, 1955). Of these five were first nursed in tank respirators until bulbar paralysis, developed; tracheostomy was then performed and the patients ventilated by IPPR. Two severe cases in children both under the age of 2 years were treated in the face-down position without tracheostomy, in a tank specifically designed to allow the use of this position. There were two deaths in this group of 9, both being adults with severe bulbospinal encephalitis.

Children. The treatment of bulbospinal polio in children is somewhat more controversial. It has been suggested by Rossi (1958) that these patients should be treated by intermittent positive pressure respiration (IPPR). Of 13 patients under 10 years of age, whom he treated in this way, seven died. Using IPPR in four patients of average age of 2 years all died, and similar results were obtained with tracheostomy plus tank respirators.

In view of these discouraging results, the tank respirator alone is used without tracheostomy. All patients are nursed on the face with the tank tilted into the head-down position except for ¾ to 1 hour after feeding. The stomach is intubated for feeding purposes with a narrow polythene tube passed via the nose. The airway is kept clear by suctioning and tilting. Weaning is carried out as previously described. During 1964

Table 18.6

Poliomyelitis. Cases and Deaths by Classification and Treatment and by Age

African cases and deaths

Age (years)	B	BS	Abd	Sp	Total	Posture etc.	Posture $+O_2$	Tank	Tracheostomy	Deaths
0– 1	2	0	3	10	15 (3)	5	5 (1)	5 (2)	0	3
1– 2	1	1	1	12	15 (4)	3	5	6 (3)	1 (1)	4
2– 5	0	2	0	4	6	2	2	2	0	0
5–15	0	0	0	3	3 (1)	0	2 (1)	1	0	1

European cases and deaths

Age (years)	B	BS	Sp	Total	Posture etc.	Tank	IPPR	Deaths
1– 2	0	1	0	1	0	1	0	0
5–15	1	0	0	1	1	0	0	0
20–30	1	5	5	11 (2)	4	2	5 (2)	2
30–50	2	2	2	6	3	1	2	0

Asian cases and deaths

Age (years)	PE	BS	Sp	Total	Posture etc.	IPPR	Deaths
0– 1	0	0	1	1	1	0	0
1– 2	0	0	1	1	1	0	0
2– 5	1	0	1	2	2 (1)	0	1
5–15	1	1	0	2	1	1	0

All cases and deaths

Age (years)	PE	B	BS	Abd	Sp	Total	Posture etc.	Posture $+O_2$	Tank	IPPR	Tracheostomy	Deaths
0– 5	1 (1)	3	4	4	29 (7)	41	13 (1)	12 (1)	14 (5)	0	1 (1)	8
5–15	1	1	1	0	3 (1)	6	2	2 (1)	1	1	0	1
20–50	0	3	7 (2)	0	7	17	7	0	3	7 (2)	0	2
Total:	*2 (1)*	*7*	*12 (2)*	*4*	*39 (8)*	*64*	*22 (1)*	*14 (2)*	*18 (5)*	*8 (2)*	*1 (1)*	*11*

PE = Polioencephalitis. *B* = Bulbar paralysis. *BS* = Bulbospinal paralysis. *Abd* = Paralysis of abdominal muscles, without intercostals or diaphragm. *Sp* = Paralysis of intercostals and/or diaphragm with or without abdominal muscles. *Posture, etc.* = Prone position, elevation of foot of bed, pharyngeal suction. *Posture* + O_2 = Above plus oxygen tents. Deaths in brackets.

(By courtesy of the Editor, *South African Medical Journal.*)

Table 18.7

Poliomyelitis. Respiratory Cases (Average Age Two Years)

Year	Type of disease	Tank	Tank plus tracheostomy	IPPR	Deaths	Average time on respiratory aid (days)
1959–60	Spinal	54			19	20
	Bulbospinal	7			2	42
	Bulbospinal		3		3	
	Bulbospinal			4	4	
1961–62	Spinal	7			2	25
1963	Spinal	9			0	37
	Bulbospinal	7			0	60

(By courtesy of the Editor, *East African Medical Journal.*)

nine consecutive patients of an average age of $2\frac{1}{2}$ years were treated with this method without a death. The average duration of respiratory care was 60 days and swallowing was resumed within 3 weeks. Another 11 patients were also treated earlier in this way with three deaths.

Abdominal Paralysis

These patients need aid when there are râles in the lung. If these are not extensive we make it our practice to put a pad and binder on the lower abdomen and nurse on the face with or without an oxygen tent. If difficulties arise, they can be nursed on the face in a tank as for the bulbospinal cases.

Hypothermia

Hypothermia of varying degree may be used in cases showing hyperpyrexia (temperature of over 104°F) where previous experience has shown that a high mortality rate could be expected (Engström, 1954). Lassen (1953) found a mortality rate of over 90 per cent in these cases.

Cross-Infection

Considerable inconvenience has been encountered by cross-infection. A *Staphylococcus aureus* phage-type 80 was isolated among other bacteria from tracheostomy wounds, bronchial secretions, and infected urines. Four members of the staff developed acute septic conditions of the hands; three were of a serious nature. Again a *Staph. aureus* phage-type 80 (penicillin-resistant) was isolated from each case. This emphasizes the need for strict aseptic precautions.

Differential Diagnosis

Among the cases admitted as suspected poliomyelitis were the following:

Landry's paralysis in two cases showing bulbar spinal paralysis; these were successfully treated with steroids; one case required respiratory aid. *Herpes zoster* in a middle-aged European with an abnormal CSF; the predominant features were severe pain in one leg with paralysis followed by the typical herpetic eruption. Three cases of *benign lymphocytic chorio-meningitis*. A case of *postmumps encephalitis* in a European adult. Two cases of *pertussis encephalitis* in African infants. Two *hemiplegics*, both being young African males. Two African infants showing *osteomyelitis of the femur*. A European adult female with a *Coxsackie infection*, who had severe pain of the intercostals and diaphragm which embarrassed respiration. A fatal case of *pneumococcal meningitis* with a normal CSF in a European schoolboy. A European adult with *cerebral malaria*. An African adult with *transverse myelitis*. Two European adult females with *hysteria*.

CSF Findings

Some of the CSF findings did not fit into the so-called classical picture. The cell count ranged from 5 to over 1000. In cases showing these extremes of the cell count poliomyelitis was not diagnosed unless typical paralysis was evident.

Causes of Death

Out of the 315 paralytic cases there were 156 with life-threatening disease. This high incidence was occasioned by the selective nature of our admissions; the great majority of cases from hospitals outside Nairobi were of a serious nature. Of the 156, 38 died, three deaths occurring in the European and Asian groups.

Post-mortem examinations were performed in 10 cases, in seven of which there was obstruction to respiration in the lower respiratory tract due to mucopus in six cases and to inhaled milk in the seventh. In one other case the predominant findings were in the brain, no other obvious cause of death being found. One case, who died within 24 hours of the cessation of induced 'mild hypothermia' (Delorme, 1956), showed a massive thrombosis in the right auricle extending through the tricuspid valve into the right ventricle and from there into the pulmonary artery.

Another case died during induced 'moderate hypothermia' (Delorme, 1956), and showed changes not dissimilar to those described in experimental animals by Knocker (1955) and Gray (1954).

Of the eight deaths in African children, four occurred while the children were in tanks and four in cases treated by posture, suction, antibiotics, and oxygen tents. One of these latter cases had a tracheostomy.

Respiratory Obstruction by Secretions

The most serious difficulty in the treatment of life-threatening poliomyelitis in African infants during this epidemic was not the poliomyelitis *per se* but the lower respiratory tract obstruction caused by the accumulation of secretions. In three infants who died the main respiratory muscles involved were the abdominals, while involvement of the intercostal muscles or diaphragm was minimal. In many of these cases it was difficult to decide whether or not a respiratory aid was necessary. All had raised respiratory rates and some were slightly cyanosed. Tracheostomy was performed on one of these infants to facilitate suction; this was one of the three infants who died.

In cases of 'wet lung' where evidence of respiratory paralysis was insufficient to warrant the use of a respiratory aid, treatment by posture, abdominal binders to help coughing and nursing in an oxygen tent seemed reasonably effective.

Improvement in Mortality Rate

In the past 5 years the mortality rate for life-threatening poliomyelitis has declined. Among the factors responsible for this can be listed the introduction of IPPR by Bjorn Ibsen (1954 *a* and *b*, 1955).

It has been suggested by Trueta (1956) that tracheostomy should be avoided if possible in acute poliomyelitis in infants, not because the mortality rate is increased, but because weaning is made more difficult. In our experience tracheostomy with IPPR in adults is sometimes a life-saving measure, though this method carries its own specific complications and difficulties and requires considerable experience to achieve success. This is possibly shown by figures from our own unit. In our first season we treated five adults with IPPR with three deaths (60 per cent mortality), whereas the following season eight adults were so treated with two deaths (25 per cent mortality). Other factors that may have contributed were more detailed investigation of electrolyte and fluid balances and an improvement in hypothermic techniques.

In our hands, the treatment of choice for bulbospinal paralysis in very young children is the tank respirator plus postural drainage and suctioning. It has proved vastly superior to tracheostomy and IPPR, and tracheostomy plus a tank respirator.

In our first season three patients showed hyperpyrexia, and all three died. Subsequently, seven patients showed sustained temperatures of over 104°F; they were all treated with hypothermia and two of them died.

Hypertension in acute poliomyelitis may be alarming, e.g. a systolic pressure of over 220 mm Hg. In many cases this would appear to be central in origin, or at least not due to hypercapnia, for in three of our cases who showed high blood pressure readings the arterial CO_2 levels were normal. Lassen (1953) stated that the mortality rate is increased in cases showing hypertension. Our three cases were treated with subcutaneous pentolinium tartrate, which effectively reduced the blood pressure. All cases survived.

NUTRITIONAL DISORDERS

Pellagra

Pellagra is not frequently encountered in Kenya now but several years ago a large number of cases were seen among detainees in prisons. The clinical features of the pellagrous neuropathy are well known and consist of a peripheral neuropathy with loss of peripheral sensitivity to painful stimuli, vibration and position sense, together with evidence of pyramidal involvement and sometimes a spinocerebellar ataxia. These signs tend to improve with nicotinic acid, vitamin B_{12} and thiamine and, of course, skin lesions clear. Patients in whom the skin lesions have cleared but who have residual cord signs may resemble spastic cord syndromes or even subacute combined degeneration of the cord, especially if a clear history is not forthcoming.

Subacute Combined Degeneration of the Cord

Pernicious anaemia is uncommon among Africans (Foy, Kondi, and Manson-Bahr, 1955). The occurrence of subacute combined degeneration is a distinct rarity so the following patient warrants description.

Case 1. A female Kikuyu aged 18 years (non-pregnant) was admitted to hospital with weakness, dyspnoea, limb pains and instability on walking. She had a typical megaloblastic anaemia with histamine-fast achlorhydria. Her gait was spastic with exaggerated reflexes and extensor plantar responses. There was absence of vibration and position sense in the legs. There were no other abnormalities in the central nervous system. Tongue raw and smooth. Gastroscopy showed a normal mucosa with no gastric atrophy. Serum B_{12} level 20 $\mu\mu$g per ml before treatment, rising to 98 $\mu\mu$g after administration of penicillin but falling again to 40 $\mu\mu$g and rising once more to 132 $\mu\mu$g after administration of vitamin B_{12} 80 μg by mouth. There was a submaximal increase in the reticulocytes, the red cell count, and the haemoglobin after administration of penicillin followed by a decrease. After administration of vitamin B_{12} 80 μg by mouth the reticulocytes increased to the expected maximum, and the red cells and haemoglobin to 4 020 000 per cu mm and 13 g per 100 ml respectively.

The responses to penicillin and to vitamin B_{12}, 80μg by mouth, indicate the presence of intrinsic factor, although perhaps in diminished amounts. The megaloblastic anaemia, the histamine-fact achlorhydria, the definite but early signs of nervous involvement, and the high excretion of radioactive vitamin B_{12} (78 per cent of administered dose) all suggest a pernicious anaemia in its very early stages. The absence of gastric atrophy as shown by gastroscopy could also be explained on the assumption that the disease was in its early stages. Perhaps a gastric biopsy would have shown some atrophy. The amount of vitamin B_{12} made available after administration of penicillin was probably insufficient, with the diminished amount of intrinsic factor, to maintain blood regeneration, whereas the greater quantity of vitamin B_{12} available after administration of vitamin B_{12}, 80 μg, led to a higher rise in the serum B_{12} level and a more sustained blood regeneration.

Nutritional Spastic Paraplegia

Nutritional cord syndromes are much less frequent than in West Africa, which may be accounted for by the fact that maize is the usual staple food in Kenya. However, the occurrence of six cases in non-cassava-eaters is of importance. These patients ate a staple diet of maize with beans and meat, vegetables and milk. Some improvement occurred with vitamin B_{12} in large doses.

Case 2. A typical example was a 24-year-old male Kikuyu complaining of difficulty in walking of 1 month's duration. He was unable to walk without the support of a stick. He had a spastic paralysis of the legs with brisk reflexes and extensor plantar responses, and slight loss of vibration sense. There were no other abnormalities in the central nervous system. His tongue was smooth and he had an angular stomatis. Investigations included haemogram, bone-marrow examination, fractional test-meal, examination of the spinal fluid, serology, serum pyruvate and hunts for parasites, with no abnormalities. Multivitamin preparations produced little change but after prolonged administration of vitamin B_{12}, 100 μg daily over 3 months, there was considerable improvement. He was able to walk quite well although his gait was still slightly spastic.

Nutritional Spinal Ataxia

Only two cases of this condition were seen with the following typical findings.

Case 3. A male Luo aged 40 years was admitted with a recent history of difficulty in walking and when seen needed the support of two people. Apart from sluggish reflexes and a slight tremor towards the end of movement in the arms, the abnormalities were confined to the lower limbs which were hypotonic with good power, absent reflexes and flexor plantar responses. There was loss of vibration sense up to the iliac crests and loss of position sense. Touch and pin-prick sensibility were slightly impaired over the feet. There was some ataxia on heel-toe testing and Romberg's test was positive. His muscles were not tender. Investigations were completely unhelpful. He was treated with vitamin B_{12}, 100 mg daily for 6 weeks. There was some return of vibration sense and he was able to walk well though he still had loss of position sense, and Romberg's sign remained positive.

The following description of an obscure nutritional disorder is included as the prominent feature of a black tongue and black pigmentation of the feet and hands had not previously been seen by the author.

Case 4. A male child 13 years old (Kikuyu) was admitted with severe anaemia and inability to stand. The relevant clinical findings were of severe anaemia, with pale discs, and a black tongue, while both the palms and backs of the hands and the soles and dorsum of the feet were black—much darker than the remainder of the skin though the skin was smooth and quite unlike that in pellagra. There was a neurological disturbance with areflexia, peripheral sensory loss, marked ataxia of a cerebellar type and extensor plantar responses. Investigations revealed a megaloblastic anaemia, haemoglobin 6 g with a megaloblastic marrow and histamine-fast achlorhydria. The anaemia responded well to B_{12} and a high-protein diet and reached 15 g after 5 weeks, followed by disappearance of the pigmentation of the tongue, hands and feet after 6 weeks of treatment. There was some improvement in the neurological status on this regime but until nicotinic acid was added 3 weeks after admission, improvement was slow. After a further 9 weeks the child was able to run about the ward and showed considerable remission of physical signs. The pigmentation of the tongue was similar to that described in dogs with a diet deficient in nicotinic acid and did not in fact disappear until nicotinic acid was added to the B_{12} therapy.

COMMENT

It is evident from the statistics presented that epilepsy is the most frequent disease seen by neurologists in Eastern Africa, although from previous comments it can be seen that much remains to be done in the follow-up of patients and in the education of employers who are loath to give work to these unfortunates and also of their own people who tend to reject them.

The figures presented do not, however, give proper emphasis to the considerable numbers of acute infections of the central nervous system, in the form of meningitis: tuberculous meningitis which is common and not infrequently seen in adults, and cryptococcal meningitis which with its various focal signs may resemble the former.

Cerebrovascular disease is surprisingly common in a racial group in which coronary artery disease is practically non-existent, and it is equally interesting that the majority of these patients are in a relatively young age-group. Several patients with carotid artery stenosis have been seen but in the majority of these young people no aetiological factor is found. There is quite a lot of evidence, unrelated to neurology, which indicates the possibility that oestrogens are responsible; this could be a fruitful line of research. Other conditions towards which research efforts could be fruitfully directed are the common cerebellar ataxias of unknown origin, as in Kenya these appear high on the list of intractable disabling disorders, following close after cerebrovascular diseases and Parkinson's disease. One of the interesting features of Parkinson's disease in Africans is the relatively young age-group in which it is seen, although in none of our patients was there any unequivocal evidence of a viral origin. Only one case of trypanosomiasis was seen but this disease does not occur in the Nairobi area and all cases are reported from Nyanza Province which borders on Lake Victoria, where from time to time there are upsurges of the disease.

Rheumatic chorea is quite common in the highland areas of Kenya and is not infrequently complicated by valvular disease. This is in contrast to acute rheumatic arthritis which is much less common; the latter is itself the most usual mode of presentation.

It used to be said that most cerebral tumours in Africans were tuberculomas, and indeed antituberculous therapy was a popular treatment once the diagnosis of a tumour had been made. It is apparent from the figures presented that this assumption was incorrect and, in fact, these figures give the cerebral tumour incidence at about 4·5 per cent of neurological disorders seen in the medical wards; this may be underestimating the situation.

Only three cases of Pott's paraplegia are recorded but these patients usually gravitate to the orthopaedic surgeons and comprise one of the most common forms of spinal cord compression.

The report of two probable examples of multiple sclerosis may renew interest in the search for this disease but it may well be that the presentation in Africans is not classical and may be modified by genetics, other disease, and diet.

Muscle disorders, once thought to be as rare as multiple sclerosis, are being reported with increasing frequency.

Hysterical reactions are of considerable frequency and interest and deserve further study. This is illustrated by the study of a male patient with a paralysed arm. The skin temperature in this arm was found to be several degrees lower than that on the normal side, reverting to normal when the paralysis cleared up. This may explain the absence of bleeding and possibly the insensitivity to pain in some of the self mutilating procedures that are practised under the hysterical trance state.

All in all, further statistics are needed in Africa, which still remains an untapped field for research in neurology with modern techniques.

References

CLIFFORD, P., OETTGEN, H. G., BEECHER, J. L., BROWN, F. P., HARRIES, J. R., and LAWES, W. E. (1963) Nitrogen mustard therapy with aortic occlusion in nasopharyngeal carcinoma, *Brit. med. J.*, 1, 1256.

DELORME, E. J. (1956) Discussion on the application of hypothermia to surgical procedures, *Proc. roy. Soc. Med.*, 49, 368.

ENGSTRÖM, C. G. (1954) Treatment of severe cases of respiratory paralysis by the Engström Universal Respirator, *Brit. med. J.*, 2, 666.

FOSTER, R. M., and HARRIES, J. R. (1970) Multiple sclerosis in the African, *Brit. med. J.*, 2, 628.

FOY, H., KONDI, A., and MANSON-BAHR, P. E. C. (1955) Penicillin in megaloblastic anaemias of Africans. Effect on serum B_{12} levels and absorption of radioactive vitamin B_{12}, *Lancet*, ii, 693.

GRAY, T. C. (1954) Reflections on circulatory control, *Lancet*, i, 383.

GREENWOOD, B. M., and FRANCIS, T. I. (1967) Myasthenia gravis in Africans, *W. Afr. med. J.*, 16, 97.

HARRIES, J. R. (1956) A case of myasthenia gravis occurring in an African, *E. Afr. med. J.*, 33, 45.

HARRIES, J. R. (1969) Myasthenia gravis in Kenya, *Trans. roy. Soc. trop. Med. Hyg.*, 63, 680.

HARRIES, J. R., and LAWES, W. E. (1955) Intermittent positive pressure respiration in bulbo-spinal poliomyelitis. Use of the Radcliffe Respiration Pump, *Brit. med. J.*, 1, 448.

IBSEN, B. (1954*a*) The anaesthetist's viewpoint on the treatment of respiratory complications in poliomyelitis during the epidermic in Copenhagen, 1952, *Proc. roy. Soc. Med.*, 47, 72.

IBSEN, B. (1954*b*) The epidemic of poliomyelitis in Copenhagen, 1952, *Proc. roy. Soc. Med.* 47, 67.

IBSEN, B. (1955) The management of respiratory and bulbar paralysis in poliomyelitis, in Poliomyelitis, *Wld Hlth Org. Monogr. Ser.*, No. 26, p. 157.

IDOWU, C. A. (1967) Myasthenia gravis in a Nigerian, *W. Afr. med. J.*, 16, 96.

KNOCKER, P. (1955) Effects of experimental hypothermia on vital organs, *Lancet*, ii, 837.

LASSEN, H. C. A. (1953) Preliminary report on 1952 epidemic of poliomyelitis in Copenhagen with special reference to treatment of acute respiratory insufficiency, *Lancet*, i, 37.

MACRAE, J., MCKENDRICK, G. D. W., SEFTON, E. M., and WALLEY, R. V. (1954) Positive-pressure respiration: management of patients treated with Clevedon respirator, *Lancet*, ii, 21.

MEHTA, S., PATEL, K. C., JINDANI, A., and HARRIES, J. R. (1970) Benign intracranial hypertension, *E. Afr. med. J.*, 47, 333.

ROSSI, E. (1958) in *Poliomyelitis: Papers and Discussions Presented at the Fourth International Poliomyelitis Conference*, Philadelphia, p. 505.

SMITH, A. C., SPALDING, J. M. K., and RUSSELL, W. R. (1954) Artificial respiration by intermittent positive pressure in poliomyelitis and other diseases, *Lancet*, i, 939.

TRUETA, J. (1956) in *Handbook on Poliomyelitis*, eds. Trueta, J., Wilson, A. B. K. and Agerholm, M., Oxford, p. 82.

19 Neurosurgery in Rhodesia

L. F. LEVY and J. AXTON

INTRODUCTION

Rhodesia is a landlocked territory in the southern part of Africa; to the south is the Republic of South Africa, to the north the Republic of Zambia, eastwards lies Mozambique and westwards, Botswana. Most of the country lies at or above 4000 feet on a central plateau where the climate is subtropical, although many tropical diseases such as malaria, bilharzia, trypanosomiasis and cysticercosis are seen. To the north this plateau drops sharply to the Zambesi river valley, while to the south it slopes away less abruptly to the Limpopo river, both of which form natural boundaries to the country. Rainfall in the east is approximately 32 inches per year, in the west it is about 25 inches, all of it falling between the months of November and March when the country is green. During the remaining 7 months the country becomes dry and brown and bush fires are common. The two largest towns are Salisbury in the east (350 000 Africans, 120 000 Europeans), and Bulawayo in the west (170 000 Africans, 40 000 Europeans) situated at more or less opposite ends of the plateau. Six other towns of up to 60 000 people scattered throughout the country comprise the main centres of population and industry. Economically the country is dependent upon agriculture, light industry and mining.

The population can be split into two basic groups, approximately 5 000 000 people of African descent and slightly over 200 000 of European descent, with a further 10 000 of mixed and 10 000 of Asian descent. There are another 100 000 Europeans in neighbouring territories, some of whom attend for medical treatment. The African population is divided into two main groups: the Mashona—descendants of the original southerly migrating tribes who settled in the east of the country; and the Matabele—Zulus who doubled back and migrated northwards under Mzilikazi in the middle of the last century—who live in the west, although increasing urbanization of the population has tended towards a mixing of the groups. Constant raids by the Matabele on the Mashona punctuated the lives of these people and the animosity so engendered is still echoed in a certain amount of intertribal rivalry. In addition there is a fair leavening of Malawians migrating south, usually on a temporary basis to work, who then return to their homeland after a number of years. Living habits and diet are essentially similar in all areas.

The disease patterns among the European population are similar to those of Europe or the United States of America, and their living standards do not differ greatly. By contrast, although many live in towns, a large proportion of Africans live in Tribal Trust Lands or Reserves and many still adhere to the tribal way of life. Indeed, of the urban people very few can be said to have completely severed their rural connexions and to be considered totally detribalized town-dwellers. In the rural areas the houses are usually circular and consist of poles and wood lined with mud with a thatched roof, although occasionally brick or stone is used. In the towns, houses comprise anything from a formal brick or prefabricated house to a tin shanty, depending upon the location. The diet in many areas is poor, consisting mainly of mealie meal (maize)—over 80 per cent of the calories are derived from this source—flavoured with meat and vegetables. A very small percentage of the calories is derived from fats. In addition to overt malnutrition or subnutrition many patients suffer from the consequences of overcrowding and poor hygiene—parasitic infestation, tuberculosis, anaemia and vitamin deficiencies, in addition to their neurological disorder.

Hospital facilities comprise two large central hospital groups in Salisbury and Bulawayo, each with a wide range of specialist services. Rural hospitals and clinics in the smaller towns and country areas, both government and missionary, supply local medical and surgical services and refer such patients as they think require it to the larger centres. Neurological surgery is located in Salisbury and most cases requiring surgery are transferred there.

The Godfrey Huggins Medical School of the University of Rhodesia is located in Salisbury and is centred on the Harare Central Hospital. Graduating between 35 and 40 students per year this medical school is being supervised until 1975 by the University of Birmingham whose degrees will be awarded until that date.

The central hospital patient population therefore varies tremendously from the sophisticated town-dweller to the rural agriculturalist and many have little idea of the factors which may cause disease. The belief is still widely held that the Mudsimu or ancestral spirits, who must be properly respected and placated, can cause disease if displeased, while spells cast by other living persons are also held responsible for much ill health. For this reason most patients still consult the nganga or herbalist (sometimes called the witch doctor) first, in an effort to get these matters settled before presenting at a clinic or hospital, unless the complaint is obviously one about which the latter can do little, for example a broken bone or other results of trauma. The nganga stands in relation to his local population in much the same way as the true general practitioner does to his patient elsewhere. He is a combination of father confessor, religious mentor, seeker-out of evil spirits and interpreter of their wishes, and simple physician. He treats a variety of conditions and has success with many mild illnesses especially those of functional origin, but in attempting to treat more serious diseases he may delay the patient's eventual progress to hospital. Rarely does he give any treatment that is not connected in some way with the mystical.

Once the patient decides to take himself to a clinic or hospital his troubles are far from over. The distance to the nearest clinic may be many miles and he may not possess money for the bus fare even if such transport exists. Once at an outlying clinic there may be delays before transport can be arranged on to a major medical centre. Having eventually arrived at such a centre, further difficulties such as the natural reluctance of many rural people to consent to an operation on the head, the nature of which is difficult to understand, may cause further delays and almost invariably such a decision has to be a family affair.

Neurosurgery has now been performed as a speciality in Salisbury for 16 years and inevitably, as the unit and service become better known throughout the community, so the work steadily increases. Over the 11 years from January 1957 to December 1967, 1676 operations were performed on African patients and 1230 on European patients. The fact that there have been almost as many 'European' operations as 'African', when the populations are so disparate, is explained partly by the fact that only a very small percentage of the African population requiring therapy actually reached the Neurosurgical Unit, but also by the fact that disease patterns vary between the races. For example, as the African population is so heavily weighted towards youth, diseases of old age are not nearly so common as they are in other peoples. None the less, once having reached the age of 40 a person's expectation of life is virtually equal in the two races and as 15 per cent of the African population are over 40 years (75 000 people) there should be a considerable number of patients presenting themselves at hospital with degenerative complaints. However, although atherosclerosis, for example, is a major degenerative and killing disease among Europeans it is almost unknown among Africans. This is shown by the fact that the internal carotid artery has only once been explored in an African patient, while it was explored 16 times during the same period in Europeans, and this may also have some bearing on the apparent rarity of Parkinson's disease and some other degenerative disorders.

NEUROSURGICAL PROCEDURES

Table 19.1

Synopsis of Neurological Procedures Performed in Salisbury: January 1957 to December 1967

Operations	*European*	*African*
Head trauma		
Depressed fracture of skull	60	173
Subdural haematoma	98	191
Epidural haematoma	13	18
Aspiration of intracerebral haematoma	21	17
Gunshot wound of skull and brain	6	3
CSF fistula	1	3
Caroticocavernous fistula	—	2
Cranioplasty	39	35
Space-occupying lesions		
Brain tumours	241	136
Intracranial abscess	32	65
Tuberculoma of brain	—	32
Orbital decompression	2	9
Cysticercosis of brain	2	5
Mucocele of sinuses	1	5
Diagnostic burr-holes		
Ventriculography: head injury, brain biopsy	91	192
Cerebrovascular disorders		
Cerebral aneurysm	45	17
Cerebral angioma	7	1
Exploration internal carotid artery	16	1
Temporal arteritis	4	—
Congenital disorders		
Hydrocephalus	44	155
Meningocele	12	88
Craniostenosis	1	—
Spinal disorders		
Operations for spinal decompression (traumatic paraplegia and tetraplegia and other decompressions)	49	142
Herniated lumbar intervertebral disc	108	17
Spinal cord tumours	29	93
Anterolateral and other vertebral body resections for tuberculosis	—	57
Skull traction for cervical injuries, etc.	8	24
Cervical disc and fusion for trauma	18	13
Gunshot wounds and stab-wounds of spine	5	12
Spinal arachnoiditis	4	9
Operations for cervical osteoarthritis	27	5
Spinal fusion	1	1
Scoliosis	1	1
Wiring of cervical spine	1	2
Cysticercosis of spine	—	1
Operations for pain		
Fifth nerve procedures—various	50	4
Cordotomy	17	2
Posterior root section	25	2
Peripheral nerve operations		
Anastomosis, lysis, etc.	27	7
Anterior root section	—	7

Operations	*European*	*African*
Obturator neurectomy	1	5
Sympathectomy	2	—
Carpal tunnel syndrome	2	—
Psychosurgery and epilepsy surgery		
Leucotomy	14	11
Cortical resection	6	2
Stereotaxic surgery		
Parkinson's disease and athetosis	28	24
Pituitary stalk resection for carcinoma	3	—
Sequestrectomy for osteomyelitis and infected bone flap, etc.	24	27
Basal meningitis	2	5
Miscellaneous	11	17
Tenotomy	—	1
Tracheostomy	31	37

Cerebral Tumours

Tumour surgery forms a very large proportion of the work of neurosurgeons in Europe and North America, and malignant primary neoplasms constitute the largest group of these. These tumours tend to occur in patients over the age of 40 and it is for this reason that they are not nearly so frequently seen in African practice where only 15 per cent of the population exceeds that age compared with 32 per cent among the Europeans. It is partly this that has given rise to the belief that 'brain tumours do not occur in Africans'. That they do is shown by the fact that over the last 10 years 172 have been seen and operated upon by us, but this is a small proportion of those occurring in the African population of 5 000 000. By contrast, 152 brain tumours were seen over the second 5 of these 10 years in a European population of slightly over 200 000 [TABLE 19.2]. The malignant glioma is the tumour most commonly seen among Europeans—55 in a total of 152 (36

Table 19.2

152 *Brain Tumours Seen in Europeans over* 5 *Years Compared to* 172 *Brain Tumours Occurring in Africans over* 10 *Years on the Neurosurgical Units at the Harare Central and Salisbury Central Hospitals*

Tumour	*European*	*Percentage*	*African*	*Percentage*
Astrocytoma: Grade I	7		8	
Grade II	7	36·00	7	20·00
Grade III	20		3	
Grade IV	21		15	
Craniopharyngioma	1	0·65	5	3·00
Cerebral metastases	41	26·50	9	5·30
Ependymoma	3	1·95	11	6·55
Meningioma	19	12·50	34	20·2
Pituitary tumour	10	7·10	14	8·35
Eighth nerve tumour	3	1·95	1	0·60
Third ventricle tumour	1	0·65	1	0·60
Oligodendroglioma	1	0·65	—	
Medulloblastoma	8	5·50	11	6·55
Oligo-astrocytoma	1	0·65	—	
Astrocytoma of cerebellum	2	1·30	3	1·80
Glioma unclassified	4	2·60	—	
Haemangiosarcoma	1	0·65	—	
Melanoma	2	2·20	—	
Neuriloma (source undiagnosed)	—		1	0·60
Pontine glioma	—		2	1·20
Posterior fossa tumour (undiagnosed)	—		2	1·20
Tuberculoma[1]	—		32	19·00
Granuloma—blastomycosis	—		1	0·60
Plasma cell myeloma of skull	—		1	0·60
Squamous cell carcinoma	—		1	0·60
Haemangio-endothelioma	—		1	0·60
Carcinoma of nasal sinus	—		2	1·20
Yeast granuloma	—		1	0·60
Cysticercosis of brain	—		5	2·80
Benign cyst of brain	—		1	0·60
Total:	*152*		*172*	

[1] The tuberculoma has been included in this group as a 'brain tumour' because it is a space-occupying lesion frequently indistinguishable from a neoplasm before operation and occasionally only after histological examination.

per cent). By contrast, 33 cases (20 per cent) were seen among Africans, and although the absolute number on percentage occurring in Europeans far exceeds those occurring among Africans, in both groups the more malignant Grade IV lesion predominates. Among Europeans, cerebral metastases form the next largest group, with 41 cases (26·5 per cent), while nine cases were seen among Africans (5 per cent). This, like the malignant glioma, is a function of the age structure of the two populations. The majority (but not all) of these metastases in Europeans were the first sign of neoplasia—all were the first sign in Africans. By contrast, 34 meningiomas (20·2 per cent) were seen in the African group compared with only 19 (12·5 per cent) in the European group. The benign meningioma is therefore more commonly seen than other growths but even this benign tumour has its disadvantages. Even in the most developed countries patients are seen in whom a tumour has been present for many years and under those circumstances it may have interwoven itself among, but not invaded, many vital structures of the brain—for example the carotid artery and optic nerves, and cannot be removed without doing severe damage to them. This unfortunate state of affairs is commonly seen in any centre but seems more common in Africa. Such a tumour, histologically benign, assumes a quasi-malignancy as a result of this infiltration which makes total removal difficult or impossible and recurrence very likely.

Tuberculoma of the Brain

An accurate pre-operative diagnosis of the nature of any cerebral space-occupying lesion is desirable and is made necessary by the occasional occurrence of masses which the surgeon would rather not remove immediately if it can be avoided. One such mass is the tuberculoma, which constitutes 19 per cent of our cold space-occupying lesions, a figure commensurate with the Indian experience of Ramamurthi (1961 *a*), Ramamurthi and Varadarajan (1961), Dastur and Iyer (1966), Dastur and Desai (1965), and Sinh, Pandya, and Dastur (1968), and slightly greater than that of Odeku and Adeloye (1969) in Nigeria who found 12·5 per cent and Collomb *et al.* (1963) in Senegal with 14 per cent. Cabieses (1961) noted 17 per cent in Peru.

Delay before surgery is undertaken in these cases is desirable because on several occasions a massive 'flare-up' of the tuberculous process has followed their too early removal. In these cases craniotomy had either been forced by the patient's clinical state, or else the nature of the lesion was not apparent before operation so that antituberculous therapy was not given pre-operatively to provide antibiotic cover. In a number of cases the mass will subside on suitable chemotherapy and surgery will be obviated although epilepsy from brain scarring is likely to remain and cause some problem. If possible, a course of INH, PAS, and streptomycin should be given first and surgery only embarked upon if the pressure signs become more marked and demand urgent relief. Not every case, however, will respond to antituberculous therapy and one patient who was followed up for a year prior to requiring surgery died from this encephalitis despite the fact that he had been receiving antituberculous therapy throughout the period. The factors responsible for determining which mass can and which cannot be removed safely are as yet unclear. Ramamurthi and Varadarajan (1961) feel that 2 weeks of chemotherapy should show a marked improvement in the patient's condition, and they use this as a therapeutic test for tuberculoma—our experience is that a longer period is required before the patient may show benefit.

The pre-operative diagnosis of tuberculoma may not be easy. A Heaf or Mantoux test should be performed in every case, although occasionally it will not be helpful while a search for TB foci elsewhere must be undertaken. X-ray of the skull is not very revealing in our experience as only the old and virtually healed lesions show calcification. Cerebral arteriography will indicate the presence of a space-occupying lesion, the histology of which may be divined from its total avascularity in the majority of cases. In regions where tuberculosis and parasitic diseases of the brain are uncommon, the surgeon would probably refrain from lumbar puncture in the presence of a manifest increase in intracranial pressure, but it has been our policy to carry out this test on patients suspected of harbouring such a lesion. Provided the test is done carefully, with a very small needle, and only up to 4 cc of cerebrospinal fluid is removed we believe that the information gained outweighs the dangers and indeed we have had no untoward results with the test. The fluid may show a few lymphocytes and an elevated protein; if many lymphocytes are present this suggests that some degree of tuberculous meningitis is also present, an additional reason for delaying surgery as long as possible.

At operation the tuberculoma is usually seen to be greyish, or greyish-yellow and may appear not to infiltrate the brain on the surface. For this reason it can be mistaken for a meningioma, although it is rare for the tumour not to involve the brain at some point. Inside, the tumour may be rubbery or firm and removal of the centre of the mass, if this is necessary to collapse it and allow complete excision, may be very difficult.

Generally speaking, the long-term results of successful removal of these masses is good but there are still many problems to be overcome at the actual time of surgery. Of our 32 cases, one was cured by antibiotics alone, while of the remainder the mortality was 53 per cent among the early operation/no antibiotic group, but was still 33 per cent in the delayed operation/antibiotic group.

Brain Abscess

Frank brain abscess is not nearly as common as one might expect. Over the 11 years in question 65 such lesions were seen in African patients and 32 in European patients. Brain abscesses as seen in Africans tend to be of the solitary type, and the acute diffuse fulminating abscesses that one sometimes sees in European patients do not seem to occur. It is believed that this is because the really severe infection, which one might expect to produce multiple abscesses if it was treated early, does not receive treatment in time with the result that the patient dies from the acute fulminating meningitis, instead of surviving at the expense of several foci of pus formation as happens in many European cases who seek immediate treatment. African patients suffering lesser infections which produce solitary abscesses as their complications are the ones who come for treatment (Pennybacker, 1956; Levy, 1963). An abscess is suspected if a patient presents with signs of meningitis associated with focalizing neurological signs or if a localized infection close to the brain (middle ear, sinus) is noted with meningitic extension and clinical deterioration. Arteriography is undertaken as soon as the abscess is suspected, although for abscesses thought to be in the posterior fossa ventriculography or exploratory needling may be required. These abscesses are treated by repeated needling through a burr-hole until all pus has been removed and the inflammatory process has settled down. Arteriography or pneumoencephalography is then employed to determine whether a space-occupying capsule remains. If there is no capsule or the capsule is completely collapsed, no further therapy is given except to ensure that the primary focus has been adequately treated; should an abscess capsule remain and cause a ventricular shift, it is removed by craniotomy.

Solitary brain abscess carries with it a relatively low mortality; in contrast to this subdural abscess, which is by no means uncommon, is associated with seizures usually of a Jacksonian nature although they often progress to a generalized convulsion or status epilepticus. This condition, also treated by drainage through several burr-holes, has a very high mortality.

Head Trauma

Trauma plays a very large part in the work of the hospital, and the neurosurgical department is no exception. All types of head injury are seen, associated with motor accidents or crimes of violence, and 50 per cent of our beds are occupied by such cases. No surgeon can avoid a wide experience in the treatment of such injuries. In the 11 years from 1957 to 1967, 442 operations for head trauma were undertaken on Africans and 238 on Europeans [TABLE 19.1]. There appears to be no significant difference in the results of head trauma in these two groups.

Spinal Cord Tumours and Non-Traumatic Compression

In contradistinction to brain tumours, which are much more commonly seen among Europeans than among Africans (although the incidence of the neoplasm in either group cannot be estimated), spinal cord tumours in Africans greatly outnumber those seen in Europeans. One hundred and ten compressive spinal cord lesions (excluding trauma and spinal column tuberculosis) occurred in Africans during the period under review compared with 34 such lesions in Europeans [TABLE 19.3]. These cases consist only of those in which the spinal cord symptoms were the primary manifestation of disease. The most salient difference lies in the part played by infection in Africans and the same situation seems to hold good in India (Ramamurthi, 1961*b*). Of particular interest are the nine granulation tissue masses and the 15 cases of arachnoiditis (localized pial-arachnoidal scarring with cord compression) neither of whose aetiologies could be determined. In the former a mass is found lying in the extradural space, frequently attached to the dura mater and compressing the spinal cord. This mass is usually somewhat firm in consistency and appears totally removable at operation. Histologically a chronic granuloma is observed. Some of these granulomas are typically tuberculous, while in other cases no aetiology can be ascribed. Grossly, those that are frankly tuberculous on histological examination are indistinguishable from those in which the infective agent cannot be elucidated. Clinical improvement usually results from their removal and most patients are treated for tuberculosis even though this aetiology cannot be proven.

The cause of arachnoiditis is quite obscure in the majority of our own and other people's cases (Rodgers and Cruickshank, 1962). The patient presents with a history of progressive weakness and pain or even total paraplegia. The arachnoiditic process which binds the spinal cord or nerve roots tightly in a pial-arachnoidal fibrous scar lies at any, and often quite a restricted, level of the spinal cord or cauda equina. Lumbar puncture may demonstrate a complete block to the passage of cerebrospinal fluid with high protein and some cells, usually lymphocytes. Myelography using oil or air (Jacobson, 1969) shows the obstruction. It is presumed that the neurological defect results from compression of the nerve fibres and vessels. Attempts to free the scar tissue have not met with great success, although the dissecting microscope may make this possible. Improvement following radiotherapy (Feder and Smith, 1962) and steroids (Rodgers and Cruickshank, 1962) has been reported.

Pott's Disease of the Spine

Tuberculosis of the spine is very common and in former years, before the development of antituberculous drugs, prolonged sanitorium treatment was the only therapy that could be offered.

Table 19.3

Non-Traumatic Spinal Cord Compression in Europeans and Africans

	European 34 *cases*	*African* 110 *cases*
Benign tumours		
Neurofibroma	5	12
Meningioma	2	4
Haemangioma	1	1
Angioma of bone	—	1
Haemangiopericytoma	—	2
Aneurysmal bone cyst	—	1
Calcified cyst, type unknown	1	—
Osteoma	1	—
Chondroma	1	—
Ependymoma	2	—
Malignant tumours		
Primary:		
Sacrococcygeal chordoma	—	1
Astrocytoma of cord	1	3
Ganglioneuroblastoma	—	1
Type unknown	2	2
Secondary:		
Myeloma	—	4
Haemangio-endothelioma	—	1
Carcinoma, primary site unknown	4	6
Thyroid carcinoma	—	4
Parotid carcinoma	1	—
Prostate carcinoma	1	—
Lung carcinoma	1	—
Hepatoma	—	1
Seminoma	—	1
Fibrosarcoma	—	1
Lymphosarcoma	5	7
Hodgkin's disease	—	2
Lymphoma	—	1
Reticulum cell sarcoma	—	1
Infections		
Acute bacterial—epidural abscess	—	1
Tuberculous granulation tissue	—	3
Granulation tissue	1	9
Tuberculomata	—	2
Cysticercosis	—	1
Hydatid disease	—	1
Arachnoiditis	—	15
Congenital		
Arachnoidal cyst	—	3
Dermoid cyst	2	3
Spinal cord compression (cause unknown)	3	15

Frequently this failed to result in a resolution of the paraplegia which complicates a considerable number of cases. Surgical intervention was not regarded favourably in these cases because of the frequency of secondary infection and the danger of miliary spread of the disease throughout the body. With the introduction of antituberculous drugs, however, a new approach to tuberculous paraplegia has been permitted, in that it has now become possible to sterilize the diseased area and resect that part of the spinal column which has collapsed and is causing pressure on the spinal cord. This is done by means of an anterolateral (Alexander, 1946; Dott, 1947), transthoracic (Hodgson and Stock, 1960), or anterior cervical (Cloward, 1958) approach. The abscess cavity is opened and the pus and diseased bone resected until healthy vertebral bodies are exposed above and below, and all the necrotic tissue is removed from the dura, which is completely decompressed. A healthy strut of bone is then removed from the iliac crest and grafted in to fill the gap between the vertebrae.

The anterolateral approach, in which the operator comes obliquely down onto the vertebral body from a point about 2 inches lateral to the midline, exposing the intercostal nerve and the pedicle on the way to the vertebral body, is satisfactory in the thoracic and lumbar regions, and particularly so if there is a marked kyphos present angling the spine out towards the operator. None the less, even in these circumstances it is still difficult to see round the corner to the dura mater and to remove the tissue from the anterior surface of the dura without damage. This is particularly so if calcification has taken place and a bony posterior ridge has formed. The anterolateral approach cannot be used in the cervical region, nor in the approach to the body of L5 nor at the upper end of the sacrum. The transthoracic approach, which is made through the front of the chest and involves cutting one or two ribs (or possibly even resecting one subperiosteally), allows very good access to the thoracic vertebrae from T3 to T10. Once the thoracic cage is opened, the pleura is incised and the lung collapsed. The mediastinal structures are pulled across out of the operator's way and the abscess cavity, lined by parietal pleura and fibrous tissue, is exposed. Care must be taken when the intercostal arteries are sectioned as they can produce brisk bleeding, but this route provides a very good approach to the vertebral bodies and the posteriorly lying dura, which the operator may look at straight from the front instead of round the corner as in the anterolateral approach. The cervical region is best approached from the front, as described by Cloward. The most difficult areas are the fifth lumbar vertebra, second, third and fourth thoracic vertebrae, and the first and second cervical vertebrae. The fifth lumbar vertebra can best be approached from the front using an extraperitoneal approach. A paramedian abdominal incision is made, and the parietal peritoneum and its contained viscera are moved sideways to expose the body of the fifth lumbar vertebra. Care must be taken to demonstrate the ureter and the large vessels of this region. The upper end of the thoracic cage can be approached through the axilla, the operator passing his instrument between the second and third ribs at their most lateral aspect. The apex of the lung is pushed downwards, if possible extrapleurally, and the lateral aspects of the vertebral bodies are exposed. The best approach to the upper end of the cervical spine is still a matter of debate—the transoral route through the pharynx has been recommended, as has the retropharyngeal route. The odontoid process is the most commonly affected point in the upper cervical region and many prefer to treat this conservatively, because of the difficulty of operating on it and also because it does not commonly lead to paraplegia. Fusion of the C1–C2 joints would be preferred by many rather than a direct attack on the disease process.

It has been our practice to treat the majority of tuberculous paraplegics by resection of the diseased region with extremely gratifying results in that their hospital stay is reduced and the final outcome greatly improved; the majority make a complete recovery. It seems that if a patient has a paraplegia without spasticity and hyper-reflexia, he has a good chance of making a complete recovery; if he has some spasticity he will probably be left with some disability. The exact mechanism of this is not clear at the present time.

Spinal Cord Trauma

In the treatment of spinal cord trauma it has been our policy to decompress the majority of such patients by laminectomy where cord pressure can be demonstrated. We have felt that in the lumbar region this is particularly important, because there the nerves are 'peripheral' and should possess the same regenerative ability as their more distant branches in the arms and legs. Even if these are anatomically intact they may be prevented from recovering by pressure from dislodged discs, a fractured vertebral body or laminae. This pressure produces a neurapraxia and traumatic inflammation which may proceed to an adhesive arachnoiditis. Our observations suggest that this adhesive process constricts the nerve fibres and prevents recovery of function, and therefore our object is to remove the pressure and to separate these compressed nerve fibres as far as possible, while allowing them to float freely in their bath of cerebrospinal fluid, so that the inflammation will subside and function will be restored. In the thoracic and cervical regions we practise decompression if we feel that there is any chance that complete destruction of the cord has not occurred because we feel that this must be the logical therapy, even though it is often demonstrated that the cord is irrecoverably damaged. No patient has been made worse by this process, and rarely has the spine become unstable. The ultimate solution to this problem can only be the resection of a vertebral body with end-to-end anastomosis of the cord, so far practised on several cases without success, or spinal cord transplantation to fill in the defect. Nothing can be successfully done about spinal cord grafting or suturing until the problem of spinal cord regeneration and the ability of the recovering fibres to cross the gap between the upper and lower segments of the cord has been solved (Turbes and Freeman, 1953). However, with poor rehabilitation facilities and often desperate home conditions, the problem of spinal cord regeneration is greater in Africa than in other countries.

Herniated Lumbar Intervertebral Discs

Prolapse of a lumbar intervertebral disc is very common in the white races but extremely uncommon among Africans. In the course of 9 years only 21 discs were removed from the entire African population whereas during the same period over 1000 discs were removed from the European population of our own and surrounding territories. The majority of patients were males and the L4–L5 disc was most constantly involved in contradistinction to the L5–S1 disc seen in most Europeans. The patients always presented with extremely severe symptoms; indeed five were admitted with paraplegia or paraparesis although only four gave a history of trauma. It is believed that this condition occurs less frequently in Africans than in Europeans because of the increased mobility of the lumbar spine in the former group. Tests have shown that the range of flexion and extension of the spine in young Africans is much greater than it is in Europeans, and presumably it is this mobility which protects the patients from extensive disc herniation (Levy, 1967).

Porter's Neck

This is trauma to the cervical spine caused by carrying heavy articles on the head, which is a widespread practice in Africa. These articles range from small packages and pots and pans, to long sticks being carried for firewood, and heavy sacks. In Rhodesia alone over 8 000 000 bags of mealie meal are grown annually quite apart from the innumerable sacks of other foodstuffs, fertilizers, etc., which are produced. The vast majority of these sacks, which sometimes weigh as much as 200 lb are carried on a porter's head at some point in their journey to the consumer, if not more than once. It is a testimony to the strength of the cervical vertebrae, discs and muscles, that over the course of the last 10 years only 14 cases of severe injury to the neck resulting from carrying such sacks have been seen in the Neurosurgical Unit at the Harare Hospital. Other milder cases have reported to the Outpatients' Department but none the less they are relatively few compared with the number of sacks transported. It is interesting to note that whereas most injuries to the neck which require hospitalization and which result from a fall on the head associated with acute flexion or extension of the neck involve the vertebrae and discs at the level of C4–C5 downwards, in this type of injury the majority involve the region C1–C4. It is interesting, too, that whereas injury to the lower cervical regions results in tetraplegia, or near-tetraplegia in 50 per cent of cases, injury to the upper vertebrae rarely involves the spinal cord at all. We believe that the reason is that the injury is not one of flexion alone, as it is in a diving accident, but is a mixture of flexion and rotation because the porter carries the sack on his head, balanced by his arms but with the head embedded in the sack as it sags around him. The head, therefore, cannot move without moving the sack which has considerable weighty resistance to sudden movements, while the sack cannot be moved without moving the head. If the porter is unfortunate and slips while walking, either on the flat or up or down steps, and one leg gives way, he will not only fall forward but tend to twist to the weak side as well, imparting a flexion as well as a rotatory movement to his cervical vertebrae. As a result it is the upper two or three vertebrae that are strained as the body turns, rather than the lower ones. Injury to the cervical cord is less likely to happen when the upper cervical vertebrae are involved than when the lower are affected because the cross-sectional area of the vertebral canal in the region of the atlas is 4·66 sq cm while that of C2 is 3·09 sq cm. The lower vertebrae have a cross-sectional area which averages only 2·6 sq cm, so when movement does occur there is considerably less room available for the spinal cord and it is therefore more easily damaged. This is not the whole story, however, because, oddly enough, the narrowest part of the cervical canal is at the C3–C4 level (2·5 sq cm) which is the region of minimal cord damage (C1–C4) so that factors other than pure cross-sectional area of the affected segment must play a part. Injury to the neck seems to be a slightly different entity when a weight on the head is involved compared with an injury inflicted by a fall (Levy, 1968).

The Rehabilitation of the Paraplegic and Tetraplegic Patient

Care of paraplegic and tetraplegic patients poses a tremendous problem. In the main, cases are traumatic, neoplastic or tuberculous in origin. Of these, a certain number of patients will recover all or part of their functions. The first problem, therefore, is to provide adequate nursing and physiotherapeutic facilities so that the patient can survive his period of paraplegia without suffering irreparable damage to his physique, while the opportunity is given for his spinal cord to recover from the agent causing his paralysis. For those who do not recover, extensive rehabilitation procedures must be undertaken if all the surgery and therapy spent on them is not to be wasted, not to mention the necessity for giving the patient the maximum opportunity of living his life to the full. Rehabilitation centres do not exist *per se* in most parts of Africa and hospitals must learn to do the best they can with physiotherapy and other staff available. None the less much of this work is in vain if patients are ultimately discharged to their homes, often far away in the country. How difficult, indeed impossible, it is for a man living in a small hut miles away in the country, with a minimum of education and a maximum of insanitation, to learn to cope with paraplegia, to avoid decubitus and to cope with his bladder and bowels, and many of these unfortunates perish at home after strenuous efforts to help them in hospital have only produced purely medical treatment and no social solution to their problems. These paraplegics can only be helped in the long run by the provision of a residential paraplegic centre near a hospital where they can be properly cared for and at the same time hold down a suitable job in a nearby industrial complex, having their families to live with them if desired (Kelly and Levy, 1962).

Parasitic Infestation of the Central Nervous System

Unhygienic conditions predispose to the infestation of the body with parasites, and intestinal helminths of all sorts are extremely common. As a corollary to such insanitary conditions as are found in Africa the contamination of food with faecal matter is not uncommon. This may result in the ingestion by humans, not merely by cows or pigs, of the oncospheres of the tapeworm. In the stomach the shells and embryophores are digested and the hexacanth embryos freed. These bore into the gut wall (mistaking the human for their normal secondary host) and enter the blood or lymphatic vessels whence they are carried as emboli round the body. Becoming trapped in one of the smaller vessels they bore through the walls and enter the neighbouring tissue. This tissue is frequently muscle, but any other of the body structures may be affected and the brain or spinal cord is no exception. Once embedded the hooks are cast off and the embryo develops into a sac-like 'bladder worm' or cysticercus which may be anything up to a centimetre in diameter. This cysticercus then waits for the secondary host to be eaten. Needless to say this does not often occur in man and usually after several years the cyst dies and becomes surrounded by a calcified, or partially calcified, fibrous tissue wall. In the brain, which is not uncommonly involved, the majority of these cysticerci are found on the surface lodged in the cortex, or else closely adherent to, or within, the walls of the ventricles. It is uncommon to find cysticerci deep in the white matter. Possibly this is associated with the size of the embolic hexacanth embryos which travel along the larger vessels on the outside of the brain and then lodge at the point where the vessel becomes too small for further passage. At this point the embryo bores through the vessel wall, entering the surrounding tissue. When the surface of such a brain is examined at craniotomy or post-mortem the examiner cannot fail to be impressed by the enormous numbers of cysticerci that are present. For example, over a small area of the parietal lobe in a child of 5 years the authors once encountered 36 of these cysts lying on the surface, while on another occasion it was estimated that 2500 were present in the whole brain of a heavily contaminated adult. When there are as many as this pressure effects are marked; more commonly, however, the cysts manifest themselves by focal or generalized epilepsy from cortical irritation. At present these cysts are untreatable by medical means, in the sense that nothing is available to destroy and dissolve them, so that the epilepsy has to be controlled by routine anticonvulsants. In the course of time, as these cysticerci calcify and become less irritating, smaller amounts of anticonvulsant medication are required; however, it is probable that the tendency towards seizures never completely dies away. Only a few of these cases are amenable to surgery—occasionally a cyst may block an interventricular foramen and relief can be obtained by its removal—sometimes a particularly irritating small group may be removed to help control seizures (Mendelow, 1968). Usually, however, large groups of cysticerci lodge in the cerebral cortex and surgical removal without causing widespread damage appears impossible. Where large numbers of cysts cause pressure by their volume the problem of treatment is particularly difficult. Wide decompression by freeing large bony flaps and ventricular drainage into the auricle or great veins (ventriculo-atrial shunt) is only partially successful. Although the cysticerci appear within the substance of the brain they have only once been noted by us actually within the spinal cord. Possibly this is due to the fact that the branches of the anterior spinal artery are too small to permit the emboli to enter. Paraplegia has been caused by a group of cysts pressing on the spinal cord and in a recent case, on opening the dura mater, we found that enormous numbers of cysts were extruded from the subdural and extradural spaces. Education and increasing standards of hygiene are all that are required to control what is a very considerable problem.

Bilharzia most commonly affects the bowel (*Schistosoma mansoni*) or bladder (*S. haematobium*) but migrant worms have been found in many other parts of the body. El Gazayerli (1939) found a male *S. haematobium* in the circumflex branch of the coronary artery, while Badir (1946) removed a tumour from the conjunctiva of the left eye and found a pair of worms in a branch of the ophthalmic vein. Funjanami and Nakamura (1913) discovered a male worm in the middle cerebral vein of an experimentally infected monkey (*S. japonicum*). Raper (1948) reported seeing an adult fluke in the extradural veins of the spinal cord. Ova have also been found in emigrant sites. Gelfand (1950) examined the brains of 50 patients suffering from bilharzia who came to autopsy and found ova in 28 of them. By contrast, 25 spinal cords were examined from bilharzial subjects and only one was found to contain ova. On one occasion we have mistaken a thickened granular arachnoid caused by histologically verified bilharzial ova surrounded by scar tissue for the same tissue affected by the metastatic growth for which we were searching. In all these cases the patients appeared to have been asymptomatic. How the ova got to this site and why they caused no trouble is a matter for conjecture.

By contrast, at times the ova can cause severe damage by their presence. Bilharzial paraplegia is an established entity due to multiple small granulomata appearing around ova which have been deposited in or adjacent to the spinal cord or nerve roots (Levy and Taube, 1969; Levy, 1969; Odeku, Lucas, and Richard, 1968). Presumably these ova are living and irritate the surrounding nervous tissue which they may destroy by direct toxic action or as a result of the granuloma which forms. The presence of these granulomata and their irritating contents destroys nerves and disrupts their function so that permanent or temporary paralysis appears. Most of the cases reported in the literature seem to have had a rapid onset of paraplegia and it is our impression that this paraplegia makes its appearance early in the course of the bilharzial infestation, towards the end of the stage of dissemination of the cercariae throughout the body prior to their lodgement in the liver. The symptoms usually develop rapidly, pain usually being the first to make its appearance, followed by difficulty with micturition, weakness and numbness in varying degrees; these usually take only a few days to progress to total paraplegia. During the acute phase the diagnosis may be hard to establish, although most of the patients show an eosinophilia of the blood and in a number an eosinophilia or lymphocytosis of the cerebrospinal fluid as well—occasionally there are no spinal fluid changes. Energetic treatment with antibilharzial drugs affords relief in cases which are treated early and actively enough. Other cases have remained permanently disabled, and clearly only partial recovery can occur if the granulomata are well established even though the ova may be destroyed.

Bilharzia may attack the brain, although its mode of action is at present obscure. It would, however, appear to do so in the following ways. In the first place solitary granulomata may be produced inside the skull. This is particularly prone to occur in infestation by *S. japonicum* which, when it invades the central nervous system, appears to show a predilection for the brain as opposed to *S. haematobium* and *S. mansoni* which prefer the spinal cord. No case of a solitary large intracranial granuloma has been seen due to *S. haematobium* or *S. mansoni* and, as mentioned earlier, the only case we have seen where ova have been found in the brain during life consisted of only a mild thickening of the arachnoid without the production of physical signs or symptoms.

It is clear that bilharzia can also produce encephalitis or at least an encephalopathy. In these cases there is a lowered level of consciousness possibly associated with focal neurological impairment, and an EEG compatible with a diffuse encephalopathy. Very high eosinophil counts may be noted in the blood but the CSF may be normal. This condition also seems to make its appearance during the stage of acute invasion. It responds to determined antibilharzial therapy and would appear to be either a direct inflammatory lesion or some sort of an allergic manifestation. The pathology of this condition is by no means clear at present, likewise the relationship of bilharzial infection to epilepsy. Possibly there is no relationship here but a number of cases have been seen, particularly in European patients, in which the bilharzia appeared to have triggered off the attacks—probably it has flared up a latent epilepsy—and the latter improved once the bilharzia was treated. In view of the fact that bilharzia can produce such a profound upset as acute encephalopathy, it is not impossible that lower levels of toxicity caused by less severe infection could produce epilepsy, particularly if living ova are deposited in the brain by migrant flukes.

Both sleeping sickness (trypanosomiasis) and cerebral malaria intrude into the field of neurosurgery at times by the sudden onset of coma and the possibility that this has a surgical basis.

Atherosclerosis of the Cerebral Vasculature

Atherosclerosis is extremely uncommon in Africans. Harare Hospital in Salisbury is a general hospital of approximately 1000 beds. It serves an African population of over 500 000 and as a referral hospital for a further population of over 1 000 000. Yet during the last 2 years there has only been one case of coronary thrombosis diagnosed in this hospital. In the last 12 years there has not been a single case of amputation of the lower limbs for arteriosclerotic gangrene, apart from the occasional case associated with diabetes mellitus. No procedure for clearing out the region of the bifurcation of the common carotid artery has ever been performed, and only very rarely has a total occlusion of that artery been observed and this is not believed to have been due to atherosclerosis. One attempt was made in the 11 years under review to clear the internal carotid artery of blood clot above the carotid siphon intracranially. We do not think that this failure to undertake surgery on these vessels is due to lack of investigation, as many patients and certainly all young ones suffering from hemiplegia or hemiparesis are subjected to arteriography with this condition in mind—it is simply that large vessel atherosclerosis is extremely rare in this population (Levy, 1971).

Examination of the figures listing the principal factors of mortality for the City of Salisbury for the years 1964–65–66–67 shows that there is a significant difference in the death rate of the African and European populations over 45 years of age for the following conditions:

Arteriosclerotic and degenerative heart disease
$0{\cdot}001 > P$.

Vascular lesions of the central nervous system
$0{\cdot}01 > P > 0{\cdot}001$.

Hypertension without heart disease
$0{\cdot}001 > P$.

If the 'cause of death' study is carried further and only the population over the age of 60 years is considered (i.e. 2 per cent of the African population and 7·7 per cent of the European population) the same picture can be seen very clearly indeed [TABLE 19.4].

Table 19.4

Causes of Death in 100 African and 100 European Patients over the Age of 60 (Non-Traumatic)
(Department of Statistics, Rhodesia, 1969)

Cause	*African percentage*	*European percentage*
Coronary thrombosis	3	25
Hypertensive heart disease	3	11
Cerebral haemorrhage and thrombosis	6	14
Generalized arteriosclerosis	3	7
Congestive cardiac failure, etc.	—	5

Dietary factors must play a considerable part in the relative immunity of this population to atherosclerosis since fats form a very small portion of the diet, of which mealie meal (ground maize) is the main constituent. An investigation into the rural man's diet conducted in a reserve near Umtali, Rhodesia, showed that both men and women took in just over 1900 calories of food per day of which only 15 per cent was derived from fat. This was compared with the Europeans diet of 2500 calories which derived 35–40 per cent of its energy from fat.

Although atherosclerosis is rare, a number of cases have been seen in which it was extremely severe when present and not all these cases were older patients, so that other factors than diet must play some part. One thing seems strange, however, and that is that despite the fact that we find little atherosclerosis in the coronary and cerebral vessels and almost never make the diagnosis of coronary thrombosis, we often diagnose cerebral thrombosis and cerebral haemorrhage. This aspect of the situation requires further investigation. In addition, a considerable number of patients with thrombosis of the middle cerebral artery or its branches are seen—the aetiology of this is likewise obscure; sometimes it is related to pregnancy, never to the 'pill', but whether it actually is more common than in other races remains to be seen. Much work has to be done on this condition.

Just as cerebral atherosclerosis is relatively uncommon so are cerebral aneurysm and subarachnoid haemorrhage. This is a condition severe enough to bring a sufferer to hospital, yet over the 7 years from 1962 to the end of 1968 only 63 cases of primary subarachnoid haemorrhage were admitted to the Mpilo Hospital, Balawayo, Rhodesia, and three were brought in dead. Of these, 27 had no abnormality while 24 had aneurysms, two had angiomata and 13 had no arteriogram—this is from a hospital of 750 beds admitting 15 000 patients per annum (Levy, Rachman, and Castle, 1973; Odeku, 1968; Ramamurthi, 1969; Collomb *et al.*, 1966). The figures from Harare Hospital are similar. Vascular disease of all sorts is therefore comparatively rare.

Hydrocephalus and Myelomeningocele

The difficulties encountered in the management of the majority of African patients is probably best illustrated by considering the associated problems of myelomeningocele and hydrocephalus in children. In Europe, referral to the neurosurgeon is usually rapid and the widely accepted practice of operation soon after birth is now routine, except where the child has multiple congenital defects in addition to the myelomeningocele. The African baby born with a myelomeningocele is usually less fortunate, unless he happens to be born at one of the larger hospitals. If the child is born at home, traditional remedies may be applied to the spinal defect in the form of poultices of various sorts, before the child is taken to the nearest clinic, which may be several hundred miles away from the two centres where definitive treatment is possible. Ambulances with special incubators are not available and further deterioration in the infant's condition may occur during the journey (Sharrard *et al.*, 1963).

Once the decision to operate has been taken it follows that the hydrocephalus which develops in a large percentage of cases must also be treated. During the months and years following the shunt insertions many African children are lost to follow-up and fail to turn up for review or shunt revision. In a recent follow-up survey of over 150 African children treated with the Pudenz tube we found that 80 per cent had died, presumably because the valve became obstructed and the children failed to attend for review. In so far as many of these valves have not been recovered to be used again one has to admit that all the effort and money involved in the procedure has been wasted. Although the work involved in inserting these valves is not grudged, they are extremely expensive items and in the context of African medicine with its tight budgets, one has to ask oneself whether such procedures are justified and whether the money could not be used to some better purpose.

Depressed Skull Fractures in Infants

Depressed fractures or congenital moulding depressions of the skull in the newborn are uncommon but do occur from time to time, and in the course of 6 years 36 cases were seen on the Neurosurgical Unit. Some infants were delivered in the Maternity Department while others were delivered in outlying clinics or in their homes. In only three cases was there any obstetrical intervention and in each of these it is doubtful that the intervention caused a depression. An estimated incidence of one case in 4000 births has been made, while during a similar period one instrumentally produced depression was observed in 6000 deliveries of European women. It seems, therefore, that spontaneous moulding depressions are relatively common in this country. Characteristically, the condition consists of a depression of small or large dimensions which may indent the entire half of the frontal bone on the one side. This saucerization does not pass behind the coronal suture, although from time to time the parietal bone may be involved instead. These are not true fractures but indentations. In more than 50 per cent of cases the depression lies in the frontal region on the same side of the head as that to which the occiput pointed during the first stage of labour, and in these and other cases in which the parietal bone is involved rather than the frontal region, it is believed that the depression was caused by the pressure of the sacral promontory as the head descended past it to enter the pelvis. In other cases it was clear that pressure from a deformed pubic ramus was the cause. Pelvimetries were performed on 34 of the mothers and all were found to be abnormal in some way or other in size or shape. On the other hand, there was nothing to suggest that the children themselves were larger than normal in so far as the birthweights of these children showed no statistical difference from those of children without skull depressions. However, the head circumference, suboccipitofrontal and interparietal diameters were all found to be significantly larger when compared with a control group of 25 full-term normal deliveries. The most significant difference was that in interparietal diameter. It seems likely that an increase in the head size aggravates a relative cephalopelvic disproportion but that abnormality of the pelvis is the basic cause. The average length of labour was no greater in these cases, and only four depressions occurred in first-born infants. Probably this is due to an increase in the size of the foetus with successive pregnancies, although weight alone is not the only factor since in at least one case a previous baby of the same weight as the affected one was born without a depression. Frequently, subsequent children have been born unaffected. It is possible that multiparous women push harder in labour and that this gives less time for the head to mould, while the possibility of the pelvis altering its shape with the passage of time must be borne in mind. Some of these cases can only be accounted for on the basis of failure of asynclitism (Axton and Levy, 1965; Chassar Moir, 1956).

Elevation of these fractures is advised, if they have shown no spontaneous improvement by 1 month, in order to minimize the possibility of brain scarring from pressure, for cosmetic reasons and to exclude co-existent subdural effusions. However, we have never seriously pressured the parents over this because the majority of depressions do correct themselves over the course of several months, and since this prognosis is apparently well known to the parents it has not always been possible to obtain permission for an operation. In point of fact no subdural haematoma has been found in any of the operated cases and this suggests that the depression is a form of moulding without attendant danger to the venous sinuses. Recently, the repositioning of these depressions by sucking them out with a vacuum extractor has been suggested.

Meningitis and Subdural Effusions

Meningitis caused by *Haemophilus influenzae* or streptococcal pneumonia is common in African children under 5 years of age. Frequently, the children are brought to hospital late in the course of the disease, or after partial treatment in outlying clinics. The incidence of subdural accumulations of fluid is high and is suspected when one or more of the following is present: failure of the temperature to fall with adequate treatment; secondary rise in temperature; continuing tension of the fontanelle beyond the third or fourth day; the onset of vomiting or persisting neck stiffness. Diagnostic and relieving taps are made and if the fluid continues to accumulate, burr-holes are made followed by removal of the underlying membranes present (Ingraham and Matson, 1944).

Pain Problems

It is rare for the surgeon to undertake a procedure for pain on an African patient and the reason for this is obscure. During the 11 years in question 50 procedures for fifth nerve pain, 17 cordotomies (for malignant growths or causalgia), and 25 posterior root sections were performed on European patients, while only eight operations in all were performed on Africans. Only one case has ever been seen in which a definite diagnosis of trigeminal neuralgia has been made in an African, although it is a common diagnosis among Europeans. Although traumatic amputation of the limbs occurs, only one case of causalgia has been seen in a woman whose arm was bitten off by a hippopotamus and she refused a surgical procedure for its relief.

Parkinson's Disease

Parkinson's disease occurs frequently among Europeans—it is rare among Africans and no explanation is offered for this. Athetosis and other similar conditions associated with cerebral palsy are seen and a number of stereotaxic procedures have been performed on these patients in an effort to relieve the abnormal movement, though without much success.

CONCLUSION

The most important medical problems of Africa lie in the field of preventive medicine. If bilharzia, intestinal parasites, malaria and tuberculosis could be eradicated, much chronic ill health would be removed. Inevitably, however, the treatment services get the lion's share of any health budget because the problems with which they deal are so much more real and obvious to the man in the street. None the less, this money also has to be allocated in such a way as to produce the maximum result: there is little doubt that the most economical doctor in the context of Africa is one who can practise midwifery, paediatrics and a little simple general surgery. Such a doctor can run a rural hospital a long way from skilled help and get the best out of it. Further down the line of priorities come the specialist paediatricians, obstetricians and gynaecologists, general surgeons and general physicians. Finally, there are the plastic surgeons, orthopaedic surgeons, cardiologists and other specialist physicians, with the thoracic and neurological surgeons trailing behind, because they depend upon expensive equipment and highly trained personnel. None the less, as soon as a country reaches the stage at which it can afford these specialities, whole new fields of therapy are immediately opened up. Those working in such a speciality find that a formal training acquired in a well-developed country is only partly applicable to the new situation. In the developed countries the parasitic diseases and tuberculomas are not encountered, nor are brain tumours of the size seen in Africa, where every case reaches the doctor so much later than in Europe, so that not only are new diagnostic problems posed to the new specialist but others which tax his surgical technique to the limits are also encountered. Strangely, too, some diseases which are frequently seen in Europe will not be encountered at all. In the neurological field, headache, a common problem elsewhere, will rarely be complained of and when it is, it very frequently has a serious cause. Migrainous symptoms have only once been noted in 11 years and this was in a very well-educated African lady; they have not been noted among the rank and file attenders at casualty departments or the specialist clinics. Trigeminal neuralgia and all the other psychological types of atypical face pain are never complained of, and surely cannot exist because the pain of tic douloureux is such as to bring any sufferer to a hospital in a desperate search for relief; only one case has been seen in 11 years. Temporal arteritis, a not very common type of headache in Europe, has never been seen by us nor have Sluder's neuralgia, Horton's cephalalgia, and cluster headache. A survey is currently being carried out in the local townships to assess the size and nature of the headache problem, if it exists at all. To date, with only several hundred people questioned, one is surprised at the number who lay claim to having fairly frequent headaches yet who have not apparently sought help for them either from conventional medicine or traditional healers. Many more interviews must be conducted before the results can be classified.

Degenerative diseases are not common in Africa. This is partly a function of the age structure of the population which is exploding rapidly, but it cannot be the only cause because there are 75 000 people over the age of 40 and even this population should produce quite a sizable number of coronary thromboses, strokes and other vascular disorders. That these disorders are rare provides food for thought, and current beliefs based on our own investigations here and those of others elsewhere is that the low fat content of the diet is primarily responsible, though since the diet also contains only very small amounts of refined sugar, this too could be playing some part. Dietary and nutritional studies are continuing.

Parkinson's disease is seen but rarely—possibly this too could be an aspect of the absence of vascular disorders of the brain.

Nowhere is the problem of introducing a highly specialized field of medicine into a poor country better illustrated than in relation to the two main problems of paediatric neurosurgery—hydrocephalus and myelomeningocele. To achieve success with either of these conditions, continuing close observation of the patient postoperatively is essential, with well-developed rehabilitation services to help the patient throughout all the stages of development. Ventriculoperitoneal shunting for hydrocephalus was attended by a very high failure rate, and when a supply of Pudenz tubes became available an attempt was made to treat all patients with hydrocephalus with this valve. Eighty per cent of patients so treated have died. Clearly great discrimination has to be exercised in selecting those cases which can be treated successfully from those which cannot. Similarly, closure of the myelomeningocele is usually a forlorn hope since most parents do not have the ability to cope with such deformed children. It is usually performed to render nursing easier for the mother and to permit the discharge of the patient from hospital. The long-term outlook, however, is very poor. Attempts have been made to develop a locally produced valve for the treatment of hydrocephalus but this has had to be abandoned because of lack of suitable materials. The procedures of neurosurgery, therefore, can only be satisfactorily carried out in a well-developed environment and the neurosurgeon introducing the subject to a developing country must be prepared to see and treat cases for which his training did not prepare him. At the same time he must be able to refuse to do anything to those cases for whom it would be impossible to carry out the whole treatment satisfactorily, rather than waste money and effort on what in the long run will not give an adequate return.

References

ALEXANDER, C. L. (1946) Discussion on Pott's paraplegia, *Proc. roy. Soc. Med.*, 39, 730.

AXTON, J. H., and LEVY, L. F. (1965) Congenital moulding depressions of the skull, *Brit. med. J.*, 1, 1644–7.

BADIR, G. (1946) Schistosomiasis of the conjunctiva, *Brit. J. Ophthal.*, 30, 215–21.

CABIESES, F. (1961) Discussion of a paper by Ramamurthi, in Proceedings of the Second International Congress of Neurological Surgery, October 1961, *Excerpta med. Amst., Int. Congr. Ser.*, 36, S13, E21.

CHASSAR MOIR, J. (1956) in *Operative Obstetrics*, 6th ed., ed. Munro Kerr, J., London, p. 962.

CLOWARD, R. B. (1958) Anterior cervical spine fusion, *J. Neurosurg.*, 15, 602.

COLLOMB, H., COURSON, B., DUMAS, M., LEMERCIER, G., and TAP, D. (1966) La part des malformations vasculaire dans les accidents haemorrhagiques cérebraux, *Bull. Soc. méd. Afr. noire Langue franç.*, 11, 243.

COLLOMB, H., COURSON, B., PHILLIPE, Y., CARAYON, A., CAMAIN, R., and DUMAS, M. (1963) Tumeurs cérébrales chez l'Africain (apropos de 43 cas). *Bull. Soc. méd. Afr. noire Langue franç.*, 8, 261.

DASTUR, D. K., and IYER, C. G. S. (1966) Pathological analysis of 450 intracranial space-occupying lesions, *Indian J. Cancer*, 3, 105–15.

DASTUR, H. M., and DESAI, A. D. (1965) A comparative study of brain tuberculomas and gliomas based upon 107 case records of each, *Brain*, 88, 375–96.

DEPARTMENT OF STATISTICS, SALISBURY (1969) Personal communication.

DOTT, N. M., (1947) Skeletal traction and anterior decompression in the management of Pott's paraplegia, *Edinb. med. J.*, 54, 620.

EL GAZAYERLI, M. (1939) Unusual site of schistosome worm in the circumflex branch of the left coronary artery, *J. Egypt med. Ass.*, 22, 34.

FEDER, B. H., and SMITH, J. L. (1962) Spinal arachnoiditis, *Radiology*, 78, 192.

FUNJANAMI, A., and NAKAMURA, H. (1913) Studies on schistosomiasis japonica in infected animals and the infectivity of the horse, *Kyoto Igarkai Zasshi* (*J. Kyoto med. Ass.*), 10, No. 3. (Japanese text with German abstract.)

GELFAND, M. (1950) *Schistosomiasis in Southern Africa*, Cape Town.

HODGSON, A. R., and STOCK, F. E. (1960) Anterior spinal fusion for treatment of tuberculosis of the spine. The operative findings and results in treatment of first 100, *J. Bone Jt Surg.*, 42, 295–310.

INGRAHAM, F. D., and MATSON, D. D. (1944) Subdural haematoma in infancy *J. Pediat.*, 24, 1.

JACOBSON, H. H. (1969) The diagnosis of spinal arachnoiditis by air myelography, *Acta neurol. scand.*, 45, 376–9.

KELLY, M., and LEVY, L. F. (1962) Rehabilitation of the paraplegic, *Cent. Afr. J. Med.*, 8, 226–31.

LEVY, L. F. (1963) Intracranial abscess: the shape of things to come? *Brit. med. J.*, 1, 1455–8.

LEVY, L. F. (1967) Lumbar intravertebral disc disease in Africans, *J. Neurosurg.*, 26, 31–34.

LEVY, L. F. (1968) Porter's neck, *Brit. med. J.*, 2, 16–19.

LEVY, L. F. (1969) Bilharziasis of the spinal cord, *Cent. Afr. J. Med.*, 15, 223–4.

LEVY. L. F. (1971) Atherosclerosis in Rhodesia. A paper presented at the Atherosclerosis in Africa Conference, Marseilles, 13–17 December, *Afr. J. med. Sci.*, 2, 229–38.

LEVY, L. F., RACHMAN, I., and CASTLE, W. (1973) Subarachnoid haemorrhage in Africans, *Afr. J. med. Sci.*, 4, 77–86.

LEVY, L. F., and TAUBE, E. (1969) Two further cases of spinal bilharziasis, *Cent. Afr. J. Med.*, 15, 52–5.

MENDELOW, H. (1968) Personal communication.

ODEKU, E. L., and ADELOYE, A. (1969) Cerebral tuberculomas in Nigerian patients, *Trop. geogr. Med.*, 21, 293–304.

ODEKU, E. L., LUCAS, A. O., and RICHARD, B. A. (1968) Intramedullary spinal cord schistosomiasis, *J. Neurosurg.*, 29, 417–23.

ODEKU, L. (1968) Intracranial vascular anomalies in Nigerians, *J. Nigeria med. Ass.*, **60**, 173–9.

PENNYBACKER, J. (1956) Brain abscess, *Ann. roy. Coll. Surg. Engl.*, 7, 105.

RAMAMURTHI, B. (1961 *a*) Tuberculosis of the brain, in Proceedings of the second International Congress of Neurological Surgery, October 1961, *Excerpta med. (Amst.), Int. Cong. Ser.*, **36**, S13, E20–1.

RAMAMURTHI, B. (1961 *b*) Spinal arachnoiditis, *Indian J. med. Sci.*, **15**, 776.

RAMAMURTHI, B. (1969) Incidence of cerebral anaeurysm in India, *J. neurol. Sci.*, **30**, 154–8.

RAMAMURTHI, B., and VARADARAJAN, M. G. (1961) Tuberculomas of the brain, clinical and radiological correlation, *J. Neurosurg.*, **18**, 1.

RAPER, A. B. (1948) Cerebral schistosomiasis, *E. Afr. med. J.*, 25, 262.

RODGERS, P. B., and CRUICKSHANK, E. K. (1962) Spinal arachnoiditis, *W. Indian med. J.*, **11**, 164.

SHARARD, W. J. W., ZACHARY, R. B., LORBER, J., and BRUCE, A. M. (1963) A controlled trial of immediate and delayed closure of spina bifida cystica, *Arch. Dis. Childh.*, 38, 18–22.

SINH, G., PANDYA, S. K., and DASTUR, D. K. (1968) The pathogenesis of unusual intracranial tuberculomas and tuberculous space-occupying lesions, *J. Neurosurg.*, 29, 149.

TURBES, C. C., and FREEMAN, L. W. (1953) Apparent spinal cord regeneration following intramuscular trypsin, *Anat. Rec.*, 117, 228.

20 Neurological Disorders in Rhodesia

I. RACHMAN

INTRODUCTION

Mpilo Hospital, situated in Bulawayo—the main city of the Matabeleland Province—is the only large Rhodesian hospital, apart from the present teaching hospital in Salisbury, to provide full consultant service. Apart from the infectious diseases and tuberculosis hospitals, and a mental hospital, it is the only one available to the African population of Bulawayo and its immediate environs (approximately 205 000 people). It further serves as a referral hospital for another 1 200 000 people.

Excluding the Maternity Department, there are 580 beds—during 1969 the average daily number of patients was 603, a bed occupancy of 103·9 per cent. Admissions for the year were 15 102, and the male to female ratio was 1·2 : 1. There are no specific neurological wards—patients are admitted to the general wards under the care of a general physician, surgeon or paediatrician—although because of my special interest in neurology, most referred cases are admitted to my wards. I see most of the interesting, unusual or difficult neurological cases admitted under other consultants. In 1969, 561 patients of neurological interest were admitted, i.e. 3·6 per cent of total admissions.

Patients vary from the sophisticated, educated city-dweller to the illiterate superstitious rural African. In these circumstances the making of a correct diagnosis in the field of neurology is often a very difficult process, and even more patience is required than is in any case so necessary for the neurologist. Accepted concepts of, for example history taking, have often to be reconsidered.

Many patients suffer from more than one disease. The patient with cirrhosis of the liver—a very common condition—who presents with weakness of the lower limbs, is much more likely to have spinal tuberculosis than some very uncommon complication of the hepatic disease. Similarly, it cannot be assumed that because a patient has bilharzial ova in the urine—a common finding in the indigenous rural population—the cause of his paraplegia has been established.

History taking can be very difficult. As there are various dialects, one often has to use an interpreter and the well-known disadvantages of this need not be considered further. Then there may be inherent deficiencies in the language itself—for instance, there seems to be only one word for 'fast', 'big' and 'deep'. The word for 'pain' may be used to mean anything from a mild discomfort to paraesthesia or even weakness.

The patient's background may profoundly affect the history. Sometimes he feels that it is only good manners to give the answers he thinks will please the doctor—whether they are correct or not. He may deliberately give wrong information; for instance an illness which has been slowly progressive, for which many witch doctors have been consulted, may be described as of recent sudden onset because the patient fears he may be scolded for not having come earlier for treatment. He may deny any previous illnesses, probably because once they were over there was no need to remember them and they have been genuinely forgotten, even though serious. This will always make the diagnosis of a condition such as multiple sclerosis difficult, although at present there is no evidence at all to suggest that this condition occurs.

Very often the patient will only give information he considers relevant or essential; for instance I have seen a patient referred for 'painful ulcer' of the tongue. The fact that the tongue had been bitten during an epileptic fit was not mentioned because 'I had not been asked'. At times the complaint will be a misleading one of pain, because many only consider a condition serious if it is painful, and therefore fear that the doctor may not give their disease the necessary attention if pain is not complained of. In these circumstances leading questions, so contrary to one's training, become invaluable—but the interpretation of answers requires experience and judgement. One must beware of asking questions in the negative. In answering 'yes' to the question, 'Have you not had any headaches?', the patient will say, 'Yes, I have not had any'.

Family history, too, may often be very difficult to obtain. It is not easy for a city worker to maintain contact with his illiterate family in some inaccessible village.

The examination, too, requires much care. Sensation is especially difficult to elicit. Again the patient may say what he thinks will please the doctor, or what he thinks he should or should not be feeling; or a language difficulty may arise, as sometimes there is only one word for pain and not one that denotes merely sharpness. A pinprick that is still sharp may therefore be described as 'not painful'. Oddly enough, in bare-footed persons light touch with cotton wool is often not appreciated on the dorsum of feet which appear otherwise normal. With some patients we at first had great difficulty in getting them to understand the concept of vibration, until it was accidentally discovered that if the word which normally means 'thunder' is used, they immediately understand. On the other hand it is usually easier to detect non-organic sensory loss. The unsophisticated often falls for the well-known method of asking a patient to say 'no' when he cannot feel the touch of cotton wool.

Plantar responses are, of course, notoriously difficult to elicit in thick insensitive soles, and at times one has to use the other well-known methods of eliciting this response. There may also be some difficulty with the pupillary reaction to light. Pupils are very often smaller than a European's; for a reasonable response to be detected one should examine them away from the usually bright daylight.

Examination of the mental state will produce further difficulties. The fact that the week of the month is not known is hardly surprising in one who has no calendar and only measures time by ploughing seasons. Nor is his intelligence necessarily affected because he does not know the name of the Prime Minister. There are as yet no standard tests to replace tests like the serial subtraction of 7 from 100.

Finally a word about treatment. It is not much good ordering a drug to be taken every 4 hours if the patient has no watch and no idea of time, but with some common sense one can usually come to a sensible arrangement. Generally it is better to use drugs which need be given once daily, or morning and evening only—especially for the worker who is away from home all day.

THE SPECTRUM OF NEUROLOGICAL DISEASE

As has been mentioned, diseases of neurological interest formed about 3·6 per cent of all admissions during 1969. This figure includes cases not primarily neurological, such as spinal tuberculosis, but only those with neurological complications. Probably, a smaller proportion of neurological as opposed to other diseases reach hospital, as many people still consider conditions which result in fits or paralysis to be due to witchcraft, and therefore not illnesses for white doctors to treat.

The case-notes of all those patients who were admitted in 1969 have been reviewed, and the various conditions seen will now be briefly discussed.

Infections of the Nervous System

As in all developing countries, infections are responsible for a great deal of morbidity, and this applies to the nervous system as well.

TABLE 20.1 gives the number of cases admitted with infection. It should be noted that the seven patients with intracranial abscess all had meningitis, and are also included in the group with acute pyogenic meningitis.

Table 20.1
Infections of the Nervous System

Infection	*No. of cases*
Meningitis:	
Acute pyogenic	63
Viral	3
Tuberculous	10
Other	4
Intracranial abscess	7
Leprosy	10
Syphilis[1]	20
Tetanus:	
Neonatorum	26
Other	9
Tuberculosis of spine (with neurological signs)	39
Acute anterior poliomyelitis	1
Viral encephalitis	6
Cysticercosis	8
Cerebral malaria	7

[1] Possible cases: *see* text.

As will be seen from TABLE 20.2, 63 out of 80 cases of meningitis had purulent cerebrospinal fluids. Although the proportion of negative cultures is steadily being reduced, nevertheless there were 24 such cases. In some, at least, this was because patients had received antibiotic therapy prior to admission.

The four young adult males with meningococcal meningitis all did very well.[1] The mortality in the other cases of pyogenic meningitis in which organisms were cultured was, however, still very high, at 50 per cent (in *Haemophilus influenzae* infection) or higher. Many of these were young children who died soon after admission. Those in whom no organisms were cultured did somewhat better, 62·5 per cent surviving. This group probably included some cases with meningococcal meningitis.

Two patients had had previous episodes of meningitis and both recovered. In one patient no organisms were cultured on either occasion. The other was a child whose first infection was due to *H. influenzae* while the second was pneumococcal. This child was one of the two cases of acute pyogenic meningitis (the other also a pneumococcal infection) who were left with brain damage after recovery.

Despite modern chemotherapy a great improvement in mortality is unlikely until patients come to hospital earlier.

[1] In the latter half of 1970 there was an epidemic of meningococcal meningitis. Fifty-two cases were seen—nearly all in young adult males who made good recoveries.

Table 20.2
Pyogenic Meningitis

Organism	*Sex* Male	Female	*Age span*	*Outcome*
Meningococcal	4	0	22–30 years	All recovered
Pneumococcal	10	9	1 month–50 years	7 recovered
Streptococcal	1	4	3 weeks–17 years	1 recovered
Haemophilus influenzae	4	2	4 months–6 years	3 recovered
Other	4	1	4 days–24 years	1 recovered
No growth	17	7	5 days–70 years	15 recovered

Included in the 63 cases of pyogenic meningitis, were seven cases who, though presenting as meningitis, also had cerebral abscesses. In one infant this arose from an infected haematoma; in an adult male it followed a traumatic perforation of the roof of an orbit. The third case, a 70-year-old man, had three cerebral abscesses at autopsy.

The remaining cases are of particular interest, as they illustrate a problem which is seen from time to time. Young males, usually in their teens, with subdural abscesses, osteitis of the skull, and occasionally a sinus infection, present with fulminating meningitis progressing to rapid death. Four young males aged between 16 and 21, of whom one had a sinus infection, presented in this way during 1969. In the two cases from which organisms were cultured, streptococci were responsible.

No other abscesses were seen in 1969, but in most years some occur after mastoiditis.

Non-pyogenic (Viral and Tuberculous) Meningitis

Only three cases of viral meningitis, a child of 8 months and two adults aged 27 and 38, were seen. Recovery was uneventful.

Despite an excellent tuberculosis service, tuberculous meningitis is still very prevalent, and since tubercle bacilli are rarely seen or cultured in the cerebrospinal fluid, it is wise to regard all cases with a mononuclear pleocytosis as tuberculous, if cerebrospinal fluid sugar content is low. The occasional case of cryptococcal meningitis, which presents similarly, has usually been readily diagnosed.

Six children aged between 9 months and 4 years and four adults aged between 35 and 70 years were admitted with tuberculous meningitis. Only one survived. After the initial period of illness these patients are usually transferred to the Tuberculosis Hospital. Perhaps because of the insidious onset, patients tend to present very late, especially children, and again this is responsible for many deaths. A further difficulty is that there may be a delay in diagnosis because the cerebrospinal fluid may occasionally be atypical. The cells may be predominatly polymorphonuclear, or rarely there may be virtually no increase, and the sugar may also be normal.

Other Cases of Meningitis

Four patients referred to in TABLE 20.1 presented with the sequelae of an untreated illness which was almost certainly meningitis. In two patients with raised intracranial pressure, chronic basal meningitis was in fact confirmed either at operation or at autopsy. Other sequelae seen included mental retardation, opisthotonus, seizures, and hemiplegia.

Leprosy

Leprosy is rare in the region drained by this hospital and the cases seen are usually from the distant Zambezi valley. Most cases are admitted direct to the Infectious Diseases Hospital, but 10 patients were admitted here in 1969. Four of these were known cases under treatment who came for surgical treatment of infected lower limb ulcers. A fifth case, also a known leper, was admitted with paraplegia due to neoplastic disease.

A further five patients, four males and one female aged between 29 and 50 were diagnosed in hospital. One had a septic foot and was found to have thickened ulnar and common peroneal nerves. The other four presented with ulnar nerve palsies, although other nerves were also involved in most cases. Two of these patients had previously undergone surgical operations, one for carpal tunnel syndrome and the other for cervical spondylosis. Neither had shown much improvement, and it is very likely that leprosy was to blame for their original symptoms.

Syphilis

The diagnosis of neurological syphilis is not easy. In a population where multiple pathology is common, positive serological tests do not necessarily imply that this is the cause of the neurological symptoms and signs. The 20 cases in TABLE 20.1 had positive serology, but it is not possible to say that this was definitely the cause of the neurological disturbance in all of them.

The commonest mode of presentation was as cerebral thrombosis, nine cases having hemiplegia and one hemianopia. Atherosclerosis is generally much rarer than in Europeans and the incidence of syphilitic arteritis may partly explain why cerebrovascular disease is relatively common, while coronary artery disease is extremely rare. The 10 cases of cerebral thrombosis with positive serology were on average younger than those without evidence of syphilis. An eleventh case, a two-year-old boy with hemiplegia, may perhaps be included in this group also. The boy (and his mother too) had positive serology with no abnormality in the cerebrospinal fluid, but was not further investigated.

Of the other nine cases, six males and two females aged between 28 and 65 years, all had abnormalities in the cerebrospinal fluid—a mononuclear pleocytosis between 30 and 315 cells/c mm and protein between 41 and 144 mg/100 ml, but the Lange test did not always show a characteristic curve, nor did the cerebrospinal fluid (as opposed to the blood) always give a positive Wassermann reaction. Two of these patients had early optic atrophy, three had hemiparesis, one hemiparesis and seizures, one seizures, and one a sudden onset of paraplegia with retention of urine and a sensory level. In all cases the cerebrospinal fluid showed considerable improvement after treatment with penicillin, and apart from the two patients with optic nerve involvement, there was also great clinical improvement. The ninth case was a young male with epilepsy, a positive blood serology, but a normal cerebrospinal fluid.

General paralysis of the insane has occasionally been seen, although there were no cases in 1969. Tabes dorsalis has not been seen at all.

Tetanus and Tetanus Neonatorum

Twenty-six patients, aged between 3 and 13 days, were admitted with tetanus neonatorum. In contrast to the patients with meningitis, the majority were admitted within 1 or 2 days of the onset of the illness. This condition is known to have a grave prognosis, but 10 recovered.

Nine other patients, aged between 4 and 73 years were admitted with tetanus and five of these recovered. In both groups the ratio of males to females was approximately 4:1.

Tuberculosis of the Spine

This is a common condition, and a total of 84 patients (including those with no neurological deficit) were seen. However, as this hospital is taking part in a Medical Research Council trial, a disproportionately large number of cases may have been referred. Thirty-nine of these 84 had evidence of neurological involvement which varied from hyper-reflexia in a very few, to severe paraplegia in 14 cases. It was exceptional for there to be evidence of tuberculosis elsewhere in the body.

There were 24 males and 15 females, of ages varying from 3 to 71 years, in this group of 39 patients. Those with paraparesis were usually first seen in medical wards, and when the diagnosis was established they were transferred to our surgical colleagues.

Poliomyelitis

Immunization is now more widespread, and most patients are admitted direct to the infectious diseases hospital. Only one acute case, a 2-year-old boy, was admitted in 1969, but a large number of cases are still being admitted by our orthopaedic colleagues for correction of deformities resulting from old infection, frequently in infancy.

Encephalitis

Viral encephalitis was diagnosed when patients presented with headache, fever and impaired consciousness with or without other neurological signs, and with no evidence of malaria, frank meningitis or other cause. Unfortunately a virus laboratory is not as yet available.

This condition was diagnosed in five children aged between 1 and 8 years and in one adult of 33. Three of these patients also had seizures and one of them a hemiparesis. Four made complete recoveries, but one, a year later, was mentally retarded and had seizures. Another who had shown evidence of mental deterioration, was steadily improving when last seen.

Herpes Zoster

Patients suffering from this condition are not usually referred to consultants, and it is difficult to know how common it is. Only one patient was admitted, a male of 40 with involvement of the first and second divisions of the trigeminal nerve.

Parasitic Disorders

Cysticercosis. Eight cases of epilepsy in patients with cysticercosis were seen and these will be further discussed in the section on epilepsy. Although the occasional case of hydrocephalus or meningitis due to cysticercosis has been seen, none with these complications was admitted in 1969.

Cerebral Malaria

Although it is not as a rule seen in Bulawayo, malaria is still very prevalent in outlying districts. The incidence varies greatly, depending on the rainfall. During the rainy season, patients admitted for other reasons often have malarial parasites (*Plasmodium falciparum*) in their blood, but the presence of these does not always indicate that malaria is the cause of the neurological deficit.

1969 was a year of relative drought and there was less malaria about. Seven cases were admitted with a diagnosis of cerebral malaria. There were five males and two females aged between 2 and 26 years, and all presented with fever, headache and depression of consciousness. Two also had seizures and two developed focal signs. All responded well, but one patient with aphasia still had difficulty in speaking when discharged.

Bilharzia of the Nervous System

Bilharzia is very common in the community but compared to other parts of the country blessed with a better rainfall, the infection in each patient is comparatively light and mostly due to *Schistosoma haematobium.* The condition is not mentioned in TABLE 20.1 as no cases of neurological deficit due to this condition were seen in 1969, despite the fact that 1897 autopsies (including many deaths from outside the hospital) were performed in that year at this hospital. Well over 90 per cent (95 per cent in 1969) of all deaths have autopsies (although the spinal cord is examined only when indicated), but only one case of bilharzial granuloma in the spinal cord (and none elsewhere in the central nervous system) has been found since this hospital first opened in 1958.

Cerebrovascular Disease

Atherosclerosis

As has been stated, atherosclerosis is relatively rare. In 1969 seven patients with cerebral infarction died—all had macroscopic evidence of atherosclerosis at autopsy. Sixteen patients with cerebral haemorrhage died and atherosclerosis was found in four of the 13 patients on whom autopsies were performed.

Cerebral Thrombosis

This diagnosis was made in 29 adults, 24 males and five females aged between 19 and 72 years, and was also the presumptive diagnosis in three children aged 9 months, 2 years, and 10 years. The great majority presented with hemiplegia—with or without aphasia. One patient had the typical signs and symptoms of posterior inferior cerebellar artery obstruction; two others also had evidence of brain stem ischaemia and a third had hemianopia alone.

Although arteriography was usually only performed in younger patients, the clinical picture suggested middle or anterior cerebral artery ischaemia in the vast majority of patients. It is presumed that the patient with hemianopia had involvement of the posterior cerebral artery only. An extracranial site was shown in two patients, one in the internal carotid, while the other had a large left vertebral artery and an obstructed right vertebral. Two other patients, one with a bruit over the carotid, and another with transient ischaemic episodes were also thought to have extracranial lesions.

Only one patient had a history of transient ischaemic attacks. It is difficult to know how accurately this reflects the rarity of the condition. Most patients who have such short-lived episodes would probably either not bother to seek medical advice or blame their episodes on witchcraft.

As has been mentioned, 10 of the 29 adults had positive serological tests for syphilis, and these 10 were on average younger (mean age 40·7 years) than the other 19 (mean age 57·3 years). Despite the small numbers, the difference is statistically significant at the 1 per cent level, using the student's t test ($t = 3{\cdot}39$).

Intracerebral Haemorrhage

This condition had a very high mortality, with 16 out of 19 patients dying. One was a 5-month-old baby in whom the cause of the haemorrhage was not discovered. There was also a 40-year-old man in whom the bleeding was caused by myeloid leukaemia.

The remaining 12 males and five females were aged between 30 and 70 years and all but five had definite evidence of hypertension. Four patients had pontine and two had cerebellar haemorrhages—the others were all supratentorial.

It is, of course, not always easy to distinguish between cerebral thrombosis and haemorrhage, and it is possible that cases of the latter should in fact have been included in the thrombosis group. In addition to those mentioned above there were 10 cases in whom it was not possible to decide into which of the two groups they fell. In most of these patients, all males aged between 45 and 68 years, the difficulty of diagnosis was caused by the considerable delay occurring between the cerebrovascular accident and the patient's admission.

Subarachnoid Haemorrhage

Apart from two neonates born outside the hospital in whom haemorrhage was probably due to birth injury, there were nine cases with subarachnoid haemorrhage. One was a 5-year-old boy, another a 67-year-old man, while the other seven (four males, three females) were all between 28 and 35 years. Once diagnosed and if permission for surgery is granted (this is fairly frequently refused) these patients are handed over to our surgical colleagues.

Subdural Haematoma

Although this survey does not include cases due to trauma, subdural haematoma must be briefly mentioned as such cases often present to the physician. Diagnosis depends on a high index of suspicion. Head injury is very common among the population, and is often soon forgotten by the patient, especially if it was sustained at a 'beer drink'. Often the relatives have not been informed and consequently any history of head injury is strongly denied. It is therefore the practice of this hospital to have angiography or burr-holes done in any patient in whom there is even a slight suspicion of subdural haematoma. Inevitably, there have been patients in whom bleeding was not found, but on the other hand several lives have been saved.

Cerebral Embolism

Rheumatic heart disease is common and cerebral embolism certainly occurs. Unfortunately, because of shortage of staff, only the principal condition—in this instance the heart disease—has been recorded in the past and the exact incidence is not available. Certainly, enough of these cases are seen to make one suspect underlying heart disease in every young patient with a sudden neurological deficit such as hemiplegia.

Sinus Thrombosis

The only case of sinus thrombosis was a 50-year-old man with pneumococcal meningitis who subsequently died. His superior sagittal sinus was thrombosed.

Hypertensive Encephalopathy

Two patients, a girl of 15 and a man of 40, were admitted with fits and impaired consciousness. Both were severely hypertensive with diastolic blood pressures ranging from 150 to 180 mm Hg. However, neither of these patients had the expected advanced retinopathy. Hypertension is fairly common, but retinopathy is only occasionally seen in the African, and a diagnosis of hypertensive encephalopathy should perhaps be accepted in the absence of such changes.

Epilepsy

Epilepsy is one of the commonest conditions seen in the medical wards. In 1969, 146 such cases were admitted. However, some of these were admitted overnight only and full records are not available. More comprehensive details are available from a previous survey (Rachman, 1970) of all new cases, both in- and outpatients, seen in 1967.

One hundred and thirty-two patients were investigated, 86 males and 46 females. All age-groups from infancy to 80 were represented but in 78 patients (63 per cent) the age of onset was between 11 and 40 and in another 30 (24 per cent) it was under the age of 11. In 80 patients a full family history was available, and in only 10 of these was there definite epilepsy in another member of the family.

One patient had focal fits only, and another 15 had focal jerking before the generalized convulsion. There were premonitory symptoms in 36, although many of these patients were at first reluctant to admit bizarre visual or auditory aurae—probably because they feared ridicule or that their sanity would be queried.

Serological tests for syphilis were positive in the blood of 14 out of 84 cases. The cerebrospinal fluid was examined in 76 patients. Seven had a raised protein of between 48 and 90 mg/100 ml, two had increased cells, and three had positive Wassermann tests.

Birth trauma was thought to be the cause of the epilepsy in nine patients, and other head injuries in another nine. Evidence of cysticercosis was found in 11 cases. In one of these, the calcified cysts were seen only in the chest X-ray, in three in both chest and thighs, and in the other seven in the thighs only. Radiographs of the thighs appeared to be the one single investigation which gave most positive results. Air encephalography revealed cerebral atrophy to be the cause in one patient; in another, where electroencephalography, air encephalography, and arteriography all suggested a space-occupying lesion, but at a later date had returned to normal, a haematoma was suspected. In another patient, who had previously had a hemiplegia of sudden onset, the fits were considered to be due to cerebral atherosclerosis.

A history of alcoholic intake was not always sought or admitted to, but in six patients there was a definite relationship to drinking. The attacks usually occurred during the morning after a drinking bout; the known hypoglycaemic affect of alcohol was probably aggravated by the tendency of many to go to work without breakfast.

Eight of the 46 women insisted that seizures occurred only during pregnancy or in the puerperium.

Petit mal is not commonly encountered in hospital practice. In this 1967 series, however, two of the patients with generalized convulsions also had petit mal. (In one case there was no history of this, but electroencephalography was typical). Another child had petit mal only. In 1969 the diagnosis was made in one case—an 11-year-old girl.

No cases of narcolepsy were seen in 1967, but in 1969 this condition was thought probable in four patients. All were males between the ages of 28 and 32 years.

Febrile Convulsions

In 1969 this diagnosis was made in seven children aged between 2 months and 2 years. This figure consists only of those patients who presented because of the convulsions—and not those who had one or two convulsions while undergoing treatment for known infections.

Syncope

Although patients suffering from syncopal attacks are not as a rule admitted to hospital, there were some cases in which the diagnosis was in sufficient doubt to warrant hospitalization for observation or investigation. Three girls, aged between 11 and 16 years, and one 17-year-old male in whom syncope was the eventual diagnosis, were admitted in 1969.

Tumours

Intracranial

The incidence of brain tumours in Rhodesia is dealt with elsewhere [p. 225]. Here I shall only refer to those cases which did not reach the neurosurgeons.

The diagnosis of primary intracranial tumour was made in nine patients; three of these refused surgery and a fourth died soon after admission. A woman of 42 and a man of 74 presented with loss of vision due to optic atrophy. Pituitary fossa tumours were diagnosed, and these two cases, together with a 37-year-old male with a hemiparesis who was shown on angiography to have a space-occupying lesion, all refused further treatment.

The one patient who died was a 30-year-old man with a hemiplegia and papilloedema. At autopsy an oligodendroglioma of the left frontal lobe was found.

Metastases

Of the five patients with metastases only one reached the neurosurgeons. The youngest of the other four was a 17-month-old female child with a neuroblastoma and multiple extradural metastases with invasion of the skull and orbits. Two males aged 42 and 65 years both had carcinoma of the bronchus with metastases in the right parietal lobes. The fourth patient, a 45-year-old female, was admitted with carcinoma of the cervix. She had been treated for a melanoma on the foot 3 years previously, and at autopsy was found to have numerous widely scattered melanotic intracranial metastases.

Tumours Outside the Cranium

Three patients, boys of 7 and 9 years and a male aged 34, were seen with neurofibromatosis. The adult had a sarcoma of the leg in addition. Two other males with neurofibrosarcomas were seen aged 18 and 32.

Four patients presented with paraplegia. In one case, a 50-year-old male, this was due to carcinoma of the oesophagus which appeared to have spread directly to the vertebral column. A 52-year-old man with known leprosy had metastases from a hepatoma. A 13-year-old boy was found to have an aneurysmal bone cyst. The fourth patient, a 32-year-old male, was found on laminectomy to have an 'invasive and adherent tumour', but microscopy showed only fibrous tissue.

One male aged 58 presented with cranial nerve palsies (ninth, tenth, and eleventh nerves) due to nasopharyngeal carcinoma.

Congenital, Hereditary and Degenerative Diseases

Hydrocephalus

Patients with this condition often present very late, and only those who are willing to undergo surgery and can be helped by it are admitted. Five such patients were admitted in 1969. A girl, who was 3 months old when first seen, was found to have stenosis of the aqueduct. In the other four cases, one boy and three girls aged between 1 and 5 months, all ventricles were dilated. In two of these air encephalography showed very little cerebral cortex, and in another there appeared to be almost complete failure of development of one cerebral hemisphere.

Microcephaly

Patients with microcephaly are not usually admitted, but two girls and one boy aged between 1 month and 2 years were in hospital because of other abnormalities.

Meningoceles and Encephaloceles

Four males and three females with meningoceles were seen—of these four were, in fact, meningomyeloceles. The majority of patients were seen within a few days of birth, but three presented at 2 weeks, 4 months, and 7 years respectively. Three had no neurological deficit (although one of these developed hydrocephalus later), one had some sensory loss and hypotonic lower limbs, and the other three were paraplegic.

One 5-day-old infant presented with an encephalocele and meningitis from which she did not recover.

Cerebral Palsy

Seven children, six males, and one female aged between 10 months and 14 years, with spastic limbs were seen in hospital. Four of these were considered to be mentally retarded. One 13-month-old infant was admitted because of pneumonia, and three others because of epilepsy.

An 11-month-old male with no spasticity but with marked choreo-athetosis and mental retardation was also admitted.

Mental Retardation

Thirteen patients with mental retardation were admitted in 1969. Five of these with cerebral palsy and one with microcephaly are considered above. One male aged 20 had Down's syndrome. Four were admitted because of epilepsy. The other two patients with mental retardation were admitted prior to transfer to an institution.

There were also four other patients in whom it was possible that the mental retardation followed an illness such as meningitis or encephalitis, though details were difficult to obtain. A fifth patient, a girl aged 7 had had a severe head injury 15 months previously. Her mental state prior to the head injury was, however, doubtful, and it may be of significance that her mother suffered from severe epilepsy.

Although no cases of mental retardation due to tuberous sclerosis were seen in 1969, mention of this condition is made because a few known patients are referred from time to time from the local mental hospital, usually because of intercurrent infection.

The Hereditary Ataxias and Related Diseases

No patients suffering from these conditions were admitted in 1969, but cases of Friedreich's ataxia and other hereditary cerebellar ataxias, familial spastic paraplegia, and peroneal muscular atrophy have all been seen at times. However, such conditions are uncommon; consanguinity is extremely unusual in the local population.

Infantile Spinal Muscular Atrophy

Two patients with this condition were seen. One, a 3-month-old boy, had two other siblings who had died with this disease, and two normal siblings. The other patient was a 3-year-old girl with a less severe form and no family history.

Motor Neurone Disease

Three males and two females aged between 46 and 70 years were seen. One of these had progressive bulbar palsy only and another appeared to have primary lateral sclerosis. The other three all had mixed pictures, with bulbar palsy the predominant manifestation in one and progressive muscular atrophy in the other two.

Myasthenia Gravis

This condition is only seen very occasionally. In 1969 one 18-year-old girl with ocular involvement alone was seen.

Muscular Dystrophy

Only one case, a 10-year-old boy with the Duchenne type of muscular dystrophy, was seen in 1969. There was no family history. Other types have very occasionally been seen in other years.

Parkinsonism

This condition is very uncommon. Three cases were seen in 1969 and this is about average. One 80-year-old man with rigidity, bradykinesis and tremor subsequently died and was found to have widespread atherosclerosis. In the other two patients, males aged 55 and 73, the aetiology could not be established. Tremor was the dominant feature in both.

Disorders of Cranial and Peripheral Nerves and Spinal Cord

Optic Neuritis and Atrophy

Excluding patients discussed in other sections, in whom optic involvement was but part of the neurological picture, the optic nerve alone was affected in seven patients. Four males and one female—all aged between 15 and 25 years presented with optic or retrobulbar neuritis. Investigations were negative and all showed some improvement before discharge.

One male aged 32 and one female aged 38 presented with optic atrophy for which no cause could be established.

In all these seven cases the lesion was unilateral—the left side being affected in only one. No doubt some of these would be considered as cases of possible multiple sclerosis elsewhere, and this will be discussed in the paragraph on demyelinating disease.

One other patient, a 50-year-old female, presented with right optic atrophy and a third nerve palsy on the same side. The cerebrospinal fluid showed a protein of 63 mg/100 ml and the right anterior cerebral artery failed to fill on angiography. The patient left hospital before a final diagnosis was made. By this time the third nerve lesion had much improved.

Oculomotor, Trochlear and Abducens Nerve Lesions

In most years we see a few cases of unexplained third or sixth nerve lesions, including some with the characteristics of unilateral 'painful ophthalmoplegia', but apart from the patient mentioned above, who also had optic atrophy, only two cases with sixth nerve palsy were seen in 1969. Curiously enough both were bilateral. In an 8-year-old girl the condition cleared up completely—no cause being found. A 44-year-old man, who was admitted with mastoidis, also had bilateral sixth nerve palsies. However, this man had had a lumbar puncture (which revealed no abnormality) and it is not known whether the palsy was present before this was done.

Paresis of ocular muscles associated with proptosis is not uncommonly seen, but in 1969 only one such case was admitted. At operation a 'fibrous granuloma' was removed.

Facial Nerve Palsies

Bell's palsy is not infrequent, but such patients are not normally admitted. Those seen in hospital are usually cases referred from elsewhere with lower motor neurone seventh nerve palsies which have not cleared up after several months. A 3-year-old girl and two males aged 36 and 39 with palsies of five to twelve months' duration were seen. No other abnormalities were found.

Another 39-year-old female was also admitted because of a seventh nerve palsy but was found to have chronic suppurative otitis media. Her palsy cleared up completely.

Other Cranial Nerve Lesions

Other cranial palsies were not seen in isolation—and those cases in which they occurred are discussed in the relevant sections. It is of interest that only one case of trigeminal neuralgia has been seen in the last 10 years.

Peripheral Nerve Lesions

Radial nerve lesions ('Saturday-night palsy') are not infrequently seen in outpatient clinics, but the only case admitted was a patient whose radial nerve was accidentally injured by an injection.

All the ulnar nerve lesions seen were due to leprosy. Common peroneal nerve pressure palsies are also seen, but there was none in 1969.

Carpal Tunnel Syndrome

Although no cases were admitted in 1969, a few are usually seen each year. This condition is certainly less common than in the local white population.

Prolapsed Intervertebral Disc

Thirty-one cases of prolapsed intervertebral discs were admitted but only 10 of these presented with neurological symptoms and signs and are included in this review. There were eight males and two females, and the ages varied from 25 to 71 years, although only two patients were over 50.

One patient had a cervical (C5–C6) protrusion, in another it was at L3–L4. L5–S1 was the commonest site (five cases) and L4–L5 the next (three cases). All but three of the patients underwent surgery.

Peripheral Neuropathies

Excluding the Guillain-Barré syndrome, four patients with peripheral neuropathy were seen. In a 70-year-old man with uraemia, who had motor signs and pain but no objective sensory loss, the neuropathy was almost certainly precipitated by nitrofurantoin. In two patients, a man of 33 and a woman of 35 with both motor and sensory signs, no cause was established. Both showed considerable improvement. The fourth case was a 69-year-old male with a predominantly sensory neuropathy. Only the lower limbs were affected. It was thought that this probably had a nutritional origin.

A few cases of arsenical, alcoholic, carcinomatous and diabetic polyneuropathy have been seen in recent years.

Four cases were considered to be due to the Guillain-Barré syndrome. There were two males and two females aged between 20 and 42 years. The cerebrospinal fluid protein content was 186 mg in one case, and in the other three between 420 and 540 mg. One patient who had had a previous episode showed only slight improvement.

Myelopathies

Six patients presented with paraplegia of subacute onset. Three of these, two males aged 14 and 21 and a woman of 35, were considered to have transverse myelitis. One was still severely disabled on discharge, but the other two made excellent recoveries.

Three patients were more difficult to classify. A 13-year-old boy was suspected of having an epidural abscess, but neither this nor the apparent block on myelography were confirmed at operation. His clinical state remained unchanged. A 39-year-old man with paraplegia was found to have a healing fractured femur. He was very evasive about the duration of his disability, and denied any injury, though this was strongly suspected. The third patient, a 38-year-old woman, had bilateral nerve deafness, posterior column loss and a spastic paraplegia. It was thought that the aetiology might be nutritional, but both this patient and the man with the fractured femur were discharged from hospital before a definite diagnosis had been established.

Miscellaneous

Migraine

Migraine is very uncommon, even among outpatients, and only one or two cases are seen each year. One 38-year-old nurse was admitted because of the severity of her symptoms. All the cases seen have been females with such occupations as teaching or nursing.

Psychoneurosis

Six patients, three of each sex aged between 10 and 48 years, with symptoms which included hysterical fits, 'dizziness', headaches, blindness and hemianaesthesia were seen. No patients with hysterical paralysis were admitted in 1969, although such cases are seen from time to time.

Nutritional

It is always difficult to be sure whether neurological deficits are due to nutritional deficiencies. One case mentioned above, of nerve deafness, posterior column loss, and spastic paraplegia and another with peripheral neuropathy, probably were of nutritional origin. No other such syndromes were seen in 1969. However, in other years patients with a mild spastic paraparesis, often associated with pellagra and responding to dietary treatment, have occasionally been seen and were considered to be nutritional.

Drug Overdosage

Attempted and successful suicides are fairly common, but drugs are not usually used. Two such patients were admitted in 1969. One man, a known epileptic, took an overdose of primidone, and one woman took phenobarbitone.

Iatrogenic

Two known epileptics were admitted with nystagmus and ataxia due to phenytoin. In another patient with vertigo, streptomycin was considered to be the cause.

The only other patient with drug-induced symptoms was the case already discussed with peripheral neuritis due to nitrofurantoin.

Sydenham's Chorea

Rheumatic fever is very common, but only one case of chorea, in an 18-year-old girl, was seen in 1969.

Choreo-athetosis

One 13-year-old boy, with a 6-year history of choreo-athetosis, was seen in 1969. There was no family history and the onset was thought to be too late for the child to be included in the cerebral palsy group.

Cerebellar Lesions of Unknown Aetiology

One woman of 28 and one man of 29 presented with cerebellar ataxia affecting the lower limbs in particular. The only abnormality found on investigation was a raised cerebrospinal fluid protein (varying between 210 and 500 mg/100 ml in the woman, and 54 mg in the man). The man recovered completely, but there was little improvement in the other case.

Polymyositis

Two men presented with proximal muscle weakness, the clinical picture and muscle biopsies being consistent with polymyositis. Both responded to steroids, but one relapsed later.

Demyelinating Disease

Multiple sclerosis has not been diagnosed in any African in Bulawayo, although it has been seen in Rhodesian-born whites. One patient, a male of 35, presented with bilateral retrobulbar neuritis and a few days later he developed a paraparesis. At this stage he was considered to be a case of neuromyelitis optica, but after another week cerebellar signs appeared. He gradually improved, although when last seen still had some visual loss and ataxia. He has been classified as a case of acute disseminated encephalomyelitis.

Because of the apparent absence of multiple sclerosis in the indigenous population, it is felt that cases of retrobulbar neuritis and patients with paraplegia of subacute onset are most unlikely to be due to multiple sclerosis. Unless this disease becomes more common, the diagnosis should be reserved for cases with the classical distribution of lesions both in space and time.

Reference

RACHMAN, I. (1970) Epilepsy in African hospital practice, *Cent. Afr. J. Med.*, 16, 201.

21 Neurological Complications of Parasitic Disease

M. GELFAND

CEREBRAL MALARIA

Although there is no doubt that cerebral malaria is a recognized pathological state, its clinical recognition is by no means always easy since a certain number of patients suffer from a cerebral state or acute encephalopathy with confusion, restlessness and even convulsions, while others with parasites in their blood are not afflicted. The fact that acute mental disturbance may occur in any severe infection makes the diagnosis more difficult. We cannot often perform a cerebral biopsy and confirm the presence of parasites plugging the cerebral capillaries. If a patient with malarial parasites in his blood is in coma one would be justified in attributing this state to the parasites, provided other causes of coma have been excluded. Thus, we can say with reasonable assurance that such a patient has cerebral malaria, but one with precoma, showing the features of an acute encephalopathy, may not have cerebral malaria. The major problem facing the clinician is to decide what are the essential criteria for accepting a diagnosis of cerebral malaria. One criterion would be a history of exposure to the infection or the knowledge that the patient is or has been living in an infected region. Secondly, one would expect the blood smears to be positive. Although it might well happen occasionally that the peripheral blood smears are negative in a patient with cerebral malaria, one has always to exclude other causes of cerebral disorders in such a patient when the parasites are not demonstrable.

Recovery following the administration of specific treatment, although suggestive, would still not be sufficient grounds for a firm diagnosis. On the other hand we know that a patient may be ill with another condition, such as encephalitis, typhoid fever or meningitis, and yet the blood smears may be positive. The parasites may be present coincidentally. Therefore one cannot rely entirely on the positivity or otherwise of the smears, but must take the entire picture into account—the history, the presence of splenomegaly, the absence of localized cerebral symptoms, a usually normal spinal fluid, and the response to treatment. To have malaria when pregnant may be a serious event. It is quite possible that a pregnant woman's resistance to malaria is reduced and if she is infected with it the cerebral form may appear. In 58 cases of cerebral malaria in the Harare African hospital, Rhodesia, 23 were female; of the 15 of these women who were between the ages of 17 and 38 years, eight were pregnant. The baby was saved in two cases, aborted in three and born prematurely in three cases. One of the premature babies died but the other two survived and none of them had malaria. Again, the finding of falciparum parasites in a non-immune subject, such as a European in whom a chronic parasitaemia must be extremely rare, would favour malaria as the primary cause rather than a coincidental occurrence.

Out of 51 589 admissions to Harare Hospital during 1967–69, there were 58 recorded cases of cerebral malaria. Ten of these were not definitely positive and were thus not included in the series; 16 out of 48 patients with positive blood smears died, giving a mortality rate of 33 per cent.

Workers on falciparum cerebral malaria in East Africa stress that the blood smears usually show numerous rings (Rothe, 1956; Hutton, 1956). They emphasize the high parasitaemia which results in a rapid drop in the red cell count. Muwazi and Trowell (1944), also in East Africa, considered that cerebral malaria is always due to an intense blood-stream infection and they stated that usually at least 5 per cent of all red cells are infected. Furthermore, Rothe pointed out that *schizonts* are rare in contrast to the ring forms, since the division takes place in the capillaries of the internal organs like the brain or kidney. Because of the usual distribution of red cells and probably also because of a direct hepatitic effect, a slight or mild degree of yellowness of the conjuctivae may be found. In all their cases ring forms of *Plasmodium falciparum* and/or gametes of *P. falciparum* were found. Musoke (1966) also supports the view that the blood slides usually reveal a heavy infection with *P. falciparum*. More valuable evidence on the severity of the blood infection comes from Edington (1954), who records a case of a child in whom no parasites were present in the peripheral blood vessels yet malarial granulomata, containing parasites, were demonstrable at autopsy. Again the parasitaemia may be slight.

The age incidence of cerebral malaria in the 58 cases at Harare Hospital showed that the majority were in the 0–10 years age-group.

Age group in years	*Number of cases*
0–10	29
11–20	10
21 and over	18

From Thailand we have the experience of Chipman, Cadigan, and Benjapongse (1967) who reported on 22 cases of malaria showing involvement of the nervous system. Of the 22 cases, six were aged up to 20 years, five were between 21 and 30, and five more were between 31 and 40. Beyond the age of 40 there were comparatively few cases.

In endemic regions cerebral malaria is largely a disorder affecting childhood although no age-group is exempt. In the African we can expect to meet fewer and fewer cases with increasing age, and beyond the age of 55 in an immune population cerebral malaria is likely to be diagnosed very rarely. In East Africa involvement of the central nervous system is a symptom complex which attacks children, whereas in the Sarabui province of Thailand it tends to appear in young adults rather as it does in the non-immune adult (e.g. Caucasian) in Central Africa. One can expect more cases among children in a population living in a malarial zone, since a child would be in the process of establishing its tolerance. Rothe (1956) also noted from Kenya that the gradual acquisition by Africans of a relative immunity renders them less susceptible to cerebral malaria with increasing age (Hutton, 1956; Musoke, 1966; Bergeret, 1950). In a non-immune population this difference in age structure would not apply as the disease is common, especially in the adult between the ages of 20 and 60 years. In this particular population it is generally the adult—policemen, miners, prospectors and soldiers—who is likely to contract cerebral malaria (Gelfand, 1957).

The disease may attack either sex. Although more cases may occur in the male this is probably because of the greater risk of exposure. In Chipman, Cadigan, and Benjapongse's series of 22 cases with involvement of the nervous system 14 were males and 8 were females. In another of their series cerebral malaria appeared with almost the same frequency—25 males as compared with 13 females.

Gelfand, Rothe, and Hutton all stress that the cerebrospinal fluid is always clear, its cell count normal or low, without any biochemical change, and the pressure usually normal. Musoke (1966), in East Africa, emphasizes that the cerebrospinal fluid is normal in children. In the 58 cases of cerebral malaria in Harare Hospital the fluid was mostly normal, but in eight it showed a leucocyte count slightly above normal with a protein level of over 40 mg/100 ml; one case had a low sugar level. Guyer (1943) gave a detailed report on a European soldier in East Africa with cerebral malaria whose fluid contained 24 lymphocytes per cu mm. Muwazi and Trowell (1944) were not so definite about a normal fluid; they pointed out that it is normal apart from a rise in pressure and possibly a slight increase in globulin. Further, they found that the cell count in the cerebrospinal fluid may increase up to 20 cells, although in the large majority of patients it is normal. Bergeret (1950) in West Africa, writing on cerebral malaria in children, reported that while the lumbar puncture always gives a clear fluid it is usually under tension with a slightly increased cell count, although the protein content remains normal.

The brain is said to have a suggestive macroscopic appearance. It is of a grey colour, and on section minute deep brownish-red spots, due to thrombi or haemorrhage, are visible throughout the brain substance. On section, the capillaries are seen to be plugged, and scanty ring forms or sporulating parasites are visible. The malarial pigment of these parasites stands out as bright pin-point spots and this constitutes a highly diagnostic feature. Also, a varying number of malarial granulomata are described within the central subcortex (Guyer, 1943). It is believed that the symptoms of cerebral malaria are due to the parasitized erythrocytes sticking to the capillary endothelial walls, mechanically plugging the lumen of small vessels and causing infarction in the surrounding cerebral tissue (Chipman, Cadigan, and Benjapongse, 1967). Edington (1954) carried out autopsies on four children who died of cerebral malaria in the Gold Coast (Ghana). In the livers of all four there was much malarial pigment in the Kupffer cells. Autopsies were performed on 11 of the patients who died at Harare Hospital; they tended to have the same results in all cases. Malarial pigment was found deposited in the spleen, in the Kupffer cells of the liver, and occasionally in the brain itself. It was usually found in the small vessels of the brain, and small haemorrhages were often seen as well.

Clinical Features

One may best describe cerebral malaria as a serious acute febrile encephalopathy in which, for practical purposes, localizing signs can be said to be absent and malarial parasites of *P. falciparum* can as a rule be demonstrated in the peripheral blood smear. There should be a history of the patient's having been exposed to an environment in which malaria is known to occur. If recovery takes place it is generally complete. There are two main ways in which the disease may manifest itself. The first, perhaps less frequent way in which the state is ushered in, is as an acute cerebral disturbance in a patient who was previously well. He is strange in manner, refuses to eat or cooperate, his eyes are staring, and his lips and tongue tremulous. The picture is that of an acute irritative cerebral condition in which convulsions may figure largely. The onset of the coma may be fairly sudden. Headache is a very prominent symptom and the patient may be confused or difficult to control. Mental irritability and photophobia are two symptoms that are stressed (Muwazi and Trowell, 1944). Bergeret (1950) mentions that the patient, often a child, is brought to hospital in a state of coma with conjugate deviation of the head and eyes. Changes in mood, mental clouding, non-purposeful actions, and bed-wetting are other symptoms which should be noted as a warning of the development of cerebral malaria (Ransome, 1950). In the Harare Hospital cases a common symptom of cerebral malaria was the occurrence of fits. Before admission 31 patients had one or more generalized convulsions, often followed by incontinence, 20 complained of severe headache. On admission, 10 patients were unconscious, 12 were described as semiconscious, 5 were drowsy, and 15 mentally confused.

The second way in which the disease manifests itself is as an acute febrile state, during or even after which the patient suddenly or subacutely passes into a cerebral state. Fever was found in all the cases in the Harare Hospital series. In 28 patients it was over 102°F, while in the others it was less. In the early stages of the disease many of the patients suffered from weakness, chills, and rigors. They vomited frequently or had diarrhoea. A large number were dehydrated on admission. Five patients were jaundiced. It is impossible to predict whether a patient will develop this complication. I have seen it in the young, in the middle-aged and even in the elderly. There would almost appear to be a sudden breakdown in the immune processes of the body by which the balance of resistance was maintained, when for no obvious reason, despite a course of treatment, the body's powers seem to be overwhelmed.

It is as well to stress that the patient very soon—within a matter of a few days of the course of cerebral malaria—begins to show signs of stress; loss of flesh is quickly apparent, the patient appears sallow and perhaps pale.

The coma is usually deep and convulsions may be expected. The patient is mostly quiet, seldom restless or confused at this stage. Usually there are no signs in the nervous system apart from some abnormality of the pupils. Bergeret, in West Africa, reports that a hemiplegia, monoplegia or ophthalmoplegia is not uncommon. Guyer (1943), while pointing out that recovery is the rule in cerebral malaria, mentions that permanent cerebral damage is possible and this might take the form of a monoplegia, hemiplegia or mental effect. Chipman, Cadigan, and Benjapongse (1967) recorded a case with global aphasia, a spastic right hemiplegia and conjugate deviation of the eyes to the left; they attributed these effects to occlusion of the lumen of the small cerebral vessels.

It is probable that in cerebral malaria the spleen is palpable in over half the cases, which is a useful finding, although the absence of splenomegaly should not rule out a diagnosis of malaria. The spleen is best described as a full, tense organ, slightly or even moderately enlarged, but one should hesitate to diagnose malaria on an enlarged spleen alone. A hard, stony spleen is more likely to be a sign of portal hypertension. The liver may also show simultaneous involvement with the brain; there may be some degree of jaundice, sometimes marked, and the liver is likely to be enlarged.

The illness usually lasts a matter of days. The cerebral state is an acute and relatively short-lived disorder in which, with correct treatment, recovery may occur fairly rapidly and the patient pass out of danger. In some patients the state of coma may continue for 2, 3 or more days, but if there is going to be any response to treatment one can begin to detect a lightening in the cerebral state before full consciousness is restored. In the great majority of cases the comatose state should have passed over within 10 days. In malarial areas like the west coast of Africa, people are known to develop cerebral malaria and after being in a coma for some days recover spontaneously. This also happened in early colonial days when parenteral quinine therapy was not available. How often this happy result occurred one cannot say, but it is unlikely to occur without quinine or other specific therapy in more than a minority of cases.

There are at least two important disorders in Africans which must be mentioned in discussing cerebral malaria. It would appear that the disease is unlikely to develop in a child with kwashiorkor or the sickle-cell trait. There is good evidence to show that while malaria may occur in those who have this abnormal haemoglobin, very few actually succumb to cerebral malaria itself. This is more surprising with kwashiorkor because one would have expected a child with such a low resistance to be prone to malaria, especially its severe forms. Yet it is incorrect to believe that cerebral malaria cannot occur in a child with sickle-cell disease. Rey, Quenum, and Guerin (1967) quote such an example. A boy aged 10, born in Dakar, presented with all the features of cerebral malaria. The blood showed *P. falciparum*. He died despite treatment. Red blood cells were demonstrated in the capillaries of the brain and the sickle cells contained *P. falciparum* schizonts.

Chipman, Cadigan, and Benjapongse (1967), when describing the involvement of the nervous system in malaria in Thailand, emphasize the frequency with which seizures occur, as well as disturbances of consciousness and behaviour, and memory defects. By far the most common symptom they encountered was a severe headache experienced mostly in the occipital and bitemporal regions. These workers also refer to the occasional localized paralysis which may occur in cerebral malaria. Again, Musoke (1966), in Uganda, while noting that if recovery takes place in cerebral malaria it is generally complete, also mentions that occasionally such a patient is left with a monoplegia or other form of paralysis.

The diagnosis of cerebral malaria is made from the knowledge that the patient has been exposed to the malarial parasite and from the usual presence of the ring forms of *P. falciparum* in the blood, the enlarged spleen, the absence of localizing signs and the generally normal cerebrospinal fluid. One must be careful to remember that in an endemic region it is not uncommon for a patient to be harbouring parasites in his blood, yet to be suffering from an entirely different disorder, such as acute meningitis, typhoid fever or lobar pneumonia. Important disorders which may closely mimic cerebral malaria, especially in the child, are acute meningitis, chronic meningitis, particularly in its tuberculous form, acute encephalitis, brain abscess and trypanosomiasis.

Since the patient with cerebral malaria is in coma one has to remember the many other causes of coma. In a country like Central Africa, malaria must never be dismissed without careful consideration, although the recognized causes of coma can be expected.

Where the clinician is in doubt, specific treatment should always be given, but, even if the patient recovers fairly rapidly after it, one must be careful not to ascribe the coma to malaria in case he has recovered from some other state which was not recognized, such as spontaneous hypoglycaemia. Nevertheless, it is true to say that if a patient has cerebral malaria and quinine is administered the response is usually quite rapid.

Treatment

Once the diagnosis of cerebral malaria is made, treatment consists of the selection of the antimalarial drug and injection and administration of intravenous fluids. My drug of preference in Central Africa is quinine dihydrochloride. Its action is fairly quick and if care is exercised no untoward reaction should occur. Others prefer chloroquine by the intravenous route. As I have not conducted any controlled therapeutic trials it would be wrong to state that chloroquine is not helpful. My own reasons for not favouring it for a disorder like cerebral malaria are that it appears to be rather slow in its action, and it can cause grave reactions, such as collapse, when given by the intravenous route, and, in the patient with a glucose 6-phosphate deficiency, I believe it may precipitate a haemolytic anaemia with haemoglobinuria.

The first procedure is to administer intravenous fluid in a generous amount. When this has been started quinine (or chloroquine, if preferred) must be introduced. Perhaps the best method is to inject it into a bottle containing 100 ml of fluid and to give this first; this should take about 15 minutes. Then the rest of the fluid can be given in the usual way. The quinine is given every 6 hours, again using a small bottle of fluid with the drug in it. If this is not possible, it can be injected into the rubber connexion near the needle and the vacolitre dripper regulated to about 10 to 15 drops per minute for about 10 minutes, by which time the quinine should have begun to circulate; after this the rate of administration can be increased. The amount of quinine should not be less than 600 mg for an adult and half this amount for a child. For an infant one can given between 3 and 6 grains. The quinine therapy is continued until the patient shows signs of regaining consciousness, after which the next injection may be by the intramuscular route; thereafter it is taken by mouth in doses of 10 grains of the hydrochloride salt, three or four times a day. It is good practice at the stage when the patient can swallow to give chloroquine as well.

Lambert (1961) in the Congo recommends glucose saline infusions with 500 mg of quinine in 500 ml given twice or three times in the 24 hours. To each infusion is added 25 mg hydrocortisone. Woodruff and Dickinson (1968) recommend the use of dexamethasone in cerebral malaria. The rationale of dexamethasone is that there is usually cerebral oedema, associated with many petechial haemorrhages in the brain, caused by damage to the vessels brought about by anoxaemia which results from shock and occlusion of the vessels with erythrocytes. It is suggested that the oedema causes further pressure on the blood vessels. Should acute renal failure develop, as first pointed out by Jackson and Woodruff (1962), haemodialysis must be seriously considered.

If anaemia is present with a haemoglobin of 60 per cent or less, a blood transfusion should be considered. If the clinician prefers, he might also give intravenous steroids, which may have some value, although it is difficult to be certain on this point. The same would apply to the use of adrenaline (Ascoli treatment). For cases with threatening coma the treatment just outlined is recommended, or intramuscular quinine may be given if the doctor considers the patient's condition is less serious and circumstances are such that fluid cannot be administered intravenously.

Dennis and his colleagues (1967) refer to the depletion of coagulation factors which may occur in severe falciparum malaria. Indeed, Spitz (1946) found many thrombi in cerebral vessels as well as glomerular congestion and thrombosis. Thus we can expect in the severe forms of malaria the state now referred to as diffuse intravascular coagulation (DIC) with an accompanying reduction in platelets, prothrombin and fibrinogen levels, as well as the presence of fibrin degradation products in the blood. If these factors are present the clinician may wish to consider the use of heparin. On the other hand Eales (1972) considers that bleeding in acute malaria might result from the accompanying renal failure rather than from a thrombotic coagulopathy and that heparin under these circumstances should not be given.

References

BERGERET, C. (1950) Quoted in Cerebral malaria in children, *Trop. Dis. Bull.*, 47, 9.

CHIPMAN, M., CADIGAN, F. C., and BENJAPONGSE, W. (1967) Involvement of the nervous system in malaria in Thailand, *Trop. geogr. Med.*, 19, 8.

DENNIS, L. H., EICHELBERGER, J. W., INMAN, M. M., and CONRAD, M. E. (1967) Depletion of coagulation factors in drug-resistant *Plasmodium falciparum* malaria, *Blood*, 20, 713.

EALES, L. (1972) Imported malaria in Cape Town. A life-threatening hazard, *S. Afr. med. J.*, 46, 2053.

EDINGTON, G. M. (1954) Cerebral malaria in the Gold Coast, *Ann. trop. Med. Parasit.*, 48, 300.

GELFAND, M. (1957) *The Sick African: A Clinical Study*, 3rd ed., Cape Town, p. 64.

GUYER, O. K. G. (1943) Report on a case of cerebral malaria, *E. Afr. med. J.*, 20, 139.

HUTTON, P. W. (1956) Neurological disorders in Uganda, *E. Afr. med. J.*, 33, 209.

JACKSON, R. C., and WOODRUFF, A. W. (1962) The artificial kidney in malaria and blackwater fever, *Brit. med. J.*, 1, 1367.

LAMBERT, C. (1961) Quoted in notes on the treatment of algid cerebral malaria in adults, *Acta trop. (Basel)*, *Trop. Dis. Bull.*, 58, 773.

MUSOKE, L. K. (1966) Neurological manifestations of malaria in children, *E. Afr. med. J.*, 43, 561.

MUWAZI, E. M. K., and TROWELL, H. C. (1944) Neurological disease among African natives of Uganda. A review of 269 cases, *E. Afr. med. J.*, 21, 2.

RANSOME, G. A., (1950) Quoted in notes on the management of cases of cerebral malaria, *Trop. Dis. Bull.*, 47, 317.

REY, M., QUENUM, C., and GUERIN, M. (1967) Quoted in a death from malaria in a patient with sickle cell anaemia, *Trop. Dis. Bull.*, 64, 1188.

ROTHE, H. (1956) 100 cases of cerebral malaria, *E. Afr. med. J.*, 33, 405.

SPITZ, S. (1946) The pathology of acute falciparum malaria, *Milit. Surg.*, 99, 555.

WOODRUFF, A. W., and DICKENSON, C. J. (1968) Use of dexamethasone in cerebral malaria, *Brit. med. J.*, 3, 31.

SLEEPING SICKNESS

Human trypanosomiasis is an African disease which follows the distribution of certain species of tsetse fly (Chesterman, 1952). We speak further of two forms—the Rhodesian and the Gambian. According to parasitologists the trypanosomes of these two forms of sleeping sickness are distinct. Gambian sleeping sickness is carried by *Glossina palpalis* and *G. tachinoides*, which are found amidst the vegetation lining the banks and streams, rivers and lakes. Both species are often encountered in heavily populated areas where there is no game. Rhodesian sleeping sickness is carried mainly by *G. morsitans* and to a lesser extent by *G. pallidipes* and *G. swynnertoni*, which are closely associated with an abundance of wild game. However, clinicians may remain a little puzzled as to the finer clinical differences between the Rhodesian and Gambian forms. In countries south of the Luapula River, in Zambia, Rhodesia, Angola and Tanzania, this problem does not arise as only the Rhodesian form exists there. In West Africa, Kenya, Uganda and French Equatorial Africa other forms may be seen but the Gambian variety seems to be paramount. Nevertheless, to the clinician the difference between Rhodesian and Gambian sleeping sickness may not be as impressive as was formerly believed, and for practical purposes the two forms are indeed one and the same. There seems to be little doubt of the role of the animal as a reservoir in the transmission of Rhodesian trypanosomiasis, but of the reservoir of *Trypanosoma gambiense* there is considerable doubt; it is generally accepted that man forms the only reservoir. There is also much argument about the relationship of the three polymorphic trypanosomes. One authority, Hoare, considers that they are all three biological races of a single species. *T. brucei* is morphologically identical with *T. rhodesiense* and the latter's ability to infest man is the only means of distinguishing the two. *T. gambiense* and *rhodesiense* probably represent the opposite extremes of one species.

The human has gradually become adapted to *T. gambiense* and this explains the milder course which this type assumes in man in contrast to the more acute course of *T. rhodesiense*. Still, the picture is by no means clear cut, as there are different degrees of virulence in the strains of either trypanosome. In *G. palpalis* areas trypanosomiasis assumes the Gambian form only, whereas the Rhodesian type is seen only in association with *G. morsitans* or *pallidipes*.

Lester (1945) broadly divided Gambian sleeping sickness into three categories, mild, nervous and toxaemic. But a high percentage of deaths occur in the milder forms of the disease. A man may be suffering mildly from the infection for months or years, when, for reasons not definitely known, there is a sudden flare-up with high fever and toxaemia and a more or less rapid progression to death.

Mulligan (1955) noticed that in Gambia the disease carried by *T. gambiense* is clinically of the mild type in local inhabitants; glandular enlargement may be an early and prominent symptom of the disease. As it occurs only where *G. palpalis* is present, and is absent where this species does not occur but where *G. morsitans* may be prevalent, there can be no reasonable doubt that *G. palpalis* is the sole vector. Mulligan considers that *T. gambiense* is the only species responsible for human trypanosomiasis in West Africa. He believes that estimation of the protein content of the cerebrospinal fluid is one of the most valuable single tests for the assessment of a sleeping sickness case. The ESR is generally increased as well as the gamma globulins.

Waddy (1956) agreed with Mulligan, and reported that the type of trypanosomiasis now seen in Ghana is almost always very mild. Subjects may not feel ill and therefore do not report for treatment until the infection has reached a late stage with cerebrospinal fluid changes and no trypanosomes in the blood. The patient may be in good health with considerable cerebrospinal fluid changes. The mortality Waddy found to be low. McLetchie (1948) reported that in Gambian sleeping sickness some of the mild cases may live 9 to 15 years. The mild infection may be slowly progressive with regard to involvement of the nervous system, but sudden breakdown with high fever and toxaemia occurs in patients who have had the usual minor manifestations of the disease for months or even years; most of these cases die unseen and untended. He emphasized the importance of seeking out and treating these mild cases. In Uganda, Gambian infection has also been described as mild but fatal (Brown, 1938; Shore, 1960). Duggan (1959) believes that the course assumed in African trypanosomiasis is governed by a changing host-parasite relationship. In the later stages there is involvement of the nervous system. He emphasizes the variation in the progress of the disease in different patients and even goes so far as to state that spontaneous cure may occur, even when there are early cerebrospinal fluid changes.

In the Zambesi valley, Blair, Burnett-Smith, and Gelfand (1968) described three categories of the Rhodesian type of cases:

1. The healthy carrier.
2. The subacute case with early neurological signs.
3. The acute case with a rapid course if early treatment is not given.

The *healthy carrier* will be found to have lived in a tsetse fly-infected area for a considerable period, and the patient is only rarely a woman or child. The illness usually begins with a febrile disorder from which recovery is made, and the patient then returns to his normal occupation. Despite the presence of trypanosomes in his blood he is able to work hard and walk considerable distances.

The *subacute case with early neurological signs*: the patient is constantly bitten by tsetse flies, and then develops an illness of subacute severity, with a history of several months with loss of weight and inability to carry on with his work. He is largely confined to his village.

The acute case with rapid deterioration: this type is seen not only in persons who live in fly areas but also in those who have only paid short visits to them and become ill with an acute pyrexial illness. The patient is often a European who has not been in a tsetse fly area before or who only visits it from time to time. Involvement of the nervous system probably occurs even in the healthy carrier sooner or later, although it is not possible to be dogmatic on this point, since such a patient is given treatment whenever he is found.

According to Ormerod (1961), Rhodesian sleeping sickness is a new disease which has evolved during the past century. No evidence exists of major outbreaks before the present century when the disease arose and spread northwards. In its wake it left endemic disease in Rhodesia, Malawi and Tanzania; the epidemic appears to be passing through Uganda today. *T. gambiense*, on the other hand, according to Ormerod, is associated with the chronic form of sleeping sickness seen also in West Africa and along the shores of Lake Victoria, where originally it was the only type of the disease present before the arrival of *T. rhodesiense* in this area in about 1940.

One of the interesting features of Rhodesian sleeping sickness is the relatively small number of cases seen in the regions in which the causative trypanosome is found, despite the great density of *Glossina morsitans. G. pallidipes* and perhaps other tsetse flies which transmit *Trypanosoma rhodesiense* to man. In an area like the Zambesi valley only a few to several cases are described each year. One asks the question, why? While only a handful of cases occur among the indigenous Africans living in these areas there are perhaps one or two Europeans, mostly hunters or visitors in the region, who contract the disease shortly after entering the infected zone, in contrast to the hundreds of visitors there each year and the thousands of indigenous tribesmen inhabiting the areas.

It is also interesting that, whereas in the European visitor the disease is characterized by an acute onset with high fever, in the African, although many do conform to this pattern, a number seem to develop a mild chronic illness, or what Blair and his colleagues refer to as the 'carrier state of the disease'. Many are seen with so few symptoms as not to be recognizable as an illness even by the patient. As far as we are aware, this occurs only in the indigenous population. Some of these patients are able to work normally but sooner or later, perhaps even years later, they develop signs of involvement of the nervous system after which the course is probably a slow downhill one, but so far our knowledge of the natural history of the disease in these cases is scant. The disease often has a typical onset and course and it is as well to draw attention to the milder forms.

There are subacute cases too—once again Africans who live in endemic regions—who are ill but do not necessarily require admission to hospital. They are affected by bouts of fever, headache and poor health, the illness running upwards of some months or perhaps even extending into a year or more. These patients, it is believed, eventually succumb to involvement of the nervous system although it is possible that the latter has already been invaded by the trypanosomes although the effects are relatively mild for a long time.

There is no doubt as to what happens in the acute illness in a non-immune subject. Four to 6 weeks after the onset of the acute infection, there is a very good chance that the brain becomes involved in the encephalitic process and after a few months every untreated case probably passes into the cerebral stage.

Clinical Features

In a typical case within a few or more days after the sting, there appears a red nodule which increases in size for a few days until it becomes an itchy, painful, brawny lump resembling a carbuncle but filled with a greyish fluid (Gelfand, 1966). If at this stage the nodule is punctured and fluid removed and examined microscopically, the trypanosomes may be seen in fairly large numbers even before they can be detected in the blood stream. At the time this primary sore appears the patient develops a high temperature with constitutional symptoms, and may shiver and vomit. Unless one is aware of the sore on the leg or other part of the body—and especially when it is not present—the onset of the illness is indistinguishable from acute malaria, usually also endemic in regions in which trypanosomiasis occurs. Furthermore the spleen may enlarge. Perhaps a useful sign is the jaundice which is found in about a quarter to one-third of these cases. Jenkins and Robertson (1959) drew attention for the first time to the occurrence of jaundice and hepatic dysfunction in Rhodesian trypanosomiasis. They recorded that 4 per cent of their cases in Uganda developed jaundice. However, although jaundice itself was an uncommon sign, 83 per cent of their cases showed an excess of urobilin in the urine and a high proportion also showed bilirubin, both clearing within a week or so. Gelfand and Friedlander (1963) confirmed the presence of this sign in Rhodesia.

Within several days the lymph nodes draining the chancre enlarge, and it is not unusual for the patient to develop a generalized lymphadenopathy. At this stage the blood smears are often positive although occasionally they are negative. This negative finding should not lead one to exclude trypanosomiasis in the face of a strong supportive history as the trypanosomes may be present in scant numbers. Manson-Bahr and Charters (1963) from Kenya reported on the occurrence of myocarditis in two cases of African trypanosomiasis. The main features were generalized cardiac enlargement, a gallop rhythm and signs of congestive cardiac failure. Both these cases they thought conformed more to *T. rhodesiense* infection than to *T. gambiense*.

Involvement of the nervous system may become evident in the acute general illness, as it continues into its third or fourth week, with the patient becoming mentally confused or delirious with a corresponding reduction in the level of his consciousness. The speed with which this happens and the interval after the time of infection vary greatly from case to case. The decline may be insidious, the patient slowly developing a change in his personality in contrast to the more rapid form already described. When the brain is involved the encephalopathy is striking; the patient is drowsy, unable to concentrate for long, and characteristically falls asleep after filling his mouth with food and has to be roused again. Taube and Nixon (1958) emphasized that if an African patient, living in a sleeping sickness belt such as in Zambia, is seen with a clouded mind and emaciation in association with a parkinsonian picture, trypanosomiasis must be considered. A further characteristic feature of this type of the disease is the absence of localizing signs. These are extremely rare. In contrast to tuberculous meningitis or even viral encephalitis one seldom meets with localized paralysis or palsies. The drowsiness or stupor may continue with shorter and shorter periods of consciousness or improvement in the conscious level, until eventually the patient passes into a deep coma and after a while finally succumbs. At the same time he may assume a rather myxoedematous appearance or may begin to lose flesh and become cachectic. In some cases the heart probably begins to fail at the same time. Convulsions may intrude. Some patients are moderately febrile, whereas in others little or no fever is noted. At the same time the lymph nodes may remain swollen and discrete. The longer the process has continued with involvement of the brain the less likely is recovery to take place. In the early stages of the encephalitis there is no doubt that full and lasting recovery may ensue but once the patient relapses after treatment, or if the encephalitis has become severe, the chances of cure are virtually hopeless.

Acres (1950) in West Africa reminds us of some of the clinical features of the disease in young children. He states that the affected child is backward or retrogressive in behaviour and character due to the meningoencephalitis. The child who has begun to stand up no longer does so, but is content to sit or even to lie down. He postulates that a meningovascular stage, passing to that of meningoencephalitis, is much more rapid than in the adult and hence the presence of signs indicative of severe nervous involvement (neck rigidity). Strabismus, conjugate ocular deviation and nystagmus are commoner in the child. Acres emphasized that in endemic regions in the Congo the more elderly adult may complain only of lumbar backache and stiffness but, on lumbar puncture, one is surprised to find a very high cell count with trypanosomes in the fluid.

Once a diagnosis of cerebral trypanosomiasis is made, treatment must be directed towards administration of a drug which will reach the central nervous system; as far as I know the only remedy likely to be of help is *Mel B* or perhaps tryparsamide (Duggan, 1959, 1962). Whichever of these is chosen the patient or family should have the risks explained. Actually, we have seldom encountered any untoward effect with *Mel B* and the results in about half our cases have been satisfactory.

Sleeping sickness, as seen in Rhodesia, is predominantly a disease of the working age-groups (16 to 44 years) as was reported by David Scott (1957) in West Africa. In 11 cases in Harare Hospital, from 1967 to 1969, the ages ranged from 12 to 51; there were no young children amongst them, although I have encountered the disease in European children between the age of 5 and 12 years, in whom the clinical picture (all early cases) was typical. Ten of the cases in Harare Hospital were male and one female.

There are important changes in trypanosomiasis once the brain barrier has been penetrated. In the early stage of blood infection there are apparently none, particularly in the protein or cell content. It is possible, however, for trypanosomes to appear in the cerebrospinal fluid in the earlier phases of the disease without this carrying a serious prognosis (Keevil, 1928; Maclean and Fairbairn, 1932). When the nervous system is affected one can expect a slightly raised pressure in the spinal fluid together with an increase in the number of cells. At first the count rises to about 10 to 20 cells or more per c mm, the increase being in lymphocytes and other cells, especially monocytes and plasma cells. The count may increase later to a few hundred cells. At this stage, too, the total protein count of the fluid is elevated from about 40 to 100 mg. Again, it is not uncommon to demonstrate the trypanosome in the spinal fluid, or in a rat after inoculating it with the fluid. No constant relationship exists between the presence of trypanosomes in the cerebrospinal fluid on the one hand and the cell and protein levels on the other hand. Deckelbaum and Lowenthal (1970) of Zambia refer to a patient suffering from Rhodesian sleeping sickness who had a CSF cell count of 300 per c mm without trypanosomes, while in another case trypanosomes were present in the fluid—the cell count being 32.

In 9 of the 11 cases seen at Harare Hospital, there were signs of involvement of the nervous system. In all of them the cerebrospinal fluid showed high numbers of leucocytes and raised protein levels, the leucocyte count varying between 38 and 320 leucocytes per c mm. Four of the patients were drowsy.

Treatment

The treatment of trypanosomiasis, before the nervous system is involved, is relatively straightforward; *Antrypol* (suramin or *Bayer* 205) is probably the treatment of choice; the dose is 1 G intravenously once a week for about 10 weeks. Another method of treatment with suramin is to give a total adult dose of 5 G and a total dose of tryparsamide of from 12 to 30 G. Tryparsamide is given in injections every 5 days or once a week up to a total of 8–15 injections (Duggan, 1959, 1962). Other clinicians may prefer a course of pentamidine isethionate, given intramuscularly once a day for 10 days, the course thus being shorter. Both treatments are given in my wards.

Once the nervous system shows signs of infection, as evidenced by changes in the spinal fluid, the course of treatment must be different. Here perhaps the best drug is melarsen oxide (melarsen, one of the melaminyl compounds developed by Friedheim, is a pentavalent arsenical disodium 2:4-diamino-1:3:5-triazinyl-6-aminophenylarsenate). It has an arsenic content of 20 per cent, which although toxic, especially to the brain and perhaps to the cranial nerves, is perhaps the only drug achieving a fair degree of success. Other workers, such as Duggan, prefer tryparsamide, considering it safer and possibly more effective in advanced Gambian sleeping sickness and malaria.

The commonly chosen dosage of melarsen, is 3·5 mg/kg bodyweight for 4 days; then after an interval of 10 to 14 days the course is repeated. With melarsen oxide some cases may develop an arsenical encephalopathy or a Herxheimer-like reaction with an exacerbation of the encephalitis. Others again relapse. Sometimes the relapses are curable with a further course of *Mel B*, but others are extremely refractory to repeated courses of it. The efficacy of a trypanocidal drug may be judged by whether there is deterioration of either the objective symptoms of the patient or in the state of the cerebrospinal fluid within 2 years after the end of treatment. Melarsen may very occasionally result in exfoliative dermatitis, acute mania, dimness of vision, headache and mild gastrointestinal symptoms.

Butler, Duggan, and Clarkson (1957), treating Gambian trypanosomiasis, reported that 50 per cent of advanced cases, 80 per cent of intermediate cases and 100 per cent of early cases were cured with melarsen.

References

Acres, J. S. (1950) A study of sleeping sickness in the endemic area of the Belgian Congo over a period, *Trans. roy. Soc. trop. Med. Hyg.*, **44**, 77.

Blair, D. M., Burnett-Smith, E., and Gelfand, M. (1968) Human trypanosomiasis in Rhodesia, *Cent. Afr. J. Med.*, 14 (Suppl.), 1.

Brown, A. A. F. (1938) *Trypanosomiasis gambiense.* Some observations in Uganda and their bearing on prophylaxis, *J. trop. Med. Hyg.*, **41**, 200.

Butler, G. C., Duggan, A. J., and Clarkson, M. R. (1957) Melarsen in the treatment of trypanosomiasis, *Trans. roy Soc. trop. Med. Hyg.*, **51**, 69.

Chesterman, C. C. (1952) Trypanosomiasis, in *British Encyclopaedia of Medical Practice*, 2nd ed., Vol. 12, London, p. 329.

Deckelbaum, R., and Lowenthal, M. N. (1970) Trypanosomiasis in Ndola Central Hospital, *Med. J. Zambia*, 4, 187.

Duggan, A. J. (1959) An approach to the clinical problems of Gambian sleeping sickness, *J. trop. Med. Hyg.*, **62**, 268.

Duggan, A. J. (1962) A survey of sleeping sickness in Northern Nigeria from the early times to the present day, *Trans. roy. Soc. trop. Med. Hyg.*, **55**, 439.

Gelfand, M. (1966) The early clinical features of Rhodesian trypanosomiasis with special reference to the chancre, *Trans. roy. Soc. trop. Med. Hyg.*, **60**, 376.

Gelfand, M., and Friedlander, J. (1963) Jaundice in Rhodesian sleeping sickness. Report on two cases, *Trans. roy. Soc. trop. Med. Hyg.*, **57**, 290.

Jenkins, A. R., and Robertson, D. H. H. (1959) Hepatic dysfunction in human trypanosomiasis, *Trans. roy. Soc. trop. Med. Hyg.*, **53**, 524.

Keevil, A. J. (1928) *Trypanosoma rhodesiense* infection treated with 'Bayer 205', *Trans roy. Soc. trop. Med. Hyg.*, **22**, 83.

Lester, H. M. O. (1945) Further progress in the control of sleeping sickness and hygiene, *Trans. roy. Soc. trop. Med. Hyg.*, **38**, 425.

Maclean, G., and Fairbairn, N. (1932) Treatment of Rhodesian sleeping sickness with 'Bayer 205' and tryparsamide on 719 cases, *Ann. trop. Med. Parasit.*, **26**, 157.

McLetchie, J. L. (1948) The control of sleeping sickness in Nigeria, *Trans. roy. Soc. trop. Med. Hyg.*, 41, 445.

Manson-Bahr, P. E. C., and Charters, A. D. (1963) Myocarditis in African trypanosomiasis, *Trans. roy. Soc. trop. Med. Hyg.*, 57, 119.

Mulligan, W. H. (1955) Recent investigations on trypanosomiasis in British West Africa, *Trans. roy. Soc. trop. Med. Hyg.*, 49, 197.

Ormerod, W. E. (1961) The epidemic spread of Rhodesian sleeping sickness, 1908–1960, *Trans. roy. Soc. trop. Med. Hyg.*, 55, 525.

Scott, D. (1957) The epidemiology of human trypanosomiasis in Ashanti, Ghana, *J. trop. Med. Hyg.*, 60, 257.

Shore, H. (1960) An epidemic of sleeping sickness in the Lango district of Uganda, Part III, *E. Afr. med. J.*, 37, 255.

Taube, E., and Nixon, L. C. (1958) The treatment of advanced *Trypanosomiasis rhodesiense* with Mel B, *Cent. Afr. J. Med.*, 4, 141.

Waddy, R. B. (1956) Organization and work of the Gold Coast medical field units, *Trans. roy. Soc. trop. Med. Hyg.*, 50, 313.

AMOEBIC CEREBRAL ABSCESS

Although in 1904 Kartulis found 11 instances of brain abscess among 384 cases of liver abscess, 10 of which followed 'dysenteric liver abscess', few series of reported cases would perhaps support so high a figure (quoted from Wilmot, 1962). Since Kartulis reported them about 90 further instances have been recorded. The majority were seen in association with liver and pulmonary lesions, although in about 10 per cent no forms of the disease could be found elsewhere. It is suggested that the amoebae may reach the brain via the paravertebral plexus of veins.

The prognosis was usually bad in cases in which *Entamaoeba histolytica* was demonstrated in the brain abscess, and recovery has only once been recorded (Powell and Neame, 1960). The symptomatology varies, depending largely on the site and extent of the lesion. The picture is often not distinct. The lesion is essentially a liquefactive one without a clear capsule, the pus being brown and creamy. The abscess, too, may rupture within the subarachnoid space. Drug therapy, including emetine and chloroquine, has proved disappointing. What effect metronidazole may have on the lesion is, in my opinion, still uncertain.

Powell and Neame (1960) describe an interesting case of amoebic brain abscess. The patient was an African male aged 35 years, presumably in good health, who suddenly developed a right hemiparesis. The CSF protein was 200 mg/100 ml and the cell count 128 lymphocytes and polymorphs. Trophozoites of *E. histolytica* were seen in the fluid. The patient died, and at autopsy a localized yellow exudate was found in the meninges of the left parietal lobe which contained a large abscess. The wall of the abscess was ragged and of a yellowish-grey colour and in the abscess itself could be seen strands of necrotic brain tissue. In the wet preparation of the abscess motile forms of *E. histolytica* were seen. On microscopy the sections revealed a central area of necrosis surrounded by neutrophils, lymphocytes and mononuclear cells in which amoebae were evident.

Powell and Neame also mention two other cases of brain abscess of amoebic origin. One was in a male infant aged 5 months and the other in a 47-year-old man. Both died.

That cerebral amoebiasis is possibly not as rare as is supposed is propounded in an article by Odungo (1969), of West Africa, who found four brain abscesses in 135 autopsy cases with intestinal amoebiasis. They were single and situated in the cerebral hemispheres. In one there was an abscess in each hemisphere. The patients were all between 5 and 12 years of age. The largest abscess measured 8 cm in diameter. *E. histolytica* was demonstrated in only one case but in all of them there were intestinal lesions due to that organism.

Emetine, metronidazole and chloroquine can be used effectively for amoebiasis of the liver but for an amoebic brain lesion there is little evidence that these drugs reach it in sufficient concentration to be of value.

References

Odungo, E. O. (1969) Cerebral amoebiasis, *W. Afr. med. J.*, 17, 117.

Powell, S. J., and Neame, P. B. (1960) A case of amoebic brain abscess, *Brit. med. J.*, 2, 1136.

Wilmot, A. J. (1962) *Clinical Amoebiasis*, Oxford.

BILHARZIAL EFFECT ON THE NERVOUS SYSTEM

The clinician in Central Africa is becoming increasingly aware of the effects of bilharziasis on the nervous system, especially since the discovery that lesions may develop unexpectedly in the early phase of the illness. Until recently we regarded the appearance of lesions in the brain or spinal cord as typical of the later stages of the disease. However, the later granulomatous masses seem to be much less frequent in Central Africa despite the many references in the literature to inflammatory cerebral masses resembling tumours, due especially to *Schistosoma japonicum* or *S. mansoni.*

In Central Africa the attack on the nervous system, including both the brain and spinal cord, usually appears fairly early—often only a matter of some weeks or months from the time the disease has been contracted. In Rhodesia this early phase is referred to as the Katayama syndrome, which is a febrile illness appearing mostly in the young Caucasian adult or child and is characterized by urticarial swellings, a high blood eosinophilia, and a self-limiting course of a few or several weeks. Shortly after the onset of the disease ova appear in the stool but less often in the urine (Clarke, Warburton, and Blair, 1970). The spleen is often palpable. It is curious that the brunt of the attack falls on one organ in one patient (such as the lungs) while in another patient it affects only the brain. On rare occasions the brain or spinal cord is principally affected in this early phase, and the patient develops either an encephalopathy with or without localizing signs such as hemiplegia, or a myelitis with weakness and sensory loss in the lower limbs and sphincter disturbances.

The effects of bilharzial disease on the nervous system assume two main forms, one on the brain and the other on the spinal cord or its roots.

Cerebral Bilharziasis

The cerebral form usually reveals itself as an encephalopathy. Another way is the formation of a granuloma which gives rise to symptoms indistinguishable from those of tumour, but this has not been described as yet in Central Africa.

In the first there is an acute or subacute encephalopathy in which the patient develops clouding of the mind, stupor or even coma, together with a varying degree of fever and often an eosinophilia (Zilberg, 1967 *b*, 1970). The condition may easily be mistaken for a viral encephalitis, cerebral malaria, subdural haematoma, confused states or acute or chronic meningitis. The cerebrospinal fluid is clear, perhaps under pressure, but as far as we are aware there is always a pleocytosis which may consist mainly of lymphocytes and/or polymorphs or even on occasion of many eosinophils; the protein is moderately raised. While no localizing signs may be seen in the acute stage, these may develop, especially a hemiplegia. I saw such a case for Dr. James Montgomery of Umtali in a European boy aged 15 years, who suddenly developed a left-sided hemiplegia. He had active urinary bilharziasis and made a very good recovery with treatment. More recently I saw a European patient who had an acute encephalopathy, a mild eosinophilia, and a history of exposure to infected waters; he had developed a severe hemiplegia during this state. He was found to have *S. mansoni* in his rectum, and made an excellent recovery (Clarke, Warburton, and Blair, 1970).

What would happen to these cases if left untreated is not clear. It is possible that a number would recover slowly, but now that the clinician in these regions is aware of cerebral bilharziasis he is likely to make a careful search for ova. Those treated have generally recovered fully. A case recorded by Zilberg (1967 *a*) is well worth referring to briefly. A European boy aged 7 years developed abnormal behaviour; he became stuporous over 2 days and showed opisthotonos. There was mild stiffness and the plantar reflexes were extensor. Raper (1948) records his findings in an autopsy he performed upon an East African Askari, whose history was not available. The brain and meninges were congested and the substantia reticularis of the pons was occupied by what appeared to be an area of diffuse capillary haemorrhage. Histologically all the capillaries and venules were blocked by thrombi. Digestion of the brain tissue showed the presence of eggs of *S. mansoni*. Raper postulates that this patient died from vascular blockage either by an adult fluke or by ova outside the range of the section.

In contrast to the acute encephalopathy, bilharzial granulomas of sufficient size to give rise to the symptomatology of cerebral tumour have been recorded, notably in the Far East and South America. So far as I am aware no one has seen such cases in Central Africa. I believe it must be rare in contrast to glioma or tuberculoma.

Allusions have been made to the possible role of bilharziasis in the causation of epilepsy, but proof is lacking. In 1948 the author drew attention to the great frequency with which epilepsy occurred in the Africans of South-Central Africa but found it difficult to say how often bilharziasis was responsible. He recently digested portions of frontal and parietal lobes in KOH in 40 consecutive adult autopsies showing bilharziasis of the bladder or rectum but failed to find ova in a single case.

Bilharziasis of the Spinal Cord

Bilharzial Paraplegia

The paraplegia which occurs in the disease appears to be of two types. The first is seen in a patient who has presumably had the infection for a long time—possibly for years—who develops a granulomatous process in the spinal cord. This type, as far as my experience is concerned, is very uncommon and hitherto I have failed to demonstrate such an event in the living. In the second type the paraplegia is found in the non-immune subject, such as the European. The patient is usually a young adult who has exposed himself in infected waters several or more weeks previously. The diagnosis is established by finding the ova in the stools and perhaps in the urine, although in some cases they may be difficult to find and a rectal biopsy may be necessary.

In both forms of bilharzial paraplegia, where it develops soon after the infection has been acquired or much later in the disease, the onset seems to be similar, namely an acute or subacute weakness involving both lower limbs and the bladder. The factor determining the onset of the acute symptoms is not clear. Possibly at some point there is a critical disturbance of the spinal cord blood supply in the affected region, by ova or even by an adult schistosome; or possibly it is due to an allergic or hypersensitive reaction causing swelling and oedema. It is not difficult to explain how the ova may reach the spinal cord. Batson (1940) showed that communications exist between the common iliac veins and the inferior vena cava through the vertebral venous plexus of veins. He showed that by raising the intra-abdominal pressure blood will flow from the iliac veins into this system and that this is the probable route taken by metastases to the cord in malignant disease of the prostate. That adult schistosomes themselves may enter the spinal canal, presumably by this route, has been demonstrated by Raper (1948). The adult schistosomes may deposit ova in the veins which are in close proximity to the spinal canal. In the second type of paraplegia there is a rather diffuse and negative bombardment of the cord by ova via the vertebral venous plexus—a state that would more easily arise with *Schistosoma haematobium* infection. We might at this stage attempt to classify bilharzial disease of the spinal cord as described below.

Transverse Myelitis. There appear to be two forms of this. In the first, the onset occurs soon after exposure to infection for the first time in a non-immune subject. In the second type the myelitis develops months or years after the infection was contracted. In both, the onset appears to be rapid or subacute.

The onset of symptoms in the first group is typically fairly sudden and often a complete paraplegia is evident within a matter of days or weeks. This happened in the case reported by Abbott and Spencer (1953). The patient, an African indigenous to the Sudan, experienced pains in his back and in 24 hours was completely paralysed in both legs with retention of urine. He died, and at autopsy granulomatous lesions with bilharzial ova were found in the segment of the cord from D11 to L2; the ova were those of *S. mansoni*. Hutton and Holland's case (1960) from Uganda is also of interest. A European male aged 33 became completely paralysed over 15 days. He eventually died, and at autopsy bilharzial tubercles with many bilharzial ova were evident in the lumbar and lower thoracic cord; *S. mansoni* was responsible. These two cases are worth mentioning because both developed rapid paraplegia, and in each pathological proof of its bilharzial origin was provided at autopsy. One can ask how soon in the course of the illness these ova are deposited in the nervous tissues. This is not clear from the cases so far described.

Perhaps at this juncture it is worth referring to the cases of bilharzial paraplegia which are now being recorded from Central and South Africa. Although in the majority actual proof that the cord was invaded by the schistosome adult or its ova is not forthcoming, there is very strong presumptive evidence. A case of Zilberg's (1967 *a*) is of interest, for he described how a European female child developed an attack of diarrhoea and 4 weeks later complained of pains in her legs; within several days she was unable to pass urine and walking was difficult. She developed a flaccid paralysis as well as a partial sixth nerve palsy. Her blood showed a 36 per cent eosinophilia, the bilharzial fluorescent antibody test was positive and the cerebrospinal fluid showed 63 lymphocytes per c mm; protein 80 mg/100 ml. The second specimen of spinal fluid revealed a well-marked eosinophilia. Ova of *S. mansoni* were found in the stools. There was no improvement in the paraplegia 4 months after the completion of treatment.

A similar case is reported by Levy (1969) and by Levy and Taube (1969) in a European child who developed a sudden weakness in his legs. A 42 per cent blood eosinophilia was discovered. In the cerebrospinal fluid there were 80 leucocytes per c mm, mainly monocytes. The protein was 120 mg per cent. Viable ova of *S. haematobium* were discovered in his urine; with a course of *Ambilhar* he made a very good recovery. They described a second rather similar case in a European male who developed a sudden paraplegia with urinary retention. In the spinal fluid a pleocytosis was noticed, 50 per cent of the cells being eosinophils. He had *S. mansoni*, but made a good though somewhat slower recovery.

Bilharzial Radiculitis chiefly Affecting the Nerve Roots of the Cauda Equina. Bird (1965) described this condition in a European man of 34 years of age who had grown up in an endemic bilharzial area and had frequently exposed himself to the infection. In February 1963 he slipped, hurt his hand and developed a low back pain. Four weeks later he noticed wasting in his right calf muscle. He next experienced increasing difficulty in voiding urine and became impotent. A laminectomy (D12–L1) was performed; a small portion of nerve root with surrounding tumour was removed for biopsy, and bilharzial granulomata containing terminal-spined ova were found. He was given a course of sodium antimonyl gluconate and lucanthone hydrochloride and made a complete recovery including full return of bladder control and sexual potency.

A similar condition, also of fairly rapid onset, was reported by Pepler and Lombard (1958) in an African boy aged 8 years. Within a matter of 2 days he started to complain of weakness of the legs and pain in the lower back and thighs. He had symmetrical weakness of the lower limbs; all sensory modalities appeared to be intact except for some slight hypaesthesia over the groins. There was a marked increase in protein in the cerebrospinal fluid as well as of lymphocytes. A myelogram showed a complete hold up at the upper border of L1. At operation a tumour 2½ cm by 1 cm was removed from within the cord, firmly attached to an anterior root—probably D12. On histological examination, numerous granulomata were seen as well as eggs of *S. haematobium*. Thus, a solitary granuloma was proven. It is suggested that the ova were produced locally by a worm or worms which migrated outside their normal habitat. It is not certain how ova reach the cord. They may be discharged by a gravid worm into the pulmonary blood stream, from which they are disseminated as arterial emboli. Another suggestion is that the adult worm is localized in the pelvic venous plexus and the ova are conveyed via anastomoses between the pelvic veins and the vertebral venous plexus, and between the systemic pelvic and haemorrhoidal veins. A third possibility is that a gravid schistosome worm finds its way into the cerebral venous plexus and so enters the intravertebral space of the spine (Bird, 1965).

Raper (1948) suggests how adult schistosomes may enter the spinal canal. He quotes the instance of an Askari of East Africa, who developed sudden pain in his legs with difficulty in walking. A spastic paralysis of both legs with wasting and sensory changes was found and the cerebrospinal fluid showed the loculation syndrome. A laminectomy was performed and a dense, white plaque of fibrous tissue was found lying extradurally and compressing the cord; its removal was followed by complete recovery. Sections of this fibrous matter showed that it had been laid around an adult fluke. An acute episode 2 years previously had probably heralded the arrival of the worm in the spinal canal.

References

Abbott, P. H., and Spencer, H. (1953) Transverse myelitis due to ova of *Schistosoma mansoni*, *Trans. roy. Soc. trop. Med. Hyg.*, 47, 221.

Batson, O. V. (1940) The function of the vertebral veins and their role in the spread of metastases, *Ann. Surg.*, 112, 138.

Bird, A. V. (1965) Spinal cord complications of bilharziasis, *S. Afr. med. J.*, 39, 158.

Clarke, V. de. V., Warburton, B., and Blair, D. M. (1970) The Katayama syndrome, *Cent. Afr. J. Med.*, 16, 123.

Gelfand, M. (1948) Cysticercosis of the brain in the African of Rhodesia, *E. Afr. med. J.*, 25, 110.

Hutton, P. W., and Holland, J. (1960) Schistosomiasis of the spinal cord. Report of a case, *Brit. med. J.*, 2, 1931.

Levy, L. F. (1969) Bilharziasis of the spinal cord, *Cent. Afr. J. Med.*, 15, 223.

Levy, L. F., and Taube, E. (1969) Two further cases of spinal bilharziasis, *Cent. Afr. J. Med.*, 15, 52.

Pepler, W. J., and Lombard, C. M. (1958) Spinal cord granuloma due to *Schistosoma haematobium*. Report of one case, *J. Neurolpath. exp. Neurol.* 17, 656.

Raper, A. B. (1948) Cerebral schistosomiasis, *E. Afr. med., J.*, 25, 262.

Zilberg, B. (1967 *a*) Bilharzial paraplegia in a child. A case report, *S. Afr. med. J.*, 41, 783.

Zilberg, B. (1967 *b*) Cerebral and cardiac abnormalities in Katayama fever, *S. Afr. med. J.*, 41, 598.

Zilberg, B. (1970) Unusual manifestations occurring in the early stages of bilharziasis in children, *Cent. Afr. J. med.*, 16, 524.

22 Neurological Disease in Natal

J. E. COSNETT

INTRODUCTION

The province of Natal in the Republic of South Africa extends from the Indian Ocean in the east to the Drakensberg mountains in the west. In the south-west it borders on the Transkei territory and in the north it adjoins Portuguese East Africa. In size it is some 35 000 sq miles, which is three times the size of Belgium, twice the area of Denmark, and slightly larger than Portugal or the whole of Ireland.

Lying between latitudes 27° and 31°S its coastal climate is subtropical, although its northern division of Zululand is nearly tropical. With altitudes which range from over 9000 feet in the Drakensberg to sea-level the climate shows great variation. Along the coast, popular for its seaside resorts, heat and humidity are pronounced in the summer and frost is never experienced in the winter. Further inland in the capital, Pietermaritzburg, humidity is less but temperatures still reach 100°F (38°C) in the summer. In the Natal midlands temperate conditions prevail and frost is likely for 60 to 90 days in the year. The average annual duration of sunshine is 60 per cent to the possible maximum of 70 per cent. Rain falls mainly in the summer when the usual pattern consists of hot days frequently relieved by brisk thunderstorms in the evening. More rain falls at the coast than inland and the mean annual rainfall for the province varies from 30 to 45 inches.

From the foothills of the Drakensberg, best known for its mountain resorts and nature reserves, the country flattens in the midlands, which contain fertile undulating grassland used primarily for dairy farming and agriculture. At the coast sugar-cane is the principal crop, but this is being increasingly propagated inland. In addition to agriculture, forestry occupies large areas in the midlands. The only mineral found in any quantity in Natal is coal. Flourishing industries are growing up around Pietermaritzburg, the capital, and Durban, South Africa's busiest seaport.

Population

The present population of Natal is composed of the descendants of three waves of immigrants. As far as is known the area was originally, before about AD 1300, populated solely by pygmy hunters called Bushmen. These were first driven from the coastal areas and plains into the shelter of the Drakensberg mountains, and finally eliminated by successive waves of invaders and immigrants.

The first invaders were the Negro people who came from Central Africa and whose descendants are today the Zulu- and Xhosa-speaking Bantu of Natal and the surrounding territories.

During the age of exploration Natal was visited sporadically by passing ships, mainly Portuguese. The name, Natal, is derived from such a visit by Vasco da Gama on Christmas day, 1497. The first permanent European settlers arrived in 1824 and subsequently the second wave of immigration, mainly settlers from England, gathered momentum. European settlement was reinforced by the arrival, overland, of Boers (Dutch farmers) from the Cape Province who undertook the Great Trek to escape from the strictures of the Cape Government.

The third group of immigrants consisted of indentured labourers brought from India to work in sugar-cane plantations. The first arrived in 1860, and organized Indian immigration continued intermittently until 1911. In the wake of the labourers came Indian shopkeepers and traders.

Thus the present population of Natal consists of Bantu who are predominantly Zulu-speaking and who number about 2·25 million. There are some 350 000 people of European descent, and about 400 000 Indians. A smaller number is of mixed Bantu and European origin, called 'coloureds'.

Traditionally, the Bantu of Natal have a tribal society. This system is perpetuated in the reserves or homelands where the land belongs, by tradition, to a tribe with trusteeship vested in a chief. Each family or group of families, under a headman, has an allotment of land for cultivation and one for residence. The cattle are herded, usually by small boys, on a common pasturage. The women are mainly responsible for cultivation of crops such as maize and kaffir-corn (sorghum).

Two principal factors have distrupted the traditional tribal system. One is the poverty of the homelands where the balance has been upset by the increase in population relative to the land available. Unscientific and primitive practices in agriculture and animal husbandry have contributed to deterioration of the land and of the quality of cattle. In the reserves cattle still represent wealth, and still constitute a form of currency when *lobola* must be paid for a bride. Unfortunately it is by the quantity, rather than the quality, that the price is usually measured.

A further influence which has disrupted the tribal system is that this lack of productivity in the homelands makes it necessary for many active men to seek their fortunes in the towns and cities, attracted by the wages that may be earned. Wives and families often remain in the reserves while the men go to live and earn in the cities. As a result of this migration to towns and towards industries, an urban Bantu proletariat is developing. Huge townships are being built on the outskirts of the cities, as well as many in proximity to the border industries which the Government fosters at the margins of reserves.

This process of urbanization has given rise to two social groups, a class of more primitive people who live in the reserves and adhere to the tribal system and an increasing group of urbanized, more progressive, people who live in townships adjacent to the industries in which they are employed. Shopkeepers, tradesmen, teachers and professional personnel naturally follow this migration to urban and industrial areas.

While steps have been taken for many years to improve methods of agriculture and animal husbandry in the reserves, a vicious cycle of deterioration has been in progress and it will be some time before these efforts at improvement bear fruit. Malnutrition is therefore more prevalent in the reserves than among those who live in the periurban townships.

Religion and Witchcraft

In this preface to Bantu neurology one other factor needs emphasis. This is the power that superstition and witchcraft exerts on the community and the individual. This influence is seen not only among the rural Bantu, but also among the moderately sophisticated urban population. Many types of witch doctor are in practice, which is often very lucrative. There are the medicine-men (*nyanga*) who treat illness; there are those who divine, prophesy and diagnose (*isangoma*); and those who exorcize spirits and cast spells. Furthermore, some degree of specialization may occur. A witch doctor may confine his practice to the treatment of mental illness, or he may gain a reputation for the efficacy of his love potions. Neither the *nyanga* nor the *isangoma* has any concept of pathology in the scientific sense and treatment of illness is directed at relief of predominant symptoms. A large number of unidentified remedies is used; many of these are herbal; some of them are harmless, others are distinctly toxic. Bryant's authoritative work on Zulu medicine (republished in 1970) lists 240 plants which are used medicinally, together with their uses.

The clinical picture of a disease may be obscured by the effects of treatment administered by a witch doctor, or by the patient himself, before he arrives at the hospital. A common method of treatment is to make superficial incisions or scarifications over a part which is thought to be the seat of the illness. The fact that a large proportion of patients attending hospital have such scarifications is evidence of the competition which the witch doctors offer, and of the fact that many patients have greater initial faith in witchcraft than in scientific medicine.

Traditionally, the Zulu's religion is based on ancestor worship. While a single God is acknowledged, the tribal Zulu believes that most of his fortunes and misfortunes are subject to the whims of the spirits of his ancestors, some ancestors being more influential than others. Most misfortunes, such as illness, are attributed either to the wrath of the ancestors or to witchcraft, such as a spell being invoked by an enemy or rival. In the event of illness the *isangoma* is consulted to divine the cause and the *nyanga* may be required to recommend treatment. If the diagnosis is ancestral displeasure, some sacrifice may be necessary, or a feast may be considered propitious. If the misfortune is due to a spell, some countermeasure may be indicated, or herbal or medicinal treatment prescribed.

This background of superstition and belief in the power of witchcraft offers certain obstacles to the efficient practice of scientific medicine. It is not uncommon for a patient to refuse an urgent operation until such time as the ancestors have been consulted, through the medium of a witch doctor, and their wrath appeased. The treatment of a prolonged illness, where hospital treatment does not offer a dramatic cure, may be interrupted or discontinued because relatives have consulted a witch doctor. The advice may be that a feast should be held, and this demands the presence of the patient outside hospital. The result, when the patient suffers from a cerebral tumour or meningitis, may be disastrous. Largely, this persistence of belief in witchcraft is evidence of lack of education. Only among the generation who are now children is there any consistent effort at education. Complete lack of education and illiteracy are common among the older generations, especially in the reserves.

About half of the Bantu population profess Christianity in some form. The accepted faiths such as Roman Catholicism and the Methodist, Presbyterian, Anglican, and Dutch Reformed churches, have, through their mission schools and hospitals, considerable influence. There are, however, a number of independent sects which profess Christianity, but these are adulterated, to a greater or lesser extent, by traditional belief in witchcraft and ancestral worship. It is probably because they allow some recognition of traditional beliefs that these independent churches have unexpected support, especially among the semi-literate. Traditional beliefs die hard; even among the educated a catastrophe may provoke a return to the more primitive religion as a source of advice and means of comfort.

Diet

In the homelands the staple diet is *puthu*, a thick porridge made from mealie (maize) meal. This diet may be supplemented with meat or vegetables, but the incidence of pellagra and protein malnutrition indicates that *puthu* is often eaten to the exclusion of any other foodstuff. Milk is taken when it is available, often in a soured form called *maas*. This is a popular beverage. Another, commonly fed to babies, is *machewu* a slightly fermented porridge made from kaffir-corn (sorghum). Among the urban or periurban Bantu population the dietary habits of Europeans are being increasingly adopted.

The traditional alcoholic beverage is Zulu beer, made from fermented kaffir-corn. From this basic product other more potent liquors are made either by distillation or by the addition of various substances. Some of the additives, such as methylated spirit or metal polish, are highly toxic if taken in quantity. Herbs or tissue of animal, or even human, origin may be added to the brew for the sake of flavour or potency. European liquors such as brandy, cane spirit, or beer are consumed by the more sophisticated urban people. True alcoholism is rare, except among the latter group; civilization seems to foster alcoholism.

Medical Services

Each province in the Republic of South Africa is divided into Magisterial Districts centred around towns or villages. Every district has its magistrate and district surgeon. The latter, employed by the State Health Department, is responsible for public health measures, treatment of infectious diseases such as tuberculosis and syphilis, the treatment of indigent patients, and for forensic medical work. Clearly the district surgeons, some of whom are also in private practice, have difficulty giving adequate cover to all aspects of their work. Nevertheless, they are the representatives of an organized medical service, even in the most remote areas.

In such areas other most useful purveyors of medical services are the mission hospitals. These were mostly established by various denominations in the early years of the century. Their main function in the medical field is therapeutic, but they are responsible for training many Bantu girls as nurses or auxiliary nurses. While they are still staffed by the religious orders, most of them are heavily subsidized by the South African Government, with regard to both capital expenditure and running costs.

Each town of moderate size has its own hospital, administered by the provincial Government. These provincial hospitals are able to supply general hospital services to all races, and in some, specialist services are available.

The teaching hospital of the University of Natal Medical School, King Edward VIII Hospital, is situated in Durban. It provides undergraduate training for Bantu, Indian and coloured students. Its postgraduate training facilities are open to all races. With its ancillary hospitals, such as Wentworth Hospital, it is able to offer all modern medical facilities including open heart surgery and neurosurgery.

Edendale Hospital is in a relatively unique position. Situated 6 miles outside Pietermaritzburg, it is just within a large Bantu area or reserve. As such its administration falls, not under the aegis of the provincial Government, but under the State Health Department. With accommodation for over 1400 inpatients and a medical staff of about 100 doctors, including full-time specialists, it is the largest general hospital in any of the Bantu reserves in South Africa. It admits over 35 000 patients, and treats over 250 000 outpatients annually. The annual budget is over R3 million (£1·8 million). The functions of the hospital are twofold: first, it supplies general medical services to the large Bantu population in the neighbouring reserves; secondly, it provides specialist services to the Bantu and Indian population of a large area of inland Natal. As a reference centre for specialist services, patients may be referred from remote areas, perhaps as far as 150 or 200 miles distant. Draining this large area, roughly 300 miles long and 100 miles wide and containing agricultural areas and Bantu reserves, the hospital has a clientele which is generally less sophisticated than that of other large hospitals. In a recent article from Edendale Hospital, Fernandes (1970) has outlined the work of the hospital with particular reference to the interaction between scientific medicine and traditional Zulu beliefs. Neurology falls within the scope of the Department of Medicine, while specialist neurosurgeons visit from Durban, or patients are sent to Durban for their attention.

NEUROLOGICAL PRACTICE IN NATAL

Among the white population, neurological practice is similar to that in Europe, with the single important exception of the relative rarity of multiple sclerosis. The same generalization applies to the Indian population, whose spectrum of disease is similar to that of the white races. The Bantu, however, show numerous differences in disease incidence and presentation. For this reason this account will refer principally to the Bantu races, most of whom, in Natal, are Zulu-speaking.

Difficulties in Neurological Practice

Neurology, perhaps more than most medical disciplines, requires a considerable degree of rapport between doctor and patient. Where the patient and doctor share neither language nor culture, and especially where history and physical signs must be elicited through the medium of an interpreter, such rapport is difficult to achieve. The lack of it is clearly disadvantageous to accurate diagnosis.

Sometimes the patient may expect from the doctor an approach which is more in keeping with that of the traditional witch doctor. Some patients, albeit the more primitive, expecct no history to be taken; the doctor should be able to describe the patient's symptoms and their causes at the conclusion of the examination, without the benefit of any questions to the patient or his relatives. A doctor who needs to ask questions may be considered to lack proficiency. Clairvoyance commands great respect. Other patients, out of respect for the doctor and in an effort to please, may answer all questions in the affirmative, thus rendering the history valueless. Similarly, in examination, a patient may, through humility, feel obliged to present the signs which are more compatible with his concept of the disease. This fallacy is especially prevalent in the case of sensory examination.

The very nature of neurological disease with its symptoms of strokes, fits, paralysis, and involuntary movements, provokes, in the patient's mind suspicion of witchcraft, spells and other occult practices: a disease with such dramatic symptoms might need an equally sudden and dramatic cure. A doctor who resorts to prolonged and apparently unfruitful treatment such as physiotherapy may be considered ineffective. The patient, perhaps abetted by relatives, may decide to leave hospital to seek a witch doctor's advice. He may ultimately return in a deteriorated state when all else has failed.

While the demand for hospital services increases constantly, some less sophisticated patients are reluctant to attend hospitals until late in their illness when all other remedies, self-administered herbs, and witchcraft have been of no avail. Many patients still come, or are brought, to hospital in the terminal stages. They may be suffering not only from the effects of their illness but also from the effects of prior treatment by witch doctors. In the case of cerebral disease this often means that the patient is stuporose, comatose or mentally disturbed when he reaches hospital. This renders history taking difficult, especially as reliable witnesses of the onset and progress of the disease may not, by reason of distance or expense, be able to accompany the patient to hospital.

Assessment of intellect, and particularly of its deterioration, is most difficult in the totally illiterate patient. Even the most intelligent person will not be able to subtract 'serial sevens' or perform arithmetical calculations if he has never been to school. Tests of memory and orientation are difficult to devise when a patient is unaware of world events or personalities. Tests of writing and drawing are invalid if the patient has never held a pen. Psychiatry, even more than pure neurology, suffers most in these circumstances.

Geography and distance also lead to difficulty. In the more remote areas communications and transport facilities are relatively poor, and distances correspondingly great. A patient may not be able to attend hospital more than once in the course of his illness. If an adequate diagnosis and effective treatment are not available at the first visit the patient may not, for reasons of economy and distance, be able to return. In cases of neurological illness this may be a particular handicap as the patient may not be able to use what public transport is available. The value of serial observation is limited by this difficulty of repeated visits to hospital.

Another factor which impedes refinement in neurology is the handicap of overcrowded clinics and congested wards containing all varieties of acute illnesses. Acute medical emergencies must take precedence over chronic illness, and time may not permit the extended examinations which are necessary for accurate neurological diagnosis. The relative lack of specialized diagnostic services, especially in the fields of radiology and clinical pathology, makes one more reliant on the patella hammer, the pin and the ophthalmoscope as instruments of diagnosis. When specialized diagnostic services are available they are, of necessity, first provided to the acutely and curably ill, with the result that procedures of a more academic nature must be sacrificed.

Physical Signs

While most physical signs and their interpretation are identical with those in European neurological cases, there are a few features of difference produced by racial factors, or the result of modification by local circumstances. These peculiarities deserve mention.

The Zulus are, by tradition, a pugnacious race. Faction fights and tribal skirmishes still occur. Quarrels are frequently settled by violence, and assaults are common. The weapons are usually heavy sticks with clubbed ends ('knob-kerries') or knives, with the result that blunt head injuries and stab-wounds are very common. While the acute injuries are not in the province of the neurologist, their delayed effects form an appreciable proportion of the neurological cases seen in medical wards. In this community it is almost rare to find an adult scalp which is unscarred by previous injury. Because the late effects of such traumata are frequent causes of neurological disability, history or signs of previous injury assume greater importance in diagnosis. Palpation of the scalp sometimes reveals an old depressed fracture, hidden under the hair, which explains epilepsy or other symptoms.

Another feature which is, of course, common to all neurological practice, but more obvious in primitive societies, is the frequency with which the cause of neurological illness is to be found in disease of other systems. The reason for this greater emphasis on systemic disease is that the primary disease is often neglected until it has some catastrophic, perhaps neurological, complication. It goes without saying that physical examination must be total. Sudden hemiplegia may, for example, be easily explained by signs of neglected rheumatic heart disease or bacterial endocarditis. The cause of an expanding intracranial lesion may be found on chest X-ray which shows a lung abscess or carcinoma. The search for a cause of meningitis need sometimes go no further than the finding of miliary tuberculosis on X-ray, or enlarged lymph nodes in the neck.

The plantar (Babinski) reflex appears to be more difficult to elicit and to have less significance in some Bantu people, especially those from rural areas. Stroking of the sole of the foot frequently results in no response or in an equivocal reaction. This is probably the result of thickening of the soles consequent on the habit of wearing no shoes from childhood. In addition to the thickening of the soles, it is possible that lifelong exposure of the feet to sensory stimuli renders them less sensitive to stimulation.

One sign, peculiar to Africa, is the presence of multiple superficial incisions made by witch doctors over the diseased part, or over the site of pain. These incisions are usually 0·5 to 1 cm in length. Their clinical value is that they may indicate the situation of pain, and the degree of healing may give some indication of the duration of the illness. A patient with cerebral disease, brought to hospital unconscious, may have almost healed incisions indicating that the illness is not of very recent onset.

In pigmented races the ocular fundi have an appearance which differs in certain respects from that in Europeans. The greater pigmentation of the retinae produces greater contrast between the optic disc and the retina with the result that the disc appears unduly pale and distinct. Those inexperienced in African ophthalmoscopy may mistakenly interpret this appearance as being due to optic atrophy. By contrast, the optic fundus in light-skinned races appears pink and hyperaemic and may even be construed as early papilloedema. A tigroid appearance of the retina is common among Africans.

A further peculiarity of the eyes of pigmented races is their relative insensitivity to mydriatic drugs. The practitioner in Africa who wishes to dilate his patient's pupils prior to ophthalmoscopy often finds that he must use larger amounts of mydriatics, in higher concentrations, than is usual in light-skinned people.

A characteristic which has been observed in Bantu races is the relative infrequency of pineal calcification on X-ray of the skull. The sign of pineal displacement is, therefore, less likely to be helpful than it is in Europe.

EPIDEMIOLOGY AND PUBLIC HEALTH

As in all underdeveloped populations, especially in warm climates, a large proportion of the disease among the Natal Bantu is the result of infection, either bacterial or parasitic, and thus, ideally preventable. The most common causes of admission to a general hospital include pneumonia, tuberculosis, and other respiratory infections; and intestinal infections such as bacillary and amoebic dysentery, and typhoid. Cardiac conditions such as rheumatic carditis and a local variety of cardiomyopathy are also common.

Of the infections of the nervous system tuberculous, meningococcal, and pneumococcal meningitis are the most common. Meningococcal meningitis occurs sporadically and has not been known, recently, to occur in epidemic form. The high incidence of tuberculosis is augmented by the great difficulties in control and treatment in rural areas, and by malnutrition. While syphilis is common its incidence has declined during the past decade.

The State Health Department is responsible for the control of infectious diseases which are notifiable to that department. Singular success has been achieved in the control of two diseases. Malaria, until 35 years ago endemic even as far south as Pietermaritzburg, never occurs unless it has been imported from elsewhere. Poliomyelitis, once occurring in devastating epidemics, has virtually been eliminated by nationwide oral vaccination. Acute poliomyelitis is rarely seen, and those cases which do occur are the result of parental negligence rather than the unavailability of vaccination. The elimination of acute poliomyelitis has been one of the features of the past decade in South Africa.

As in all fields of medicine, so in neurology there are noteworthy differences between the incidence of certain diseases in Europe, in white people living in South Africa, and in other racial groups in South Africa. Documentation of these differences is difficult. The factors necessary for accurate epidemiological studies are often impossible to achieve. One relies on impression, which, even though based on long experience, is not acceptable to the rigid discipline of statisticians.

The three prerequisites for accurate epidemiological studies are: knowledge of the population at risk, precise diagnosis, and accurate knowledge of the disease incidence among the population. Circumstances in Africa make it impossible to obtain some of this information. While estimates of the regional population may be accurate, it is impossible to assess what proportion of this population will seek medical advice or attend hospital when they fall ill. Clinical diagnosis may be reasonably accurate, but pathological proof unavailable. Certain features inherent in chronic neurological illness make it unlikely that autopsy material will be available. Patients with such disease cannot be kept in hospital indefinitely. Follow-up is sketchy when communications and transport are poor and social circumstances are medieval.

Despite these difficulties it is possible to form distinct impressions of the incidence of various diseases. Unfortunately these impressions are often rejected by those who maintain, for example, that the reason brain tumours appear rare is that cases do not attend hospital for this condition and thus escape recording. This may be true to a small extent, but comparison with other diseases will show fallacies in this argument.

For, in this example, why should patients frequently attend hospital with chronic subdural haematoma, brain abscess, or secondary tumour, but not for primary tumours? Impressions of the rarity of certain diseases are also sometimes countered by the argument that the disease occurs, but is not diagnosed. However, if the circumstances and facilities do not permit the diagnosis of multiple sclerosis, why should the diagnoses of such diseases as neurosyphilis, tuberculous meningitis, and motor neurone disease be possible under the same circumstances?

COMMON NEUROLOGICAL DISEASES AND DEVIATIONS FROM THE USUAL PATTERN

A survey of consecutive hospital admissions from 1959 to 1962 aimed at determining the relative incidence of neurological diseases (Cosnett, 1964). It was found that the most common presenting features of neurological disease were stroke, fits, symptoms of intracranial infection, mental disturbance and disorders of the lower limbs. When the final diagnoses of 1302 consecutive neurological cases were analysed the incidence of common disorders was as shown in TABLE 22.1. These cases were drawn from some 59 500 general hospital admissions. No more recent comprehensive surveys have been made, but the present incidence is similar, with one exception. It is our impression that neurosyphilis has become less common during the past decade.

Table 22.1

Analysis of 1302 Neurological Admissions, Edendale Hospital, 1959–1962

Diagnostic category	*Percentage (of all neurological cases)*
Cerebral vascular disease	29·0
Epilepsy and allied disorders	15·9
Meningitis	10·3
Neurosyphilis	8·1
Other intracranial infections	3·8
Psychiatric	4·9
Peripheral neuropathy	4·7
Spinal cord disorders	3·1
Undiagnosed and unusual	7·6
Miscellaneous	12·5

Cerebral Vascular Disease

Cerebral vascular disease accounts for about one-third of all neurological admissions to hospital. Most of these patients present the clinical picture of a stroke, frequently with sudden disturbance of consciousness and the development of hemiplegia. While the clinical features are similar to those in Europeans there are certain facets in the pathogenesis which show local peculiarities. The most common varieties of cerebral vascular disease are cerebral haemorrhage, occlusion of intra- or extracerebral arteries by thrombus, and cerebral embolism.

Among South African whites there is a high incidence of coronary and cerebral vascular disease attributable to atherosclerosis. These conditions are similarly prevalent among the Indian population. In the Bantu, by contrast, coronary thrombosis and ischaemic heart disease are exceptionally rare. During a survey of cardiac disease at Edendale Hospital (Cosnett, 1962) it was found that myocardial infarction acounted for only six patients among 1000 cases of heart disease. This number was representative of some 25 000 general hospital admissions. In comparison, among some 60 000 admissions there were 378 cases of cerebral vascular disease. It would appear that cerebral vascular disease is about 27 times as common as myocardial infarction in the Bantu population.

While atherosclerosis undoubtedly occurs in the Bantu there is little doubt that its degree and extent are less than is found in Europeans of comparable age. This observation has been documented by several workers. Wainwright (1961), in a survey of atheroma of the aorta and coronary vessels, showed that the degree and extent of involvement were considerably less in the Bantu than in the European. Similar observations have been made in respect of cerebral atheroma (Wainwright, 1968). Furthermore, it was noted that the severity of cerebral atheroma was related to hypertension and to the age of the patient. Atheroma had a low incidence in non-hypertensives of both sexes. There is no doubt that hypertension is very common in the Bantu. The reason for the striking difference in the incidence of coronary and cerebral vascular disease is not known. The elucidation of this problem may contain the clue to the pathogenesis of occlusive arterial disease, and deserves closer study.

Strokes in the Bantu are not confined to the aged or the hypertensive. During a survey of strokes in young people at Edendale Hospital (Cosnett, 1969) there were 28 patients, between 10 and 40 years old, in whom the cause of the stroke could not be clearly defined. In many of these, angiography showed occlusion of the internal carotid, middle cerebral, or anterior cerebral arteries, but none of the recognized predisposing causes of vascular disease could be found. Some cases of occlusion of the internal carotid or intracranial arteries followed blunt injuries to the head or neck.

Cerebral embolism is a common cause of strokes in the young Bantu, and usually follows in the wake of rheumatic heart disease, with or without bacterial endocarditis. The high incidence of rheumatic heart disease is related to underpriviledged circumstances and the difficulty of adequate prophylaxis. An unusual variety of cerebral embolism is that which occurs in association with the cardiomyopathy which is prevalent among the Bantu (Cosnett and Pudifin, 1964). This variety of cardiomyopathy appears to be peculiar to South Africa and it accounts for 25 per cent to 30 per cent of cases of heart failure among the Bantu (Cosnett, 1962; Kallichurum, 1969). One pathological feature of this disease is the development of endocardial or mural thrombi in one or both ventricles. From this source emboli become detached and cause infarction of the spleen, kidneys, lungs or brain. Cerebral infarction of this type is one of the varieties of cerebral vascular disease observed in this population (Cosnett, 1964).

Neurosyphilis

In the Edendale survery of neurological diseases, neurosyphilis was found to account for 8 per cent of cases. The majority of these were diagnosed as meningovascular syphilis on the grounds of otherwise unexplained cerebral vascular occlusion in patients with positive serological tests in blood or cerebrospinal fluid (CSF). Other patients presented features of subacute meningitis, isolated cranial nerve palsies, or spinal cord lesions.

Many South African observers have noted the extreme rarity of parenchymatous forms of neurosyphilis, despite the relative frequency of other forms of syphilitic affection in the Bantu. The series of 1302 neurological cases included only one case of tabes dorsalis and a few cases diagnosed as general paralysis. The total number of cases of parenchymatous syphilis accounted for less than 1 per cent of all neurological cases.

In some other cases it was thought that syphilis was responsible for a more acute encephalopathy associated with mental disorder and epileptic fits (Cosnett, 1965 *a*), which responded to treatment with penicillin. In the absence of opportunity for autopsy studies, however, one cannot be certain that these were not examples of some toxic or nutritional encephalopathy occurring coincidentally in patients with positive serological tests.

There is little doubt that the incidence of all forms of late syphilis has decreased during the past 15 years. This decrease is probably attributable to the advent of penicillin and to the earlier treatment of primary and secondary infections.

Epilepsy

Epilepsy of recent onset accounts for about 20 per cent of neurological admissions to hospital. In about 70 per cent of these no cause can be found for the epilepsy, and they are classified as idiopathic. Regarding these idiopathic epileptics, it is likely that genetic factors play an important part in aetiology, as has been indicated by a study of Bantu residents on the Witwatersrand (Hurst, Reef, and Sachs, 1961). In a survey of male Bantu mineworkers from the same area Bird, Heinz, and Klintworth (1962) found cerebral trauma and cysticercosis to be important aetiological factors. In the Edendale series 17 per cent of epileptics admitted to hospital were regarded as post-traumatic on the grounds of a history of severe head injury or the presence of old depressed skull fractures. These patients were almost invariably men, the trauma resulting from fighting or assaults.

Several workers have commented on the rarity of petit mal in the African. From experience based largely on hospital admissions, it is impossible to provide statistical proof of this observation, but it does appear that petit mal is rare in this population. It is possible, however, that such a minor complaint may not lead the patient to attend hospital, and thus may not appear in hospital records. On questioning, Bantu school-teachers and nurses have stated that they have not been aware of cases of petit mal among children of their acquaintance.

Cerebral cysticercosis accounts for a proportion of cases of otherwise unexplained epilepsy. This diagnosis is impossible to prove in most cases, but tapeworm infestation is common and cerebral cysts are sometimes found at autopsy when their presence has not been suspected during life.

For reasons detailed above the long-term control of epilepsy is difficult in this community. Patients tend to regard freedom from fits as an indication to discontinue treatment. Superstition, witchcraft, and geographical and economic factors all militate against adequate and conscientious long-term anticonvulsant treatment.

Meningitis

Approximately 22 per cent of all neurological cases admitted to hospital are suffering from infections of the nervous system. Of these meningitis is the most common. In about two-thirds of cases the infection is a pyogenic one but, unfortunately, precise identification of the organism is often not possible. When organisms are identified these are usually either meningococci or pneumococci. When bacteriological identification is not available the diagnosis and treatment are based on the nature of the pleocytosis and the chemical characteristics of the CSF.

About one-third of cases of meningitis are tuberculous. Again, bacteriological proof of diagnosis is often difficult to obtain. The value of chest X-ray and the detection of tuberculosis of other sites has often been shown. One feature of the CSF in many cases of tuberculous meningitis, which is not well documented, is the frequent preponderance of polymorphs in the early stages of the disease. Such preponderance may lead to diagnostic confusion, but the number of polymorphs does not usually exceed 300 per c mm and the glucose content is not as low as occurs in pyogenic meningitis. Later in the course of the disease lymphocytes predominate. Provided that treatment is sought before the patient is moribund the results of treatment with streptomycin, isoniazid and PAS are good. There seems, today, to be little place for the use of intrathecal streptomycin. Adrenocortical steroids are often of great value in late cases, or those in whom cranial nerve palsies or very high CSF protein levels develop.

Expanding Intracranial Lesions

The most common causes of raised intracranial pressure in this community are haematomas: subdural, extradural, or intracerebral. Inflammatory masses, either abscess or tuberculoma, are also common. Raised pressure consequent on obstruction to CSF pathways by inflammatory exudate or parasitic cysts is also seen. Brain tumours, especially primary neoplasms, are relatively rare.

Subdural and Extradural Haematoma

The high incidence of blunt head injuries resulting from assaults and fighting has its aftermath in many cases of intracranial haematomas both acute and chronic. In the diagnosis of these conditions a high index of suspicion and subsequent carotid angiography have been shown to be most important.

Brain Abscess

The frequency of cerebral abscess reflects inadequate and delayed treatment of lung abscesses, bronchiectasis, and otitis media. The stoicism of many patients leads them to neglect the primary suppuration until cerebral complications appear. In addition to delayed presentation, a further feature which contributes to the high mortality rate is the presence of multiple abscesses. It is not unusual to diagnose and treat one abscess, only to find at autopsy that several other abscesses are present in other parts of the brain.

Brain Tumours

Of all the intracranial neoplasms encountered in this community the majority are secondary growths. These usually arise from bronchial carcinoma, which is one of the most common malignant tumours, and one which is frequently neglected until it reaches an advanced stage. We have also encountered secondary cerebral deposits in cases of choriocarcinoma, carcinoma of the cervix, primary hepatic carcinoma, and ovarian carcinoma.

There is little doubt that primary intracranial tumours of all types are considerably less common in the Bantu than in people of European stock. In the series of 1302 consecutive neurological cases reviewed only 0·7 per cent were cases of primary tumour. Both meningiomas and gliomas are rare, but it is our impression that meningiomas are more common than gliomas. Furthermore, it appears that childhood gliomas, especially the pontine type, occur more frequently than gliomas in adults. In a busy general hospital such as this, years may pass without an adult supratentorial glioma being encountered.

Confirmation of our observations comes from a Cape Town survey of supratentorial gliomas and meningiomas in three race groups: European, coloured, and Bantu (Louis and Keet, 1964). While the number of Bantu residing in the Western Cape Province is small, the authors show that the incidence of these tumours is considerably higher in whites that in the Bantu, with the coloureds occupying an intermediate position. This remarkable observation has, so far, received little attention, but it deserves more. It is sometimes asserted that this racial discrepancy is due, not to any real difference in incidence, but to the belief that the Bantu do not present for diagnosis or that the diagnosis is missed. That this explanation is unlikely is illustrated by the fact that they do not hesitate to attend hospital for secondary tumours, subdural haematomas, and epilepsy. Furthermore, if the diagnosis was missed the tumours would surely be found at autopsy. This difference in racial incidence seems to be a fruitful field for further epidemiological study.

Neurofibromatosis

This condition, in all its forms, is relatively common among the Bantu, and it is probably the most common primary tumour of the nervous system in this race. Some cases have been seen with gross spinal deformity, and others with intraspinal and intracranial neurofibromata.

Peripheral Neuropathy

Although the survey (Cosnett, 1964) indicated that peripheral neuropathy was responsible for 4·7 per cent of neurological admissions, it is likely that its true incidence is considerably higher. Because of its relatively undramatic nature, especially when the patient suffers from some other disease in addition, the diagnosis of peripheral neuropathy often escapes recording in hospital statistics. Many patients admitted for malnutrition, tuberculosis, diabetes and gastrointestinal infections have the subsidiary complaints of paraesthesiae in the legs, weakness and sensory loss. Examination reveals diminished or lost deep reflexes and peripheral anaesthesia. It is likely that about one-third of all patients admitted to general medical wards have some such symptoms and signs, while only the major diagnosis will be recorded for statistical purposes. Common causes of peripheral neuropathy are malnutrition, alcoholism, and diabetes, while chronic hepatic and renal failure, malignant disease, and isoniazid therapy account for a proportion of cases.

A further variety of neuropathy, which appears to be a distinct entity, has been observed. The patient usually complains of intense dysaesthesia in the feet. This is usually a burning sensation which is worse at night, to the extent that he cannot tolerate the weight of the bedclothes on his feet. There is often excessive sweating of the feet and hands, with the result that these feel moist and soggy. The third characteristic feature is exaggeration of the deep reflexes, although the plantar reflexes remain flexor in response. This condition closely resembles that described in other tropical countries (Spillane, 1947), and is sometimes called the 'burning foot syndrome'. Some authors also mention the burning dysaesthesia, hyperidrosis, and hyperreflexia as being characteristic features. The condition undoubtedly occurs in a setting of malnutrition and alcoholism. It is infrequently associated with pellagra, but often with a dermatosis of the face which includes dyssebacea, cheilosis, and angular stomatitis. This is similar to the follicular hyperkeratosis described by other authors. The condition responds to several weeks' treatment with improved diet, abstinence from alcohol, and vitamin B complex. The exaggeration of the deep reflexes and the hyperidrosis may indicate that the pyramidal tracts and autonomic fibres are involved, rather than the peripheral nerves only.

Porphyria

The variety of porphyria which is common in this community is that known as porphyria cutanea tarda which results from chronic liver disease, invariably due to abuse of the various alcoholic liquors which are brewed, often illicitly. For this reason it is also called symptomatic or hepatic porphyria. While the usual neurological manifestations of acute intermittent or variegate porphyria are not observed, workers in Durban (Asmal, Vinik, and Joubert, 1970) have drawn attention to a peculiar sensory disturbance which occurs in porphyria cutanea tarda. The main feature is impairment of superficial sensation on the face and peripheral parts of the limbs, without evidence of motor involvement. It is suggested that this is a form of neuropathy caused by the disturbance in porphyrin metabolism.

Leprosy

About 80 to 100 new cases of leprosy are admitted annually to the Amatikulu Leper Institution in Zululand (Welsh and Pretorius, 1970). This institution receives all cases of leprosy notified in Natal, so this figure probably reflects the incidence in the province with reasonable accuracy. About one-quarter of these cases are referred from Edendale Hospital. Apart from a higher proportion of cases of tuberculoid leprosy, indicating a greater natural resistance, these cases do not differ from lepers elsewhere. All varieties of neural involvement are observed. The frequent involvement of branches of the facial nerve is a feature which, from our experience, needs emphasis. Cases of pure neural leprosy, without florid cutaneous lesions, occur occasionally and create difficult diagnostic problems.

Spinal Cord Disorders

It is probably the experience of every neurologist that cases of spinal cord disorder occur which defy all investigation and are subsequently classified as idiopathic. In Europe and North America some such cases are probably labelled as multiple sclerosis or other demyelinating disease. In South Africa, however, where multiple sclerosis is rare, it seems less likely that such cases can be so diagnosed. The most common causes of paraplegia in this community are trauma, spinal tuberculosis, transverse myelitis, syphilis, and secondary tumours. Less common causes are vascular lesions, primary tumours, especially neurofibromas, parasitic cysts, and epidural abscesses.

Nutritional and Toxic Myelopathy

Among the spinal cord syndromes which have been recognized occasionally are nutritional myelopathy, and a toxic myelopathy associated with acute infections. The nutritional myelopathy is usually associated with pellagra or other evidence of vitamin B complex deficiency. The patient shows features of pyramidal and sensory tract involvement which improves with the nutritional state. A similar, fortunately transient, form of cord disorder has occasionally been observed during the convalescent stages of typhoid fever and dysentery. It is possible that this also represents a nutritional defect, unmasked by the severe infection.

Unexplained Spastic Myelopathy

During the survey of neurological disease at Edendale Hospital it was noticed that an undue number of unexplained cord lesions was recorded, and that these had certain features in common. Forty-one such cases were seen during a 5-year period, and their records were analysed retrospectively (Cosnett, 1965 *b*). Most of the patients were young (10 to 50 years) with a peak incidence in the third decade. They usually presented a clinical picture of spastic weakness of both legs, developing over several months. The physical signs were those of pyramidal tract involvement with exaggerated tendon reflexes and ankle clonus. The arms were not usually affected. The majority of patients had no sensory disturbance but some had distal sensory loss, interpreted as being due to peripheral neuropathy; and a few showed features of posterior column involvement.

Investigations did not reveal the cause. X-rays of the chest and spine and serological tests were negative. The CSF was usually normal. A few patients had slight pleocytosis (fewer than 20 cells per c mm) and slight elevation of the protein content (less than 100 mg per cent). Myelography was negative in the 22 cases in whom it was performed. Some patients were found to have eosinophilia of the peripheral blood. This may have been due to coincidental parasitic infestation. In most cases the disease was not progressive, and the disability improved slowly without specific treatment. It was never known to be fatal.

Similar cases have been observed at the King Edward VIII Hospital, Durban (Hill, 1970). In both centres it appears that the condition has become less common in the last 3 years. This fact would indicate that, whatever the cause, it is no longer operating to the same extent. These cases resemble the larger group of cases from Jamaica (Montgomery *et al.*, 1964) described as spastic myelopathy. Cases resembling the ataxic type of neuropathy have not been observed in Natal. Our cases also show features similar to lathyrism, described in India. It seems likely that the cause of this spastic myelopathy is some toxic factor, possibly dietary in origin. An undue proportion of our cases were from rural areas, particularly those of Northern Natal. Inquiry did not, however, enable us to relate this incidence to any known dietary factor.

Bilharzial Myelopathy

This condition undoubtedly occurs in Natal where bilharzia, especially infestation by *Schistosoma haematobium*, is endemic (Bhagwandeen, 1968). It is, however, impossible to define its true incidence with any accuracy. This difficulty arises from the fact that the existence of a bilharzial lesion of the spinal cord cannot be proved unless the patient is subjected to exploration and biopsy, procedures which are not undertaken unless there is good evidence of cord compression.

The usual clinical problem is of a young patient who has signs of a cord lesion and is found to be suffering from bilharzia. Eosinophilia is commonly present, and myelography negative. Serological tests are unhelpful where as many as 41 per cent to 67 per cent of the Bantu population are infested with the parasite (Bhagwandeen, 1968). Therapeutic trials with anti-bilharzial drugs are not likely to be conclusive, since damage to the cord is not quickly repaired, whatever the cause. Even dead worms may occlude spinal veins or cause other inflammatory reaction. Although some patients with bilharzial myelopathy show myelographic abnormality, a normal myelogram does not exclude vascular lesions of bilharzial origin. In these circumstances, therefore, it is difficult to make a firm diagnosis of bilharzial myelopathy although doubtless some cases do occur.

Intrathecal Tuberculous Granuloma

All varieties of tuberculosis are exceptionally common in this community. Spinal tuberculosis is one of the most frequent causes of paraplegia. The entity of intrathecal granuloma without vertebral disease (Arseni and Samitca, 1960; Rose-Innes, 1969) has also been observed here. Commonly, the patient has evidence of tuberculosis elsewhere, especially pulmonary or glandular tuberculosis; but the absence of such evidence does not exclude the condition. The patient usually presents with the symptoms and signs of a slowly progressive spinal lesion, mimicking a spinal tumour. The CSF shows slight lymphocytic pleocytosis and slight elevation of protein content. X-rays show normal vertebrae. Myelography may reveal varying degrees of abnormality.

As in the case of bilharzial myelopathy, precise proof of diagnosis can only come from exploration and biopsy. Yet one is reluctant to advise this course when the patient has a small or equivocal myelographic abnormality. When the patient has evidence of tuberculosis elsewhere, and signs of a cord lesion without block, he may be treated by means of tuberculostatic drugs in the first instance. The neurological signs have been known to improve considerably in these circumstances. A therapeutic trial of tuberculostatic drugs probably has a place in such cases.

Scurvy, Osteoporosis, and Vertebral Collapse

A recently recognized and distinct clinical entity, which sometimes has neurological manifestations, is osteoporosis associated with scurvy and siderosis. The condition appears to be peculiar to Bantu men, and it occurs in most parts of South Africa, especially in the Transvaal and Natal. Elegant studies carried out in Johannesburg (Seftel *et al.*, 1966) have revealed its pathogenesis. The main determining factor is iron overload which results from prolonged excessive consumption of iron. The source of this iron is probably the popular Zulu beer which is brewed in iron containers. Siderosis, or excessive iron deposition in many organs, results in such complications as hepatic portal fibrosis, cirrhosis, porphyria cutanea tarda, pancreatic siderosis, and diabetes.

In addition, the iron deposits have been shown to interfere with metabolism of ascorbic acid. This situation, combined with dietary lack of ascorbic acid, leads to latent or florid scurvy. Scurvy, in turn, leads to osteoporosis, since the vitamin is necessary for the formation of osteoid. Support for this concept of its pathogenesis comes from the observation that scurvy and this variety of osteoporosis are rare among Bantu children and adult women. Neither of these groups consume Zulu beer in such large quantities as do the men.

While this condition has many facets, its neurological interest lies in the fact that the patient may present with symptoms of nerve root compression by collapsed vertebrae, with features resembling those of a disc syndrome, or with signs of spinal cord compression. Its incidence is confined largely to those who have been heavy drinkers of Zulu beer for many years, and whose diet is deficient in vitamin C. The diagnosis is based on the clinical features of siderosis and scurvy with osteoporosis and vertebral collapse on X-ray. Once it is established the condition is difficult to treat, but help can be had from rest, orthopaedic appliances, and correction of diet. Unfortunately the nature of the cause militates against cure. Unless one is able to modify the lifelong drinking and dietary habits of the patient reversal of the metabolic changes and improvement of the osteoporosis is unlikely.

Psychiatric Disorders

Although, as a general hospital, Edendale does not cater specifically for psychiatric disorders, about 9 per cent of all neurological cases admitted have mental disorder as their predominant feature (Cosnett, 1964). Of these, almost half are found to have underlying organic disease, and the remainder are ultimately classified as psychotic or psychoneurotic. The detection or exclusion of organic disease is an important function of the general hospital in respect of such cases.

Among the common identifiable conditions which may produce mental disorder are malnutrition, especially vitamin B complex deficiency; alcoholic intoxication; post-traumatic states and subdural haematoma; acute infections such as typhoid and meningitis; uraemia; and cerebral vascular disease. Many other less common organic disorders and intoxications have been known to produce psychotic symptoms.

Psychoneurosis

All types of neurosis are considerably less common among the Bantu than among people of European or Indian origin. When they do occur they often illustrate how the degree of civilization and development determines the prevalent types of neurosis. Anxiety neurosis is only seen among the more sophisticated classes such as nurses and school-teachers. Obsessive-compulsive neurosis has never been observed in a Bantu patient at Edendale.

In contrast, true hysteria is relatively common, especially among young girls. These usually have somatic symptoms such as paralysis of limbs; tremors and involuntary movements; various types of convulsion; and aphonia or blindness. The bizarre nature of the symptoms, together with the dramatic suddenness of recovery, leaves no doubt that their nature is truly hysterical.

Widespread belief in witchcraft leads to certain specific types of neurotic disorder which are recognized among the Bantu and regarded as peculiar to the race. *Ufufunyana* is a variety of neurotic behaviour resulting from bewitchment, which leads the victim to wander aimlessly about the veld, to mutter incoherently to himself, and to imitate wild animals in noise and action. *Uka-hayiza* is a form of hysteria affecting young girls which causes them to cry out continually, *hayi-hayi-hayi*. This affection is said to be the result of an unwanted suitor having used love potions on the unfortunate victim, or in other ways pressing his unsolicited attentions on her. These specific varieties of neurosis are well recognized by the Zulu people. It is equally well recognized that their cure is not within the competence of 'white medicine', but demands the services of *isangoma* (the diviner) and *nyanga* (the witch doctor). Even in the case of other psychiatric disorders it is not uncommon for relatives to declare that it is a 'Bantu disease' which will not respond to hospital treatment, and requires the services of a witch doctor. In many cases this is true, but, unfortunately, some cases of remediable organic disease are similarly diagnosed, with dire results.

Psychosis

Of the psychoses the most common varieties are schizophrenia and the organic dementias. Depressive states are rare, and suicide is very uncommon. A year may pass without one suicidal attempt in a Bantu being treated. When suicide does occur it is usually in one who is above the average in education and sophistication. Among Indians, on the other hand, suicidal attempts are common.

Cases of psychosis requiring certification are admitted to one of the four large mental hospitals in Natal. Of these two are situated in Pietermaritzburg, one in Howick, and one in Newcastle, Northern Natal. All modern forms of psychiatric treatment are available for such cases.

Cerebellar Disease

While cerebellar disease is not infrequent, the rarity of such conditions as multiple sclerosis, primary tumours, and the heredofamilial ataxias, leads one to interpret signs of cerebellar disorder differently in this community. Inflammatory conditions such as abscess and tuberculoma are the most common identifiable causes of cerebellar disorder. Occlusive vascular disease is sometimes responsible for the signs of posterior inferior cerebellar artery occlusion. This may occur in association with atherosclerosis and hypertension, but the syndrome has been observed in association with strongly positive blood and CSF Wassermann reactions. In these cases the vascular occlusion must be presumed to result from meningovascular syphilis.

Cases of cerebellar degeneration also occur. Some are associated with carcinoma or alcoholism, but in a few cases it has occurred sporadically without any discoverable cause, and in the absence of any family history of similar disease. The precise nature of such cerebellar degeneration is not clear. These appear to be sporadic cases of primary cerebellar degeneration.

UNUSUALLY RARE CONDITIONS

The observation that a disease is rare is sometimes met with scepticism, especially where the community is such that there is little hope of providing statistical proof. The observation is countered, for example, with the argument that the disease occurs but is not diagnosed, or that the patients fail to attend hospital with that disease. Certain of these arguments may be valid but long experience does, it is felt, permit one to make certain observations in this respect. Rarity of a condition in a certain population may, from the aspect of epidemiological research, be as important as an unduly high incidence. Even in the absence of statistical proof such observations cannot afford to be ignored.

Multiple Sclerosis

The epidemiology of multiple sclerosis (MS) and its relative rarity in tropical and subtropical regions is well documented. Of all the differences between European and South African neurology this is the most striking. The epidemiological details are discussed elsewhere [CHAPTER 23, p. 277]. While well-documented cases have been reported among indigenous white South Africans (Thomson and Ames, 1965; Wright *et al.*, 1965), the majority of cases of MS seen in South Africa are imported, or occur in people who have lived in Europe. A proved Bantu case has never been reported in South Africa. A few reports of cases have appeared but either these were not proved, or they were shown subsequently to have other conditions (Kaufmann and Lipschitz, 1962). A firm diagnosis of MS has not been made in a single case at Edendale hospital in 11 years. Patients suspected of having MS have subsequently been shown to have other diseases. Other forms of demyelinating disease are also very rare, although Devic's disease has been diagnosed occasionally.

Primary Cerebral Tumours

The relative rarity of primary cerebral tumours has been mentioned previously. Meningiomas appear to be slightly more common than gliomas; no more than 2 or 3 cases of glioma are admitted to Edendale Hospital in a year. Since this is a busy general hospital of some 1400 beds, serving a population of at least half a million in a specialized capacity, it does seem that this incidence is considerably lower than would be expected in a European hospital of similar dimensions. When gliomas do occur they are almost invariably infratentorial tumours in young people. Supratentorial tumours in older people are exceptionally uncommon.

Disc Syndromes and Spondylosis

Another unexpected finding in this community is the relative rarity of neurological syndromes due to spondylosis and disc protrusion. While radiological evidence of spinal osteoarthritis is common, associated neurological lesions have a low incidence. The classical syndromes of cervical spondylosis and lumbar nerve root compression are uncommon, but the reason for the relative immunity of the Bantu to such lesions is not obvious. All the supposed predisposing causes such as heavy manual labour and spinal trauma are operating to a high degree. It is possible that lifelong manual work and physical exertion condition the individual to stresses which provoke damage in those less accustomed to such stress. Hutton (1956) and Trowell (1960) have commented similarly on the low incidence of these conditions among Africans.

Nerve Entrapment Syndromes

The carpal tunnel syndrome and allied disorders are unexpectedly rare. Years may pass without one of these conditions being diagnosed in a Bantu patient. Rheumatoid arthritis, myxoedema, and other auto-immune diseases are rare in this population (Zoutendyk, 1970), but this alone would not account for the virtual absence of the carpal tunnel syndrome in the Bantu.

Migraine

Migraine is also exceptionally uncommon. The few cases which are seen are invariably among the more privileged and sophisticated members of the population, such as students, teachers, and nurses. In several years the diagnosis of migraine has not been recorded in a tribal Bantu at this hospital.

Trigeminal Neuralgia

While other organic causes of facial pain, such as antral carcinoma, sinusitis, dental abscess, and herpes zoster are common, true trigeminal neuralgia has not been diagnosed in a Bantu patient at Edendale hospital in over 11 years. Unlike most of the conditions which are unduly rare in the Bantu, the rarity of trigeminal neuralgia seems to extend to the European population of South Africa, though perhaps to a lesser extent. This geographical, as opposed to racial, distribution might suggest that trigeminal neuralgia is aetiologically related to multiple sclerosis, which has a similar epidemiological behaviour.

Ménière's Syndrome

Organic causes of deafness and vertigo are not unusual, but a typical case of Ménière's syndrome has not been observed in a Bantu patient at Edendale hospital in 11 years.

Parkinson's Disease

Extrapyramidal syndromes, such as Sydenham's chorea, congenital athetosis, parkinsonism and hemiballismus due to vascular lesions, occur with normal frequency. True idiopathic Parkinson's disease or paralysis agitans is, however, rare. When it does occur the accent is more on the akinesia and rigidity than on tremor, which is usually minimal. It is tempting to speculate that this rarity in pigmented races may be linked with the known, but hitherto unexplained, disturbance of metabolism of melanin and its precursors which may be involved in the pathogenesis of paralysis agitans.

Petit Mal

Epilepsy of the grand mal type is common, occurring either idiopathically or in response to organic lesions or trauma. Petit mal, on the other hand, is rarely diagnosed in the Bantu. Unlike certain other conditions mentioned above it is possible that petit mal attacks are considered too trivial to warrant attendance at hospital, although it is surprising that it is not observed by school-teachers (who have been questioned in this respect) and by the more sophisticated and educated parents. My impression is that it is a genuinely rare disease.

Other neurological conditions which appear to be extremely rare among this Bantu population are Huntington's chorea and Wilson's disease. Cases of these two diseases have not been seen at this hospital in 11 years. Heredofamilial ataxias of the Friedreich type have been seen very occasionally. These and other peculiarities of disease incidence in this population are summarized in TABLE 22.2.

While it is not possible to provide statistical proof of their low incidence the rarity of the conditions mentioned above is so striking that it deserves more attention. Hidden in this field of epidemiology may lie the germs of fruitful research.

Table 22.2
Relative Incidence of Neurological Disorders

<table>
<tr><th colspan="3">Incidence Similar to that in Europe</th></tr>
<tr><td colspan="3">Cerebral vascular disease
Epilepsy
Intracranial aneurysm
Angiomatous malformation
Infective polyneuritis
Motor neurone disease
Muscular dystrophy
Encephalitis
Syringomyelia
Transverse myelitis
Subacute combined degeneration
Primary cerebellar degeneration</td></tr>
<tr><th colspan="3">Deviations from European incidence</th></tr>
<tr><th>Unduly Common</th><th>Unduly Rare</th><th>Not Encountered</th></tr>
<tr><td>Post-traumatic epilepsy
Meningovascular syphilis
Peripheral neuropathy
Brain abscess
Tetanus
Sydenham's chorea
Tuberculous meningitis
Subdural haematoma
Cerebral tuberculoma
Leprosy
Organic psychoses
Hysteria</td><td>Tabes dorsalis
Primary cerebral tumours
Cervical spondylosis
Lumbar disc syndromes
Carpal tunnel syndrome
Petit mal
Migraine
Paralysis agitans</td><td>Multiple sclerosis
Trigeminal neuralgia
Ménière's syndrome
Huntington's chorea
Wilson's disease</td></tr>
<tr><th colspan="3">Syndromes which are largely peculiar to the Bantu</th></tr>
<tr><td colspan="3">Embolic complications of cardiomyopathy
Nutritional encephalopathies
Nutritional neuropathies: 'burning foot syndrome'
Unexplained spastic myelopathy
Bilharzial myelopathy
Intrathecal tuberculous granuloma
Siderosis-scurvy-osteoporosis syndrome with nerve involvement
Porphyria cutanea tarda with neuropathy</td></tr>
</table>

References

ARSENI, C., and SAMITCA, D. C. (1960) Intraspinal tuberculous granuloma, *Brain*, 83, 285.

ASMAL, A. C., VINIK, A. I., and JOUBERT, S. M. (1970) A neurological disturbance in porphyria cutanea tarda, *S. Afr. med. J.*, 44, 781.

BHAGWANDEEN, S. B. (1968) *The Clinico-pathological Manifestations of Schistosomiasis in the African and the Indian in Durban*, Pietermaritzburg.

BIRD, A. V., HEINZ, H. J., and KLINTWORTH, G. (1962) Convulsive disorders in Bantu mine-workers, *Epilepsia*, 3, 175.

BRYANT, A. T. (1970) *Zulu Medicine and Medicine-men*, Cape Town. (Reprinted from *Annals of the Natal Museum, Pietermaritzburg*, Vol. II, Part I, pp. 1–103.)

COSNETT, J. E. (1962) Heart disease in the Zulu: especially cardiomyopathy and cardiac infarction, *Brit. Heart J.*, 24, 76.

COSNETT, J. E. (1964) Neurological disorders in the Zulu, *Neurology (Minneap.)*, 14, 443.

COSNETT, J. E. (1965 *a*) Acute cerebral syphilis in the African, *Centr. Afr. J. Med.*, 11, 103.

COSNETT, J. E. (1965 *b*) Unexplained spastic myelopathy, *S. Afr. med. J.*, 39, 592.

COSNETT, J. E. (1969) Strokes in young people: experience in a Bantu hospital, *S. Afr. med. J.*, 43, 501.

COSNETT, J. E., and PUDIFIN, D. J. (1964) Embolic complications of cardiomyopathy, *Brit. Heart J.*, 26, 544.

FERNANDES, D. B. (1970) Medicine and the Zulu, *Practitioner*, 205, 73.

HILL, J. (1970) Personal communication.

HURST, L. A., REEF, H. E., and SACHS, S. B. (1961) Neuropsychiatric disorders in the Bantu, 1. Convulsive disorders: a pilot study with special reference to genetic factors, *S. Afr. med. J.*, 35, 750.

HUTTON, P. W. (1956) Neurological disorders in Uganda, *E. Afr. med. J.*, 33, 209.

KALLICHURUM, S. (1969) Major aetiological types of heart failure in the Bantu in Durban, *S. Afr. med. J.*, 43, 250.

KAUFMANN, J. C. E., and LIPSCHITZ, R. (1962) Trigeminal neurofibroma: review and follow-up report of a case in a Bantu mimicking disseminated sclerosis, *S. Afr. med. J.*, 36, 872.

LOUIS, S., and KEET, P. C. (1964) A survey of supratentorial gliomas and meningiomas, *S. Afr. med. J.*, 38, 949.

MONTGOMERY, R. D., CRUICKSHANK, E. K., ROBERTSON, W. B., and MCMENEMEY, W. H. (1964) Clinical and pathological observations on Jamaican neuropathy: a report on 206 cases, *Brain*, 87, 425.

ROSE-INNES, A. P. (1969) Tuberculous paraplegia without radiological bone changes, *S. Afr. med. J.*, 43, 1327.

SEFTEL, H. C., MALKIN, C., SCHMAMAN, A., ABRAHAMS, C., LYNCH, S. R., CHARLTON, R. W., and BOTHWELL, T. H. (1966) Osteoporosis, scurvy, and siderosis in Johannesburg Bantu, *Brit. med. J.*, 1, 642.

SPILLANE, J. D. (1947) *Nutritional Disorders of the Nervous System*, Edinburgh.

THOMSON, J. G., and AMES, F. R. (1965) Disseminated sclerosis in a white South African, *S. Afr. med. J.*, 39, 389.

TROWELL, H. C. (1960) *Non-infective Disease in Africa*, London.

WAINWRIGHT, J. (1961) Atheroma in the African (Bantu) in Natal, *Lancet*, i, 366.

WAINWRIGHT, J. (1968) Personal communication.

WELSH, N. H., and PRETORIUS, M. (1970) The ocular signs in leprosy: results of a survey in a leper institute, *S. Afr. med. J.*, 44, (Suppl.), 9.

WRIGHT, K. B., VIVIERS, G. J., PROCTOR, N. S. F., KAUFMANN, J. C. E., and BRUNING, E. G. H. (1965) Multiple sclerosis in a South African born white man and woman, *S. Afr. med. J.*, 39, 386.

ZOUTENDYK, A. (1970) Auto-antibodies in South African whites, coloured, and Bantu, *S. Afr. med. J.*, 44, 469.

23 Porphyria Variegata and Multiple Sclerosis in South Africa

G. DEAN

Porphyria and multiple sclerosis differ greatly in their prevalence among white South Africans when compared with the United Kingdom and Europe. A Mendelian dominant porphyria, porphyria variegata, is extremely common among the white South African-born, although it is very uncommon in Europe, while on the other hand multiple sclerosis, which is the commonest disease of the nervous system to affect men and women in the prime of life in Northern Europe, is uncommon among the white South African-born, particularly the Afrikaner, and is extremely rare among the Coloured and Asian and has not yet been seen in South Africa's 16 million Bantu. These two diseases are outstanding examples of the way in which genetic and environmental circumstances have determined the prevalence of a neurological disorder in a subtropical country.

PORPHYRIA VARIEGATA

In 1937 Waldenström described a form of Mendelian dominant porphyria in Sweden which he called intermittent acute porphyria (Waldenström, 1937). In Sweden, acute attacks of porphyria usually occurred after the patients had taken certain drugs, generally barbiturates or sulphonamides. The skin did not abrade unduly easily and sores and blisters did not occur. In the Swedish type of porphyria Ehrlich's aldehyde reagent, when added to the urine, caused a purple coloration and this colour did not pass down in chloroform—the Watson–Schwartz test (Watson and Schwartz, 1941). There is usually increased porphyrin in the urine, particularly if it is left to stand for some hours, but little or no increase in the stool porphyrin.

Starting practice in South Africa in 1947, I was called to see a series of patients, usually young women, who had become emotionally disturbed after a thiopentone anaesthetic or after taking barbiturates. They complained of abdominal and muscle pain, had attacks of vomiting and a rapid pulse, and showed marked weakness due to peripheral neuritis. Their urine was dark in colour and gave the brilliant pink fluorescence of porphyrin when examined in ultraviolet light with a Wood's filter.

The family histories of these patients were traced and, wherever possible, all members of the family were contacted and asked to provide specimens of urine and stool for examination. It was found that many members of the family, particularly on the male side, had a sensitive skin on the back of the hands that abraded easily when it was knocked and a number of scars of previous sores could often be seen [PLATE 25*a*]. This skin was frequently described as the 'van Rooyen skin'. The first family studied was one by the name of van Rooyen and 574 descendants of the great-grandfather of the patient, who had acute porphyria and who was born in 1814, were traced; their urine and later their faeces were examined for increased porphyrin excretion. Seventy-four of this group were found to have porphyria and at least 16 had died from acute porphyria (Dean and Barnes, 1955). On average, half the children of a patient with South African porphyria inherited the disorder. There was a high concentration of porphyrin in the liver but not in the bone marrow of those who had inherited prophyria, and there was nearly always a high excretion of porphyrin in the stool. The stool, when dissolved in a solvent consisting of equal parts of amyl alcohol, glacial acetic acid and ether, would fluoresce in ultraviolet light. The stool porphyrin consisted of a mixture of more or less equal parts of copro- and protoporphyrin [FIG. 23.1].

Over a period of 10 years, 32 similar family groups were studied and traced back to the beginning of the eighteenth century. About half of these were descendants of 5 of the 11 children of Cornelius van Rooyen who came from Gorkum in 1711 and married Jacomijntje the daughter of Gerrit in 1720. Jacomijntje was born in 1692. Other families were traced back to Jacomijntje's sister, Aletta Gerritsz, who was born in 1700 and had married Pieter Willem Nel in 1725. Still other family groups were traced back to both the first and second marriage of another sister, Johanna Margrieta Gerritsz, and other family groups traced back to the first and third marriage of a brother, Jacobus Gerritsz. Four of the eight children of Gerrit, the son of Jan, had porphyria; Gerrit came from Deventer and married Ariaantje, the daughter of Jacob, who was one of the eight orphans sent by the 'Lords Seventeen' from Rotterdam on the ship *China* to be wives for the first free burghers. Gerrit Jansz and Ariaantje married in 1688 and one of them must have carried the gene for porphyria. The porphyrics alive today are of the twelfth to sixteenth generations of this family (Dean, 1971) [FIG. 23.2].

Porphyria of the South African type has been called porphyria variegata to distinguish it from intermittent

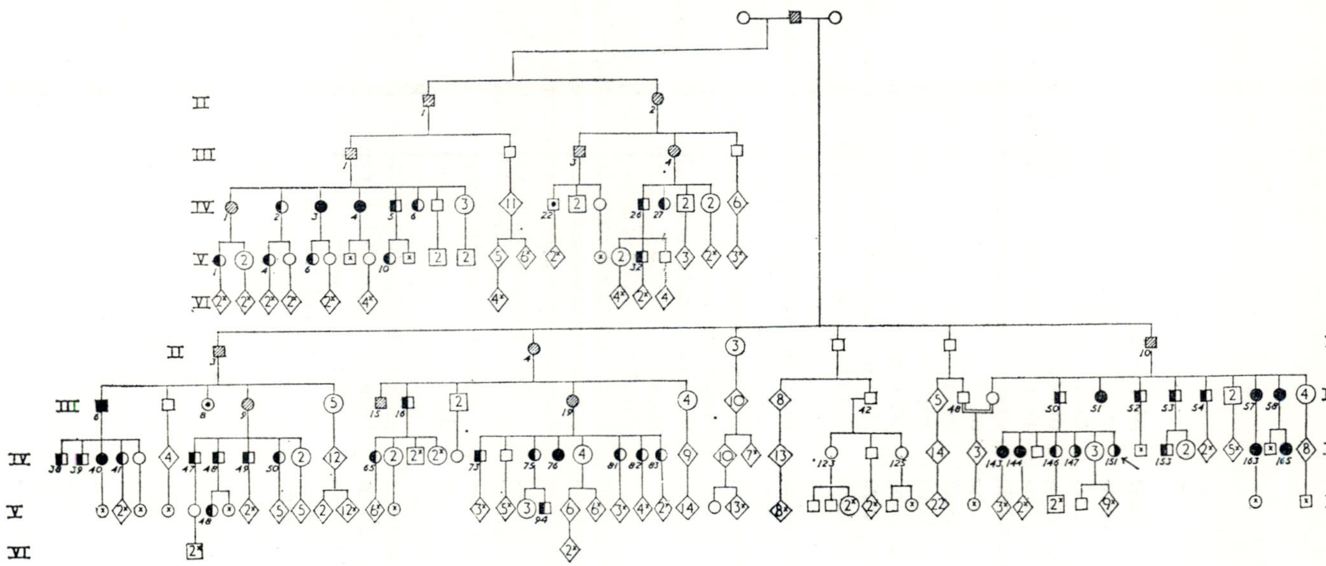

Males and females with a sensitive skin who died before the survey. Histories obtained from relations, occasionally confirmed by doctors. Urine not examined.

Urine positive for porphyrin, no clinical manifestations. Latent cases.

Skin fragile or lesions present. No acute symptoms.

Acute episode (s), no skin fragility or lesions.

Affected skin and acute episode (s).

x Within a symbol indicates members under 18 years of age in 1955.

◇ With a number inserted indicates siblings of both sexes.

All the porphyrics alive now have had the diagnosis of porphyria confirmed by examination of their faeces.

Fourteen further porphyrics have been found in the younger generations since 1955.

FIG. 23.1. Genealogical tree of G. R. van Rooyen, born 1814.

acute porphyria because it can present in a variety of forms—in acute attacks, with skin lesions, or with neither acute attacks nor skin lesions but with only raised stool porphyrin (Dean and Barnes, 1959).

Today there are over 9000 white South Africans who have inherited porphyria variegata, and prevalence studies show that the incidence of porphyria variegata is highest in the Eastern Cape Province, as the early porphyrics were among the Boers who trekked eastwards from Cape Town with their cattle and sheep (Dean, 1960); in Port Elizabeth the incidence of porphyria variegata is also common among the coloured people of South Africa. Among these settlers it has been traced back to Gerrit, the son of Jan, or his wife Ariaantje.

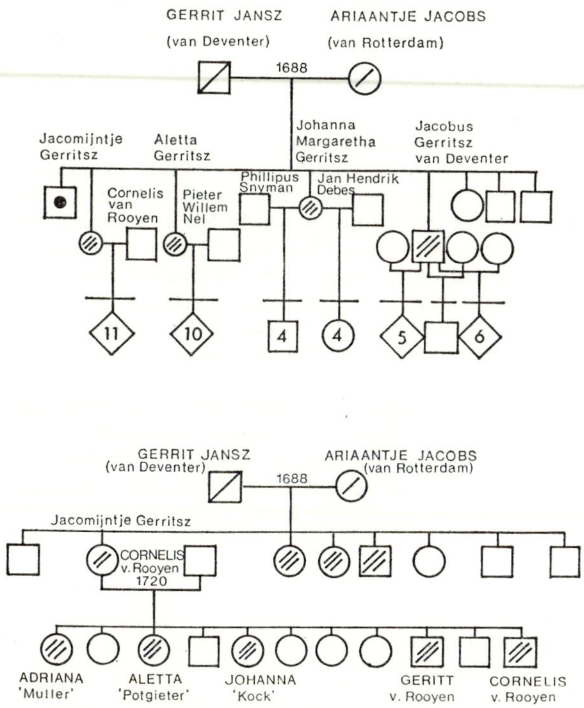

FIG. 23.2. Porphyria variegata traces back to four of eight children of Gerrit Jansz and Ariaantje Jacobs. □ = male. ○ = female. ▨ ⊘ = porphyric line of descent.

The high prevalence of porphyria variegata among the white South African population is an outstanding example of the founder effect: the disease is so common because a small number of early settlers increased very rapidly and became a people. They married young and had large families, there was no malaria at the Cape and armed with the horse and the gun they were more than a match for the indigenous population, the Hottentots and Bushmen. It was only in 1790, when they had advanced 600 miles eastwards from Cape Town, that the Boers met another race of invaders, the Bantu, who were entering the country which is now South Africa from the north.

It is perhaps easiest to understand how the small group of early settlers increased by studying family names. In South Africa 500 000 of the 4 million white population hold 20 family names and derive these names from 20 original free burghers. The commonest names are Botha (49 000) and van der Merwe (35 000).

Studying the genealogies of the porphyric families, it is quite clear that they had as large families, on average, as the other early settlers and as good an expectation of life until the introduction of barbiturates and sulphonamides in the twentieth century. There is no higher prevalence of porphyria variegata in the mental hospital populations that have been studied in the Eastern Cape than there is in the general population, and the mental disturbances that occur with acute porphyria disappear when the acute attack subsides.

Acute Porphyria Variegata

Acute porphyria, with emotional disturbance, abdominal and muscular pain, a rapid pulse, constipation, often vomiting, and finally generalized peripheral neuritis and paralysis, may be inadvertently precipitated by certain drugs, most commonly by barbiturates and sulphonamides, in three types of Mendelian dominant porphyria: intermittent acute porphyria, porphyria variegata, and coproporphyria. It has already been explained why porphyria variegata is so common among white South Africans. Intermittent acute porphyria and coproporphyria have also been seen in South Africa but these two forms of the disease are rare, although in Britain, Europe, and North America the former type is considerably more often the cause of acute porphyria than porphyria variegata. Besides the barbiturates and sulphonamides, certain less commonly used drugs can also occasionally precipitate acute attacks, e.g. chloroquine diphosphate, griseofulvin and the sulphones. Women who have inherited porphyria variegata sometimes suffer from minor abdominal pain, especially in the premenstrual period and during pregnancy when they are especially liable to be given a barbiturate sedative and, if their pains increase, to have an exploratory laparotomy, perhaps under a thiopentone anaesthetic. The oral oestrogen-progesterone contraceptives may precipitate an increase in porphyrin production in porphyria variegata, which will result in a great increase in skin blistering due to the high level of circulating porphyrin (Dean, 1965).

Treatment of Acute Porphyria Variegata

Prevention of attacks is the most important aspect of treatment. Once a patient has been diagnosed as having inherited the disease, all the relatives on the affected side of the family should be traced and their stools and urine tested for porphyrin. In this way many who have inherited the gene can be warned to avoid the drugs that will precipitate an acute attack. The Watson–Schwartz test on the urine is only positive during the acute attack and is of no value for routine testing.

In an attack of acute porphyria the patient's life is in great danger and he should therefore be nursed in a special care unit in hospital, or if this is not available, in a single-bedded room, because the emotional disturbance makes it difficult to control such a patient without a very high level of nursing. During the acute attack there is often a marked fall in the blood electrolytes and calcium. Salt is lost in the urine, perhaps due to excessive antidiuretic hormone, although this has not yet been proved. Additional salt must be given, intravenously if necessary, because it may be essential to keep the stomach empty for a while by Wangensteen's method because of vomiting. Calcium gluconate (1 G 12-hourly intramuscularly) lessens the risk of convulsions, and chlorpromazine (50 mg 8-hourly) is a good tranquillizer in acute porphyria. Digitalis is not very effective in slowing the pulse and the chelating agents have not proved to be of help in this type of porphyria.

A tracheostomy should be performed without delay and a mechanical respirator such as the Bird's or Engström machine used if respiration is embarrassed, because the peripheral neuritis may cause respiratory involvement quite rapidly. Patients have been treated on a respirator for 3 months and eventually made a good recovery. The assistance of a respiratory unit can be of the greatest help in treating patients with acute porphyria and they should be brought into consultation before respiratory paralysis occurs. Every effort to keep the patient alive is worthwhile, because if the vital functions can be maintained the acute attack will subside and eventual recovery is usually excellent, although it may take some months (Dean, 1967 *a*).

The skin sensitivity which usually affects the exposed skin, particularly on the hands, and more often affects men than women, is treated by protecting the exposed skin from sunlight as much as possible, for instance by using gloves and a hat out of doors. Excessive and long-continued use of alcohol can increase porphyrin production and aggravate the tendency to blistering of the exposed skin.

Those who have inherited porphyria variegata, intermittent acute porphyria, or coproporphyria, should carry a letter stating this fact, mentioning the extreme danger of barbiturates and sulphonamides. They should be strongly advised to show this letter to any doctor they consult.

In conclusion, porphyria variegata in South Africa is, as already mentioned, an outstanding example of founder effect—a gene that is uncommon in Europe was brought by chance to South Africa by one of the early settlers who, living in ideal conditions, have many thousands of living descendants after 12 to 16 generations. The gene for porphyria variegata until the introduction of modern drugs, quite clearly did little harm, except perhaps in the tendency of some of those who inherited it to have skin which abraded unduly easily when exposed. Acute porphyria variegata results from the interaction of inheritance and environment, the seed and the soil, and the study of this disease in South Africa has required the study of the formation of a people and goes back to the Lords Seventeen, the

Table 23.1

Prevalence of Probable Multiple Sclerosis in South Africans (1960)

White South Africans	*Population at Risk per 1000*			*Probable MS*			*Rate 100 000*	*Age corrected to population of England and Wales*
	Male	*Female*	*Total*	*Male*	*Female*	*Total*		
South African-born	1374	1389	2763	46	112	158	5·7	6·9
Afrikaans-speaking	927	910	1837	20	37	57	3·1	3·6
English-speaking	446	479	925	26	75	101	10·9	12·7
Unspecified language group	0·4	0·4	0·8					
Immigrants	159	154	313	37	86	123	39·0	
Born United Kingdom	63	66	128	26	39	65	50·8	40·3
Born Central and Northern Europe	53	49	102	7	42	49	48·0	
Born South Europe	15	10	26	1	3	4	15·4	
Born elsewhere	27	29	57	3	2	5	8·8	
Birthplace not known	0·9	0·9	1·9					
Total:	*1534*	*1544*	*3078*	*83*	*198*	*281*	*9·1*	11·0
Coloured	751	758	1509	1	2	3		
Asian (Indian and Chinese)	242	235	477	3	3	6		
Bantu	5512	5416	10928	—	—	—		
Total:	*8039*	*7953*	*15992*	*87*	*203*	*290*		

directors of the East India Company, who first decided to settle free burghers at the Cape to provide vegetables and meat for their ships trading with the East, and may be traced to the eight girls whom they sent out in the ship *China* in 1688 as wives for these early founders of a nation.

MULTIPLE SCLEROSIS

On settling in South Africa in 1947, I learned that multiple sclerosis (MS) was thought to be uncommon among white South Africans. In that year, in the four teaching hospitals, there were only 27 white patients in whom the diagnosis could be accepted as probable out of all the patients admitted during the previous 10 years. Fourteen of the 27 were immigrants from the United Kingdom or Europe, although immigrants formed less than 10 per cent of the white population at risk. Among the South African-born white population the disease was clearly very uncommon (Dean, 1949).

A detailed study of the annual incidence, prevalance and mortality of MS was made during the years 1956 to 1969. Every practical means was used to discover and investigate patients who might possibly have the disease.

At the 1960 census, South Africa had a white population of just over three million, of whom 313 000 were immigrants. There were 2 763 000 South African-born, two-thirds of whom (1 837 000) were Afrikaans-speaking, and the remainder (925 000) English-speaking [TABLE 23.1]. The Afrikaners have, on the whole, much closer contact with non-whites, who have a low standard of hygiene, than the English-speaking South African-born.

The prevalence of MS in 1960 was high among immigrants from Europe. The prevalence of probable MS in the English-speaking white South African-born was between one-third and one-quarter, and in the Afrikaans-speaking white South African-born only one-eleventh, of the prevalence in the immigrants from the United Kingdom and North and Central Europe. Immigrants from Northern Europe had a prevalence of MS three times greater than that of immigrants from the Mediterranean countries, while the white immigrants from other African states had a low risk (Dean, 1967 *c*).

Among the immigrants from the United Kingdom the female to male ratio of 1·6:1 for the population at risk is much the same as that found in other studies. The average estimated by Acheson is 1·4:1 (McAlpine, Lumsden, and Acheson, 1965). Among 69 000 male immigrants from continental Europe there were only nine MS patients and among 59 000 female immigrants there were 43 with MS. The Registrar General of England and Wales (1951), Miller, Ridley, and Schapira (1960), and Beebe *et al.* (1967) have reported that MS is more frequent in the higher social classes, and male immigrants from continental Europe are very often unskilled single men, unlike most of the male immigrants from the United Kingdom. Unskilled men would not be likely to emigrate if they already had symptoms of MS.

No difference in MS prevalence between urban and

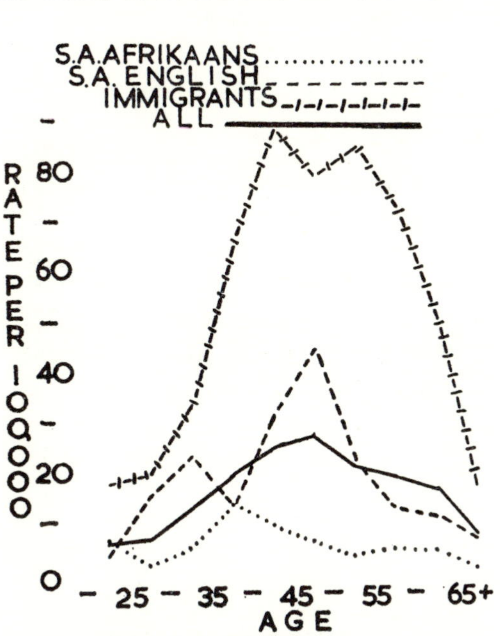

FIG. 23.3. Multiple sclerosis in white South Africans, prevalence rates 1960.

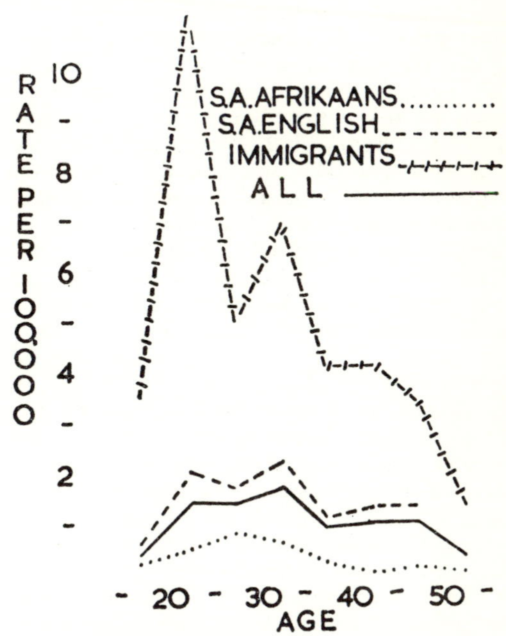

FIG. 23.4. Multiple sclerosis in white South Africans, average annual incidence, 1945–54.

Table 23.2

Average Annual Incidence of Probable Multiple Sclerosis (1945–54) per 100 000, Actual and Age Corrected for the Distribution of England and Wales

White South Africans	*Actual*	*Age corrected*
Immigrants from United Kingdom and Europe	1·9	2·1
White immigrants from elsewhere	0·5	0·7
English-speaking South African-born	0·5	0·5
Afrikaans-speaking South African-born	0·2	0·2
All white South Africans	0·4	0·4

rural areas was found in South Africa, nor was any significant difference found for the various groups of white South Africans among the provinces, that is between the temperate Cape, the high-veld Transvaal, and subtropical Natal. The high prevalence and average annual incidence [TABLES 23.1 and 23.2, and FIGS. 23.3 and 23.4] of MS among immigrants from the United Kingdom and Northern Europe is still very apparent if only those patients are considered who had their first symptom after leaving Europe.

An environmental factor would, therefore, appear to be mainly responsible for MS and this environmental influence may be associated to some extent with latitude. Barlow believes that geomagnetic latitude has a closer correlation with the frequency of MS than has geographic latitude (Barlow, 1960). Nevertheless, this does not accord well with the hypothesis that it is due to direct action of the climate on the body in the same sense that frost-bite or cancer of the skin is directly related to climate. For instance, the coldness of winter is closely related to the distance from the ocean but this is not correlated with the prevalence of MS. Swank has suggested that MS is related to consumption of large quantities of animal fat deficient in unsaturated fatty acids (Swank, 1961). That this is unlikely to be true can be shown in South Africa, where there is a very low prevalance of MS among the white South African-born, who eat a diet rich in animal fat and have a very high death rate from coronary thrombosis.

Age at Immigration

With evidence of differential risk in migrants from a high-frequency MS region to a low-frequency region, it was considered necessary to seek an answer to the question of whether age at immigration was a factor.

There was a marked scarcity of immigrants with MS who had immigrated below the age of 15 or 16, and in the 15–19 age-group there were six to seven times as many immigrants represented as for any younger 5-year period. Those under the age of 20 came, of course, before MS was considered. There are more cases aged 25–29 and 30–34 at immigration than at any other age. Numbers, of course, decline in the older groups.

Table 23.3

Prevalence of Multiple Sclerosis per 100 000 Immigrants from the United Kingdom and from All of North and Central Europe

Age at Immigration	*United Kingdom*	*All North and Central Europe*
0–14	12·8	12·9
15–19	66·1	81·1
20–29	45·7	44·9
30–39	58·2	52·4
40–49	57·7	62·4
50+	70·5	80·8

The overall corrected prevalence for immigrants from the United Kingdom was 48 per 100 000 of the general population while for all Northern Europeans it was 49 per 100 000 [TABLE 23.3]. The prevalence for immigrants under the age of 15 was 13 per 100 000 but prevalence for those aged 15–19 at immigration was 81. For immigrants from the United Kingdom only it was 66 per 100 000. Such a difference in risk of MS above and below the age of 15 is in the order of 5 to 1. A prevalence of 13 per 100 000 is quite similar to that previously recorded for the native-born English-speaking white South Africans—11 per 100 000. We have therefore strong evidence that the age of about 15 is critical.

If we take only the immigrants whose onset of MS was after immigration to South Africa the same pattern persists.

Table 23.4

Actual and 'Expected' Number of Immigrants with MS Aged 35 and Over by Age at Immigration. The 'Expected' Number Calculated by Age (35–49 and 50+) and by Sex

All Immigrants		
Age at Immigration	*Number of MS cases (MRA study)*	*Actual number of MS cases*
0–15	25·8	6
16–20	9·8	12
21–30	30·7	32
31–40	24·7	34
41+	17·0	24
Total:	*108·0*	*108*

The number of MS patients (6) who had immigrated before the age of 16 is less than a quarter of the 'expected' number (25·8). $P < 0{\cdot}001$.

Table 23.5

English-Speaking South African-Born with Probable MS who had Visited Europe (1969). *Actual and 'Expected' Number*

Age	*Before Onset*	*After Onset*	*Total MS*	*'Expected' Number MRA Survey 1969*
Male				
25–34			4	1·1 (204)[1]
35–49	4	1	11	4·2 (277)
50+	5	1	14	6·7 (302)
Total:	*9*	*2* [1][2]	*29*	*12·0 (781)*
Female				
25–34	3	2	13	2·7 (235)
35–49	6	5	35	7·6 (323)
50+	17	5	44	13·7 (353)
Total:	*26*	*12* [6][2]	*92*	*24·0 (911)*

[1] Numbers in parentheses are sample size.
[2] Numbers in brackets visited Europe for medical consultation for MS symptoms.

A Study of Immigrant Controls 1968–69

In order to confirm our findings that there was a low risk of MS among young immigrants to South Africa from Europe, we compared the MS patients with randomly chosen controls (1968–69). The 'expected' number of MS cases (25·8) who immigrated below the age of 16 was more than four times the actual number who immigrated before this age (6) and the difference is statistically highly significant [TABLE 23·4]. It is still significant if only those MS patients are considered who developed their first symptoms after arrival in South Africa.

Visiting Europe

Only two Afrikaans-speaking MS patients had visited Europe. Among male English-speaking white South African-born, 11 out of 29 had visited Europe and the 'expected' number, calculated from the MRA study, was 12 [TABLE 23.5]. One of the 11 had visited Europe in order to have the diagnosis of MS confirmed. Among women, 38 out of 92 had visited Europe and the expected number was 26, but six of these 38 had visited Europe specifically for treatment of the symptoms of MS or to have the diagnosis confirmed, and they state that this was the reason why they visited Europe. There was therefore no significant difference in the risk of developing MS between the white South African-born who stayed in South Africa and those who had visited Europe (Dean, 1970; Kurtzke, Dean, and Botha, 1970; Dean and Kurtzke, 1971).

In recent years most workers who have contemplated MS from its epidemiological features have concluded that it is an acquired exogenous disorder. Alter and his group have also shown that MS is much commoner among Jewish immigrants from Northern Europe than among the Israeli-born, and is less common in European immigrants to Israel who immigrated under the age of 15 than in those who immigrated after this age (Alter, Leibowitz, and Speer, 1966).

The theory that best fits the facts, in the writer's opinion, is that MS is normally an infection of infancy or childhood, perhaps a viral gastrointestinal disorder. When the level of hygiene is low this early infection would be the rule. If, however, childhood infection does not occur there will be susceptibility to a later infection which may, in certain people, result in a precarious balance between the infectious agent and immunity which produces the syndrome we call multiple sclerosis. Poskanzer has made the same analogy for MS as for paralytic versus non-paralytic poliomyelitis (Poskanzer, Schapira, and Miller, 1963). It is interesting that in South Africa paralytic poliomyelitis in adults was formerly twice as common among immigrants from Northern Europe as in the white South African-born, and much more common among the white South African-born than among the non-white (Dean, 1967 *b*).

Let us consider how MS fits this theory. In MS the prevalence is high among immigrants from Northern Europe to South Africa or Israel, unless they immigrate below the age of 15 or 16. It is only one-quarter as common among the English-speaking white South African-born as among the immigrants, and only one-eleventh as common among the Afrikaans-speaking white South African-born who, as a whole, have close contact in childhood with the non-white population and have, on the whole, a lower standard of hygiene than the English-speaking. MS is extremely rare among the Coloured or half-caste people of the Cape and those of Asian stock, and no MS patient has yet been found among the 16 million Bantu people in South Africa. In Australia, which does not have an indigenous native population looking after the children of the white population, there is no such difference between the immigrant group and the Australian-born (Rischbieth, 1966). There is also good evidence that visiting Europe does not increase the risk of MS among the white South African-born.

Multiple sclerosis, therefore, is undoubtedly due in the main to the environment. A virus infection appears at present to be the most likely aetiological agent, perhaps one of the newly discovered class of slow or latent viruses.

References

ALTER, M., LEIBOWITZ, U., and SPEER, J. (1966) Risk of multiple sclerosis related to age at immigration to Israel, *Arch. Neurol. (Chic.)*, 15, 234.

BARLOW, J. S. (1960) Correlation of geographical distribution of multiple sclerosis with cosmic ray intensities, *Acta psychiat. scand.*, 35, Suppl. 147, 108.

BEEBE, G. W., KURTZKE, J. F., KURLAND, L. T., AUTH, T. L., and NAGLER, B. (1967) Studies on the natural history of multiple slcerosis, *Neurology (Minneap.)*, 17, No. 1.

DEAN, G. (1949) Disseminated sclerosis in South Africa, *Brit. med. J.*, 1, 842.

DEAN, G. (1960) Routine testing for porphyria variegata, *S. Afr. med. J.*, 34, 745–51.

DEAN, G. (1965) Oral contraceptives in porphyria variegata, *S. Afr. med. J.*, 39, 278.

DEAN, G. (1967 *a*) The porphyrias, in *Current Therapy*, ed. Conn, H. F., Philadelphia, p. 346.

DEAN, G. (1967 *b*) Poliomyelitis among white immigrants to South Africa, *S. Afr. med. J.*, 41, 294.

DEAN, G. (1967 *c*) Annual incidence, prevalence and mortality of multiple sclerosis in white South African-born and in white immigrants to South Africa, *Brit. med. J.*, 2, 724.

DEAN, G. (1970) The multiple sclerosis problem, *Scient. Amer.* 223, 40.

DEAN, G. (1971) *The Porphyrias: A Story of Inheritance and Environment*, 2nd ed., London.

DEAN, G., and BARNES, H. D. (1955) The inheritance of porphyria, *Brit. med. J.*, 2, 89.

DEAN, G., and BARNES, H. D. (1959) Porphyria in Sweden and South Africa, *S. Afr. med. J.*, 33, 246.

DEAN, G., and KURTZKE, J. (1971) On the risk of multiple sclerosis according to age at immigration to South Africa, *Brit. med. J.*, 3, 725–9.

KURTZKE, J., DEAN, G., and BOTHA, D. P. J. (1970) A method for estimating the age at immigration of white immigrants to South Africa, with an example of its importance, *S. Afr. med. J.*, 41, 663.

MCALPINE, D., LUMSDEN, C. E., and ACHESON, E. D. (1965) *Multiple Sclerosis. A Reappraisal*, Edinburgh.

MILLER, H., RIDLEY, A., and SCHAPIRA, K. (1960) Multiple sclerosis. A note on social incidence, *Brit. med. J.*, 2, 343.

POSKANZER, D. C., SCHAPIRA, K., and MILLER, H. (1963) Multiple sclerosis and poliomyelitis, *Lancet*, ii, 917.

REGISTRAR GENERAL'S DECENNIAL SUPPLEMENT, ENGLAND AND WALES (1951) *Occupational Mortality*, Part II, Vol. 1, *Commentary*, London, H.M.S.O., p. 33.

RISCHBIETH, R. H. (1966) The prevalence of disseminated sclerosis in South Australia, *Med. J. Aust.*, 1, 774.

SWANK, R. L. (1961) *A Biochemical Basis of Multiple Sclerosis*, Springfield, Ill.

WALDENSTRÖM, J. (1937) Studien über Porphyrie, *Acta med. scand.*, Suppl. 82, 1.

WATSON, C. J., and SCHWARTZ, S. (1941) Simple test for urinary porphobilinogen, *Proc. Soc. exp. Biol. (N.Y.)*, 47, 393.

Part Three

SOUTH-EAST ASIA

See PLATES 25–28

24 Neurological Disorders in Singapore

A. L. GWEE and G. A. RANSOME

INTRODUCTION

The island of Singapore—some 225 sq miles in area—is separated from the southernmost tip of the Malay peninsula by a narrow stretch of water and linked to it by the Johore Causeway. It was acquired by the British East India Company in 1819. The population of the city now approaches two million, the majority being Chinese, then Malays, Indians, Eurasians and Europeans.

The Medical School, now the Faculty of Medicine of the University of Singapore, opened in 1905. For some time it was known as the King Edward VII Medical College. University chairs in the major medical subjects were established in the twenties, but there is still no separate university hospital. Teaching takes place in the government hospitals and the university units in medicine and surgery are operated by a mixed staff of university and government officers. The three main government hospitals are the Thomson Road General Hospital (396 beds), the Tan Tock Seng Hospital (1324 beds), and the Outram Road General Hospital. One hundred and twenty students take the M.B., B.S. degree each year, and recently a new professional degree of Master of Medicine has been introduced. This is based on the London Membership examination with particular reference to local conditions. Apart from chest physicians, there are no true specialists in the full sense, but there are general physicians with a special interest in neurology and cardiology, and there are plans for full specialization in due course.

There is a Department of Neurosurgery, but no special Department of Neurology. There are, however, several physicians with an interest in neurology, and an active neurological group.

THE PATTERN OF NEUROLOGICAL DISEASE

Before the Second World War, syphilis, beriberi, tuberculosis, and meningitis in all its forms, dominated clinical neurology. Even lead poisoning was not uncommon. Most of these diseases have now largely disappeared, and Singapore has now become a tropical island with no tropical disease, but with all the ravages of the neurological disorders of temperate countries. But there are still remarkable differences. Multiple sclerosis and vitamin B_{12} neuropathy are extremely rare. Encephaloceles, intracranial angiomas, and perhaps hydranencephaly are much commoner than in Western countries and there are aspects of cerebrovascular disease which merit attention.

Intracranial Arteriovenous Malformations in Singapore

It is generally acknowledged that by far the commonest cause of subarachnoid haemorrhage in Western countries is intracranial aneurysm. Angiomas are usually found to be responsible for only a very small proportion of cases (from 2 per cent to 10 per cent). Among Asians the proportions are reversed. Although there are no published statistics, Spillane (1969) recently quoted several observations and personal communications suggesting that the incidence of arteriovenous malformations was four to six times greater than aneurysms in patients with subarachnoid haemorrhage in Thailand and Malaysia. We have made similar observations in Singapore.

The present study is based on 50 cases of arteriovenous malformations seen between 1962 and 1969 at hospitals in Singapore. There were 33 males and 17 females. A breakdown of the ethnic groups of these 50 patients reflected only the general proportion of these groups in Singapore [TABLE 24.1]. Clinical manifestations most commonly occurred during the second decade of life, with the next highest incidence occurring in the third and fourth decades [TABLE 24.2]. Two-thirds of the patients were below 30 years of age.

In all cases the diagnosis was made by arteriography. Two were later confirmed at operation and three at autopsy. The indications for arteriography were intracranial haemorrhage in 34, epilepsy in 10, and suspected brain tumour in six cases.

Initial symptomatology could be classified into four groups; subarachnoid haemorrhage in 34 per cent; intracerebral haemorrhage in 30 per cent; epilepsy in 24 per cent, and symptoms and signs of raised intracranial pressure in 12 per cent.

An orbital bruit was heard in six instances; there were no cranial bruits.

Of the 17 patients presenting with subarachnoid haemorrhage, eight bled during the second decade. Of the 15 presenting with an intracerebral haemorrhage, 10 bled during the second and third decades. Only two patients died of haemorrhage. Among the survivors recurrent haemorrhages occurred in seven of the patients who presented with haemorrhage. Five of these had one recurrent bleed; two others had two recurrent bleeds. The intervals between these haemorrhages ranged from 2 months to 11 years. None of

Table 24.1
Intracranial AVM in Singapore 50 Cases: 1962 to May 1969

Sex: Male 33	*Female 17 (Ratio ♂:♀ = 2:1)*		
Race	*Cases*	*Percentage*	*Singapore Population Percentage*
Chinese	42	84	75
Others	3	10	15
Malays	5	6	10

them were fatal and disability was slight. TABLE 24.8 shows the length of survival of these patients. Thus, bleeding from an arteriovenous malformation was more benign than from an aneurysm.

Table 24.2
AVM in Singapore: Age at Onset of First Symptom

Age in years	*No. of cases*	*Percentage*	
0–10	3	6	66
11–20	19	38	
21–30	11	22	
31–40	10	20	34
41–50	6	12	
51–60	1	2	
Total:	*50*		*100*

In contrast to the haemorrhagic onset, patients presenting with epilepsy were evenly distributed in the second, third and fourth decades. Small malformations accounted for only two of the 12 cases, the rest being medium (7) or large (3). It would appear that if perchance a small malformation did not bleed while the patient was young, it eventually grew larger with age and might then produce symptomatic epilepsy. The frequency of epileptic attacks in such patients was very variable. Two patients who survived 20 years after the first fit had only three or four fits each during all this while, without treatment. Conversely, another patient surviving 19 years after onset had increasing frequency of fits despite anticonvulsant treatment. Owing to this variability in the course of the illness, it would be difficult to assess the results of medical or surgical treatment.

Of these 50 arteriovenous malformations, 26 were found in the right hemisphere, 22 in the left, and 2 in the midline. The location of these malformations is illustrated in FIGURE 24.1: 70 per cent were found in the frontal or parietal lobes, so that the anterior and middle

Table 24.3
Arterial Supply in A-V Malformations

	Cerebral Arteries					
Lobes	*Anterior*	*Middle*	*Ant. and Mid.*	*Posterior*	*Mid. and Post.*	*Total*
Frontal	12	4				16
Frontoparietal	1	4	1			6
Parietal	5	7	3	1	1	17
Parieto-occipital			1	2		3
Occipital		1		1		2
Parietotemporal		1				1
Temporal		4				4
Midbrain				1		1
Total:	*18*	*21*	*5*	*5*	*1*	*50*

Table 24.4
Size and Position of A-V Malformations

	Size			Position	
	Small <2 cm	Medium 2–6 cm	Large >6 cm	Superficial	Deep
No. of cases	19	24	7	17	33
Percentage	38	48	14	34	66

cerebral arteries supplied the majority [Table 24.3]. Whereas the anterior cerebral artery supplied predominantly those malformations in the frontal lobe, the middle cerebral artery had a much wider distribution, supplying malformations in parietal, frontal, temporal and even the occipital lobes; 66 per cent of the malformations were deep seated, while 34 per cent were superficial, involving the brain convexity. The malformations were small, medium-sized or large. Medium-sized malformations measuring between 2 and 6 cm formed 48 per cent of the series; 38 per cent were small, and 14 per cent were large [Table 24.4].

Thus, in comparison with Western figures there seems to be a preponderance of arteriovenous malformations among patients in Singapore. As these malformations and aneurysms are both congenital lesions, the preference of the former or the latter to one particular race must be regarded as genetically determined.

LOCATIONS OF THE A–V MALFORMATIONS

	Right	Left	Midline
No. of cases	26	22	2
Percentage	52%	44%	4%

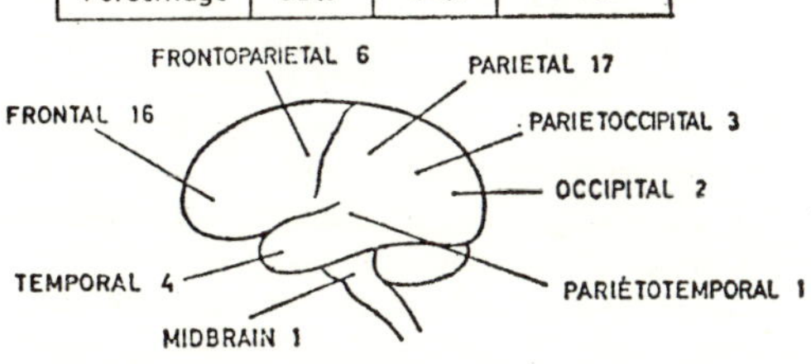

78% FOUND IN FRONTAL AND PARIETAL LOBES

Fig. 24.1. Locations of the arteriovenous malformations.

One of the major differences between Western cases and our patients is the much higher incidence of intracranial haemorrhage in the present study. In the majority of Western series, subarachnoid haemorrhage is much commoner than intracerebral haemorrhage, whereas in our patients there were equal numbers of both. Moreover, in our series the angiomas were more often smaller and deeper in location. It is also interesting to note that in our series there was a higher proportion of frontal lobe malformations (44 per cent) as compared with the predominant parietal lesions in Western series (Mackenzie, 1953; Paterson and McKissock, 1956; Sharkey, 1965; Svien and McRae, 1965; Henderson and Gomez, 1967). But we have not performed vertebral arteriography routinely, so these figures may not be accurate. Orbital bruits were uncommon in our series probably because there were so few large malformations. It is the size and not the position of the lesion that determines the presence of an audible bruit.

The ratio of four malformations to one aneurysm certainly suggests that genetic factors may be important.

We have also found that bilateral carotid arteriography in intracranial haemorrhage, intracerebral or subarachnoid, only reveals the presence of an aneurysm or an arteriovenous malformation in less than 10 per cent of all cases. In the investigation of cases with intracranial haemorrhage, with and without hypertension, we customarily carry out arteriography 14 days after the haemorrhage. Ninety-five per cent of our cases have only a bilateral carotid arteriogram, yet our figures seem to be remarkably low with regard to the incidence of aneurysm. As the quality of our arteriography is satisfactory, we suspect that it is reflecting a genuine low incidence of these lesions. The difference between our figures and those of centres in the West is such a large one that clearly more thorough investigations will be necessary in the future.

For various reasons we have never been able to complete an adequate study of a series of consecutive cases of subarachnoid haemorrhage admitted to hospital. Such figures as we possess indicate that the ratio of arteriovenous malformation to aneurysm is 4:1. But we suspect that if we included the cases not admitted to

Table 24.5
Eyeball Bruits in AVM

Eyeball		*Malformation*			
		Side	*Lobe*	*Size*	*Position*
1	Left	Left	Parietal	M	Superficial
2	Left	Left	Parietal	L	Superficial
3	Left	Left	Parietal	L	Deep
4	Left	Left	Frontoparietal	L	Deep
5	Right	Right	Frontal	S	Deep
6	Right	Right	Temporal	M	Deep

Table 24.6
The Initial Symptoms in A-V Malformations, Overall Series

Series	*Mackenzie* (1953)	*Paterson and McKissock* (1956)	*Svien and McRae* (1965)	*Henderson and Gomez* (1967)	*Singapore*
Cases	50	110	95	70	50
Haemorrhage					
Subarachnoid	24%	39%	47%	75%	34%
Intracerebral	6%	3%	6%	—	30%
Epilepsy	32%	26%	46%	16%	24%
Headache	24%	21%	34%	—	6%
Paresis	12%	7%	21%	1%	4%
Bruits	66%	39%	25%	50%	12%

Table 24.7
Initial Symptoms in A-V Malformations, Singapore Series

Symptom	*No. of cases*	*Percentage*
Subarachnoid haemorrhage	17	34
Intracerebral haemorrhage	15	30
Jacksonian epilepsy	7	14
Generalized epilepsy	5	10
Headache	3	6
Weakness	2	4
Dementia	1	2
Total:	*50*	*100*

hospital, the figure would be 2:1. We know there is a tendency for the patient with a subarachnoid haemorrhage to be kept at home for the first 3 days before admission to hospital is agreed. The mortality rate is considerable.

Multiple Sclerosis

In Singapore, acute demyelinating disorders and acute encephalitis are common. We also see neuromyelitis optica, primary lateral sclerosis and acute transverse myelitis of unknown aetiology. But we do not encounter multiple sclerosis.

In 1965 an inquiry on this subject unearthed only one case (Gwee and Toh, 1970). This inquiry included consultations with all consultants in government hospitals and private practice who saw neurological cases, a review of autopsies in the Pathology Department of the teaching hospital and a follow-up of all cases of retrobulbar neuritis diagnosed between January 1964 and December 1966. These patients were traced, re-examined and assessed.

No cases of multiple sclerosis were forthcoming from the first and second lines of inquiry. On the other hand the incidence of neuromyelitis optica in the Singapore Hospitals was about one case every 2 or 3 years.

There were 20 cases of retrobulbar neuritis: 18 were in Chinese, 2 in Indians, and there were 9 males and 11 females. No Malay patients were found, the

Table 24.8
AVM: Length of Survival

No. of Patients presenting with	*Total*	*Died*	*Survival in years (to 1969)*			*Defaulted*
			1–5	6–10	>10	
Subarachnoid haemorrhage	17	1	11	2	1	2
Intracerebral haemorrhage	15	1	5	4	2	3
Epilepsy	12	1[1]	3	2	4	2

[1] Not attributable to AVM.

reason for which was hard to formulate, but it is difficult to believe that only Malay patients with sudden loss of vision would not seek hospital advice. The clinical features of these 20 patients with acute retrobulbar neuritis, are outlined in TABLE 24.9.

One of them was actually thought to be suffering from multiple sclerosis (Case 14) until the findings of neuromyelitis optica were obtained at autopsy. Case 20 was also finally considered to be an example of neuromyelitis optica. Only four cases (Cases 3, 9, 11 and 12) could be followed and examined; they were all well. Five patients had already died, and at autopsy in four of them characteristic features of acute encephalitis were established. Of the 11 cases who were not available for re-examination, 10 had had steroid treatment and had improved or recovered. None had anything suggesting remission, relapse, or new neurological complaint. It would seem that multiple sclerosis of the classical type must be either very rare or unknown among Singaporians.

But during the course of the investigation, in 1967, a Chinese female of 26 was seen with classical multiple sclerosis. The disorder began with acute retrobulbar neuritis with recovery, followed a year later by diplopia and subsequently by paraplegia. Her progress has been followed over a period of 5 years and the characteristic remitting and disseminated features of the disorder have been witnessed. We think she is the first authentic case of the disease among the Singapore Chinese.

Nasopharyngeal Malignancy

The high incidence of this disease in Singapore has been known for many years; it is literally confined to the Chinese. The cause is not known and there is little to support the many speculations concerning the eating of spicy food, the use of snuff, opium smoking, the inhalation of incense or smoke of a domestic origin, and the topical applications of traditional Chinese medicine. The strong racial preponderance would suggest a genetic factor.

The tumour is of epithelial origin and commonly spreads from the nasopharynx to involve the base of the skull, characteristically producing intractable headaches and multiple cranial nerve palsies. Metastatic deposits within the nervous system, in the brain and spinal cord, are exceptional. Metastasis usually takes the form of an extradural en plaque lesion. The lesions are extremely radiosensitive but unfortunately bone is frequently invaded and improvement is often only temporary.

The high incidence of nasopharyngeal carcinoma in South-East Asia was first stressed by Digby, Fook, and Che (1941) in Hong Kong, who found that it accounted for 27·2 per cent of 419 cases of neoplasia.

In Singapore, Mekie (1949) quoted an incidence of 16·41 per cent in 530 cases.

Nasopharyngeal carcinoma is therefore one of the first suspicions in a Chinese from Singapore with one or more recurrent cranial nerve palsies.

Hydranencephaly

This congenital malformation is characterized by a complete or near complete absence of the cerebral hemispheres, with preservation of the cerebellum, which is often malformed, a brain stem and intact meninges, and a cranium filled with cerebrospinal fluid. It is a very rare anomaly. The majority of published reports refer only to isolated cases. In Singapore, Yong (1969) reported the clinical, radiological, electroencephalographic and autopsy features in nine cases. The youngest was 2 days old and the oldest 8 months at the time of diagnosis. There were seven Chinese, one Malay and one Sino-Malay. There were six males and three females.

The commonest mode of presentation is with progressive enlargement of the head, which is usually

Table 24.9
Retrobulbar Neuritis: 20 Cases, 1965

Case No.	*Race*	*Age*	*Sex*	*History suggestive of DS*	*Feature of DS other than optic involvement*	*PM findings*
1	Ch.	32	F	—	—	Alive
2	Ch.	53	F	—	—	Alive
3[1]	Ch.	12	F	Giddiness	—	Alive
4	Ch.	15	M	—	—	Leukaemia with secondaries in brain
5	Ch.	30	F	Squint, difficulty in passing urine	—	Alive
6	Ind.	37	F	—	—	Alive
7	Ch.	28	F	—	—	Alive
8	Ind.	35	M	—	—	Alive
9[1]	Ch.	31	M	—	—	Alive
10	Ch.	27	F	—	—	Alive
11[1]	Ch.	19	M	—	—	Alive
12[1]	Ch.	47	M	—	—	Alive
13	Ch.	30	F	—	—	Alive
14	Ch.	16	F	Cerebellar sign, nystagmus, micturition difficulty	Transverse myelitis	Died Neuromyelitis optica
15	Ch.	60	M	—	—	Died, bronchogenic cancer with secondaries
16	Ch.	6	F	—	—	Alive
17	Ch.	6/12	F	—	—	Alive, ?Schilder's disease
18	Ch.	9	M	Headache	Ataxia	Alive
19	Ch.	6	M	Weakness of legs	(L) Babinski positive	Dead No PM final diagnosis Encephalitis
20	Ch.	?30	M	Dribbling of urine, weakness of legs	Bilateral positive Babinski sensory level T2	Alive, diagnosed neuromyelitis optica finally

[1] Cases responded to recheck call-up in 1966.
Source: Gwee, A. L. and Tob, C. S. (1970) A search for disseminated sclerosis in Singaporeani, *Far East med. J.*, 6, 51.

obvious at birth, but may develop later. Hydrocephalus and subdural haematoma are often initially suspected. The baby is fretful and restless, usually able to move all four limbs, but posture soon becomes abnormal. The upper limbs are flexed with clenched fists and the lower limbs extended, as in the decorticate preparation in monkeys. There are tonic neck reflexes. During sleep the decorticate posture is relaxed. There is usually a coarse tremor affecting one or more limbs. Spasms are frequent. Convulsions are not witnessed. The pupils react normally, but vision is not apparent in the majority. The optic discs are often malformed and white, and there is usually nystagmus. The infant appears to be able to hear and can certainly smile.

Transillumination of the skull is a useful and simple diagnostic procedure. Using an ordinary torch held against the head and making sure that no stray light interferes with the observation, it is possible to pemonstrate in a darkened room that the head lights up a brilliant red, like a Chinese lantern. The falx stands out as a midline linear shadow; the presence of the cerebellum casts a shadow in the lower portion of the posterior fossa.

A subdural tap through the lateral angle of the anterior fontanelle extracts cerebrospinal fluid. Air introduced into the intracranial cavity will confirm the absence of cortical tissue. The electroencephalogram is characteristically flat.

It may be that this congenital anomaly is more common in Singapore than in the Western world, but clearly this is only a preliminary observation as yet.

Local Diseases: Amok, Latah, and Koro

Amok

This complaint is overwhelmingly a Malay one, although Chinese cases have been reported. *Amok* in Malay means madness and the general idea conveyed by it is to die fighting. It is also said that the word *amok* was once a battle cry of Malay pirates and that 'to run amok' may be the Malay way of committing suicide. 'Europeans commit suicide, Malays run amok.'

In recent years the incidence of this disease has decreased. The manic activity is short-lived and entirely murder-bent. A number of these patients have had to be shot during the furore.

Latah

This is also an essentially Malay disorder mainly of females. The phenomenon can be brought on by a sudden act, such as a tap on the shoulder or a shout, when the patient will immediately become confused and emulate whatever action her 'tormentor' is making. The disturbance is short-lived and followed by complete amnesia and recovery. It is thought to be a fright neurosis with hysterical elaborations. It has many forms, such as the sudden use of obscene language, coprolalia, echolalia and various compulsive movement and speech disorders. In general, Malays consider it to be a form of personal peculiarity rather than a disease.

Koro

This is an affliction of the Chinese, but it is occasionally seen in the Malay. It affects only males, usually young adults. The patient is seized with a sudden notion that his penis is retracting into this abdomen and should this materialize he would surely die. In his desperation he employs every physical means at his disposal, manual or mechanical, to prevent this retraction [PLATE 25b] and frequently he is assisted by his relatives. It is not peculiar to the Malaysian peninsula and has been known in Southern China for many years (Gwee, 1963).

The three behaviour disorders described above are all decreasing in incidence and may be regarded as forms of hysteria in which the symptomatology has a cultural basis.

CEREBROVASCULAR DISEASE IN SINGAPORE

In all developing countries, the control of diseases such as the infectious fevers, malaria, and malnutrition changes the pattern of mortality, and certainly, too, of the morbidity in a country. Hence, the place of cerebrovascular disease in mortality is often underestimated. Furthermore, the morbidity of cerebrovascular disease is far greater than that of other diseases because of the relatively longer survival of affected cases, and the greater inadequacy in physical ability that follows. Besides, the present mode of population planning tends towards the creation of an ageing society with an increasing proportion of old people at the expense of the young, and hence it is safe to say that cerebrovascular disease must inevitably become the most important factor, apart from accidents, both in mortality and in morbidity.

Incidence represents a major aspect of epidemiology, and in Singapore the important question is what proportion of cerebrovascular accidents are seen in the hospital population. It has been observed that the hospital utilization rate varies from race to race. This rate varies also for sex and for individual disease. In general, a case of acute illness with severe pain, such as tetanus, or a major nursing problem such as coma, is likely to be sent to the hospital irrespective of race, sex and disease bias, provided that the patient will survive for at least a few days. Where the survival is expected to be of a short duration, Chinese and Malays usually keep the patient at home. On the other hand, where the disability is not too great, and the demand for care not too exacting, the utilization rate is also likely to be very different. Thus, when considering hospital figures, one must accept that whereas figures for cerebral and subarachnoid haemorrhages are likely to be close to the true incidence among the population and to be relatively free from utilization bias, those for cerebral thrombosis and transient ischaemic attacks must differ considerably from the true incidence. An attempt was made to show locally that the racial breakdown of cerebrovascular accidents has some resemblance to, and is therefore a reflection of, the racial breakdown of the population, but since cerebrovascular accidents affect principally those in the fifth and sixth decades, the comparison should in fact be with the same groups in the population; when this is done, it will be seen that the racial proportion of 7·5 : 1 : 1·5 for Chinese : Indian : Malay no longer holds good [FIGS. 24.2 and 24.3]. In fact, taking the age-group 50–69, the ratio is 21 : 1 : 7·5. The fall in the Indian figure for cerebrovascular accidents is chiefly because Indians generally return to India when they retire from active work. Some of the Chinese also return to China but the figure is small. However, the adult Chinese population are less stable than Malays, as they are apt to migrate to Malaysia in search of employment, whereas the Malays, being mostly public service employees or fisherman, are less liable to move out. Surveys in other countries show varying figures (Stallones, 1965). The figure may well be lower in Singapore because we have a younger population and hence fewer similar cases, and secondly, our doctors are less aware of the entity of transient ischaemic attacks.

In fact, a more accurate picture may be obtained by comparing the annual mortality figures of the hospital

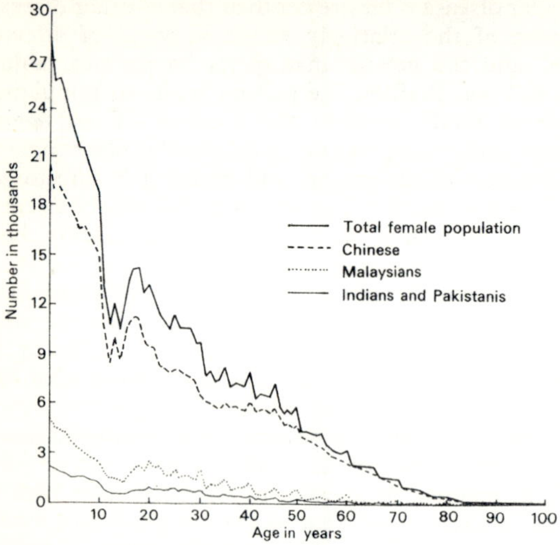

FIG. 24.2. Age distribution (in single years) 1967: females.

and the nation as a whole. Bearing in mind that probably almost all cerebral and subarachnoid haemorrhages are admitted, and the total mortality in our general hospital is about 300 a year, then it seems likely that in the bleeding cerebrovascular accident, the hospital figure is a good and reliable index of the population incidence, being almost the bulk of the disease. The same cannot unfortunately be said for cerebral thrombosis, embolism and ischaemic diseases, and the true incidence must await a planned population survey. A sample survey carried out in 1966 of a population of 10 116 people showed an incidence of neurological illness of 14 per cent in the chronic sick population. If we exclude cases under 40 years of age (most of these cannot be cases of cerebrovascular accident, apart from a very few embolic cases) then the figure would be 0·9 per cent or 90 per 10 116 i.e. 89 per 10 000. This, of course, would represent only surviving cases, and taking into account an immediate mortality of about 30 per cent, the true incidence seems likely to be round about 120 per 10 000. However, this figure must await confirmation by a planned survey on a greater scale.

The relationship with hypertension has been a subject of interest in the past. It is generally agreed that cerebral haemorrhage is a frequent mode of termination of malignant hypertension. On the other hand, the place of hypertension as a contributory factor in the incidence of cerebral thrombosis is not well established. In computing figures, we must be careful of at least two things. First, hypertension is a not uncommon finding in the age-group we are dealing with, namely the fifth and sixth decades, although for obvious difficulties the exact proportion of hypertensives to normotensives at this period of life is difficult to decide, especially as we are by no means agreed as to what constitutes the range of normal blood pressure at this period. Secondly, a large number of patients in this age-group are labile when hypertensive and their blood pressure readings change within wide limits. Furthermore, it is common to have a rise of blood pressure during the acute cerebral vascular catastrophe, and then a fall with the

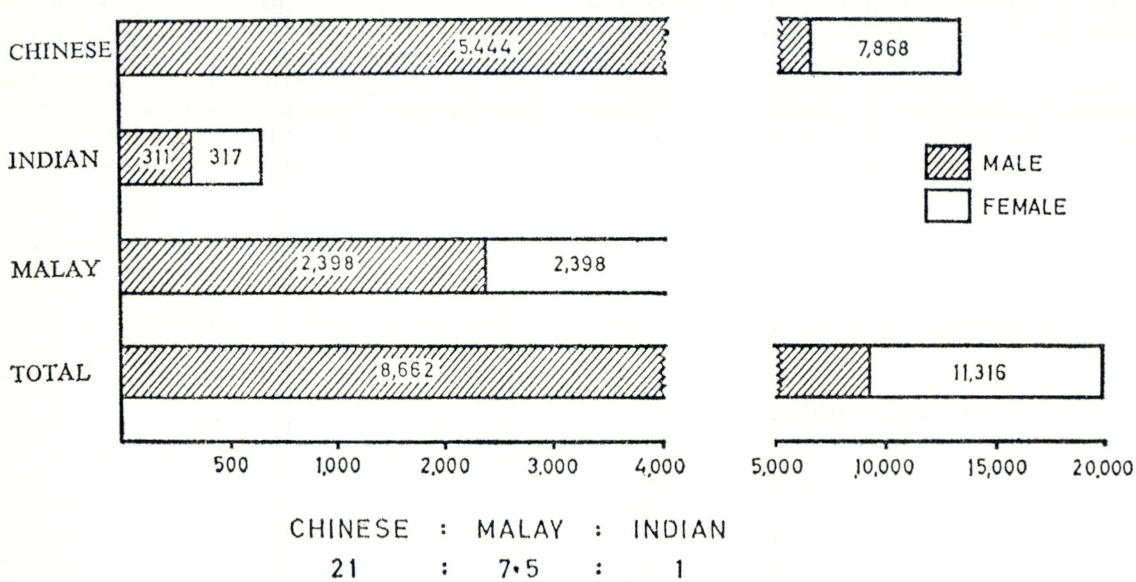

FIG. 24.3. Population distribution at the fifth and sixth decades, Singapore, 1967 (census figure).

subsequent enforced state of rest and dietetic restriction. Thus, unless the premorbid blood pressure reading is known, the figures recorded at admission and subsequently during convalescence are suspicious, and cannot be relied on implicitly.

Finally, it has always been suspected that a number of cases of cerebrovascular accident may have died before admission, and it is not uncommon for doctors whose series showed a higher mortality to claim that they admitted such patients earlier in the acute episode—thus showing a higher mortality. We thought it would be interesting to search our hospital records for cases brought in dead to see how many did in fact die before admission, particularly as we had found that the mortality figure we had for the present series was low by comparison with those for other series. Looking through the records of 1967—the year in question—we were able to find only 45 cases in this category. Assuming an even distribution between three medical units this would put our deaths up by 15 only, i.e. from 72 to 87 deaths (giving an adjusted mortality of 35 per cent). This is still a very respectable figure, particularly as cerebral and subarachnoid haemorrhages, with high mortality, accounted for 48 cases, i.e. more than half of our total mortalities.

A second moot point is the question of statistics for survival after the acute episodes. This sort of study is beset with difficulties in Singapore and we have reliable figures up to 1 year only, when the death rate is about 19 per cent. We must take this into account, together with the fact that it is uncommon to elicit a history of previous episodes of cerebrovascular accident in our cases (<8 per cent). If recurrence is common among the survivors, then a significant number of patients should give an account of a previous episode. This will of course depend on the patients' awareness of illness, and minor ischaemic episodes occurring locally are likely to be ignored and forgotten. Taking all these factors into account, the conclusion would seem to be that recurrence of cerebrovascular accident is not a serious problem locally, either because recurrence is not common or because most of the cases have perished from other causes in the meantime. This could mean that aftercare is defective, and death from bedsores, urinary infection and other results of impaired mobility is significant. The following account is based on an analysis of admissions to hospital during 1967.

Cerebral Thrombosis

All patients admitted between 1 January 1967 and 31 December 1967 in whom a diagnosis of cerebral thrombosis was made are included in the study. A non-haemorrhagic spinal fluid is taken as a *sine qua non* of the diagnosis.

The age-group, sex and race distribution of the 141 patients can be seen in TABLE 24.10. There is an equal sex distribution of 71 males and 70 females, although the hospital admission has a bias of M:F = 2:1. The Chinese have the highest incidence but this is due to population distribution. More than half of the patients with cerebral thrombosis are in the 50–70 age-group (65 per cent).

The prognosis for life in relation to age at the time of admission is shown in TABLE 24.11. A feature of this table is that two-thirds (67 per cent) of the patients

Table 24.10

Age-Group, Race and Sex Distribution in Cerebral Thrombosis

Age in Years	*Males*				*Females*				*Total*
	Chinese	*Indian*	*Malay*	*Others*	*Chinese*	*Indian*	*Malay*	*Others*	
<30	—	—	—	—	—	1	—	—	1
31–40	3	—	—	—	—	—	—	—	3
41–50	3	2	3	—	3	—	—	1	12
51–60	21	2	2	—	15	1	1	—	42
61–70	19	1	2	—	26	—	2	—	50
71–80	13	—	—	—	16	—	—	—	29
>80	—	—	—	—	4	—	—	—	4
Total:	*59*	*5*	*7*	—	*64*	*2*	*3*	*1*	*141*

Source: Gwee, A. L., Tam, N. B., Chee, K. H., and Chew, L. S. (1970) Cerebrovascular disease- epidemiological and clinical considerations, *Singapore med. J.*, 11, 2.

Table 24.11
Prognosis for Life in Relation to Age at Time of Admission to Hospital

Age in Years	*Males*			*Total*	*Females*			*Total*
	Improved	*Same*	*Dead*		*Improved*	*Same*	*Dead*	
<30	—	—	—	—	1	—	—	1
31–40	3	—	—	3	—	—	—	0
41–50	4	2	2	8	3	1	0	4
51–60	16	4	5	25	12	4	1	17
61–70	17	3	2	22	17	7	4	28
71–80	8	1	4	13	10	3	3	16
>80	—	—	—	—	4	—	—	4
Total:	*48*	*10*	*13*	*71*	*47*	*15*	*8*	*70*

Source: Gwee, A. L., Tam, N. B., Chee, K. H., and Chew, L. S. (1970) Cerebrovascular disease: epidemiological and clinical considerations, *Singapore med. J.*, 11, 2.

showed improvement of the hemiplegic state in spite of differences in age. The overall mortality in this series was 15 per cent with a higher death rate in the older age-group of patients. Eighteen per cent of the patients showed no improvement during the initial hospitalization.

For the purpose of this study hypertension was defined as a diastolic pressure of 100 mm Hg or above [Table 24.12]. The table shows that 71 patients were hypertensives, of whom 37 were males and 34 were females. There is no significant difference in the incidence of non-hypertensive cerebrovascular disease between men and women. There is also no increased mortality in the hypertensive (13 per cent) over the non-hypertensive (16 per cent) group of patients.

Tables 24.13 and 24.14 show some related findings. It is interesting to note that diabetcs and hypertension were not uncommon, while the recurrence rate was 8 per cent.

More than half the deaths [Table 24.15] succumbed

Table 24.12
Comparison of Diastolic Blood Pressure in Survivors and Patients Who Died

Age in Years	*Males*				*Females*			
	Diastolic Pressure <99 mm Hg		*Diastolic Pressure >100 mm Hg*		*Diastolic Pressure <99 mm Hg*		*Diastolic Pressure >100 mm Hg*	
	Alive	*Dead*	*Alive*	*Dead*	*Alive*	*Dead*	*Alive*	*Dead*
>30	—	—	—	—	1	0	—	—
31–40	1	0	2	0	—	—	—	—
41–50	3	2	5	0	2	0	2	0
51–60	15	3	10	2	5	1	12	0
61–70	10	2	12	0	15	2	13	2
71–80	5	1	8	1	9	0	7	3
>80	—	—	—	—	4	0	—	—
Total:	*34*	*8*	*37*	*3*	*36*	*3*	*34*	*5*

Source: Gwee, A. L., Tam, N. B., Chee, K. H., and Chew, L. S. (1970) Cerebrovascular disease: epidemiological and clinical considerations, *Singapore med. J.*, 11, 2.

Table 24.13

Some Clinical and Laboratory Findings Associated with this Series. Cerebral Thrombosis

Sex	*Diabetes Mellitus*		*Blood Kahn Positive*	*Cerebrospinal Fluid*		*Renal Disease*	*Diseases*		*Valvular Heart Disease*	*PTB*	*Others*
	Treated	*Poorly or un-treated*		*Kahn Positive*	*Kahn Nega-tive*		*Coron-ary Heart*	*Cardiac Arrhy-thmia*			
Male	5	6	6	1	62	5	6	8	1	3	5
Female	3	6	0	0	61	11	6	0	0	1	4
Total:	*8*	*12*	*6*	*1*	*123*	*16*	*12*	*8*	*1*	*4*	*9*

Source: Gwee, A. L., Tam, N. B., Chee, K. H., and Chew, L. S. (1970) Cerebrovascular disease: epidemiological and clinical considerations, *Singapore med. J.*, 11, 2.

Table 24.14

Incidence of Recurrent Thrombosis and its Relation to Age, Sex, Blood Pressure and Mortality

Age in Years	*Sex*		*Blood Pressure*		*Time Interval between Initial and Second Thrombosis*							*Alive*	*Dead*
	M	*F*	*Diastolic <99 mm Hg*	*Diastolic >100 mm Hg*	*<6 mths*	*>6 mths*	*1 yr*	*2 yrs*	*3 yrs*	*4 yrs*	*>4 yrs*		
41–50	—	1	—	1	1	—	—	—	—	—	—	1	—
51–60	2	1	2	1	1	—	—	—	—	—	2	3	—
61–70	3	3	2	4	1	—	2	1	—	—	2	5	1
71–80	—	1	1	—	1	—	—	—	—	—	—	1	—
Total:	*5*	*6*	*5*	*6*	*4*	*0*	*2*	*1*	*0*	*0*	*4*	*10*	*1*

Source: Gwee, A. L., Tam, N. B., Chee, K. H., and Chew, L. S. (1970) Cerebrovascular disease: epidemiological and clinical considerations, *Singapore med. J.*, 11, 2.

Table 24.15

Causes of Death

Sex	*Time of Death*				*Persistent Coma*	*Deepening Coma*	*Renal Failure Uraemia*	*Cardiac Failure*	*Respira-tory Failure*	*Others*
	1 Day	*1 week*	*1 mth*	*>1 mth*						
Male	3	4	6	—	5	3	—	3	2	—
Female	—	6	1	1	3	—	2	—	1	2
Total:	*3*	*10*	*7*	*1*	*8*	*3*	*2*	*3*	*3*	*2*

Source: Gwee, A. L., Tam, N. B., Chee, K. H., and Chew, L. S. (1970) Cerebrovascular disease: epidemiological and clinical considerations, *Singapore med. J.*, 11, 2.

in the first week of admission with three patients (14 per cent) dying within 24 hours of admission. These resulted from either a persistence of coma or a deepening coma (55 per cent) arising from the cerebrovascular accident.

Comment

The immediate mortality from cerebral thrombosis in this series is 15 per cent, with a higher death rate in the older age-group of patients. This is somewhat lower than the 20–30 per cent mortality stated by Marshall (1968). Among the major factors which contributed to the mortality of the patients (in 55 per cent of cases) were the state of consciousness on admission and its persistence or subsequent deterioration.

It is generally believed that the vast majority of episodes of cerebral thrombosis occur in patients whose blood pressure is elevated above the mean for their age-group. The blood pressure of the remainder is elevated to varying degrees. Seventy patients were non-hypertensive whereas 71 were regarded as hypertensives on this criterion. Furthermore, the immediate mortality of the hypertensive group was not increased over that of the non-hypertensive group.

Cerebral Haemorrhage

In 1967, 52 patients with primary intracerebral haemorrhage were seen in the Unit, accounting for 22 per cent of all forms of cerebrovascular accidents admitted in that year. TABLE 24.16 shows the sex, race and age of the patients. The youngest patient was 31 years old and the oldest 80.

Mortality

Forty patients (77 per cent) died in this series. The times of their deaths in relation to the times of admission are shown in TABLE 24.17. As most of the patients were admitted soon after the onset of symptoms, this corresponds quite closely to the time of onset.

Of those who survived, four were alive 1 year after discharge, two alive 2 years after discharge and six were presumed dead as they could not be traced in the subsequent follow-up.

Table 24.17
Time of Death in Relation to Time of Admission

Time	*No. of cases*
Within the first 24 hours	14 (35%)
1 day	10 (25%)
2 days	4 (10%)
3 days	3
4 days	1
5 days	0
6 days	2
7 days	0
8 days to a month	6

Source: Gwee, A. L., Tam, N. B., Chee, K. H., and Chew, L. S. (1970) Cerebrovascular disease: epidemiological and clinical considerations, *Singapore med. J.*, 11, 2.

Clinical Features

The clinical features of the patients who died and of those who survived are outlined in TABLES 24.18 and 24.19.

Management

All the patients were conservatively treated. Conservative management consisted of nursing care, control of cerebral oedema and pulmonary complications, and treatment of hypertension, if severe. No tracheostomy was performed in any of the patients.

Table 24.16
Sex, Race and Age Distribution in Cerebral Haemorrhage

Sex	Male	= 34	Female = 18
Race	Chinese	= 48	
	Indian	= 4	
Age	<40	= 1 (female)	
	41–50	= 8 (male = 7, female = 1)	
	51–60	= 18 (male = 12, female = 6)	
	>60	= 25 (male = 15, female = 10)	

Source: Gwee, A. L., Tam, N. B., Chee, K. H., and Chew, L. S. (1970) Cerebrovascular disease: epidemiological and clinical considerations, *Singapore med. J.*, 11, 2.

Table 24.18

Clinical Features of Those who Died from Cerebral Haemorrhage

Clinical Features	*Hypertensive (19) 70 per cent*		*Normotensive (21) 80 per cent*	
Age: 41–50	M (71%)	F (69%)	M (78%)	F (87%)
	3 (75%)	0	2 (67%)	1 (100%)
51–60	7 (88%)	2 (67%)	3 (75%)	1 (10%)
>60	2 (50%)	5 (72%)	12 (92%)	2 (67%)
Coronary disease	1		0	
Arrhythmia	0		0	
Valvular disease	0		0	
Diabetes mellitus	1		1	
Level of consciousness:				
Conscious	1		0	
Coma I	0		2	
Coma II	3		1	
Coma III	4		7	
Coma IV	11		11	
Unilateral signs	R = 3 L = 7		R = 1 L = 4	
Bilateral signs	9		11	
Alcohol	1		2	
Severe strain	1		0	

M = Male F = Female L = Left R = Right

Source: Gwee, A. L., Tam, Chee, K. H., and Chew, L. S. (1970) Cerebrovascular disease: epidemiological and clinical considerations, *Singapore med. J.*, 11, 2.

Comment

In this series of 52 patients with primary intracerebral haemorrhage, more males than females were seen, the ratio being 2:1. The patients were mostly in the sixth decade and beyond. An interesting feature to note is the absence of Malay patients.

One-third of the deaths occurred within the first 24 hours of admission. The majority of patients (70 per cent) died within the first 2 days. Thereafter the mortality rate showed an appreciable decline. In the hypertensive females in the seventh decade and beyond, the mortality was observed to be somewhat higher than that of the hypertensive males of the same age-group.

A study of the clinical features reveals a few factors that were important in influencing prognosis. Age had no significant effect up to the age of 70, after which the mortality rose steeply. Hypertension did not significantly affect the mortality. A very significant prognostic factor was the level of consciousness at the end of the first 24 hours. The mortality of those in deep coma (coma IV) was 100 per cent, coma III, 84 per cent, coma II, 67 per cent, and coma I, 50 per cent. Only one (14 per cent) of the seven patients who were conscious died.

Primary Subarachnoid Haemorrhage

Twenty-two patients with subarachnoid haemorrhage were admitted to the Unit in 1967, forming 9 per cent of all forms of cerebrovascular accidents seen in the Unit in the same year. There was a preponderance of male patients, numbering 15. Twenty patients were Chinese, one Indian and one European. No Malay patients were encountered.

Table 24.19

Clinical Features of Patients who Survived

Clinical Features	*Hypertensive (8)*	*Normotensive (4)*
Age: <40	1	0
41–50	1	1
51–60	2	1
>60	4	2
Coronary disease	1	0
Arrhythmia	0	0
Valvular disease	0	0
Diabetes mellitus	1	0
Level of consciousness:		
Conscious	3	3
Coma I	1	1
Coma II	2	0
Coma III	2	0
Coma IV	0	0
Unilateral signs	R = 2 L = 5	R = 1 L = 3
Bilateral signs	1	0
Alcohol	1	0
Severe strain	1	1

R = Right L = Left

Source: Gwee, A. L., Tam, N. B., Chee, K. H., and Chew, L. S. (1970) Cerebrovascular disease: epidemiological and clinical considerations, *Singapore med. J.*, 11, 2.

Age

The youngest patient was 23 years old and the oldest 68.

Mortality

Nine patients (41 per cent) in this series died, six within 24 hours, while the others survived for months.

One was presumed dead 1 year after discharge as he was not traceable in the subsequent follow-up. A patient who died on the ninetieth day had associated coronary thrombosis.

Carotid Arteriography

Six patients had carotid angiograms. No abnormality was detected in two patients. Berry aneurysms were shown in two; arteriovenous malformation was present in one. Another patient had atheroma of both carotid arteries but no detectable bleeding source.

Comment

The mortality of 41 per cent is about half that in intracerebral haemorrhage. The majority of the patients died within the first 24 hours.

The source of bleeding was revealed by carotid angiography in two patients, one due to an aneurysm and the other due to arteriovenous malformation. In the majority of cases, the cause of the bleeding was not known, as no carotid angiograms were performed on them. A history of a focal lesion such as a third nerve palsy prior to the subarachnoid haemorrhage, or of a haemorrhage without a stroke, may suggest the possibility of an aneurysm as the source of bleeding, but there were no such helpful clues in our patients apart from one who had a previous history of subarachnoid bleeding. The age of the patient may be of some help. In the case of patients in the third and fourth decades a stroke associated with subarachnoid bleeding is likely to be due to a ruptured aneurysm. In Pakkarinen's series (1967), 76 per cent of patients were found to have aneurysms, 2 per cent had arteriovenous malformation, and in 22 per cent no cause was found.

Nine patients (1 per cent) in this series had hemiparesis but none had hemiplegia.

The presence of neurological deficit did not significantly affect the mortality. Hypertension was observed to have had an adverse effect on the prognosis. All those who died were hypertensive. It is well known that hypertension tends to precipitate the rupture of an aneurysm. Another significant factor influencing the prognosis was the level of consciousness on the first day of admission. None of those who were conscious or only drowsy died, whereas 75 per cent of those in coma III and IV succumbed.

Transient Cerebral Ischaemia Attacks

Transient attacks of cerebral ischaemia are defined as disturbances of neurological function, usually lasting a few minutes only. This definition is primarily based on the clinical features, which are presumed to be due to temporary interruption of part of the cerebral circulation, however caused. The main features, besides their brief duration, are spontaneous recovery without residual signs, and the tendency to recur.

In our series we have extended the arbitrary temporal criterion even further, our choice being 1 week, while fully adopting the other criteria. In defence of our amended definition we propose the following reasons. First, the time limit is arbitrarily fixed by different authors in any case, and the difference between 1 day and 1 week is, in an important sense, no greater than the difference between 1 hour and 24 hours. Secondly, patients with cerebral infarcts or haemorrhages are very unlikely to recover completely in 1 week. Thirdly, in our series of 26 patients, 14 recovered completely within 24 hours, and 12 within 1 week, and there was no significant difference between these two groups.

The true incidence of transient cerebral ischaemia attacks is extremely difficult, if not impossible, to determine, for their nature is such that a large if not the major proportion of people afflicted do not seek medical aid. According to Glynn (1956), transient ischaemia attacks constitute 6 per cent of cerebrovascular accidents. In our series, the proportion of transient ischaemia attacks was 10·6 per cent.

The number of our TIAs totalled 26 and analysis showed that:

1. The racial distribution of our Chinese cases corresponded closely with the local racial structure, which consists of 72 per cent Chinese, 25 per cent Malays and 3 per cent Indians in the 50–69 age group [FIGS. 24.2 and 24.3], whereas there were more Indian and fewer Malay cases than would be expected.
2. Males predominated over females in a ratio of 1·6 : 1, which was much lower than the ratio of 3·8 : 1 in the series studied by Acheson and Hutchinson (1964), especially when it can be shown that our hospital admission has a M : F = 2 : 1 bias, chiefly due to bed distribution.
3. The risk of developing TIAs increased with advancing age, with the vast majority (77 per cent) occurring after 50 years of age. The average age of the female cases was significantly higher than that of the male cases (66·0 years against 53·3 years).
4. Those who had hypertension were in the minority (27 per cent), and hypotension played little or no part in the pathogenesis.
5. The incidence of ischaemic heart disease (15 per cent) was exactly the same as that found by Acheson and Hutchinson (1964).

The commonest presenting clinical feature was hemiplegia (46 per cent), followed by cranial nerve involvement, impairment of consciousness and vertigo (27 per cent each). By comparison, in Marshall's series (1964), vertigo was the commonest feature, followed by hemiparesis, hemianaesthesia and visual field disturbance.

In our series the cerebrospinal fluid was normal in the majority of cases, but it may be worth noting that 38 per cent of the cases showed a rise in protein and 11 per cent showed a pleocytosis.

The majority (58 per cent) of our TIAs could not be definitely localized to any part of the brain. Of the rest, more occurred in the vertebrobasilar territory than in the carotid territory (31 per cent as opposed to 11 per cent).

Regarding prognosis, 62 per cent of our patients remained well for at least 1 year after discharge from hospital, and 38 per cent were dead or presumed to be dead because they could not be traced despite every effort. Acheson and Hutchinson (1964) found 52 per cent of their patients developed strokes on average about 13 months after they were first seen, and these strokes carried a mortality of 29 per cent. Thus, our series had a somewhat lower morbidity rate but a much higher mortality rate.

Cerebral Embolism

As we had only three cases in our series, two being due to mitral stenosis and one to atrial fibrillation of uncertain cause, no analysis is meaningful beyond the fact that they constituted just over 1 per cent of our cerebrovascular accidents, compared with 2 per cent in the series studied by Glynn (1956), and 5 per cent in the series studied by Groch, McDevitt, and Wright (1961).

THYROTOXIC PERIODIC PARALYSIS

Although Singapore is a multiracial society, thyrotoxic periodic paralysis occurs exclusively in the Chinese. Eighteen patients were seen over a period of 10 years (1961–70) in a total of 1022 thyrotoxic patients of all ethnic groups. The condition occurs in about 5 per cent of Chinese patients with thyrotoxicosis. Of our 18 patients only one was female, although there were 782 females in the whole series. The age of onset is usually between 20 and 30 years and bouts of flaccid paralysis usually develop with the onset of thyrotoxicosis or shortly afterwards.

The usual story is that following a period of rest, sitting in a chair or lying in bed, the patient has difficulty in rising. Attacks vary both in frequency and severity. In a mild attack there may only be a transient weakness of a group of muscles which soon subsides. But in a severe attack there may be almost complete paralysis. The patient may wake in the early hours and find himself unable to move his limbs or trunk, but able to talk, swallow and breathe normally. The attack may last several hours or persist for a few days. During the day a mild attack may be warded off by exercising the weak muscles. Lower limbs are usually affected first and in severe cases facial, bulbar and respiratory muscles are the last to become paralysed.

As in the familial form of the disease, the most important predisposing factors are prolonged rest after vigorous exercise or a heavy meal. A large meal of rice may result in an attack of paralysis. The patient usually sweats during the attack and sometimes cannot urinate. In the majority of cases the tendon reflexes are impaired or absent during the paralysis. As in the familiar form of the disease, there are the same biochemical changes; hypokalaemia and retention of water and sodium. In thyrotoxicosis the occurrence of paralysis is related neither to the duration nor to the severity of the endocrine disorder. The attacks of paralysis subside when the patient becomes euthyroid and cannot then be induced. Clinical evidence of thyrotoxicosis is usually present but may be minimal. The characteristic effects of hypokalaemia are seen in the electrocardiogram; prominent U waves, flattening of the T waves, prolongation of the PR, QRS and QT intervals, with depression of the RST segment.

Attacks of paralysis may be precipitated by intravenous glucose and insulin, but this is dangerous and fatalities have been reported. Treatment during paralysis is with oral or intravenous potassium chloride. Fresh oranges and bananas are a good source of potassium.

Thyrotoxic periodic paralysis is well known in Japan, where it was first described, and where the majority of cases have been reported. It is also well known in Hong Kong and Thailand, but is rare in the West.

References

ACHESON, J. E. C., and HUTCHINSON, E. C. (1964) Observations on the natural history of transient cerebral ischaemia, *Lancet*, ii, 871.

DIGBY, K. H., FOOK, W. L., and CHE, Y. T. (1941) Nasopharyngeal carcinoma, *Brit. J. Surg.*, 28, 517.

GLYNN, A. A. (1956) Vascular disease of the nervous system. A series of 315 cases, *Brit. med. J.*, 1, 1216.

GROCH, S. N., MCDEVITT, E., and WRIGHT, I. S. (1961) A long-term study of cerebral vascular disease, *Ann. intern. Med.*, 55, 358.

GWEE, A. L., (1963) Koro—a cultural disease, *Singapore med. J.*, 4, 119.

GWEE, A. L., TAM, N. B., CHEE, K. H., and CHEW, L. S. (1970) Cerebrovascular disease: epidemiological and clinical considerations, *Singapore med. J.*, 11, 2.

GWEE, A. L., and TOH, C. S. (1970) A search for disseminated sclerosis in Singaporeans, *Far East med. J.*, 6, 51.

HENDERSON, W. R., and GOMEZ, R. de R. L. (1967) Natural history of cerebral angiomas, *Brit. med. J.*, 4, 571.

MACKENZIE, I. (1953) The clinical presentation of the cerebral angioma: a review of 50 cases, *Brain*, 76, 184.

MARSHALL, J. (1964) The natural history of transient ischaemia, cerebrovascular attacks, *Quart. J. Med.*, 33, 309.

MARSHALL, J. (1968) *The Management of Cerebrovascular Disease*, 2nd ed., London.

MEKIE, D. E. C. (1949) Lymphoepithelioma, *Malay. med. J.* 3, 236.

PAKKARINEN, S. (1967) Incidence, aetiology, prognosis of primary subarachnoid haemorrhage, *Acta neurol. scand.* 43, Suppl. 29.

PATERSON, J. H., and MCKISSOCK, W. (1956) A clinical survey of intracranial angiomas with special reference to their mode of progression and surgical treatment: a report of 110 cases, *Brain*, 79, 233.

SHARKEY, P. C. (1965) Intracranial arteriovenous malformations; a partial community study, *Arch Neurol.*, (*Chic.*), 12, 546.

SPILLANE, J. D. (1969) Tropical neurology, *Proc. roy. Soc. Med.*, 62, 403.

STALLONES, R. A. (1965) Epidemiology of cerebrovascular disease; a review, *J. chron. Dis.*, 18, 859.

SVIEN, H. J., and MCRAE, J. A. (1965) Arteriovenous anomalies of the brain. Fate of patients not having definitive surgery, *J. Neurosurg.*, 23, 23.

TAY, C. H., OON, C. L., LAI, C. S., LOONG, S. C., and GWEE, A. L. (1971) Intracranial arteriovenous malformations in Asians, *Brain*, 94, 61.

YONG, C. K. (1969) Hydranencephaly, *Proceedings of the Fourth Singapore-Malaysia Congress of Medicine*, Vol. 4, Singapore, p. 115.

25 Neurological Disorders in Malaysia

R. SELBY

INTRODUCTION

The former Federation of Malaya with the states of Sarawak and Sabah, located on the island of Borneo, constitutes Malaysia. West Malaysia, the previous federation, occupies the southern portion of the Kra Peninsula which extends from Thailand. It is shaped like a scimitar. East Malaysia (Sarawak and Sabah) is located along the entire northern coast of Borneo, separated from one another by the state of Brunei.

The climate is tropical, with a relatively high constant temperature, high annual rainfall, and a humid atmosphere. The country does not experience the extremes of temperature found in continental tropical and subtropical areas. The climate is largely controlled by the country's exposure to the sea.

Malaysia has a population of approximately ten million people, slightly over half of whom are Malays or of Malay stock. Approximately 40 per cent are Chinese. The remainder are mostly from the subcontinent of India including Ceylon. There are approximately 50 000 Orang Asli who are regarded as the descendants of the original human inhabitants of the peninsula. There are smaller numbers of Eurasians and Europeans.

The capital, Kuala Lumpur, has a population of approximately 350 000 people. There has been a steady increase in the urban population throughout the country. Although the primary sources of revenue are rubber, palm oil and tin, there has been a substantial increase in the growth of secondary industries following the end of the Second World War. The expansion of industrial development and the Communist Emergency which existed between 1948 and 1960 have been largely responsible for urban growth. The Chinese tend to live in the cities and the Malays in small towns and rural areas, but there has been a distinct increase in the numbers of Malays moving to the cities. The ancestors of the modern Malays are believed to have migrated to the peninsula from the north, possibly from South-western China, in about 2000 BC. Their descendants have intermarried over the centuries with people from Sumatra, Java, India and Arabia. The Malays are mostly farmers, but many have entered government service. By religion they are Muslim.

The Chinese have come to Malaysia over several hundreds of years, and the chief immigration occurred between 1880 and 1920. Most of them arrived from Southern China. Their main dialects are Cantonese, Hokkien, Teochew, Hakka, and Hylam. While some are Buddists or Christians, most of the Chinese follow the customs of traditional Chinese religion.

For the most part, the Indians were immigrants from Southern India, and towards the turn of the century came to the country because of the development of the rubber industry. Many still work on the rubber estates but a sizable number have entered business, the professions and the Civil Service. A goodly number of Ceylonese have been employed in the railways but large numbers have also entered the professions and government service. Most of these two groups are Hindu. Sikhs frequently came to serve in the armed services and with the police.

The peoples of Sarawak and Sabah are rather numerous. There are the Dyaks, Kayans, Kenyahs, Kelabits, and Muruts, while in Sabah there are Kadazans, Suluks and Bajaus, to name but a few. They share certain features in common both in culture and language.

The more common medical problems in the past have been tuberculosis, malaria, and yaws. However, malaria is now almost absent from the major cities, and an extensive eradication programme is underway. Yaws, too, is no longer a serious problem, and tuberculosis is being brought under satisfactory control. Of the three, probably malaria remains the most serious, affecting most of the rural areas. However non-toxic goitre, nutritional problems, iron-deficiency anaemia, and intestinal parasities are encountered rather frequently. Certain viral infections such as dengue and poliomyelitis are endemic.

Arteriosclerosis, hypertension, cerebrovascular disease, myocardial infarction, and diabetes are also seen. It is difficult to gauge their frequency in comparison with Western countries. Because of the predominance of Chinese and Indians in the cities and because more complete medical facilities are available there, these diseases may only *appear* to be more common in those groups than among the Malays. However, there do seem to be fewer cases of such illnesses among the latter, a fact which may be related to dietary habits and possibly genetic factors. There is very little alcoholism.

The government medical services are maintained by the Ministry of Health of the Federal Government. While there are only a few private hospitals, there has been a substantial increase in the number of nursing homes established by private practitioners. There is also a Faculty of Medicine with a university hospital located near the capital of Kuala Lumpur. Nevertheless most of the doctors are employed by the Government. At the time of Independence in 1957 there were very few specialists, but the numbers have substantially increased both in government and in private practice.

The major diagnostic facilities and the greater number of specialists are to be found in the general hospitals. Each of the major cities has a general hospital. Smaller cities have district hospitals, in some instances staffed by specialists, in others by medical officers. In still smaller towns there are district health centres, and in the rural areas there is an extensive health clinic programme. The rural health clinics and centres are staffed by hospital assistants and midwives.

Patients from the rural areas are referred to general hospitals from the district hospitals and rural clinics. Those from smaller cities may be referred by private practitioners as well. In the larger cities consultations from private practitioners are more frequent. Referrals and consultations are generally requested when diagnostic or therapeutic means are required which go beyond those available in the other facilities.

Whether a patient will come to a general hospital depends on several factors. Distance alone may make it unlikely; some patients in rural areas may never have ventured very far from their homes. A husband may be accompanied by his family to a district hospital, but it may be extremely difficult for them to accompany him should he require transfer to another hospital located many miles away from their home. Transportation and facilities for the family may be lacking. Moreover, there may be small children in the family who cannot be left alone and are too small to travel. In the case of a wife becoming ill the husband may be forced to leave his work and the family's source of income becomes curtailed.

Another factor is the fear that many have of dying far from their homes. Some, such as the Orang Asli, may have the superstition that if they were to die away from their homes their souls would not be able to find their way back to the village. Others may feel that they would not be permitted entry into heaven. Some, preferring to be buried at home, may refuse transfer to another hospital because they know that if they were to die, there would be no funds available for the transport of the remains back to their homes; and ordinarily no agency would pay for such a thing.

Yet another factor is the accumulative effect of being transported not only to an alien city, perhaps leaving loved ones behind, but also into an alien world of medicine where language barriers may be considerable, and where medical methods are not understood. The individual may feel himself utterly lost.

Sometimes the patient, at other times the family or friends, may postpone consulting a doctor trained in Western medicine. Medicine-men of other disciplines may be consulted. Some of these may engage in Shamanism, others may use herbs, acupuncture or astrology. Some patients or their families consult their religious authorities and advisers.

These factors have delayed early diagnosis and treatment of patients for many years. Even though the pattern is slowly changing for the better, many patients still seek medical treatment only very late in their illness. Because there is very little to be done at such a late stage, and in some instances a high percentage of the patients die, the family and friends may remain convinced that Western medicine has little to offer.

Moreover, once the patient has been hospitalized certain problems still exist in arriving at a diagnosis. While the history of the illness is of great importance, it is often incomplete. The relative lack of seasonal variations in weather makes it difficult to judge time. But of greater importance is the problem of language. Although Malay is the most common means of communication between races many specific terms referring to the body are absent from the language or are unknown to non-Malays. In some instances the patient may not know basic Malay adequately, and the history must be obtained in his own language by translation. This is particularly difficult in some of the Chinese dialects which may be understood by very few. The patient's history may be erroneously translated from one dialect to another. The physical examination therefore assumes a very great importance, much greater than in Western countries where more reliance is placed on the history of the illness.

Laboratory and X-ray procedures also become of great importance in arriving at an accurate diagnosis in a patient who is admitted quite late in the course of his illness. However, facilities for these procedures may be very limited in certain of the hospitals. Clinical acumen, often based on inadequate history, is required to establish the most probable diagnosis and to serve in the rapid initiation of treatment.

If the patient were to be found suffering from a surgical condition, effective treatment would have to be delayed because of the shortage of blood for transfusions, inadequate anaesthesia coverage, and the general medical status of the patient which may be quite poor. The patient may be found to be suffering from pulmonary tuberculosis, intestinal parasites, chronic malnutrition, iron-deficiency anaemia or a combination of any of the above. Surgery may have to be delayed for several weeks or cancelled altogether. But in emergency situations surgery often has to be undertaken with acceptance of these compromises.

Autopsies in the past have been more customarily obtained after death from trauma. Seldom is it possible to obtain an autopsy of a Muslim. Moreover, it is often difficult to obtain consent for autopsies on adults of other races and religions, with the exception, however, of Chinese children. It is thought by many of the more traditionally oriented Chinese that if a child dies he is demonstrating ingratitude to his parents—for the child is supposed to attend his parents at their deaths, failing which he will go to hell. If the child dies away from home, he cannot be held responsible by God because he cannot recognize his parents, and is therefore permitted to go to heaven. Therefore, Chinese parents often may not claim the body of their child and autopsy becomes possible.

NEUROLOGICAL PRACTICE IN KUALA LUMPUR

The following report is based on the investigation and treatment of approximately 5700 patients in Kuala Lumpur, Malaysia, seen over a period of 7 years. For the most part the patients came from urban areas and predominantly by referral from other general and district hospitals. Initially, approximately 50 to 60 per cent were Chinese, 30 per cent Indian with the remainder Malays. These ratios changed slowly to approximately 40 per cent Chinese, 30 per cent Indian and 30 per cent Malays, a fact indicative of a slow but progressively increasing number of patients admitted from rural areas.

Diagnosis was facilitated by the ability to carry out routine X-ray examinations and contrast studies, by the establishing of a neuropathology laboratory in March 1964, by the opening of an electroencephalography laboratory in 1966, and by the availability of an arboviral laboratory. A medical neurologist was not available, however, and may account for the lack or reduced numbers of observations of certain neurological disorders. It was generally the custom for doctors not to refer patients to the neurosurgical service unless it was felt that they were harbouring surgical lesions. In spite of this a number of medical problems were encountered.

Epilepsy

Hypsarrhythmia was not seen at all. Only rarely were consultations requested for electroencephalography of babies with 'spasms'.

Petit Mal

This was uncommon. Prior to the opening of our electroencephalography laboratory, several patients thought to be suffering from petit mal failed to respond to treatment adequately, and were subsequently found to be suffering from psychomotor seizures. It is possible that the mild episodes of petit mal either were not observed by the family or did not alarm them sufficiently to bring the patient to a doctor. It was usually when the seizures continued into adult life and changed their pattern that consultation occurred.

Centrencephalic Epilepsy

This was found on only one occasion. Other patients who presented with the picture on their initial EEGs were found on subsequent recordings to have focal epilepsy. Grand mal epilepsy was commonly seen and was of the idiopathic variety in approximately half the patients. About 50 per cent of those investigated with the adult onset of grand mal epilepsy proved to have a symptomatic form.

Grand Mal

Two common types of *grand mal* epilepsy were encountered which proved to be quite puzzling. One was that of a child or young adult experiencing both seizures and mental retardation. Frequently, behavioural disturbances were present and often to a marked degree, disrupting the family life. Both the seizures and behavioural disturbances were difficult to control. Only in approximately 20 per cent could a history be obtained of a probable cause such as birth trauma or neonatal injury or infection. Prenatal factors were seldom seen and toxoplasmosis was encountered only once. Microcephaly was seen on six occasions. It was not possible to carry out genetic studies, but the family histories received were non-contributory. As none of these children ever came to autopsy and they were only referred after several years, the aetiologies of approximately 80 per cent of them are unknown.

The second and even more baffling problem was that of several children who were referred with the development of seizures from 2 to 5 years of age followed by the subsequent onset of progressive psychomotor deterioration, usually associated with behavioural disturbances. The electroencephalogram would generally show multiple seizure foci superimposed on the moderately or markedly low background activity. In only one case was it possible to arrive at a probable aetiology. A cortical biopsy in that instance showed changes compatible with a viral encephalitis, consisting of glial shrubs and perivascular lymphocytic cuffing. Pneumoencephalography generally demonstrated varying degrees of cerebral atrophy. Family histories were uniformly unhelpful except for a familial history of epilepsy in three instances. None of these children came to autopsy.

Psychomotor seizures were seen frequently. This was the group in which the electroencephalogram was of the greatest help. We found approximately 50 per cent of such patients to have a surgical lesion such as a tumour, abscess or arteriovenous malformation.

Focal Sensory or Motor Seizures

These were quite commonly seen. With the exception of evidence of an inflammatory origin in approximately 25 per cent of such patients the other aetiologies were found in approximately the same percentage as in Western countries.

All patients with seizures would have an electroencephalogram, chest and skull X-rays, and appropriate blood chemistry determinations. All adults were admitted to the hospital for a lumbar puncture and a pneumoencephalogram was performed. If focal slow wave activity was found, the patient would ordinarily have angiography as well as pneumoencephalography. Brain scans were not available for the first several years, and subsequently only on a monthly basis.

The author had been told by several doctors that therapy with diphenylhydantoin and phenobarbital did not require the large dosages administered in Western countries, and that this same sensitivity to smaller amounts was also true for a number of other drugs. This could not be confirmed for the anticonvulsants, however, except that it was seldom necessary to administer more than two anticonvulsants and never more than three simultaneously. One disturbing complication of therapy with diphenylhydantoin was seen on several occasions; this was severe exfoliative dermatitis. It was seen on three occasions, involving the mucosae as well. No explanation of this could be found except for a presumed hypersensitivity to the drug. Samples of the drug were analysed in the United Kingdom and were found to be pure. These reactions occurred at dosage levels of 50 mg twice a day to 100 mg three times a day.

Congenital Malformations

Craniospinal Dysraphism

This was seen quite commonly. However, it was not possible to show that this occurred more commonly among any particular race or in any geographical area of the country. It was seen quite as often in Chinese as in Malays and Indians, whether they came from rural or urban areas.

Encephaloceles

These were usually nasal in location, similar to those found in Thailand, but unlike those found in Western countries, which tend to be occipital. Seldom was the lesion threatening to the life of the child affected but instead constituted a cosmetic defect and a potential threat to vision. The lesions were well covered by skin and were associated with a sizable defect in the region of the nasion, and extending for variable distances posteriorly through the cribriform plate, and bilaterally. At surgery the optic chiasma was frequently inspected, and both optic nerves were often found to be smaller than normal and quite pale. Frequently, adhesions were found in the region of the chiasmatic cistern, and some of these children had communicating hydrocephalus. With the absence of inflammatory reaction in the arachnoid, a possible explanation may be that the cisterns had failed to develop normally leading to the subsequent development of hydrocephalus. A few of these children also had seizures. A shunting procedure would ordinarily be required. Because of the young age of these patients it was not possible to evaluate their eyesight and visual fields adequately. In two or three older children and adults the visual fields appeared to be intact, as was the acuity, but this was in association with smaller lesions. The only ocular abnormality present was hypertelorism.

Occipital Encephaloceles

These were also encountered. These tended to be much larger in size with very thin skin coverage. The lesions seen did not involve the structures of the posterior fossa, but instead were supratentorial and always included an extension from the lateral ventricle of one side. The neck of the lesion contained choroid plexus and the lesion itself often consisted of loculated collections of brown or a xanthochromic fluid. These cysts and choroid plexus would be surrounded by a thin layer of dysgenetic cortex. Hydrocephalus was not present in these patients. Their eyesight and visual fields could not be adequately evaluated because of their age, but no gross defects were evident.

Meningomyeloceles

These were frequently encountered but were often referred too late for corrective surgery as damage had already been allowed to occur with the presence of meningitis which invariably ended in death. In those who survived and escaped this complication closure was carried out, but required the sacrifice of the neural plaque. Very few of these children had any appreciable function of the lower limbs or anal sphincter. Only four newborns were referred in whom surgery could be carried out within the first 96 hours of life. These four patients all survived and the plaque was spared. With one exception the lesions were located in the lumbosacral region.

No pure meningocele was encountered in infancy but several were encountered in older children and young adults. Lipomas were frequently found in association. These lesions usually extended from the subcutaneous tissue through the dural defect and were multilobulated. In general, they were bound to the roots of the cauda equina and required considerable dissection for removal. A 6-year-old child who had a well-covered lesion in the upper thoracic region had developed progressive paraplegia. The lesion was found to have a narrow stalk of fibrous tissue extending to the surface of the cord, associated with a subpial intramedullary lipoma at the verebral level of T4.

In those patients who were not experiencing neurological dysfunction, the lesions were often corrected for cosmetic purposes.

The patients with meningoceles never manifested hydrocephalus; on the other hand, those suffering from meningomyeloceles uniformly did. Contrast studies were performed shortly after surgery of the spinal lesion and invariably hydrocephalus was found to be present, often of a marked degree whether the head was enlarged or the anterior fontanelle appreciably tense. Shunting procedures would then be performed.

Pathological findings in babies dying with meningomyelocele revealed a small percentage with Arnold–Chiari malformation but a much larger percentage with forking of the aqueduct.

It was the author's impression that *craniospinal dysraphism* occurred more commonly than in the West, apparently without relation to racial difference and bearing distinct similarity to those lesions seen in Thailand. An epidemiological survey is required to establish the true incidence and pattern of such lesions and their possible relationship to genetic, toxic or nutritional factors.

Hereditary Disorders

No patients were found suffering from either suspected or proven *cerebral lipidoses.*

A few patients with *Laurence–Moon–Biedl syndrome* were seen. One family of boys had polydactyly of the toes.

Tuberous Sclerosis

This was more commonly encountered and on one occasion was found in association with von Recklinghausen's disease. One patient suffered from a subependymal giant cell astrocytoma obstructing the foramen of Monro on the right side. Although the lesion was resected, he developed recurrent signs of increased intracranial pressure 3 years later. At autopsy there was not only extensive recurrence of the tumour within the right ventricle but also an equally large neoplasm, apparently distinct from it, within the left lateral ventricle

The patient manifesting signs of both von Recklinghausen's disease and tuberous sclerosis had no family history of either illness. He had pituitary dwarfism and suprasellar calcification measuring 2 cm in diameter. He had developed progressive weakness of the legs and was found to have both an intradural and extradural neurinoma at the vertebral levels of T5 and T6. The chest X-ray had shown the presence of numerous large to moderately sized paraspinal shadows. The spinal cord tumour was resected. At the time of bilateral thoracotomy the paraspinal lesions were found to be multiple neurinomas. The child died following his chest operation, and at autopsy he showed the presence of several dozen neurinomas involving the paraspinal axis and the coeliac and mesenteric plexuses. None of these lesions was malignant. The calcified lesion was found to be a meningioma of the third ventricle. A smaller meningioma was found lying within the island of Reil subcortically.

Sturge–Weber Syndrome

This was seen on several occasions. However, it was more common to find the naevus of the face with no intracranial calcification or seizures.

Von Recklinghausen's Disease

This was by far the most common of the phacomatoses seen. In spite of close questioning and the occasional opportunity to examine other members of the family, very few patients were found to have members of their family affected, and even in those affected only cutaneous manifestations could be identified. The author does not feel that too much reliance should be placed on this observation, because family histories in general were difficult to obtain. Nevertheless, it may mean that there is less penetrance of the gene for the disease than is found in Western countries. Sometimes, in the examination of patients suffering from other illnesses, several *café au lait* spots would be identified, some of which were extremely large in size, but were not associated with neurinomas affecting the nervous system, nor with any other manifestations of von Recklinghausen's disease. One patient was found to be suffering from a malignant intradural neurinoma and he subsequently died with disseminated disease. X-ray therapy had not been of any appreciable benefit to him.

Von Recklinghausen's disease affected Chinese predominantly, but Indians were affected frequently. Although it was identified on several occasions in Malays the illness was decidedly less frequent in this group. No patients were found with phaeochromocytoma.

The types of tumour encountered consisted for the most part of spinal cord lesions. It is remarkable that none of the patients suffering from acoustic neurinomas or brain stem gliomas was found to be suffering from von Recklinghausen's disease. An optic nerve glioma was encountered twice. Several orbital neurinomas were found, sometimes in association with scalp tumours. Two lesions of the greater occipital nerve were seem; the tumour had eroded through the skull, and in one instance had produced a bruit because of the defect overlying the transverse sinus with kinking of the sinus. These latter lesions were plexiform in type.

Wilson's Disease

This was encountered twice, but no family history could be elicited and the families were not available for investigation. Both patients responded well to DL-penicillamine.

Laboratory facilities did not permit the examination of children for amino-aciduria. *Phenylketonuria* was never seen and was said not to exist. However, newborn babies were usually not examined for it.

No patients with the *parkinsonian-dementia complex* were encountered. However, several Chinese were seen suffering from *amyotrophic lateral sclerosis.* There was no positive family history. The illness tended to occur in older age-groups.

Although haemangioblastoma and other vascular neoplasms of the central nervous system were seen in a proportion larger than in the West, no cases of von Hippel–Lindau disease were encountered.

Friedreich's ataxia was seen on two occasions. Three patients with demonstrable atrophy of the pons and cerebellum, as confirmed by air studies and with the clinical manifestations of *olivopontocerebellar degeneration*, were seen. None of these patients ever came to autopsy, and pathological confirmation is therefore absent. None of them had a positive family history.

'Degenerative' Disorders

Multiple Sclerosis

The possibility of *multiple sclerosis* occurring in Malaysia and Singapore has been considered and discussed by a number of doctors for many years. However, there has never been autopsy confirmation of the presence of the disease. Nevertheless, it was the experience of several doctors that a small number of patients presenting with neurological signs would undoubtedly have been interpreted as suffering from multiple sclerosis if they had been seen in Western countries. This may be indicative of the readiness to make this diagnosis in Western countries in the face of unusual presentations, when in reality other pathological processes may be responsible. A still smaller number of patients presented with signs that were suggestive. The author saw two such patients, both of whom were Chinese. One was a 16-year-old boy who presented with sudden onset of a left fourth nerve palsy with monocular nystagmus. Spinal fluid findings were normal and there was no evidence to suggest an inflammatory process. His signs completely disappeared after 3 months. The second patient was a young Chinese girl who experienced her first attack (dysarthria, ataxia, diplopia and pyramidal signs) while undergoing higher studies in the United Kingdom. On her return she had a second similar episode, 2 years later.

Neuromyelitis Optica

Multiple sclerosis appears to be decidedly less frequent in Malaysia than in other countries located in temperate climates. However, patients with *neuromyelitis optica* were more commonly seen. For the most part these patients were also Chinese. The patient usually presented with bilateral retrobulbar neuritis or optic neuritis with almost total, and in some instances complete, blindness, and the development within a 6-month period of transverse myelitis. Sometimes the presenting signs were reversed in order. In two patients blindness had been present for an appreciable length of time, several years before the onset of the transverse myelitis. No autopsy studies were possible. The visual loss and paralysis were permanent. It must be borne in mind that a very high percentage of all the patients were Chinese, perhaps giving a false impression of the racial incidence. Furthermore, bilateral optic neuritis or retrobulbar neuritis were quite common, as was transverse myelitis, occurring independently of one another.

Infective Disorders

Brain Abscess

Sinusitis with mixed bacterial infection was quite common. The majority of patients suffering from *brain abscesses* had developed them as a sequela of sinusitis. Most were found to be located in the temporal region resulting from infection of the middle ear. Often the abscess would be connected by a stalk to the petrous bone. Some of the patients required surgery for the abscess before mastoidectomy could be carried out, and a few of these lesions recurred. A small number of patients were found with subdural empyema, but only rarely with epidural abscess. Two patients were found with a combination of thrombosis of the sagittal sinus, intracerebral abscess and subdural empyema. Both of these were children and survived. No children suffering from the long-term effects of venous sinus occlusion were found.

On three occasions brain abscesses were found unexpectedly. One had developed 14 years after a penetrating wound to the skull. Usually it was not possible to determine the source of infection when sinusitis was not present. In such patients endocarditis could not be found, nor active pulmonary disease.

Because of the frequency of brain abscess, contrast studies were often performed shortly after admission to determine whether one was present. If a child or young adult was admitted by referral with the possibility of abscess and the finding of increased intracranial pressure, an electroencephalogram would be obtained as quickly as possible through the use of needle electrodes. If focal slow wave activity was identified, an angiogram would be performed on that side. However, diffuse abnormalities were usually found. If the patient was moderately or markedly lethargic, a right carotid angiogram would be carried out immediately to determine the presence of hydrocephalus. The right side would be chosen in the absence of localized signs, because if complications from angiography were to occur, leading to hemiparesis, they would not affect the patient's dominant side and speech in most instances.

If the angiogram demonstrated changes compatible with hydrocephalus and the patient was moderately or markedly lethargic, a shunting procedure was performed as an emergency. The ventricular fluid would be studied. Indian ink preparations, protein and sugar levels would be determined. If the protein was elevated in an inflammatory process, there was a strong likelihood that cryptococcal meningitis would be found. Shortly after the shunting procedure, the lumbar puncture would be done and complete studies obtained. If the patient failed to show improvement following a shunting procedure in which hydrocephalus had definitely been present, the patient usually did not benefit from medical therapy and shortly died. By that time the disease was well advanced.

Most of the shunting procedures were ventriculo-atrial in type. In none of the patients who had presumed tuberculous meningitis and on whom shunting was performed, before or shortly after the commencement of antituberculous therapy, was there subsequent development of signs of miliary tuberculosis. It was felt that the shunting procedure could be safely performed in the presence of active tuberculous meningitis without jeopardizing the patient's life. In fact it was often a life-saving procedure in those patients who were suffering as much from increased intracranial pressure and the effects of hydrocephalus as from the inflammatory process itself.

Bacterial Meningitis

This would occasionally be seen either because of the referral for possible brain abscess, or because of symptoms and signs of increased intracranial pressure. The most disturbing aspect for the author, and for other specialists too, were the children or adults who had received some form of antibiotic therapy before coming to hospital and whose spinal fluid was free of organisms on smear and culture. The spinal fluid sugar in such cases would range from 20 to 40 mg per cent. The spinal fluid cell count would be between 100 and 500, with 50 per cent to 90 per cent polymorphonuclear leucocytes. Because of the prevalence of tuberculosis and the confusing spinal fluid findings, many of these patients would initially be started on therapy for bacterial meningitis as well as tuberculous meningitis. Because BCG was used in the country a positive skin test was seldom of any help.

Tuberculous Meningitis

Tuberculous meningitis was seldom proved by the culture of the organism or by smear, but was presumed to be present by the favourable response and recovery with the use of antituberculous medication. The therapy consisted of INH, streptomycin and PAS, with steroids administered whenever the spinal fluid protein was elevated more than 100 mg per cent. Steroids were not administered intrathecally. Vitamin B_6 was given routinely even though the author had been told that no patient with peripheral neuropathy from pyridoxine deficiency had ever been seen. The latter was again interpreted by several doctors as a Western manifestation of antituberculous therapy and quite uncommon in the tropics.

Following the recommendations and practice of other physicians in the country, the usual form of antibiotic therapy for bacterial meningitis would be penicillin, chloramphenicol and sulpha drugs. The author never detected the presence of aplastic anaemia or agranuloctyosis in any patients who received chloramphenicol nor did he learn of any such cases from other physicians.

On only one occasion was the tuberculous organism actually cultured from the spinal fluid. In that particular case six lumbar punctures were performed before finding the organism. On the other hand, pellicle formations were used as a strongly confirmatory test. Likewise, the spinal fluid chloride level was usually found to be low. This was used as an aid in diagnosis, and perhaps without much justification, but it was found to be lower than in patients with bacterial meningitis. The level of chloride did not seem to be dependent on vomiting. A low-grade fever would generally be present. If the fever was higher than 102°F and the patient was in coma the outcome was usually fatal. Steroids would be administered in large doses in such situations but without success.

Tuberculoma of the Brain

Seven patients with *tuberculomas of the brain* were encountered, considerably less than one might expect. It was thought that perhaps they were being overlooked. However, this is not likely to be the case. Although one tuberculoma was found in an aborigine child (Orang Asli), the others were in Indians. The author had thought that, as in the different types of leprosy encountered among the Malays, Chinese and Indians, tuberculosis might also have a more varied form of presentation dependent on the host reaction to the organism. Indians might therefore be more inclined to develop tuberculomas than other groups.

Extradural Abscesses of the Spinal Cord

These were seen on several occasions, more commonly occurring in younger adults. Some of the patients had survived the initial acute episode and presented with chronic extradural granulomas. The tissue contained staphylococci. These patients were usually completely paralysed on admission and would not recover. There was one exception to this. Even though surgery had been performed approximately 1 week after the onset of paraplegia, he subsequently regained his ability to walk, bladder control returned, and the sensory findings disappeared. He was left with mild spasticity. Those patients presenting more acutely had better results. In every instance the illness had begun with systemic symptoms of infection with a high fever. There was often an ascending progression of the lesion.

Metastatic Osteomyelitis of the Spine

This was seen on several occasions and was generally found to be staphylococcal in origin. One suspected case of brucellosis was operated upon but the aetiology could not be proven.

Tuberculous Involvement of the Spine

This was frequently seen, and more often than not involved the thoracic region. However, one case was seen in which the infection had destroyed the dens, and three patients were found with lesions of the lower lumbar vertebrae.

Cryptococcal Meningitis

This was found frequently. Many cases were seen and treated by physicians, but a sizable percentage were referred as patients with possible brain abscesses. Close questioning of the patients and their families failed to elicit any common denominator among environmental factors. The illness was encountered in those living in cities or rural areas alike; alike among those raising farm animals, such as chickens, and those who did not, and equally distributed among the three races. But, geographically, more patients were encountered from the north-western portion of Malaysia. The author had the initial impression that the structural appearance of the organism on Indian ink preparations differed from what he was accustomed to seeing in the United States, but serological studies on specimens submitted to laboratories in the United States and Switzerland failed to show any difference in strain.

Most of the patients were treated with amphotericin B, several requiring shunting procedures for hydrocephalus. Four patients were treated with 5-fluorocytosine alone and three in combination with amphotericin B. Three cases of cryptococcal granuloma were encountered; one presented initially with spinal fluid negative for the organism on both Indian ink preparation and culture, and was initially treated with antituberculous medication for over 1 year. During the early stages of his illness, when deterioration was occurring rapidly, he was given amphotericin B empirically for 1 week. Substantial improvement occurred in his level of consciousness, but the drug had to be discontinued because of adverse reaction. Further deterioration in his status lead to a second week's therapy with a similar improvement, after which the patient steadily improved while receiving antituberculous medication. Approximately 14 months later he appeared with a rapid onset of left hemiplegia. Angiography revealed a right temporal mass and surgery showed this to be a firm granular encapsulated lesion which proved to be a granuloma containing numerous cryptococci.

A second patient presented with seizures and personality alterations. Contrast studies revealed no abnormalities and the spinal fluid was normal. He was started on anticonvulsant medication. Within 2 months he was admitted to the hospital again. A history was obtained of head injury. An angiogram revealed a right temporal lesion and at surgery an intracerebral haematoma was evacuated. However, his condition failed to improve substantially except that he regained the use of his left side. There was no evidence of increased intracranial pressure until 2 months after discharge, when the left hemiparesis recurred and the patient became delirious. A repeat angiogram showed a space-occupying lesion in the right temporal lobe. Surgery on that occasion showed there to be a loculated cystic lesion containing some old blood pigment in the walls; it was a firm mass which histologically and on Indian ink preparation was found to contain many cryptococci.

It was not found helpful to rapidly increase the dose of amphotericin B if the patient's neurological status was rapidly deteriorating and hydrocephalus was not present. Such patients all died. The post-mortem examinations showed multiple cystic lesions in the substance of the brain with minimal inflammatory reaction here but a more marked inflammatory reaction at the base. The patients who responded satisfactorily were followed closely with serial lumbar punctures. It was found to be more helpful to take the spinal fluid sugar, protein and cell count as indicators of the activity of the disease, rather than the absence, persistence or reappearance of organisms. Serological tests were not available. It was found that the prognosis was considerably better the more rapidly the spinal fluid protein fell; however, a low spinal fluid sugar might persist for a considerable length of time, even though clinically the patient showed steady improvement. If few organisms were found on Indian ink preparation, but the spinal fluid sugar continued to be quite depressed, therapy was maintained. Amphotericin B was administered for 7 days with an interruption for a further 7 days before another course. This was felt to be more desirable than continuous administration on alternate days. If the spinal fluid protein progressively increased, it generally meant that hydrocephalus was developing. The patient would be observed closely for manifestations of increased intracranial pressure. If such signs appeared, a right carotid angiogram was performed. A shunting procedure followed if angiographic changes compatible with hydrocephalus were found, or if the vascular changes were questionable or lacking while the clinical suspicion of hydrocephalus was great.

In the patients receiving 5-fluorocytosine, it was found that budding forms and many organisms would be found for several weeks after the beginning of therapy when using this agent alone. Nevertheless, the clinical status of the patient would steadily improve although the spinal fluid sugar remained extremely low and was in some instances less than 10 mg per cent. Quite suddently, after 4 to 8 weeks of therapy, budding forms would cease to be seen and the numbers of organisms precipitously dropped. 5-Fluorocytosine was not used in patients who were severely ill.

A subcutaneous and extradural granuloma from *Allescheria boydii* was encountered in a Malay woman. This was located in the thoracic region and was apparently secondary to a remote fall with injury of her back.

One brain abscess secondary to *Candida albicans* infection was identified. This was apparently secondary to an infection of the middle ear.

One woman, who had been diagnosed as having *sarcoidosis* of the central nervous system and whose spinal fluid had been negative for cryptococci on several occasions, was subsequently admitted for increased intracranial pressure. She had been receiving high doses of steroids. She was found to be suffering from hydrocephalus and cryptococcal meningitis. It is presumed that the large doses of steroids used in treating her initial illness resulted in her subsequent contracting of cryptococcal meningitis.

No case of fungal infestation of the nervous system was encountered in patients receiving immunosuppressive therapy, but this form of treatment was not used widely.

Japanese Encephalitis

Of the *viral encephalitides*, Japanese encephalitis was by far the most common. The diagnosis was established on the basis of the demonstration of a fourfold or more rise in the titre of antibodies present in the blood. The organism was seldom cultured from spinal fluid. Even if the patient was only seen some time after the onset of the illness, it was occasionally possible to establish the probably aetiology by demonstrating a fall in the titre. Such titres generally persisted for 6 months.

The mortality rate of *Japanese encephalitis* was approximately 10 per cent and the prognosis was more favourable in children than in older people or Europeans. For the most part the disease was seen in Malaysian children and European adults. It was presumed that most children developed variable degrees of resistance to the disease through exposure, so that it was seldom encountered in adult life.

A number of other *arboviruses* have been isolated but they have not yet been found to be associated with any neurological disease, and in many instances with no evidence of clinical disease of any type. A new strain of Japanese encephalitis virus was isolated.

Herpes Simplex Virus

This was isolated from one patient in Malaysia, and to the author's knowledge it is the only proven case thus far. It occurred in a 10-year-old Chinese boy who presented with progressive coma, and sudden and marked fever with progressive collapse. There were no localizing signs and no evidence of a space-occupying lesion. Within 2 days he had died. The isolation was made from brain tissue obtained at post-mortem. Histological examination of the brain confirmed changes compatible with herpetic encephalitis.

Kkru

No patients resembling those described with *kuru* have been seen.

Leptospirosis

This has been extensively studied in Malaysia for many years. Although it is known to be associated with meningismus and other symptoms of central nervous system involvement only one patient was encountered in the Department of Neurosurgery. He was a laboratory assistant working with the organism daily. More serious neurological complications, including transverse myelitis, had been described previously by several authors but we were unable to identify any of these.

Acute Transverse Myelitis

This was seen perhaps four or five times per year. Over half the cases occurred in childhood. The disease would develop suddenly, sometimes preceded by fever for 1 to 2 days and usually immediately preceded by the onset of interscapular pain, followed quite shortly by the rapid progression of paraplegia. No space-occupying lesion could be identified, and the spinal fluid examinations were usually normal with the occasional finding of a mild increase in the protein and cell counts. It was in this group of patients that all the known infectious agents that have been described as producing this type of pathology were looked for; none were found. This included schistosomiasis and scrub typhus.

Arachnoiditis

Adhesive arachnoiditis of the spinal cord, and less frequently of the posterior fossa, was seen in 23 patients who eventually went to surgery. The most common denominator, accounting for 14 of these patients, was a previous history of tuberculosis, even in the absence of tuberculous meningitis. Two patients had a history of tuberculous meningitis, and following surgery on one of them the tuberculous meningitis recurred. The leptomeninges and the adhesions were not cultured on any of these cases. The arachnoiditis appeared to occur in three stages. In the earliest lesions rather delicate adhesions were present, and were responsible for progressive cord compression, these were avascular and could in most instances be readily broken up. In the second stage the adhesions were more numerous, thicker and vascularized to a mild degree. Complete lysis was more difficult and time-consuming, but could still be achieved in many instances. In the third stage the adhesions were extremely dense and fibrous with considerable collagenous components and a rich vascularity binding the spinal cord down to where it appeared as a cord or rope. In these instances not only was dissection almost impossible but there was also the fear that these vessels might possibly be supplying the spinal cord itself, and that interruption of them to any considerable degree would compromise cord function. When the author was less experienced with this particular stage of arachnoiditis two patients were made worse by surgery. In all these patients the arachnoiditis extended over several segments, and in a few involved the entire spinal cord including the cauda equina. The posterior fossa arachnoiditis occurred only in one patient, and had followed an undiagnosed inflammatory process of the meninges for which the patient had received some unknown form of therapy. He was treated with a shunting procedure.

One of the above patients was found to have arachnoiditis involving two vertebral levels in the lower thoracic region in association with a large subcutaneous granuloma in which colonies of *Allescheria boydii* were seen. Severe pachymeningitis was also present at the same level. In view of this finding, the material removed from other patients with arachnoiditis is being studied to determine whether a mycotic infection could have been responsible.

The above cases do not include those seen following trauma to the spine, nor the very localized arachnoiditis occasionally encountered about roots in the lumbar region; nor do they include one patient in whom an arachnoid cyst was found.

Eosinophilic Meningitis

Because of the recent interest in *eosinophilic meningitis* occurring in the Pacific and South-East Asian areas, the syndrome was looked for intensively in the department. The vector and the parasite, *Angiostrongylus*, are known to exist in West Malaysia. However, this specific disease has not yet been encountered at Kuala Lumpur. On the other hand, there have been case-reports from Sarawak, although only one patient with eosinophilic meningitis has been seen in West Malaysia between 1965 and 1970. This patient, a Chinese male of approximately 38 years of age, had complained of chronic dull aching headaches for several weeks before being seen. He had a progressive rise in spinal fluid protein, and a persistent increased cell count consisting of 40 to 60 per cent eosinophils with the rest being lymphocytes. Over repeated admissions various tests were carried out after sending blood samples to three different centres. The spinal fluid was also examined on many occasions with the withdrawal of large amounts of fluid. Syphilis, trichinosis, ascariasis, cysticercosis, sarcoidosis, toxoplasmosis, filariasis and gnathostomiasis were ruled out. It was the feeling of several investigators in other countries, as well as of the parasitologist of the Institute for Medical Research in Kuala Lumpur, that the patient in all likelihood did not have *Angiostrongylus* infestation because of the chronicity of his illness. When last seen approximately 1 year after the onset of his symptoms, his headaches were unchanged and the spinal fluid protein was approximately 140 mg per cent. He had received steroid therapy for several months without any appreciable effect on the protein level. No additional neurological signs had appeared in the meantime. The aetiology of his illness remains unknown, and the true extent of this syndrome in Malaysia is unknown. In view of the large number of cases that have been described in Thailand and the few case-reports from East Malaysia, it would be remarkable if the syndrome were not encountered more frequently and the specific illness of *Angiostrongylus* infestation diagnosed.

Cysticercosis and *echinococcosis* were not encountered.

Vascular Disorders

Cerebral Thrombosis

Cerebrovascular disease, with or without hypertension, was more commonly found in Chinese, Indians and Sikhs than in the Malays. The type of lesion most commonly found was that of *cerebral thrombosis*. Many patients with cerebrovascular accidents were not referred to the neurosurgical service unless there was a suspicion that they had sustained primary subarachnoid haemorrhage. For this reason the actual situation with regard to racial predominance and types of pathology is not known. Carotid artery disease was encountered but always when the vessel was completely occluded. *Intracerebral haemorrhage* was seldom seen.

Congenital Intracranial Aneurysms

These were very uncommon. Excluding those found in Europeans they were almost entirely confined to the Chinese. The lesion in this condition was frequently fusiform in shape, involving one or more branches, and usually affecting the middle cerebral artery. In those lesions removed at surgery, as well as from observation of those which were only clipped, there was extensive arteriosclerosis of both the aneurysm and the parent vessel and branches. Only two patients with mycotic aneurysms were investigated, and both were found to be suffering from endocarditis.

The few congenital aneurysms were usually located on the internal carotid artery at the point of bifurcation with a smaller number present at the trifurcation of the middle cerebral artery. Only one aneurysm of the anterior communicating artery was found, and a giant aneurysm of the internal carotid artery was found in another patient.

Congenital intracranial aneurysms are uncommon throughout South-East Asia. The author thought that perhaps sociological factors might be partially responsible. A 'stroke' was commonly known as an illness of adult life and accepted as untreatable. The adult would either die, be treated at home by members of the family, or be seen by a doctor who might also be content with the diagnosis of 'stroke', particularly if the patient had hypertension. On the other hand, a child or young adult sustaining something similar to a 'stroke' would be treated with more alarm, and perhaps eventually found to have an arteriovenous malformation. The older adult would recover or die without angiography. Although this might account for some of the discrepancy in the incidence between the East and West, neurological and neurosurgical centres throughout the area have consistently reported few aneurysms.

Arteriovenous Malformations

These outnumbered the aneurysms 10 to 1. Approximately two-thirds of these lesions had bled. They tended to manifest themselves first between the ages of 10 and 30 years. Those which bled were usually small in size, measuring up to 4 cm in diameter. Whenever possible they were treated by excision. The larger lesions produced symptoms either of seizures or of progressive neurological deficit. When associated with progressive hemiparesis they were treated with embolization, and on occasion by the subsequent ligation of some of their major feeding vessels. The patients experiencing controllable seizures were not operated upon. No arteriovenous malformations of the spinal cord were found.

Neuropathies

Diabetes

Diabetes was encountered in Chinese, Malays and Indians. Peripheral neuropathy, particularly of the oculomotor and femoral nerves often would occur before systemic manifestations. *Leprosy* was the most common neuropathy in the country but not the most common seen in the Department. Instead, *diabetes* was more often encountered, and frequently before other clinical manifestations of the disease. The diagnosis would be made on the basis of an initial blood sugar study, a glucose-tolerance test using 50 g of glucose, and subsequently of the administration of 1 g of glucose per kg of body weight.

The Guillain–Barré Syndrome

This was seen on many occasions. Steroid therapy was usually instituted but no controlled study was carried out. The youngest patients tended to make a more complete recovery than the older ones. In almost every instance the illness was preceded by a mild upper respiratory tract infection. Relapses were seen several times, particularly in two patients whose steroids had been discontinued. Improvement again became evident when steroid therapy was recommenced.

Subacute Combined Degeneration

This, together with peripheral neuropathy secondary to vitamin B_{12} deficiency, was said not to occur. *Megaloblastic anaemia of pregnancy* was seen frequently, however. We were never able to prove or disprove the presence of pernicious anaemia itself, nor did we encounter a patient with the more typical manifestations of subacute combined degeneration. The author learned that the diagnosis had been made in two or three patients in Singapore.

Tapioca (Cassava) Poisioning

This was suspected in one patient, an aborigine woman who had experienced recurrent ulnar neuropathy on three occasions before presenting with weakness of both legs of a flaccid type and minimal sensory changes. The spinal fluid was non-contributory. Because all new admissions were placed on vitamin therapy we could not make the diagnosis. Cyanide levels of the blood and urine were normal. This disease may very well occur in Malaysia, particularly among the Orang Asli, because of this group's high dietary intake of tapioca, or cassava.

Leprosy

Although most of the patients with leprosy were referred for surgical procedures to relieve pain, or in one instance for the debridement and drainage of an extensive abscess, a few patients were seen in whom the diagnosis had not been made before. One such patient was a 7-year-old Chinese girl who had developed a progressive and ultimately total ulnar nerve palsy. She was found to have a left supracondylar firm mass, measuring about 2 cm in diameter, which on soft tissue X-ray revealed a small amount of calcification. This was found to be a granuloma containing very few acid-fast organisms. It had destroyed the entire substance of the ulnar nerve. There were a few skin manifestations in the left hand. Another patient, a young adult Chinese male, had evidence of a carpal-tunnel syndrome. There were no skin manifestations of the disease nor any other peripheral nerve involvement. At surgery, on transecting the carpal ligament, the nerve was found to be soft, swollen and yellowish in colour. A small biopsy was taken and showed necrosis with one giant cell. No acid-fast organisms were found. A lepromin skin test was strongly positive. Antileprous medication was administered for over 3 years with no progression of the disease and almost total recovery of function.

A third patient was referred because of the presence of painless ulcers and wounds of the feet. This 11-year-old Chinese boy had stocking distribution of sensory loss of both legs. He had no cutaneous manifestations of leprosy. Diagnosis was made by sural biopsy and the lepromin skin test. No organisms were found. He was started on therapy, and the ulcers healed. He had no evidence of arthropathy. One elderly Indian male presented with the clinical manifestations of tardy ulnar nerve palsy and was found to have borderline lepromatous leprosy. Most patients presenting to the neurosurgical service, and subsequently found to be suffering from leprosy, had the tuberculoid form of the disease with minimal or no cutaneous manifestations.

Collagen Diseases

The collagen diseases are said to be much less frequent than in Western countries, perhaps on a genetic basis or due to the lack of exposure to antigenic substances.

Lupus Erythematosus

Lupus erythematosus was found to be present in three patients; all three were women. One presented with marked progressive lethargy and bilateral third nerve involvement closely resembling the clinical description of von Economo's encephalitis. Nine positive LE preparations were obtained. Steroid therapy was employed, after which she made a complete recovery. Another young woman presented with left hemiparesis. Her angiogram demonstrated a sausage-like deformity of the middle cerebral artery with evidence of obstruction in its midportion as well as collateral filling. Although lupus erythematosus was looked for frequently it was very seldom found.

Polyarteritis

This was proven in only one patient. He was a European male who presented with ulnar neuropathy. Diagnosis was established by cutaneous biopsy of a nodular red lesion of the thumb. He became asymptomatic on steroids. The author did not encounter any Malaysian patients with this disease.

On the other hand a baffling case was encountered in 1969 affecting a young Chinese male adult, who had injured his left ankle and had developed an ulcer at the site of injury which had failed to heal. He worked for the Department of Fisheries in bacteriological research but we were not able to learn the exact type of research in which he was engaged. The ulcer of the ankle became associated with severe pain and diffuse swelling of the entire foot requiring his admission to another hospital where the lesion was incised. No biopsy or culture was made. Antibiotics were administered. Five days later he was found by his father in bed, lethargic, complaining of severe headache and with marked swelling of his entire face and neck. A doctor on examining him found papilloedema and referred him to Kuala Lumpur. Other evidence of superior vena cava occlusion was observed but there were no other findings. The ulcer measured only $1\frac{1}{2}$ cm in diameter, had a granulating base, and turned-in edges. It was shallow. A biopsy of the lesion revealed only chronic inflammatory reaction. Stains and cultures for bacteria and fungi were negative. A right carotid angiogram failed to reveal any abnormalities, including venous sinus thrombosis. No studies were made of the superior vena cava. A chest X-ray was entirely normal, and a bone-marrow aspiration was negative. However, the patient had a peripheral white count of approximately 12 000 and a markedly elevated sedimentation rate. Quite suddenly he developed right hemiplegia with aphasia. A left carotid angiogram showed an avascular mass in the left temporal lobe, which at surgery was found to be an intracerebral haematoma measuring approximately 6×10 cm in surface area. A biopsy was made from the wall and showed evidence of panvasculitis with necrosis of some of the vessel walls and varying stages of occlusion and recanalization of the lumina. Despite steroid therapy he died, and no post-mortem examination was permitted. The family and the patient had been questioned closely about drug therapy, recent immunizations, and histories of allergy, skin rashes, etc. No causative agent was identified and it was assumed that he was suffering from a diffuse vasculitis, necrotizing in type, possibly of bacterial origin.

Myopathies

Muscular Dystrophy

Patients with *muscular dystrophy* were seen primarily by the paediatric and orthopaedic services. Nevertheless, they were occasionally seen by the Department of Neurosurgery. They did not appear to differ in type from those found in Western countries. The incidence and racial patterns are not known.

Myasthenia Gravis

This was seen on only two occasions. It is not known whether this illness is more or less common than it is in Western countries, since ordinarily such patients would have been seen by the Department of Medicine. In speaking with physicians, the author was told on several occasions that their experience with the disease was quite limited and that very few patients had been encountered.

Polymyositis

Polymyositis of the clinical types familiar to Western doctors was seen in three male patients over this period of 7 years, and in varying degrees of severity. Two of them responded quite well to steroid therapy but one of the patients, a young Indian male, had a more chronic involvement and continued to show progression. However, muscle biopsy was not diagnostic, and it is quite possible that he had some other form of myopathy.

Giant Cell Arteritis

This was only encountered once, and then in an elderly Chinese male who was rapidly losing the sight of his left eye. Steroid therapy reversed this. He experienced a perforated peptic ulcer but survived. It was necessary to withdraw steroid therapy. He was lost to follow-up, and we do not know the eventual outcome.

Trauma

Most of the patients seen had suffered from motor vehicle accidents, although a number were seen who had fallen from trees, particularly during the fruit seasons. Alcoholism was rare and the same was true of acute alcoholic intoxication associated with head injuries.

Extradural Haematoma

Extradural haematoma of the brain is said to be quite uncommon in American Negroes. It has been suggested that perhaps variations in the shape and thickness of the skull would produce a different incidence among various populations. Skull variations are certainly present among the Malays, Indians, and Chinese but do not appear to affect the incidence or manifestations of the lesions. Such haematomas were seen frequently in all population groups in Malaysia, and did not differ in any respect from those found in Western countries. Venous extradural haematomas arising from tearing of one of the major venous sinuses or from extensive bleeding from the diploë were also seen.

The mortality rate in extradural haematoma was generally related to delays in diagnosis and surgery.

However, the high mortality rate in acute subdural haematoma appeared to be independent of these factors. The mortality and morbidity rates quite closely parallel those reported from Western countries. The autopsy presentation of such cases was almost stereotyped. The source of bleeding was almost always from severe maceration and contusion of the orbital surfaces of the frontal lobe and both temporal lobes. This was often equal but sometimes asymmetrical. Such patients would generally be admitted with small fixed pupils showing a progression within 24 to 48 hours to bilateraly fixed, dilated pupils. Their coma would persist. They would frequently develop a very high fever shortly after admission. This was difficult to control. It was not like that seen with hypothalamic lesions, where the extremities are cold, with peripheral vascular constriction. Instead there would be profuse sweating. A few patients benefited from surgery, with the removal of subdural clot. Emergency angiography was not available for the first 5 years of the period in question. Burr-holes and subtemporal craniectomies were performed from the clinical findings.

Several children and adults were seen with massive post-traumatic haematomas of the scalp, and with a history of easy bruising. When diagnostic facilities became available, these patients were found to be suffering from haemophilia.

Intracerebral Haematoma

Isolated post-traumatic *intracerebral haematomas* producing progressive neurological deficit were rare. None of the patients coming to autopsy with acute head injuries demonstrated an isolated intracerebral haematoma. Even though haematomas were present in the temporal lobes, in many instances they occurred in association with marked maceration and laceration of the entire undersurface of the frontal lobes and the rostral portion of the temporal lobes.

One patient who presented with coma and fixed, dilated pupils following a head injury was an adolescent Chinese boy who had been struck at the vertex of the skull with a volley ball. We found a fibrosarcoma which had eroded through the bone. The volley ball had struck this tumour causing sudden massive haemorrhage leading to an acute vertical bilateral extradural haematoma.

Penetrating injuries of the skull and spine from missiles were seen infrequently. Military ammunition was usually involved. They were managed on the principles established during the Second World War and the Korean conflict.

Spinal Injuries

These were identical to those found in Western countries with the exception of injuries sustained in falling from trees while picking fruit. The patient, usually a child or young adult, would land on his buttock and sustain a compression fracture or a fracture-dislocation, sometimes with lateral displacement, of the lower thoracic or upper lumbar vertebrae, with involvement of either the conus medullaris or cauda equina. They were usually operated upon to determine the extent of injury to the neural elements and to remove any blood clots that might be present. Surgery probably played little role in the patient's subsequent recovery. Nevertheless, the observations at surgery did serve as an indicator of the likely degree of recovery.

Toxic Disorders

There was only one patient seen by the author who may possibly have died of an exogenous toxic compound. He was a 35-year-old Chinese male who was admitted with progressive coma, high fever, and focal seizures which eventually became generalized. His fever rose to 105° and 106°F, progressing to profound coma with bilaterally fixed, dilated pupils. Angiography had revealed no space-occupying lesion. Burr-holes were made to determine whether there might be appreciable ventricular enlargement and to institute constant ventricular drainage. No hydrocephalus was found, but cerebral oedema was marked. Steroids and intravenous urea were administered. He died 3 days after admission. At autopsy multiple petechial haemorrhages were found throughout the substance of the white matter, particularly in the corpus callosum but also extending into the cortex. On questioning the family it was learned that he had been taking drugs obtained from a traditional Chinese doctor. Since a number of drugs used by such practitioners contain arsenic, a search was made for his medications only to find that they had been discarded. Unfortunately no material had been obtained for viral isolation. There was no evidence of malaria.

Neoplasms

A higher percentage of benign tumours of the central nervous system was encountered than in Western countries. This was particularly noticeable for the 3 years following the opening of the Department of Neurosurgery, but there was subsequently a slow increase in the percentage of malignant tumours. This perhaps indicated that a number of potential patients had died before reaching the Department or before facilities were available for their diagnosis and treatment. This was certainly true for adults, but in the case of children malignant tumours predominated. In addition to the difference in the ratio of benign to malignant neoplasms there was also the added factor that certain types of tumours were apparently more common than in the West. For instance it is difficult to explain why so many patients with clinical manifestation of von Recklinghausen's disease were seen unless the illness is more common in Malaysia. The same is also true of the brain stem gliomas and primary intracranial sarcomas.

Meningiomas Total: 65

1. *Location*			
Intracranial		*Spinal*	
Parasagittal	18	Thoracic, upper	3
Sphenoid wing	10	Thoracic, lower	2
Convexity	8	Cervical	1
Falx	8		
Pterion	4		
Olfactory groove	3		
Tentorium	3		
Cerebellopontine angle	2		
Intraventricular (lateral)	2		
Tuberculum sellae	1		
Total:	*59*	*Total:*	*6*
2. *Sex*			
Female	36	Female	5
Male	23	Male	1
3. *Race*			
Chinese		*Chinese*	
Female	22	Female	3
Male	11	Male	1
Malay		*Malay*	
Female	9	Female	1
Male	8		
Indian		*Indian*	
Female	5	Female	1
Male	2		
Orang Asli			
Male	1		
Sikh			
Male	1		
4. *Average age*			
47 yrs		51 yrs	

The patients subsequently found to have intracranial meningiomas would frequently be seen and treated at a very late stage of their illness. A few were too ill to be operated upon, and in some instances would refuse surgery. The incidence of blindness secondary to increased intracranial pressure and chronic papilloedema was approximately 35 per cent. Dementia, profound hemiplegia, marked lethargy, or semiconsciousness were often the immediate manifestations at the time of admission.

Histologically most of the meningiomas proved to be of the meningotheliomatous and fibroblastic types. There were two invasive lesions of the skull and scalp but without evidence of malignancy. Only one demonstrated malignant changes.

Gliomas

A. Ependymomas—Total: 35

1. *Location*		*Spinal* 0
Intracranial		
4th ventricle	26	
3rd ventricle	5	
Lateral ventricle	2	
Septum pellucidum	1	
Cerebellar hemisphere	1	
Total:	*35*	
2. *Sex*		
Female	13	
Male	22	
3. *Race*		
Chinese		
Female	9	
Male	14	
Malay		
Female	2	
Male	5	
Indian		
Female	1	
Male	2	
Iban		
Female	1	
Kenyah		
Male	1	
4. *Average age*		
11 yrs		

Ependymomas

Because of the frequency with which this tumour was found, the histology of the lesions was re-examined on several occasions. They conformed to the histological appearances of the ependymoma. Those children with lesions of the fourth ventricle would seldom present with blindness. Their histories would be of short duration, in some instances only a few days. They would manifest lethargy, papilloedema, cerebellar signs, and stiffness of the neck. The patients in whom the lesion was located within the third ventricle presented greater diagnostic problems. Chronic papilloedema or primary optic atrophy with varying degrees of visual impairment, and not infrequently slight manifestations of unilateral motor impairment, were noted. In general, lesions of the third ventricle were found to be more frequent than has been reported in Western countries. In the absence of signs referable to the posterior fossa, a lesion of the third ventricle would be looked for closely.

B. Medulloblastomas—Total: 6

1. *Location* *Intracranial* 4th ventricle	 *6*
2. *Sex* Female Male	 1 5
3. *Race* Chinese Indian	 5 1
4. *Average age*	3 yrs

In contrast to the ependymomas the children with medulloblastomas were very few and considerably younger. The author has no explanation for this difference in incidence.

C. Oligodendrogliomas—Total: 4

1. *Location* Laterial ventricle 3rd ventricle *Total:*	 2 2 *4*
2. *Sex* Female Male	 1 3
3. *Race* *Chinese* Female Male *Iban* Male	 1 1 2
4. *Average age*	27 yrs

As noted above these lesions were found within the ventricular system. Mixed gliomas containing oligodendroglial elements were seen, but are listed elsewhere. The tumours of the lateral ventricle would be extremely large in size before producing symptoms of increased intracranial pressure and focal neurological findings. Those within the third ventricle would produce hydrocephalus. Even though they probably arose from the region of the diencephalon, focal neurological signs were usually absent.

D. Astrocytomas—Total: 18

1. *Location* *Intracranial* Cerebral hemisphere 3rd ventricle Optic nerve Lateral ventricle *Total:*	 9 5 1 1 *16*	 *Spinal* Thoracic Conus *Total:*	 1 1 *2*
2. *Sex* Female Male	 5 11	 Male	 *2*
3. *Race* *Chinese* Female Male *Malay* Male *Indian* Male *Thai* Female *Kadazan* Male	 3 6 3 2 1 1	 *Chinese* Male	 2
4. *Average age* 27 yrs			

Only a very small number of benign astrocytomas were found affecting the supratentorial region. Again, the rather large number of lesions encountered within the third ventricle should be noted. The one tumour affecting the optic nerve occurred in association with von Recklinghausen's disease.

E. Cerebellar Astrocytomas—Total: 14

1. *Sex* Female Male	 3 11
2. *Race* *Chinese* Female Male *Malay* Male *European* Male	 3 4 6 1
3. *Average age*	11 yrs

These lesions have been separated from the astrocytomas affecting the supratentorial region because of their more distinctive symptomatology and their occurrence at a much younger age. While the cerebral astrocytomas were found more frequently in the Chinese, the cerebellar astrocytoma was found almost as frequently in the Malay. One lesion demonstrated the histological appearance of glioblastoma.

F. Glioblastomas—Total: 22

1. *Location*		*Spinal* 0
Intracranial		
Cerebral hemisphere	21	
3rd ventricle	1	
Total:	*22*	
2. *Sex*		
Female	8	
Male	14	
3. *Race*		
Chinese		
Female	7	
Male	8	
Malay		
Female	1	
Male	3	
Indian		
Male	2	
European		
Male	1	
4. *Average age*		
33 yrs		

The racial predominance of the Chinese is still manifest, as is the larger number of males affected. With the exception of the mixed gliomas the ratio of male to female for all the gliomas was 2 or 3 : 1.

The author separated the gliomas affecting the brain stem from the astrocytomas and glioblastomas occurring elsewhere in order to demonstrate the rather high incidence. All but one of the tumours has been confirmed histologically. All but two were malignant. A small number demonstrated a mixed cellular composition. Sixteen of the lesions were grossly haemorrhagic at autopsy.

In contrast to the experience in Western countries, the children would present with manifestations of increased intracranial pressure and hydrocephalus. Two or more cranial nerve palsies would be identified in association with long tract findings. A shunting procedure would be performed for the relief of hydrocephalus. Approximately half of the patients were treated with X-ray therapy. Only one patient survived longer than 1 year, and radiation therapy did not seem to be of benefit. The degree of haemorrhage and necrosis could not be correlated with antecedent administration of X-ray therapy. It has been noted that von

G. Gliomas of the Brain Stem—Total: 19

1. *Sex*	
Female	6
Male	13
2. *Race*	
Chinese	
Female	6
Male	11
Indian	
Male	1
Sikh	
Male	1
3. *Average age*	11 yrs

H. Mixed Gliomas—Total: 7

1. *Location*		*Spinal* 0
Intracranial		
Lateral ventricle	4	
Subependymal		
Cellular types:		
Ependymoma:		
Astrocytoma	2	
Ependymoma:		
Oligodendroglioma	2	
Cerebral hemisphere	2	
Cellular type:		
Astrocytoma:		
Oligodendroglioma	2	
Cerebellum	1	
Cellular type:		
Astrocytoma:		
Ependymoma	1	
2. *Sex*		
Female	5	
Male	2	
3. *Race*		
Chinese		
Female	5	
Male	2	
4. *Average age*		
23 yrs		

Recklinghausen's disease was commonly seen, but it is remarkable that none of the children suffering from gliomas of the brain stem revealed any manifestations of von Recklinghausen's disease.

The tumours tended to contain an ependymal element when located near or within the ventricle, and an astrocytic component when located further away from the ventricular system. The mixed glioma was found more commonly in females, in contrast to the other gliomas, and they were seen entirely in Chinese.

Craniopharyngiomas—Total: 17

1. *Sex*	
Female	4
Male	13
2. *Race*	
Chinese	
Female	2
Male	12
Malay	
Female	2
Male	1
3. *Average age*	16 yrs
below age 16–10 yrs	12 patients
above age 16–31 yrs	5 patients

Almost all these lesions were calcified. One was located entirely within the third ventricle, and another was encountered completely within an extremely large sella with destruction of the sphenoid sinus. The Babinski-Fröhlich syndrome was found twice. Hydrocephalus was usually marked. Visual impairment of a moderate to marked degree was associated with primary optic atrophy.

Pituitary Adenomas—Total: 15

A. Chromophobe—9

1. *Sex*	
Female	4
Male	5
2. *Race*	
Chinese	
Female	4
Male	2
Indian	
Male	2
Malay	
Male	1
3. *Average age*	41 yrs

B. Eosinophilic—1

1. *Sex*	
Male	1
2. *Race*	
Eurasian	1
3. *Average age*	57 yrs

C. Mixed—5

1. *Sex*	
Female	3
Male	2
2. *Race*	
Chinese	
Female	2
Male	2
European	
Female	1
3. *Average age*	28 yrs

The mixed adenomas tended to occur at a younger age. The patients manifested signs of pituitary insufficiency. One presented with acromegaly, and the lesion was mixed in cellular type.

Choroid Plexus Papilloma—Total: 4

1. *Location*	
Lateral ventricle	2
Third ventricle	1
Fourth ventricle	1
2. *Sex*	
Female	1
Male	3
3. *Race*	
Chinese	
Male	2
Malay	
Female	1
Male	1
4. *Average age*	22 yrs

One of these tumours showed histological evidence of malignancy, ultimately recurred, and was fatal. The lesion located within the fourth ventricle produced intermittent symptoms of increased intracranial pressure and was found only through the repetition of contrast studies.

Neurinomas—Total: 70

1. *Location*			
Intracranial		*Spinal*	
Posterior fossa	*36*	Cervical	6
Acoustic	33	Thoracic	18
Jugular foramen	1	Lumbar	4
5th nerve root	1		
12th cranial nerve	1		
2. *Sex*			
Female	18	Female	7
Male	18	Male	21
3. *Race*			
Chinese		*Chinese*	
Female	10	Female	4
Male	12	Male	10
Malay		*Malay*	
Female	4	Female	2
Male	5	Male	7
Indian		*Indian*	
Female	1	Female	1
Male	1	Male	4
Eurasian			
Female	1		
Orang Asli			
Female	1		
Sikh			
Male	1		
4. *Average age*	39 yrs	37 yrs	
1. *Location*			
Orbit	4		
2. *Sex*			
Female	1		
Male	3		
3. *Race*			
Chinese			
Female	1		
Male	1		
Malay			
Male	2		
4. *Average age*	18 yrs		
1. *Location*			
Occipital nerve	2		
2. *Race*			
Indian			
Male	1		
Malay			
Female	1		

The neurinoma was the most common tumour. Only two patients suffering from acoustic neurinomas showed evidence of von Recklinghausen's disease; whereas nine of those with spinal cord tumours manifested the disease. The one patient with a tumour affecting the fifth nerve root had several *café au lait* lesions of the skin. The ratio of male to female was equal in those having intracranial lesions, but males predominated in those with spinal cord tumours.

Four of the tumours occurred within the orbit. Two were found in association with von Recklinghausen's disease. Two lesions affected the greater occipital nerve and had eroded through the skull.

Phaeochromocytomas were not found. Of the spinal cases, one of the patients had a malignant neurinoma and subsequently died with multiple malignant lesions of the abdomen. Approximately half of the spinal cord tumours were extradural for the most part or entirely, with the other half well-circumscribed, intradural lesions. They tended to be more necrotic than the acoustic neurinoma. Special stains for mast cells revealed them to be abundant when necrotic changes were extensive.

Haemangioblastomas—Total: 10

1. *Location*			
Intracranial	*9*	*Spinal*	1
Posterior fossa	7	Cauda equina	1
2. *Sex*		*Chinese*	
Female	5	Male	1
Male	2		
3. *Race*			
Chinese			
Female	5		
Male	1		
Indian			
Male	1		
4. *Average age*	38 yrs		
1. *Location*			
Cerebral	2		
2. *Race*			
Chinese			
Male	2		
3. *Average age*	25 yrs		

No patients with von Hippel–Lindau disease were found. The family histories were negative for the disease. Even though most of the tumours were solid polycythaemia was never found.

Metastatic—Total: 33

Primary	
1. *Prostate*	2
Thoracic	1
Lumbar	1
Race	
Chinese	2
Average age—65 yrs	
2. *Lymphoma*	3
Thoracic	1
Lumbar	2
Sex	
Male	3
Race	
Chinese	1
Malay	1
Indian	1
Average age—33 yrs	
3. *Bronchogenic carcinoma*	8
Cerebral	5
Cerebellum	1
Parietal bone	1
Thoracic	1
Sex	
Female	1
Male	7
Race	
Chinese	
Male	7
Orang Asli	
Female	1
Average age—51 yrs	
4. *Thyroid, follicular*	4
Cervical	1
Thoracic	1
Sex	
Female	2
Male	2
Race	
Chinese	
Female	1
Male	2
Malay	
Female	1
Average age—42 yrs	
5. *Cervix*	1
Lumbar	1
Race	
Chinese	1
6. *Breast*	3
Cerebral	3
Race	
Chinese	3
Average age—42 yrs	
7. *Melanoma*	1
Thoracic	1
Race	
Chinese	
Male	1
8. *Choriocarcinoma*	2
Cerebral	2
Race	
Chinese	1
Indian	1
9. *Myeloma*	1
Thoracic	1
Race	
Chinese	
Female	1
10. *Neuroblastoma*	3
Scalp	1
Skull	1
Thoracic spine	1
Race	
Chinese	
Male	2
Malay	
Female	1
11. *Primary unknown, squamous*	6
Cerebral	2
Thoracic	1
Lumbar	3
Sex	
Female	1
Male	5
Race	
Chinese	
Female	1
Male	2
Malay	
Male	3
12. *Primary unknown, adenocarcinoma*	3
Frontal bone	1
Cerebral	2
Race	
Chinese	
Female	2
Male	1

Bronchogenic carcinoma was the most common metastatic neoplasm to be seen. However, unlike the Western countries where metastatic tumours of the nervous system are being seen with increasing frequency, examples of such tumours are not seen so commonly in Malaysia.

Miscellaneous

1. Lipoma, falx	1
2. Giant cell tumour, spine	2
3. Chondrosarcoma, spine	1
4. Ewing's sarcoma, skull	1
5. Fibrous dysplasia, skull	2
6. Amyloidoma, orbit	1
7. Cerebellar sarcoma	11
8. Chordoma, intracranial	2
9. Colloid cyst of third ventricle	3
10. Pinealoma	8
11. Teratoma, intracranial	7
12. Epidermoid, intracranial	2
13. Epidermoid, spinal	1
14. Dermoid, intracranial	1
15. Dermoid, spinal	1
16. Primary sarcomas of the nervous system:	23
Intracranial:	*21*
Dural	2
Leptomeningeal	7
Vascular (perithelial, endothelial)	12
Spinal:	*2*
Vascular	2
17. Unclassified	7

The numbers of pinealomas and intracranial teratomas exceeded the percentage reported from Western countries. The most frequent cause of death in cases of pinealoma was sudden massive intraventricular haemorrhage from erosion of the internal cerebral vein, or of the great vein of Galen. The teratomas occurred either at the base, or in the vicinity of the pineal gland.

Primary sarcomas of the nervous system occurred so commonly that the author entertained serious doubts as to the histological diagnoses. The slides were reviewed once and sometimes on two occasions with a neuropathologist who established or confirmed the diagnosis. The reason for the high incidence in Malaysia is not known. In the period in question, these sarcomas tended to occur in childhood and in young adult life. Most frequently they were located over the cerebral convexity. One was found in association with an ependymoma.

Without entering into the controversy over the nomenclature of cerebellar sarcoma, the histological appearance of this lesion was encountered in 11 patients. Reticulin was prominent. Cerebellar sarcomas were more frequently seen in older children and young adults, and they frequently metastasized, but no spread was found outside the nervous system.

Nasopharyngeal carcinoma is not included in the tabulated data because diagnosis was established by biopsy by the Department of Otolaryngology. This neoplasm is common in Chinese males but is seen in Malays. It is the most common cause of multiple cranial nerve palsies, and indeed the infiltrative form may reveal no other manifestations. When the intracranial structures became involved, X-ray therapy would generally result in a merely transient improvement.

Miscellaneous Disorders

Uveomeningo-encephalitis

One example of *uveomeningo-encephalitis* was seen. This patient was a young Chinese seamstress who had noted the onset of blindness of the left eye followed within 2 weeks by blindness of the other eye. She had begun to behave peculiarly, and someone had administered phenothiazines without examining her. She had then noted the onset of weakness of her legs. On admission to hospital she was mildly demented, had evidence of peripheral neuropathy of both legs, uveitis, and bilateral retinal detachment. The spinal fluid examination showed a large number of cells consisting almost entirely of lymphocytes, and a protein of several hundred milligrams. The cell count slowly subsided, but the spinal fluid protein progressively rose to over 1 g. Contrast studies were normal. Repeated cultures of her blood and spinal fluid for bacteria, tuberculous bacilli, and fungi were negative. Repeated searches were made for *Cryptococcus*. Blood, spinal fluid, and stool specimens were collected for viral isolation and serologies. Her EEG was grossly abnormal and showed diffuse dysynchrony and marked slow wave activity. Although the retinae reattached, vision did not return. Steroid therapy and large amounts of vitamin B complex were administered but had no appreciable effect. Delirium occurred periodically and the dementia grew progressively worse. At autopsy a specimen was obtained for viral studies, and a virus was isolated, but has not yet been identified. Histologically there was considerable thickening of the arachnoid and scattered areas of demyelination with minimal inflammatory reaction.

Transverse Myelitis

As previously mentioned, *transverse myelitis* was often seen unassociated with any evidence of cord compression or of changes in the cerebrospinal fluid. This occurred without antecedent or subsequent neurological signs or symptoms. The illness affected children and young adults. It would strike suddenly, and would be associated with interscapular or midthoracic pain with the onset of paraplegia within a few hours, and little or no subsequent recovery. These patients were investigated for rickettsial infection, schistosomiasis, leptospirosis, poliomyelitis, and other viruses as well as surgical lesions. All of these studies were negative. A baffling aspect was the occasional relationship of the onset to a sudden fever of 101° to 102°F, that would rapidly subside following the appearance of the neurological deficit. This syndrome was commonly experienced in hospitals.

A similar syndrome was seen in three instances in postpartum aborigine women who shortly after delivery would develop a flaccid weakness of both legs and usually an indefinite sensory level which would be gradual in its zone of transition. No evidence of an inflammatory process or a neurosurgical lesion could be found. Their spinal fluid examinations were normal. It was postulated that perhaps the position for delivery was related to this lesion; squatting is common in some races. However, aborigine women assume the usual lithotomy position. The syndrome was not seen in women delivered in hospital but only in those delivered in the jungle by members of the family or other members of the tribal group. No nutritional basis was established. Recovery was slow but usually satisfactory. The author does not know whether any of these patients subsequently experienced recurrences on other deliveries. Large doses of vitamins were administered to these patients. It is possible that pelvic involvement of the lumbosacral plexus was responsible but this is only conjecture.

Sarcoidosis

Sarcoidosis affecting the nervous system was seen in four patients. The case-histories and slides of biopsies from the Kveim skin test were reviewed by the investigators of the International Sarcoidosis Survery who confirmed the diagnosis. One patient, an Indian woman aged 32, presented with an 8-month history of progressive cranial nerve palsies affecting the left third through the twelfth cranial nerves. A second patient presented at the age of 37 with a history of diplopia for 2 months associated with paraesthesiae of the left side of his face for 2 weeks. He was found to have a left third, fourth and sixth cranial nerve palsy with involvement of the first and second divisions of the fifth nerve on the left side. He was subsequently readmitted with the chief complaint of progressive involvement of the right side of his face with right third, fourth, and sixth cranial nerve palsies, and a suggestion of a mild right seventh nerve paresis of the peripheral type. A third patient, a young Chinese woman, complained of recurrent episodes of facial palsy.

Some people regard sarcoidosis as non-existent in Malaysia, and others as extremely rare. In the period in question, physicians at a hospital for chest diseases reported that they had seen it as clinical manifestations in four or five instances.

Bell's Palsy

This was seen, usually in older individuals. Some patients were found to be suffering from mild diabetes mellitus. The Guillain–Barré syndrome seldom presented in this fashion. ACTH therapy was employed and with excellent results if it was started shortly after the onset of the illness. Taste was found to be involved in approximately one-third of the patients. The lumbar punctures were normal. The Ramsay Hunt syndrome was not seen.

Vestibular Neuronitis

This was a troublesome condition for several patients, mostly young adult males. Most episodes were self-limited, but a few would experience two or three recurrences. Although no auditory component could be found, it is possible that some were suffering from Ménière's disease. In two patients with identical symptomatology, but with headache, the protein of the lumbar spinal fluid was found to be elevated, and required several months to return to normal. In view of the sudden onset, the headache, the generalized malaise, and the elevated protein, a possible viral agent was suspected. However, all attempts at identification of such an aetiology were unsuccessful.

Optic Neuritis and Retrobulbar Neuritis

These were baffling problems. Not only were they relatively common, but also often bilateral. The vision would sometimes be permanently impaired and occasionally lost. The author usually encountered this condition in young people, teenagers, or young adults. The great majority were women. There were no preceding symptoms of neurological disease, and the spinal fluid would be non-contributory. Steroids or ACTH would occasionally be of benefit to the patient. This was confirmed in two patients who had experienced considerable improvement in visual acuity after receiving steroids (dexamethasone) for approximately 1 week. When the drug was withdrawn, the visual acuity again deteriorated, only to show subsequent improvement on the recommencing of steroid therapy. None of these patients ever returned with additional neurological symptoms.

Meningismus

Several adults presented at clinic with headache, *meningismus*, and occasionally vertigo. The patient might have a low-grade fever of 99° to 100°F. There would be no systemic manifestations of an infectious process. The lumbar puncture would reveal a normal sugar, an elevated protein of 40 to 80 mg per cent, and 10 to 20 lymphocytes. Viral studies and other investigations were of no help in arriving at an aetiology except by exclusion. The headache might persist for several weeks, and the protein level of the spinal fluid might remain elevated for several weeks to 2 or 3 months. In the latter situation, more comprehensive investigations would be carried out but with negative findings. The patients would eventually make a complete recovery.

Acute Lumbar Disc Protrusion

This was more commonly encountered among individuals who were overweight and sedentary. It may, however, occur more frequently among those employed in manual labour than appeared to be the case because of certain economic situations. Many of the labourers were paid daily and lacked provision for hospitalization insurance. With the threat of potential economic hardship and the possibility of the loss of a job, hospitalization may have been postponed except in the case of more severe attacks of pain and the development of motor impairment.

Cervical Spondylosis

This was seen more frequently and irrespective of social class. However, those from the upper economic levels more commonly sought consultation because of pain, while the economically poorer patient more frequently presented with objective neurological findings.

Whip-lash Injuries

Whip-lash injuries of the cervical spine were seldom seen, and only then in the urban and more affluent individuals. For the most part, the syndrome was seen in Europeans. The low incidence is difficult to explain. Automobile accidents were common, and of the type known to be associated with this syndrome. Most automobiles afforded no special protection. Neck rests and seat belts have only become popular within the last few years.

CONCLUSION

The foregoing presentation represents the introductory phase of the investigation of neurological illnesses occurring in Malaysia. Much of the data is incomplete and many questions remain unsolved. Further lines of investigation will concern perhaps the establishing of the true incidence of the neurological and neurosurgical conditions, their degree of importance, racial predilections, and aetiologies. More detailed information is required with regard to congenital malformations, demyelinating diseases, cerebrovascular disease, the causes of mental retardation, the reasons for the high incidence of von Recklinghausen's disease, and the infrequency of congenital aneurysms.

While the various racial groups all live within the same country, their immediate environments are not necessarily identical, and cultural and religious patterns may also be contributing factors. Epidemiological surveys are required in some instances, whereas in others improvements of laboratory facilities would be of great assistance. One of the most difficult problems is the maintenance of detailed and accurate records.

26 Leprosy

J. H. S. PETTIT

INTRODUCTION

In recent years there has been a tendency to think of leprosy as a tropical disease, but it must be remembered that the condition was not originally limited to the warmer climates, and indeed until comparatively recently it was endemic in many countries even in the most northerly parts of Europe and Asia. The name 'Hansen's disease' serves as a reminder that not only was pioneer work performed in Norway but that it was also performed on Norwegian patients with leprosy.

The disease is of extremely ancient origin and excellent descriptions of leprosy existed in India 2500 years ago (Andersen, 1969). There is increasing doubt whether the word 'leprosy' that is so frequently used in the Old Testament refers to the true disease at all, as the original word (*tsaraath*) (Goldman, Moraites, and Kitzmiller, 1966) probably indicated a state of ritual defilement of the scaly human skin and of cloth or leather or the walls of houses (Browne, 1970). It is also probably true that the word 'leprosy' in the New Testament is not accurately translated, because the Greek medical term for the condition was 'elephantiasis'. Despite the fact that leprosy is known to leave diagnostic mutilations in bone (Möller-Christensen, 1961), there have been no cases of bony abnormality attributable to leprosy discovered in extensive studies both in Egypt and in Jericho of skeletal remains dating back to 600 BC; moreover, leprosy was probably unknown in Greece and the Western world before about 300 BC. There is evidence to suggest that the disease was brought to the Mediterranean by soldiers of Alexander the Great returning from the Indian campaign in 326 BC.

The disease was well established in Denmark in the Middle Ages (Möller-Christensen, 1953), but for reasons which are none too clear endemic leprosy seems to have disappeared from Europe prior to the dissemination of effective antileprosy medication, although a few cases of endogenous leprosy persisted in Norway and Iceland until recent years. It may be that the eradication of the disease from Europe was due to the rigidly applied policy of total segregation from the community which has left an atavistic fear of leprosy ingrained in many Europeans, but even in areas of the world which have not been affected by European thought fear of leprosy moves deeply back into the past, particularly in China (Skinsnes, 1964). The spread of Christianity did not help the eradication of these irrational fears, as it brought with it further misconceptions due to mistranslations of both Old and New Testaments. It is possible that the deeply ingrained prejudice that is so widespread is a reaction to the fact that leprosy is rarely rapidly fatal. In a disease where neurological signs frequently predominate, and where the destruction of the hands and feet may cause a patient to be unable to feed himself, let alone follow a gainful occupation, the social implications are enormous. A family may well accept the responsibility of maintaining such a member, but as the years go by the motivations of kindness slowly atrophy, and the unfortunate patient becomes an increasing burden on the originally sympathetic relations who gradually develop a resentment against him; this all too human reaction must indeed play a very great part in perpetuating fear of the disease, because each individual who sees his own sympathy waning will dread the possibility of finding himself in a similar situation.

GEOGRAPHICAL INCIDENCE

Leprosy is still a major problem in most countries between the tropics of Cancer and Capricorn and, although in the past maps have been published showing different degrees of incidence of leprosy in different countries, we are not offering such a map in this chapter as it seems highly probable that the areas which were previously shown as having a low incidence simply had a low recognition of the condition. The World Health Organization (*Leprosy Review*, 1969) has recently claimed that in tropical Africa, since 1965, 150 000 new cases have been registered, and in Burma the number of registered cases of leprosy has risen from 12 000 to over 170 000 in a few years. There are probably some 16 000 000 cases of leprosy in the world, and as the index of clinical suspicion is still regrettably low in many physicians, it is to be expected that further cases will be discovered in large numbers as the improvement in medical services continues in developing countries.

An unexplained feature of the geographical distribution of the disease is the fact that the predominant type of leprosy seems to vary markedly in different parts of the world; in the West African the incidence of tuberculoid disease is extremely high, while in the Asian (particularly the Chinese) there seems to be a very much higher incidence of lepromatous leprosy. This suggests that various races have different degrees of susceptibility to the disease, but it is unwise to discuss genetic variation in a condition which is caused by bacteria, until it is perfectly certain that such variation is in the patient and not in the causative organism. Unfortunately, the present standard of knowledge concerning *Mycobacterium leprae* is such that it cannot be said with certainty that there are not different types of organisms occurring in different areas, and until this has been disproved it will be impossible to determine whether the different incidences of the various types of disease are due to the individual or the infecting agent.

A further variation in geographical distribution which must be mentioned here is the very high incidence of diffuse lepromatosis (Franken, 1963) which is found among Spanish-Americans, particularly in Central America. Again it remains to be seen whether it is a genetic variant produced by the patient or by the organism.

One of the most unhappy divergences found across the world is due neither to the patient nor to the mycobacterium, but to the authorities of different countries whose regulations concerning the handling of leprosy patients are so enormously variable that one can only view with horror the apparent inability of some governments to accept advice from medical authorities. In certain countries, e.g. South Africa (Schulz and Pentz, 1970) lepromatous patients are compulsorily kept in institutions until smears have been negative for 12 consecutive months, while in others (e.g. Malaysia) the bacteriological condition of the patient is scarcely considered in the assessment of whether or not hospitalization is necessary; and some authorities (Gauntlett, 1969) have come to the conclusion that 'the evils engendered by admission to a leprosarium might be greater than the effects of the disease itself'; increasing emphasis is therefore laid on outpatient treatment.

It is to be hoped that evidence of the great advances in leprosy research which have been made in the past decade will penetrate to the desks of the authorities, and so ensure that the benefits of hard-won knowledge are transmitted to the patients and not relegated to the library.

CLASSIFICATION

In order to understand the various forms that leprosy can take it is necessary to explain briefly the theory that at present holds, concerning the relationship of host and parasite in the disease. Even in areas of highest endemicity, no more than 5 per cent of the population show clinical manifestations of disease and so it is clear that many people who come into contact with the infecting agent must be able to obliterate the organism shortly after it has invaded the body, and thus no disease will occur. A percentage of other people, however, will have a high but incomplete resistance to the infection and the earliest forms of lesion will develop.

It is now recognized that leprosy is primarily a neurological infection and that *Myco. leprae* has a specific affinity for cells originating from the neuro-ectodermal crest. Lesions are therefore rarely found outside the nerves and the skin until late in the progress of the disease. Although the earliest damage almost certainly occurs in nerves, this is not associated with any recognizable symptom or sign (it has occasionally been said that 'pins and needles' is a prodromal sign of leprosy but it is unwise to base a diagnosis solely on such a frequent and non-specific complaint) and usually the earliest lesion will be found on the skin. This is called indeterminate leprosy and as its name suggests the appearance is not of very great help to a physician seeking to reach a firm diagnosis. At this stage the patient may overcome the infection spontaneously, the patch will disappear, the individual will produce no classical lesion, and more often than not nobody will ever know that there was a temporary invasion of the body by the leprosy organism.

Some people fail to resist the infection in its early stages, and according to their degree of resistance they will produce a more classical disease picture. If they have a high but incomplete resistance a tuberculoid lesion will develop, while those with no resistance at all will become lepromatous. The tuberculoid and lepromatous types are the 'polar' aspects of this spectrum of reaction, and there has been a widespread search for other names to describe stages between the two poles. Most leprosy workers now accept the phrase 'borderline leprosy' as covering those conditions which are not polar; such patients have a degree of resistance which is less than complete but is high enough to enable them, at least in the first instance, to avoid developing lepromatous disease. In some centres names such as 'indeterminate' and 'dimorphous' are still used but the word 'borderline' was recommended at the Eighth International Congress of Leprosy (*Leprosy Review*, 1964).

Ridley and Jopling (1966) have suggested a classification of leprosy and while originally recommending this for research purposes, have found since, as have many others, that it is a simple and practical method for all workers in the field. Continuing the analogy of the spectrum, of which tuberculoid and lepromatous disease occupy the visible ends while borderline leprosy has now taken its place in the centre, two further 'colours' have been added known as 'borderline tuberculoid' and 'borderline lepromatous'; for ease of reference these five basic types are usually referred to as TT, BT, BB, BL and LL. It must be remembered that a patient may well be found whose clinical appearance does not fit exactly into any one basic type, and in leprosaria which have accepted the Ridley-Jopling classification it is quite common to find patients diagnosed as BT/BB or BL/LL thus showing their exact position in the spectrum.

This classification explains most of the clinical findings. As the patient's resistance diminishes his clinical appearance will approach the lepromatous, and the lepromin test (an intradermal injection of killed leprosy bacilli, freed as much as possible from the tissue elements that are at present unavoidable in its preparation), which is simply a manifestation of this resistance, will be strongly positive in tuberculoid disease and uniformly and persistently negative in pure LL. According to the patient's resistance the number of bacilli will naturally vary, and in patients where there is no resistance at all *Myco. leprae* reproduction will be completely uninhibited; the spectrum will therefore show an increase of bacterial number in each lesion and in the patient as a whole; similarly, the number of actual lesions present on the patient will increase as resistance diminishes.

An additional complication of clinical leprosy is that patients whose diagnosis lies in the wide borderline range may show alteration of clinical appearance following a change in resistance. Reasons for this are not fully understood but it is not uncommon to see a case with BL or LL dramatically acquiring a high resistance with consequent change of the histology towards the tuberculoid end of the scale; this usually occurs under the influence of treatment. The obverse is also seen where resistance collapses, so producing a patient who originally had plaques which were tuberculoid in nature but finishes with lepromatous disease; this usually occurs before treatment is fully established. Many workers do not believe that the true polar types (TT and LL) can take part in this change of classification, but all are uniform in agreement that the borderline types may show lability throughout the clinical course of the disease. This can lead to confusion in diagnosis because a patient may show clinical signs of more than one type of the disease.

CLINICAL APPEARANCE

Indeterminate Leprosy

Leprosy patients not infrequently say that before they were diagnosed as having leprosy a patch appeared somewhere on the skin, and such lesions are also sometimes discovered in sociological and epidemiological studies. The macule is usually scaly and hypopigmented, although complete achromia is never found. In some cases it will progress to a recognizable leprosy lesion but more frequently it simply disappears.

It is exceedingly difficult to be sure that such patches are really early leprosy in the absence of recognizable diagnostic features, and indeed if such features were present the condition would no longer be 'indeterminate' and would deserve a more established traditional name. The only way of being sure that the patient has indeterminate disease is to recognize the presence of the acid-fast bacilli in a lesion and this is only rarely done with routine methods of staining (Lara and Nolasco, 1956).

Pure Tuberculoid Leprosy (TT)

In this condition the patient usually has a small number of lesions which are asymmetrical and somewhat hypopigmented; classically, they have a well-defined outer border which is usually somewhat raised [Plate 25c]. The skin is dry and scaly and there is anaesthesia to touch, pain and temperature within the lesion. In such patients the lepromin test is strongly positive and skin scrapings will reveal no bacilli. In most cases of this type neurological involvement is easily recognized, and enlargement, nodularity or dysfunction of the pre-auricular, radial, ulnar or common peroneal nerves are seen. As this is the type of disease with fewest lesions, the invasion of bacteria having to a great extent been combated by the patient's resistance, it is possible that only one lesion may develop and this could be either in the skin or in a nerve. The latter occurrence is the usual cause of the so-called pure neural leprosy [p. 327].

Borderline Tuberculoid (BT)

This still maintains many features of tuberculoid leprosy although a lessened resistance of the patient will probably be associated with rather more skin lesions, and scrapings taken from them will demonstrate the presence of a few bacilli. The patches are still rather scaly but may be more erythematous and indurated than before, while the classical anaesthesia which is so easily demonstrated in TT cases has diminished and may not be entirely uniform throughout the the plaques [Plate 27b]. In many of the largest lesions there is a tendency to central clearing. Peripheral nerves may still be involved although usually less severely than in TT.

Borderline Leprosy (BB)

The classical borderline lesion is no longer scaly or anaesthetic but red, and raised. Small lesions are quite obviously not of the tuberculoid type and if the lesions are large there is often central clearing to produce an annular appearance [Plate 26a]. Such annular lesions may be found both in BT and BB cases but are easily differentiated in that the tuberculoid lesions show a well-demarcated *outer* margin while the inner border is diffuse, and in BB cases there is the well-demarcated *inner* margin giving a punched-out appearance. The borderline type may show a considerable number of lesions all over the body and there is a tendency, particularly among the small maculopapules, towards symmetry. Such lesions are rarely anaesthetic and it is relatively unusual to find signs of neurological involvement in the early uncomplicated stages of this type.

Borderline Lepromatous (BL)

This is perhaps the least well defined subgroup on the Ridley-Jopling scale. Although some patients have considerable numbers of lesions, most of which are maculopapular or nodular, there are less of these than in the typical well-established lepromatous case and the distribution has not yet attained the classic symmetry. It is not infrequently seen that BL cases have a number of annular lesions with the central clearing that has been described as typical of pure BB, and this is because such patients started with a borderline condition but a diminution in their resistance caused the lesions to become more classically lepromatous. The histology and clinical appearance of the lesions will therefore be diagnostic of BL, and smears in these patients will show large numbers of organisms in all lesions. The lepromin test is almost invariably completely negative.

Lepromatous Leprosy (LL)

In this type of disease the host has no resistance to the invading organisms which therefore cause a vast number of lesions all containing very many *Myco. leprae*. The lepromin test is invariably negative. There are two recognized types of pure lepromatous leprosy: the diffuse lepromatous type which is commoner in Central and Southern America, and the nodular lepromatous type which is commoner elsewhere. It is probable that the diffuse type of disease is a manifestation of total absence of resistance *ab initio*, and that the nodular form is found in people who originally have a small amount of resistance which later collapses.

Diffuse Lepromatous Leprosy

This is often very difficult for a non-specialist to recognize, above all in a patient who is only in the early stages of infection. The whole of the skin is diffusely thickened and infiltrated with lepromatous pathology [PLATE 27d], and as this frequently does no more than to eradicate wrinkles on the face of a middle-aged person it has been given the name in Mexico of 'pretty' leprosy. In both forms of lepromatous disease there is a fairly early loss of the outer part of the eyebrows; this *madarosis* is one of the classical signs of both forms of LL but it is often the only sign that is obvious at a distance in a case of diffuse infection.

Nodular Lepromatous Disease

This is perhaps the more classical condition in the sense that it is the type that is more commonly thought of when the word 'leprosy' is 'mentioned [PLATE 27a]. The patient has a large number of infiltrated erythematous nodules and plaques scattered all over the body. They are particularly noticeable on the face and extensor surfaces in general, and the only areas that are usually free from infiltration are the scalp, the axillae and the groins. There is a marked tendency to symmetry in the smaller lesions and smears taken from any site will reveal a very high concentration of acid-fast bacilli. It is unusual to find nodular or asymmetrically involved nerves, but as all neuro-ectodermal tissue is inundated with bacilli lepromatous pathology will invade peripheral nerves and in the later stages there will be clinical signs of bilateral nervous involvement of a generalized nature. This is discussed more fully below.

REACTIONS IN LEPROSY

During the course of leprosy and its treatment a number of rather strange complications may occur, and although these have been more commonly noticed since the advent of efficient antileprosy treatment they had all been described prior to the introduction of sulphone therapy. There is a superficial similarity between these reactions which has caused a considerable amount of diagnostic confusion, and regrettably even today there is very little international agreement concerning even the names of these reactions while theories as to their causation are vehemently attacked and defended at most meetings of leprologists. The conditions all present with an eruption of red nodules or plaques, but while in certain cases this erythema and oedema seems to be associated with pre-existent lesions, another form of complication produces erythematous nodules which do not necessarily occur in the leprosy patches. Unfortunately the name 'lepra reaction' has been applied to both types by various authorities at different times, and in a recent attempt to persuade leprologists to think about this more clearly Jopling (1970) has suggested that the different reactions be simply called Type I and Type II. This has not, however, attained universal acceptance and probably the most frequent practice at present is to describe Jopling's Type I as 'acute exacerbation' and Jopling,s Type II as 'erythema nodosum leprosum'; and it is these latter names that we intend to use in this chapter.

Acute Exacerbation (Jopling Type I)

This is most commonly seen within the first 6 months of the establishment of active treatment for leprosy, but workers in the larger centres of disease are conversant with such a reaction occasionally occurrnig prior to the onset of therapy, in which case the sudden change in appearance usually causes the patient to seek medical advice.

The primary complaint is almost invariably of a sudden explosion of oedema and erythema occurring in the sites of the leprosy lesions [PLATE 26b]. This is particularly commonly found at the tuberculoid end of the scale, and although an acute exacerbation of borderline lepromatous nodules has frequently been recorded it probably never occurs in pure lepromatous (LL) disease. The condition is usually afebrile and the skin lesions are rarely painful although occasionally an extensive oedema makes the skin so tight that it may actually burst open to produce a ragged ulceration.

Not infrequently small red nodules appear on the limbs or the trunk in association with this acute exacerbation, and it was thought that this contradicted the theory that such lesions occurred in previously existent patches. This suggestion is discounted by other workers, particularly dermatologists who are not unused to the theory of 'invisible' skin diseases (Gougerot, 1949), who point out that not all leprosy lesions in the dermis are large enough to produce macroscopic signs and that the apparently spontaneous nodules are simply a reaction in previously sub-macroscopic lesions.

Ridley (1969) has suggested that this clinical type of reaction with the apparent worsening of the condition can be subdivided into two types. It is postulated that the acute oedema in the lesions may be either a 'reversal' or a 'downgrading' reaction. The reversal reaction is associated with an improvement in the patient's resistance to the organism, which may either occur naturally or under the influence of therapy, and such patients are found afterwards to have changed their clinical and histological appearance towards the tuberculoid end of the scale [PLATE 26c]. The downgrading reaction is associated with a decline of immunity and corresponding increase in the number of bacilli. This is likely to be found only in untreated patients, and is probably the type of acute exacerbation which causes a patient to seek medical advice for the first time.

Both these subtypes of the acute exacerbation are relatively easy to treat, but particular attention must be paid to the dangers of neurological involvement; this can cause an acute paresis which if ignored may become permanent.

Erythema Nodosum Leprosum (Jopling Type II)

This occurs, in contrast to the acute exacerbation, specifically at the lepromatous end of the scale [PLATE 26d]. Originally described by Murata in 1912 (Murata, 1912) it has become much more common in the past 30 years and recent work seems to have confirmed Murata's suspicion that the reaction is due to the degeneration of dead bacilli and a subsequent release of antigenic material. The resulting condition can be extremely serious. In the first few attacks small, painful, red nodules appear in the skin; these are transient and at most mildly pyrexial, but later the most severely affected patients have a debilitating high fever for many months or even years associated not only with painful skin nodules but with manifestations of vascular sensitization occurring in the joints, the uveal tracts, the reticulo-endothelial system, and indeed almost any part of the body. Occasionally, the skin nodules become extensive, confluent and necrotic (Waters and Ridley, 1963) and such patients have been known ultimately to develop amyloid disease. Histologically, the changes are those of a Herxheimer reaction.

This condition has become much more frequent since the advent of sulphone therapy and many workers unfortunately consider that it is actually caused by sulphone. We find it impossible to accept this theory, however (Pettit and Waters, 1967), in view of the facts that it was described and named 30 years before the sulphones were used and that it is also seen in patients treated with other antileprosy drugs. It is almost certainly due to the release of bacterial toxins from the killed bacilli producing an allergic vasculitis, and the condition lasts a long time because of the unusual bacteriological fact that *Myco. leprae* do not disintegrate quickly after they have been killed. Patients who are being satisfactorily treated do not become smear negative for many years after the onset of therapy, and therefore the individual who has become sensitive to bacterial toxins will of necessity have to suffer a long period of reaction while the killed organisms slowly disintegrate after death. It cannot be too strongly emphasized that the habit of stopping antibacterial therapy for severe ENL is an emotional and retrogressive step, and will do no more than permit still viable organisms to multiply and so lead inexorably to further ENL when treatment is finally re-established and the organisms again start to disintegrate.

Lucio Phenomenon

In Spanish America where diffuse lepromatous disease is so much more frequent, a reaction is seen, limited to such patients, which is known as the 'Lucio phenomenon'. The condition usually begins on the lower legs with an ill-defined pinkish macule which becomes darker and is then surmounted by a flaccid haemorrhagic blister containing necrotic material (Franken, 1963). When this blister breaks it leaves an irregular punched-out ulcer which scars to form a hypopigmented scar surrounded by darker ichthyotic skin. It is a matter of some doubt whether this condition is ever seen elsewhere in the world; it is probably simply a more severe variant of allergic vasculitis, precipitated for the same reasons as the ENL lesions with which it is sometimes clinically associated. Cases of acute neurological involvement in this reaction have not come to our attention but are theoretically possible and presumably will ultimately be recognized.

NEUROLOGY OF LEPROSY

Introduction

Leprosy is a neurological disease and every leprosy patient has some involvement of the peripheral nerves; but although about 20 per cent of patients suffer major motor or sensory damage, the study of the peripheral nerve lesions has lagged behind studies of the bacteriology and the dermatological aspects of the disease. *Myco. leprae* has a special relationship with the Schwann cell (Lumsden, 1964) and it is believed that the bacilli reach these cells via the lymphatic spaces inside nerves (Carayon, 1968). In nerves, as elsewhere, clear distinction must be drawn between the presence of the bacilli and the damage caused by them, for although bacilli may be found in many nerve trunks and have occasionally been reported in dorsal ganglia and even in the central nervous system, damage seems to be confined to the peripheral nerves (Brand, 1964). The reason for this is not fully understood but there is some evidence that *Myco. leprae*, like *Myco. ulcerans* and *Myco. balnei*, prefers to grow at a relatively low temperature, and probably the limitation of damage to peripheral nerves is associated with their relative coolness (Sabin and Ebner, 1969). This is supported by the fact that even in peripheral nerves the pathology is limited to segments lying near the skin and when such nerves return deeper into the body of the limb the pathology usually disappears. For example, although the ulnar nerve is frequently involved, damage is usually limited to areas at the elbow and just above the wrist; similarly, the median nerve shows lesions at the front of the wrist, while the radial is most commonly affected about 2½ inches above the elbow just below the point of its emergence from under cover of the triceps. On the face, the zygomatic branch of the facial nerve is usually involved in the region of the zygoma; the remainder of the facial nerve limits its pathology to the bony facial canal. In the leg the common peroneal is damaged at the level of the knee or near the neck of the fibula, and the posterial tibial may be affected a few inches above the ankle. These are the only motor nerves that are damaged and paralysis of muscles not supplied by these nerves is exceptionally rare.

Anaesthesia follows the same pattern, but in addition to the nerves already mentioned sensory change can be produced by infection of the long cutaneous nerves that run down to supply the distal parts of the limbs. Other areas of patchy anaesthesia can be found particularly in tuberculoid patients but this is usually exceedingly superficial and does not affect deep sensation.

Direct Involvement of Nerves in Leprosy

Tuberculoid Leprosy

When a patient presents with two or three fairly well-demarcated lesions that are hypopigmented and somewhat scaly, the possibility of tuberculoid leprosy should be considered and the diagnosis will be confirmed if there is anaesthesia. In such cases peripheral nerves must be examined with particular care. Ideally, leprosy may be suspected if one of the superficial peripheral nerves is enlarged; but unfortunately, in practice most physicians are not in the habit of routinely palpating these nerves and so are unable to say whether or not they have enlarged since a previous examination of the patient. Involvement of the nerve can therefore be suspected only if it is grossly larger than normal, but the presence of hardening or nodularity will be easier to elicit. The rigidity may be so marked that on some occasions the nerves at the wrist can be mistaken for tendons. Such signs are of considerable aid in making a clinical diagnosis, and although it is usually unnecessary a small biopsy from the affected nerve will show that most of it has been heavily infiltrated by a granuloma which is indistinguishable from the classical tuberculoid pathology, with foci of epithelioid cells surrounded by a dense cloud of lymphocytes; Langhans' giant cells are usually present in the border between the epithelioid cells and the lymphocytes. In skin lesions it is often impossible to find any sign of a nerve bundle histologically, but as Pearson, Weddell, and Palmer (1968) have shown, even though most of the nerve is replaced by a granuloma and the axons totally destroyed there is a relatively normal perineurium in the larger nerves. The smallest nerves present in the skin are frequently completely invisible and the area will be anaesthetic.

In patients who have borderline tuberculoid disease the nerves may be similarly affected, but anaesthesia is usually incomplete as the granuloma is not as totally destructive as it is in the polar type of the disease.

It has already been shown that there are relatively few lesions in patients with tuberculoid leprosy and so these are almost always asymmetrically distributed; similarly, not all superficial nerves will be involved. Usually only one or two are found to be affected, most often in close anatomical association with the site of the skin abnormality, but it is not rare for a nerve lesion to be found in a limb where there is no skin lesion visible.

Destruction of motor nerves will result in muscle damage but it must not be expected that muscle weakness, wasting and the consequent paralysis will occur early in the course of the disease. As time goes on weakness of denervated muscle will unbalance its antagonists and, as Brand (1964) has pointed out, this leads to permanent shortening in response to prolonged tonic contraction; muscle ability will be greatly handicapped and disuse atrophy will occur. Similarly, loss of power in one group of muscles will unbalance the ligaments of a joint and lead to a loss of movement which diminishes the nutrition; the cartilage will slowly be replaced by fibrous tissue, and ultimately the joint is permanently deformed usually producing a classical claw hand in tuberculoid cases [PLATES 28a and b].

Lepromatous Leprosy

At the lepromatous end of the scale the patient has no resistance to infection and the mycobacterium is master of the situation. The pathological reaction shows very few lymphocytes and the granuloma is composed of histiocytic cells which may resemble epithelioid cells; in pure lepromatous disease (LL) the granuloma consists almost entirely of such histiocytes with a number of giant cells of multinucleate nature which are quite different from the Langhans cells seen in tuberculoid disease.

It is quite obvious that the patient is unable to make satisfactory antibacterial response and the nerve changes such as are found at the tuberculoid end of the scale are non-existent here. The resistance of the perineurium, which caused it to be clearly demarcated from the endoneurium in tuberculoid leprosy, is missing in lepromatous disease (Pearson, Weddell, and Palmer, 1968), and the nerve may contain enormous numbers of acid-fast bacilli both in the perineurium and the endoneurium; the amount of reactive granuloma, however, is small and axons are still recognizably present. In long-standing cases of untreated lepromatous disease this mixture of granuloma and bacilli will ultimately lead to anaesthesia, and as the infection will be widespread in all the nerves that have been listed above, the clinical picture will not be of a regional anaesthesia but more of 'stocking and glove' type. In long-standing cases of untreated lepromatous disease it may be found that almost the whole of the body has become anaesthetic (Sabin and Ebner, 1969). Similarly, motor paralysis in the lepromatous patient develops insidiously and bilateral claw hands and claw feet are frequently seen together.

Borderline Leprosy

The intermediate types of leprosy that lie between the polar extremes usually show less nervous involvement, as there is neither the gross destruction of a segment of nerve which is found in the tuberculoid lesion nor yet the high degree of bacterial infiltration which causes such widespread damage at the lepromatous end of the scale. Pearson and his colleagues have found no specific pathology in the borderline neurological lesions which they have biopsied, and claim that they show either the tuberculoid or the lepromatous picture. Usually, neither anaesthesia nor muscle wasting plays a very great part in the condition unless there has been a clinical change towards one of the poles, in which case the typical abnormalities will be found.

Neural Leprosy

This is the term that has been used for many years to signify a clinical condition in which the signs and symptoms of leprosy are confined to the peripheral nervous system and there is no visible change in the skin. The diagnosis of this condition is frequently difficult and there is consequent disagreement among authorities as to its incidence. Litalien *et al.* (1960) think that it is not exceptional and one of their group collected 90 cases in Vietnam alone, but in 1965 Jopling and Morgan Hughes (1965) commented on the scant references to this type in the literature and could not persuade themselves that any previous report that they had met proved the existence of a pure neural form of tuberculoid leprosy. In an extensive study of over 11 000 leprosy patients seen in the Leprosy Research Department in Calcutta, Kundu and Ghosh (1970) could only find 34 cases that were classified as primary polyneuritic leprosy; unfortunately they failed to confirm the diagnosis histologically.

As we have shown above, patients with little or no resistance to the organism will develop lepromatous disease and it is theoretically highly unlikely that leprosy infection in such people can ever be confined entirely to the nerves. In the borderline condition it is not surprising that occasional cases may be limited to the nerves for a fairly long period before dermatological manifestations present themselves (Jopling, 1956). The more highly resistant tuberculoid-prone patients can be expected occasionally to show a clinical picture where all lesions are confined to the nerves.

All 34 patients reported from Calcutta were smear negative and most were lepromin positive. These findings underline the diagnostic problems in this type of disease as it is difficult to confirm the diagnosis of an infectious disease when the infecting organism is not found. One would expect neural cases to have a strongly positive lepromin reaction but this reaction can be positive in members of the general public, even in countries where there is little likelihood of their ever having come into contact with leprosy. Ideally, no case should be diagnosed as neural leprosy without a nerve biopsy which shows the classical tuberculoid histology within the perineurium, but unfortunately this too can be confusing as tuberculoid disease inside a nerve is frequently caseous; there are very few credible reports of caseation occurring in tuberculoid leprosy other than in nerves. At present no explanation is available.

Neural leprosy is usually first noticed by the patient because of a diminution in cutaneous sensation in a small area. This anaesthesia increases and is followed by a gradual loss of power in a group of muscles. This is reported most frequently in association with the ulnar nerve but it is expected that increasing awareness of the condition will allow the detection of more cases in other nerves. The physical signs are not surprising. A hard peripheral nerve, often large and nodular, is associated with varying degrees of wasting of the muscles it supplies and with anaesthesia to touch, pain, and temperature over the distribution of its cutaneous branches. Skin scrapings from the anaesthetic lesions will be negative but the lepromin test will be strongly positive, and it is suggested that if the latter is found to be negative the diagnosis should be reconsidered.

Although in pure neural disease there will be no leprotic lesion on the skin, it must not be forgotten that the anaesthetic areas frequently show hypoidrosis or anidrosis and many such areas develop a secondary ichthyosis.

Complications of Leprosy Involvement in Nerves

Anaesthesia

Although this is the most common result of neurological involvement it is not found in all patients with leprosy and many people have remained undiagnosed simply because physicians expect all leprosy cases to show areas of anaesthesia. Regional or segmental anaesthesia is associated with leprosy at the tuberculoid end of the scale, and diffuse anaesthesia of the hands and feet is found in long-standing (usually untreated) cases of lepromatous disease. This means that most borderline cases and all early lepromatous cases will *not* be anaesthetic; if a physician waits for the appearance of anaesthesia before he takes other steps to confirm the diagnosis, treatment will be dangerously delayed.

Surprisingly frequently, a patient is unaware of a certain degree of anaesthesia in his hands and will therefore submit them to trauma that might otherwise be avoided. In the hands this frequently takes the form of burns produced by smokers who do not realize that the cigarette has burnt down to the fingers, and in many cases the presenting symptom has been 'spontaneous' blisters on the sides of the fingers. In the feet, trauma that is painless to the patient may be followed by infection which can penetrate to the bone causing an osteomyelitis, which is also painless. Consequent absorption of bone produces the classical deformities associated with long-standing disease of the feet.

The trophic changes consequent to anaesthesia may affect the skin, the joints of the bones.

Trophic Changes of the Skin. Although the smooth and unused appearance of skin which is found in a paraplegic limb can also be seen in leprosy, this form of trophic wasting is not particularly usual, and the two commoner forms of dermatological complications are ichthyosis and ulceration. In most cases of leprosy, sweating is absent from the anaesthetic areas for reasons which are not completely clear. The amount of moisture passing through the epidermis other than in the sweat is almost insignificant and this moisture alone cannot be expected to hydrate keratin adequately. As a result of such anidrosis, the keratin becomes dehydrated and appears clinically as a secondary xeroderma.

Trophic ulcers are probably the greatest single problem of leprosy management, and this is particularly distressing in view of the fact that with adequate education a very large degree of deformity and crippling can be avoided. Most ulcers start in an anaesthetic area following external trauma (e.g. persistent unwise carrying of excessively heavy objects with an anaesthetic hand, or prolonged walking in unsuitable footwear) but it is possible that certain ulcers may arise due simply to ischaemic necrosis of subcutaneous tissue without actual damage through the epidermis. If the patient does not report for treatment immediately, further trauma and later infection will enlarge the ulcer which, if it remains unnoticed, can penetrate deeply leading to osteomyelitis. Although leprosy can itself infect a bone this usually produces only minor damage until infection reaches it from extension of a skin ulcer; the bone will, of course, be more than usually prone to necrosis and the presence of necrotic fragments of bone can frequently be recognized clinically by inserting a probe deep into the sinuses leading from foot ulcers. Once a patient has developed an ulcer he will be more prone to repeated ulceration in the same area, not only because of persistence of the conditions which cause the ulceration but also because the original ulcer will heal by fibrosis and such scar tissue is more liable to damage. Ulceration will therefore occur repeatedly for increasingly trivial reasons.

Trophic Changes in Joints. These will follow muscle paralysis and the consequent antagonal imbalance. As the joint becomes increasingly useless there will be absorption of the neighbouring bones as well as fibrosis and consequent destruction of the joint itself. Such changes finally lead to a claw hand, for example, which is originally mobile on passive movement becoming fixed in a distorted position.

In recent years there has been increasing realization that Charcot joints can be seen in leprosy [PLATE 28c]. It is probable that this recognition was delayed because of the relative infrequency of adequate radiological facilities in many leprosaria. The changes may occur in small joints or in the upper limbs but are most frequently limited to the ankle and the foot. In 38 cases recently described (Matsuda, 1969), 19 were limited to the ankle joint, 3 showed destruction of all tarsal bones and the other 16 cases were scattered among the various joints of the foot.

This condition starts with a mild swelling and warmness near the affected joint which is naturally painless. The first sign in the ankle is usually a degree of compression of the talus producing a 'parrot-beak' shadow of the posterior part of the bone [PLATE 28d], but later sclerosis of a rather haphazard type appears and the long bones of the leg seem slowly to push their way through the foot. The articular surface of the lower end of the tibia remains intact much longer than might be expected. By this time the ankle will be markedly swollen and there will be a lateral instability of the joint. Charcot changes in the tarsal area, while producing various deformities on X-ray, do not usually lead to an unstable foot in addition.

It is a matter of some doubt whether *trophic changes of bone* actually occur as a primary complication of anaesthesia or indeed of leprosy involvement of nerves. A case can be made that the osteoporosis and absorption so frequently seen is a result of immobility secondary to joint involvement and aggravated by anaesthesia.

Nerve Pain

Neurologists are not unused to treating symptoms of various paraesthesiae, but patients outside the field of leprosy who complain of acute pain which actually originates inside a nerve are rare. In uncomplicated leprosy, intraneural granulomata may stretch the perineurium to an extent which causes local discomfort, but usually this does no more than produce a dull ache in an affected nerve. During the course of the lepra reactions, both Type I (AE) and Type II (ENL), it is not unusual to see a patient who complains of pain and tenderness in one or more areas. In both subgroups of Type I acute oedema in the lesions will, if the nerve is involved, unavoidably produce signs or symptoms similar to those of ischaemia of nerves; the clinical emphasis here is on motor change, and severe pain is relatively unusual.

The most extreme form of pain occurs in association with severe erythema nodosum leprosum. Even a small skin nodule of early and mild ENL is inflamed and tender and those unfortunate patients whose lesions become extensive or necrotic cannot reasonably hope that their nerves will escape damage. The ulnar nerve at the elbow (as usual) is most frequently involved, and sometimes this pain reaches a severity which can only be conjectured by those fortunate enough not to have the disease if it is realized that patients actively welcome the additional pain caused by intraneural injection in an attempt to obtain a few hours' relief. The actual diagnosis is not difficult as other symptoms of ENL are present; occasionally the nerve pain is the major symptom and seems to be disproportionately severe in relation to the minor ENL found elsewhere. The symptoms are rarely associated with acute motor changes but recurrent attacks of pain in the same nerve may be associated with a slowly developing atrophy of the muscles it supplies.

Paralysis

Leprous involvement of peripheral nerves will, if a sufficient number of axons are destroyed, slowly be followed by paralysis. Sometimes an acute muscular dysfunction is complained of but this is rarely seen in non-reactional cases. In a few areas (e.g. the carpal tunnel) simple enlargement of a nerve within limited confines may alone be sufficient to produce enough pressure to cause either pain or paralysis. Most frequently, however, acute paralysis is found while the patient is in Type I reaction and it is irrelevant to our present purpose whether these symptoms are precipitated by a reversal or a down-grading form of reaction. The clinical picture that is most commonly seen is of a relatively sudden swelling and erythema of the pre-established lesions associated with a sudden loss of function either in the foot or the wrist. Wrist-drop or foot-drop can surprise a clinician not previously aware of the presence of damaged nerves and the paralysis may develop rapidly over the course of 1 or 2 days with little subjective discomfort, although sometimes there will be nerve pain in the area of reacting pathology. In patients with visible tuberculoid leprosy of the face and neck and involvement of the great auricular nerve, Type I reaction is sometimes complicated by a sudden facial palsy [PLATE 27c], and although most attacks of acute paralysis in a limb will recover, facial paralysis seems much less likely to respond to treatment; because of this many leprologists are more than usually careful in cases of leprosy of the face.

The acute onset of wrist-drop varies in incidence in certain parts of the world and although Brand (1964) says that it appears 'very occasionally' in Malaysia, we have had the experience of hearing an international authority stand in a ward where there were five cases of wrist-drop, and claim that he has never seen a case before. There seems to be no explanation of this extraordinary clinical diversity.

Paralysis of a limb may also develop slowly in any form of leprosy and it is one of the leprologist's greatest frustrations to watch a patient continue to develop weakness in a hand or foot despite successful antibacterial treatment. Probably this is due to fibrosis replacing the original infection, and there seems to be no way of arresting this; while education, physiotherapy, and sometimes active surgical intervention may diminish the effects of this fibrosis, it is a regrettably frequent occurrence to find weakness or paralysis of muscles and joints as a residual abnormality in what would otherwise be a cured patient. If such structural weakness is also associated with anaesthesia, the mutilations which gave leprosy its bad name will almost certainly follow in patients who do not take care.

Nerve Abscesses

One of the least well-known complications of leprosy is the spontaneous appearance of an abscess in one of the superficial nerves. This was probably first described in 1924 (Muir, 1924) and since then leprosy literature has been studded with reports of occasional cases which are usually found in tuberculoid patients. The presenting symptom is of severe pain in a localized area radiating down a limb. On examination, the patient's leprosy looks quiescent and non-reactional but the area of pain is swollen and tender, and an associated muscle weakness can be detected. This needs to be explored surgically; usually a single intraneural abscess is found, but cases have been reported where the superficial nerve showed gross oedema and abscess formation in two or three separate areas. Histologically, there will be a tuberculoid pathology including caseation, and often the centre of the nerve contains frank pus. If it is incised, drained, and antileprosy therapy is maintained, more particularly with one of the newer antileprosy drugs (clofazimine or rifampicin), not only should the lesion heal quickly but the muscle weakness may also disappear with physiotherapy.

Cases have been reported of an abscess occurring in a nerve in association with non-tuberculoid disease (Sehgal, Tuli, and Dube, 1967; Job and Bhaktaviziam, 1967; Enna and Brand, 1970), but these cases, both of BL and LL type leprosy, seem always to be found in association with severe erythema nodosum leprosum. The incidence of necrotic lesions in ENL is known (Waters and Ridley, 1963) and it is presumed that a 'lepromatous nerve abscess' is really a necrotic ENL lesion which has fortuitously occurred within a nerve.

We have to decide whether the words 'nerve abscess' in leprosy simply describe tissue breakdown associated with inflammation, in which case they can be used in any type of the disease, or whether the phrase should be limited to its original meaning, in which case it would imply a lesion associated with *tuberculoid* leprosy. At present there seems to be no real agreement on nomenclature, but as nerve abscesses are very rare and those lesions which occur in lepromatous disease are even rarer, the problem remains somewhat academic.

MEDICAL TREATMENT

Treatment of Uncomplicated Leprosy

Although Hansen recognized the presence of an infecting agent in tissue removed from leprosy patients 100 years ago, and so started the science of bacteriology as applied to human disease, it was a long time before a drug was discovered which seemed to have incontrovertible success in ameliorating active disease, and for many years after this it was not realized that even when dead the leprosy bacillus took an unusually long time to disintegrate and disappear from the body. The discovery that the *Myco. leprae* would multiply when injected into the foot-pad of mice (Shepard, 1960, 1962) made it possible to confirm Hansen's original suggestion that bacilli which did not stain uniformly were no longer viable. Previously it had only been possible to recognize the presence of acid-alcohol-fast bacilli in skin but now, by counting the percentage of solidly staining organisms present in smears of tissue fluid taken from the lesions, it can be determined how many bacilli are alive. This percentage, which is known as the morphological index (MI), can be used as an assessment of the success of antibacterial therapy even before the bacilli have begun to disappear from the patient (Waters and Rees, 1962).

When drug trials had to be dependent on observation of clinical change or bacterial disappearance, they took a long time to perform; many cases of lepromatous leprosy do not become smear negative for several years after the onset of treatment. It is now known that the MI falls to zero within the first few months of therapy, and this demonstration of the efficacy of a remedy can be used to reduce the time needed for drug trials to be performed. Confirmation that newer medications are efficacious—clofazimine (Pettit, Rees, and Ridley, 1967), rifampicin (Leiker and Kamp, 1970)—was made much more rapidly than would previously have been possible and the same technique has proved that in the past unnecessarily high doses of sulphone were given to patients.

It is increasingly accepted that routine antileprosy therapy should be diamino-diphenyl sulphone (DDS) and that 50 mg twice weekly is a perfectly adequate dose for routine usage, but as in practice patients may forget to take tablets which are so infrequently needed, it is wiser to ask them to take 100 mg tablets twice a week. As there is a feeling in some circles that even 5 mg of DDS twice weekly might be a sufficient dosage it can be seen that our recommendation verges on the conservative side of therapy. Other drugs are sometimes used (diphenylthiourea, thiambutosine, sulphamethoxypyridine) but there are two which have recently come to the fore. Clofazimine, originally known as B663, is a phenazine derivative which has been shown to be as efficacious as DDS in doses of 100 mg two or three times a week, while rifampicin, in a rather higher dosage, also produces a rapid negation of the MI. These two drugs are of great value in cases of sulphone-resistant disease (Sheskin and Convit, 1969), but until their cost is reduced to a level comparable with sulphone they will necessarily take second place in the leprologist's armamentarium.

Treatment of Reactions

Acute Exacerbation (Jopling Type I)

The skin manifestations of this type of reaction are usually relatively painless and with the exception of simple analgesics there is no indication for change of treatment. It has in the past been a regrettable habit of many leprologists to blame this reaction on the medication that is being provided and an unfortunate habit has arisen of stopping the antileprosy drug. We believe most strongly that this is ill-advised and that continuation of sulphone will not hinder the patient's chance of recovery from reaction.

If the patient's leprosy is on the face and there are enlarged preauricular nerves, it is sometimes considered a wise precaution to start the patient on 15 or 20 mg of prednisolone daily in an attempt to diminish the chance of facial paralysis secondary to a neural reaction. This may not be truly prophylactic, but when one is confronted with a patient who may develop a permanent facial palsy there is no harm in doing everything possible to prevent it.

Erythema Nodosum Leprosum

There has probably been more confusion concerning the aetiology of this reaction than in any other field of leprosy, but the author and his colleagues are in total disagreement with those who teach that the reaction is precipitated by sulphones and that the treatment of ENL necessitates the cessation of antibacterial treatment (Pettit and Waters, 1967). Not only was this reaction described 30 years before the introduction of sulphone therapy but it also occurs in patients who have never been treated with sulphone. We believe that no case of ENL persists after the patient has become bacterially negative, and as bacterial cure is one of the aims of therapy, antileprosy treatment should not be interrupted simply because of the onset of ENL. It has been our habit to continue the antileprosy treatment at all times.

The early symptoms of ENL are relatively trivial

and need no more than symptomatic therapy; mild sedatives are of some value while chloroquine sulphate and antimonials are frequently recommended, but as the condition increases in severity steroids must be administered; in many parts of the world it is still unfortunately necessary to treat prolonged febrile reactions with high doses of steroids or ACTH. Although these drugs undoubtedly help the patient, such large doses are needed that complications of steroid therapy are all too frequent.

In recent years it has been shown that thalidomide is probably the best available treatment for this condition (Sheskin and Convit, 1969). In varying doses, rarely exceeding 25 mg per day, thalidomide has been shown to suppress most of the symptoms and signs of reaction in an amazingly short time. Unfortunately this drug has no antibacterial effect nor is it 'curative' of ENL, in the sense that it is continually needed to suppress the symptoms and if the drug is stopped the symptoms not infrequently return, especially in those who have previously suffered from severe reactions. It is regrettable to have to note that at present in many parts of the world the emotional reaction to thalidomide's unfortunate history is such that many leprologists are unable to obtain suitable supplies for their patients.

Treatment of Neurological Complications

Anaesthesia

Patients who have suffered from either neural or tuberculoid leprosy without having had the opportunity or desire to consult a doctor may undergo spontaneous recovery (the 'burnt-out case' of the pre-sulphone era), but sometimes such patients will come to a doctor many years later complaining of anaesthesia. This is always too late to help. However, if symptoms are of recent onset and therapy is started within a year or so of the recognition of anaesthesia, it can reasonably be hoped that the area of sensory loss will diminish with treatment. Improvement of sensation will be particularly marked around the periphery of the lesion, and although this is most commonly found at the tuberculoid end of the scale sometimes patients with the 'glove and stocking' type of anaesthesia, associated with long-standing lepromatous disease, will feel a subjective improvement at the upper level of the anaesthetic zone, although this can rarely be confirmed clinically. It is presumed that the improvement in these patients is due to the disappearance of bacteria and pathology from those parts of the nerves which had not been totally destroyed before the diagnosis was made and this seems to confirm the suggestion that early nerve lesions are of an ischaemic nature and axons are not immediately destroyed.

Nerve Pain

All nerve pain is due basically to the stretching of the perineurium by intraneural pathology, and in many cases specific treatment is too slow to give rapid symptomatic relief. Although sedatives are often helpful in mild cases of nerve pain, there remains a large group of patients whose discomfort is not helped by simple medication and who are in need of some form of surgical intervention. As most severe cases of nerve pain are associated with ENL it is possible, if thalidomide returns to general favour, that the number of patients who need operation will diminish, but at present there is still some place for non-medical therapy. Very often in the past leprologists have been compelled to inject a painful nerve with a local anaesthetic, while more recently this has been combined with injectable forms of steroids. Hyaluronidase has also been added to the injection in the hope that it will facilitate spread of medication within the perineurium. Unfortunately, paraneural injections are relatively unhelpful but direct intraneural injections may dramatically relieve pain for several days; and despite the considerable discomfort of the procedure patients frequently ask for further injections when the pain returns. Sometimes after several attacks it becomes obvious that the nerve has been permanently damaged and muscle wasting and paralysis develop; it would be comforting to the leprologist to be quite sure that none of these sequelae was due to the injections, but there remains an unpleasant suspicion that the therapy itself might be responsible for at least some of the residual fibrosis.

If intraneural injections do not control nerve pain, there are various surgical methods to reduce intraneural tension. Nerve stripping, that is, the total removal of a segment of nerve sheath, is no longer favoured as such an operation removes some of the blood supply to the damaged nerve and may enhance the possibilities of further paralysis. This operation alleviates nerve pain immediately, but it would seem wiser to limit its use to patients whose severe pain is associated with a recognizably permanent paralysis. In such cases there is nothing to lose.

Slightly less drastic surgery is probably safer, and although a simple slit along the nerve sheath would seem to be logical this is often followed by herniation of oedematous nerve tissue through the incision, and the consequent danger of further nerve damage. The best technique is to make a linear incision and lift off the sheath as medial and lateral flaps, leaving it attached to the deep surface of the nerve and thereby both releasing pressure and maintaining blood supply (Brand, 1964).

Treatment of Paralyses

In most cases of paralysis associated with leprosy the condition only reaches the surgeon's attention when a nerve is irreparably damaged. The various techniques of treatment of the resulting paralyses of the hands, feet and face are not discussed here, and we shall limit this section to consideration of the treatment of acute paralysis.

Foot-drop and wrist-drop usually associated with the

Type I reaction may occur acutely and can frequently be cured. Splinting of the affected limb in a position of rest was in the past the only possible measure, and many cases who were treated in this way recovered normal muscle power in 6 to 8 weeks as the reaction subsided. Although the supplemental administration of prednisolone in doses of 15 to 25 mg a day has become routine there seems to have been no controlled study to determine whether the addition of steroids increases the speed or the number of cures. If the acute paralysis is associated with nerve pain, modified nerve stripping, supplemented by splinting of the affected muscles, may be a more advantageous treatment.

Nerve Abscess

There is no medical therapy for these abscesses. In the true nerve abscess associated with tuberculoid disease operation is invariably needed with evacuation of the pus and caseous material. In the so-called lepromatous nerve abscess, where there is no caseation, it can be presumed that thalidomide would be as successful here as it is in all other forms of erythema nodosum leprosum. The rarity of the condition is such, however, that there seems to be no report at present of the use of thalidomide and it must be presumed that the drug would only be successful if used prior to the development of necrosis. If caseation or pus formation has occurred surgical incision will be necessary.

Trophic Problems

Ichthyosis due to the destruction of sweat ducts cannot be helped by the simple application of a greasy ointment, as such treatment only helps to soften the skin by retarding the evaporation of sweat and so encouraging hydration of keratin. In leprosy, secondary xeroderma will need a different approach and it is necessary to hydrate the keratin by soaking the affected area in water for 15 minutes and then covering the part with a greasy ointment which will postpone evaporation for at least a few hours. More permanent forms of treatment cannot be expected.

Prevention of ulcers on the hands and feet is entirely dependent on the standard of self-awareness of the patient, and it is in this field of education that much remains to be done. Every method should be used to remind the patient of the complications that are possible as a result of his anaesthesia. If he insists on smoking he should use a cigarette holder, if he comes from a part of the world where shoes are not usually worn he should be encouraged to wear shoes at all times. An anaesthetic foot ought to be examined every day for signs of trauma, and the shoe itself must also be inspected to ensure that there is nothing which is liable to cause damage. This routine is most important as an ulcer, once formed, is rarely a unique event; it can only heal by fibrosis and as such tissue is more easily damaged by subsequent trauma repeated ulceration becomes more and more likely.

When an ulcer has developed it should be fully explored to determine whether or not there are any sinuses extending deeply; X-rays are necessary to assess bone damage. Often, these ulcers have already affected the depth of the foot and bone fragments should be removed, the sinus curetted and the lesion treated by rest and antibiotics in an effort to encourage it to heal from below. Usually this necessitates rest, either in bed or at least with a walking plaster, which is so arranged that no weight is placed on the affected area. When the ulcer has finally healed, special footwear should be provided for the patient which spreads the weight of the body evenly over the unscarred areas. Recently, there has been a tendency to substitute a plastic foam (Mondl, Gardiner, and Bisset, 1969) for the microcellular rubber inner soles which were previously used.

There is little that can be done to prevent a Charcot joint from developing, but the patient should be made aware that a twisted ankle or ricked foot in an anaesthetic limb is dangerous, and in addition to the foot drill recommended to guard against the onset of an ulcer it is urged that patients should be taught that swelling and redness in the region of the ankle is a serious sign and that they should immediately seek advice. Although neuropathic lesions of the foot joints do not always produce an unstable foot, the commonest type (affecting the ankle joint) will leave a foot which is not stable and so will increase the likelihood of ulceration of parts of the foot not normally weight-bearing.

NEUROSURGERY AND PHYSIOTHERAPY

This is not the place for a detailed account of the large part that physiotherapy and surgery can play in the treatment of leprosy complications, but it may not be out of place to remind the reader that claw hands and claw feet can often be restored to a reasonable state of function by the combined efforts of the physiotherapist and the surgeon [PLATES 28a and b]. If contracture of muscles is not complete physiotherapy will prevent the development of joint deformity, and later, when the disease has been rendered inactive, tendon transplants will give a new lease of life to the hand and foot. Interested readers are recommended to refer to the relevant chapters in Cochrane and Davey's textbook on leprosy.

OCULAR LEPROSY

There are three major ways in which the eye can be involved in leprosy.

In non-lepromatous disease the eye is most at risk following facial paralysis due to Type I reaction; lagophthalmos will lead to the permanent uncovering of a cornea which is frequently already anaesthetic due to concomitant trigeminal involvement; resulting corneal ulceration will lead at best to scarring and at worst to infection and destruction of the eye.

In lepromatous disease complications are due directly to the presence of bacilli. Seventy-five per cent of lepromatous patients show biomicroscopical abnormalities in the first 5 years of their disease (Brand, 1968), and often these changes are the first detectable signs of leprosy. Macroscopically, the first sign is the appearance of asymptomatic nodules in the upper outer quadrant of the cornea associated first with non-vascular infiltration and later with the appearance of an interstitial keratitis. Later still, there is chronic inflammation of the iris with synechial formation causing adhesion to the lens. Unfortunately, all these changes may occur before the patient has noticed anything wrong with his vision and it is the leprologist's responsibility to ensure regular examination of the eyes in all cases that are under treatment.

The eye may also be involved in erythema nodosum leprosum reactions, giving an acute diffuse iritis with pain and photophobia. At present, this is usually treated with atropine and anti-inflammatory drugs but it is hoped that more widespread use of thalidomide will reduce the incidence of ocular complications of ENL.

In the eye, as elsewhere, surgical intervention should not take place until the leprosy is quiescent but when this has occurred corneal transplantation, lens extraction, and iridectomy have all been performed with advantage in suitable cases, while tarsorrhaphy and plastic manoeuvres may be called upon to protect the exposed cornea in lagophthalmos.

LEPROSY OF THE CENTRAL NERVOUS SYSTEM

There have been few reports concerning the brain and spinal cord in leprosy, and while it is not surprising that in heavily bacilliferous patients scanty *Myco. leprae* have occasionally been found in the CNS, no microscopic changes were found in a detailed study of 20 cases, most of whom showed extensive involvement of the peripheral nervous system (Ermakova, 1936). It is a strange fact that while a proportion of dorsal root ganglia seem to be destroyed by leprosy without the agency of actual invasion of acid-fast organisms (Lumsden, 1964), there is a complete failure of any form of pathology to extend into the cord. This is only explicable by the fact that the passage of bacilli along the column of Schwann cells is centripetal; the reason for this is not known.

Spastic Paralysis in New Caledonian Leprosy Patients

Attention has recently been drawn (Brody *et al.*, 1969) to a number of patients in New Caledonia who, while having leprosy, also showed a degree of spastic paralysis with pathologically hyperactive reflexes in the lower limbs. No patient had sustained clonus. In a nearby tuberculosis sanatorium no cases of hyperreflexia were detected in a group of Melanesian and European patients.

Such cases have never been described elsewhere, and although the authors seem to suspect that the condition is associated with sulphone therapy further information must be obtained before comment can be made on this unique group.

References

ANDERSEN, J. G. (1969) Studies in the mediaeval diagnosis of leprosy in Denmark, *Dan. med. Bull.*, 16, Suppl. 9, 1.

BRAND, M. (1968) *Early Ocular Change in Leprosy*, Paper presented at the Ninth International Congress of Leprosy, London.

BRAND, P. (1964) in *Leprosy in Theory and Practice*, 2nd ed., eds. Cochrane, R. G., and Davey, T. F., Bristol, p. 447.

BRODY, J. A., YASE, Y., CHEMIER, G., and PHILIPPE, Y. (1969) Hyperreflexia and spastic paralysis among New Caledonian leprosy patients, *Amer. J. trop. Med. Hyg.*, 18, 132.

BROWNE, S. G. (1970) How old is leprosy? *Brit. med. J.*, 3, 640.

CARAYON, A. (1968) *Direct Surgical Treatment of Large Nerve Trunks in Leprosy*, Paper presented at the Ninth International Congress of Leprosy, London.

ENNA, C. D., and BRAND, P. (1970) Peripheral nerve abscess in leprosy: report of three cases in dimorphous and lepromatous leprosy, *Leprosy Rev.* 41, 175.

ERMAKOVA, N. (1936) Studies on leprosy: central, sympathetic and peripheral nervous systems, *Int. J. Leprosy*, 4, 325.

FRANKEN, J. H. (1963) *Diffuse Leprosy of Lucio and Latapi*, Netherlands Antilles.

GAUNTLETT, S. L. (1969) Leprosy control in the Southern Province of Zambia, *Leprosy Rev.*, 40, 223.

GOLDMAN, L., MORAITES, R. S., and KITZMILLER, K. W. (1966) White spots in biblical times. A background for the dermatologist for the participation in discussions of current revision of the Bible, *Arch. Derm.*, 93, 744.

GOUGEROT, H. (1949) Lepres invisibles, *Int. J. Leprosy*, 17, 13.

JOB, C. K., and BHAKTAVIZIAM, C. (1967) Nerve abscess in lepromatous leprosy: report of a patient, *Leprosy Rev.*, 38, 243.

JOPLING, W. H. (1956) Borderline (dimorphous) leprosy maintaining a polyneuritic form for eight years: a case report, *Trans. roy. Soc. trop. Med. Hyg.*, 50, 478.

JOPLING, W. H. (1970) Reactions in leprosy, *Leprosy Rev.*, 14, 62.

JOPLING, W. H., and MORGAN-HUGHES, J. A. (1965) Pure neural tuberculoid leprosy, *Brit. med. J.*, 2, 799.

KUNDU, K. K., and GHOSH, S. (1970) Observations on clinical manifestations of primary polyneuritic type of leprosy, *Indian J. Derm.*, 15, 45.

LARA, C. B., and NOLASCO, J. Q. (1956) Self-healing, or abortive, and residual forms of childhood leprosy and their probable significance, *Int. J. Leprosy*, 24, 245.

LEIKER, D. L., and KAMP, H. (1970) First results of treatment of leprosy with 'Rifadin', *Leprosy Rev.*, 41, 25.

LEPROSY REVIEW (1964) Report on the Round Table on

Borderline and Interminate Leprosy, 8th Int. Cong. Lepr. 1963, *Leprosy Rev.*, 35, 15. (Special supplement.)

LEPROSY REVIEW (1969) Proceedings of World Health Organization No. 169, *Leprosy Rev.*, 40, 64.

LITALIEN, F., HARTER, P., DON, T. T. K. M., and DANH, N. T. (1960) Cutaneous determination of Hansen's disease in pure neural leprosy patients under the influence of sulfone treatment, *Bull. Soc. Path. exot.*, 53, 943.

LUMSDEN, C. E. (1964) in *Leprosy in Theory and Practice*, 2nd ed., eds. Cochrane, R. G., and Davey, T. F., Bristol, p. 221.

MATSUDA, H. (1969) Charcot-like changes in leprosy, *La Lepro*, 38, 167.

MÖLLER-CHRISTENSEN, V. (1953) *Ten Lepers from Naestved in Denmark*, Copenhagen.

MÖLLER-CHRISTENSEN, V. (1961) *Bone Changes in Leprosy*, Bristol.

MONDL, A., GARDINER, J., and BISSET, J. (1969) Use of plastazote in footwear for leprosy patients. A preliminary report, *Leprosy Rev.*, 40, 177.

MUIR, E. (1924) Nerve abscess in leprosy, *Indian med. Gaz.*, 59, 87.

MURATA, M. (1912) Über Erythema Nodosum Leprosum, *Jap. Z. Derm. Urol.*, 12, 1013.

PEARSON, J. M. H., WEDDELL, A. G. M., and PALMER, E. (1968) *Sensory Changes and the Histopathology of Nerve Fibres Before and During the Treatment of Leprosy*, Paper presented at the Ninth International Congreess of Leprosy, London.

PETTIT, J. H. S., and REES, R. J. W. (1966) Studies on sulfone resistance in leprosy, 2. Treatment with a riminophenazine derivative (B.663), *Int. J. Leprosy*, 34, 391.

PETTIT, J. H. S., REES, R. J. W., and RIDLEY, D. S. (1967) Chemotherapeutic trials in leprosy. 3 pilot trials of a riminophenazine derivative B.663 in the treatment of lepromatous leprosy, *Int. J. Leprosy*, 35, 25.

PETTIT, J. H. S., and WATERS, M. F. R. (1967) The etiology of erythema nodosum leprosum, *Int. J. Leprosy*, 35, 1.

RIDLEY, D. S. (1969) Reactions in leprosy, *Leprosy Rev.*, 40, 77.

RIDLEY, D. S., and JOPLING, W. H. (1966) Classification of leprosy according to immunity. A five group system, *Int. J. Leprosy*, 34, 255.

SABIN, T. D., and EBNER, J. D. (1969) Patterns of sensory loss in lepromatous leprosy, *Int. J. Leprosy*, 37, 239.

SCHULZ, E. J., and PENTZ, H. H. L. (1970) Leprosy control in South Africa, *Leprosy Rev.*, 41, 15.

SEHGAL, V. N., TULI, S. M., and DUBE, B. (1967) Leprotic nerve abscesses in Northern India, *Int. J. Leprosy*, 35, 60.

SHEPARD, C. C. (1960) The experimental disease that follows the injection of human leprosy bacilli into foot-pads of mice, *J. exp. Med.*, 112, 45.

SHEPARD, C. C. (1962) Multiplication of *M. leprae* in the footpad of the mouse, *Int. J. Leprosy*, 30, 291.

SHESKIN, J., and CONVIT, J. (1969) Results of a double blind study of the influence of thalidomide on the lepra reaction, *Int. J. Leprosy*, 37, 135.

SKINSNES, O. K. (1964) Leprosy in society, II. The pattern of concept and reaction to leprosy in oriental antiquity, *Leprosy Rev.*, 35, 106.

WATERS, M. F. R., and REES, R. J. W. (1962) Changes in the morphology of *Mycobacterium leprae* in patients under treatment, *Int. J. Leprosy*, 30, 266.

WATERS, M. F. R., and RIDLEY, D. S. (1963) Necrotizing reactions in lepromatous leprosy. A clinical and histologic study, *Int. J. Leprosy*, 31, 418.

27 Neurology in Thailand

A. VEJJAJIVA

INTRODUCTION

Thailand, formerly known as Siam, is situated in South-East Asia between the 5th and 20th parallels of the North Latitude. In terms of land area, the country is about twice the size of the United Kingdom. On the north-west it is bounded by Burma, on the north-east by Laos, on its eastern side by Cambodia and South Vietnam, and in the southern peninsular region by Malaysia. The capital city of Bangkok is located in the central region, the economic and political heart of modern Thailand. This region comprises a shallow trough, bounded on the east and west by a forested wilderness of hills and mountains. The fertile central plain is drained and irrigated by many rivers, the most important being the Chao Phya which flows south into the Gulf of Thailand. High mountain ranges dominate the country's northern and western borders, while the north-east is an unspectacular sandstone plateau.

With the exception of the western side of the peninsula of Thailand, where there is no long dry season, the entire country experiences the marked seasonal variation in rainfall typical of the tropics. The rainy season lasts from May until October, followed by a cool dry season from November to February, and a hot dry season with rising humidity from March until the onset of heavy rains 3 months later. The annual mean temperature is 80° to 85° Fahrenheit, dropping as low as 60° in December and rising as high as 98° in April.

The word *Thai* means 'free'. The original Thais migrated south from Yunnan province in south-west China some 1200 years ago. With the continuous intermingling of Indian and Chinese cultural elements, a distinctive culture has developed in the kingdom over the ensuing centuries, centring on the Chao Phya basin. Europeans first arrived in the seventeenth century and established commercial footholds. However, unlike most other South-East Asian countries, Thailand has never at any time been under the domination of a Western power.

Thailand's current population is approximately 35 million, of whom some 3 million live in Bangkok. The rate of population increase is in excess of 3 per cent per year. Over 50 per cent of the population are under the age of 20, while only 4 per cent are aged 60 or more. Despite its size and its uneven geographic distribution, the population is more culturally homogeneous than in many parts of South-East Asia, and there is virtually no friction between the various ethnic groups. The Chinese, who constitute the largest minority group and are active in all forms of commerce, number about 3 million. Only about one-tenth of these Thai Chinese were born in China, and immigration from mainland China is now prohibited. Malays are the second largest ethnic minority, numbering about 1 million and living for the most part in the southern provinces. Finally, there is a small and diverse group of immigrants from Laos, the Vietnams and Cambodia, mainly settled in the North-East region, and a significant group of about 10 000 Europeans and Americans living primarily in Bangkok. Buddhism is the chief religion of the people. It is as dominant a force in Thailand as is Roman Catholicism in such countries as Spain and the Republic of Ireland.

Still predominantly agricultural, the economy of the country hinges on the production of rice. Four-fifths of the Thai people depend on farming for their livelihood. Rice alone occupies nearly 70 per cent of the land used for farming, leaving the remainder, about 6 million acres, for vegetable gardens, coconuts, rubber and fruit trees, maize and all other field crops, and for livestock grazing. Tin-mining and rubber-planting in the southern provinces, teak forestry in the north and the manufacture of silk on hand-operated looms are the important industries. Compared with many Western nations, Thailand is an underdeveloped country. The *per capita* gross national product at mid-1965, with a population of approximately 30 million, was U.S. $120.00, whereas that of the United Kingdom, with a population of 54·5 million, was U.S. $1550.00. The corresponding figures for Nigeria (population approximately 10 million) and India (487 million) were U.S. $80.00 and $90.00 respectively (Bryant, 1969).

Except for an affluent group in the capital who have adopted a Western style of living, the diet of the average Thai contains a high percentage of carbohydrates, with rice as the mainstay, and a relatively low amount of animal proteins and fats. Fresh fruits and vegetables are abundant.

There are at present four medical schools in the country, three in Bangkok and one in Chiang Mai, the largest city in the North. The oldest school, the Faculty of Medicine at Siriraj Hospital, is over 80 years old, while the newest and most modern faculty, at Ramathibodi Hospital in Bangkok, graduated its first group of students in early 1971. There is a serious shortage of medical man-power, particularly in the rural areas. For Thailand as a whole, the ratio of doctors to population is 1 to 7600. In Bangkok it is 1 to 940, but in many remote areas it is less than 1 to 200 000.

Until recently in Bangkok, neurology has been entirely a part of the practice of general physicians. The emergence of modern and well-equipped neurological and neurosurgical units and the formation of the Neurological Association of Thailand have only occurred within the past 10 years. However, in all except one medical school, these units are divisions within departments of Internal Medicine and Surgery, and neurologists must spend a minor part of their time in general medical care. Neurosurgeons, on the other hand, generally limit themselves to neurosurgery. The situation in the provinces is totally different in that there is not a single hospital with a neurological unit or a specialist in this field, with the sole exception of the Faculty of Medicine at Chiang Mai in the North. Thus, a large number of patients attending neurological clinics in Bangkok come from various parts of the country, imposing a heavy service load on the available neurologists whose total number does not exceed twenty. It is expected that the certification of neurology as a separate specialty by the recently formed postgraduate examination board of the Thai Medical Council will help to recruit young neurologists and to relieve the present heavy demands placed on specialists in this field.

NEUROLOGICAL DISORDERS IN THAILAND

Ready acceptance of patients from all social strata throughout the country and the provision of free medical care to those who cannot afford to pay give neurologists a good opportunity to treat the wide variety of neurological disorders prevalent in the country. A series of patients treated by the author during a 2-year period (1965–67) may be taken as an illustrative sample. Analysis of 865 patients by diagnosis is as shown in TABLE 27.1. Since many patients are seen directly by neurosurgeons, statistics are also given for in-patients on a university neurosurgical service with two consultant neurosurgeons [TABLE 27.2].

Table 27.1
Neurological Diseases Seen by the Author During a 2-Year Period

Diseases	*No. of Cases*	*% of Total*
CVA	346	40·0
Infection of nervous system	97	11·2
Epilepsy	76	8·7
Spinal cord diseases	48	5·6
Tumour	36	4·2
Demyelinating diseases	31	3·6
Peripheral neuropathies	45	4·9
Neuromuscular disorders	31	4·0
Degenerative diseases	18	2·0
Miscellaneous	137	15·8
Total	865	100·0

Table 21.2
Statistics of Inpatients for 3 Years (1962–1965), Section of Neurological Surgery, Chulalongkorn Hospital

Diseases	*No. of Cases*	*% of Total*
Head injuries	491	32·2
Spinal injuries	92	5·9
Nerve injuries	22	1·4
Intervertebral disc disorders	200	13·1
Tumour	184	12·1
Infection	113	8·4
Congenital malformations	90	5·9
Vascular diseases	77	5·0
Miscellaneous	254	16·0
Total	1523	100·0

Source: *Clinical Bulletin* (1965) Neurology, neurological surgery and psychiatry, Chulalongkorn Hospital and Medical School, Bangkok.

Cerebral vascular accidents formed 40 per cent of neurological admissions, while head injuries headed the list of neurosurgical patients. It is noteworthy that some 10 per cent of the patients had nervous system infection —a high figure compared to the prevalence of such diseases in the Western hemisphere. Outpatient statistics reveal a pattern different from that of inpatients, with relatively minor ailments such as migraine, tension headache and neuralgia forming the majority of cases. Many patients with epilepsy and intervertebral disc disorders are treated in Thailand as outpatients, so that the true prevalence of these particular disorders is far higher than is suggested by inpatient statistics. A thorough epidemiological survey of the prevalence of neurological diseases has not yet been made in any community in Thailand. In view of the inadequate neurological facilities outside Bangkok, the lack of uniformity of hospital standards throughout the country, the generally poor records kept by private practitioners, and the unreliability of official government health statistics, it is unlikely that the true epidemiological picture could be accurately defined without an extensive, detailed, and well-coordinated survey.

Cerebrovascular Disease

From the inpatient statistics, cerebral vascular accidents ranked first among neurological admissions, accounting for 40 per cent of the total. Of these, two-thirds were due to vascular occlusion. Intracerebral haemorrhage formed a quarter of the cases, and about 5 per cent were due to primary subarachnoid haemorrhage (Vejjajiva and Fazekas, 1968). A great majority of cases with occlusive vascular diseases were due to atherosclerosis, and the incidence increased with age. Nearly two-thirds of such patients were found to be hypertensive with a diastolic blood pressure of over 110 mm Hg, and about 40 per cent were diabetic, while in only 20 per cent was neither disease present. There appeared to be no significant difference in the incidence of occlusive vascular disease among various socio-economic groups, but this clinical observation awaits epidemiological confirmation. It is also worth noting that although the diet of the low-income group contains a small amount of fat with a relatively high proportion of unsaturated fat, the average serum cholesterol level is no lower than that found in Western white populations. In a group of 160 patients between the ages of 60 and 90, with no clinical manifestations of cerebral vascular disease, the mean serum cholesterol was 213 ± 45 mg per cent, with a range of 168 to 258 mg (Snyder, 1968). This group resided in a home for the indigent aged and were thus limited to a traditional Thai diet. The frequent presence of atherosclerosis as an important cause of cerebral vascular occlusion among the Thai is thus similar to that found in Western countries. However, the incidence of extracranial cerebral vascular occlusion appears to be less common. An angiographic study of 129 patients with acute stroke revealed the presence of internal carotid occlusion in less than 5 per cent (Hongladarom *et al.*, 1962). This contrasts with the series in England reported by Bull, Marshall, and Shaw (1960), who found an incidence of 17 per cent in 80 cases studied. Another point of note with regard to degenerative vascular disease is that the incidence of acute myocardial infarction from coronary occlusion appears to be significantly less than that in Europe and the United States. This discrepancy between the high incidence of cerebral vascular disease and the low incidence of coronary occlusion in Thailand is similar to that observed in the Japanese. Part of this discrepancy may be due to the fact that coronary artery disease in the Thai often presents as atherosclerotic congestive cardiac failure rather than as acute myocardial infarction. Detailed pathological studies of coronary vessels among the Thai have not been made, but it is likely that the incidence of atherosclerosis is high and not significantly different from that found in cerebral vessels. The factor which ultimately determines the cardiac insult, namely thrombosis, may, for some as yet unexplained reason, be less frequent in the Thai and the Japanese. The distinct rarity of deep vein thrombosis and pulmonary embolism, as generally experienced by physicians in these two countries, would support such a hypothesis. Another plausible but as yet unexplored mechanism is that the process of fibrinolysis may be more efficient in the Thai and the Japanese, and it is possible that this is dietary or genetic in origin. Non-infective cerebral venous sinus thrombosis is exceedingly uncommon in Thailand, perhaps for the same reason. Thrombo-embolic phenomena associated with oral contraceptives have not as yet been documented in Thai women, although these drugs have been in use on a wide scale in Bangkok for over 5 years. The differences from the American and European experience are striking.

Apart from atherosclerotic occlusion, some cases of acute stroke are due to meningovascular syphilis. Such patients presenting with acute stroke and showing angiographic findings of vascular occlusion have been recorded (Vejjajiva and Hongladarom, 1969). In the young adult with non-embolic occlusion, two other diagnoses deserve mention. In young females, the onset of acute stroke may be the presenting feature of Takayasu's arteriopathy, a disease which is frequently seen in Thailand. In all such cases with an acute cerebral vascular accident, angiography has revealed either marked stenosis or occlusion of one or more extracranial cerebral vessels. The entire common carotid or innominate artery may be involved, and there have been cases with subclavian stenosis and angiographic demonstration of subclavian steal syndrome. Involvement of the extracranial cerebral vessels may be part of a diffuse process involving the aortic arch and the descending aorta, or it may be the only finding. Cases have also presented with features of renal vascular hypertension, with narrowing of the aorta and renal arteries. In some of these cases, study has revealed stenosis and sometimes occlusion of extracranial cerebral vessels without clinical evidence of neurological deficit. A detailed pathological study of Thai patients with Takayasu's arteriopathy has been reported (Vinijchaikul, 1967). Another group of young patients was observed with occlusive vascular disease distinct from Takayasu's and consisted predominantly of males aged 20 to 30. In all these cases, there has been no evidence of valvular heart disease, syphilis, diabetes, hypertension or any other systemic disease predisposing to thrombosis. Angiographic studies have revealed occlusion of the middle cerebral artery, or one of its branches, with apparently normal extracranial vessels. The cause of this syndrome is undetermined.

Cases of cerebral embolism form a small proportion of those with occlusive vascular disease. The main aetiological factor is rheumatic valvular heart disease, and most cases are due to non-septic emboli. A peculiar feature of this disease in Thailand is the occurrence of tight mitral stenosis in early adult life, in contrast to the natural history of mitral disease as seen in the West. In one series of 303 patients with mitral stenosis who underwent valvulotomy, 24 per cent were aged 20 or under and most of these cases were severely incapacitated by dyspnoea (Jumbala *et al.*, 1968). This experience appears to be similar to that in India and Israel (Cherian *et al.*, 1964; Borman *et al.*, 1961). Cerebral embolism may thus be encountered very early in the course of the disease.

Intracerebral haemorrhage is usually seen in association with hypertension, although some normotensive cases are due to arteriovenous malformation, blood dyscrasias, or nervous system invasion by the parasite *Gnathostoma spinigerum*. The incidence of primary spontaneous subarachnoid haemorrhage among cases admitted with acute cerebral vascular accidents is comparable to that in Western series, but the incidence of the causative factors appears to be different. Among 94 patients with subarachnoid haemorrhage seen during a 5-year period (Suwanwela *et al.*, 1969*a*), 40 had bleeding secondary to intracerebral haemorrhage, neoplasms, cerebral infarction or parasitic invasion. Of the remaining 54, 20 were due to ruptured aneurysms of which 17 were congenital and 3 mycotic. Arteriovenous malformations were found in 14 cases, and in the remaining 20, the cause was undetermined. The incidence of congenital berry aneurysms is relatively low, although still more common than that of arteriovenous malformation, unlike the experience in Malaysia (Selby, 1968). The number of patients in the series quoted is not sufficient for definite conclusions to be drawn. Complete four-vessel angiography was not carried out in all patients and cases of 'unknown cause' may have been due to rupture of small aneurysms. Indeed, in an angiographic and pathological study by Bunyaratavej (1970) of cases with primary subarachnoid haemorrhage, 52 cases of aneurysm were found. Among these, five cases were found to have peripheral aneurysms. This experience differs from that in the United Kingdom, Europe and the United States, and this interesting discrepancy deserves further study.

Infections of the Nervous System

As in many other tropical countries, one of the major medical problems in Thailand is the diverse manifestations of infectious diseases. Nervous system infections due to bacteria, parasites and viruses are common. Spirochaetal and fungal infections are less frequent. These infections often present distinctive local problems, as exemplified by tuberculosis. Tuberculous meningitis is commoner than pyogenic meningitis in adults, but in young children it is less common. In spite of national public health campaigns advising BCG vaccination, enthusiastic antituberculous programmes, and readily available and free treatment for pulmonary tuberculosis, the disease is still very common. In many cases, inadequate or delayed treatment has led to serious neurological sequelae such as arachnoiditis or arteritis, giving rise to focal deficits and cranial nerve palsies. A curious feature of tuberculous infection of the nervous system in Thailand is that tuberculomas are exceedingly rare, while tuberculous meningitis is common. This contrasts with clinical experience in many parts of India where tuberculosis is similarly abundant and intracranial tuberculoma is relatively common. This difference merits further study. Perhaps genetically determined immunological mechanisms are involved. Pyogenic meningitides from meningococci, pneumococci and other bacteria are occasionally seen. Widespread use and early recourse to antibiotics, and ready access to these drugs even without a doctor's prescription have probably reduced the incidence of pyogenic meningitis in our community. However, the illness still carries a depressing prognosis. A recent study of acute bacterial meningitis in 24 Thai children (Duangmani *et al.*, 1970) showed a mortality rate of 47·6 per cent. The commonest organisms were *Diplococcus pneumoniae* and *Haemophilus influenzae*. Syphilitic diseases involving the nervous system are not uncommon and all forms of neurosyphilis are seen. In a series of 35 patients recently reported over half belonged to the meningovascular type. Unusual presentations such as acute syphilitic myelitis, localized basal meningitis involving the cerebellopontine angle and acute carotid occlusion at the siphon were cited. It is perhaps noteworthy that the incidence of meningovascular syphilis was reported to be much higher than that of tabes dorsalis and general paresis in Africans (Gelfand, 1957). Accurate diagnosis of neurosyphilis in Thailand has been greatly facilitated by the use of refined tests such as the Reiter Protein Complement Fixation and the fluorescent treponemal antibody and absorption (FTA, FTA-Abs) methods, and the determination of spinal fluid gamma globulin which has been found to be invariably high, over three times the normal value, in patients with neurosyphilis even when the total protein content is slightly elevated or normal (Vejjajiva, Boongird, and Vejjajiva, 1967). Leptospirosis is another endemic disease in all parts of the country, but meningeal involvement is rare and patients with this disorder hardly ever present to neurologists for diagnosis or treatment. Cryptococcosis of the nervous system, although uncommon, may present an urgent diagnostic problem. Six cases have been encountered by the author during the past 5 years and about 20 have been reported in Thailand. Most of these cases closely simulated tuberculous meningitis but occasionally patients have presented with the symptoms and signs of a focal cerebral expanding lesion. Diagnosis was often made late in the course of the disease and the mortality has understandably been high. However, increasing clinical awareness and examination of cerebrospinal fluid with Indian ink stain as a routine in suspected cases has permitted more frequent and earlier diagnosis in less disabled patients. This, together with the use of amphotericin B and the new and highly effective agent against cryptococcosis, 5-fluorocytosine, have contributed to the successful treatment and complete recovery.

Among virus diseases of the nervous system in Thailand, rabies has deserved foremost attention. The disease is still endemic and relatively common (*vide infra*); outbreaks of encephalitis from Japanese B virus have recently occurred in the northern part of Thailand.

The mortality rate is about 20 per cent and neuro-psychiatric sequelae are common among survivors (Sitasuwan and Ramayodhin, 1970). Encephalitis complicating Thai haemorrhagic fever caused by the dengue and chikungunya viruses is also worth mentioning. This disease tends to occur seasonally, being highly prevalent during the rainy season when mosquitoes breed readily, and is widespread throughout the country including Bangkok. Virus encephalitides are common but at present little is known of the organisms responsible. In a recent investigation of children admitted to hospital with the diagnosis of encephalitis, aseptic meningitis or poliomyelitis, assessment included home-visits on the admission day for environmental study and mosquito collection (Bourgeois *et al.*, 1970 *a*). Enterovirus, ECHO, CMV and coxsackie were isolated from some of the patients but there was little evidence that arborvirus plays a significant role. Cases of subacute sclerosing panencephalitis or Dawson's inclusion-body encephalitis were first reported in Thailand in 1967 (Boongird and Vejjajiva, 1967). The diagnosis was based on clinical features, electroencephalographic findings, the presence of high cerebrospinal fluid gamma globulin levels and the characteristic histopathological findings at brain biopsy. Since then, sporadic cases have been encountered in children from various parts of the country.

Epilepsy

Epilepsy of all forms accounts for just over 8 per cent of the total neurological hospital admissions, but comparable clinical impressions from outpatient practice indicate that the disorders are at least as frequent as in the West. However, some differences are worthy of comment. Petit mal, with characteristic three-cycle-per-second wave and spike activity in the electroencephalogram, is distinctly uncommon among Thais. This low incidence is as yet unexplained. As there is a distinct possibility that such cases are not brought for medical advice and so remain undetected, it would be premature to entertain other hypotheses at present. Idiopathic, or the so-called centrencephalic, grand mal is common but is less frequently encountered than focal or symptomatic epilepsy. The latter is commonly found to be due to cerebral cysticercosis, the diagnosis of which has been made more difficult by the very low incidence of both intracranial and subcutaneous calcification. Curiously, *Taenia saginata* infestations are common whereas *T. solium* is said to be rare. It is also noteworthy that calcification of the pineal gland is much less frequent among Thais than in the white population; approximately 14 per cent as compared with 50 per cent in the West (Suwanwela, Charuvorn, and Arthachinta, 1966). The two observations may be unrelated, but they may be due to the low calcium content in the diet of Thai people, or may reflect some genetical difference in the metabolism of calcium (Spillane, 1969).

Tumours of the Nervous System

A detailed study was recently made of 309 cases of neoplasms of the nervous system in Thailand (Shuangshoti, Tangchai, and Netsky, 1969 *a*). Intracranial neoplasms were the most common. In order of decreasing frequency were tumours of the cranial and peripheral nerves, the spinal cord, the retinal primordium, the sympathetic ganglia and the paraganglionic cells. As in Western countries, the commonest intracranial neoplasms were gliomas. Among intracranial gliomas, astrocytoma was most frequently encountered, occurring twice as often as glioblastoma multiforme. They were slightly more common in women than in men, while in the West experience indicates the reverse (Shuangshoti, Tangchai, and Netsky, 1969 *b*). In a study of 40 cases of astrocytomas, these authors also found that more than half occurred in the first two decades of life, while the peak occurrence in Western reports was between the ages of 20 and 45 years (Levy and Elvidge, 1956). Five of the 21 supratentorial astrocytomas were located in the optic nerve and chiasm—a high incidence in contrast with 3 out of 121 cases reported by Levy and Elvidge (1956).

The similarity between the Thai and Japanese series of intracranial neoplasms is further evident in the analysis of glioblastoma multiforme (Shuangshoti and Tangchai, 1969 *a*). This tumour has an unusually high incidence in children, is relatively frequent subtentorially in both countries, and is thus different in both aspects to that found in the European studies. The reason for the East-West differences is as yet undefined.

In Thailand, meningioma is the second most common intracranial neoplasm, as in the Western hemisphere and Japan, but its occurrence on the cerebral convexity is much more frequent than in studies reported from the West (Shuangshoti, Tangchai, and Netsky, 1968). Intraspinal tumours comprise about 15 per cent of all neural neoplasms in Thailand; the ratio is 3 : 1 of intracranial to intraspinal tumours (Shuangshoti and Tangchai, 1969 *b*). The site and type of tumours do not significantly differ from those found in the West. The similarities and differences of the various aspects of neoplasms of the nervous system in the Eastern and Western hemispheres cited above should not be regarded as conclusive until a larger number of cases are studied.

Multiple Sclerosis

Multiple sclerosis is generally believed to be very rare or even non-existent among the population of Thailand and other South-East Asian countries including Singapore (Gwee, 1968), Malaysia, Vietnam and Burma. Thus, among 865 consecutive patients admitted to the Neurological Unit of Chulalongkorn Hospital under the author's care during a 2-year period (1965–67), only three patients were diagnosed as having multiple sclerosis. All three patients were Thais who had never travelled abroad. They were aged 28, 36 and 40. One patient died and the diagnosis was confirmed at autopsy (Vejjajiva, 1970). Clinical features in the two living cases belonged to the optic—brain stem—spinal form which is also the most common presentation in Japan (Kuroiwa, 1968), and diagnoses were based on classical histories of multiple symptoms and signs with relapse and remission, by spinal fluid examination and special neuroradiological procedures. Lack of a confirmatory laboratory test has limited the accuracy of all epidemiological studies of multiple sclerosis, for clinical methods even in the most experienced hands are not absolute. For example, a 31-year-old Thai woman showing neurological features suggesting the presence of multiple lesions, and showing relapses and remissions characteristic of multiple sclerosis, had at autopsy findings of chronic disseminated non-specific meningo-encephalomyelitis without evidence of demyelinated plaques (Vejjajiva, 1970).

By contrast, patients with acute transverse myelitis are relatively common and some also have bilateral optic neuritis and can readily be classified as Devic's disease. Although many recover completely, a few show subsequent relapse with signs indicating involvement of other parts of the central nervous system such as brain stem, cerebral cortex and cerebellum. This illness is clinically indistinguishable from multiple sclerosis. The course, however, tends to be shorter with death ensuing in a few years. An unusual clinical feature, which appears to be common in Thai patients with this disorder, is tonic seizures of spinal or brain stem origin. These were seen in no less than 3 out of 15 Thai patients diagnosed by the author as multiple sclerosis—my total experiences of this disease in Thai patients. This has also been the experience in Japan where Kuroiwa, Araki, and Katsuki (1965) reported an incidence of 13 per cent. In a series of 600 patients, Espir and Millac (1970) from the United Kingdom found only five to have tonic seizures. Among Thai patients the value of carbamazepine (*Tegretol*) in promptly controlling tonic seizures was confirmed.

Optic neuritis is a common problem in Thailand. It is more often synchronously bilateral and tends to be monophasic. Although in many instances causative factors such as toxins and nutritional deficiencies cannot be entirely excluded, some are almost certainly due to demyelination since spinal cord or brain stem involvement may subsequently develop. A long-term follow-up of these cases has not been made, but it is likely that a small number will eventually turn out to be unequivocal examples of multiple sclerosis. The figure would probably be somewhere nearer to the 13 per cent found by Kurland and his colleagues (1963) among United States Army personnel, and less than the 30 to 50 per cent reported by Lynn (1959), and Hierons and Lyle (1959) in England. The prevalence rate of multiple sclerosis has not been determined in Thailand, but it appears to be very low, at least when clinical diagnostic criteria based on the patterns of Western experience are used. However, the possibility that climatic and environmental factors (Acheson, 1963; Kurland, Stazio, and Reed, 1965) in a low-prevalence area may, in some instances, modify the disease process by promoting the spontaneous tendency to lasting remissions cannot be dismissed, and the true prevalence may indeed be much higher than is apparent at present.

Miscellaneous Disorders

'Degenerative' disorders such as motor neurone disease and parkinsonism are seen, but their prevalence rates have not yet been estimated. The clinical patterns seem to be similar to those in the West, except that motor neurone disease appears to occur in a slightly younger age-group. In 1963, a solitary outbreak of parkinsonism occurred in employees of a flash-light battery factory in Bangkok. The disorder was the result of the excessive inhalation of manganese in dry dust form (Sukonthabhand, cited by Allison, 1965). Myelopathy of undetermined aetiology is sometimes encountered; convincing evidence of vitamin deficiency or toxic causes is lacking, however. Cervical myelopathy associated with spondylosis is common. The latter has been found to be highly prevalent in Thailand. In a radiological study of 400 patients suffering from other disorders, cervical spondylosis was diagnosed in 40 per cent. The majority of these patients were aged over 40 (Chienpradit *et al.*, 1969).

Cases of Wilson's disease and porphyria have been encountered but pernicious anaemia with subacute combined degeneration of the cord has not so far been reported. The extreme rarity of vitamin B_{12} deficiency in Thais has been noted by many physicians. No reasonable explanation has been offered and the problem awaits further study.

Peripheral neuropathies are common. Although neuropathies from arsenical poisoning are occasionally seen, since the element is often present in both traditional Thai and Chinese medicine. Apart from leprosy, the spectrum of known aetiologies appears to be the same as in the West. Beriberi is hardly seen nowadays in Bangkok, although some mild cases are still common in the north-east of Thailand. Chronic alcoholism accounts for certain cases of peripheral neuropathy and also rarely presents as cerebellar degeneration, but curiously Wernicke's encephalopathy has not yet been reported.

Multiple cranial nerve palsies, on the other hand, are frequently encountered. They are commonly due to invasive carcinoma arising from the nasopharynx. The incidence of this neoplasm is high among Chinese and Thai-Chinese inhabitants, but appears to be less common in the traditional Thai population. The high frequency with which it occurs and the fact that it readily spreads to involve cranial nerves at the base of the skull ranks carcinoma of the nasopharynx high in the differential diagnosis of any adult Thai or Chinese patient presenting with single or multiple cranial nerve palsies. The oculomotor and trigeminal nerves are most often affected, but the entire 12 cranial nerves and the upper cervical nerve roots may be involved. Cervical lymphadenopathy is often but not invariably present. In advanced cases distant metastases, such as spinal extradural masses, causing cord compression and cauda equina syndromes have been encountered. We also see the syndrome of recurrent multiple cranial nerve palsies described by Symonds in England in 1958. Headache nearly always precedes the abrupt onset of isolated or multiple cranial nerve palsies. The oculomotor and facial nerves are the most frequently involved. In a series of 14 Thai patients studied by Steele and Vasuvat (1970), the age of the patients ranged from 18 to 77 years with the majority being in the fifth decade. There was no sex preponderance and patients came from various parts of the country. Symptoms are self-limited and corticosteroids hastened recovery in the majority of cases. Recurrence after many months or years is not uncommonly seen and different cranial nerves may be affected. Involvement of peripheral nerves or other parts of the nervous system has not been encountered. Apart from the frequently raised erythrocyte sedimentation rate, no other eivdence of co-existing systemic disease is present. The cerebrospinal fluid cell count is usually normal, but the protein is often slightly or moderately elevated—not more than 100 mg per cent—while the gamma globulin level is within the normal range or slightly raised. This is in contrast with the spinal fluid findings of patients with carcinoma of the nasopharynx in which the gamma globulin content is invariably high; for example, in a series of 11 patients seen by the author with cranial nerve palsies from invasion by the carcinoma the average cerebrospinal fluid protein was 53·5 mg per cent, of which 24·9 per cent was gamma globulin. This simple test serves as a useful aid in differentiating these two common conditions. High spinal fluid gamma globulin values so strongly favour carcinoma of the nasopharynx that initial negative nasopharyngeal examination and biopsy should be serially repeated. The syndrome of cranial polyneuropathy seen in Thai patients does not significantly differ from those reported by Ratanavale from Ceylon (1968), and by Symonds (1958) and Hunt *et al.* (1961) from the West, although there is suggestive evidence that it is commoner in the East. The aetiology remains unknown. A single post-mortem study reported (Tolosa, 1954) revealed granulomatous inflammation of the dura adjacent to and involving the perineurium of cranial nerves; but it is still undetermined whether the syndrome is a distinct disease due to the direct effect of a single agent, as yet unidentified, or whether it is a specific and local hypersensitivity reaction to various agents.

Neuromuscular syndromes associated with hyperthyroidism are commonly encountered. Myasthenia is relatively common and the same relationship with thyrotoxicosis as documented in Western literature is seen here. A much more striking association occurs, unique to the Thai, Chinese and Japanese, of hypokalaemic periodic paralysis and hyperthyroidism. In Europe and the United States, this combination is rarely seen but periodic paralysis has been reported to occur in some 2 per cent of all thyrotoxic patients in Japan (Okinaka *et al.*, 1957) and a similar incidence has been described among the Chinese living in Hong Kong (MacFadzean and Yeung, 1967). Twelve such patients have been seen by the author during the past 5 years; the clinical features were similar to those reported in the Chinese and Japanese literature (Vejjajiva, 1968 *a*). In all cases, there was no family history of periodic paralysis and the ages of onset were higher than encountered in the familial hypokalaemic variety. Over 80 per cent of the patients reported in the literature were between 20 and 40 years of age; there was a preponderance of males, the sex ratio being estimated to be between 6:1 and 20:1 (Engel, 1961; Satoyoshi *et al.*, 1963). All patients were free from attacks when the euthyroid state was restored and attacks nearly always recurred when the hypermetabolic state returned. During paralysis, serum potassium levels always fell to below normal and in most instances the fall was proportional to the extent and severity of weakness. Attacks could be induced in most patients by any means which would lower the serum potassium such as the combination of a high carbohydrate intake and the administration of insulin. Attacks varied widely in severity and ranged from slight weakness of the proximal lower limb muscles lasting a few hours to a total paralysis of all muscles from the neck downwards lasting up to 2 days. Respiratory failure, speech and swallowing difficulties did not occur. In both spontaneous and induced attacks, electrocardiographic changes almost invariably developed. Atrial and ventricular extrasystoles were commonest (MacFadzean and Yeung, 1967) but prolongation of the P-R interval and second degree atrioventricular block of the Wenckebach pattern also occurred. It has been suggested that the disturbance of atrioventricular conduction is the result of a combination of transient changes in the conducting fibre of the cardiac muscle due to hypokalaemia and the effects of increased thyroxine production (Muenthongchin, Vejjajiva, and Jumbala, 1970). The unusual susceptibility of Japanese, Chinese and Thai, all members of the Mongolian race, to hypokalaemic periodic paralysis, associated with hyperthyroidism, suggests that genetic factors must be implicated in the pathogenesis of this interesting phenomenon.

Unlike thyrotoxic periodic paralysis, the familial hypokalaemic variety is rare. Indeed, only one family with two affected siblings has been seen by the author during a 7-year period; experience in Taiwan and Japan has been similar. Chen, Hung, and Lin (1965) found two out of 28 cases with familial occurrence, and in a series of 119 patients reported from Japan (Okinaka *et al.*, 1957) only one such case was present. In a series seen by the author, four patients had sporadic hypokalaemic periodic paralysis without hyperthyroidism, all of whom were males over 25 years of age. One patient aged 28 presented with severe paralysis of all limbs with marked involvement of the proximal muscles and respiratory distress necessitating tracheostomy and artificial respiration. The serum potassium at the height of paralysis was 1·9 milliequivalent per litre. He made a dramatic and complete recovery 6 hours after beginning oral and intravenous potassium administration. In this patient, attempts to induce attacks by trying to lower the serum potassium failed, and diseases and factors that might have caused hypokalaemia such as aldosteronism, nephritis, gastrointestinal disturbance and the intake of local medicinal herbs were excluded. Thyroid function tests were normal and when last examined 3 years after the single attack, he had remained well.

NEUROLOGICAL MANIFESTATIONS OF SYSTEMIC DISEASES

Common in Thailand are cirrhosis of the liver and systemic lupus erythematosus (SLE). The former is usually due to viral hepatitis and the latter seems to occur unduly frequently. Up to 20 patients with SLE were seen annually at a large teaching hospital in Bangkok (Wasi, 1970) and in a personal series of 41 patients (Muenthongchin and Vejjajiva, 1969), 12 were found to have one or more neurological abnormalities including epilepsy, hemiplegia, extrapyramidal syndromes, subarachnoid haemorrhage, encephalomyelitis, polyneuropathy and psychosis. In most of these patients, neurological features developed at a late stage of the illness when other systems had already been involved and when LE cell preparations were invariably positive. In a few, however, the presenting symptoms were neurological, as illustrated by a woman of 31 (Vejjajiva, 1965) who, following an upper respiratory infection, developed acute disseminated encephalomyelitis which cleared after a week of corticosteroid therapy. A month later she returned with the classical features of SLE.

Malaria with central nervous system involvement still occurs in some parts of Thailand where the disease is endemic. In a study by Chipman, Cadigan, and Benjapongse (1967) of patients with malaria admitted to a 180-bed hospital in Saraburi province, some 60 miles north of Bangkok, 22 patients with neurological manifestations were seen during 13 weeks. These manifestations included seizures, disturbances of consciousness, acute psychoses, memory deficits and hemiplegia. All patients were infected by *Plasmodium falciparum*. Unlike East Africa, where the majority of such patients are children, 16 of the 22 Thai patients were aged over 20. Almost all had previously had uncomplicated attacks of malaria. Cerebral complications tended to occur in cases with severe parasitaemia. One death occurred in a patient with increased cerebrospinal fluid pressure, who probably died from brain stem compression, but the exact pathogenesis of brain symptoms in malaria remains obscure. Thrombosis has been incriminated as the important factor but, at necropsy, evidence of intravascular fibrin has seldom been found (Maegraith, 1948). Knisely, Eliot, and Bloch (1945) described red blood cells coated with a glassy precipitate considered to be fibrin, a pasty sludge formed in blood vessels. In monkeys with *Plasmodium knowlesi* infections, heparin prevented the red blood cell coating and sludge formation. The monkeys then remained active despite extremely high parasite counts, and died only when almost all their haemoglobin had been consumed (Knisely *et al.*, 1964). A recent investigation of six patients with *P. falciparum* infection and two normal controls (Devakul, Harinasuta, and Reid, 1966) using radioactive iodine (125-I)-labelled fibrinogen demonstrated precipitous falls in plasma fibrinogen in two patients, suggesting intravascular coagulation. These two patients were severely infected and their illnesses were resistant to chloroquine. The authors postulated that intravascular coagulation may be important in both the pathogenesis of severe malaria and in drug resistance. However, since the antimalarial drugs including chloroquine and quinine are known to enhance fibrinolytic activity, it is possible that chloroquine resistance primarily maintains intravascular coagulation, rather than that intravascular coagulation restricts access of chloroquine (Hetherington, 1966).

NEUROSURGERY

Among the local neurosurgical problems, the following are worthy of mention. Cerebral trauma ranks first as a cause for admission to any hospital taking neurosurgical emergencies. The majority of head injuries are due to road accidents. Apart from those admitted to the few neurosurgical centres in Bangkok, the great bulk of head injuries is still managed by general surgeons. Trauma to the nervous system sustained in the unique Thai-style boxing, in which the contestants not only use their gloved fists but are allowed to kick, to deliver blows with the point of the flexed elbow and to hit their opponents with flexed knees, includes cerebral concussion, contusion, intracranial haematoma and common peroneal nerve palsy. 'Boxing encephalopathy' is perhaps less common among the Thai-style boxers than conventional pugilists, because the former tend to rely much less on punches and fight without making fists. There is a possibility that direct kicks damage the carotid artery and cause subsequent occlusion, but the author has not come across such an instance.

Another common neurosurgical problem in Thailand is *fronto-ethmoidal encephalomeningocele* (Suwanwela and Hongsaprabhas, 1966), a condition rarely encountered in Europe and the United States. During a 7-year period, 82 such patients were treated by Suwanwela and his colleagues (1969 *b*). Among 21 071 live-births in the maternity ward of Chulalongkorn Hospital in Bangkok, during a 2½-year period, four cases were found; in a survey of a rural community of Nong Ree district, Kanchanaburi province in Western Thailand, one case of fronto-ethmoidal encephalomeningocele was found among a population of 6124 (Suwanwela *et al.*, 1969 *c*). The cause of this congenital anomaly is unknown. The hereditary factor appears to be insignificant, since only one of a pair of identical twins has been affected; and two affected siblings have not so far been recorded. Chromosome studies in five patients revealed no abnormality in four and a questionable trisomy in one (Dharmkrong-At, 1968). However, the condition seems to be much more common in the Thai population than in Chinese or Indian immigrants. There is no correlation with the mother's age and parity, and no evident history of trauma, infection or metabolic disturbance during the mother's pregnancy. The possibility of toxin present in the traditional Thai medicine which may be taken by the mother during her pregnancy has not been excluded.

PARASITIC INFECTIONS

The first report in Thailand of meningitis with marked eosinophilic pleocytosis was in 1957 (Khwanmitra, Bodhidatta, and Punyagupta, 1957). One of the four cases described was believed to have been caused by *Gnathostoma spinigerum*, a tissue nematode. In 1962, Punyadasni and Punyagupta reported two patients, brother and sister, who developed eosinophilic meningitis following the ingestion of raw *Pila* snails presumably infected with the rat lungworm, *Angiostrongylus cantonensis*. Since then several reports on this disorder have followed. At present, the clinical features of patients infested by those two parasites seem to be quite distinct.

Eosinophilic Meningitis due to

Angiostrongylus cantonensis

The third-stage larvae of the parasite, the metastrongylid lungworm of rats, were first recovered from the cerebrospinal fluid of a patient who died in Taiwan in 1944 (Nomura and Lin, 1945). Subsequently, parasites were demonstrated in the brains of patients who died from eosinophilic meningitis in Honolulu, Vietnam and Thailand (Rosen *et al.*, 1962; Jindrak and Alicata, 1965; Tangchai, Nye, and Beaver, 1967).

The disease is widely distributed throughout the country but is particularly prevalent in the northeastern and central regions. It appears to be confined to traditional Thai people of the lower socio-economic groups and the rarity among the Chinese and their first-generation descendants is noteworthy. In some areas such as Bangkok, seasonal occurrence has been evident. A large number of cases occur during the rainy season when *Pila* snails breed and are readily available. Most patients give a history of having eaten raw or undercooked *Pila* snails within a month before the onset of their symptoms. The incubation period ranges from 3 days to 5 weeks with an average of about 2 weeks. It is not uncommon to encounter several affected patients, a week or two after they have enjoyed a common meal consisting of *Pila* snails which are considered to be a great delicacy. However, in less than one-fifth of cases, no definite source of infection could be incriminated.

A clinical analysis of 484 typical cases of *A. cantonensis* infestation made by Punyagupta, Juttijudata, and Bunnag (1970) showed that the disease occurred in all age-groups but was most common in the third and fourth decades; males were affected slightly more than twice as often as females. The disease took a benign and self-limited course, the mortality rate being less than 1 per cent. Indeed, only one of those 484 cases studied, a 2-year old boy, died of the illness.

Fever is uncommon and, when present, is of low grade, rarely exceeding 38°C, and lasting only a few days. Headache is the commonest presenting symptom and occurs in almost all cases. It usually begins in and is often localized to the occipital region, although bitemporal and retrobulbar headaches may occur. When severe, it tends to be generalized. It is often throbbing or bursting in nature, usually intermittent in the beginning, but soon becomes persistent and is often associated with nausea and vomiting. Stabbing pains in the head and paraesthesia of the scalp are occasionally present. Rarely, mental confusion and generalized convulsions occur and a few patients complain of generalized weakness of the extremities. Examination reveals neck stiffness and Kernig's sign in practically all cases. In the majority of cases seen, no other abnormal neurological signs were noted, but in 16 per cent of cases visual acuity was found to be impaired and in 12 per cent visual blurring and swelling of optic discs were present (Punyagupta, Juttijudata, and Bunnag, 1970). These abnormal findings are of some importance in that although visual impairment gradually improved in the majority, complete blindness was an occasional sequel. Optic neuritis may be explained on an allergic basis, but living parasites trapped in between the optic nerve sheath and nerve fibres have been found in an experimentally-infected rat, and a Thai patient with ocular angiostrongyliasis but without central nervous system involvement has been documented (Prommindaroj, Leelawongs, and Pradatsundarasar, 1962).

Occasionally, slight swelling of both eyelids and cranial nerve involvement, usually of the sixth and seventh nerves, are seen. Diplopia from the ocular palsy often clears early and could well be secondary to increased intracranial pressure. Hyperaesthesia of a limb or the trunk is detected in about a third of cases. This may be the result of migration of worms in the nerve roots and spinal cord. It is remarkable that spinal cord symptoms and signs are noticeably lacking in this disease, although the parasite has been demonstrated in the spinal cord of a patient who succumbed (Yii *et al.*, 1968).

The spinal fluid is often under increased pressure, particularly in those with severe headache. The fluid is usually turbid and is likened to water after washing rice grains. The white cell count is over 500 per cubic millimetre in 75 per cent of cases. Eosinophilia of 20 to 70 per cent of the total cells is common, and over 90 per cent has been recorded; the remaining cells are neutrophils and lymphocytes. There seems to be no connexion between blood and spinal fluid eosinophilia. Blood leucocytosis of over 10 000 per cubic millimetre is common, and in the majority of cases eosinophilia of over 10 per cent is present. Spinal fluid eosinophils tend to be high between the second and fourth weeks after the onset of clinical symptoms, then decline, only to climb again during the sixth and eighth weeks, usually disappearing at the end of the third month (Punyagupta, Juttijudata, and Bunnag, 1970).

Cerebrospinal fluid protein is often elevated but is usually less than 100 milligrams per cent. The gamma globulin content is always disproportionately high and remains so for some time. This is a helpful diagnostic point in cases with suggestive clinical features and in whom the fluid is examined at a stage when eosinophil count is low. The sugar content in the cerebrospinal fluid is normal, although slight decrease has been observed in a few cases.

Despite several earlier attempts to recover the parasite from the spinal fluid at lumbar puncture, this was unsuccessful until recently, when Bunnag and his associates (1969) identified several male and female living fifth-stage *A. cantonensis*, measuring about 0·5–1·5 cm in length, from the spinal fluid of a 29-year-old Thai male on three occasions. Isolation of the parasite from the fluid had hitherto been more successful in Taiwanese children under 10 years of age. This could well be related to the intensity of infestation, because the African snail *Achatina fulica*, the suspected host for the parasite in Taiwan (Cross, 1967), was much more heavily infected than *Pila* snails in Thailand.

Other investigations including chest and skull X-rays are normal, and the electoencephalogram often shows generalized, non-specific abnormalities.

Treatment is symptomatic. Prompt and dramatic relief of headache occurs following the release of spinal fluid, and repeated tappings are often necessary. In severe cases, corticosteroids have been tried, but efficacy is doubtful. Rarely, optic atrophy with visual impairment or blindness is found. Most patients make a complete recovery within a month or two, but long-term follow-up will be necessary, since late-onset epilepsy and impaired mental function may develop.

Autopsy findings on cases from which *Angiostrongylus cantonensis* were identified in the brain included the presence of track-like lesions containing necrotic tissue debris and scattered inflammatory cells, mostly histiocytes and neutrophils, and generalized vascular congestion. Large numbers of Charcot-Leyden crystals were present in the meninges, indicating a massive response by eosinophils to the dead parasites (Tangchai, Nye, and Beaver, 1967).

Nervous System Invasion by *Gnathostoma Spinigerum*

Although the first case of human gnathostomiasis, a Thai girl from Bangkok. was reported by Levinsen as early as 1889, awareness of nervous system involvement in this disease has been recent. The parasite, a tissue nematode—first removed from a tiger's stomach—is widely distributed in nature in the South-East Asian countries, particularly Thailand. The adult worms are inhabitants of the stomach wall of cats and dogs. The mature female worms produce fertilized ova which are excreted with the host's faeces. Flushed by rain into ponds, canals and rivers, ova hatch into first-stage larvae which are then ingested by *Cyclops*, the first intermediate host. There, the larvae develop into the second stage which is distinguished morphologically by a well-defined head with four rows of spines. Infected *Cyclops* are eaten by fishes, shrimps, frogs and eels, and the larvae penetrate their intestines to become encysted in their flesh or visceral organs and develop into the third-stage larvae which are infective. Thai people of all income groups are very fond of eating undercooked or even raw freshwater fishes and shrimps and it is not surprising that infestation by gnathostomiasis is highly prevalent in Thailand. The third-stage larvae, which may be ingested by man, migrate and soon transform into immature worms, each of about $\frac{1}{2}$–1 cm in length with four or eight rows of cephalic spines, and capable of burrowing and migrating. Most of the clinical manifestations of human gnathostomiasis are due to the high motility of the adult immature worm. However, a new symptom complex, consisting of fever, malaise, mild abdominal pain and liver tenderness, dry cough, chest pain and marked eosinophilia, labelled the 'abdomino-pulmonary hypereosinophilic syndrome', has recently been described and there is evidence indicating that this is due to an inapparent migration of the infective third-stage larvae (Punyagupta, 1967). Theoretically, this symptom complex should occur in all infested patients, but it may be mild and thus goes unrecognized or perhaps misdiagnosed. The adult immature worm, on the other hand, commonly causes painless, migratory, subcutaneous swelling which usually lasts a few days and subsides spontaneously. The swelling may recur several times a year and the course of the disease may last several years. Migration of the worm into the eye, the lung and pleura, the intestine, urinary tract, and the uterus has been encountered. Involvement of the central nervous system has been suspected but was never proven until Chitanondh and Rosen (1967) identified the immature worm in the spinal cord of a fatal case of ascending myelitis. Further clinicopathological and epidemiological studies of this human parasitic infestation have led to the recognition of a clinical entity, eosinophilic myeloencephalitis (Punyagupta *et al.*, 1968; Bunnag, Comer, and Punyagupta, 1970).

The clinical picture differs from that due to invasion by *A. cantonensis*. Here, the presenting neurological symptom is usually severe, sharp agonizing pain due to irritation of a nerve root, located in the trunk or extremities. This is often followed in a day or two by sudden onset of paraplegia with urinary retention. In some cases, impairment of consciousness follows progressing to deep coma and death. Less commonly, patients present with features of acute intracerebral haemorrhage and die within 2 or 3 days. Recently, a patient presenting with fever, signs of meningeal irritation and hemiparesis, and in whom electroencephalogram and radioactive brain scan strongly suggested the presence of a temporal lobe lesion, was found at craniotomy to have cerebral gnathostomiasis (Bunyaratavej and Vejjajiva, 1970). The peripheral blood count of this patient prior to operation was within normal limits, but the spinal fluid contained 95 cells, of which 10 per cent were eosinophils. In general, practically all cases show a moderate to marked eosinophilia in the peripheral blood, greater than that seen in eosinophilic meningitis due to *A. cantonensis*. The spinal fluid often shows moderate pleocytosis with a high eosinophil count. Sometimes, the fluid is xanthochromic and occasionally bloody with a deceptively low leucocyte count. This could mislead one into diagnosing spontaneous subarachnoid or intracerebral haemorrhage from aneurysm or arteriovenous malformation. The history of ingesting raw or undercooked freshwater fishes, prawns or shrimps, a remote story of migratory subcutaneous swellings, and the absence of hypertension in a young adult presenting with a stroke should alert the physician to the possibility of cerebral gnathostomiasis. The condition is a major health problem for this country, since the eating habit which leads to the invasion by this parasite is nationwide and prevails among Thai people of all social strata. Unlike the disease due to *A. cantonensis*, the mortality rate from nervous system involvement is significant and the morbidity is high. Permanent paraplegia is not uncommonly seen and no specific treatment is available. In patients presenting with acute intracerebral haemorrhage or an expanding cerebral lesion, craniotomy and evacuation of blood clots, surgical decompression, together with high doses of corticosteroids to relieve cerebral swellings, may be life-saving.

Neuropathological findings include multiple haemorrhagic and necrotic areas. In some cases, massive intracerebral, subarachnoid or intraventricular haemorrhages may be seen. The characteristic findings on macroscopic examination are visible tortuous tracks in the brain and spinal cord which are the result of worm migration. Gnathostomas were isolated from the brains of two out of nine fatal cases studied by Bunnag, Comer, and Punyagupta (1970). It is believed that the worm continues to migrate after the death of the patient, leaving no trace of vital reaction in the brain and thus adding to the difficulty in finding the parasite. Worms have been recovered in three instances from the conjunctivae and eyelids of patients who originally presented with symptoms and signs of eosinophilic myeloencephalitis (Punyagupta and Juttijudata, 1967; Bunnag, Juttijudata, and Punyagupta, 1968). This suggests that in many cases, fatal or otherwise, the parasite may leave the central nervous system through the optic foramen, possibly via the optic nerve (Bunnag, Comer, and Punyagupta, 1970).

Udorn Encephalopathy (*Encephalopathy and Fatty Degeneration of the Viscera in Thai Children*)

This condition has been recognized for a number of years by physicians in Udorn, a north-eastern province of Thailand, and is known locally as 'Udorn encephalitis'. A study by Bourgeois and his colleagues (1969) of 139 patients with this syndrome, admitted to the provincial hospital, revealed that the condition was identical to that described by Reye, Morgan, and Baral in 1963 in Australia, but in Thailand the disease is most common during the rainy season and over 80 per cent of the patients were under 7 years of age, the age range being 3 months to 14 years. All of the 67 patients in whom the diagnosis was proven at autopsy or biopsy (Bourgeois *et al.*, 1970 *b*) appeared well-nourished and had no skin rash. They presented with coma of sudden onset and convulsions. Fever was an initial finding in about half of the patients and in some, mild prodromal symptoms such as abdominal pain, vomiting, diarrhoea and headache were present for less than 24 hours. Hepatomegaly was found in about a quarter of cases; three patients were jaundiced and three had gross irregularities in cardiac rhythm. There were no focal neurological signs on admission, save for one patient with meningeal irritation. Thirty-one of the 43 patients with seizures were in status epilepticus and about a third of the total 67 patients displayed intermittent decerebrate posturing. Blood glucose was generally lower than 50 mg per cent and the spinal fluid, although clear and showing no increase of cells, had a low glucose content —less than 40 mg per cent. Serum glutamic oxaloacetic transaminase (SGOT) was nearly always elevated. The mortality was slightly over 80 per cent, death occurring within 3 days of onset. Those who survived generally improved within 48 hours of admission. At autopsy, the brain was markedly oedematous with flattened gyri, mild uncal grooving and tonsillar pressure cones. Microscopically, oedema was evidenced by perivascular and pericellular clear spaces; fat vacuoles within the walls of cerebral vessels were common. No evidence of inflammation was seen. The liver was increased in weight and microscopically its architecture was preserved, but the cytoplasm of the hepatocyte was almost completely replaced by small droplets of Oil Red O positive lipid. The kidneys were swollen and pale, and similar fat droplets were found in the epithelium of the proximal convoluted tubules. Invariably, the abdominal lymph nodes were increased in size and number and the thymus was prominent. These lymphoid tissues showed an increase in histiocytes, most of which contained similar lipid material. Analyses revealed the increased hepatic lipids to be predominantly triglycerides and free fatty acids. Viral studies showed no evidence of recent arbor, dengue or chikungunya infections, but chemical analyses of autopsy tissues for aflatoxins gave positive results in over 90 per cent of cases (Bourgeois *et al.*, 1970 *b*). Monkeys receiving a lethal dose of the same toxin developed clinical and pathological changes similar to patients with Udorn encephalopathy.

SNAKE-BITE

There are about 2500 species of snakes, of which some 200 are poisonous to man. Being a tropical country, Thailand abounds in snakes of great varieties, poisonous as well as harmless. The poisonous ones encountered belong to four families or subfamilies: the Elapinae, which include cobras and coral snakes, the Viperinae (true vipers), the Crotalinae (pit vipers) and the Hydrophidae or sea-snakes. During a 3-year period, out of 8921 patients admitted to the medical wards of Chulalongkorn Hospital (Kaeowplung, 1960), 148 suffered from snake-bites. About 80 per cent of those patients were bitten by vipers; cobras accounted for 15 per cent, while the remaining 5 per cent were bitten by sea-snakes. Several factors affect the outcome of snake-bite (Bennett, 1966). The age, size and health of the patient are significant. Thus, envenomation in children is usually serious and a fatal outcome more likely than in adults. Bites on extremities or into adipose tissues are less dangerous than those on the trunk or face or those penetrating blood vessels, while the size of the snake and the dose of venom discharged are important. Moreover, exercise or exertion such as running immediately after the bite hastens systemic absorption of toxin.

Snake venom is a mixture of several toxic proteins and enzymes. For example, the venom of the Indian cobra, *Naja naja*, contains a neurotoxin, a haemolysin, a cardiotoxin, a cholinesterase, phosphatases, a nucleotidase and a potent inhibitor of cytochrome oxidase. However, its action is usually predominantly neurotoxic. In cobra poisoning the early constitutional symptoms are generalized weakness, drooping of eyelids and difficulties of speech, swallowing and breathing. Death results from respiratory paralysis, probably due to damage to the brain stem, and to a curariform interference with transmission at the neuromuscular junction. The venom of a viper, on the other hand, acts mainly on blood and blood vessels. The bite produces severe local pain and swelling with ecchymoses. In severe viper poisoning, widespread haemorrhages into the skin and mucous membranes, epistaxis, haematemesis and blood diarrhoea resulting in circulatory collapse are usually seen, and death may occur in 6 to 48 hours. Survival may be attended by massive local tissue loss from gangrene and secondary infection. In sea-snake poisoning, muscular symptoms are the main clinical features (Reid, 1961); muscle movement pain usually occurs half an hour after the bite and often precedes weakness or paralysis by several hours, even in rapidly fatal cases. Neck, back and proximal limb muscles are affected early and paresis is usually more pronounced. Trismus is a common finding, while fibrillation and fasciculation are absent. Widespread necrosis of muscles results in myoglobinuria and death is attributed to renal failure, hyperkalaemia or respiratory paralysis.

In the management of a patient with snake-bite, an attempt should be made to determine with certainty whether or not the bite is that of a poisonous snake. Absence of distinct fang punctures and failure of local pain, oedema, numbness or weakness to appear within 20 minutes are strong evidence that the bite has not been inflicted by a venomous species. Treatment includes immobilization, application of tourniquet above the bite, incision and suction, administration of antivenin, application of ice packs to the affected area, measures to combat infection and general support. The maintenance of respiration by manual or mechanical aids is important in patients bitten by the elapine snakes. The results of corticosteroid theapy for lessening local necrosis or systemic intoxication have been inconclusive. In a recent study on sea-snake poisoning (Sitprija *et al.*, 1971), haemodialysis appeared to be a useful alternative method of treatment to antivenom administration.

RABIES

With better public health measures, human rabies has become a rarity in the Western hemisphere, but in South-Central and South-East Asia the disease is still endemic, and half of the cases reported in recent years have been from this part of the world. Unfortunately, Thailand is still one of the few countries where the disease is highly endemic: rabies accounts for about 300 deaths each year. At Chulalongkorn University Hospital in Bangkok, during a 4-year period (1963–66), there were 152 cases (Vejjajiva and Tamthai, 1967).

Rabies is one of the oldest communicable diseases known to man. The word 'rabies' comes from the old Indian root *rabh*, to 'make violent'. The transfer of infection from the saliva of a mad dog to rabbits and roosters was successfully performed by Zinke in 1804. Nine years later, Magendie propagated the disease from a human victim to a healthy dog using the patient's saliva. The well-known Pasteur treatment was introduced in 1884 (Dupont and Earle, 1965).

It is now known that the rabies virus particle is RNA in nature. It is thus degraded by lipid solvents, surface active agents and proteolytic or lipolytic enzymes. Electron microscopic study shows the virus to be bullet-shaped with one rounded and one flat end. Its length is up to 180 μ and its diameter from 75 to 80 μ (WHO, 1968).

Among 152 Thai patients studied (Vejjajiva and Tamthai, 1967), 145 gave histories of transmission of the disease from dogs. In two patients, cats were responsible and in five no history of animal exposure was obtained. Other animals known to be responsible for the transmission of the disease in other countries include wolves, jackals, skunks, mongooses, foxes and insectivorous bats. Indeed, the rabies virus may potentially be transmitted by any warm-blooded animal (Tierkel, 1963). While amphibians and reptiles are known to harbour the inoculated fixed virus for up to 1 year, there is no record of their bites having transmitted the disease (Dupont and Earle, 1965). A recent field study (Phuangsab *et al.*, 1967) in northern Thailand has indicated that rats and ground squirrels may represent a potential source of virus and could be the constant reservoir of infection which is intermittently conveyed to dogs.

Animals with rabies generally appear ill or show clinical manifestations of the disease within a week, but bats may carry and transmit the disease while asymptomatic (Pawan, 1936). In addition to transmission by animal bites, the disease may be passed on to animals and man by airborne inoculum (Constantine, 1962; Tierkel, 1963). Man-to-man transmission has not been unequivocally reported, except for the case mentioned in Lubinski and Prausnitz's review (1926): a gentleman kissed his maid who, in retrospect, was in the early stages of clinical rabies. Both died with the disease. Fear of contact with a rabid patient may, on the whole, cause the physician unnecessary concern.

Once inoculated, rabies virus is believed to spread centripetally via peripheral nerves through the endoneurial spaces, which is more likely by a passive than by an active process. Nothing is known about the pathophysiological changes that take place in the affected nerve during the spread of the virus from the site of infection to the central nervous system. There is ample evidence that virus is not transmitted in the blood. Viraemia following experimental rabies infection has been reported, but this seems to occur only after infection with high doses (WHO, 1968). The prolonged symptom-free period of infection followed by overt disease and death is still a major biological puzzle. In 24 cases studied by Tangchai, Yenbutr, and Vejjajiva (1970), the shortest incubation period was 12 days and the longest about 180 days. The shortest period was encountered in patients with facial and head wounds, with an average of 23 days for five out of 24 patients, as compared to 47 days for eight patients with wounds of the upper extremity, and 63 days for seven patients with wounds of the lower extremity. However, a 12-year-old boy with a wound of the left foot had the shortest incubation period (12 days). By contrast, two patients with incubation periods of about 180 days also had wounds located in the extremities. Incubation periods of up to 2½ years have been recorded (Hogyes, 1897).

Of 152 patients reported by Vejjajiva and Tamthai (1967), the male to female ratio was approximately 2:1. This male preponderance is consistent with the world literature on rabies. It is also noteworthy that a male to female ratio of 7:1 has been reported in rabid dogs (Remlinger and Bailley, 1938). The age of the 152 patients ranged from 2 to 89 years, with approximately 50 per cent under 20. Younger animals have been found to be more susceptible to rabies (Tierkel, 1958).

The most frequent presenting symptom is that of itching at or near the location of the animal bite. The itching may be so severe that it is misdiagnosed as neurodermatitis or some other primary skin disorders. This may be the only symptom for the first 24 to 48 hours, before other classical features of rabies appear. In some cases, itching is followed by pain either of a neuritic type or one similar to causalgia. An anxious-looking patient rubbing the inoculated limb with cold towels to obtain relief from pain is a picture not uncommonly encountered. Early in the disease, low-grade fever, mild headache, malaise, nausea and vomiting are seen. These are soon followed by mental excitement and difficulty in swallowing. These ill-defined complaints have sometimes led the unwary physician to a diagnosis of upper respiratory infection. The well-known symptom of hydrophobia is nearly always present at some stage and is due to pharyngeal spasms. A helpful sign due to the same mechanism and frequently appearing early on in the clinical course is that of aerophobia—the patient bending his face and body away from a current of air intentionally blown at him by the use of a fan, and gasping. Other rare presenting symptoms are nervous irritability, hiccough, dysuria, spermatorrhoea, and paralysis of the lower limbs. Except in those very rare cases with signs of a transverse cord lesion, neurological examination may fail to reveal any definite objective sensory loss or hyperaesthesia. As the disease advances, mental excitement may be followed by lethargy and exhaustion. There is excessive salivation and fever increases. Coma and sometimes convulsions supervene. The disease is invariably fatal and the clinical illness usually lasts approximately 1 week. The longest clinical course recorded was 38 days (Dupont and Earle, 1965). There are sporadic reports of apparent recovery from rabies, but they are unconvincing.

The histopathology of human rabies encephalomyelitis consists of three main features, namely:

1. The inflammatory cellular reaction.
2. The inclusion bodies.
3. The vascular changes (Tangchai, Yenbutr, and Vejjajiva, 1970).

The inflammatory reaction is present in about two-thirds of cases and is characterized by perivenous leucocytic infiltration in both grey and white matter, particularly in the thalamus, hypothalamus, brain stem and the anterior part of the spinal cord. Meningitis is uncommon, being present in four of the 24 cases studied, all of whom were children. The exudate is composed mainly of lymphocytes and large mononuclear cells, but in cases with a short clinical course the presence of polymorphonuclear cells is striking. Intracytoplasmic inclusion bodies (Negri bodies) are present in 70 to 95 per cent of cases. These inclusions are round or oval, commonly located at the junction between the cellular cytoplasm and the axon, and are clearly recognized in ordinary formalin-fixed and paraffin-embedded section stained with haematoxylin and eosin. They may be found in nerve cells at any site of the central nervous system except in the granular cells of the cerebellum. They may be single or multiple, large or small. The larger the inclusion bodies, the more distinct is the internal ring structure. The latter is absent in tiny acidophilic bodies, and is believed to be elementary protein material derived from virus organism. It is probably the forerunner of the typical Negri bodies. These bodies are also observed extracellularly, perhaps left *in situ* from previously viable cells which have been destroyed by the infection. In addition, inclusion bodies very similar or identical to Negri bodies are also seen in astrocytes in some cases. These are always single and are found mostly in the floor of the third ventricle, paraventricular areas and occasionally in the brain stem. Recent electron microscopic study (Morecki and Zimmerman, 1969) shows that cytoplasmic inclusions with the optical characteristic of Negri bodies do not contain virus particles. Conversely, sites of viral synthesis can be easily identified with the electron microscope but are not visualized optically. On the basis of staining characteristics and fine structure, Negri bodies appear to contain nucleoproteins, probably ribonucleoproteins. It has been suggested that they may represent sites where nucleoproteins are stored and modified until a proper template for virus assembly is formed. Such adaptation would appear necessary following inoculation with the street virus which, at least at the time of transmission, is replicating in salivary glands of the host. In contrast, the fixed virus strain has been well adapted to neuronal replication during its preparation by animal passage in laboratory animals, and thus there is no need for any further adaptation. This could account for the absence of Negri bodies in animals inoculated with the fixed rabies virus. The vascular changes in the brain and spinal cord of human cases (Tangchai, Yenbutr, and Vejjajiva, 1970) are unusually prominent and are characterized by thrombosis of the capillaries and venules, extreme hyperaemia in both arteries and veins, and frank haemorrhages and haemorrhagic necrosis. Other changes found in the central nervous system such as neuronophagia, satellitosis, glial nodule formation, and vascular proliferation are probably non-specific.

Histopathological changes in peripheral nerves and corresponding ganglia have recently been studied in nine cases (Tangchai and Vejjajiva, 1971). Degeneration was seen in nerve ganglia in over 50 per cent of these cases, and similar changes were observed in the axons of peripheral nerve trunk in seven instances. Other findings included leucocytic infiltration and non-specific vascular congestion.

For adequate confirmation of the diagnosis of rabies encephalitis in man, the histopathological examination should be accompanied by virus isolation through mouse passage, the serological virus neutralization test or the fluorescent antibody technique.

Once the disease is clinically evident, there is no specific therapy and death invariably occurs in about a week. No authentic instance of recovery in man has been established.

Preventive measures following a rabid-suspect animal bite have been clearly outlined (WHO, 1966). Bites and scratches should be cleaned thoroughly and immediately with strong soap solution for 15 minutes. Cauterization with nitric acid or other corrosive chemicals is no longer advocated. In face, neck and deep wounds, local infiltration with rabies antiserum is recommended. A course of 14 daily subcutaneous injections of antirabic vaccine, each of 2 ml, should be promptly instituted. Rabies antiserum is also recommended in patients with facial and deep wounds. At least 40 International Units per kilogram body weight should be given intravenously within 24 hours of exposure. Only one instance of death from rabies has been recorded among those cases promptly treated with antiserum and vaccine (Anderson, Daly, and Kidd, 1966). The overall mortality in patients with wounds at all sites is in the region of 40 per cent. For pre-exposure immunization, two doses of 1 ml of duck embryo vaccine given subcutaneously 1 month apart followed by a third dose 6 months later are recommended. Satisfactory neutralizing antibody is obtained in 90 per cent of vaccinees 1 month after the third dose. If more rapid immunization is required, three injections of the vaccine at weekly intervals followed by a fourth dose 3 months later would be satisfactory. Adequate antibody response is then found in 80 per cent of those vaccinated (*Annals of Internal Medicine*, 1967). If a patient who already has antibody is exposed to rabies, one booster dose should suffice after mild exposure and after severe exposure five daily doses of vaccines followed by a booster dose 20 days later. If it is uncertain whether the exposed person has had antibody or not, the complete postexposure antirabies treatment should be given.

Neurological Sequelae of Vaccination Against Rabies

It is unfortunate that, in Thailand, Semple's vaccine prepared from fixed virus grown in sheep brain and inactivated with phenol is still widely used in the treatment of individuals exposed to rabies. Because of its high cost, the use of the duck embryo vaccine which is free of neural tissue is limited to very few cases. At the Pasteur Institute in Bangkok, the number of people receiving Semple vaccine amounts to about 4000 a year. The incidence of neurological complications following its use has been estimated at 1 in 500. During a 4-year period a series of 35 patients with such complications was studied (Vejjajiva, 1968 *b*); their ages ranged from 4 to 73 years. In over 60 per cent of these patients, neurological symptoms occurred between the eighth and the fourteenth day after the initial injection; the shortest interval from the commencement of vaccination to the onset of neurological involvement was 3 days and the longest 26 days. Clinically, four main types of neurological complication were recognized; namely, meningo-encephalitis, meningo-encephalomyelitis, transverse myelitis and polyradiculoneuropathy. Twelve out of the total 35 patients had meningo-encephalitis with moderate fever, headache, drowsiness and signs of meningeal irritation. Two patients showed aggressive behaviour and one of them remained apyrexial throughout the illness. In none of the 12 patients was there any significant impairment of motor or sensory function of the limb. Meningo-encephalomyelitis was the commonest complication, being encountered in 14 patients. Neurological symptoms were more severe; two patients were comatose on admission and all showed evidence of spinal cord involvement with partial or complete paralysis of both lower limbs, segmental sensory impairment and sphincter disturbances. In eight patients the mental state was unaffected and clinical features were those of transverse myelitis. Only one case of polyradiculoneuropathy was seen. Unilateral or bilateral facial palsy was occasionally observed, but optic neuritis was not encountered. In almost all patients, the cerebrospinal fluid was abnormal; the pressure was abnormally high in less than one-third of cases while the number of cells was increased, being predominantly lymphocytes, in over 90 per cent of patients. The protein content was normal, or slightly to moderately increased, often to not more than 90 mg per cent, but the gamma globulin content was invariably high. Corticosteroids were given to almost all patients except a few with mild symptoms. Recovery was complete in 60 per cent of cases, while about 20 per cent showed slight residual disability. The overall mortality rate was 17 per cent, and pathological studies of the brains of patients who died from this disorder showed widespread perivenous demyelination and perivascular mononuclear cell infiltration. Spontaneous recurrence of symptoms has not been observed in any patient who has completely recovered from the neuroparalytic accident. Reports from Japan (Uchimura and Shiraki, 1957; Shiraki and Otani, 1959) of some instances of rabies postvaccinal encephalomyelitis, with chronic symptoms and signs and with pathological appearances strikingly reminiscent of multiple sclerosis, are indeed unique.

References

Acheson, E. D. (1963) The geography of multiple sclerosis, *Med. J. Aust.*, 1, 556.

Allison, R. S. (1965) *On Nervous Disease in Thailand*, Scott-Heron Lecture at the Royal Victoria Hospital, May 1965, London.

Anderson, J. A., Daly, F. T., Jr., and Kidd, J. C. (1966) Human rabies after antiserum and vaccine post-exposure treatment. Case report and review, *Ann. intern. Med.*, 64, 1297.

Annals of Internal Medicine (1967) Rabies prophylaxis. Recommendation of the United States Public Health Service Advisory Committee on Immunization Practices, *Ann. intern Med.*, 67, 159.

Bennett, I. L., Jr. (1966) Snake bite, in *Principles of Internal Medicine*, 5th ed., eds. Harrison, T. R. *et al.*, New York, Section 263, p. 1462.

Boongird, P., and Vejjajiva, A. (1967) Subacute inclusion body encephalitis, *J. med. Ass. Thailand*, 48, 806.

Borman, J. B., Stern, S., Shapira, T., *et al.* (1961) Mitral valvotomy in children, *Amer. Heart J.*, 61, 763.

Bourgeois, C. H., Jr., Keschamras, N., Comer, D. S., *et al.* (1969) Udorn encephalopathy. Fatal cerebral oedema and fatty degeneration of the viscera in Thai children, *J. med. Ass. Thailand*, 52, 553.

Bourgeois, C. H., Jr., Gould, D., Olson, L., *et al.* (1970 *a*) Combined investigation of central nervous system infection in Bangkok children, in *The Annual Progress Report*, The SEATO Medical Research Laboratory, Bangkok, Thailand, April 1969–March 1970, p. 23.

Bourgeois, C. H., Jr., Comer, D. S., Cotton, R. B., *et al.* (1970 *b*) Encephalopathy and fatty degeneration of the viscera in Thai children, in *The Annual Progress Report*, The SEATO Medical Research Laboratory, Bangkok, Thailand, April 1969–March 1970, p. 175.

Bryant, J. (1969) *Health and the Developing World*, Cornell University, Ithaca, N.Y p 21.

Bull, J. W. D., Marshall, J., and Shaw, D. A. (1960) Cerebral angiography in the diagnosis of the acute stroke, *Lancet*, i, 562.

Bunnag, T., Benjapong, W., Noeypratimanond, S., and Punyagupta, S. (1969) The recovery of *Angiostrongylus cantonensis* in the cerebrospinal fluid of a case of eosinophilic meningitis, *J. med. Ass. Thailand*, 52, 665.

Bunnag, T., Comer, D. S., and Punyagupta, S. (1970) Eosinophilic myeloencephalitis caused by *Gnathostoma spinigerum*, neuropathology of nine cases, *J. neurol, Sci.*, 10, 419.

Bunnag, T., Juttijudata, P., and Punyagupta, S. (1968) Two cases of eosinophilic meningoencephalitis with evidence of gnathostomiasis, *J. med. Ass. Thailand*, 51, 813.

Bunyaratavej, S. (1970) Personal communication.

Bunyaratavej, S., and Vejjajiva, A. (1970) Cerebral gnathostomiasis presenting as a space-occupying lesion, unpublished ms.

Chen, K. M., Hung, T. P., and Lin, T. (1965) Periodic paralysis in Taiwan, *Arch. Neurol. (Chic.)*, 13, 165.

Cherian, G., Vytilingan, K. I., Sukumar, I. P., and Gopinath, N. (1964) Mitral valvotomy in young patients, *Brit. Heart J.*, 26, 157.

CHIENPARADIT, K., VEJJAJIVA, A., SUWANWELA, C., and HONGSAPRABHAS, C. (1969) *Cervical Spondylosis in Thailand*, Paper presented at the Annual Meeting of the Medical Association of Thailand, Songkla.

CHIPMAN, M., CADIGAN, F. C., and BENJAPONGSE, W. (1967) Involvement of the nervous system in malaria in Thailand, *Trop. geogr. Med.*, **19**, 8.

CHITANONDH, H., and ROSEN, L. (1967) Fatal eosinophilic encephalomyelitis caused by the nematode, *Gnathostoma spinigerum*, *Amer. J. trop. Med. Hyg.*, **16**, 638.

CONSTANTINE, D. G. (1962) Rabies transmission by nonbite route, *Publ. Hlth Bull. (Wash.)*, 77, 287.

CROSS, J. H. (1967) *Review of Angiostrongyliasis in Taiwan*, Seminar on Helminthiases and Eosinophilic Meningitis, Noumea, New Caledonia.

DEVAKUL, K., HARINASUTA, T., and REID, H. A. (1966) 125-I-labelled fibrinogen in malaria, *Lancet*, **ii**, 886.

DHARMKRONG-AT, A. (1968) *Chromosome Studies in Various Congenital Anomalies*, M.Sc. thesis, Univ. Med. Sci., Bangkok, quoted by Suwanwela, C., *et al.*, 1969 *a*.

DUANGMANI, C., NOYES, H. E., KASEMSARN, P., and SUNAKORN, P. (1970) Acute bacterial meningitis in Thai children, in *The Annual Progress Report*, The SEATO Medical Research Laboratory, Bangkok, Thailand, April 1969–March 1970, p. 78.

DUPONT, J. R., and EARLE, K. M. (1965) Human rabies encephalitis, *Neurology (Minneap.)*, **15**, 1023.

ENGEL, A. G. (1961) Thyroid function and periodic paralysis, *Amer. J. Med.*, **30**, 327.

ESPIR, M. L. E., and MILLAC, P. (1970) Treatment of paroxysmal disorders in multiple sclerosis with carbamazepine (Tegretol), *J. Neurol. Neurosurg. Psychiat.*, **33**, 528.

GELFAND, M. (1957) *The Sick African: A Clinical Study*, 3rd ed., Cape Town, p. 567, quoted by Spillane, J. D. (1970).

GWEE, A. L. (1968) Neurological pattern in Singapore, *Proc. Aust. Ass. Neurol.*, **5**, 375.

HETHERINGTON, R. J. (1966) Fibrinogen in cerebral malaria, *Lancet*, **ii**, 971.

HIERONS, R., and LYLE, T. K. (1959) Bilateral retrobulbar neuritis, *Brain*, 82, 56.

HOGYES, A. (1897) *Lyssa*, Vienna, quoted by Dupont, J. R., and Earle, K. M. (1965).

HONGLADAROM, T., BUNNAG, T. S., KAOPARISUTHI, V., and CHIENPRADIT, K. (1962) Cerebral angiographic study of cerebro-vascular accidents, *Thai J. Radiol.*, **2**, 4.

HUNT, W. E., MEAGHER, J. N., LE FEVER, H. E., and ZEMAN, W. (1961) Painful ophthalmoplegia—its relation to indolent inflammation of the cavernous sinus, *Neurology (Minneap.)*, **11**, 56.

JINDRAK, K., and ALICATA, J. E. (1965) A case of parasitic eosinophilic meningoencephalitis in Vietnam, probably caused by *Angiostrongylus cantonensis*, *Ann. trop. Med. Parasit.*, 59, 294.

JUMBALA, B., SUKUMALCHANTRA, Y., VICHITPAN, P., TONGMITR, V., PRACHUABMOH, K., and CHATIKAVANIJ, K. (1968) Juvenile mitral stenosis in Thailand, in *Cardiology: Current Topics and Progress, Symposia of the Fourth Asian Pacific Congress of Cardiology*, eds. Eliakim, M., and Neufeld, N. H., London, pp. 184.

KAEOWPLUNG, M. (1960) Analysis of cases of snake-bite, *Chula. med. J.*, 7, 13.

KHWANMITRA, S., BODHIDATTA, P., and PUNYAGUPTA, S. (1957) Report of four cases of eosinophilia in cerebrospinal fluid, *J. med. Ass. Thailand*, **40**, 341.

KNISELY, M. H., ELIOT, T. S., and BLOCH, E. H. (1945) Sludged blood in traumatic shock, I. Microscopic observations of the precipitation and agglutination of blood flowing through vessels in crushed tissues, *Arch. Surg.*, **51**, 220.

KNISELY, M. H., STRATMAN-THOMAS, W. K., ELIOT, T. S., and BLOCH, E. H. (1964) Knowlesi malaria in monkeys, IIa, *Angiology*, 15, 411.

KURLAND, L. T., AUTH, T. L., BEBBE, G. W., *et al.* (1963) Studies on the natural history of multiple sclerosis, **2**. Progression from optic neuritis to multiple sclerosis, *Trans. Amer. neurol. Ass.*, 88, 231.

KURLAND, L. T., STAZIO, A., and REED, D. (1965) An appraisal of population studies of multiple sclerosis, *Ann. N.Y. Acad. Sci.*, **122**, 520.

KUROIWA, Y. (1968) Clinical features of demyelinating disease in Japan, *Proc. Aust. Ass. Neurol.*, **5**, 341.

KUROIWA, Y., ARAKI, S., and KATSUKI, S. (1965) Clinical features of demyelinating diseases in Japan, in *Proceedings of the Eighth International Congress of Neurology*, Vienna, p. 83.

LEVINSEN, G. M. R. (1889) *Medd. Donsk. Naturh. Foren i. kjbenhaven. f.*, p. 323.

LEVY, L. F., and ELVIDGE, A. R. (1956) Astrocytoma of the brain and spinal cord—a review of 176 cases, *J. Neurosurg.*, **13**, 413.

LUBINSKI, H., and PRAUSNITZ, C. (1926) Lyssa, *Ergebn. Hyg. Bakt.*, **8**, 164, quoted by Dupont, J. R., and Earle, K. M. (1965).

LYNN, B. H. (1959) Retrobulbar neuritis, *Trans. ophthal. Soc. U.K.*, **79**, 701.

MACFADZEAN, A. J. S., and YEUNG, R. (1957) Periodic paralysis complicating thyrotoxicosis in Chinese, *Brit. med. J.*, **1**, 451.

MAEGRAITH, B. G. (1948) *Pathological Processes in Malaria and Blackwater Fever*, Oxford.

MORECKI, R., and ZIMMERMAN, H. M. (1969) Human rabies encephalitis, *Arch. Neurol. (Chic.)*, **20**, 599.

MUENTHONGCHIN, N., and VEJJAJIVA, A. (1969) Neurological manifestations of systemic lupus erythematosus, *J. med. Ass. Thailand*, **52**, 673.

MUENTHONGCHIN, N., VEJJAJIVA, A., and JUMBALA, B. (1970) Disturbance of atrio-ventricular conduction in a patient with thyrotoxic periodic paralysis, *J. med. Ass. Thailand*, **53**, 814.

NOMURA, L., and LIN, P. H. (1945) First case report of human infection with *Haemostrongylus ratti*, Yukogawa, *Taiwan No. Ikai*, **3**, 589.

OKINAKA, S., SHIZUME, K., IINO, S., WATANABE, A., IRIE, M., NOGUCHI, A., KUMA, S., KUMA, K., and ITO, T. (1957) The association of periodic paralysis and hyperthyroidism in Japan, *J. clin. Endocr.*, **17**, 1454.

PAWAN, J. L. (1936) Rabies in the vampire bat of Trinidad, with special reference to clinical course and latency of infection, *Ann. trop. Med. Parasit.*, **30**, 401.

PHUANGSAB, A., PANAS-AMPOL, K., LAWHASWASDI, K., and LE BEAU, L. (1967) Rats as a reservoir of rabies in Chiengmai, *J. med. Ass. Thailand*, **50**, 26.

PROMMINDAROJ, K., LEELAWONGS, N., and PRADATSUNDARASAR, A. (1962) Human angiostrongyloidiasis of the eye in Bangkok, *Amer. J. trop. Med. Hyg.*, **11**, 759.

PUNYADASNI, V., and PUNYAGUPTA, S. (1962) *Two cases of Eosinophilic meningitis following the Ingestion of Raw Snails Possibly Due to Angiostrongylus Cantonensis*, paper presented at the meeting of the Medical Association of Thailand, October 1962.

PUNYAGUPTA, S. (1967) Recent knowledge on clinical gnathostomiasis, *J. med. Ass. Thailand*, **50**, 686.

PUNGYAGUPTA, S., and JUTTIJUDATA, P. (1967) Gnathostomiasis in a case of eosinophilic myeloencephalitis, *Roy. Thai Army med. J.*, 20, 367.

PUNYAGUPTA, S., JUTTIJUDATA, P., BUNNAG, T., and COMER, D. S. (1968) Two fatal cases of eosinophilic myeloencephalitis, a newly recognized disease, caused by *Gnathostoma spinigerum*, *Trans. roy. Soc. trop. Med. Hyg.*, 62, 801.

PUNYAGUPTA, S., JUTTIJUDATA, P., and BUNNAG, T. (1970) Eosinophilic meningitis in Thailand, 1. Clinical studies of 484 typical cases probably caused by *Angiostrongylus cantonensis*. Personal communication.

RATANAVALE, G. (1968) Cranial polyneuritis—a distinct clinical entity, *Proc. Aust. Ass. Neurol.* 5, 527.

REID, H. A. (1961) Sea-snake poisoning, *Brit. med. J.*, 1, 1284.

REMLINGER, P., and BAILLEY, J. (1938) Etudes sur la rage, *Monogr. Inst. Pasteur*, Paris.

REYE, R. D., MORGAN, G., and BARAL, J. (1963) Encephalopathy and fatty degeneration of viscera: a disease entity in children, *Lancet*, ii, 749.

ROSEN, L., CHAPPELL, R., LAQUER, G. L., *et al.* (1962) Eosinophilic meningoencephalitis caused by a metastrongylid lung-worm of rats, *J. Amer. med. Ass.*, 179, 620.

ROSEN, L., LOISON, G., LAIGRET, J., and WALLACE, G. D. (1967) Studies on eosinophilic meningitis, 3. Epidemiologic and clinical observations on Pacific islands and the possible etiologic role of *Angiostrongylus cantonensis*, *Amer. J. Epidemiol.*, 85, 17.

SATAYOSHI, F., MURAKAMI, K., KOWA, H., *et al.* (1963) Periodic paralysis in hyperthyroidism, *Neurology (Minneap.)*, 13, 746.

SELBY, R. (1968) quoted by Spillane, J. D. (1969).

SHIRAKI, H., and OTANI, S. (1959) Clinical and pathological features of rabies post-vaccinal encephalomyelitis in man, in *Allergic Encephalomyelitis*, ed. Kies M. W., and Alvord, E. C. Springfield, Ill.

SHUANGSHOTI, S., TANGCHAI, P., and NETSKY, M. G. (1968) Intracranial meningioma in Thailand, *J. med. Ass. Thailand*, 51, 741.

SHUANGSHOTI, S., and TANGCHAI, P. (1969*a*) Special features of intracranial glioblastoma multiforme in Thailand, *Far East med. J.*, 5, 29.

SHUANGSHOTI, S., and TANGCHAI, P. (1969*b*) Intraspinal neoplasms in Thailand, *J. med. Ass. Thailand*, 52, 217.

SHUANGSHOTI, S., TANGCHAI, P., and NETSKY, M. G. (1969*a*) Neoplasms of the nervous system in Thailand, *Cancer*, 23, 493.

SHUANGSHOTI, S., TANGCHAI, P., and NETSKY, M. G. (1969*b*) Intracranial astrocytoma in Thailand, *Far East med. J.*, 5, 114.

SITASUWAN, C., and RAMAYODHIN, T. (1970) Psychiatric symptoms due to encephalitis, *J. psychiat. Ass. Thailand*, 15, 10.

SITPRIJA, V., SRIBHIBHADH, R., BENYAJATI, C., and TANGCHAI, P. (1971) Haemodialysis in sea-snake bite poisoning, *Brit. med. J.*, 3, 218.

SNYDER, D. (1968) Personal communication.

SPILLANE, J. D. (1969) Tropical neurology, Presidential address, *Proc. roy. Soc. Med.*, 62, 403.

STEELE, J. C., and VASUVAT, A. (1970) Recurrent multiple cranial nerve palsies. A distinct syndrome of cranial polyneuropathy, *J. Neurol. Neurosurg. Psychiat*, 33, 828.

SUKONTHABHAND, S. (1965) cited by Allison, R. S. (1965).

SUWANWELA, C., and HONGSAPRABHAS, C. (1966) Fronto-ethmoidal encephalomeningocoele, *J. Neurosurg.*, 25, 172.

SUWANWELA, C., CHARUVORN, T., and ARTHACHINTA, S. (1966) Incidence of calcified pineal body at Chulalongkorn Hospital. A study of 500 skull roentgenograms, *J. med. Ass. Thailand*, 49, 11.

SUWANWELA, C., SUWANWELA, N., HONGLADAROM, T., and HONGSAPRABHAS, C. (1969*a*) Subarachnoid haemorrhage, aneurysms and arterio-venous malformations of the brain in Thailand, *Chula. med. J.*, 14, 56.

SUNWANWELA, C., HONGSAPRABHAS, C., SRIKASIKUL, S., *et al.* (1969*b*) Fronto-ethmoidal encephalomeningocoele, *Chula. med. J.*, 14, 179.

SUWANWELA, C., BOONYATHITI, T., SUWANWELA, N., *et al.* (1969*c*) Medical experience at Nong Ree District, Kanchanaburi Province, *Chula. med. J.*, 14, 22.

SYMONDS, C. P. (1958) Recurrent multiple cranial nerve palsies, *J. Neurol. Neurosurg, Psychiat.*, 21, 95.

TANGCHAI, P., NYE, S. W., and BEAVER, P. C. (1967) Eosinophilic meningoencephalitis caused by angiostrongyliasis in Thailand. Autopsy report, *Amer. J. trop. Med. Hyg.*, 16, 454.

TANGCHAI, P., YENBUTR, D., and VEJJAJIVA, A. (1970) Central nervous system lesions in human rabies. A study of twenty-four cases, *J. med. Ass. Thailand*, 53, 471.

TANGCHAI, P., and VEJJAJIVA, A. (1971) Pathology of the peripheral nervous system in human rabies. A study of nine autopsy cases, *Brain*, 94, 299.

TIERKEL, E. S. (1958) Recent developments in the epidemiology of rabies. Introduction, *Ann. N.Y. Acad. Sci.*, 70, 445.

TIERKEL, E. S. (1963) *Diseases Transmitted from Animal to Man*, Springfield, Ill., Ch. 9.

TOLOSA, E. (1954) Periarteric lesion of the carotid siphon with the clinical features of a carotid infraclinoidal aneurysm, *J. Neurol. Neurosurg. Psychiat.*, 17, 300.

UCHIMURA, Y., and SHIRAKI, H. (1957) A contribution to the classification and the pathogenesis of demyelinating encephalomyelitis, with special reference to the central nervous system lesions caused by preventive inoculation against rabies, *J. Neuropath. exp. Neurol.*, 16, 139.

VEJJAJIVA, A. (1965) Systemic lupus erythematosus presenting as acute disseminated encephalomyelitis, *Lancet*, i, 352.

VEJJAJIVA, A. (1968*a*) Thyrotoxic periodic paralysis in Thailand, *J. med. Ass. Thailand*, 51, 235.

VEJJAJIVA, A. (1968*b*) Neurological sequelae of anti-rabic inoculation, *Proc. Aust. Ass. Neurol.* 5, 367.

VEJJAJIVA, A. (1970) Multiple sclerosis in Thailand, *Clin. Neurol. Japan*, 10, 36.

VEJJAJIVA, A., BOONGIRD, P., and VEJJAJIVA, S. (1967) Spinal-fluid gamma-globulin in various neurological disorders in Thailand, *J. med. Ass. Thailand*, **50**, 173.

VEJJAJIVA, A., and FAZEKAS, J. F. (1968) The incidence of cerebral vascular and associated diseases in Bangkok, *Far East med. J.*, 4, 278.

VEJJAJIVA, A., and HONGLADAROM, T. (1970) Neurosyphilis with reference to cases with diagnostic problems, *J. med. Ass. Thailand*, 53, 117.

VEJJAJIVA, A., and TAMTHAI, B. (1967) Human rabies. An analysis of 152 cases, *J. med. Ass. Thailand*, **50**, 796.

VINIJCHAIKUL, K. (1967) Primary arteritis of the aorta and its main branches (Takayasu's arteriopathy). A clinicopathologic autopsy study of eight cases, *Amer. J. Med.*, 43, 15.

WASI, P. (1970) Personal communication.

WORLD HEALTH ORGANIZATION (1966) Fifth Report of the Expert Committee on Rabies, *Wld Hlth Org. techn. Rep. Ser.*, No. 321.

WORLD HEALTH ORGANIZATION (1968) The present and future in rabies research, *Wld Hlth Org. Chron.*, **22**, 199.

YII, C. Y., CHEN, C.Y., FRESH, J. W., CHEN, T., and CROSS, J. H. (1968) Human angiostrongyliasis involving the lung, *Chinese J. Microbiol.*, 1, 148.

Part Four

OCEANIA

See Plates 29–31

28 Amyotrophic Lateral Sclerosis and Parkinsonism-Dementia in Guam

J. A. BRODY and L. T. KURLAND

The striking concentration of amyotrophic lateral sclerosis (ALS) and parkinsonism-dementia (PD) among the Chamorro people of Guam has attracted the attention of the medical world since the early 1950s (Brody and Chen, 1969; Brody, Hirano, and Scott, 1971). Extensive studies conducted over the past 20 years have not revealed the causes of these diseases and the reasons for their remarkable concentration on Guam. Approximately 1 in 10 Guamanian deaths over age 25 is from ALS, and another 1 in 10 dies of PD. ALS still occurs approximately 50 times more frequently on Guam than in the continental United States.

Advances in virological and biochemical techniques, and long years of study, appear to be leading us to a point where some of the problems will be resolved. Here we shall attempt to review the pertinent background information and summarize the data and observations up to the present time.

HISTORICAL BACKGROUND

Guam, a territory of the United States, is the largest of the Mariana Islands which, together with the Caroline, Marshall, and Gilbert Islands, make up the geographic island grouping of Micronesia (Reed, Plato, Elizan, and Kurland, 1966). Guam lies within the Tropic of Cancer at 13° North latitude and 145° East longitude. The island is approximately 30 miles long and 4 to 9 miles wide [FIG. 28.1].

The natives of Guam and of the other Mariana Islands belong to the Chamorro linguistic group. They are descendants of aboriginal people whose origins are not completely known, although they appear to be closely related to the people of Malaysia, the Philippines, and Polynesia. Intermarriage with Spaniards, Filipinos, Mexicans, Orientals, and Europeans over the past four centuries has so modified the genetic pool that it is unlikely that any 'pure' Chamorros exist today. In 1970 the indigenous population of Guam was approximately 40 000. In addition there were about 40 000 transient American military and civilian personnel and dependents, 6000 Filipino contract workers, 600 Carolinians, and a few hundred persons of various other nationalities.

Before the Second World War the population was concentrated in and around the centrally located capital city of Agana. During the Second World War there was a dramatic emigration from Agana to the relatively unpopulated regions of the island, but mostly to the central and northern areas. These newly established communities have now become permanent villages. The population in the southern areas of Guam has been more stable, and until recent years was relatively isolated from the rest of the island.

Although Guam is a small island, it contains distinct geologic regions. The northern one-third is a coralliferous limestone plateau, the central one-third is a blend of limestone flats into low volcanic hills, and the southern one-third is volcanic massif.

The unusual prevalence of a 'hereditary paralysis' on Guam was first reported in the medical literature in 1900 (cited by Elizan *et al.*, 1966*b*). The diagnosis of 'progressive muscular atrophy' was recorded on local death certificates as early as 1904, and the diagnosis of ALS first appeared on a death certificate in 1931. In 1945 Zimmerman reported the diagnostic confirmation at autopsy of two of seven ALS patients seen during a period of 1 month at the local hospital. Clinical and epidemiological studies from 1949 to 1954 established the phenomenal frequency of amyotrophic lateral sclerosis on Guam (Arnold, Edgren, and Palladino, 1953; Koerner, 1952; Tillema and Wijnberg, 1953; Kurland and Mulder, 1954).

In discussions with older people on Guam it appears that ALS occurred at least 40 years before 1900 and possibly the illness has existed for many hundreds of years. The word for ALS in the Chamorro language is *lytico* which is derived from the Spanish word *paralytico*. The disease has been well recognized by the population and there are myths and legends concerning its origin.

In the course of their studies of ALS, Mulder, Kurland, and Iriarte (1954) observed a number of patients with 'parkinsonism', many of whom appeared confused and demented. It gradually became apparent that a second chronic fatal neurological disease existed on Guam. This disease, which involves severe organic dementia and extrapyramidal signs, was called parkinsonism-dementia. It was first described in the medical literature by Hirano *et al.* (1961) and Hirano, Malamud, and Kurland (1961), although a case-report by Okaya in Japanese (Okaya, 1936) possibly described a PD Patient. In contrast to ALS, PD is less clearly defined as an entity by Guamanians. The disease appears primarily among people in their fifties and sixties as a gradual slowing down of mental and physical functions. Hence

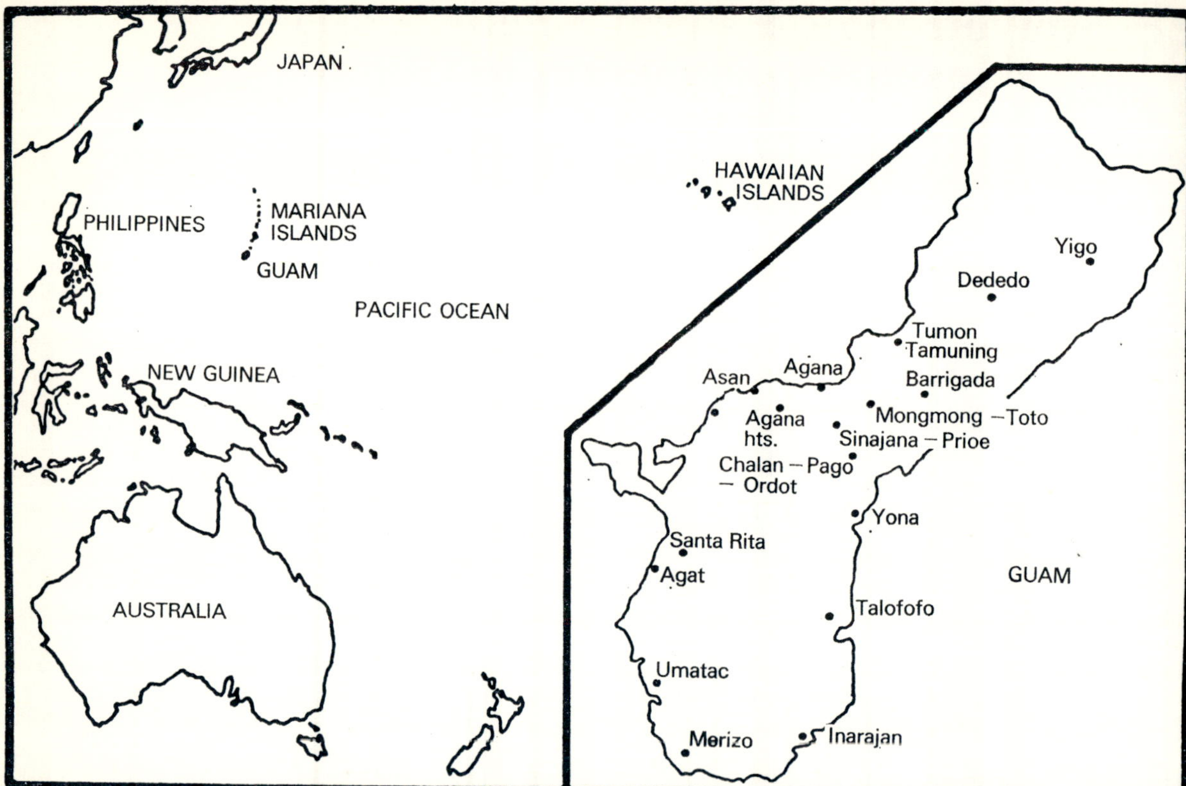

FIG. 28.1. Map of Guam and the Western Pacific region.

the words for this condition in Chamorro are nonspecific and are frequently those words used in jest to describe a person who is lazy or detached.

Guam has fairly sophisticated medical facilities. The Government of Guam maintains the Guam Memorial Hospital, a modern 250-bed hospital with approximately 20 fulltime physicians. Since 1956 the Epidemiology Branch, C & FR, National Institute of Neurological Diseases and Stroke (NINDS), National Institutes of Health, has maintained the NINDS Research Center on Guam. The Research Center is devoted exclusively to the study of ALS, PD, and other neurological disorders in the community.

EPIDEMIOLOGY

Since 1945 we have confirmed a total of 492 cases of ALS and PD [TABLE 28.1]. There is some clinical overlap between the diseases, as is indicated on this table. While 445 of the 492 patients had either clinical ALS or PD, 15 had features of clinical parkinsonism only. In addition, 10 patients whose primary symptoms were those of ALS had some features of PD and 22 patients whose primary illness was PD had features of ALS. ALS appears in three Guamanians who had one grandparent who was non-Chamorro [TABLE 28.2], in eight Guamanians of whom one parent was non-Chamorro, and in four non-Chamorro Filipinos. PD

Table 28.1

Confirmed Cases of ALS and PD Since 1945

Diagnosis	*Male*	*Female*	*Total*
ALS	204	107	311
PD	100	34	134
P	14	1	15
ALS/PD	4	0	4
ALS/P	5	0	5
ALS/D	1	0	1
PD/ALS	15	5	20
P/ALS	2	0	2
	345	*147*	*492*

appeared in three Guamanians of whom one parent was non-Chamorro. Clinical parkinsonism appeared in two Filipinos and in one person who was only one-fourth Chamorro.

In TABLE 28.3 all known patients with ALS and PD are presented by year of death in 5-year groupings since 1945, plus those who died in 1970, and those who were still alive at the time of writing (1971). In parentheses are shown the numbers of mixed cases which were included in the totals by their primary disease. The number of deaths from ALS for males and females has been relatively stable for each 5-year period from 1950 to the present time. The number of known ALS deaths from 1945 to 1949 was considerably less, and probably represents a failure to make the diagnosis prior to the establishment of the hospital and the NINDS Research Center on Guam. We have evidence that this occurred, since in questioning families we have learned of probable cases in people who died in those years of postwar reconstruction but on whom no medical information was available (Brody and Chen, 1969). Most of the subsequent analyses of ALS are based on patients dying between 1950 and 1969, who had any degree of Chamorro ancestry.

PD was not well recognized until late in the 1950s as is suggested by the figures in TABLE 28.3. From 1955 to 1959 there were 20 deaths from PD among men, while the disease was diagnosed in only one woman. As awareness of PD grew, the reported number of deaths from PD has increased and the disease is being diagnosed increasingly among women. Most of the subsequent analyses of PD are based on Chamorro patients dying between 1960 and 1969, although even in this group we recognize limitations because of probable incomplete ascertainment of this disease.

Age

In FIGURE 28.2 are presented the age-specific death rates per 100 000 individuals who died of ALS between 1950 and 1969, in terms of the population at risk at the beginning of each 10-year period (based on United States Census Bureau statistics). Slightly more than

Table 28.2
Racial Descent of Cases

Diagnosis	*Chamorro*	*¾ Chamorro*	*½ Chamorro*	*¼ Chamorro*	*Filipino*	*Total*
ALS	297	(2 Filipino) 3 (1 Chinese)	8 (4 Filipino) 8 (3 Japanese) (1 Caucasian)	—	4	311
PD	131	—	(2 Filipino) 3 (1 Japanese)	—	—	134
P	12	—	—	1 (Caucasian)	2	15
ALS plus PD	10	—	—	—	—	10
PD plus ALS	20	—	—	—	—	20
P plus ALS	2	—	—	—	—	2

Table 28.3
ALS and PD Deaths Since 1945 and Living Cases

Years of Death	*1945–49*	*1950–54*	*1955–59*	*1960–64*	*1965–69*	*1970–?*	*Total*
ALS							
Male	22	42	48(3)	42(3)	35(4)	25	214(10)
Female	9	21	19	18	20	20	107
Total	*31*	*63*	*67*	*60*	*55*	*45*	*321(10)*
PD							
Male	1	5	20(1)	53(19)	40(8)	12(3)	131(13)
Female	1	2	1	18(3)	15(3)	3	40(6)
Total	*2*	*7*	*21*	*71*	*55*	*15*	*171(37)*
Total	*33*	*70*	*88*	*131*	*110*	*60*	*492*

( ) = Mixed cases which are included in totals.

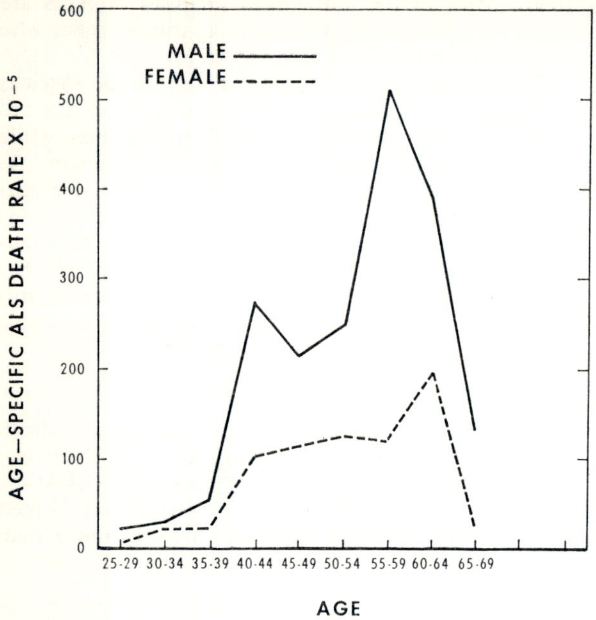

FIG. 28.2. Age-specific ALS death rate $\times 10^{-5}$.

10 per cent of deaths from ALS occurred before the age of 40 in both sexes. Rates among men over 40 remained high until the early seventies, with the highest rates (514 per 100 000 per year) occurring in the 55 to 59 year age-group. For women, the rates after the age of 40 remained high and then peaked in the 60 to 64 age-group, 5 years later than the peak for men. The mean age of death for all women was 50·0, while for all men it was 51·2.

PD death rates for 1960 to 1969 appear in FIGURE 28.3. There were a few cases before age 45. Among women from age 50 on, the rates were relatively stable; among men, however, there was an enormous increase up to age 60 to 64. During this 5-year age span 0·75 per cent of the entire male population died each year of PD.

Sex

The ratio of men to women for ALS was 2·5 : 1 for all deaths from 1950 through 1969 [TABLE 28.4]. The ratio between men and women did not vary much from age 30 through 64. Thereafter, however, the rate among men was over five times that for women.

The overall ratio of men to women for PD based on deaths occurring between 1960 and 1969 [TABLE 28.4] was 3·35 : 1. Since the numbers involved are relatively small, there was more variation among different age-groups.

Table 28.4

Sex Ratio of Age-Specific Death Rates for ALS and PD

Age Group	No. of Males/No. of Females *ALS*	*PD*
25–34	1·60	—
35–44	2·49	1·76
45–54	1·88	2·60
55–64	2·92	4·48
65+	5·30	3·58
All	2·48	3·35

Area

It is not known whether village of birth or village of onset was more closely related to factors causing ALS or PD. As mentioned earlier, until the Second World War approximately half of the Guam population lived in the capital city of Agana. It was customary for people to own farms in outlying areas and commute daily and on weekends from Agana. During the war, people dispersed to the sites of present villages in the north and

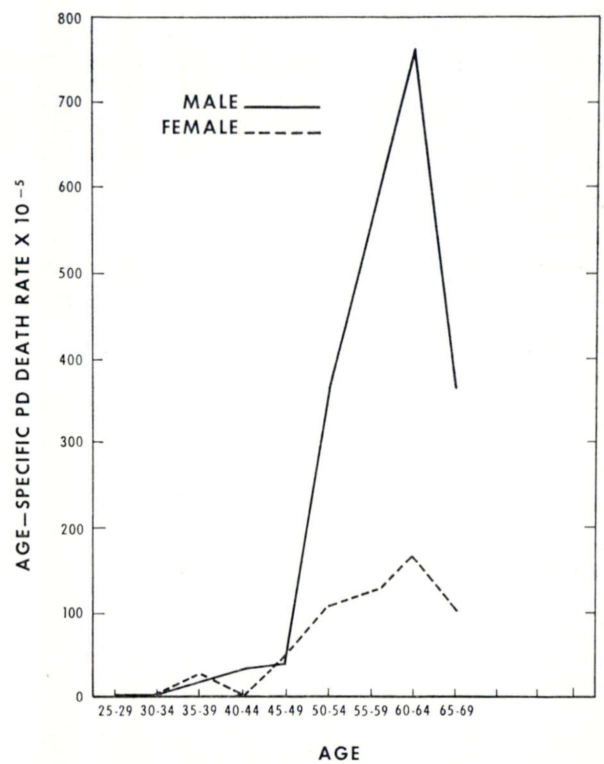

FIG. 28.3 Age-specific PD death rate $\times 10^{-5}$.

Table 28.5
Death Rate by Geographic Area and Village $\times 10^{-5}$

	1960 Census M	1960 Census F	Males ALS	Males PD	Females ALS	Females PD
Northern	494	530	233	304	38	75
Central	2915	3584	129	158	50	42
Western	991	1259	45	71	40	8
Southern	710	814	338	282	111	111
Northern						
1. Yigo	166	157	241	361	0	127
2. Dededo	328	373	229	274	54	54
Central						
3. Agana*	878	1133	47	80	9	26
4. Barrigada*	1018	1235	152	196	73	49
5. Sinajana*	767	903	248	287	78	44
6. Yona	252	313	119	238	64	96
Western						
7. Asan	215	262	70	0	38	0
8. Piti	153	216	65	0	23	0
9. Agat*	623	781	32	128	51	13
Southern						
10. Talofofo	171	199	263	175	75	50
11. Inarajan	238	271	210	420	111	0
12. Merizo	193	228	363	52	0	0
13. Umatac	108	116	694	556	388	690
All	*5110*	*6187*	*152*	*172*	*55*	*47*

Calculation: ALS: $\frac{\text{No. deaths in 20 years (1950–69)}}{20 \times \text{1960 count}}$

PD: $\frac{\text{No. deaths in 10 years (1960–69)}}{10 \times \text{1960 count}}$

* Includes environs.

central parts of Guam, leaving Agana a relatively small town. The villages in the south, in which ALS and PD incidence rates were highest, were comparatively unchanged by this migration. Higher rates in individual villages were similar when analysed either by village of onset or village of birth. Although we recognize the possible bias, data are presented here only in terms of place of onset.

The village of Umatac [Fig. 28.4 and Table 28.5] had the highest rates for both men and women with ALS and PD. Of striking interest was the village of Merizo, which borders Umatac. Here, although we encounter the second highest rate of ALS among men, there were no female cases of ALS or PD and only one male PD case.

Death rates in northern and southern villages were higher for men with ALS and for both sexes for PD. ALS death rates for women were higher in the southern villages only. Variation in rates was observed in the central villages while western villages had consistently low rates for both sexes for ALS and PD. While temporal variations were noted in given areas, no overall secular trend was detected during the years of study. To date we have no satisfactory explanation for these observed geographic patterns.

CLINICAL APPEARANCES

ALS

In our series of 321 patients with ALS [Table 28.1] 311 had only motor neurone disease while in 10 some features of dementia or extrapyramidal disease were encountered. These mixed cases will be discussed later.

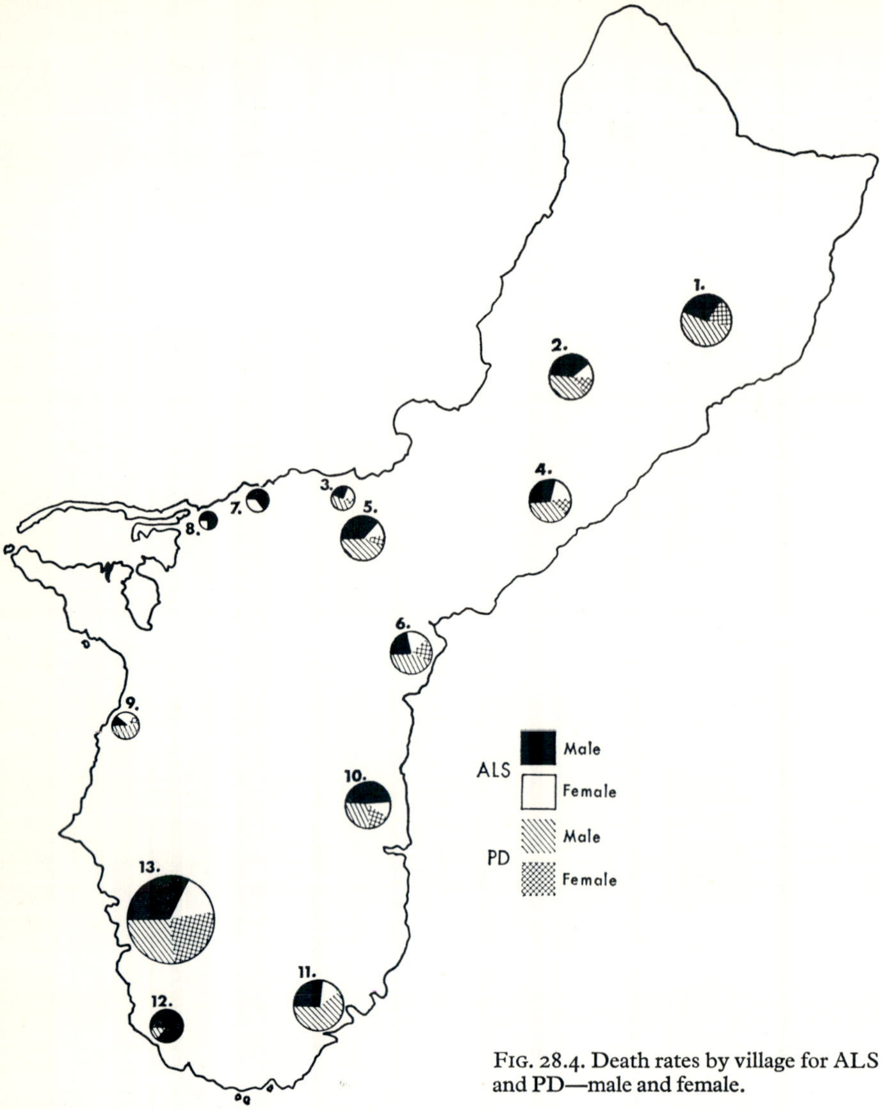

FIG. 28.4. Death rates by village for ALS and PD—male and female.

Clinically, the ALS of Guam conforms closely with the classical syndrome as described by Charcot and Joffray (1869) and in most subsequent studies (Elizan *et al.*, 1966 *b*). Signs of upper and lower motor neurone lesions of pseudobulbar, bulbar, and spinal areas developed almost invariably during the course of the illness. The presenting symptom was muscle atrophy in about half of the patients, while in 15 per cent spasticity appeared first, and in the remainder atrophy and spasticity appeared to develop concomitantly. In less than 5 per cent of the cases spasticity had not appeared by the time of death and clinical involvement was confined to muscle atrophy at the bulbar or spinal level. When autopsies were performed on these patients, however, histological evidence of upper motor neurone involvement was invariably present (Elizan *et al.*, 1966 *b*; Hirano *et al.*, 1966). Age of onset of patients ranged from 20 to 72. The mean duration of survival among 177 men in whom date of onset was reliable was 4·1 yr, and among 94 women it was 4·3 yr [FIG. 28.5]. There was a slight tendency, particularly among young women, to survive longer but in general age of onset did not affect survival appreciably; 21 per cent of men and 34 per cent of women survived more than 5 years after onset while 10 per cent of men and 17 per cent of women lived for 10 years or more (calculated by the life table method of Cutler and Ederer, 1958).

No weakness of extra-ocular muscles or of urinary and bowel sphincters was noted. Objective sensory deficits were absent in all cases.

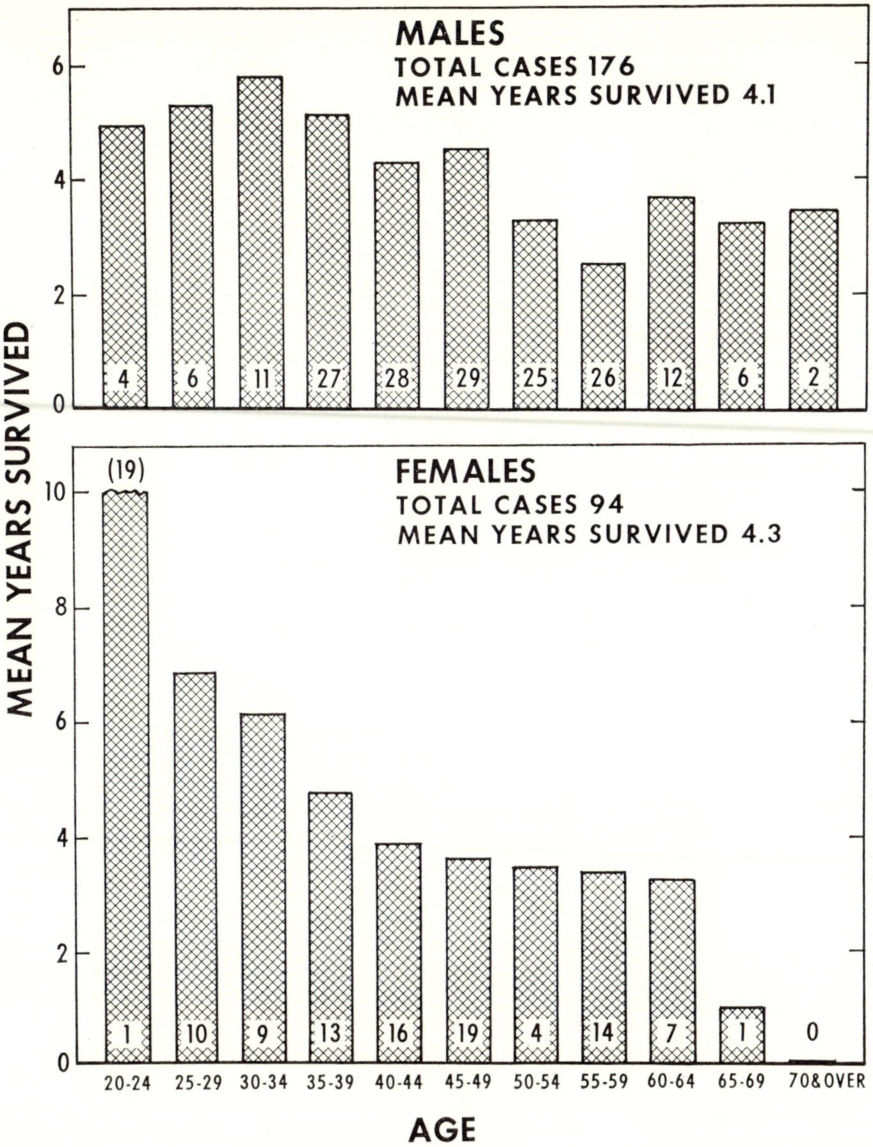

FIG. 28.5. Mean years survived —ALS.

PD

PD is an invariably fatal disease characterized by an insidiously progressive organic mental deterioration and extrapyramidal dysfunction in the form of bradykinesia, rigidity, or tremor. Dementia or organic mental syndrome was the most common single initial feature of the illness, occurring in approximately 30 per cent of cases. Bradykinesia occurred alone initially in 15 per cent of cases, rigidity in 8 per cent and tremor in 5 per cent. Various combinations of these signs were noted at onset in the rest of the cases. Ultimately, all patients developed some degree of mental deterioration, 85 per cent had bradykinesia, 75 per cent had rigidity, and 65 per cent had tremor.

Of the 169 Chamorro patients who fell into the general classification of PD, mixed or incomplete clinical syndromes were observed. Thirteen died with only extrapyramidal involvement in the absence of organic mental changes, and in two more instances extrapyramidal features in the absence of mental changes preceded the development of ALS. A total of 20 patients with the full syndrome of PD developed unmistakable motor neurone disease. Mixed cases and those with only extrapyramidal features will be discussed later. PD is apparently a unique disease found only among Chamorros, and a more extensive description of the clinical findings will therefore be presented, based primarily on the observations of Elizan *et al.* (1966 *b*).

Dementia

In almost a third of the cases, dementia was the only feature of the disease for a variable period of time. Memory deficits and disorientation for time, place, or person were the presenting signs of dementia in almost all cases. Changes in personality or behaviour pattern were present initially in about a third of the cases, and consisted of one or more of the following: apathy, depression, irritability, restlessness, agitation, childishness, loss of insight, incontinence, and violent behaviour. Hypersomnia or insomnia at some phase of the illness has been reported by the patients' families in about one-quarter of cases. Inaccuracies in simple calculation and reversals, slowness in comprehension of even the most concrete ideas, marked difficulty in simple reasoning, increasing confusion, and apathy became more obvious as the disease progressed. Depression was a major feature of the disease in a few instances but the majority of patients remained emotionally indifferent to their illness, even during the early phase when insight was still fairly intact. Nine patients exhibited violent antisocial behaviour. There was no instance of suicide. Hallucinations were reported in three patients during the last phase of the illness. In contrast to ALS there was suggestive decrease in libido early in several of the younger patients. No changes in eating habits were noted.

Bradykinesia

Generalized slowness or difficulty in initiating and maintaining voluntary motor activities, with marked diminution in spontaneous or associated movements, was the most common extrapyramidal dysfunction, occurring in 85 per cent of the patients. Slurring and sluggishness of speech and slowing down of gait with diminished associated movements were usually early signs. The festinating gait of classical paralysis agitans was observed in only one case in this series. Propulsion and retropulsion with imbalance were seldom observed. The patients' strides usually remained fairly normal in size but were slowly and laboriously executed. Alternating movements usually retained their amplitude but were done slowly and hesitantly. Handwriting was tested in many cases, and no micrographia was observed. Ability to perform skilled and fine movements was markedly reduced. The combination of bradykinesia and rigidity became increasingly obvious in the later phases of the disease.

Rigidity

Seventy-five per cent of the patients developed objective rigidity in the course of the illness. Facial 'masking' with diminished spontaneous eye blink and a 'stare' was an early sign. More overt postural rigidity occurred later in the disease, most marked in the flexor muscles of the trunk and neck. Rigidity of the extremities was usually symmetrical and started proximally, and later involved the entire limb with the flexors and extensors being similarly involved. The upper limbs were usually affected earlier than the lower. Stiffness interfered with fine voluntary hand movements quite early in some cases. Initially the rigidity of trunk and limbs was more apparent than real—i.e. patients looked more rigid from their overall appearance than they actually were on clinical testing. Later, lead-pipe rigidity or occasional cogwheel resistance was unequivocal. Unusual rigid postures of the upper limbs resembling those seen in catatonic states were observed in some patients. Marked rigidity of the fingers sometimes resulted in flexion contractures of the hand. Concomitant spasticity of the limbs was often difficult to distinguish from rigidity, especially in the presence of generalized hyper-reflexia, a frequent sign in these cases. Rigidity of bulbar muscles occurred in advanced cases, with increasing difficulty in mastication, swallowing, phonation, and articulation. Generalized rigidity and relative immobility were not uncommon in the terminal stages.

Tremor

Tremor was noted in 65 per cent of the patients. It was usually localized in the hands and was mild, fine, and regular at a rhythmic frequency of 4 to 7 per second. It was present at rest, with change of posture, or with movement of limb. Occasionally, it disappeared with repose; often, it became accentuated with movement or with emotional excitement. The typical 'pill rolling' tremor of paralysis agitans was observed rarely. Movements at the wrist or elbow were usually flexion and extension or lateral displacement. The tongue was affected in a third of the cases. Eyelid tremor was noted in several patients; jaw tremor and head tremor were rarely seen, and an isolated foot tremor was not observed. Tremor was never a prominent or an incapacitating feature at any stage of the disease, and in many instances it lessened considerably or even disappeared in the later phase of illness as rigidity increased.

EEG abnormalities were marked and progressive in almost all PD patients within 6 months before death (Chen, Abrams, and Brody, 1968). The EEG pattern was a progressive slowing of background alpha rhythms, which were gradually replaced by 5 to 7 c/sec diffuse low to medium voltage waves and diminished reactivity over a 2- to 3-year period. About 28 per cent of cases showed focal delta activity in the frontotemporal areas. No epileptiform activity was noted. The degree of EEG abnormalities paralleled the clinical course, but correlated more closely with dementia than with extrapyramidal symptoms. The EEG findings in PD resembled those of Alzheimer's disease and Pick's disease, but differed from those reported in the classical Parkinson's disease. Similar changes were not encountered in ALS patients.

Duration of survival after onset of PD was difficult to determine because the cardinal symptoms of slowly progressive dementia and bradykinesia were frequently

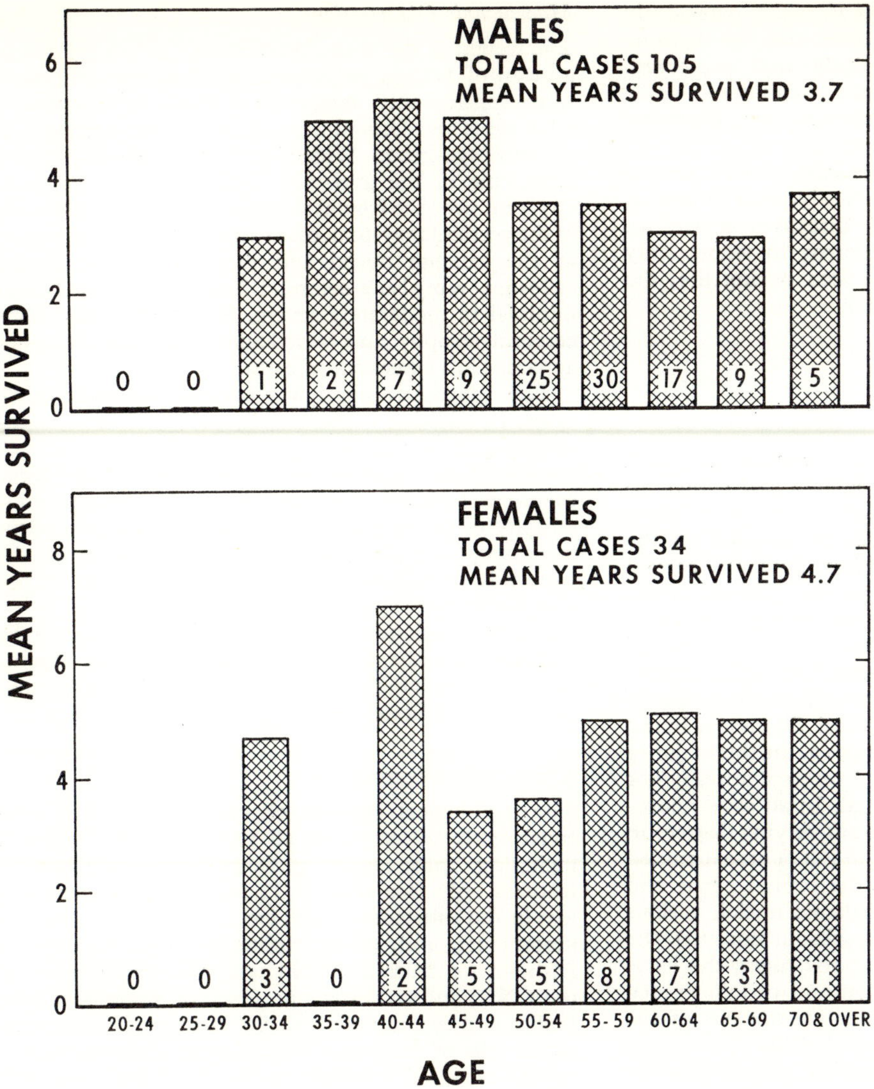

FIG. 28.6 Mean years survived—PD.

confused with normal ageing. Our most accurate data indicate that men survived an average of 3·7 years after onset and women survived 4·7 years [FIG. 28.6]. Survival did not vary appreciably with age at onset; 27 per cent of men and 39 per cent of women survived more than 5 years, while none survived 10 years.

'Parkinsonism'

During the years of study 15 patients with extrapyramidal disease developed no evidence of organic mental syndrome during life. Of these, 13 had Chamorro ancestry while two were Filipino. All 13 Chamorros have died and the brains of eight have been examined (Elizan *et al.*, 1966*b*; Hirano *et al.*, 1966). In each instance the autopsy findings were those of Guamanian PD and not those of paralysis agitans. Severe cerebral atrophy was present and there was marked cellular destruction of the substantia nigra and other areas of the basal ganglia. Neurofibrillary tangles were abundant in subcortical regions, while Lewy bodies were rare or absent. The mean age at death and the mean survival time were not significantly different from those in patients who developed the full syndrome of PD. This short survival time contrasts with that of paralysis agitans where the median duration exceeds 10 years (Nobrega, Glattre, Kurland, and Okazaki, 1967). In the one Filipino patient with paralysis agitans on whom an autopsy was performed, the neuropathological findings were those of classical Parkinson's disease and differed markedly from the findings in Guamanian PD (Hirano *et al.*, 1966). The substantia nigra was not as extensively involved as in the Chamorro cases and the neurone population was still comparatively well preserved. Neurofibrillary changes were not encountered while Lewy bodies were numerous in the substantia nigra and the pigment granules were altered.

We have not seen true Parkinson's disease among Chamorros on Guam (Chen, Brody, and Kurland, 1968). From the observations discussed above we conclude that for those Chamorros in whom only extrapyramidal symptoms were seen during life, the pathologic process was that of PD.

NEUROPATHOLOGY

ALS

The classical neuropathological changes of ALS throughout the world are well known and similar to those found in Guamanian ALS. As a result, these findings are not reviewed here. In addition to the classical neuropathological findings, however, certain distinctive changes are always present (Hirano *et al.*, 1966). These alterations are qualitatively similar to those found in PD but quantitatively less pronounced. Grossly, the mean weight of brains from ALS patients was 1235 g, which was heavier than the mean weight of PD brains but less than the normal Chamorro brain, which weighed approximately 1450 g. In the majority of cases there was no evidence of cerebral atrophy nor was the ventricular system dilated. In all cases neurofibrillary degeneration was found to varying degrees in those areas where it was present in PD. These included the cerebral cortex (especially the orbital gyrus and Ammon's horn) various hypothalamic nuclei, various basal ganglia (especially the amygdaloid nucleus), the substantia innominata, the substantia nigra, the locus caeruleus, the reticular formation and certain cranial nuclei of the brain stem, the dentate nucleus of the cerebellum, and the reticular nuclei of the spinal cord. In addition to neurofibrillary tangles, granulovacuolar bodies were almost always present, by and large confined to the pyramidal cells of Ammon's horn (Hirano, Malamud, Kurland, and Zimmerman, 1969; Malamud, Hirano, and Kurland, 1961). Eosinophilic rod-like inclusions were also observed at this site in several severely involved cases (Hirano *et al.*, 1966; Hirano, 1966) and by electron microscopy were seen to be strikingly crystalloid in structure (Hirano, 1965). In addition neurofibrillary tangles occurred in motor areas usually involved in ALS.

PD

A more extensive description of the neuropathological changes will be presented largely based on the observations of Hirano (Hirano *et al.*, 1966; Hirano, Malamud, Kurland, and Zimmerman, 1969) since this disease is apparently unique among Chamorros.

Macroscopic Observations

The weight of the brain varied from 837 to 1575 g with a mean of 1114 g. In general, the brains in PD cases were considerably smaller than those in Guamanian ALS cases and United States paralysis agitans cases of a similar age-group. Widening of the cerebral sulci and narrowing of the gyri were bilateral and were more apparent over the frontal and temporal lobes. Dilatation of the vetricular system, often associated with flattening of the caudate nuclei and thinning of the corpus callosum, was also a common feature and varied from minimal to moderately severe. However, conspicuous cerebral atrophy and ventricular dilatation were not apparent in 15 per cent of cases.

The substantia nigra was severely atrophic in all cases. In addition it was usually pale, and in some instances a brown pigment had replaced the normal black colour. It was usually difficult to identify the locus caeruleus because of advanced atrophy. Conspicuous atrophy of the globus pallidus was also often evident macroscopically. Shrinkage and discoloration of the pyramids of the medulla and lateral columns of the spinal cord were evident in 7 per cent of cases.

The major blood vessels at the base of the brain in the Guamanian cases contained remarkably fewer atheromatous plaques than are usually encountered at autopsy in the United States.

Microscopic Observations

The histological changes characteristic of PD were consistently observed in all the Chamorro patients, including those eight patients with parkinsonian features only [see above]. These included severe cell loss in the substantia nigra, locus caeruleus, substantia innominata, and, often, globus pallidus; widespread Alzheimer's neurofibrillary changes in specific parts of the CNS; and consistent presence of granulovacuolar bodies and eosinophilic rod-like inclusions in the pyramidal cells of Ammon's horn. Changes were observed in the areas of predilection in all of the cases, the topographical distribution being similar to that in the ALS cases described above. In general, the cerebral cortex and the subcortical nuclei were more severely affected in PD than in ALS cases, while in the brain stem neurofibrillary changes were occasionally more prominent in the ALS cases. The number of neurones with these changes varied from case to case and from one area to another. A simple correlation between severity of those changes and age of patient, duration of illness, or other clinical data was not found in our series. A 35-year-old woman had the most severe neurofibrillary changes, and the case with the longest clinical course in the series had the least extensive neurofibrillary change. The clinical symptoms appeared to be much better correlated with loss of neurones than with the number of neurones having neurofibrillary changes. Fibrillary tangles seemed to persist comparatively longer after the disappearance of other cytoplasmic constituents, although eventually they also disappeared completely. Thus, in the most severely affected regions the most striking feature was the paucity of neurones. This observation was well illustrated in the locus caeruleus and Ammon's horn. There, only a few neurones remained, although the number with neurofibrillary changes was, in general, much less in the PD cases than in the Guamanian ALS cases.

Aside from the changes characteristic of PD, several pathological features reminiscent of ALS were found. Involvement of the motor neurones and pyramidal tracts is the most characteristic histological feature in ALS. In the spinal cord, neuronal loss in the anterior horns associated with gliosis was seen in one-third of PD cases. Involvement of the motor neurones was extensive in one-third of these cases and moderate in the other two-thirds, and neurofibrillary changes involving only small numbers of cells were seen in two-thirds of these spinal cords. Occasionally, in areas where the neuronal population appeared to be well preserved, neurofibrillary changes were evident unassociated with any obvious neuronal alteration. In cases which had no clear anterior horn cell loss, neurofibrillary changes in the reticular formations of the posterior horns was occasionally observed. Demyelination was almost complete in the pyramidal tracts of 7 per cent of cases, and mild but present in another one-third of those examined. Eosinophilic cytoplasmic inclusions in the anterior horn cells were looked for in nine cases but were not found.

Neuropathology of Guamanian Controls

Hirano *et al.* (1966) reviewed 29 Guamanian adults who died of causes other than ALS or PD. In five of these individuals they encountered neurofibrillary changes of the same pattern which they described for the classical PD cases and ALS cases of Guam. Detailed neurological information was not available for these five cases. In 12 cases, no neurofibrillary changes were observed. The 12 remaining brains had neurofibrillary tangles only to the extent that is sometimes encountered among non-Chamorro—apparently non-neurological cases.

Brains from five of the control patients and four ALS patients were studied by Nakai (1969). The controls were a 42-year-old man who died of a myocardial infarct, a 62-year-old woman who died of amoebic dysentery, a 69-year-old woman who died of cardiovascular disease, a 69-year-old woman who died of cor pulmonale, and a 75-year-old man who died of cancer of the lung. Nakai's results agreed closely with Hirano and his colleagues (1966). Neurofibrillary changes were observed in subcortical areas of all ALS patients. Among the five controls, no neurofibrillary tangles were observed in one (the 42-year-old man). Of the four remaining cases, the numbers of neurofibrillary tangles in three were seemingly insignificant. In two of these the tangles were limited to the hippocampal gyrus in small numbers. In the third (the 69-year-old woman who died of cor pulmonale) only small numbers of these changes in the cortex and subcortical regions were seen. The final control brain (the 75-year-old man) had relatively numerous neurofibrillary tangles in the hippocampus and hippocampal gyrus, but only a small number in other areas.

Material from the brain in six control cases was studied by Richardson, and by Sangalang, at the Massachusetts General Hospital (cited by Brody, Hirano, and Scott, 1971). In a man aged 35 who died of internal injuries as a result of trauma sustained in a fall from a tractor, neurofibrillary changes were abundantly present in the frontal and sensorimoror cortex, hippocampus, basal ganglia, amygdaloid nucleus, and brain stem (locus caeruleus and median raphe of pons). A second patient was a 39-year-old man who had had myotonia dystrophica and who was a member of a large family with this disease on Guam, which was previously reported (Chen, Brody, and Kurland, 1968; Plato, Reed, Elizan, and Kurland, 1967). He died of gastro-intestinal haemorrhage. The brain was of atrophic appearance (weight 1055 g), and neurofibrillary change was observed in many nerve cells in the cerebral cortex (especially in the hippocampus, where additional cells contained granulovacuolar degeneration), thalamus, putamen, globus pallidus, substantia innominata, substantia nigra, oculomotor nucleus, and locus caeruleus. Loss of neurones was evident in the hippocampus, but was much less pronounced, if present at all, in other structures including the substantia nigra. Representative sections of the spinal cord and of several spinal nerve roots were available in this case; evidence of ALS or other abnormalities was not encountered.

In three cases, there were nerve cells with neurofibrillary changes restricted to the hippocampal region. In these cases, the distribution of the changes and their severity were such as are frequently seen in patients of advanced age in a random hospital population, with or without clinical evidence of dementia. The patients autopsied were a 72-year-old woman, a 49-year-old man, and a 58-year-old man who died of uterine carcinoma, congestive heart failure, and coronary heart disease, respectively. In one case, that of a 41-year-old man who committed suicide, neuropathological changes were absent in the brain. These important findings in control brains do not coincide with those of Hirano and his colleagues (Hirano *et al.*, 1966; Hirano, Malamud, Kurland, and Zimmerman, 1969) and Nakai (1969), and a much larger series is under investigation to clarify this matter (Brody, Hirano, and Scott, 1971).

TRENDS

The incidence rate for ALS in the United States and Canada is approximately 0·8 per 100 000 per year. Since data on Guam concerning deaths are more accurate than onset, we have calculated incidence in terms of

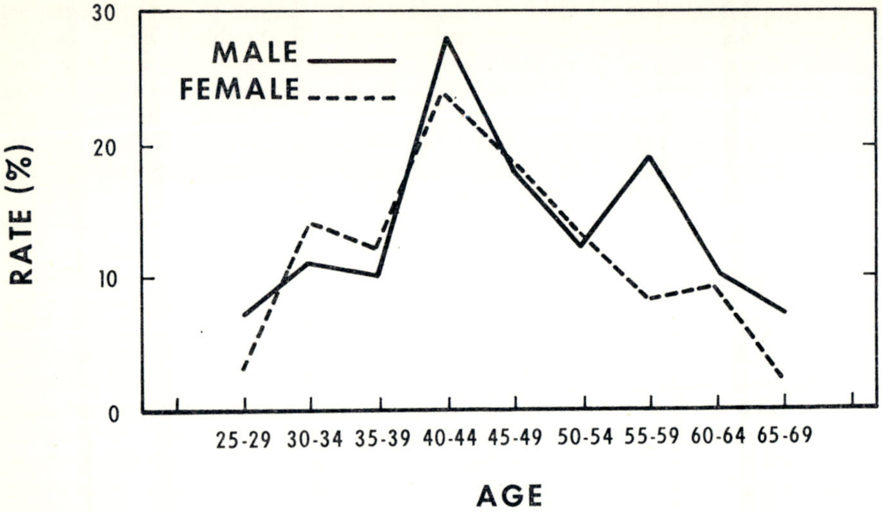

FIG. 28.7. ALS deaths/all deaths by age and sex.

deaths per year, which is valid for a fatal disease of short duration where observations were conducted over a long period of time. For the years 1950 to 1969 the incidence per 100 000 on Guam was 35. This is a minimal figure for comparison of ratios because in Guam (as in other developing areas) the percentage of people under age 20 is relatively higher than in the United States and Canada, and these people are not at risk of dying of ALS.

The true impact of ALS and PD on Guam can perhaps be better illustrated in terms of total deaths. In the United States it is estimated that there are between one and two deaths caused by ALS for each 1000 adult deaths (over age 20). Since 1950, 14 per cent of adult male deaths on Guam and 11 per cent of adult female deaths were caused by ALS; since 1960, 13 per cent of all male deaths and 8 per cent of all female deaths have been caused by PD. In FIGURES 28.7 and 28.8 are presented deaths from ALS and PD and total deaths from all causes by age. It is noteworthy that ALS caused about one-third of all deaths among people aged 40 to 45, and that approximately one-fifth of all deaths among males aged 50 to 59 were caused by PD.

A 'population explosion' on Guam has been taking place since 1930 (Brody and Chen, 1969). From the years 1895 to 1920, during which almost all of our patients were born, the Guam population increased slowly. To detect shifts in incidence of ALS on Guam, we compared the age-specific death rates for the 10-year periods 1950–59, and 1960–69 [FIGS. 28.9 and

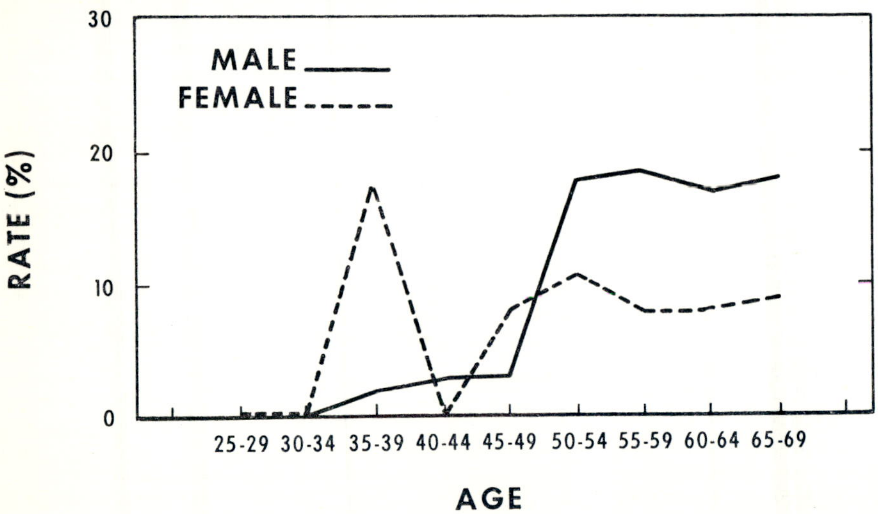

FIG. 28.8. PD deaths/all deaths by age and sex.

28.10]. The shapes of the curves for ALS among men in the two 10-year periods were surprisingly similar, with rates for all those over age 25 of 191 per 100 000 in 1950–59, and of 134 per 100 000 in 1960–69. Among women there were fewer cases and the age-specific death rate curves were less superimposable. The rates per 100 000 for the two 10-year periods were 74 and 58 (FIGURE 28.2 is a composite of these two curves, and by increasing the numbers the variations in age-groups tend to smooth out).

Thus, although a downward trend was observed in rates for ALS between 1950–59 and 1960–69, the disease persisted at a high rate. Perhaps more important was that the age-specific death rates and the ratio of ALS deaths to deaths from all causes did not change. This is evidence that we were not observing a cohort phenomenon which would have resulted from a massive early exposure or traditional but now abandoned custom or practice, because the ratio of younger cases in recent years was the same as it was in former years.

The onset of PD is vague with gradual slowing of body movements and mental processes. As mentioned earlier, the disease was not a well-recognized entity among Guamanians and could easily be mistaken for ageing. This, plus the shorter period of observation, makes it difficult for us to delineate trends for PD.

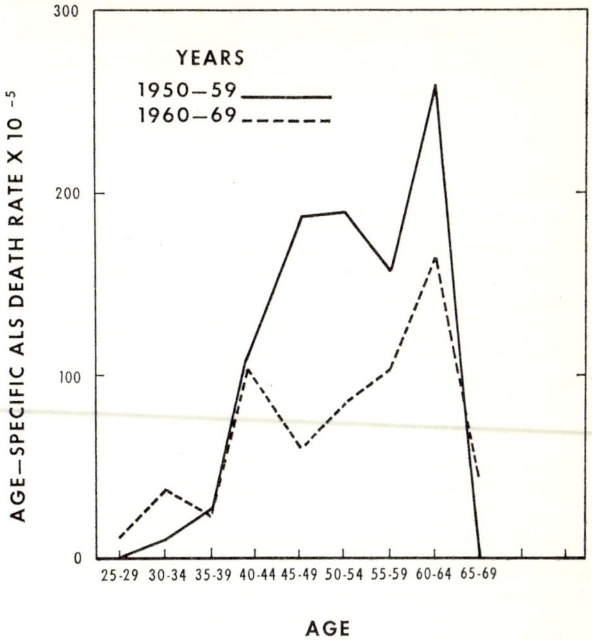

FIG. 28.10. Age-specific ALS death rate $\times 10^{-5}$—female: 1950–59 and 1960–69.

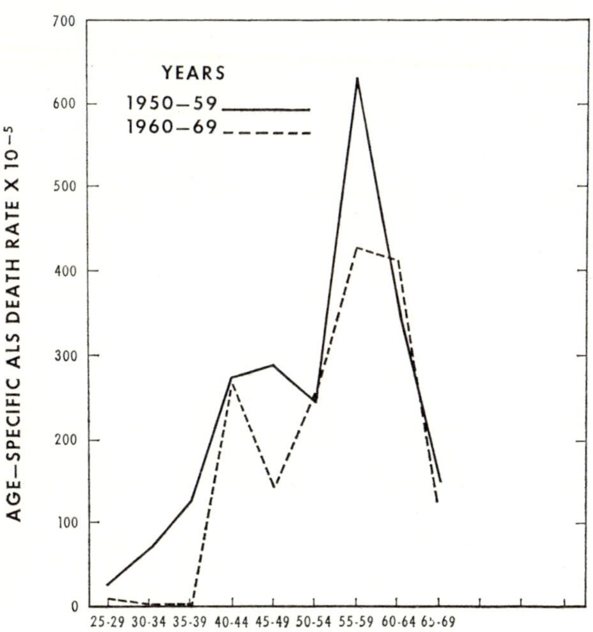

FIG. 28.9. Age-specific ALS death rate $\times 10^{-5}$—male: 1950–59 and 1960–69.

GENETICS

The role of heredity in the cause of ALS or PD remains unclear (Brody and Chen, 1969; Brody, Hirano, and Scott, 1971; Plato, Reed, Elizan, and Kurland, 1967; Plato, Cruz, and Kurland, 1969), nor were investigations of blood groupings particularly helpful (Brody and Chen, 1969; Plato and Cruz, 1967). ALS and PD tended to occur in familial clusters, but no definite pattern of inheritance was detected. Familial clustering could be an indication either of common exposure or of genetic transmission. The ALS on Guam does not resemble familial ALS seen elsewhere, but more closely resembles the sporadic cases both clinically and in terms of age of onset and duration of survival (Kurland, 1966). The male to female ratio is approximately 2 : 1, which is true for sporadic ALS seen elsewhere, but not true for familial ALS in which the male to female ratio is 1 : 1, as is encountered in most diseases transmitted as autosomal dominant traits.

It is difficult to conceive of ALS or PD being recessive traits, since we know of 11 patients in whom one parent was not Guamanian [TABLE 28.2]. If the diseases were dominant and our pedigree studies accurate, the penetrance was no higher than 20 per cent. We are now following the offspring of the first 100 patients with ALS and 100 patients with PD who have died on Guam since 1948. The bulk of the offspring are still too young for complete analysis, but in the course of the next 5 to

10 years they will be in the susceptible age-groups. In addition, we have seven instances in which two parents were affected. We are carefully following their offspring for appearance of the disease.

INFECTION

Onset of ALS or PD is not preceded by febrile illness, and a history of illness compatible with von Economo's disease was not encountered (Elizan *et al.*, 1966 *b*). Nor were disease patterns in the early life of patients different from those of Guamanian controls (Reed, Plato, Elizan, and Kurland, 1966). Since 1963, in collaboration with Drs. D. Carleton Gajdusek and Clarence J. Gibbs, Jr., of the Laboratory of Slow, Latent and Temperate Virus Infections, NINDS, we have been exploring the possibility that ALS and PD may be slow virus infections (Gajdusek and Gibbs, 1964). Material from 22 Guamanian patients has been inoculated into chimpanzees, several species of smaller subhuman primates and a wide variety of other laboratory mammalian and avian hosts. Among the chimpanzees inoculated, one has been under observation for more than 8 years and four others have been observed for more than 5 years. In no animals inoculated has neurological disease developed (Gibbs and Gajdusek, 1969 *a* and *b*). Studies using fresh unfrozen trypsinized brain material in tissue culture and lymphocyte transformation studies are also in progress, but as yet evidence of infection has not been encountered (Brody, Hirano, and Scott, 1971).

TOXINS AND OTHER ENVIRONMENTAL EXPOSURES

Most of our investigations concerning toxins have concentrated on manganese and the ingestion of the nut of cycads (Kurland, 1966). Manganese is present in high concentrations in the soil and drinking-water on Guam (Yase *et al.*, 1968). The levels are higher, however, in many areas of the world where elevated rates of ALS and PD are not encountered.

Various surveys on Guam have not revealed a food habit or other environmental exposure among patients which distinguishes them from 'controls'. This statement also applies to *Cycas circinalis* (cycad), which has been an important source of carbohydrate on the island perhaps for centuries, and was consumed heavily during the years of the Second World War and is still consumed, particularly in some of the rural households on the island. The unusual toxic features of the cycad have led to continued efforts to identify a constituent which might be of aetiological importance in the ALS and PD occurring on Guam. The observations which led to a search for such a toxic agent include a high prevalence of neurological diseases, the collagen changes which were noted in the skin of many such patients (Fullmer, Diedler, Krooth, and Kurland, 1960), and the increased presence of multiple exostoses among the Chamorro population (Krooth, Macklin, and Hilbish, 1961).

Thus, initially, some food with lathyrogenic properties was sought. In its natural form cycad is said to contain a small quantity of α-amino-β-methylamino-propionic acid which may have lathyrogenic qualities (Vega and Bell, 1967). Although neurological effects from this amino acid were noted in animals, there has been no accompanying description of neuropathological lesions (Polsky, Nunn, and Bell, 1972).

Cycad also contains a remarkable water-soluble hepatotoxic and carcinogenic agent, the aglycone of cycasin, which can be removed by thorough elution; it was the process of repeated washings, perhaps discovered centuries ago, which enabled the Chamorros to utilize this plant which grows so abundantly on the island. Several species of animals have been tested with this aglycone or methylazoxymethanol (MAM), which has some chemical similarities to the potent carcinogen dimethylnitrosoamine (*Federation Proceedings*, 1964). In large enough quantities the MAM causes hepatic necrosis and rapid death; in small quantities it produces cirrhosis; and in minute quantities it has produced hepatic, renal, intestinal, brain and other tumours after a latent period of a year or more (Laqueur, Mickelson, Whiting, and Kurland, 1963; Spatz and Laqueur, 1967; Hirono and Shibuya, 1967; Hall and McGavin, 1968).

The efforts to identify a neurotoxic agent were initially stimulated by the report that cattle in Australia and Santo Domingo fed on cycad plants developed some disturbances of gait; but the only neurological lesions noted were some changes with Marchi's stain which were thought to represent demyelination of the posterior and lateral columns of the spinal cord (Hall and McGavin, 1968; Mason and Whiting, 1966).

After several years of negative reports, the interest in the possible neurotoxic action of MAM was renewed as a result of the reports by Hirono and his colleagues (Hirono and Shibuya, 1967; Hirono, Shibuya, and Hayashi, 1969), that newborn mice and hamsters which received cycasin developed extensive necrosis of the cells of the external granular layers of the cerebellum, resulting in ataxia and other gait disturbances. Subsequently, microcephaly following antenatal administration of MAM was described (Spatz and Laqueur, 1968). In other reports (Jones, Yang, and Mickelsen, 1972; Sanger, Yang, and Mickelsen, 1972) it was noted that MAM induced cerebellar abnormalities in several other species including the dog. Hirano and Jones (1972) noted that the ultrastructural changes in the cerebellar lesions were similar to those of some viral and genetic disorders affecting the cerebellum. Hirono (1972) has also recently noted that extensive necrosis occurred in the neuroblastic layer of the retina of newborn mice and rats within 3 days of their receiving cycasin subcutaneously. Thus, MAM has neurotoxic properties but relationship to ALS and PD is still only conjectural.

Further, the experimental work cited cannot be considered sufficient to support any action with regard to the use of cycad as a food on Guam, since no toxic effect has been observed in feeding adult animals experimentally with a few samples of prepared cycad flour.

During recent years there has been a modest decline in the rates of ALS on Guam but no cohort phenomenon has been encountered. Following the Second World War the flour, which is prepared from cycad for tortillas and soups, has been used less extensively as the Guamanians' economy and food habits have become increasingly westernized (Reed, Labarthe, and Stallones, 1970). Since the use of cycad has been so widespread, one would not expect a difference between patients and controls on the question of whether they had *ever* eaten cycad and indeed no difference was found in earlier studies. However, if cycad ingested throughout the life-span of Guamanians is a causative factor of ALS and PD, there is probably a long latent period from ingestion to the beginning of symptoms; thus, reduction in its use would not be expected to result in a sudden decrease in the current incidence rates of ALS and PD. Furthermore, the failure to observe any corresponding effect on animals could be associated with the variations in response by different species and at different ages, and a possible variation in inherent detoxification mechanisms.

Cycads are also used as food in a number of other tropical and subtropical regions including Kerala, South India, and Okinawa, but to date the cycad of Guam has the highest concentration of cycasin among the cycads studied. In addition, the procedure of slicing the seed in half before soaking seems peculiar to the Chamorros; this could result in more residual cycasin than the method of pounding the seed into fine particles or meal before washing, as is the custom elsewhere.

Since there are so many variables such as seed selection, the extent of soaking, individual taste preferences, and even the use by some people of fresh cycad as a poultice for skin ulcers—and since all these could affect the quantity to which different Chamorros were exposed—it is difficult to estimate the extent of exposure to cycasin in different segments of the population of Guam. There is a familial concentration of ALS on Guam—although not to the extent of explaining the disease as a simple Mendelian trait. The possibility remains, therefore, that cycad or some other environmental exposure occurring in some families may be of aetiological importance.

STUDIES OF AMINE METABOLISM

The major catabolites of dopamine, homovanillic acid (HVA), and of serotonin, 5-hydroxyindoleacetic acid (HIAA), were consistently depressed in the spinal fluid of Guamanians with PD. HVA and HIAA levels in these patients were remarkably similar to those found in Americans with idiopathic parkinsonism (Brody, Chase, and Gordon, 1970). It is possible that the depressed cerebrospinal fluid levels of HVA and HIAA found in Guamanian patients with PD reflect a reduction in central dopamine and serotonin turnover in this disorder.

In the spinal fluid of ALS patients, HVA and HIAA levels were significantly lower than among Guamanian controls but higher than those of PD patients. Similar low levels were also found among ALS patients in the United States. This lowered level of HVA in ALS patients on Guam and in the United States is difficult to interpret, since this disorder is not known to involve dopamine-containing neuronal systems in the basal ganglia.

It was noteworthy that in one-third of Guamanians without evidence of ALS or PD, levels of HVA in the spinal fluid were markedly depressed. While this could have been an artefact, the possibility that what we were measuring represents incipient disease must be considered.

Low levels of HVA and HIAA could result from decreased synthesis of dopamine and serotonin in the central nervous system or increased utilization of these neurotransmitters. To resolve this question we administered probenecid to PD and ALS patients and controls and measured the accumulation of HVA and HIAA in the spinal fluid (Chase, Schnur, Brody, and Gordon, 1971). Probenecid prevents the absorption of HVA and HIAA from the spinal fluid. Thus, if the accumulated levels were depressed it would indicate lowered synthesis, while if they were elavated it would indicate increased utilization. In PD patients virtually no HVA was produced, while HIAA levels increased, suggesting that CNS dopamine production was compromised. HVA levels among ALS patients were intermediate between PD patients and controls. Similar findings were observed in ALS patients in the United States (Mendell, Chase, and Engel, 1971). Thus, again we encountered the puzzling observation that in ALS dopamine production in the CNS is diminished.

THERAPEUTIC TRIALS WITH L-DOPA

As a result of the above findings, eight PD patients were treated with L-DOPA using dosage schedules similar to those used for Parkinson's disease (Schnur, Chase, and Brody, 1971). Initial improvement in extrapyramidal function occurred in all patients. Although some degree of increased awareness was observed the dementia did not remit. Beneficial results were not maintained in two patients, possibly due to their inability to tolerate adequate L-DOPA dose levels, or due to the rapid progression of their illness. Specific beneficial effects of L-DOPA against rigidity and possibly against tremor were similar to those observed in patients with Parkinson's disease. Bradykinesia, on the other hand, appeared less amenable to modification by L-DOPA treatment. L-DOPA increased HVA levels in the spinal fluid in direct proportion to the dose administered. There was, however, no apparent correlation between L-DOPA-induced rise in HVA and the clinical responsivity to L-DOPA. Nor were pretreatment HVA levels or initial severity of parkinsonism signs useful in predicting clinical response to L-DOPA.

None of our patients became free of extrapyramidal signs during L-DOPA treatment. After 1 year of therapy there was some evidence of progression of the pathological condition. The long-term influence of L-DOPA on the relentlessly progressive and invariably fatal course of PD remains to be seen.

Seven ALS patients have been under treatment with L-DOPA for 2 months. After this short time it is not possible to evaluate the effects of therapy on the disease.

GUAMANIANS IN THE CONTINENTAL UNITED STATES

There are approximately 40 000 Chamorros living on Guam. Since Guam is a territory of the United States, Guamanians are United States citizens and enter the mainland without any immigration procedures in a manner analogous to residents of Puerto Rico. It is impossible, therefore, to know exactly the number and distribution of Guamanians currently living elsewhere in the United States; a reasonable estimate is that between 5000 and 10 000 reside outside Guam and that a large proportion of these are young adults and their children. Many reside in California in the areas around San Diego, Los Angeles, and San Francisco (Brody, Hirano, and Scott, 1971). Three population studies have been conducted in California (Torres, Iriarte, and Kurland, 1957; Eldridge, Ryan, Rosario, and Brody, 1969; Labarthe, Reed, Siedler, and Stallones, 1973). During the initial study only ALS patients were sought. The subsequent investigations included both ALS and PD. The individuals studied were all born in Guam and had lived in California for varying lengths of time. The major Guamanian migration has been since the Second World War, so those who were born in this country were not yet old enough to be at risk for developing ALS or PD. All three studies indicated that ALS occurs at least as frequently in California as on Guam. This suggests that hereditary factors or early environmental exposure could be responsible for this disease.

We were most impressed that in the recent California surveys we encountered only one patient with PD in whom certain atypical features were observed [see below]. Further, a review of all adult Chamorro deaths in California from 1955 to 1964 did not indicate the occurrence of PD. There were 81 adult Guamanian deaths and none had reference to parkinsonism or to the various categories which would include the severe dementias, and none of the individuals died in mental institutions. During the similar period on Guam, 1 in 10 adult deaths was from PD with the mean age at death between 55 and 60. PD is a severe progressive disease leading to death in less than 5 years in 70 per cent of the patients. The age distribution of the surveyed populations and the 81 deceased Guamanians was roughly comparable to that on Guam and, if anything, included a higher rate of individuals in the age-groups susceptible to PD. It is probable, therefore, that among Guamanians in California this disease occurred at a rate lower than that on Guam, although the limitations of survey techniques and the relative unfamiliarity of Californian physicians with this disease must be considered (Brody, Hirano, and Scott, 1971).

In one of the California surveys, two Chamorro patients with possible PD were encountered (Eldridge, Ryan, Rosario, and Brody, 1969). These patients subsequently died and autopsies were performed. The first patient lived off Guam for about 50 years except for a single 3-week visit to the island. He died at the age of 74 after a 4-year history of dementia and with parkinsonian features consisting primarily of fine pill-rolling tremor and rigidity. While these were not the typical signs of extrapyramidal involvement on Guam, this picture has been documented on the island on several occasions (Elizan *et al.*, 1966*b*). On neuropathological examination, the brain contained alterations characteristic of the PD complex as seen among the Chamorros on Guam (Brody, Hirano, and Scott, 1971). The brain was atrophic, and abundant neurofibrillary tangles were found in the characteristic distribution. No senile plaques were seen. The substantia nigra was a site of particularly severe cell loss where both frequent neurofibrillary tangles and associated, but rare, Lewy bodies were observed. Of a total of 156 PD patients we have followed to death, this man is one of five with onset over age 70 and the second oldest at time of death.

The second patient migrated to California in 1954 at age 46. After 6 years' residence in California, he developed bradykinesia and died 9 years later, at age 61, of pneumonia and other complications. At no time was he demented. Autopsy findings included rather numerous neurofibrillary changes (unassociated with senile plaques) in the cortex, hypothalamus and amygdaloid nucleus of this patient, but these changes were not observed in the brain stem. Other neuropathological findings were present but were not those encountered on Guam (Brody, Hirano, and Scott, 1971). His brain was of normal weight, and there were no neurofibrillary changes or marked neuronal loss in the substantia nigra. Instead the findings were more characteristic of those encountered in idiopathic Parkinson's disease, with Lewy bodies in classical distribution and some degree of nerve cell loss in the basal ganglia. Although we cannot ignore the neurofibrillary tangles which were present, the evidence suggests that he was suffering from idiopathic Parkinson's disease rather than the PD of Guam. If true, this finding is of considerable importance, since this would be the first documented Guamanian patient with idiopathic Parkinson's disease (Brody, Hirano, and Scott, 1971; Chen, Brody, and

Kurland, 1968). Several non-Guamanian patients with idiopathic Parkinson's disease were observed on Guam, and in at least one of these patients the clinical impression was supported by neuropathological findings (Hirano *et al.*, 1966) [see above].

OTHER NEUROLOGICAL DISEASES ON GUAM

During the years of study there was a high incidence of several genetic diseases on Guam including myotonic dystrophy, peroneal muscular atrophy, and the hereditary ataxias (Chen, Brody, and Kurland, 1968; Chen, Brody, Kurland, and Elizan, 1970). Whether hereditary diseases of the nervous system occur more frequently than would be expected in this type of population is not clear. It is tempting to relate these syndromes to amyotrophic lateral sclerosis or parkinsonism-dementia, but there is no clear evidence of this from our data.

Slightly higher rates of convulsive disorders than expected were found. We have not encountered multiple sclerosis, but the island is in the tropical belt where this illness has rarely been observed. Myasthenia gravis and progressive muscular dystrophy were not seen. These conditions are rare and their failure to appear in a population of less than 40 000 could be chance variation. Of great interest was the absence of classic paralysis agitans among the Chamorros of Guam. In one sibship of 13, four have died of different brain tumours and two have died of acute myelogenous leukaemia.

STUDIES IN OTHER PACIFIC POPULATIONS

It has been the impression among personnel assigned to the NINDS Research Center in Guam that over the years they have seen an unusually large number of ALS patients among Filipinos (Brody and Chen, 1969; Brody, Hirano, and Scott, 1971). This observation was difficult to confirm because the majority of Filipinos on Guam were not permanent residents, but were labourers hired on short-term contracts from the Philippines. The majority were men in the age bracket which is most susceptible to ALS. One Filipino man who was born in Ilocos Del Norte, Philippines, in 1911, developed ALS with no evidence of dementia or extrapyramidal signs. At autopsy neuropathological findings of classical ALS were encountered. In addition, however, neurofibrillary changes were demonstrated in a distribution essentially the same as that seen in Guamanian ALS patients. Involvement was mild, but definite. Autopsies were not performed on other Filipino ALS patients on Guam. Brains from two Filipino ALS patients, one dying in Manila and the other in California, did not contain neurofibrillary changes (Brody, Hirano, and Scott, 1971). Recently, in a survey of deaths from ALS in Hawaii, an apparent excess of this disease was encountered among Filipinos (Matsumoto, Worth, Kurland, and Okazaki, 1972). A focus of ALS has also been reported in the Kii Peninsula of Japan (Araki, Kimura, and Yase, 1966; Kimura, 1965). Japanese investigators (Nakai, 1969; Shiraki, 1969; Yase *et al.*, 1968) have noted neurofibrillary tangles in these patients in a distribution similar to that encountered among Chamorro patients. In ALS cases from other areas of Japan, neurofibrillary changes have not been described (Shiraki, 1969).

Neurofibrillary changes in characteristic distribution were not observed in three United States veterans who served on Guam during the Second World War and subsequently died of ALS (Brody, Hirano, and Scott, 1971). Further, a preliminary analysis of 12 000 white construction workers who worked on Guam for at least 1 year between 1945 and 1955 has not revealed an unusual incidence of ALS (Brody, Hirano, and Scott, 1971).

The full clinical and neuropathological appearances of PD have been documented only among the Chamorro-speaking population of Guam and the other Mariana Islands, and in the one case referred to above in California. Numerous surveys of the other islands of Micronesia have failed to uncover foci of ALS except among these people of Guam and the Mariana Islands. A small focus of motor neurone disease among Carolinian residents of Saipan has been followed by members of the NINDS Research Center since 1958 (Elizan *et al.*, 1966 *a*). In this population of less than 2000, six male patients have been observed. There have been no new cases since 1960. Spastic paraplegia was the dominant manifestation. The symptoms progressed slowly, if at all, and only two patients have died. An autopsy was performed on one patient in 1959, but most of the material was not available for study. A few slides were reviewed by Hirano *et al.* (1966) who stated that 'no definite diagnosis of ALS-PD could be made', but 'changes compatible with ALS and neurofibrillary changes in the brain stem were seen in this case'.

DISCUSSION AND CONCLUSIONS

Amyotrophic lateral sclerosis continues to occur approximately 50 times more frequently among the Chamorro-speaking population of Guam than in the United States. A second progressive fatal neurological disease, presumably a clinical variant of ALS referred to as parkinsonism-dementia (PD), occurs at a similar high rate on Guam and these diseases account for 20 per cent of deaths among Guamanians over age 20.

Clinically, Guamanian ALS resembles idiopathic ALS seen in other areas of the world. The mean age at onset and mean survival time and the excess of male patients over female patients are compatible with most other series of this disease (Kurland, Choi, and Sayre, 1969). On Guam, however, we tend to see more patients under age 40 and more patients who survive 10 or more years than elsewhere. These discrepancies can be explained in part on the basis that we are observing the full natural history of the disease by following an entire population rather than the selected population which is seen in referral centres. The differences, however, particulary in duration of survival after onset, may be real.

At the time of writing, PD appears to be a unique disease among the Chamorro-speaking people. We have observed the clinical and neuropathological syndrome only in Guam and the Marianas and in one instance in a Guamanian in California.

The finding of two major neurological diseases, occurring at extraordinarily high rates in a single small population, suggests that these diseases are related. The nature of this relationship remains conjectural since the aetiologies of ALS and PD remain unknown, and no clear genetic pattern has been discerned. The occurrence of the two diseases in the same population and the clinical and neuropathological overlap have suggested to some investigators that ALS and PD are manifestations of a broad spectrum of responses to a single aetiological entity (Elizan *et al.*, 1966*b*; Hirano *et al.*, 1966; Kurland, Choi, and Sayre, 1969). Others have interpreted these findings differently, either suggesting that the diseases are not closely related (Mulder and Espinosa, 1969), or that a genetic or environmental factor increases the susceptibility to the separate causes of these diseases, or that one disease predisposes to the other in the relationship analogous to that between herpes zoster and Hodgkin's disease, or staphylococcus and diabetes (Brody and Chen, 1969; Brody, Hirano, and Scott, 1971).

A decline in the overall rate of ALS on Guam has been observed during the past 20 years. The age-specific attack rates and the age-specific ratio of ALS deaths to deaths from all causes have not changed, however, for both men and women. This is in marked contrast to the trend observed for kuru in New Guinea, where marked shifts in attack rates for men and women in different age-groups were noted, accompanying a decline in overall attack rates (Alpers, 1970). It would appear, therefore, that the factors causing ALS on Guam are still affecting the entire susceptible age range for ALS. This probably means that the aetiological factors are still present on Guam. An alternative explanation, however, would be that an exposure early in life with a variable incubation period was involved, and that in the future we will see lower age-specific attack rates in younger age-groups. This modal has been suggested for multiple sclerosis and for classical Parkinson's disease (Poskanzer, 1968; Alter, Antonovsky, and Leibowitz, 1968; Kurtzke, Dean, and Botha, 1970; Poskanzer and Schwab, 1963).

It is difficult to detect trends for PD since we have reservations concerning the completeness of ascertainment of our case-finding, and our observations were essentially limited to one 10-year period.

Perhaps the most hopeful and significant recent finding in our Guam studies was the demonstration of depressed CNS dopamine synthesis in our cases. CNS dopamine level as measured by a major catabolite, homovanillic acid (HVA) in the spinal fluid, was markedly depressed in PD patients, at a level similar to that encountered in classical paralysis agitans. HVA levels were also significantly depressed in ALS patients as compared to Guamanian controls, although the levels were higher than those encountered in PD patients. This observation led us to the finding that CNS dopamine levels are also depressed in ALS patients in the continental United States. The implication of this observation among ALS patients is not clear, since up to the present time it was not generally thought that dopaminergic areas were involved in motor neurone disease.

Investigations of the possible aetiological role of slow viruses and other infections, and exposure to toxic products such as manganese and cycad, which have been underway for many years, have thus far failed to shed light on the cause of ALS and PD. We have accumulating evidence that exposure to the Guam environment for non-Chamorros does not result in a higher incidence of ALS or PD. In one Filipino patient, however, who died of ALS on Guam, occasional neurofibrillary tangles were observed in areas of the brain similar to those changes which were observed in Guam ALS patients. These changes have also been observed rarely among Guamanians who did not have evidence of ALS or PD at the time of death.

As a result of the observation of altered dopamine metabolism, L-DOPA was administered to PD patients with improvement in extrapyramidal function. The effect on the dementia and the natural history of this progressive disease cannot yet be evaluated. In addition, we have started ALS patients on Guam on L-DOPA, but the period of observation is still too short to evaluate the effects of treatment. Hopefully, with the observation of a metabolic abnormality among our cases, we can broaden our studies to detect possible genetic or geographical patterns of altered monoamine metabolism among residents of Guam.

On Guam, and perhaps nowhere else in the world, diseases of the motor and extrapyramidal systems and organic dementia occur with such high frequency as to be a major public health problem. Yet similar illnesses occur throughout the world and cause immense suffering and loss. Several promising leads have emerged as a result of our studies. We are optimistic that by continued investigations within the environment where the diseases occur we greatly increase the likelihood of true insight and understanding of this phenomenon. Such knowledge would not only be of vast benefit to the people of Guam but obviously have important applications in the understanding of neurological diseases throughout the world.

References

ALPERS, M. P. (1970) III. Kuru in New Guinea: its changing pattern and etiologic elucidation, *Amer. J. trop. Med. Hyg.*, **19**, 133–7.

ALTER, M., ANTONOVSKY, A., and LEIBOWITZ, U. (1968) Epidemiology of multiple sclerosis in Israel, in *The Epidemiology of Multiple Sclerosis*, eds. Alter, M., and Kurtzke, J. F., Springfield, Ill., pp. 83–106.

ARAKI, M., KIMURA, K., and YASE, Y. (1966) A histopathological study on amyotrophic lateral sclerosis in the Kii Peninsula, in *Proceedings of the Fifth International Congress of Neuropathology, Amsterdam*, eds. Luthy, F., and Bischoff, A. Excerpta Medica International Congress Series No. 100, Amsterdam, pp. 219–21.

ARNOLD, A., EDGREN, D. C., and PALLADINO, V. S. (1953) Amyotrophic lateral sclerosis: fifty cases observed on Guam, *J. nerv. ment. Dis.*, **117**, 135–9.

BRODY, J. A., CHASE, T. N., and GORDON, E. K. (1970) Depressed monoamine catabolite levels in cerebrospinal fluid of patients with parkinsonism dementia of Guam, *New Engl. J. Med.*, 282, 947–50.

BRODY, J. A., and CHEN, K. M. (1969) Changing epidemiologic patterns of amyotrophic lateral sclerosis and parkinsonism-dementia on Guam, in *Motor Neuron Diseases: Research on Amyotrophic Lateral Sclerosis and Related Disorders*, Vol. 2., eds. Norris, F. H., Jr., and Kurland, L. T., New York, pp. 61–79.

BRODY, J. A., HIRANO, A., and SCOTT, R. M. (1971) Recent neuropathologic observations in amyotrophic lateral sclerosis and parkinsonism-dementia of Guam, *Neurology, (Minneap.)*, **21**, 528–36.

CHARCOT, J. M., and JOFFRAY, A. (1869) Deux d'atrophie musculaire progressive avec lesions de la substance grise and des faisceaux anterolateraux de la moelle épinière, *Arch. physiol. norm. Path.*, 2, 354, 629, 744.

CHASE, T. N., SCHNUR, J. A., BRODY, J. A., and GORDON, E. K. (1971) Parkinsonism-dementia and amyotrophic lateral sclerosis of Guam: effect of probenecid on monoamine catabolite levels in cerebrospinal fluid, *Arch. Neurol. (Chic.)*, **25**, 9–13.

CHEN, K. M., ABRAMS, B. M., and BRODY, J. A. (1968) Serial EEGs of patients with parkinsonism-dementia syndrome of Guam, *Electroenceph. clin. Neurophysiol.*, **25**, 380–5.

CHEN, K. M., BRODY, J. A., and KURLAND, L. T. (1968) Patterns of neurologic diseases on Guam, I. Epidemiologic aspects, *Arch. Neurol. (Chic.)*, **19**, 573–8.

CHEN, K. M., BRODY, J. A., KURLAND, L. T., and ELIZAN, T. S. (1970) Clinical and genetic patterns of neurological diseases other than amyotrophic lateral sclerosis on Guam, *Neurology (Minneap.)*, **20**, 954–64.

CUTLER, S. J., and EDERER, F. (1958) Maximum utilization of the life table method in analyzing survival, *J. chron. Dis.*, 8, No. 6, 699–712.

ELDRIDGE, R., RYAN, E., ROSARIO, J., and BRODY, J. A. (1969) Amyotrophic lateral sclerosis and parkinsonism dementia in a migrant population from Guam, *Neurology (Minneap.)*, **19**, 1029–37.

ELIZAN, T. S., CHEN, K. M., MATHAI, K. V., DUNN, D., and KURLAND, L. T. (1966 *a*) Amyotrophic lateral sclerosis and parkinsonism-dementia complex: a study in non-Chamorros of the Mariana and Caroline Islands, *Arch. Neurol. (Chic.)*, **14**, 347–55.

ELIZAN, T. S., HIRANO, A., ABRAMS, B. M., NEED, R. L., VAN NUIS, C., and KURLAND, L. T. (1966 *b*) Amyotrophic lateral sclerosis and parkinsonism-dementia complex of Guam: neurological reevaluation, *Arch. Neurol. (Chic.)*, **14**, 356–68.

FEDERATION PROCEEDINGS (1964) Proceedings of the Third Conference on the Toxicity of Cycads, *Fed. Proc.*, **23**, 1337.

FULLMER, H. M., DIEDLER, H. D., KROOTH, R. S., and KURLAND, L. T. (1960) A cutaneous disorder of connective tissue in amyotrophic lateral sclerosis, *Neurology (Minneap.)*, **10**, 717.

GAJDUSEK, D. C., and GIBBS, C. J., JR. (1964) Attempts to demonstrate a transmissible agent in kuru, amyotrophic lateral sclerosis, and other sub-acute and chronic nervous system degenerations of man, *Nature (Lond.)*, **204**, 257–9.

GIBBS, C. J., JR., and GAJDUSEK, D. C. (1969 *a*) Kuru—a prototype subacute infectious disease of the nervous system as a model for the study of amyotrophic lateral sclerosis, in *Motor Neuron Diseases: Research on Amyotrophic Lateral Sclerosis and Related Disorders*, Vol. 2, eds. Norris, F. H., Jr., and Kurland, L. T., New York, pp. 269–279.

GIBBS, C. J., JR., and GAJDUSEK, D. C. (1969 *b*) Attempts to transmit subacute and chronic neurological disease to animals, with a progress report on the experimental transmission of kuru to chimpanzees, *Int. Arch. Allergy*, **36**, 539–71.

HALL, W. T. K., and MCGAVIN, M. D. (1968) Clinical and neuropathological changes in cattle eating the leaves of *Macrozamia lucida* or *Bowenia serrulata* (family Zamiaceae), *Path. Vet.*, 5, 26.

HIRANO, A. (1965) Pathology of amyotrophic lateral sclerosis, in *Slow, Latent and Temperate Virus Infections*, NINDB Monograph No. 2, eds. Gajdusek, D. C., and Gibbs, C. J., Jr., United States Department of Health Education and Welfare, Public Health Service, National Institutes of Health, Public Health Service Publication No. 1378, Washington, D.C., pp. 23–7.

HIRANO, A. (1966) Neuropathology of amyotrophic lateral sclerosis and parkinsonism-dementia complex on Guam, in *Proceedings of the Fifth International Congress of Neuropathology, Amsterdam*, eds. Luthy, F., and Bischoff, A., Excerpta Medica International Congress Series No. 100, Amsterdam, pp. 190–4.

HIRANO, A., and JONES, M. (1972) Fine structure of cycasin-induced cerebellar alterations, *Fed. Proc.*, **31**, 1517–19.

HIRANO, A., KURLAND, L. T., KROOTH, R. S., and LESSELL, S. (1961) Parkinsonism-dementia complex, an endemic disease on the island of Guam, I. Clinical features, *Brain*, 84, 642–61.

HIRANO, A., MALAMUD, N., ELIZAN, T. S., and KURLAND, L. T. (1966) Amyotrophic lateral sclerosis and parkinsonism-dementia complex on Guam: further pathologic studies, *Arch. Neurol. (Chic.)*, **15**, 35–51.

HIRANO, A., MALAMUD, N., and KURLAND, L. T. (1961) Parkinsonism-dementia complex, and endemic disease on the island of Guam, II. Pathological features, *Brain*, 84, 662–79.

HIRANO, A., MALAMUD, N., KURLAND, L. T., and ZIMMERMAN, H. M. (1969) A review of the pathologic findings in amyotrophic lateral sclerosis, in *Motor Neuron Diseases:*

Research on Amyotrophic Lateral Sclerosis and Related Disorders, Vol. 2, eds. Norris, F. H., Jr., and Kurland, L. T., New York, pp. 51–60.

HIRONO, I. (1972) Carcinogenicity and neurotoxicity of cycasin with special reference to species differences, *Fed. Proc.*, **31**, 1493–7.

HIRONO, I., and SHIBUYA, C. (1967) Induction of a neurological disorder by cycasin in mice, *Nature (Lond.)*, **216**, 1311–12.

HIRONO, I., SHIBUYA, C., and HAYASHI, K. (1969) Induction of cerebellar disorder with cycasin in newborn mice and hamsters, *Proc. Soc. exp. Biol. (N.Y.)*, **131**, 593.

JONES, M., YANG, M., and MICKELSEN, O. (1972) Effects of methylazoxy methanol glucoside and methylazoxy methanol acetate on the cerebellum of the postnatal Swiss albino mouse, *Fed. Proc.*, **31**, 1508–11.

KIMURA, K. (1965) Studies of amyotrophic lateral sclerosis in the Kozogawa District of the Kii Peninsula, Japan: epidemiological, genealogical and environmental studies, *Wakayama med. Rep.*, **9**, 177–92.

KOERNER, D. R. (1952) Amyotrophic lateral sclerosis on Guam: a clinical study and review of the literature, *Ann. intern. Med.*, **37**, 1204–20.

KROOTH, R. S., MACKLIN, M. T., and HILBISH, T. F. (1961) Diaphysial aclasis (multiple exostoses) on Guam, *Amer. J. hum. Genet.*, **13**, 340.

KURLAND, L. T. (1966) An appraisal of epidemiologic and genetic developments in amyotrophic lateral sclerosis and kuru, in *Proceedings of the Fifth International Congress of Neuropathology, Amsterdam*, eds. Luthy, F., and Bischoff, A., Excerpta Medica International Congress Series No. 100, Amsterdam, pp. 182–9.

KURLAND, L. T., CHOI, N. W., and SAYRE, G. P. (1969) Implications of incidence and geographic patterns on the classification of amyotrophic lateral sclerosis, in *Motor Neuron Diseases: Research on Amyotrophic Lateral Sclerosis and Related Disorders*, Vol. 2, eds. Norris, F. H., Jr., and Kurland, L. T., New York, pp. 28–50.

KURLAND, L. T., and MULDER, D. W. (1954) Epidemiologic investigations of amyotrophic lateral sclerosis, 1. Preliminary report on geographic distribution, with special reference to the Mariana Islands, including clinical and pathological observations, *Neurology (Minneap.)*, **4**, 355–78, 438–48.

KURTZKE, J. F., DEAN, G., and BOTHA, D. P. J. (1970) A method for estimating the age at immigration of white immigrants to South Africa, with an example of its importance, *S. Afr. med. J.*, **44**, 663–9.

LABARTHE, D. R., REED, D. M., SIEDLER, H. O., and STALLONES, R. A. (1973) Neurologic screening in the Pacific Islands and California among Micronesians. In preparation.

LAQUEUR, G. L., MICKELSEN, O., WHITING, M. G., and KURLAND, L. T. (1963) Carcinogenic properties of nuts from *Cycas circinalis* L. indigenous to Guam, *J. nat. Cancer Inst.*, **31**, 919.

MALAMUD, N., HIRANO, A., and KURLAND, L. T. (1961) Pathoanatomic changes in amyotrophic lateral slcerosis on Guam: special reference to the occurrence of neurofibrillary changes, *Arch. Neurol. (Chic.)*, **19**, 573–8.

MASON, M. M., and WHITING, M. G. (1966) Demyelination in the bovine spinal cord caused by Zamia neurotoxicity, *Fed. Proc.*, **25**, 533; also *Cornell Vet.*, 1968, **48**, 541.

MATSUMOTO, N., WORTH, R. M., KURLAND, L. T., and OKAZAKI, H. (1972) Epidemiological study of amyotrophic lateral sclerosis in Hawaii. Identification of high risk among Filipino men, *Neurology (Minneap.)*, **22**, 934–40.

MENDELL, J. R., CHASE, T. N., and ENGEL, W. K. (1971) Amyotrophic lateral sclerosis: metabolism of central monoamines and treatment with L-dopa, *Arch. Neurol. (Chic.)*, **25**, 320–5.

MULDER, D. W., and ESPINOSA, R. E. (1969) Amyotrophic lateral sclerosis: comparison of the clinical syndrome in Guam and the United States, in *Motor Neuron Diseases: Research on Amyotrophic Lateral Sclerosis and Related Disorders*, Vol. 2, eds. Norris, F. H., Jr., and Kurland, L. T., New York, pp. 12–19.

MULDER, D. W., KURLAND, L. T., and IRIARTE, L. L. G. (1954) Neurologic diseases on island of Guam, *U.S. armed Forces med. J.*, **5**, 1724–39.

NAKAI, Y. (1969) Distribution of Alzheimer's neurofibrillary changes in amyotrophic lateral sclerosis, *J. Wakayama med. Ass.*, **20**, 355.

NOBREGA, F. T., GLATTRE, E., KURLAND, L. T., and OKAZAKI, H. (1967) *Comments on the Epidemiology of Parkinsonism Including Prevalence and Incidence Statistics for Rochester, Minnesota, 1935–1966*, Vol. 1 of *Proceedings of the Second International Congress of Neuro-Genetics and Neuro-Ophthalmology, Montreal*, Excerpta Medica International Congress Series No. 175, Amsterdam, pp. 474–85.

OKAYA, N. (1936) A case of paralysis agitans observed in a Chamorro of Guam, *Tokyo med. J.*, **2997**, 2517.

PLATO, C. C., and CRUZ, M. (1967) Blood group and haptoglobin frequencies of the Chamorros of Guam, *Amer. J. hum. Genet.*, **19**, 722–31.

PLATO, C. C., CRUZ, M. T., and KURLAND, L. T. (1969) Amyotrophic lateral sclerosis/parkinsonism-dementia complex of Guam: further genetic investigations. *Amer. J. hum. Genet.*, **21**, 133–41.

PLATO, C. C., REED, D. M., ELIZAN, T. S., and KURLAND, L. T. (1967) Amyotrophic lateral sclerosis/parkinsonism-dementia complex of Guam, IV. Familial and genetic investigations, *Amer. J. hum. Genet.*, **19**, 617–32.

POLSKY, F. I., NUNN, P. B., and BELL, E. A. (1972) Distribution and toxicity of α-amino—β-methylaminopropionic acid, *Fed. Proc.*, **31**, 1473–5.

POSKANZER, D. C (1968) Etiology of multiple sclerosis: analogy suggesting infection in early life, in *The Epidemiology of Multiple Sclerosis*, eds. Alter, M., and Kurtzke, J. F., Springfield, Ill., Ch. VI, pp. 62–82.

POSKANZER, D. C., and SCHWAB, R. S. (1963) Cohort analysis of Parkinson's syndrome: evidence for a single etiology related to subclinical infection about 1920, *J. chron. Dis.*, **16**, 961–73.

REED, D., LABARTHE, D., and STALLONES, R. (1970) Health effects of westernization and migration among Chamorros, *Amer. J. Epidem.*, **92**, 94–112.

REED, D., PLATO, C., ELIZAN, T., and KURLAND, L. T. (1966) The amyotrophic lateral sclerosis/parkinsonism-dementia complex: a ten-year follow-up on Guam, Part 1. Epidemiologic studies, *Amer. J. Epidem.*, **83**, 54–73.

SANGER, V. L., YANG, M., and MICKELSEN, O. (1972) Cycasin-induced central nervous system lesions in postnatal mice, *Fed. Proc.*, **31**, 1524–8.

SCHNUR, J. A., CHASE, T. N., and BRODY, J. A. (1971) Parkinsonism-dementia of Guam: treatment with L-dopa, *Neurology (Minneap.)*, **21**, 1236–42.

SHIRAKI, H. (1969) The neuropathology of amyotrophic lateral sclerosis (ALS) in the Kii Peninsula and other areas of Japan, in *Motor Neuron Diseases: Research on Amyotrophic Lateral Sclerosis and Related Disorders*, Vol. 2, eds. Norris, F. H., Jr., and Kurland, L. T., New York, pp. 80–4.

SPATZ, M., and LAQUEUR, G. L. (1967) Transplacental induction of tumours in Sprague Dawley rats with crude cycad material, *J. nat. Cancer Inst.*, 38, 233.

SPATZ, M., and LAQUEUR, G. L. (1968) Chemical induction of microencephaly in two strains of rats, Part I, *Proc. Soc. exp. Biol. (N.Y.)*, **129**, 705.

TILLEMA, S., and WIJNBERG, C. J. (1953) 'Endemic' amyotrophic lateral sclerosis on Guam: epidemiological data, preliminary report, *Docum. Med. geogr. trop. (Amst.)*, 5, 366–70.

TORRES, J., IRIARTE, L. L. G., and KURLAND, L. T. (1957) Amyotrophic lateral sclerosis among Guamanians in California, *Calif. Med.*, 86, 385–8.

VEGA, A., and BELL, E. A. (1967) Alpha amino beta methyl-aminoproprionic acid. A new amino acid from seeds of *Cycas circinalis*, *Phytochemistry*, 6, 759–62.

YASE, Y., MATSUMOTO, N., YOSKIMASU, F., HANDA, Y., and KUMAMOTO, T. (1968) Motor neuron disease in the Kii Peninsula, Japan, *Proc. Aust. Ass. Neurol.*, 5, 335–9.

YASE, Y., *et al.* (1968) Amyotrophic lateral sclerosis studies using neutron activation analysis, *Neurology (Bombay)*, **16**, 46–50.

ZIMMERMAN, H. M. (1945) *Monthly Report to Medical Officer in Command*, U.S.N. Medical Research Unit, No. 2.

29 Kuru in the New Guinea Highlands

D. C. GAJDUSEK

Kuru is a subacute degenerative disease of the central nervous system which is caused by a virus possessing many unconventional properties. It is confined to a number of adjacent valleys in the mountainous interior of New Guinea and occurs in 160 villages with a total population of just over 35 000 [FIG. 29.1]. It is the first chronic or subacute degenerative disease of man proved to be a slow virus infection, and as such has attracted worldwide attention and stimulated the search for such virus infections as the possible cause of other subacute and chronic diseases of man. Such a slowly progressive infection of man, with an incubation period of many years and absence of any inflammatory response to the slow destruction of brain cells, was hitherto unknown. The elucidation of the aetiology of kuru has led to the discovery that presenile dementias of the Creutzfeldt–Jakob type, found throughout the world, and with a basically similar lesion at the cellular level, are also transmissible and caused by a very similar, very unconventional virus.

Kuru is characterized by cerebellar ataxia and a shivering-like tremor which progresses to complete motor incapacity and death in about 1 year from onset. *Kuru* means shivering or trembling in the Fore language. In the Fore cultural and linguistic group, among whom over 80 per cent of the cases occur, it has a yearly incidence rate and prevalence ratio of about 1 per cent of the population. During the early years of investigation, after the first description by Gajdusek and Zigas in 1957, it was found to affect all ages beyond infants and toddlers; it was common in children of both sexes and in adult females, but rare in adult males [FIG. 29.2]. This marked excess of deaths of adult females over males had led to a male to female ratio of over 3:1 in

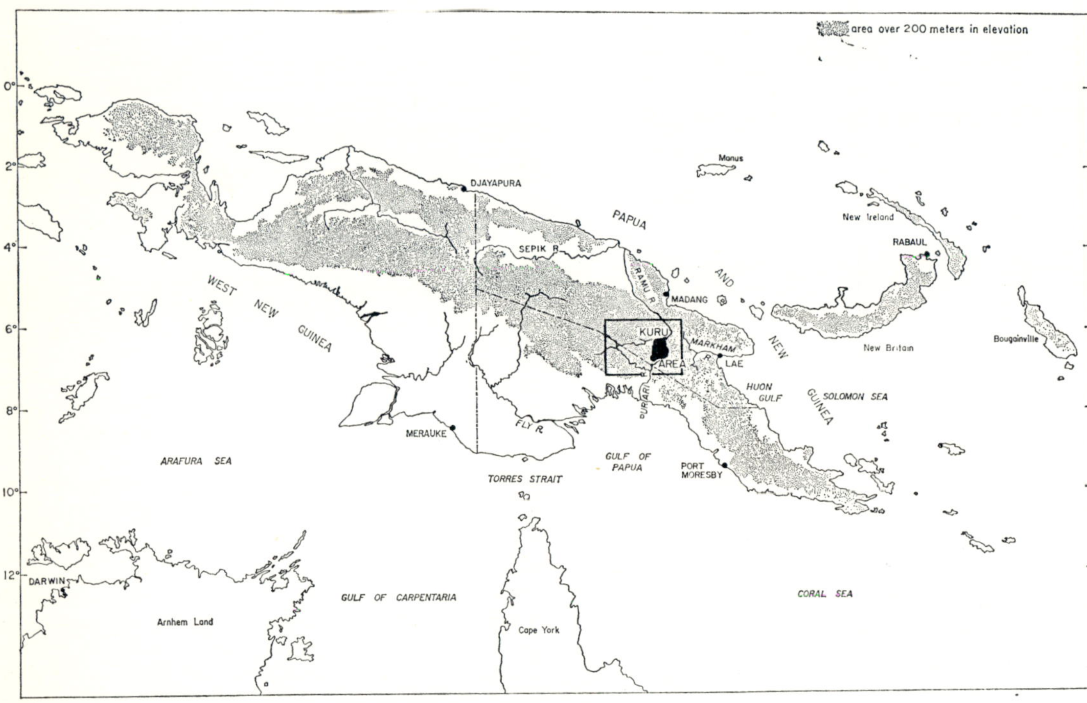

FIG. 29.1. Map of New Guinea showing in black, within the rectangle, the area from which all cases of kuru have come. It contains over 35 000 people living in 160 villages (census units) which have experienced kuru.

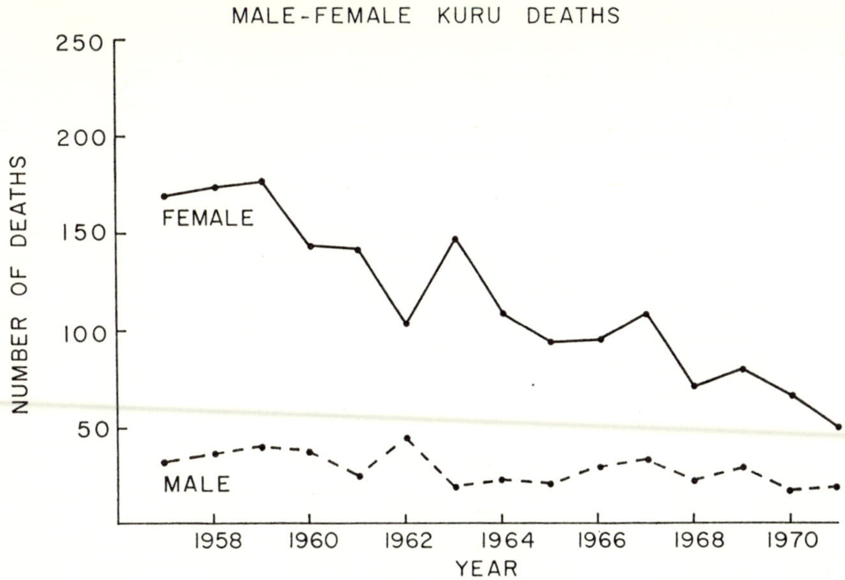

FIG. 29.2. Kuru deaths by sex 1957–71. The decline in incidence has occurred during the period of acculturation from a stone age culture, practising endocannibalistic consumption of dead kinsmen as a rite of mourning, to a modern coffee-planting society practising cash economy. Since the brain tissue with which the officiating women contaminated themselves and all their infants and toddlers contained over 1 000 000 infectious doses per gram, self-inoculation through the eyes, nose and skin, as well as by mouth, was a certainty, as was similar contamination of the younger children. The decline in incidence of disease has followed the cessation of ritual cannibalism, which occurred between 1957 and 1962 in various villages.

some villages, and of 2:1 for the whole South Fore group.

Child patients have decreased in frequency during the past decade and at present the disease is no longer seen in pre-adolescent children [FIG. 29.3]. This change in occurrence of kuru appears to be the result of the cessation of the practice of ritual cannibalism as a rite of mourning and respect for the dead kinsmen, and the resulting conjunctival, nasal, and skin contamination, mostly of women and small children, with highly infectious brain tissue.

CLINICAL PICTURE

Kuru is characterized by predominantly cerebellar symptomatology which follows a progressive and remarkably uniform course to total incapacitation and death, usually within 3 to 9 months. It starts insidiously

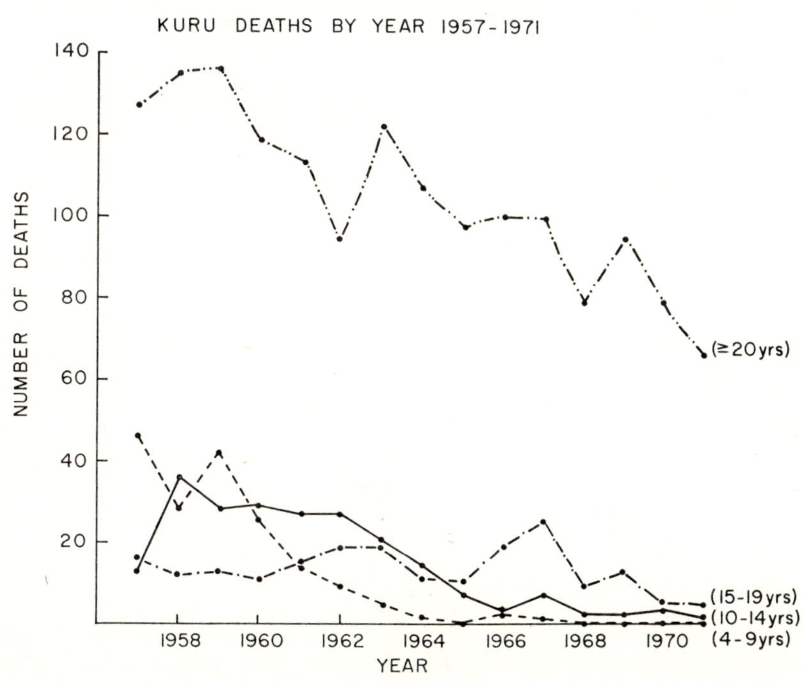

FIG. 29.3. Kuru deaths in adults, adolescents and children from 1957 through 1971. No child under 10 years old has developed kuru since 1967, and cases in pre-adolescent children have almost disappeared. From about 1959 there has been a progressive increase in the ages of the youngest patients, and a progressive decline in the number of child patients, with an overall much slower drop in the number of adult patients. These changes in the pattern of kuru incidence can be explained by the cessation of cannibalism in the late 1950s.

without acute antecedent illness, and is conveniently divisible into three stages. Some patients report prodromal symptoms of headache and limb pains.

The first, or ambulant, stage is usually self-diagnosed before others in the community are aware that the patient is ill [PLATE 29a]. There is subjective unsteadiness of stance and gait and often of the voice, hands and eyes as well. Postural instability with truncal tremor and titubation and ataxia of gait are the first signs. Dysarthria starts early and speech progessively deteriorates as the disease advances. Eye movements are ataxic, but no true nystagmus occurs. A convergent strabismus often appears early in the disease and persists. Tremors are at first no different from those of slight hypersensitivity to cold; the patient shivers inordinately. Incoordination affects the lower extremities before progressing to involve the upper extremities. Patients arising to a standing posture often stamp their feet as though angry at them. In attempting to maintain balance when standing, the toes grip and claw the ground more than usual. Very early in the disease the inability to stand on one foot for many seconds is a helpful diagnostic clue. For most of the first stage of the disease the patient usually continues to work in the garden and attempts to pursue his normal activities and take full part in village social life. In the latter part of this first stage, the patient usually takes a stick for support in order to continue to walk about the village unaided by others [PLATES 29c and 30a].

The second, or sedentary, stage is reached when the patient can no longer walk without complete support [PLATE 29B]. Tremors and ataxia become more severe and a changing rigidity of the limbs often develops, associated with widespread clonus, or sometimes shock-like muscle jerks and occasionally coarser athetoid and choreiform movements, especially when the patient is thrown into an exaggerated startle response by postural instability, or even by sudden exposure to noise or bright light. Deep tendon reflexes are usually normal; Babinski response is negative. Although muscle activity is poorly maintained there is no fasciculation or real weakness or muscle atrophy [PLATE 30b]. Emotional lability, leading to outbursts of pathological laughter, are frequent, sometimes even appearing in the first stage of the disease, and smiling and laughter are terminated slowly. This feature has given rise to unfortunate journalistic synonyms for the disease. Most patients show a resignation to, and a light-hearted attitude toward, their disease, bordering on a true euphoria. Some patients, especially adolescent and young adult males, become depressed, and a rare patient develops a pathological belligerence to all disturbances by family members or others. Mental slowing is apparent, but severe dementia is conspicuously absent. No sensory changes have been noted. The fundi appear normal.

The third, or terminal, stage is reached when the patient is unable to sit up without support, and ataxia, tremor and dysarthria become progressively more severe and incapacitating [PLATE 30c]. Tendon reflexes may become exaggerated. A grasp reflex may appear and some cases show characteristic extrapyramidal defects of posture and movement. Terminally, urinary and faecal incontinence develop and dysphagia leads to thirst and starvation. Flaccidity, inanition and signs of bulbar involvement develop, and the patient becomes mute and unresponsive. Deep decubitus ulcerations and hypostatic pneumonia appear in this stage and the patient finally succumbs, usually emaciated, but occasionally quickly enough to be still well nourished.

PATHOLOGICAL PICTURE

There is no pathological process outside the central nervous system and no gross brain lesions are noted, except for an atrophic cerebellar vermis in many of the patients. In kuru the changes in the nervous system are widespread and are characterized by marked proliferation and hypertrophy of the astrocytes throughout the brain [PLATE 31c], by mild status spongiosus of the grey matter [PLATE 31b], by diffuse neuronal degeneration which is most severe in the cerebellum and its afferent and efferent connexions [PLATE 31a], and by minimal demyelination which, though not readily seen in sections stained for myelin, can be demonstrated by the presence of neutral fat. In addition, in about three-fourths of the cases, periodic-acid-Schiff (PAS)-positive, birefringent, amyloid-containing plaques are found. Typical intracytoplasmic vacuolation is usually observed in the large neurones of the striatum. The status spongiosus is not the result of intercellular oedema, but rather of coalescing vacuolation within the pre- and post-synaptic processes of the neurones, and, to a lesser extent, in astocytes and oligodendrocytes. An occasional vessel may be cuffed with mononuclear cells, a finding compatible with the amount of tissue breakdown that is present, but this is a rare finding and the pathological process is essentially devoid of inflammatory response.

CLINICAL LABORATORY FINDINGS

Laboratory findings, like the clinical and pathological findings, have failed to suggest a conventional infectious disease. Thus, as does the afebrile clinical course (except for intercurrent or terminal infection), the lack of change in the peripheral blood smear, the absence of pleocytosis or elevated protein in the cerebrospinal fluid, and the failure to find any elevation of erythrocyte sedimentation rate, all speak against infection. There is no disturbance in renal or hepatic function tests, and endocrine function tests remain normal.

EPIDEMIOLOGY

Since the beginning of kuru investigations in 1956, a total of about 2500 cases have been recorded. All these have ended in death in under 2 years, with a few exceptions of somewhat more prolonged disease. Kuru mortality has declined significantly since the early years of investigation when over 200 patients died annually, but over 60 persons still die of the disease each year. Case-finding is complete, since the entire population of all villages in which kuru has occurred have been surveyed at least twice annually.

Epidemiological observations to date have given no evidence for its contagion. No outsiders of the kuru region have yet developed kuru after residence in the region. Cases have, however, developed in many subjects after many years of absence from the kuru region which they had left for work or study. Such persons were always found to be from families in which kuru had occurred in the past. No cases of the disease were seen in natives eating and living together with such persons in whom kuru developed, while they were away from home. Furthermore, hundreds of native peoples from elsewhere in New Guinea and from surrounding Melanesian islands have now been resident for long periods in the kuru region since early Government penetration over a decade ago. In spite of the many thousands of man-years of close contact of these immigrants with the flora, fauna, food and people of the region, no case of kuru has occurred among them. In the peripheral region of low incidence in the north and north-west of the kuru area, the few cases that have appeared are either in immigrants from villages of higher kuru incidence or in descendants of such people, although persons of such origin form but a small portion of the population of these peripheral villages of low incidence.

Soon after the discovery of kuru, patients very early in the disease were brought totally outside the kuru region and placed on a regular hospital diet; yet their disease progressed to death in typical fashion. This was also true of patients who acquired their disease after prolonged sojourn outside the region, but who never returned before death to the ecology, social surroundings, diet or drinking-water of their kuru-affected homeland.

The culture in the kuru region resembles those of surrounding kuru-free highland peoples. The pattern of the women, small children and pigs sharing the women's houses was by no means unique to the kuru region. Pigs, the principal domestic animals throughout the New Guinea highlands, had no unique relation with man in the kuru region, nor did they show any illnesses not encountered in the pigs in adjacent kuru-free regions. Adult men, who were the group least affected by kuru, ate often with the women and children, and had quite similar diets. There was no item in the Fore diet not also consumed in similar quantity by some neighbouring kuru-free groups.

Kuru was the major cause of death among the Fore; other neurological disease was rare, malaria was absent, except in a few villages, and the common causes of death, apart from kuru, were acute and chronic pulmonary disease and trauma. Yaws, tropical ulcers, scabies and intestinal parasitism were universal and leprosy common. Epidemic gastrointestinal disease was rare, and epidemics of acute respiratory disease occurred irregularly. The pattern of disease was the same, apart from kuru, in the surrounding groups. No evidence for any compensatory advantage of the Fore over their neighbours was uncovered and the death rate in the South Fore was barely balanced by the birth rate. Reprisal murders (in Fore *tukabu*) of those suspected of causing kuru sorcery, always males, was the the second commonest cause of death in some areas of high kuru incidence, and thus prevented the sex ratio from becoming yet more abnormal. Warfare, murder and suicide, and in certain areas, drowning, falls from trees, and snake bites were significant causes of death. Chronic liver failure of undetermined cause, amyloidosis and chronic glomerulonephritis occur sporadically in the region without relationship to kuru.

Kogaisantampa, a familial congenital tremor resulting in violent shaking of the hands, trunk and head, occurs in some parts of the kuru region, especially among the North Fore, Kamano, Kanite and Usurufa groups and especially in the Auyana, Tairora and Oiana groups, wherein it is distributed into villages which do not suffer from kuru. It does not interfere with life expectancy, marriage or procreation. A few patients with aseptic, apparently virus meningo-encephalitis or meningitis have been seen in the region and many cases of acute bacterial meningitis, but these appear to be unrelated to kuru. A few cases of Parkinson's disease have been found in the Eastern Highlands groups, but again, not specifically in kuru-affected villages. The scattered cases of motor neurone disease (amyotrophic lateral sclerosis) found in New Guinea have not been seen in the kuru area, and the focus of high incidence of motor neurone disease, described by Gajdusek, lies in the Jaqai and Auyu areas of southern West New Guinea. In the Western and Southern Highlands regions of New Guinea there is a chronic incapacitating neurological tremor disorder which is easily confused with kuru because of the violent tremors and myoclonus. It is very different from kuru in that there is no real ataxia other than that caused by the myoclonic jerks, and it is not rapidly progressive and fatal. This and other neurological diseases presenting a differential diagnostic problem with kuru have not been seen in the kuru region.

The mechanism of spread of kuru is undoubtedly contamination of the population during their ritual cannibalistic consumption of their dead relatives as a rite of respect and mourning. They did the autopsies bare-handed and did not wash thereafter; they wiped their hands on their bodies and in their hair, picked sores, scratched insect bites, wiped their infants' eyes, and cleaned their noses, and they ate with their hands. The brain tissue which they squeezed into a pulp with their hands and packed into bamboo cylinders was infectious at a dilution of 10^{-7} or higher. It is infectious by the peripheral routes of inoculation, and intracerebral inoculation is not necessary. The cooking of brain and other visceral tissues by steaming in bamboo cylinders at elevations of from 6000 to 7500 feet would expose them to temperatures of no more than 95°C, and would be insufficient to fully inactivate many infectious agents, especially those with such high heat stability as kuru. Women and children crowding about or in the arms of women were more exposed to the kuru-infected human tissue than were the men, who left this butchery of dead kinsmen to the women. Men rarely ate the flesh of dead kuru victims. We must presume that all children who had a close kinsman who died of kuru and whose mothers took part in the cannibalistic rite were contaminated with kuru. If a boy did not have a relative who died of the disease before he left the women's society to live in the men's house, and ate with the men at feasts, he might thereafter escape contamination—but not so for the girls.

SERIAL TRANSMISSION OF KURU BY THE INTRACEREBRAL AND PERIPHERAL ROUTES OF INOCULATION OF BRAIN AND DEMONSTRATION OF THE KURU VIRUS IN THE VISCERAL TISSUES OF AFFECTED CHIMPANZEES

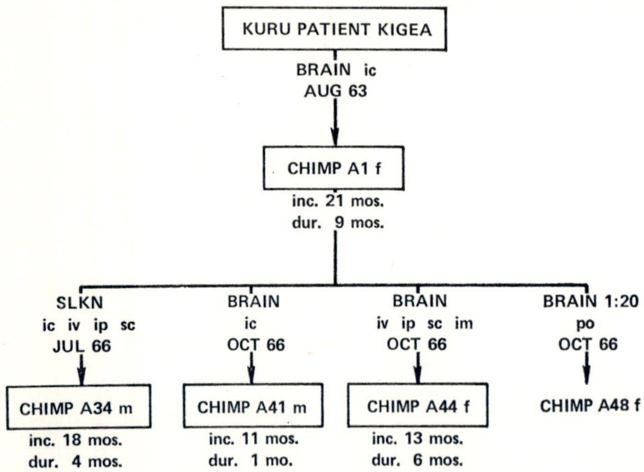

FIG. 29.4. Chimpanzees (enclosed in rectangles) have been killed in late stages of experimentally induced kuru and typical kuru neuropathology has been found in their brains. Chimpanzee A48 remains well.

f = female; m = male; ic = intracerebral; iv = intravenous; ip = intraperitoneal; sc = subcutaneous; im = intramuscular; po = oral; inc. = incubation period; dur. = duration of illness before animal was killed; mo(s) = month(s); SLKN = spleen, liver, kidney, and lymph node suspensions pooled.

AETIOLOGY

Kuru was at first thought to be an epidemic of infectious disease, because of its high prevalence. However, the absence of fever or antecedent acute disease, the absence of pleocytosis or of elevation of protein in the cerebrospinal fluid, or of alterations in the absolute or differential leucocyte count or in the erythrocyte sedimentation rate in the peripheral blood, or of changes in the urine and the total absence of neuropathological change, suggesting inflammation such as perivascular cuffing with mononuclear cells or mononuclear cell infiltration of the brain parenchyma, all suggested a 'degenerative', rather than an infectious, process. Furthermore, cases developed in youths and adults who had been away from the kuru region as labourers on coastal plantations, or as students for many years, and there were no contact cases in those with whom they had lived on intimate terms away from home. New immigrants into the kuru region did not develop kuru, even after close contact with kuru patients.

A simple genetic hypothesis seemed adequate to explain all cases: a kuru gene, K, was dominant in the adult female, rarely penetrant in the adult male, and responsible in the homozygous condition for a juvenile early-appearing form of the disease. Thus, the homozygous state (KK) would determine the disease in children of both sexes, while the heterozygous (Kk) state would determine the appearance of the disease in adult life regularly in females, but less often, because of low penetrance, in males. This hypothesis left unexplained, however, how such an enormously high gene frequency could have developed in the face of high loss of the gene in heterozygous individuals who died before the end of their reproductive period. No evidence of a sufficient compensatory reproductive advantage with increased fertility in kuru patients could be found.

In 1959, Hadlow pointed out the similarity in the neuropathology of scrapie in sheep with that of kuru in man, as reported by Klatzo, Gajdusek, and Zigas (1959), and an intensive comparative study of the two diseases was launched, along with renewed attempts to transmit kuru to laboratory animals and other species. In earlier transmission attempts, inoculated animals had been kept for only several months; now observation for many years was planned. In 1965, after 1½ years of incubation, chimpanzees inoculated intracerebrally with suspensions of human kuru brain from kuru patients developed the disease [FIGS. 29.4 and 29.5]. They were found to have the same pathological process as that in the human kuru victims.

In the interval since these first transmissions, much virological investigation has been done on the trans-

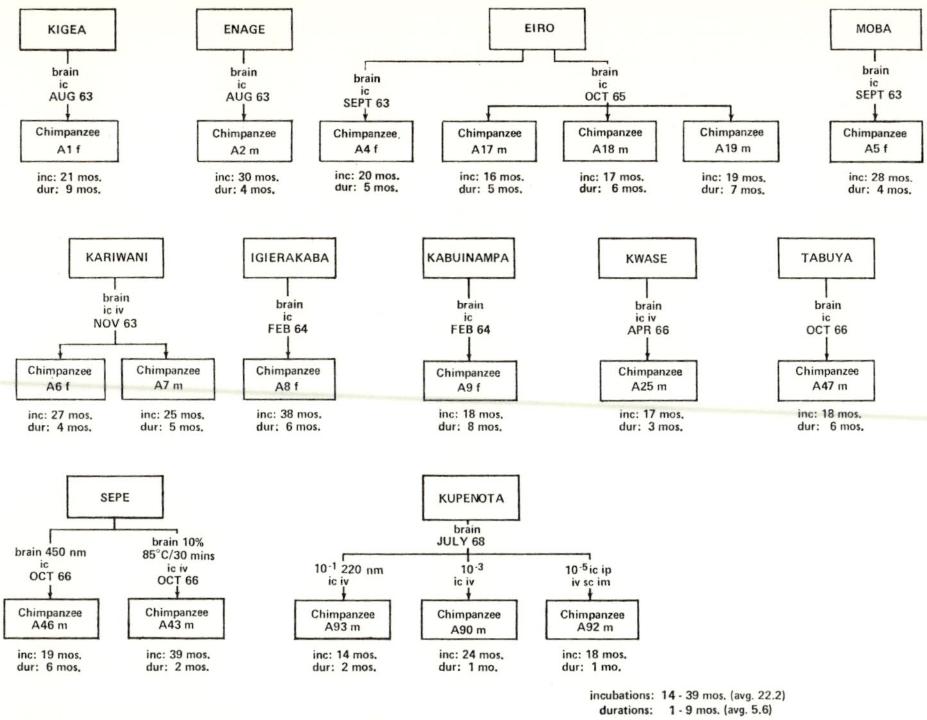

FIG. 29.5. Transmission of kuru from 11 human patients to 18 chimpanzees. All have been inoculated intracerebrally. Chimpanzee A92 received brain suspension filtered through millipore filters of 450 nm and 220 nm average pore diameter, respectively.

missible agent of kuru. Kuru is caused by a virus filterable through membranes of 220 nm minimum pore diameter; it attains a titre of over 10^7 LD_{50} per gram of brain tissue in the affected chimpanzees. The disease can be serially transmitted from chimpanzee to chimpanzee, using either suspensions of brain tissue from affected chimpanzees or visceral tissues containing no brain, and inoculated either by intracerebral or by peripheral (intravenous, intraperitoneal, intramuscular, or subcutaneous) routes. Incubation period in the chimpanzee varies from 14 to 39 months after intracerebral inoculation. On second passage in the chimpanzee it drops to about 10 to 12 months and remains at this period on further serial passage. The virus has not been found in whole blood, leucocytes, serum, urine, milk, cerebrospinal fluid, amniotic fluid or placenta from kuru victims, or from animals with experimental kuru. The disease has more recently been similarly transmitted to three species of New World monkeys, the spider (*Ateles* sp.), squirrel (*Saimiri* sp.), and the capuchin (*Cebus* sp.) monkeys [FIG. 29.6]. On primary inoculation with brain tissue from either kuru-affected man or

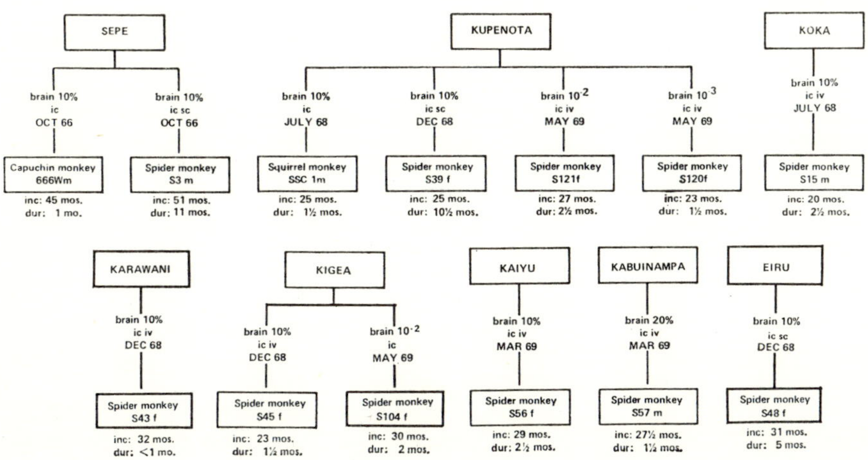

FIG. 29.6. Transmission of kuru from eight human patients to three species of New World monkeys: spider, capuchin, and squirrel monkeys. Brain tissue from two of the patients, Kaiyu and Koka, had not previously been inoculated into chimpanzees, and thus they represent the twelfth and thirteenth patients from whom the disease has been transmitted to subhuman primates. Brain tissue inoculated into spider monkey S120 was diluted 10^{-3}; the incubation period in spider monkey S3 was 51 months.

chimpanzees, the incubation period in these New World monkeys is usually 2 years or longer, but on serial passage in the capuchin monkey it has been reduced to under 1 year.

The agent remains stable on storage at −70°C for many years and on lyophilization. It is not totally inactivated by a temperature of 85°C for 30 minutes. No serological test for the virus has been found. In fact, extensive attempts to demonstrate a neutralizing, principitating or complement-fixing antibody, using tissue suspensions of high infectivity titre as antigens, and as potential antisera the sera from human kuru patients or animals with experimental kuru and from rabbits immunized with brain tissue from kuru-affected patients or animals, have all been negative. The virus has been maintained *in vitro* in tissue cultures of explanted brain fragments from chimpanzees with experimental kuru for periods of many months with or without repeated trypsinized subculture, and the virus so maintained in tissue culture has not lost its virulence for the chimpanzee.

THE TRANSMISSIBLE PRESENILE VIRUS DEMENTIA (CREUTZFELDT-JAKOB DISEASE)

With the transmission of kuru, a subacute progressive degenerative non-inflammatory disease of the CNS of man, to chimpanzees and monkeys and the demonstration of its virus aetiology, the search for further such diseases in man in less exotic populations was intensified. The similarity between kuru pathology and that of presenile dementia of the Creutzfeldt-Jakob type had been noted by Klatzo, and with the increased prominence of spongiform changes in the grey matter of the cerebral cortex in experimentally affected animals over that found in the human kuru patients, Beck and Daniel (1965) considered that this analogy was thereby strengthened. We thus sought brain biopsy and early autopsy brain tissue from patients suffering with these subacute spongiform encephalopathies of grey matter, or Creutzfeldt-Jakob disease. This disease was also found to be transmissible to chimpanzees and monkeys, and to be caused by a virus with very similar properties to that of kuru. The Creutzfeldt-Jakob disease virus also passes filters of 220 nm minimum pore diameter; it reaches infectivity titres of over 10^7 LD_{50} per gram of brain tissue in experimentally affected animals, and it resists inactivation on exposure to a temperature of 85°C for 30 minutes. The virus has also been maintained for many months *in vitro* in tissue cultures of brain cells from patients with Creutzfeldt-Jakob disease and from chimpanzees with the experimentally induced disease.

There have now been transmissions of Creutzfeldt-Jakob disease from 15 different patients to chimpanzees and New World monkeys of the same species as those susceptible to kuru. On direct transmission with human brain tissue, the incubation period in chimpanzees is only 10 to 14 months, whereas it is always longer for kuru. The basic cellular lesion, best appreciated by electron microscopic examination, is the same in both kuru and Creutzfeldt-Jakob disease: a progressive vacuolation of the dendritic and axonal processes of neurones, and to a lesser extent in astrocytes and oligodendrocytes, with slow coalescence of the vacuoles and the eventual destruction of the cell. The vacuoles are not empty, but filled with an irregular array of curled-up sheets of the same unit membrane material which forms the vacuolar wall.

The clinical picture of the transmissible disease in these patients has been one of severe dementia, advancing to death with associated motor disturbances in 3 to 18 months. The dementia is often preceded by psychiatric disturbances and disorders of higher cortical function, and is later associated with myoclonus and periodic bursts of spikes and slow waves in the electroencephalogram, and with a variety of motor abnormalities, including cerebellar, pyramidal and extrapyramidal involvement in varying degrees and often with visual symptoms, including cortical blindness.

The transmission of these presenile dementias with subacute course has permitted the evolution of the concept of transmissible virus dementias and the quest for a similar aetiology in disorders such as Alzheimer's and Pick's diseases, parkinsonism and senile dementias, and even in Huntington's chorea. One of the patients with Creutzfeldt-Jakob disease, from whose brain tissue the disease has been transmitted to chimpanzees, was from a family with the disease in three generations. A second was from a patient with the same disease in a sister. This brings into question the possibility of genetically controlled susceptibility to the agent, and re-enforces the possibility of genetic determinants, as earlier suspected, in both kuru in man and scrapie in sheep.

THE SUBACUTE SPONGIFORM VIRUS ENCEPHALOPATHIES

From the many close pathological, cytological and aetiological analogies between the two diseases, kuru and Creutzfeldt-Jakob disease, and between these two diseases of man and the two similar diseases of animals, scrapie of sheep and goats and transmissible mink encephalopathy, the concept of a related group of diseases of virus aetiology has emerged. These are all very atypical infections without associated inflammatory response and caused by viruses with very unconventional properties. In laboratory work very unusual hosts must be used in their study. This group of four diseases we have called the *subacute spongiform virus encephalopathies*, because of the characteristic vacuolating lesion in the neurones in all of them, as observed by electron microscopy and the resulting status spongiosus of grey matter, as seen by light microscopy.

The unusual properties of the viruses causing these diseases have become apparent in the study of the scrapie virus, because of the facility of using passage strains of scrapie in mice with only 3 to 6 months' incubation as an indicator of virus infectivity. A unique resistance among viruses to inactivation by ultraviolet light with an inactivation spectrum peak at 240 nm, rather than at 260 nm, has been the most disturbing property, often interpreted as indicating that the virus contains no nucleic acid. Persistent attempts to recognize the virus particle by electron microscopy in pathological sections and in zonal density gradient fractions of high infectivity have been unsuccessful, and wherever virus infectivity is concentrated only fragmented membrane structures are seen. Extreme resistance to heat inactivation and to inactivation by formaldehyde or proteolytic enzymes has been noted, and the virus has an unusually small target size in inactivation work using ionizing radiation. There remains the possibility that the virus contains a small replicating nucleic acid of under 100 000 molecular weight, such as the small plant viruses ('viroids') of Diener which cause the potato spindle tuber, chrysanthemum stunt and orange exorcosis diseases which is protected from inactivation by close binding to membrane structures.

The viruses of these subacute spongiform encephalopathies are certainly unusual in many ways, and the possibility is being considered that they may be small molecules attached to plasma membranes and acting by derepression of genetic information for their own synthesis, which is already latent, or integrated, in the host cells. Work in this direction, to investigate these possibilities, lies ahead.

SUGGESTED FURTHER READING

ALPERS, M. P. (1968) Kuru: implications of its transmissibility for the interpretation of its changing epidemiologic pattern, in *The Central Nervous System*, International Academy of Pathology Monograph No. 9, Baltimore, pp. 234–51.

ALPERS, M. P., and GAJDUSEK, D. C. (1965) Changing patterns of kuru: epidemiological changes in the period of increasing contact of the Fore people with Western civilization, *Amer. J. trop. Med. Hyg.*, **14**, 852–79.

BECK, E., and DANIEL, P. M. (1965) Kuru and scrapie compared: are they examples of system degeneration? in *Slow, Latent, and Temperate Virus Infections*, eds. Gajdusek, D. C., Gibbs, C. J. Jr., and Alpers, M. P., NINDB Monograph No. 2, Government Printing Office, Washington, D.C., pp. 85–93.

BECK, E., DANIEL, P. M., ALPERS, M., GAJDUSEK, D. C., and GIBBS, C. J., JR. (1966) Experimental 'kuru' in chimpanzees: a pathological report, *Lancet*, ii, 1056–9.

DIENER, T. O. (1972) Viroids, *Advanc. Virus Res.*, 17, 295–313.

GAJDUSEK, D. C. (1963) Motor-neuron disease in natives of New Guinea, *New Engl. J. Med.*, **268**, 474–6.

GAJDUSEK, D. C. (1972) Subacute spongiform encephalopathies, *J. clin. Path.*, **25**, Supplement, 72–83.

GAJDUSEK, D. C. (1963) Kuru, *Trans. roy. Soc. trop. Med. Hyg.*, **57**, 151–69.

GAJDUSEK, D. C., and ALPERS, M. P. (1970) *Bibliography of Kuru*, National Institute of Neurological Diseases and Stroke, National Institutes of Health, Bethesda, Md.

GAJDUSEK, D. C., and GIBBS, C. J., JR. (1971) Transmission of the two subacute spongiform encephalopathies of man (kuru and Creutzfeldt-Jakob disease) to New World monkeys, *Nature (Lond.)*, **230**, 588–91.

GAJDUSEK, D. C., GIBBS, C. J., JR., and ALPERS, M. P. (1966) Experimental transmission of a kuru-like syndrome to chimpanzees, *Nature (Lond.)*, **209**, 794–6.

GAJDUSEK, D. C., GIBBS, C. J., JR., and ALPERS, M. P. (1967) Transmission and passage of experimental 'kuru' to chimpanzees, *Science*, **155**, 212–14.

GAJDUSEK, D. C., GIBBS, C. J., JR., ROGERS, N. G., BASNIGHT, M., and HOOKS, J. (1972) Persistence of the viruses of kuru and Creutzfeldt-Jakob disease in tissue cultures of brain cells, *Nature (Lond.)*, **235**, 104–5.

GAJDUSEK, D. C., and ZIGAS, V. (1957) Degenerative disease of the central nervous system in New Guinea. The endemic occurrence of 'kuru' in the native population, *New Engl. J. Med.*, **257**, 974–8.

GAJDUSEK, D. C., and ZIGAS, V. (1959) Kuru: clinical, pathological and epidemiological study of an acute progressive degenerative disease of the central nervous system among natives of the Eastern Highlands of New Guinea, *Amer. J. Med.*, **26**, 442–69.

GIBBS, C. J., Jr., and GAJDUSEK, D. C. (1972) Isolation and characterization of the subacute spongiform virus encephalopathies of man: kuru and Creutzfeldt-Jakob disease, *J. clin. Path.* **25**, Supplement, 84–96.

GIBBS, C. J., JR., GAJDUSEK, D. C., ASHER, D. M., ALPERS, M. P., BECK, E., DANIEL, P. M., and MATTHEWS, W. B. (1968) Creutzfeldt-Jakob disease (subacute spongiform encephalopathy): transmission to the chimpanzee, *Science*, **161**, 388–9.

HADLOW, W. J. (1959) Scrapie and kuru, *Lancet*, ii, 289–90.

KAKULAS, B. A., LECOURS, A.-R., and GAJDUSEK, D. C. (1967) Further observations on the pathology of kuru (a study of two cerebra in serial section), *J. Neuropath. exp. Neurol.*, **26**, 85–97.

KLATZO, I., GAJDUSEK, D. C., and ZIGAS, V. (1959) Pathology of kuru, *Lab. Invest.*, 8, 799–847.

LAMPERT, P. W., EARLE, K. M., GIBBS, C. J., JR., and GAJDUSEK, D. C. (1970) Electron microscopic studies on experimental spongiform encephalopathies (kuru and Creutzfeldt-Jakob disease) in chimpanzees, in *The Sixth International Congress of Neuropathology, Paris*, 31 August to 4 September, Paris, pp. 916–30.

ROOS, R., GIBBS, C. J., Jr., and GAJDUSEK, D. C. (1973) The clinical characteristics of transmissible Creutzfeldt-Jakob disease, *Brain*, **96**, 1–20.

WILSON, K., ZIGAS, V., and GAJDUSEK, D. C. (1959) New tremor syndromes occurring sporadically in natives of the Wabag-Laiagam-Kundep region of the Western Highlands of Australian New Guinea, *Lancet*, ii, 699–702.

Part Five

LATIN AMERICA

See PLATES 32–40

30 Neurological Disorders in Peru

J. O. TRELLES

INTRODUCTION

Peru, on the west coast of South America and a land of 500 000 square miles, is divided into three main regions by the Andes, which stretch the entire length of the Pacific coast of South America. West of the Andes lies the Costa, a flat, dry and sandy seaboard. The Andes region is called the Sierra. Its plateaux are useful only for grazing; the valleys are fertile. East of the Andes the fertile Montana sprawls luxuriantly. It is intersected by many rivers, one of which is the Amazon. The jungle, or *selva*, comprises 72 per cent of the country and is inhabited by only one-eighth of the population. In the whole country there are 13½ million people; one-third of the population is indigenous, nearly one-third is white and the remainder are mestizo. The Indians live mainly in the Andean valleys at an elevation of 2000 to 4000 metres.

The climate varies from region to region, and seasonal changes are directly opposite to those of the Northern Hemisphere. The coastal region is subtropical but the heat is never oppressive because of the cooling influence of the Humboldt current. There is scarcely any rain but humidity is high. The Sierra region is temperate, yet there is rain in plenty; humidity is very low. In the tropical Montana, rainfall is heavy and humidity is high.

Cattle, sheep and llamas are reared on the mountain slopes and in the fertile East, coffee, tea, cotton, maize, timber and many fruits are grown.

Diet varies with the regions. On the coast it consists mainly of carbohydrates (potatoes, rice, cereals and sugar); proteins and fats tend to be deficient and there is malnutrition among the children. In the mountains consumption of fats and proteins is even lower, and this may be related to the low incidence of cerebral and coronary arteriosclerosis. In the jungle vitamin deficiencies are widespread.

Well-defined cultural groups existed in Peru in 3000 BC, the Chavin in the Sierra and the Paracas on the coast. Echoes of their artistic and technical skills are to be found in their dress designs, surgical instruments and trepanned skulls. Later cultures were the Tiahuanaco, Nazca and Chimu. By the twelfth century AD the Incas, a quechua-speaking race, ruled an empire extending far beyond the borders of Peru into Chile, Argentine and Colombia. The Spanish conquest came in 1533, led by Francisco Pizarro, and Spanish viceregal government lasted for 300 years. In the early nineteenth century the activities of men like San Martin and Bolivar led to the establishment of an independent republic in 1821.

Lima, the capital of Peru, was founded in 1535. Its population is now 3 million. It is the cultural, as well as the political and economic capital of the country. It has the oldest University of South America, the Universidad Nacional Mayor de San Marcos, created by royal letters patent signed by Emperor Charles V of Spain in Valladolid in 1551. Medical instruction began in Lima just four centuries ago in 1571. There are now four other medical schools in Peru, two in Lima and one each in Trujillo in the north and Arequipa in the south.

There are neurological departments in each of the three medical schools in Lima, and the Hospital Santo Toribio de Mogrovejo is devoted entirely to the neurological sciences.

THE NEUROLOGICAL MANIFESTATIONS OF VERRUGA PERUANA (*OROYA FEVER; CARRION'S DISEASE; BARTONELLOSIS*)

Verruga peruana is a disease found in the valleys of the Andes and caused by infection with the organism *Bartonella bacilliformis*[1]. It is transmitted by the bite of female sandflies (*Phlebotomus* sp.), and presents in two distinct forms; the first an acute febrile episode associated with anaemia (Oroya fever[2]), and the second a cutaneous form, characterized by the appearance of haemorrhagic warty lesions (verruga peruana) [PLATES 32a and b]. In both forms, principally in the first, the nervous system may be affected. In the febrile stage of the illness the organism is found in large numbers in the red cells and in the cells of the reticulo-endothelial system. There is extensive haemolysis, cutaneous and mucosal haemorrhages, and enlargement of spleen,

[1] Barton described the causative bacillus in 1905–9 and it was named after him by Strong, on the Harvard expedition to Peru in 1913.

[2] Oroya is the terminal of the Trans-Andean Railway in Peru. In 1870, when the final section was being built from Callao, 7000 workers died from the disease which therefore came to be known as 'Oroya fever'. Carrion, a medical student in Lima in 1885, studied the geographical distribution of the disease and noted that only near Oroya was it endemic. He proved that the cutaneous and malignant forms of the disease were due to the same organism by subjecting himself to an injection of wart material from a patient with the typical skin eruption. He died of the disease 38 days later and left a classical account of the symptomatology of both phases of the illness. The medical faculty of San Fernando, Lima, is named after him, as are other hospitals in Latin America.

liver and lymph glands. The bone marrow is hyperplastic.

After a varying period the haemorrhagic phase of the disease subsides and cutaneous and mucosal eruptions appear, particularly on the face and limbs. They take the form of miliary nodules which appear in successive crops, often grouped together to form warty lesions, sometimes pedunculated, haemorrhagic, and liable to secondary infection with *Salmonella* organisms [PLATES 32a and b]. They also appear in the mesenchymal tissues of the viscera, including the nervous system.

The disease was known in the pre-Colombian period; the ancient Peruvians called it *sirki*, and it was frequently portrayed on their pottery. It is thought to have affected Pizarro's soldiers. Until the end of the nineteenth century only the warty form of this disease was recognized. In 1870 the form now known as Oroya fever was identified. This was a serious, febrile epidemic associated with haemolytic anaemia, which raged during the construction of the Lima–Oroya railway.

Since Carrion's day isolated cases with nervous complications have been reported, but it was not until 1932 that their importance and frequency was established by Monge and Mackehenie (1932). Since then numerous cases have been published and today the neurological syndromes which appear during the course of the two phases of the disease are known as 'neuro-bartonellosis'.

In recent years the disease has been found in the Andean valleys of Colombia and Ecuador and also in Honduras.

In endemic areas the inhabitants contract the disease in the benign form in childhood and acquire relative immunity. People from other areas contract the lethal form.

Bartonella bacilliformis is a parasite which is found in two forms: bacillary and coccoid. A rickettsial form in vascular endothelium and a viral phase in verrucomas have also been suspected. The parasite's reservoir is not known.

The Clinical Manifestations

Suspicion is aroused when it is known that the patient has come from or visited an endemic area. The onset is acute with fever and intense headache; there is vertigo, and muscular pains occur. Nervous system involvement nearly always occurs in the haemolytic phase, seldom in the intermediate or verruga phase. There is a meningo-encephalomyelitis characterized by impairment of consciousness, convulsions, cranial nerve palsies and perhaps indications of spinal and peripheral nerve involvement.

Headache is intense; pyramidal and cerebellar signs may appear. There may be focal signs but, in general, neurological manifestations are diffuse in character. These phenomena result from neural involvement which follows vascular damage, infiltrative and thrombotic lesions, diffuse or nodular glial proliferation, and granulomas. There is also neuronal loss consequent on ischaemia, anoxia and demyelination.

These nervous complications may develop during either phase of the illness, but they are much more frequent and serious in the first. Usually, this first stage lasts from 2 to 6 weeks and is followed shortly, or some weeks or months later, by the second phase. In most cases, in addition to intense headache there are joint and muscle pains, visual and auditory impairment and vestibular symptoms and signs. In some cases there are tremors, paraesthesiae, psychic symptoms, hallucinations, delirium and perhaps disturbance of consciousness, progressing to stupor and coma.

In general, bearing in mind the localization of the lesions we can speak of cerebral, spinal and peripheral types of cases.

The cerebral form is the most frequent and serious, usually presenting as a meningo-encephalitis. Meningeal involvement is variable. There are pure meningeal forms, usually of a favourable prognosis. Likewise, the picture may be one of pure encephalitis with or without convulsions.

Spinal forms are less common, presenting as a meningomyelitis with spastic or flaccid paralysis. The latter sometimes resembles an acute poliomyelitis and is due to a predominant involvement of the arterioles in the marginal sulcus of the spinal cord.

The peripheral forms usually appear in the second phase of the disease, during the eruptive warty period, and arise from formation of granulomas in the cranial and spinal nerves. Prognosis is good.

Acute psychiatric illness, with fever and delirium, is sometimes the sole manifestation of the invasion of the nervous system. It is usually fatal.

Laboratory Examinations

A thin blood smear stained with Giemsa or Romanovsky reveals the organism in the red cells during the febrile illness. *Bartonella* organisms are Gram-negative.

There is always an acute progressive anaemia; the red cell count may fall to less than 1 million. The anaemia is macrocytic and hypochromic.

Blood culture is positive at any stage and there may be healthy carriers in endemic areas. The *Bartonella* is readily cultured in gelose with blood, and it retains its vitality for a long time in citrated blood; it is mobile and shows flagella.

In the cerebrospinal fluid, protein, especially the globulin fraction, is raised and cells are increased; *Bartonella* may be found in the cells. Positive skin reactions may be useful in diagnosis.

Pathology

The first investigations were made by Monge and Mackehenie in 1932 and they pointed out the importance of the endothelial and vascular alterations in the pathogenesis of the neuronal manifestations. The *Bartonella* organisms live and multiply in endothelial cells and give rise to thrombosis by diapedesis and adventitial proliferation. In 1939, Mackehenie and Alzamora, and Mackehenie and Encinas described subependymal haemorrhages, proliferation of the cells of the ependyma, exudates, capillary thromboses and lesions of the choroid plexus. They demonstrated the severe lesions of the meninges and hemispheres, the granulomas formed by the accumulation of neuroglia cells and perivascular histiocytes.

We have been able to study the appearances in nine cases and to verify the observations of Mackehenie and Monge, and Encinas, who stressed the importance of the cerebrovascular network. To these vascular lesions are attributed the degenerative and inflammatory developments, the reactions of the neuroglia, as well as the mobilization of leucocytes and perivascular cells.

Ependymal–Choroidal Lesions

Various lesions are seen which reflect successive phases of a process affecting the ependyma; flattening of the epithelium, proliferation, warty formation, desquamation and subependymal infiltration, sometimes with a tendency to the formation of ependymal diverticuli.

In the tela chorioidea and choroid plexus there is a characteristic infiltration by histiocytes and fibroblasts, which extend to neighbouring ependymal zones and exceptionally may lead to the formation of a glio-epithelial verrucoma. This exceptional granulomatous process is highly characteristic and has not been hitherto described in the nervous parenchyma.

Meningovascular Lesions

In the leptomeninges, perivascular lesions, oedema, and haemorrhagic infiltrations can usually be seen [PLATE 32c]. Pial melanophores are abundant, many of them of abnormal appearance. Histochemical reactions reveal the presence of iron deposition in the meninges.

The vascular lesions are of a characteristic morphological aspect and resemble those found in other organs of the body. Venule thrombosis is a feature: there are microhaemorrhages, adventitial proliferation and, exceptionally, capillary neoformation. Vessels of small calibre are mainly affected.

Neuronal Lesions

There is subacute neuronal degeneration, consequent on ischaemia, thrombosis and anaemia [PLATE 32d]. Rarely there are features of acute Nissl and Spielmeyer degeneration.

Ganglion elements are affected in various ways according to their peculiar morphology and function. The motor neurones atrophy, sometimes with Nissl protoplasmic hyperchromia without chromatolysis. Proprioceptive sensory elements suffer less, with an increase of nuclear eccentricity. Similar changes, but more marked ones, are seen in the cells of the vegetative system. Signs of microscopic necrobiosis with cellular rarefaction can be observed in the neighbourhood of thrombosed arterioles.

Glial Lesions

Lesions of the neuroglia have a varied morphopathology [PLATES 32d and e]. There is a constant subependymal gliosis with predominance of fibrotic astrocytes, many of which are hypertrophic; there is perivascular, fibroglial proliferation, marginal astrocytic fibrogliosis and oligodendroglial hyperplasia. Sometimes there is neuronal satellitosis. Microglia are hyperactive and may collect in bands or nodes. This glial proliferation, an essentially reactive phenomenon, is usually diffuse but may be nodular in distribution, a feature of some diagnostic significance.

Verrucomas

These arise in the nervous system, *sui generis*, and are composed of cells similar to fibroblasts or microgliocytic rods, in a fibrillary network admixed with histiocytes [PLATE 33a].

Presence of Bartonella in Brain

Erythrocyte parasitosis is striking; it generally reaches 90 per cent and at times 100 per cent. Thirty or more *Bartonella* may be found in one red cell. Together with endothelium parasitosis, capillary thrombosis and breaching of the blood–brain barrier, it explains the passage of *Bartonella* to the cerebral parenchyma and the reactive microglial nodular response.

Pathogenesis

It is possible that in large epidemics and after repeated passage of *Bartonella* in man, germ virulence increases or its visceral tropism is modified. Brain tissue responses may be altered as well as modification of the blood–brain barrier. Both factors of seed and soil may be involved.

Cerebral and spinal vessels carry the *Bartonella*, the parasitosed erythrocytes, products of disintegration of haemoglobin, and toxins of microbial and catabolic origin. All these factors are potentially pathogenic for the nervous system. Anoxia may result in several ways.

The meningo-encephalitis of Carrion belongs to the group of secondary encephalites of Mollaret and Schneider (1963): 'An encephalitis is secondary when it represents, not the illness itself nor a localized form, but an inconstant or exceptional complication of an illness which is perfectly autonomous'. The encephalitis is produced by the response of the vascular and reticulo-endothelial system to the invasion of the erythrocyte and its multiplication. Angiitis rather than embolism is the chief process by which the brain is implicated.

Prognosis and Treatment

There is no specific treatment, but before the antibiotic era the prognosis of verruga peruana in general and of neurobartonellosis in particular was reserved. The introduction of penicillin, and then of tetracyclines, hexacyclines, and chloramphenicol, reduced mortality and the duration of the disease. But not every case is cured. Even with modern therapy the appearance of a neurological disorder affects the outlook. This will depend on the general condition of the patient, the form of the illness, the promptness of treatment and the phase in which nervous symptoms arise. The latter are more serious in the first phase of infection.

The encephalitic form is the more dangerous and in spite of antibiotics it has the higher mortality. Convulsions and delirium are grave omens. Spinal forms have a better prognosis in regard to life but may leave invaliding disabilities. Peripheral nerve lesions tend to be chronic but not disabling; recovery is the rule.

References

BARTON, A. L. (1905) Cuerpos endoglobulares en la sangre verrucosa, *Gac. Hosp.*, 2, 46.

LASTRES, J. B. (1945) Formas comiciales de la verruga peruana, *Rev. Neuro-psiquiat.*, 8, 563–74.

LASTRES, J. B. (1945) *Las Neurobartonelosis*, Lima.

LASTRES, J. B., and ANGLAS, O. (1943) Sindrome de paraplejia espàstica en la verruga peruana, *Rev. Neuro-psiquiat.* **6**, 192–204.

MACKEHENIE, D., and ALZAMORA, V. (1939) Las lesiones anatómicas del sistema nervioso en la enfermedad de Carrión, *II Jornadas Neuro-psiquiát. Panamer.*, 2, 166–73.

MACKEHENIE, D., and ENCINAS, E. (1939) Acerca de un caso de verruga benigna complicada, *II Jornadas Neuro-psiquiát. Panamer.*, 2, 47–55.

MALDONADO, A. (1931) La verruga de los conquistadores del Perú, *Crón. méd. (Lima)*, 48, 820.

MENDEZ, M., and ANGLAS, P. (1940) Sindrome de poliomielitis anterior agudo en el curso de la enfermedad de Carrión, *Rev. Neuro-psiquiat.* 3, 88–93.

MOLLARET, P., and SCHNEIDER, J. (1963) Classification épidemiologique et virologique des encephalites humaines, *Rev. neurol.*, 108, No. 3, 225–65.

MONGE, C., and MACKEHENIE, D. (1932) Formas neurológicas de la Verruga, *Rev. méd. peru.*, 48, 523–50.

ODRIOZOLA, E. (1898) *La Maladie de Carrión ou la Verruga Peruvienne*, Paris.

REBAGLIATI, R. (1940) *Verruga Peruana*, Lima.

RICKETTS, G. (1943) *La Verruga Peruana*, Tésis de la Facultad de Medicina, Lima.

STRONG, R. P. (1930) *Report of the First Expedition to South America*, Boston, Mass (first published 1915).

TRELLES, J. O. (1955) Aspects neurologiques de la verruga péruvienne, *Rev. neurol.*, 93, 1, 357–68.

TRELLES, J. O., and ARANIBAR, Z. (1958) Las formas poliomielíticas de la verruga peruana, *An. Fac. Méd. (Lima)*, 41, 211–22.

TRELLES, J. O., PALOMINO, L., and TRELLES, L. (1968) Formas neurológicas de la enfermedad de Carrión, *Rev. Neuro-psiquiat.*, 32, No. 4, 245–306.

TRELLES, J. O., ROEDENBECK, S. D., and POLLACK, F. (1952) Contribución a la histopatología de la neurobartenelosis in *Congreso International de Neuropsiquiatria*, Vol. II, Santiago.

TRELLES, L. (1968) *Contribución a la Histopatología de la Neurobartonelosis*, Tesis de Lima.

VARGAS, FANO, J. A. (1938) Fuentes Históricas en el Estudio de la Enfermedad de Carrión, *Bol. Inform As. méd. peru. 'Daniel A. Carrión'*, 6, 18.

VEGA, G. DE LA (1944) *Historia General de Perú*, Buenos Aires.

WEISS, P. (1927) Hacia una concepción de la verruga peruana, *An. Fac. Méd. (Lima)*.

WEISS, P. (1932) Contribución al estudio de la verruga peruana o enfermedad de Carrión, *Rev. méd. peru.*, 37–38, 5–25, 55–70.

WEISS, P. (1952) Verruga du Pérou, *Encyclopédie Médico-Chirurgicale*, Paris.

NEUROCYSTICERCOSIS

The embryo of the *Taenia solium* is responsible for one of the most frequent and lethal parasitic diseases of Latin America. The study of cerebral cysticercosis is exceptionally interesting and very essential because of the extraordinary diffusion of the parasite, the problems of diagnosis, the seriousness of prognosis, and the inefficacy of treatment.

History

Known from most remote times in the pig, this disease seems to be the reason why this animal was excluded from the dietary of some Oriental countries: the Jews abstain from it and the Koran forbids it. In man, it was first described by Rumler in 1558 and its parasitic nature was determined by Malpighi in 1696.

Rudolphi called it *Cysticercus cellulosae* because of its common location in connective tissues. Van Beneden, in 1853, proved the relationship between the cysticercus and *Taenia solium*, and Zenker (1886) recognized the racemose variety (*Cysticercus racemosus*).

It was described in Argentina in 1875, in Brazil in 1881 and in Peru in 1945. Many workers in South America have studied and written about the disease in man including Tretiakoff, Pachecho, and Silva (1924), Monteiro Salles (1934), Oswaldo Lange (1935), Dimitri y Balado and Brinck and it has been systematically studied by Trelles and his colleagues for some years.

Aetiology

Frequency and Geographical Distribution

In general, cysticercosis has a worldwide distribution, mainly in countries where pork is eaten and where hygiene and sanitation are poor.

It was common in Europe until the beginning of this century as can be verified by Vosgien's thesis (1911) which was based on 800 cases. It is now rare in Europe but is still reported from Poland, Rumania, Russia, Spain and Portugal.

In Africa it is rare among Moslems. Proctor (1961), in South Africa, in an autopsy survey involving 7597 autopsies, found 71 cases of infestation by tapeworms, approximately 1 per cent; most of them were cases of cysticercosis.

In Asia, it is endemic, and it is said to be frequent in India and relatively frequent in China and Indo-China.

In North America, it is rare in Canada and the United States, but in Mexico recent statistics show a high incidence: Nieto's report (1956) was based on 168 cases; Lombardo and Mateos (1961) found it responsible for about 11 per cent of admissions to the Neurological Institute.

In Brazil, Canelas (1961) reported 276 cases of neurocysticercosis registered at the Neurological Department at São Paulo in 15 years. In Chile, Asenjo (1961) reported 145 cases seen at the Neurological Institute in 25 years. Our series comprises 77 verified cases; 27 men and 50 women.

The Parasite

Human cysticercosis is caused almost exclusively by the larvae *Cysticercus cellulosae* of *Taenia solium*.

The biological cycle of this parasite has three stages: man, pig, man. The adult *Taenia* enters the man's intestine; the expelled larvae are developed in the pig; and then man is again infested by eating pork.

The Adult Taenia. This is a segmented tapeworm, usually 2 or 3 metres in length, but sometimes as long as 8 metres. It lives in the small intestine often for several years; it consists of head, neck and body. The head is slightly thicker than the body, 2 to 3 mm in diameter and provided with four circular suckers and 25 to 50 hooks. The neck is thin, without segmentation. The body is the portion of the worm which is enormously developed and is formed by a series of rings or proglottides. Each ring has both male and female reproductive organs which perform their own fertilization; once this process is ended, the mature ring is eliminated together with others in groups of four or five; each ring encloses many (500 to 600) six-edged embryos or oncospheres, protected by several wrappings which disappear, with the exception of one, the embryophore. The embryo, 20 μ in length, is provided with four pairs of hooks; it readily changes shape to facilitate its passage through the body. It is strongly resistant to exposure and from its habitual host, the pig, it is ready to infest man and reach the adult stage.

The Cyst. Called specifically *Cysticercus cellulosae*, the cyst constitutes a new stage of the *Taenia's* cycle. Essentially it is formed by a hydropic vesicle, of variable size, with an invaginated scolex. Like the adult *Taenia*, it also has a neck, body and head, the latter provided with rostrum, suckers and hooks (24 to 32). The head and neck are folded and spiral, submerged in a magma of connective tissue which fills the invagination cavity, or receptaculum capitis. The sucker is rounded or ovoid, semitransparent, and of opaline appearance, containing a clear liquid. The size varies from very small vesicles to giant ones.

The *Cysticercus racemosus* is a particular type found in the basal cisterns of the brain, in the ventricles, and in the spinal cord, but rarely elsewhere. It consists of enormous vesicles of strange capricious morphology showing strangulations and ramifications, commonly without scolex. They may reach a considerable size; 8, 10 or 15 cm.

Modes of Infestation

The accepted view is that the ova are swallowed, and in the stomach the gastric juice liberates the embryo which penetrates the gastric and intestinal mucosa, enters the blood stream and is disseminated throughout the body.

The commonest modes of infestation are:

1. Contamination of food (usually vegetables) or water with viable ova from human excreta.
2. Accidental contamination by poor hygienic habits; anus–finger–mouth.
3. In *Taenia* carriers, massive infestation (in one of our cases there were more than 700 cysticerci in the brain) by reverse peristalsis may deposit ova in the stomach, where gastric juices release the embryos.
4. Proctor (1961) showed that among the Bantu herbalists frequently employ tapeworm proglottides in the preparation of certain medicines.

The Clinical Manifestations

There are few diseases of the central nervous system which show so many puzzling clinical pictures as cerebral cysticercosis. Because of its polymorphous symptomatology, cysticercosis may simulate many different neurological and psychiatric disorders. Such a variability depends on numerous factors, such as the number, size and location of vesicles, the kind of cysticercus, racemose or cystic, their toxic and perhaps allergic properties, not to mention the different reactions to the parasitic lesions by brain tissues.

Cerebral Cysticercosis

There is no symptom pathognomonic of cerebral cysticercosis. The association of so many and varied factors makes it difficult to classify symptoms in an adequate manner and to delineate syndromes which assist in diagnosis and prognosis. However, three groups of phenomena constitute the basis of all clinical events; intracranial hypertension, convulsions, and mental disorders. In addition to these main syndromes there are many additional minor and inconstant symptoms.

The intracranial hypertension has some special features. The onset is often not acute as in infections, nor does it increase progressively as in tumours. For long periods the headache of cysticercosis may be intermittent and then it may become very severe. For a long period it may be the only symptom of the disease. When the intracranial hypertension reaches a peak, vomiting and papilloedema ensue. However, in ventricular cysticercosis the onset may be acute, with severe headache and the rapid development of papilloedema.

Analysis of epileptic seizures may disclose features suggestive of cysticercosis. These may be patients without a family history of epilepsy and with late onset of fits. Seizures are usually focal at onset and the interval between two seizures may be as long as 15 years. Myoclonic and sensory auras are frequently observed. Loss of consciousness in fits usually occurs later. The psychic disturbances common in idiopathic epilepsy are usually lacking.

However, mental disorders are frequently seen, especially in the racemose type of the disease. Amnesia, for example, may be mild and transitory at the onset, but as time passes other symptoms make their appearance, such as disorientation in time and space; the mental picture may be indistinguishable from simple dementia. Affective disorders are also common. The mental symptoms may be more conspicuous than the neurological ones and dominate the clinical picture.

These three groups of phenomena: intracranial hypertension, epileptic attacks, and mental disorders, constitute the fundamental symptomatology of cysticercosis. In some cases, the symptomatology is heightened by the frequency and severity of reactive vascular lesions. The predominance of one of the main symptoms determines the clinical form of the illness. Sometimes there is a definite form but at other times it is transitional.

Spinal Cysticercosis

From the clinical point of view, spinal cysticercosis must be considered according to two topographical aspects:

1. Its extra- or intramedullary location.
2. Its cervical, dorsal or lumbar location.

In either case the symptomatology is similar to a compressive process determined by the level of the lesion and producing long tract and radicular symptoms. As we are dealing with a generalized infestation there are often additional symptoms of cerebral and meningeal involvement.

The longitudinal topography is interesting for nearly all spinal cases are of cervical location.

Clinical Pathology

The diagnosis of cysticercosis is facilitated by examination of blood and cerebrospinal fluid. It must be remembered that cysticercosis is a disease of long evolution with accesses of activity. Immuno-allergic reactions in blood and cerebrospinal fluid may be absent for long periods at a time.

Blood. Moderate leucocytosis may be present; diagnostic significance depends on the degree of eosinophilia: it is of moderate value when eosinophilia is 5 to 12 per cent; when it is 15 to 28 per cent, however, its diagnostic value is high.

In our first 33 cases, 24 were carefully investigated and a moderate eosinophilia (6 per cent to 12 per cent) was found in nine cases.

The complement-fixation reaction, especially in cerebrospinal fluid, is of some value.

Cerebrospinal Fluid. This is always affected to some degree in neurocysticercosis. The changes must be systematically sought because of their diagnostic value. There is increase of protein content, albumin and globulin fractions; a pleocytosis which is predominantly eosinophil; abnormal colloidal gold curves and benzoin reactions: positive complement-fixation reactions.

The different techniques of applying the Weinberg complement reaction to cysticercosis are described by Monteiro Salles (1934), Lange (1935), and others.

Spina-França (1961) has reported the most important alterations of the CSF in 62 cases. In 40 the pleocytosis ranged from 10 to 266 per c mm; of these only in 23 was there an eosinophilia, ranging from 2 per cent to 30 per cent.

Radiology

Neuroradiological studies are important. A plain radiograph of the skull may indicate the presence of intracranial hypertension. In 25 per cent of Peruvian cases abnormal calcifications are seen. Pneumoencephalography may disclose dilatation of the ventricular system and obliteration of the basal cisterns. Posterior fossa signs are less common. In some instances spherical images may be seen in the ventricles as well as in the cisterns. Angiographic findings are less significant, being only those of bilateral hydrocephalus or of posterior fossa type.

In spinal cysticercosis lumbar puncture may demonstrate a positive Queckenstedt test and CSF analysis may resemble that of tumour compression. Pneumomyelography may demonstrate filling defects.

Pathology of Cerebral Cysticercosis

Because of its presence, its toxin, and the products of its disintegration, the parasite produces defensive and inflammatory reactions in nervous tissue, generally localized, but sometimes spreading some distance, causing a panencephalomeningitis. The parasite itself undergoes changes which are determined by the reactions of the brain; it eventually dies, degenerates or calcifies.

The cysts of cysticercosis are located mainly in the cortex and the meninges [PLATES 33b and c]. They are often seen in the ventricles where they may reach considerable size, or in the brain stem.

In the cystic form, the cysticercus may be observed in its different stages, either as young small vesicles, as bigger adult bladderworms, or finally as dead vesicles which may be disintegrating while others are already calcified.

Racemose cysticercosis is most frequently noted in the cisterna chiasmatica or in the region of the brain stem [Plate 34a]. It may also infiltrate the Sylvian fissure, sometimes penetrating into the ventricles through Bichat's fissure, or into the cisterna magna, invading the fourth ventricle; it can even extend down to the spinal cord [Plates 34c and 35]. Its growth produces mechanical compression.

Macroscopic Anatomy

Affected convolutions are flattened; sometimes they appear prominent due to the distension produced by an underlying vesicle. Sectioning discloses these features more clearly, as well as revealing thinning of grey matter in some areas, a result of compression by a cyst. In some cases, small well-circumscribed haemorrhagic foci are found. They are diffusely spread with no preferential localization.

The ventricular cavities often contain cysts; they are deformed and distended, and the ependymal lining shows irregularities and, not rarely, a granulous ependymitis. In most cases the choroidal membranes and plexus are enlarged and congested, presenting a granular appearance.

The leptomeninges are opaque and thickened, especially in the racemose form in which the adherent arachnoiditis of the basal cisterns involves the cranial nerves. The parasitic vesicles may be visible on the surface of the brain.

Histology

Few conditions show patterns of such intense, varied and neat lesions along the entire cerebrospinal axis, involving all its component tissues, as does neurocysticercosis.

The neural lesions are either of a mechanical kind affecting cells or vessels and leading to degenerative changes, or they are inflammatory in character—a true cysticercous encephalitis. Axonal lesions are relatively slight, consequent on the cytological lesions rather than primary, except in the relatively rare cases of cerebral necrobiosis.

The defensive reactions are shown in proliferation of ectodermal glia as well as by intense mobilization of microglia and an increase of perivascular connective tissue.

The Parasite. On section the cysticercus presents two aspects: the body and the vesicular wall.

1. *The body* of the parasite in longitudinal sections appears with many skin folds. The head shows a face with hooks implanted in a double crown formed by an amorphous substance which stains very poorly, and the suckers, like a horseshoe, formed by a layer of large cells with central nuclei.

Three layers are noted in the body of the parasite:

(a) A cuticular external layer.
(b) A middle layer of a pseudo-epithelial appearance.
(c) A third layer with longitudinal and circular muscular fibres.

Inside there is loose connective tissue which also surrounds the body and fills the invagination cavity.

The appearance of the parasite varies according to its age and its state of preservation. Young parasites show clearly the histological features of the organs; old ones have an amorphous appearance and uniform coloration, and show impregnation with fat and calcium salts. If the process of destruction is intense it is difficult to identify the cysticercus; it may resemble a gummatous nodule or some other amorphous pathological formation. In many cases the cuticular membrane resists the process of degeneration, facilitating the diagnosis, but in other cases the cuticular membrane disappears completely.

2. *The vesicular membrane.* It was formerly thought that this was only a limiting, protective membrane and of little interest. However, Trelles and Ravens (1953) pointed out the complex texture of this membrane with its rich ciliary layer; it is highly canalized and possesses digestive ampullae. Their observations indicate the functional importance of these structures [Plate 36a].

The electron microscopic investigations of Martinez (1961) have yielded further details of the rich structure of this ciliary layer.

Tissue Reaction. When the cysticercus lodges in nervous tissue an inflammatory reaction takes place around it [Plate 34d]. The organism reacts against the injury by forming a connective tissue membrane isolating it. The membrane is made up of three concentric layers. The inner one, which is in contact with the parasite, has a fenestrated aspect and contains epithelioid cells, leucocytes, polynuclear cells, fat-containing macrophages, and sometimes multinucleated giant cells. The middle layer is essentially fibrocollagenous, with rare plasma cells and lymphocytes, the fibrosis is more severe when the parasite is older. The third layer contains blood vessels and cells; it is the mesodermal tissue which contains some eosinophils, occasional multinucleated cells, and abundant plasma cells. According to Urechia (1937), a fourth layer of astrocytic gliosis or pericystic defensive membrane may be present. It is made up of nets of argentophile fibrils which penetrate into the parenchyma, becoming part of the defensive membrane spreading from neighbouring vessels to the parasite [Plate 36b].

Meningeal Lesions. The leptomeninges show inflammatory lesions of an infiltrative type, with mononuclear cells, especially macrophages, some eosinophils, and thick precollagenous and collagenous fibres. There is marginal gliosis in the adjacent cortex. In cases in which the cysticercus is near the surface, the capsule is atypical with predominant mesenchymal proliferation [Plate 35a].

Over the convexity of the brain, the sclerotic reaction is less severe than at the base, although it always contains lymphocytic infiltration. Racemose cysticercosis frequently obliterates the subarachnoid spaces.

Vascular Lesions. Meningeal vessels show hyperplastic reactions in their walls and are rarely obliterated; capillaries show degeneration. The cranial nerves frequently show slight inflammatory signs.

All blood vessels are affected by this inflammatory process. Vessels nearer the cysts present endarterial proliferation which produces obliteration, hypertrophic sclerosis of the media of the artery, and adventitial infiltration. In advanced cases hyaline degeneration and the beginning of a parietal necrosis can be seen. The lymphocytic adventitial infiltration which is adjacent to the parasite sometimes extends for a certain distance, decreasing in severity, and gitter cells can often be seen in it. In other severe chronic cases the endarteritis is frankly fibrous and the media and adventitia are hyalinized. An absence of infiltrating phenomena reminds one of chronic vascular syphilis.

The racemose type of cysticercosis involves the basilar artery and its branches; thromboses are frequent. This is also true of the veins, although the alterations are less severe than those of the arteries.

Ependymal and Choroidal Lesions. The ventricular ependyma shows both diffuse and localized lesions caused by the cysts, which may be either free or adherent to its surface. The racemose type invades the ventricles and the epithelium shows clear signs of granular ependymitis, with fibroglial subependymal hyperplasia. The choroid plexuses are often oedematous and contain vascular lesions.

Glial Lesions. All the glial elements present hyperplastic or degenerative alterations. The most severe reaction is in the immediate neighbourhood of the parasite. In that area the protoplasmic and fibrillary astrocytic proliferation is dense and localized around the cyst. It forms the defensive pericystic membrane which arises near the granulation tissue. This reaction decreases in severity from the cysts to the parenchyma.

In the acute form of the disease the microglia act as phagocytes or degenerate. The oligodendroglia, which usually degenerate, sometimes react with moderate satellitosis in some areas of the cortex.

Neuronal Alterations. The cells are disordered and their stratification is considerably modified in the zones near the cysts. All stages of degeneration, up to neuronal disintegration, can be seen including shrunken cells, cells in granular tigrolysis, evidence of neuronophagia, and areas of cytolysis. Acute Nissl degeneration even with nucleus involvement has been observed in recent cases.

In areas of cortical lesions, the axons present diffuse demyelination, even at a certain distance from the cysts. The mesenchymal phagocytes are full of lipoids, and cholesterol crystals in giant cells have also been described.

Pathogenesis

The cysticercus embryo is invaginated inside the cyst and has no contact with its host. In the invagination zone a pore of communication with the inner digestive cavity is observed; in front of this pore the most important reactive pericystic zone is established, and it is here that the most active and intense granulation of tissue is found. In younger vesicles hardly any reactive zone may be observed in nervous tissue.

If the cysticercus cannot derive nourishment directly from nervous tissue, how and where does it obtain it in order to live? It gets it exclusively through the nutrient activity of the vesicular membrane. This membrane constitutes the close contact between parasite and host tissue: nourishment is passed on to the vesicular fluid. This membrane is the one which serves for its maintenance, ensuring its life and parasitic potency. It is only when it is ingested by the definitive host that it sheds its covers, fixes itself to the intestine wall with its hooks and nourishes itself directly, and develops into its definitive form, the tapeworm.

This fundamental activity of the cystic membrane in the larval state of the cysticercus may be appreciated by observing the evolution undergone by the cyst. In the brain all degrees of image may be found corresponding to the different stages of disintegration of the cysticercus, up to its cicatricial glioconnective or lipocalcareous transformation. At the start, one can observe the disintegration of the membrane from the outside to the inside, from the ciliary layer towards the inner fibrocanalicular layer. In parallel, turbidity of the fluid is observed. In a more advanced stage the vesicular membrane disintegrates, the vesicular fluid coagulates and precipitates. Turbidity is thus increased and disintegration of the parasite begins.

Diagnosis

The diagnosis of neurocysticercosis is nearly always a difficult matter. In the intracranial hypertensive form it resembles a tumour; in the convulsive form it may be confused with all causes of acquired epilepsy; some cases simulate an encephalitis or a psychosis. In regions where it is not frequent, eosinophilia in blood or, more importantly, in the CSF is helpful. Serum and CSF complement fixation and radiological examinations are necessary.

Because of its frequency in Peru neurologists are alert to the disease, although well-defined clinical pictures cannot be categorized. Of the 33 cases which I reported with Rocca and Ravens in 1952, laboratory tests, blood and spinal fluid examinations, skull roentgenograms, pneumoencephalograms, arteriograms, iodoventriculograms, and electroencephalograms permitted us to make a diagnosis in the majority. However, in some cases the condition is a surprise finding on craniotomy or at autopsy.

In these 33 cases skull radiography revealed interesting signs: decalcification, bulging of the posterior fossa, and Schüller impressions. The latter indicated intracranial hypertension in 19 of our cases. Pathological calcifications were present in four cases.

Ventriculograms were performed in 19 patients and showed absence, or reduced filling of the basal cisterns, ventricular displacement, hydrocephalus and partial occlusion of the fourth ventricle and cisterna magna. A pneumoencephalogram was performed in two cases without papilloedema and did not reveal the characteristic findings. In one case in which iodoventriculogeaphy was performed, we noted the typical 'bell' image caused by the involvement of the fourth ventricle. In two cases internal carotid arteriograms were performed, and showed a narrowing of the arterial system. A vertebral arteriogram in another case revealed distortion of the basilar and posterior inferior cerebellar arteries. Electroencephalograms showed slow waves of low voltage in three patients.

Prognosis and Treatment

Cysticersosis follows an extremely variable clinical course. In many cases long periods of remission are the rule while in others death occurs suddenly, when least expected. Spontaneous cures by calcification or lipoid disintegration are possible. But in the great majority of cases the disease leads to physical and mental deterioration and finally to death. The disease is one of the most serious cerebral disorders.

Spinal cysticercosis, from the clinical point of view as well as the anatomical, shows a slow evolution and a relative respect for the structure and function of the spinal tissues, so that prognosis is less grave.

No known clinical treatment, including radiotherapy, is of use at the present time. We have tried male fern (oleoresin of Aspidium), the sulphonamides, cortisone and other adrenocorticoids—all without avail.

Today, surgical treatment is the only method that offers hope and then only in cases of cystic cysticercosis. The racemose form is not amenable to surgery. Hydrocephalus produced by obstruction of the aqueduct can be temporarily alleviated by ventriculostomy. If the patient has cystic cysticercosis the success of surgery depends mainly on the number and localization of the cysts. Spinal cysts can often be removed.

References

ARANA, R., and ASENJO, A. (1950) Ventriculographic diagnosis of cysticercosis of the posterior fossa, *J. Neurosurg.*, 2, 181–90.

ASENJO, A. (1961) Neurocisticercosis, *Neurocirugia*, 19, 143.

BERNALES, S., and ENCINAS, E. (1943) Cisticercosis cerebral con sintomatología del àngulo pontocerebeloso, *Rev. Neuro-psiquiat.*, 6, 1–57.

BICKERSTAFF, E. P., BRODIE, H., CLOAKE, P. C. P., and SMITH, W. J. (1952) The racemose form of cerebral cysticercosis, *Brain*, **75**, 1–18.

CANELAS, H. M. (1961) Neurocysticercosis: its incidence, diagnosis, and clinical forms, in *Tropical Neurology*, eds. van Bogaert, L., Pereyra-Kafer, J., and Poch, G. F., Buenos Aires, pp. 149–61.

CUADRA, M. (1949) Cisticercosis cerebral y eosinofilia en L.R., *Rev. Neuro-psiquiat.*, **12**, 339–66.

FISCHER, W. (1955) Die parasitaren Erkrankungen des zentralnervenssystems und seiner Hüllen, in *Handb. spez. Path. Anat. Histol.*, Berlin.

GUCCIONE, A. (1919) *La Cisticerocosis del Sistema Nervioso Centrale Umano*, Milan.

INSAUSTI, T. (1950) Cisticercosis cerebral, *Neuropsiquiatría*, 1, 269–98.

LANGE, O. (1935) Sobre as cellulas eosinofilas de L.C.R., *Rev. Neurol. Psiquiat. S. Paulo*, 1, 421–34.

LOMBARDO, L., and MATEOS, J. H. (1961) Cerebral cysticercosis in Mexico, *Neurology (Minneap.)*, 11, 828.

MARTINEZ, A. (1961) Anatomía patológica de la cisticercosis cerebral, *Neurology (Minneap.)*, 11, 173–90.

MONTEIRO SALLES, F. (1934) *Cysticercose Cerebral*, Thesis, São Paulo.

NIETO, D. (1956) Cysticercosis of the nervous system, *Neurology (Minneap.)*, **6**, 725.

OBRADOR, S. (1948) Clinical aspects of cerebral cysticercosis, *Arch. Neurol. Psychiat. (Chic.)*, 59, 457–68.

OBRADOR, S. (1962) Cysticercosis cerebri, *Acta neurochir. (Wien)*, 10, 3, 320.

PINTO PUPPO, P., CARDOSO, W., DOS REIS, J. B., and DA SILVA, P. (1945) Sobre a cisticercosis encefálica, *Arch. Assit. Psicop.*, 10/11, 1–123.

PROCTOR, N. S. F. (1961) Problems associated with tapeworm cyst infestation of the central nervous system, in *Tropical Neurology*, Buenos Aires, p. 140.

RAVENS, R. (1950) *Contribución a la Histoparasitología del Cysticercus Cellulosae y Cisticercus Racemosus*, Thesis, Lima.

SCHMITE, P. (1928) *Les Cysticercoses du Nevraxe*, Thesis, Paris.

SPINA-FRANÇA, A. (1956) Cisticercose do sistema nervoso central, *Rev. paul. Med.*, 48–59.

SPINA-FRANÇA, A. (1961) Biological aspects of neurocysticercosis: alterations in the cerebrospinal fluid, in *Tropical Neurology*, eds. van Bogaert, L., Pereyra-Käfer, J., and Poch, G. F., Buenos Aires, pp. 183–97.

TRELLES, J. O. (1961) Cerebral cysticercosis, *Wld Neurol.*, 2, 488–97.

TRELLES, J. O. (1962) Importance de la membrane kystique dans la pathogenie de la cysticercose cerebrale, in *Libre Jubilaire Prof. van Bogaert*, Bruxelles, pp. 826–28.

TRELLES, J. O., and LAZARTE, J. (1941) *La Cisticercosis Cerebral, Monografía Rev. Neuro-psiquiat*, Lima.

TRELLES, J. O., and PALOMINO, L. (1961) Histopathology of cerebral cysticercosis, in *Tropical Neurology*, eds. van Bogaert, L., Pereyra-Käfer, J., and Poch, G. F., Buenos Aires, pp. 162–82.

TRELLES, J. O., PALOMINO, L., and CACERES, A. (1967) Histopathologie de la cysticercose cérebrale, *Acta neuropath. (Berl.)*, 8, 115–32.

TRELLES, J. O., and RAVENS, R. (1953) Estudios de neurocisticercosis: II. Lesiones vasculares, meníngeas, ependimarias y neuroglicas, *Rev. Neuro-psiquiat.*, 16, 241–71.

TRELLES, J. O., ROCCA, E., and RAVENS, R. (1952) Estudios de neurocisticercosis: I. Sobre la fina estructura de la membrana vesicular quística y racemosa. Deducciones patológicas, *Rev. Neuro-psiquiat.*, 15, 1–35.

TRELLES, J. O., and ROEDENBECK, S. D. (1954) Estudios sobre la neurocisticercosis: III. Formas clínicas poco frecuentes de cisticercosis cerebral, *Rev. Neuro-psiquiat.*, 17, 1.

TRETIAKOFF, C., PACHECO, E., and SILVA, C. A. (1924) Contribucao para estudio da cysticercose cerebral e em particulier das lesoes cerebraes toxicas a distancia nesta affeccao, *Mem. Hosp. Juquery* (*S. Paulo*), 1, 37–66.

URECHIA, C. I. (1937) Sur quelques cas de cysticercose du systéme nerveux, *Bull. Acad. Méd. Roum.*, 2, 19.

VOSGIEN, W. (1911) *Cysticercus Cellulosae chez l'Homme et les Animaux*, Thesis, Paris.

WEIMANN, W. (1930) *Cysticercus und Hirnparasiten: die Anatomie der Psychosen*, Berlin, p. 145. Vol. VII.

31 Chagas' Disease and the Nervous System

A. SPINA-FRANÇA and L. C. MATTOSINHO-FRANÇA

Chagas' disease is caused by *Trypanosoma cruzi* (Chagas, 1909), a protozoan flagellate transmissible to humans and other animals, usually by haematophagous Hemiptera of the Triatominae subfamily. Chagas' disease is also designated American trypanosomiasis, or trypanosomiasis cruzi. Within the general clinical picture neurological changes are observed. These are due to involvement of various parts of the nervous system, both as acute lesions and as sequelae.

The clinical features, the aetiological agent, the vector and natural reservoirs were all described by Carlos Chagas at the beginning of this century. His studies began in 1907, extending through 1920. Other research associates in the same general project supplemented Chagas' observations, regarding the parasitology and morbid anatomy (Vianna, Neiva, Magarinos Torres), the clinical aspects (Villela), haematology (Dias) and immunological diagnosis (Guerreiro and Machado). The initial basic knowledge of the disease cycle was complemented by Mayer and Rocha Lima, and by Brumpt. Subsequently, the aetiological agent was identified in several Latin-American countries, but with little emphasis on the identification of the disease in its various clinical forms. This was in great part due to the fact that many of the late, chronic manifestations of the disease were not recognized to be a consequence of this parasitosis, especially the chronic nervous form of the disease. From 1930 on, interest in the disease increased with the publication of the researches of the Argentinian (Romaña, Mazza, Niño), Uruguayan (Talice), Chilean (Neghme), Venezuelan (Pifano, Torrealba) and Brazilian schools (Dias, Laranja). Since then, a considerable literature has accumulated on the several aspects of the disease, mainly published by Latin-American researchers.

In this chapter, with its neurological orientation, general data on the incidence, geographical distribution, pathogenesis and laboratory diagnosis of the disease will first be presented before an account is given of the neurological aspects. The bibliographical references, although mainly in Portuguese and Spanish, will permit the reader to obtain more detailed information.

INCIDENCE AND GEOGRAPHICAL DISTRIBUTION

Involving humans and certain mammals, Chagas' disease is a zoonosis whose distribution corresponds to the spread of Triatominae adapted to human dwellings. The disease predominates in rural settings, where the houses are of adobe construction; the crevices of walls and roofing serve as the habitat of the Triatominae.

Triatominae are found in the Americas, Africa, Asia and the East Indies. Animal infection by *T. cruzi* has been reported in monkeys from Java and India. Triatominae adapted to human dwellings have only been described in the Americas. They are found between parallels 42° N and 43° S, and adaptation to houses is observed between parallels 25° N and 38° S. Human infection is largely restricted to these limits. Exceptions are British Guiana, Surinam and the Amazon Basin, where although no human cases have yet been reported infected animals, including domestic ones, have been recognized.

In South America Chagas' disease has great medical importance, due to its high incidence in rural areas among low socio-economic groups. In general, 20 per cent of the rural population of Argentina have the disease, with an incidence of 12 to 14 per cent in Chile, 8 to 15 per cent in Uruguay and 8·5 to 60 per cent in Brazil (Romaña, 1961).

AETIOLOGY AND LIFE-CYCLE

The parasite *Trypanosoma cruzi* (*Schizotrypanum cruzi*) is an elongated, tapering flagellate, with a central, ovoid nucleus, an anterior flagellum and a rounded, posterior kinetoplast. This is formed by a parabasal portion and a blepharoplast. From this originates the flagellum axonema, which borders the nucleus, delimiting an undulating membrane and emerging at the anterior end as a free flagellum. In its biological evolution, the parasite assumes all the morphological aspects of the genus, namely leishmania, leptomonas, crithidia and trypanosoma.

The parasite has two kinds of hosts, vertebrate and invertebrate.

In the invertebrate host the parasitic cycle evolves in the gastrointestinal tract, with gastric, intestinal and rectal phases. In the first phase there is regression of trypanosoma to leishmania, with loss of the flagellum; multiplication follows, and then transformation into metacyclic trypanosomes, the contaminating form. These measure 17 μ in length; they are motile and have high resistance and penetrability. They are eliminated through the rectum, in the invertebrate's faeces. This mode of transmission (posterior station) differentiates *T. cruzi* from *T. rhodesiense* and *T. gambiense*, in which the contaminating forms migrate to the proboscis of the vector and are inoculated with the invertebrate's saliva (anterior station).

In the vertebrate host *T. cruzi* can be found free in the blood stream and within the cytoplasm of cells. The circulating form in the blood stream is elongated and continuously motile on fresh examination. On staining, it is C-shaped and measures 20 μ in length, 2 μ in width, and has no divisional forms or sexual dimorphism. In tissues it assumes the leishmania form, without a flagellum, and is found exclusively in the interior of cells. The leishmania is round or ovoid, 1·5 to 4 μ in diameter, with a nucleus and blepharoplast; leishmanias form small conglomerates.

Invertebrate Host

All the important arthropods infested by *T. cruzi* are Hemiptera of the Triatominae subfamily, in which many species are found harbouring the parasite in natural conditions. The Triatominae are haematophagic and in general have a wild habitat. The species adapted to human habitat can transmit *T. cruzi* to man by means of a change in their feeding habits. Among these species the most important are *Triatoma infestans*, *Panstrongylus megistus*, *Triatoma maculata*, *Triatoma brasiliensis*, *Triatoma sordida*, *Rhodnius prolixus*, *Triatoma dimidiata*, *Triatoma protracta*, *Triatoma phyllosoma*, and *Triatoma pallidipennis*. New species are constantly being described as harbouring the parasite.

Vertebrate Host

T. cruzi is a natural parasite of several wild and domestic animals. Chagas observed this first in armadillos (*Dasypus novemcinctus*, *D. sexcinctus*). Monkeys, bats and opossum species are among the several wild animals described as natural reservoirs of the parasite. Among domestic animals, cats and dogs are commonly infected. Experimentally, *T. cruzi* is readily inoculated in a large number of mammals—guinea-pigs, mice, rats, dogs and cats. In general, young animals are more susceptible than older ones of the same species. Birds, reptiles and batrachia are resistant to inoculation by *T. cruzi*. Man is an eventual vertebrate host and from this parasitism results Chagas' disease.

Life-cycle

Infestation of the invertebrate host occurs by means of ingestion of blood from a parasitized vertebrate host. In the great majority of infected Triatominae a durable parasitism is thus established. From the ingestion of contaminated blood to the elimination of metacyclic trypanosomes in the faeces, there is a time-span of 10 to 15 days for adult insects.

Usually, the transmission of *T. cruzi* results from deposition of infective forms on the skin or mucosae of man, in faeces eliminated during or after the insect has been feeding. Man is usually stung at night, mainly on exposed areas of skin, especially the face. The metacyclic forms of *T. cruzi* penetrate the skin through the wound or through superficial abrasions caused by scratching. The mucosae are directly penetrated and are a preferential site of entry, especially the ocular conjunctivae. On passing the skin barrier the parasites, invade the reticulo-endothelial cells of adjacent tissues assuming leishmania forms which reproduce by binary division, forming pseudocysts [PLATE 37b], in a 5-day cycle. After rupture of the pseudocysts, the parasites again assume trypanosome forms, penetrate the lymph-node barrier, and invade the blood stream, achieving systemic dissemination and invading cells in other tissues where secondary foci of infection are established. Again, leishmania pseudocysts are produced and recurring cycles of blood stream distribution ensue. The parasitic cycle is common to man and other vertebrate hosts.

The biological cycle is completed when the parasitized vertebrate, including man, is stung by a young, still uncontaminated Triatomina. However, the transmission of the disease to vertebrates is not restricted to the natural form of infection, since clinical and experimental observations have disclosed transmission to foetuses through the placental barrier and to infants through maternal milk. In humans, an iatrogenic form of the disease exists, with transmission through blood transfusions.

PATHOGENESIS

The manifestations of the disease depend on the virulence of the inoculated strain, the number of inoculated parasites, the receptor's age and his immunobiological characteristics. The evolution of the disease is divided into successive phases (periods of Mazza and Jorg). In the acute phase the cardinal features are the alterations at the inoculation site (cutaneous or ophthalmolymphatic complexes), and the manifestations resulting from the establishment of secondary foci through systemic dissemination. A transitional period —somewhat debated in the literature—follows, with recurring haematogenous spread. A final chronic stage is established, with slowly progressing lesions, scarring and eventual hyperergic phenomena. Tissue parasitism in the chronic phase is minimal, in contrast with the intensity of the invasion in the acute phase.

Secondary foci are located within muscle fibres (smooth, striated and cardiac) as well as in other tissues, including the central and peripheral nervous systems. Haematogenous spread from secondary foci is not harmonious and no cyclic manifestations occur as in malaria.

According to Rassi and Amato Neto (1969), *T. cruzi* has antigenic fractions, possibly dependent on a polysaccharide-polypeptide complex isolated by Gonçalves and Yamaha, which are responsible for eliciting the antibody response of the disease. The antibodies can be identified through precipitation, agglutination and complement fixation. Non-specific lysins and heterophile antibodies are also demonstrable. The immune mechanism in Chagas' disease is mainly cellular, and the role of antibodies is to enhance phagocytosis. They are not directly involved in the destruction of parasites. This happens in the tissue phase, the inflammatory reaction and migration of macrophages occurring when the parasitized cell ruptures; leishmaniae may then be engulfed by macrophages. Phagocytosis occurs when trypanosomes change into leishmaniae. The immune mechanism also hinders the transformation of leishmaniae into trypanosomes; it is exceptional to find cysts with trypanosome transformation in the chronic form of the disease (Muniz and Freitas, 1946; Pizzi, 1961).

The defence mechanisms elicited by the parasitic infestation gradually reduce the number of circulating parasites and the intensity of the clinical reaction. In general, this occurs 2 months after the initial infection. Malnutrition and deficiency states may aggravate or prolong this initial or acute phase. In the next phase there is apparent recovery—the chronic indeterminate phase. Now the immune state is unable to completely terminate the infection, the parasite level in the blood being very low. This period may last for several years. Debatable reinfections and modifications of the immune state may lead to exacerbation of the disease, with manifestations not unlike those of the acute phase.

The clinical manifestations of the chronic phase appear from 10 to 20 years after the acute phase. The characteristics of the lesions in this phase are related, at least in part, to damage to the parasympathetic neurones which occurred in the acute phase. The neuronal lesions, being permanent, are the main substrate of many of the manifestations of the chronic phase, the Chagasic 'pathos' of Köberle (Köberle, 1961).

The various interpretations of the pathogenic mechanisms of Chagas' disease described in the literature have followed three main lines of thought. The first considers the immuno-allergic mechanisms in the production of the lesions to be of primary importance. The second considers the toxic products of parasite destruction, or of the degradation of the cell-parasite complex, to be the responsible mechanism. The third line of thought considers the focal or local action of the parasite to be the main feature (Okumura, Mattosinho-França, and Correa Netto, 1963). Despite the ardent efforts of the defenders of these various lines of thought, it is undeniable that all three groups of factors are active in the pathogenesis of the illness; no single factor can be shown to explain all the clinical, anatomical and immunobiological phenomena of this complex morbid state.

LABORATORY DIAGNOSIS

Demonstration of the parasite in the blood is possible, most often in the acute phase. Fresh and stained specimens are used. Romanovsky stains, such as Giemsa or Wright, are used in peripheral blood smears and in lymph node or bone-marrow aspirates.

Although *T. cruzi* is cultivated in special media (NNN, Bonacci) and in tissue cultures, these methods are not used in clinical practice. Preference is given to indirect methods of demonstration of the parasite, such as inoculation of laboratory animals and the so-called xenodiagnostic method. The former is performed with laboratory-bred Triatominae, free of infection, which are allowed to bite the suspected patient and after 30 to 50 days have their intestinal contents examined for *T. cruzi*. The xenodiagnositc method is employed in the chronic phase, when circulating parasites are scarce. Even with this method the results are often falsely negative, sometimes requiring from 8 to 10 trials to obtain confirmation of a suspected case.

Specific antibodies are demonstrated through complement fixation, agglutination, precipitation and immunofluorescence. The complement-fixation test (Machado-Guerreiro) yields variable results in the acute phase but is positive in almost all chronic cases. The precipitation and agglutination reactions are usually positive in the acute phase (Pedreira de Freitas, 1961). The most widely used diagnostic procedure for the identification of cases of chronic Chagas' disease is still the complement-fixation test of Machado-Guerreiro (Sanchez, Duarte, Araujo, and D'Alessandro, 1971).

CHAGAS' DISEASE AND THE NERVOUS SYSTEM

All compartments of the nervous system may be affected by Chagas' disease. The clinical, experimental and morbid anatomical data are grouped according to involvement of the central, autonomic and peripheral nervous systems.

Central Nervous System

Involvement of the central nervous system (CNS) was originally described by Chagas (1911) and illustrated by the presentation of two clinico-pathological observations. The first case was a 3-year-old patient with a spastic paraplegia, who developed fever, convulsive seizures, and died within 20 days. Autopsy examination showed meningeal thickening, chronic leptomeningitis, parasitic nests and chronic inflammation in the cerebral cortex. The second patient was a 24-year-old with a chronic encephalopathy characterized by idiocy, spastic cerebral diplegia and athetosis. The patient died due to accidental burns; the autopsy showed meningeal adhesions and chronic encephalitis, no parasites being demonstrated.

Vianna (1911) studied the morbid anatomy of the original Chagas' patients, and one acute case, and described the CNS lesions. The findings were disseminated, with foci of varying sizes both in the white and grey matter. The parasitized cells, by their nuclear characteristics, were interpreted as glial cells. Upon rupture of these cells, intense adjacent inflammatory reaction ensued. Periarteritis and leptomeningitis were also observed.

Thus, Chagas developed his concept of the involvement of the CNS in this disease which he presented in successive publications (1911, 1913, 1916 *a*), holding *T. cruzi* responsible for a wide variety of chronic encephalopathies, from mental retardation and epilepsy to permanent motor damage, with athetosis and diplegic states as the commoner manifestations. There appeared to be a chronic, progressive form of CNS involvement resulting from neuronal damage by parasites (1916 *a*). An acute meningo-encephalitic form was also described among his original 29 cases which formed the basis for the description of the acute form of the disease (Chagas, 1916 *b*).

Magarinos Torres and Villaça (1919) reported studies on the experimental production of Chagas' disease in young dogs, finding in he tacute phase small inflammatory foci in the CNS, in which macrophages, plasma cells and microglial cells surrounded cells containing leishmaniae in the cytoplasm. These foci were more numerous in the white matter. Non-specific degeneration of nerve cells was found and sometimes microglial nodules around degenerated nerve cells. Moreover, throughout the nervous system, there were parasitized cells, probably glial in nature, containing parasites. In the leptomeninges inflammatory foci were few and mainly perivascular. These authors considered the inflammatory reaction as mild and acute, the main defence mechanism being represented by microglial cells. The inflammatory reaction was always peripheral to the reactive, proliferative neuroglial process. These concepts are repeated in a review by Magarinos Torres (1923).

A *T. cruzi* strain obtained from the armadillo (*Dasypus novemcinctus*) allowed several experimental observations on involvement of the CNS. Villela (1923 *a*) inoculated two pregnant bitches with this *T. cruzi* strain. One of these had four macerated and four live pups, one of which had sparse foci of encephalitis, though no parasites were found in the CNS. This was the first observed evidence of *in utero* transmission of Chagas' disease with antenatal involvement of the CNS. The same *T. cruzi* strain yielded data suggestive of the existence of neurotropic strains. Souza Campos (1925, 1927 *a*, 1927 *b*) observed the appearance of hind-leg paralysis in inoculated animals, the pathological examination of which showed inflammatory lesions in the thoracic and lumbar regions of the spinal cord, with extensive neuronal lesions. Villela and Magarinos Torres (1925, 1926), studying a larger series of dogs inoculated with the same strain of *T. cruzi*, also observed paralytic phenomena; the inflammatory foci were small and disseminated through the brain and spinal cord. The foci contained numerous macrophages, of both microglial and vascular origin, with leishmaniae present within the cytoplasm of macrophages and astrocytes. Neuronal damage was variable and more evident in Purkinje cells, in the pyramidal cells of the cerebral cortex, and in the multipolar cells of the spinal cord. Mononuclear perivascular infiltrates were observed around these inflammatory sites. The small vessel endothelium was swollen with occasional luminal occlusion. In the leptomeninges the inflammatory reaction was also discontinuous and predominantly perivascular, with aggregates of macrophages, lymphocytes and plasma cells. Villela and Villela (1932), studying inoculated dogs and using Del Rio Hortega and Giemsa stains, demonstrated intracellular parasitism in neurones, astrocytes, microglial and endothelial cells in the CNS.

These histopathological studies of human and experimental material, completed in the first phase of investigation of Chagas' disease, thus demonstrated a meningo-encephalomyelitis in the acute form of the disease. Chronic lesions of the CNS were also admitted to be a sequel to the disseminated neuronal damage of the acute phase, a hypothesis defended in several clinical reviews (Villela, 1923 *b*; Austregesilo, 1927). Colares Moreira (1925) studied 10 cases of chronic involvement of the CNS, predominantly in children, characterized mainly by motor symptoms (pyramidal, extrapyramidal and cerebellar), and used the designation of 'trypanosomic encephalopathy'. As in most cases it was impossible to obtain a clinical history of a previous acute form of the disease, emphasis was given to the importance of the infection in antenatal life. The importance of neurotropic strains was considered as less relevant (Chagas, 1934; Chagas, 1935; Borges Fortes, 1942).

While several experimental studies had confirmed the possibility of materno-foetal transmission of *T. cruzi*, this demonstration in humans was a late achievement. According to Romaña (1961), this evidence was obtained around 1953. Lisboa (1960) demonstrated foci of granulomatous encephalitis [PLATE 37a] and of exudative leptomeningitis in six stillborn children, the mothers having chronic Chagas' disease. Couceiro (1943) considered the CNS more likely to be affected by *T. cruzi in utero* or in the first year of life, due to the lesser efficiency of the blood–brain barrier during this period. The transmission of maternal antibodies through the placenta, as demonstrated by several authors, does not convey immunological protection to the product of conception against *T. cruzi* (Rassi and Amato Neto, 1969).

The existence of neurotropic strains of *T. cruzi* has not been definitely proven at the present time (Jardim, 1968). Variations in *T. cruzi* strain virulence is admitted, since passage through certain receptors, including humans, can reduce virulence and immunologically different strains do exist (Nussenzweig, Deane, and Kloetzel, 1962). The most virulent strains would be those most likely to damage the CNS. Thus, it is difficult to envisage a chronic encephalopathy with a silent acute phase. However, a silent acute phase is recognized for other clinical forms of the disease; when there is a small number of low-virulence *T. cruzi* in the original inoculum the first clinical signs may only appear in the chronic stage of the disease (Romaña and Terracini, 1945).

The concept of a chronic encephalomyelopathy in Chagas' disease was not supported by further clinico-pathological observations; no sequelae of chronic granulomatous encephalitis were demonstrated in autopsied cases. Autopsies of four children dying of acute Chagas' myocarditis showed no CNS lesions (Cardoso, 1960). Mice inoculated with *T. cruzi* had no CNS lesions (Alencar and Elejalde, 1959). In other endemic areas no chronic encephalopathies were described, as reported by Chagas in Brazil. Such encephalopathies could be secondary to dietary and endocrine disorders, also prevalent in the endemic areas of Brazil. Chagas (1911) had already drawn attention to the importance of this differential diagnosis. In the endemic areas of Brazil consanguineous marriages are common, and heredodegenerative disorders of the CNS are likely to exist, although no pathological studies have yet been made on the subject. These aspects led the hypothesis of a chronic Chagas' encephalopathy to be considered only with reserve (Alencar, 1964 *a*; Lima Costa, 1967).

The use of more refined histopathological techniques may yet lead to the demonstration of chronic damage to the CNS by Chagas' disease. The basic acute lesion, with a parasitic pseudocyst circumscribed by inflammatory reaction, is very transient and does not lead to definite scarring. The adoption since 1955 of the classic method of neurone count in the study of the pathology of Chagas' disease by Köberle (Köberle, 1959), by quantitatively comparing the number of nerve cells in a given anatomic site in Chagas' patients and controls, led to the publication of a considerable body of literature by the pathology school of Ribeirão Preto (São Paulo). The method was adopted by Levi and his school in their study of the application of Bizzozero and Driesch laws to comparative neurohistology, as for instance in comparing neurones of animals of similar species with different body weight (Spina-França, 1951). This technique, applied to Chagas' disease, demonstrated reduction of the neuronal population in several portions of the CNS. Schwartzburd and Köberle (1959) demonstrated that in rats with chronic Chagas' disease there was a reduction in the number of neurones, predominantly in the lumbar region of the spinal cord. According to Brandão, experimental studies on the cerebellum of mice showed considerable reduction in the number of Purkinje cells (Jardim, 1967 *a*). A statistically significant decrease in cellularity was observed in the oculomotor, supraoptic, ventromedial and mammillary nuclei of infected rats (Jardim, 1968).

The data of Köberle's group confirmed that in the acute phase the foci are small, usually adjacent to vessels, and have a large number of plasma cells and marked glial proliferation. Menezes (1964) confirmed that the lesions are distributed uniformly throughout the entire CNS, with local variations in intensity. Parasites are found, in decreasing order of frequency, in the cerebrum, cerebellum [PLATE 37c], and in the cervical thoracic and lumbar regions of the spinal cord (Menezes and Alcantara, 1965). Vichi (1964) demonstrated not only frequent leishmania pseudocysts in the spinal cord of rats, but also a statistically significant decrease in spinal cord neurones of the thoracic and lumbar regions in the acute form of the disease (Vichi, 1961).

The data published by Köberle's group shed new light on the problem of chronic damage to the CNS in Chagas' disease, the mechanism being neuronal destruction in the acute phase of the disease. The sequelae and clinical picture would thus depend on the intensity and location of the damage wrought in the acute phase.

The role of congestive heart failure is also emphasized to explain the CNS damage in chronic Chagas' disease, the reduction of neuronal population being attributed to prolonged hypoxia. In chronic Chagas' cardiopathy, as in other chronic cardiopathies, the CNS lesions are similar. Cell damage, increased lipofuscin pigment content of the neurones and astroglia, and microglial infiltrates surrounding small vessels are found in the brain. Degeneration of nerve fibres and diffuse anisomorphic astroglial proliferation are seen in the white matter (Alencar, 1964 *b*). Numerical reduction of Purkinje cells, regressive changes in the remaining Purkinje cells, changes in the nerve fibres of its nests, and microglial proliferation are seen in the cerebellum (Alencar, 1967). The prolonged hypoxia is ascribed to congestive heart failure in both groups of cases which were compared.

Peripheral Nervous System

Peripheral nervous manifestations may be due not only to spinal anterior horn damage, as already mentioned, but also to direct peripheral nerve lesions. Involvement of peripheral nerves was first demonstrated experimentally in dogs by Couceiro (1943). Perivascular infiltrates were observed along the neural sheath and interfascicular spaces. In the adjacent connective tissue the inflammatory phenomena were more pronounced than in peri- and endoneurium. Vascularites were observed, with endothelial and perithelial proliferation, and luminar occlusion in the smaller vessels. Leishmania nests were found in endothelial and perithelial cells, as well as in connective tissue cells of the peri- and endoneurium. Couceiro considered the whole process as corresponding to an interstitial neuritis. Involvement of striated muscle was observed by Chagas (1916 *a*), without clinical repercussions.

Autonomic Nervous System

The importance and extent of autonomic nervous system (ANS) involvement in Chagas' disease were only definitely revealed by the method of neuronal counting introduced by Köberle and his group. The parasympathetic neurones are predominantly affected, since in the majority they are located in the walls of hollow viscera, in immediate contact with their smooth muscular coats, an elective site of location of the parasitic nests in the acute phase of the disease. The affected fibres, in smooth and especially in cardiac muscle, suffer extensive myofibrillary damage. After rupture of the parasitic nests, there is adjacent inflammatory reaction, at first granulocytic, perhaps with eosinophils. There follows intense mononuclear infiltration and occasional giant cells. Thus are formed the inflammatory granulomas, in different stages of evolution, which characterize muscular involvement, both smooth and cardiac, in Chagas' disease. Adjacent ANS structures are also involved by the inflammatory process, the neurones showing degenerative nuclear and cytoplasmic phenomena, or complete lysis. Without the use of these methods these lesions in ANS structures of the heart were not always identified (Magarinos Torres and Melo, 1958; Alencar, 1959). Köberle (1961) ascribes to Monckeberg the original observation, in 1924, of severe cardiac neurone damage in dogs inoculated with *T. cruzi*. Systematic investigations by Köberle's group, starting in 1956, had uniform results; there was always a significant reduction in the number of ANS neurones in the viscera of humans and animals with Chagas' disease, both in the acute and chronic forms.

Special mention should be made of the studies on ANS neurones in the heart, colon and oesophagus, parasympathetic ganglia, inferior hypogastric plexus, submucous and myoenteric plexuses, appendix and intramural plexuses of the stomach. Summaries on these studies were presented by Köberle (1961, 1967).

In the light of these data, Köberle formulated the concept of the pathogenesis of the main cardiac and visceral manifestations of the chronic form of Chagas' disease. The changes would be secondary to local, long-lasting autonomic imbalance, resulting from partial parasympathetic denervation in the acute phase of the disease, and leading to organ dilatation, with cardiomegaly, mega-oesophagus, and megacolon. The changes would be sequelae of multiple, disseminated ANS neurone damage in the acute phase, and not a progressively evolving inflammatory process.

Without denying the existence of a chronic Chagas' myocarditis, Köberle explains most of the cardiac lesions by parasympathetic deprivation. As further proof of his point of view, he compared human cardiac lesions with experimental lesions produced in normal rats after administration of high doses of adrenaline for several days, finding them in morphological agreement. In the same way are interpreted the dilatation and hypertrophy of walls of hollow viscera (megas), without mechanical obstruction, observed mainly in the oesophagus and colon.

Okumura *et al.* (1960) observed extensive intestinal lesions in mice inoculated with *T. cruzi*, with a 20 per cent incidence of megacolon. The inflammatory lesions in the intestinal wall, with progression to granulomas and eventually to fibrous scarring, involved not only the muscular tunic but the myoenteric plexuses as well [PLATE 37d].

Biochemical changes may precede the morphological changes. Sena and Teles Filho (1967) studied the esterase activity in the myoenteric plexus of rats with experimental Chagas' disease, the animals dying during the acute phase of the disease. The results were compared with those found in control animals. Morphological changes in Auerbach's plexus were sparse but there was a marked reduction in esterase activity.

Mechanism of Neuronal Damage

The leishmania form of *T. cruzi* reproduces within the cytoplasm of the parasitized cell, forming a pseudocyst which eventually ruptures into the extracellular medium. This mode of invasion involves not only muscle cells and macrophages but also other cells, including neurones, as already pointed out. However, in the vicinity of inflammatory foci neuronal damage may be observed but without direct neuronal parasitism. In addition to the hypothesis of possible previous parasitism, an unlikely explanation, there are two further hypotheses which have been suggested to explain these findings.

The first is the action of a toxic substance, liberated by the disintegration of parasites. This view has many supporters (Chagas, 1916*a*; Crowell, 1923; Magarinos Torres, 1941; Köberle and Alcantara, 1960). Up to the present time, however, no neurotoxic substances have been isolated, either from the parasite itself, or from the parasitized tissues.

The second view followed from the observations of Prates-Campos (1969) who studied protein synthesis in Purkinje cells, through tagged leucin (leucin $H)_3$ radioautographs, in the cerebellum of rats inoculated with *T. cruzi*. A metabolic dysfunction was observed with reduction of protein synthesis during the acute phase of the disease. The dysfunction is parallel to local parasitism of glial cells and does not depend on local inflammatory reaction or on direct neuronal parasitism. The lesions resulting in the glial cells have a secondary metabolic effect on the neurones supported by such glial cells.

The production of immuno-antibodies by immunologically competent cells, in response to parasite antigens, is in favour of the first hypothesis. The reaction of cells to the antigenic substances could, however, be diverse. In the case of nerve cells, not immunologically reactive by their own nature, the antigenic substances could act as toxins, producing the cellular lesions already described.

All these factors—direct neuronal parasitism, the more frequent neuroglial parasitism, with secondary metabolic damage of supported neurones, and the possible action of a neurotoxin—may together contribute to neuronal damage and destruction in Chagas' disease, leading by whatever predominant mechanism to the final widespread neuronal depopulation.

Clinical Picture in the Involvement of the Nervous System

The outline given above enables one to appreciate the several clinical aspects of the involvement of the nervous system in Chagas' disease. We can speak of several forms of neurological involvement. The acute form; the acute exacerbation; the chronic form, and the complications of other clinical forms of the chronic phase. This clinical systematization is based on the review of Forjaz (1967).

Acute Form

This was first identified by Chagas (1916*b*) and discussed by several authors, emphasis being given to the studies of Talice, Costa, Rial, and Osimani (1940) and of Amato Neto (1958), for their comprehensive review.

In the acute form there is fever, generalized lymph node enlargement, oedema, enlargement of liver and spleen, and cutaneomucosal manifestations.

Fever is usually intense in the first few days, but may last from 2 to 8 weeks, varying from 37·5° to 40·0°C. It may be continuous or intermittent, remittent or irregular, and is not followed by chills. The lymph nodes are usually enlarged, firm and painless, both in the primary inoculum region and in other node groups, this alteration lasting for months. Oedema occurs with variable intensity, being elastic or firm, and more frequent in the face and lower limbs. The enlargement of liver and spleen usually subsides within months.

The cutaneomucosal alterations related to the portal of entry of the primary inoculum are usually unilateral. When located in the face (Romaña sign) they are characterized by oedema and inflammation of the ocular conjunctivae, extending to adjacent tissues, by eventual lacrimal gland involvement, and by constant regional lymph node enlargement. When occurring elsewhere in the skin (inoculum chagoma) there is circumscribed, firm, inflammatory oedema of skin and underlying tissues, sometimes with central ulceration of the epidermis. The primary lesion may last from 15 days to 2 months. Secondary focal cutaneous lesions may appear in the same patient, with similar manifestations. Other cutaneous changes may also occur, unrelated to the portal of entry, being usually eruptive, and designated as schizotrypanids.

Less frequent manifestations of the acute form are carditis and meningo-encephalitis. The acute carditis is of short duration, and its clinical picture is entirely different from that observed in the chronic form of the disease.

Blood studies show hypochromic anaemia, leucocytosis, neutrophilia with shift to the left, eosinophils either increased or reduced, and increased lymphocytes and monocytes. Haemosedimentation is high, both in the acute form and in exacerbations. Serum albumin is usually reduced, alpha-2 and gamma globulins being increased (Resende, 1957, as quoted by Veronesi, 1962).

The acute form is most severe in young infants. Older children and adults have a more benign clinical course, sometimes identified only by the cutaneomucosal signs. The acute form is sometimes confused with other infectious processes, and may be wholly unrecognized.

The CNS and meningeal involvement is usually only poorly evident, the clinical signs comprising somnolence, irritability and slight meningeal signs. Rarely, there is a full-blown acute meningo-encephalitis. This is not a common complication of the acute form of Chagas' disease, but its occurrence and course are severe (Mazza, Frere and Salica, 1942; Elizalde, 1952; Ronchi and Ara, 1953). The meningo-encephalitis is of abrupt onset; there are the usual signs of meningeal irritation, but convulsive seizures and sensorial alterations are characteristic. The convulsive seizures are usually generalized, and tonic-clonic in type. Irritability, somnolence, mental confusion, stuporous states and coma appear in progression. The picture lasts for 1 or 2 weeks, ending often in death. In very young children an acute encephalitis, with recurring convulsive seizures and coma, may be fatal in a few days. The cerebrospinal fluid changes will be considered below. The pathological findings in the CNS are similar to those found in acute experimental encephalitis (Dominguez and von Gavaller, 1962).

Exacerbation Form

Acute exacerbation of chronic Chagas' disease has been attributed to changes in the immune state of the host. Pizzi (1961) ascribed these alterations of the immune state to sublethal whole body irradiation, to blockage of the reticulo-endothelial system by colloidal thorium dioxide, and to administration of cortisone in the early stages of disease. Mattosinho-França *et al.* (1969) reported a case of a patient with the chronic form of Chagas' disease, who developed chronic lymphatic leukaemia. The patient developed progressive signs of diffuse central nervous system involvement, starting with motor alterations in the lower limbs, and bilateral mydriasis. Coma ensued, followed by death. No blood transfusions had been given. On autopsy examination, besides the general findings of lymphatic leukaemia and of chronic Chagas' involvement of the heart, an acute Chagas meningo-encephalitis was present. This was characterized by leptomeningeal mononuclear infiltrate, mononuclear perivascular cuffing in the parenchyma, disseminated microglial granulomas, and leishmania pseudocysts in astrocytes. The co-existence of chronic Chagas' myocarditis, and of acute Chagas' meningo-encephalitis, unique in the literature, was interpreted as secondary to chronic lymphatic leukaemia. This could have substituted the lymphocytic clones responsible for the immunity to Chagas' disease, thus creating conditions for an acute exacerbation of the process, and the emergence of an acute meningo-encephalitis.

Chronic Form

According to the interpretation of Köberle, the nervous system manifestations in the chronic form of Chagas' disease are due to the Chagasic pathos, the sequelae to the acute lesions.

Autonomic Neuropathy. In this group are located the main alterations of chronic Chagas' disease, the chronic cardiopathy and the megas (mega-oesophagus and megacolon).

Chronic cardiopathy is a widely studied condition, prevalent in the endemic areas. The reader is referred to the review by Laranja, Dias, Nobrega, and Miranda (1956). The clinical picture of the digestive megas, not only of the oesophagus and colon, but of other hollow viscera as well, does not differ from that of megas caused by other aetiological agents. The clinical picture will not, therefore, be discussed here.

Köberle (1967) considers both the cardiac and intestinal forms as dynamic processes resulting from reduced motility. In the evolution of the cardiopathy he identifies three phases, the first of which is purely neurogenic, with disturbances of function and cardiac rhythm. On the neurogenic alterations depend the introduction and evolution of the two following phases. In the evolution of the digestive tube alterations, partial loss of cells leads to imbalance of the autonomic nervous system regulation of the contractibility of the muscular coat of hollow viscera. Alteration in peristalsis results, with slowing of the progress of the contents, visceral dilatation and progressive hypertrophy. On this basis appears digestive megas. The same pathogenesis applies to the megas of non-digestive hollow viscera.

A large number of parasympathetic neurones have to be damaged before any physiological results are produced, since the remaining neurones tend to compensate functionally for the damaged ones. Köberle considers a 90 per cent denervation to be necessary for the production of mega-oesophagus, 55 per cent for the colon, and 25 per cent for the heart.

On a similar basis Köberle also conceives forms ascribed to ANS disturbances of secretion and of absorption.

Central Nervous System. The anatomical, clinical and experimental data described in the literature on the central nervous system involvement in Chagas' disease do not support the concept of a well-defined chronic encephalopathy (Lima Costa, 1967). However, further investigations should clarify the problem, since definite lesions exist in the acute phase, with neuronal damage. Problems for investigation are many, the first of which is the existence of clinical cases of widespread damage to the nervous system, in which no aetiology other than concomitant Chagas' disease is apparent (Romaña, 1947; Levy, 1948; Mello and Mello, 1955; Pereyra-Käfer *et al.*, 1963; Romaña, 1963). Investigations on this question continue to be reported. Clinical and electroencephalographic data do not yet allow definitive conclusions to be made.

Furthermore, there are clinical indications of alterations in central neuroregulation in chronic Chagas' patients, with possible hypothalamic dysfunction. Among these are alterations in potassium control (Vieira, Mazzoncini, and Lomonaco, 1965) and of sweating upon thermal stimulation (Jardim, 1967*b*). Such changes cannot be explained by damage to the parasympathetic neurones. The finding of hypothalamic lesions in rats infected with *T. cruzi* could eventually explain homeostatic alterations in men afflicted with the chronic form of Chagas' disease (Jardim, 1971).

Cerebral Complications of Chronic Chagas' Cardiopathy

Mural thrombi in the left ventricle of the heart are very common in chronic Chagas' patients. They are often located in the apex, overlying fibrotic endocardial lesions. These are due to ischaemic necroses of the apex myocardium, with interstitial fibrosis and chronic inflammation. Fragments of the mural thrombus may become detached, migrating with the blood current, and causing embolic phenomena in distant vessels. Nussenzveig *et al.* (1953) related the occurrence of ischaemic vascular infarctions in eight patients with chronic Chagas' cardiopathy. The vascular occlusions were attributed to thrombo-embolic phenomena, originating in the left ventricle of the heart. Four of these patients died, the autopsy showing in three of them mural thrombi in the left ventricle. Andrade (1959) demonstrated the existence of embolic cerebral lesions in 10 of 93 autopsies of chronic Chagas' cardiopathy. Other authors have made similar observations, including Pereyra-Käfer *et al.* (1963) and Badim (1966).

The neurological picture in these patients is not peculiar. Successive embolic phenomena are not uncommon and death ensues due either to the cerebral lesions, or to the natural evolution of the cardiopathy.

Carotid artery thrombosis in patients with positive Machado-Guerreiro complement-fixation test in the blood (Zaclis, Ricciardi-Cruz, and Almeida, 1956) led to the hypothesis of primary vascular lesions by *T. cruzi* (Forjaz, 1967). However, no pathological or experimental proof has yet been obtained.

LABORATORY DIAGNOSIS

Immunobiological tests so far analysed do not point to any particular mode of involvement of the nervous system.

Electroencephalographic studies on patients with possible chronic Chagas' encephalopathy await wider and more accurate observations. Studies of the cerebrospinal fluid (CSF) are few and not systematized; no peculiar alterations due to the disease have been determined at present.

Chagas (1911) commented on the turbid CSF collected at autopsy in a case of meningo-encephalitis. Direct examination of CSF samples in other cases yielded no parasites upon microscopic examination. Inoculation of CSF has yielded parasites in a few cases. Villela and Bicalho (1923) related the CSF findings in six cases of the chronic form of the disease. The examination showed normal findings for appearance, colour and cytology. Globulin reactions were negative; the Machado-Guerreiro complement-fixation test was positive in four cases. In two of these, the Wassermann reaction was also positive, casting doubt upon the positivity of the Machado-Guerreiro test. In the chronic form the CSF is within normal limits regarding cells, proteins, glucose and globulin content (Basso and Basso in 1936, quoted by Elejalde, 1959). Dalma (1954) and Pedreira de Freitas and Mendes (1955) have confirmed this finding. In the acute form published results have varied. Amato Neto (1958) found normal results in 11 cases. Elejalde (1959) reported four cases: in three of these the cytology was examined, showing pleocytosis. Differential cell count was done in only one case, showing lymphocytes and monocytes. Protein was high in three cases, in one of which electrophoresis showed increased albumin. This same author refers to the findings of Dias *et al.*, who in 1925 observed normal CSF results in one case, and of Martinez-Colombres, who in eight cases of meningo-encephalitis found a positive Pandy test (the only test performed).

In some studies an elevated CSF pressure is mentioned, this being a non-specific finding.

Occasional reports of demonstration of *T. cruzi* in the CSF by animal inoculation have been made (Pedreira de Freitas, Lion, and Tartari, 1953).

The complement-fixation test of Machado-Guerreiro is usually negative in the CSF in the chronic phase (Pedreira de Freitas and Mendes, 1955; Elejalde, 1959; Pereyra-Käfer *et al.*, 1963). However, sporadic positive results of this test, in the chronic form, are described in the literature (Dias, 1950; Rodriguez, 1950). In the acute phase, Elejalde (1959) found a positive test in two of his four patients. This author considers the positivity of this test to depend on the permeation of blood antibodies of the CSF, since after normalization of the CSF findings in one of his cases the Machado-Guerreiro test also became negative.

TREATMENT AND PROPHYLAXIS

Specific treatment of Chagas' disease is required in the acute meningo-encephalitic forms. There is no actual therapeutic approach to the other forms of nervous system involvement. There is no ideal chemotherapeutic agent in Chagas' disease. Most of the agents employed yield unsatisfactory results and active research on the subject continues to be conducted. Some of the therapeutic agents have untoward collateral results. Such is the case of nitrofuran compounds, which may cause peripheral neuropathies.

Eradication of Triatominae is difficult and the wild reserves are immense. Prophylactic measures are based on the elimination of Triatominae from their human habitat. The basic task, besides education, is the improvement of socio-economic conditions of rural populations, with the construction of dwellings which prevent the harbouring and proliferation of the Triatominae. This has been pointed out since the original description of the disease, and extensive programmes have been conducted in this direction.

References

ALENCAR, A. (1959) O sistema nervoso autônomo do coração na infestação experimental do comundongo albino pelo *S. cruzi*, *An. Congr. Int. Doença de Chagas (Rio de J.)*, 12–23.

ALENCAR, A. (1964*a*) Aspectos clínicos e biológicos das manifestações nervosas e musculares da tripanisomiase americana, *Rev. Neuro-psiquiat.*, 27, 57–69.

ALENCAR, A. (1964*b*) Atrofia cortical na cardiopatia crônica chagásica, *Hospital (Rio de J.)*, **66**, 807–15.

ALENCAR, A. (1967) Alterações cerebelares em pacientes com cardiopatia chagásica crônica, *Arch. Neuro-psiquiat. (S. Paulo)*, 25, 191–8.

ALENCAR, A., and ELEJALDE, P. (1959) O sistema nervoso central na infestação experimental do camundongo albino pelo *Schizotrypanum cruzi*, *An. Congr. Int. Doença de Chagas (Rio de J.)*, 25–34.

AMATO NETO, V. (1958) *Contribução ao Conhecimento da Forma Agunda da Doença de Chagas*, Thesis, São Paulo.

ANDRADE, Z. A. (1959) Fenômenos trombo-embólicos na cardiopatia chagásica, *An. Congr. Int. Doença de Chagas (Rio de J.)*, 73–84.

AUSTREGESILO, A. (1927) Des troubles nerveux dans quelques maladies tropicales, *Rev. neurol.*, 1, 1–21.

BADIM, A. (1966) Embolia cerebral na cardiopatia chagásica crônica, *Arch. Neuro-psiquiat. (S. Paulo)*, 24, 28–34.

BORGES FORTES, A. (1942) As lesões do sistema nervoso na enfermidade de Chagas, *J. Clín.*, 23, 353–61.

CARDOSO, R. A. A. (1960) Lesões do sistema nervoso central em quatro casos infantis agudos de doença de Chagas, *Bol. Inst. Pueric. Univ. Brasil (Rio de J.)*, 17, 101–10.

CHAGAS, C. (1911) Nova entidade morbida no homem. Resumo geral de estudos etiológicos e clínicos, *Mem. Inst. Osw. Cruz*, 3, 219–75.

CHAGAS, C. (1913) Les formes nerveuses d'une nouvelle trypanosomiase *T. cruzi* inoculé par *Triatoma megista* (maladie de Chagas), *Nouv. Iconogr. Salpêt.*, **26**, 1–9.

CHAGAS, C. (1916*a*) Processos patogênicos da tripanosomiase americana, *Mem. Inst. Osw. Cruz*, 8, 5–36.

CHAGAS, C. (1916*b*) Tripanosomiase americana. Forma aguda da moléstia, *Mem. Inst. Osw. Cruz*, 8, 37–63.

CHAGAS, C. (1934) Estado atual da tripanosomiase americana, *Rev. Biol. Hig.*, 5, 58–64.

CHAGAS, E. (1935) Súmula dos conhecimentos atuais sôbre a tripanosomiase americana, *Mem. Inst. Osw. Cruz*, 30, 387–416.

COLARES MOREIRA, J. V. (1925) *A Forma Nervosa da Moléstia de Chagas*, Thesis, Rio de Janeiro.

COUCEIRO, A. (1943) Lesões do ciático na infecção experimental do cão pelo *Schizotrypanum cruzi*, *Mem. Inst. Osw. Cruz*, 39, 435–9.

CROWELL, B. C. (1923) The acute form of American trypanosomiasis. Notes on its pathology with autopsy report and observations on trypanosomiasis in animals, *Amer. J. trop. Med.*, 3, 425–59.

DALMA, J. (1954) Nota sôbre el liquido cefalorraquideo en la enfermedad de Chagas, *An. Inst. Med. region. (Tucumán)*, 4, 47–55.

DIAS, J. C. (1950) A cardiopatia crônica da moléstia de Chagas, *Resen. clín.-cient.*, 19, 2–20.

DOMINGUEZ, A., and GAVALLER, B. VON (1962) Encephalitis chagasica, *Z. Tropenmed. Parasit.*, 13, 308–12.

ELEJALDE, P. (1959) Alguns achados no líquido cefaloraquidiano na forma aguda da doença de Chagas, *An. Congr. Int. Doença de Chagas (Rio de J.)*, 491–502.

ELIZALDE, F. (1952) Enfermedad de Chagas-Mazza: meningoencefalitis aguda, *Arch. argent. Pediat.*, 38, 225–31.

FORJAZ, S. V. (1967) Aspectos neurológicos da moléstia de Chagas: sistema nervoso central, *Arch. Neuro-psiquiat. (S. Paulo)*, 25, 175–90.

JARDIM, E. (1967 *a*) Alterações quantitativas das células de Purkinje na moléstia de Chagas experimental no camundongo, *Arch. Neuro-psiquiat. (S. Paulo)*, 25, 199–208.

JARDIM, E. (1967 *b*) Sudorese em pacientes com moléstia de Chagas crônica, *Arch. Neuro-psiquiat. (S. Paulo)*, 25, 214–20.

JARDIM, E. (1968) *Estudo das Manifestações Clínicas e do Parasitismo do Hipotálamo e do Núcleo do Terceiro Par Craniano na Moléstia de Chagas Experimental Aguda no Rato*, Thesis, Ribeirão Preto.

JARDIM, E. (1971) Moléstia de Chagas aguda experimental; parasitismo do hipotálamo, *Arch. Neuro-psiquiat. (S. Paulo)*, 29, 190–7.

KÖBERLE, F. (1959) Die Chagas Krankheit: ihre Pathogenese und ihre Bedeutung als Volkssenche, *Z. Tropenmed. Parasit.*, 10, 236–68.

KÖBERLE, F. (1961) Patologia y anatomia patologica de la enfermedad de Chagas, *Bol. Ofic. sanit. panamer.*, 51, 404–28.

KÖBERLE, F. (1967) Aspectos neurológicos da moléstia de Chagas, *Arch. Neuro-psiquiat. (S. Paulo)*, 25, 159–74.

KÖBERLE, F., and ALCANTARA, F. G. (1960) Mecanismo da destruição neuronal do sistema nervoso periférico na moléstia de Chagas, *Hospital (Rio de J.)*, 57, 173–8.

LARANJA, F. S., DIAS, E., NOBREGA, G., and MIRANDA, A. (1956) Chagas' disease: a clinical, epidemiologic and pathologic study, *Circulation*, 14, 1035–60.

LEVY, H. (1948) Forma nervosa da moléstia de Chagas, *Rev. paul. Med.*, 32, 315.

LIMA COSTA, A. (1967) *Parasitoses do Sistema Nervoso*, Rio de Janeiro, pp. 127–46.

LISBOA, A. C. (1960) Sobre a forma congênita da doença de Chagas: estudo anátomo-patológico de 6 casos, *Rev. Inst. Med. trop. S. Paulo*, 2, 319–34.

MAGARINOS TORRES, C. (1923) A tripanosomiase americana e sua anatomia patológica, *Folha méd.*, 4, 25–9.

MAGARINOS TORRES, C. (1941) Sobre a anatomia patológica da doença de Chagas, *Mem. Inst. Osw. Cruz*, 36, 391–404.

MAGARINOS TORRES, C., and MELO, R. P. (1958) Sistema nervoso autônomo do coração em caso crônico de doença de Chagas não associada ao megaesôfago, *Hospital (Rio de J.)*, 54, 813.

MAGARINOS TORRES, C., and VILLAÇA, J. (1919) Encefalite e mielite causadas por um tripanosoma (*T. cruzi*), *Mem. Inst. Osw. Cruz*, 11, 80–8.

MATTOSINHO-FRANÇA, L. C., LEMOS, S., FLEURY, R. N., MELARAGNO FILHO, R., RAMOS, H. A. JR., and PASTERNAK, J. (1969) Moléstia de Chagas crônica associada a leucemia linfática. Ocorrência de encefalite aguda como alteração do estado imunitário, *Arch. Neuro-psiquiat. (S. Paulo)*, 27, 59–66.

MAZZA, S., FRERE, R. S., and SALICA, P. N. (1942) Formas meningoencefalicas primitivas e secundarias de la enfermedad de Chagas. Considerable gravedad del proceso y tratamiento adequado con 7602(Ac)Bayer, *Mission Est. Pat. Reg. argent. (MEPRA)*, 43, 36–40.

MELLO, A., and MELLO, N. R. (1955) A forma nervosa crônica da molêstia de Chagas, *Rev. Inst. A. Lutz (S. Paulo)*, 15, 194–219.

MENEZES, H. (1964) Moléstia de Chagas experimental. Lesões do sistema nervoso central na fase aguda, *Rev. bras. Med.*, 21, 21–4.

MENEZES, H., and ALCANTARA, F. G. (1965) Distribuição dos parasitas (pseudocistos) no sistema nervoso central de ratos infectados experimentalmente pelo *T. cruzi*, *Rev. goiana Med.*, 11, 21–5.

MUNIZ, J., and FREITAS, G. (1946) Estudos sobre a imunidade humoral na doença de Chagas, *Brasil-méd.*, 40, 337–41.

NUSSENZVEIG, I., SPINA-FRANÇA, A., WAJCHEMBERG, B. L., TIMONER, J., MACRUZ, R., and SERRO-AZUL, L. G. (1953) Acidentes vasculares cerebrais embólicos na cardiopatia chagásica crônica, *Arch. Neuro-psiquiat. (S. Paulo)*, 11, 386–402.

NUSSENZWEIG, V., DEANE, L. M., and KLOETZEL, J. (1962) Diversidade na constituição antigênica de amostras de *Trypanosoma cruzi* isoladas do homem e de gambás, *Rev. Inst. Med. trop. S. Paulo*, 4, 409–10.

OKUMURA, M., BRITO, T., PEREIRA DA SILVA, L. H., SILVA, A. C., and CORREA NETTO, A. (1960) The pathology of Chagas' disease in mice: digestive tract changes, with a reference to necrotizing arteritis, *Rev. Inst. Med. trop. S. Paulo*, 2, 17–28.

OKUMURA, M., MATTOSINHO-FRANÇA, L. C., and CORREA NETTO, A. (1963) Comentários sobre a patogenia da moléstia de Chagas, *Rev. Hosp. Clín. Fac. Med. S. Paulo*, 18, 151–64.

PEDREIRA DE FREITAS, J. L. (1961) Diagnóstico de laboratorio da moléstia Chagas, *Bol. Ofic. sanit. panamer.*, 51, 429–49.

PEDREIRA DE FREITAS, J. L., LION, M. F., and TARTARI, J. T. A. (1953) Resultados de uma investigação sobre a moléstia de Chagas no municipio de Marilia e outros, com estudo clínico de dois casos agudos da moléstia, *Rev. Hosp. Clín. Fac. Med. S. Paulo*, 8, 81–92.

PEDREIRA DE FREITAS, J. L., and MENDES, R. T. (1955) Investigações sorológicas na forma crônica da moléstia de Chagas entre pacientes internados em hospital psiquiátrico, *Rev. paul. Med.*, 46, 123–6.

PEREYRA-KÄFER, J., POCH, G. F., MONTEVERDE, D. A., FERNANDEZ BLANCO, E., and TARSIA, O. (1963) Neurological manifestations of the American trypanosomiasis, in *Tropical Neurology*, eds. van Bogaert, L., Pereyra-Käfer, J., and Poch, G. F., Buenos Aires, pp. 237–50.

PIZZI, P. T. (1961) Immunologia de la enfermedad de Chagas: estado actual de problema, *Bol. Ofic. sanit. panamer.*, 51, 450–64.

PRATES-CAMPOS, J. C. (1969) Radioautographic study of the protein synthesis in the Purkinje cells at the acute phase of the experimental trypanosomiasis cruzi in rats, *Rev. Inst. Med. trop. S. Paulo*, 11, 25–33.

RASSI, A., and AMATO NETO, V. (1969) Imunopatologia da doença de Chagas, in *Imunopatologia Tropical*, eds. Lacaz, C. S., Mendes, E., and Amato Neto, V., Rio de Janeiro, pp. 135–52.

RODRIGUEZ, M. (1950) Inmunidad en la enfermedad de Chagas. La reacción de fijación del complemento, *Rev. ecuat. Hig.*, 7, 65–83.

ROMAÑA, C. (1947) Encefalopatia de posible origen esquiso-tripanosico, *An. Inst. Med. region. (Tucumán)*, 2, 19–39.

ROMAÑA, C. (1961) Epidemiologia y distribucion geográfica de la enfermedad de Chagas, *Bol. Ofic. sanit. panamer.*, 51, 390–403.

ROMAÑA, C. (1963) Epidemiology of Chagas' disease (*Trypanosomiasis cruzi*), in *Tropical Neurology*, eds. van Bogaert, L., Pereyra-Káfer, J., and Poch, G. F., Buenos Aires, pp. 227–36.

ROMAÑA, C., and TERRACINI, E. (1945) Comportamiento de las infecciones de lauchas por *S. cruzi* segun la concentracion de parasitos inoculados (infecciones cronicas iniciales), *An. Inst. Med. region (Tucumán)*, 1, 141–64.

RONCHI, O. J., and ARA, C. A. (1953) Meningoencefalitis chagasica en un lactente de 45 dias, *Arch. argent. Pediat.*, 39, 268–74.

SANCHEZ, G., DUARTE, R., ARAUJO, J., and D'ALESSANDRO, A. (1971) Infeccion por *Trypanosoma cruzi* en el hombre versus enfermedad de Chagas en Tibu, norte de Santander, Colombia, *Rev. Ofic. sanit. panamer.*, 70, 463–71.

SCHWARTZBURD, H., and KÖBERLE, F. (1959) Chagas myelopathie, *Z. Tropenmed. Parasit.*, 10, 309–14.

SENA, P. G., and TELES FILHO, M. (1967) Aspectos histoquímicos do plexo mientérico na doença de Chagas experimental, *Arch. Neuro-psiquiat. (S. Paulo)*, 25, 209–13.

SOUZA CAMPOS, E. (1925) Sur la paralysie des animaux (chien, souris) infectés expérimentalement avec des cultures de *Trypanosoma cruzi*, *C.R.Soc. Biol. (Paris)*, 93, 40–2.

SOUZA CAMPOS, E. (1927 *a*) Paralisia experimental determinada pelo *Trypanosoma cruzi*, *Bol. biol.*, 2, 153–73.

SOUZA CAMPOS, E. (1927 *b*) Estudos sobre a raça neurotrópica do *Trypanosoma cruzi*, *An. Fac. Med. S. Paulo*, 2, 197–201.

SPINA-FRANÇA, A. (1951) Dimensioni e numero dei neuroni in relazione alla mole somatica. Confronti tra due roditori di mole somatica molto differente, *Z. Zellforsch.*, 36, 222–34.

TALICE, R., COSTA, R. S., RIAL, B., and OSIMANI, J. J. (1940) *Los 100 Primeros Casos Agudos Confirmados de Enfermedad de Chagas en el Uruguay*, Montevideo.

VERONESI, R. (1962) Doença de Chagas fase aguda, in *Doenças Infecciosas e Parasitárias*, ed. Veronesi, R., Rio de Janeiro, p. 488.

VIANNA, G. (1911) Contribuição para o estudo da anatomia patologica da 'moléstia de Carlos Chagas', *Mem. Inst. Osw. Cruz*, 3, 276–94.

VICHI, F. L. (1961) Estudo do parasitismo na medula espinhal de ratos na fase aguda da moléstia de Chagas, *Rev. Inst. Med. trop. S. Paulo*, 3, 37–42.

VICHI, F. L. (1964) Destruição de neuronios motores na medula espinhal de ratos na fase aguda da moléstia de Chagas, *Rev. Inst. Med. trop. S. Paulo*, 6, 150–4.

VIEIRA, C. B., MAZZONCINI, M., and LOMONACO, D. A. (1965) Variações da potassemia na forma crônica da moléstia de Chagas, *Rev. paul. Med.*, 66, 239–47.

VILLELA, E. (1923 *a*) A transmissão intra-uterina da moléstia de Chagas. Encefalite congênita pelo *T. cruzi*, *Folha méd.*, 4, 41.

VILLELA, E. (1923 *b*) Moléstia de Chagas: descrição clínica. Terceira parte: forma nervosa, *Folha méd.*, 4, 49–52.

VILLELA, E., and BICALHO, C. (1923) As pesquisas de laboratorio no diagnóstico da moléstia de Chagas, *Mem. Inst. Osw. Cruz*, 16, 13–27.

VILLELA, E., and MAGARINOS TORRES, C. (1925) Lesions histo-pathologiques dans la paralysie expérimentale a *Schizotrypanum cruzi* chez le chien. Nature des cellules contenant le parasite dans le système nerveux central, *C.R. Soc. Biol. (Paris)*, 93, 133–5.

VILLELA, E., and MAGARINOS TORRES, C. (1926) Estudo histopatológico do sistema nervoso central em paralisia experimental determinada pelo *S. cruzi*, *Mem. Inst. Osw. Cruz*, 19, 175–98.

VILLELA, E., and VILLELA, E. (1932) Elementos do sistema nervoso parasitados pelo *T. cruzi*, *Mem. Inst. Osw. Cruz*, 26, 77–82.

ZACLIS, J., RICCIARDI-CRUZ, O., and ALMEIDA, G. G. M. (1956) Obstruções das artérias carótidas e das principais arterias cerebrais, *Arch. Neuro-psiquiat. (S. Paulo)*, 14, 158–70.

32 Hydatid Echinococcosis of the Nervous System

R. ARANA-IÑIGUEZ

Hydatid disease of the nervous system is caused by the larval stage of *Taenia echinococcus* which lodges in the central nervous system (Arana-Iñiguez, 1961, 1966; Arana-Iñiguez, San Julián, Gorlero, and Fúster, 1953) or in craniovertebral bony tissues.

Although, theoretically, the hexacanth embryo may invade any part of the human body, world statistics, and also the author's own, show that the central nervous system is impaired whenever this parasite invades either the brain or craniovertebral structures.

According to Dévé's criteria (1928) there are only three examples of hyatid cyst lodging in the spinal arachnoid tissue and in the spinal cord itself. The observations, described by Carrea and Murphy (1964), by Ley and Marti (1970), and the Garcia Guelfi (1971), are the only ones in the literature in which brain or bony tissue were not directly involved.

This preliminary statement enables one to appreciate the general clinical and therapeutic features of the disease. When the parasite is located in the brain and its scolex is transformed into a vesicle, the cyst finds itself in ideal conditions for growth, surrounded by brain tissue of fluid-like consistency and placed in a cavity where no resistance develops until the cranial wall is reached.

On the other hand, craniovertebral location shows the characteristics of any hydatid bone disease. A vesicle within bone does not easily expand; it infiltrates the neighbouring tissue with brood vesicles which develop into new, small cavities within the bone, giving rise to hydatidosis of the cranium and vertebrae.

We have therefore, on the one hand, the hydatid cyst of the brain which may grow to a large size (600 or 700 g in weight), producing as a rule a well-defined clinical picture with characteristic angiographic features, and amenable to surgery. On the other hand, we have the bony hydatid lesions, diffuse and invasive, located mainly in the cranial base and vertebrae, with ill-defined clinical and radiological features, and resistant to surgical excision.

In FIGURE 32.1 are outlined the statistics of cases registered at the Instituto de Neurologia of Montevideo.

I shall deal first with aspects of general pathology and experimental study before describing the features of cerebral hydatid cyst, cranial hydatidosis and vertebral hydatidosis.

GENERAL CONCEPTS ON HYDATID DISEASE

Hydatidosis is a disease found in countries with numerous sheep, dogs, cattle and pigs.

The cycle of the parasite occurs mainly in man, sheep and dog. The dog is the host of the adult *Taenia*, which lives in its intestine, and its egg-carrying faeces contaminate water, food and skin. These eggs are directly ingested by man, and more frequently by children.

It has been shown that the most important mechanism of spread is direct contact with dogs. The child caressing a dog is contaminated, as the latter carries the *Taenia* eggs on his skin. The disease can also be transmitted by contaminated water and vegetables.

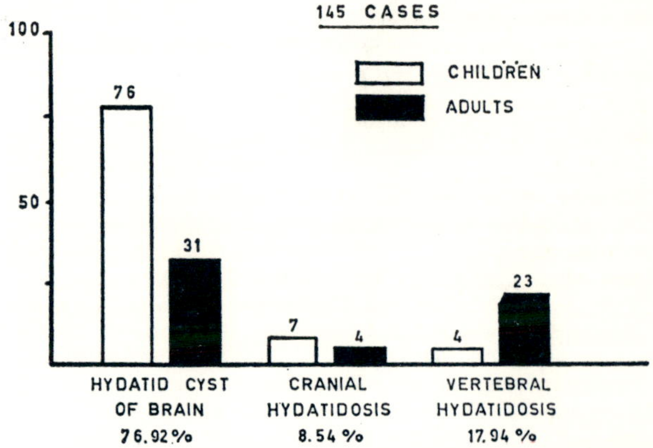

FIG. 32.1. Statistics of hydatid disease of the nervous system from the Instituto de Neurologia of Montevideo.

The hexacanth embryo thus passes to the stomach and intestine of man. It penetrates the intestinal wall, usually the duodenal wall, and—although it occasionally follows a venous, lymphatic or serous route—it is through the veins of the portal system that the embryo is transported to the liver, the lungs and the general circulation.

This cycle explains some of the facts of human pathology, the percentages of localization in the different organs being 65 per cent in the liver, 20 per cent in the lungs and the remainder in other viscera. The hexacanth embryos may be trapped in the capillaries of the liver and lungs. Nevertheless, there is some visceral tropism which influences visceral involvement.

This tropism explains the existence of animal specimens in which, although the cycle is the same as in man, the visceral distribution is different: the lungs are much more involved than the liver.

This special affinity for certain tissues may also explain why the *Cysticercus*—with a similar cycle in man—selects the brain. Although the *Cysticercus* embryo follows the same venous path as the hexacanth embryo of the *Taenia ecchinococcus*, it rarely lodges in the liver or lung and has a dominant tropism for the nervous system, the muscles and the skin.

In hydatid disease the brain is affected in 2 per cent of cases and bone localizations comprise 4 per cent. Among the latter the two localities most interesting to us—the cranial and vertebral—are found with a frequency of 2 per cent in the cranium and 50 per cent in the vertebrae. Thus, one-half of bone localizations are in the vertebrae; cranial localizations are, on the contrary, quite rare.

Dévé (1946, 1949) has described primary and secondary hydatidosis. Primary hydatidosis is the hydatid disease caused by the larval development of the hexacanth embryo. The hydatid cyst of the nervous system, as well as cranial and vertebral hydatidosis, is an example of primary hydatidosis.

Secondary hydatidosis is that form of the disease which results from the rupture of a primary hydatid cyst in an organic surrounding. In the rare cases where several hydatid brain cysts are encountered, it will be found that the heart is involved and that rupture of a hydatid cyst in the left heart chambers is responsible for the general dissemination. The rupture of this cardiac hydatid cyst liberates the elements forming part of the hydatid 'sand'—scolices, hooks and proligerous vesicles. Scolices are the most important elements determining secondary hydatidosis.

Experimental Hydatidosis of the Nervous System

The author and his colleagues (Arana-Iñiguez and Gurri, 1963) have injected hydatid 'sand' into the carotid artery of rabbits (Dévé, 1933). By sacrificing the animals at varying periods the evolution of the various stages of the disease can be examined. In further experiments we injected hydatid sand directly into the nervous system.

Although certain observations could be made on the different stages of the scolex and its transformation into a hydatid cyst, the experiments are too slow because about 6 months elapse from the injection of scolices to the formation of vesicles.

Later on, with López Fernández (Arana-Iñiguez, and López Fernández, 1967; López Fernández, Arana-Iñiguez, Velutti, Varela, and Villar, 1966; López Fernández, Arana-Iñiguez, Velutti, and Varela, 1966), direct implantation of a hydatid vesicle was performed; this vesicle was experimentally obtained from the omentum of a rat. We were thus able to observe the development of cerebral hydatid cysts in different species.

This work was mainly performed in rabbits, on which several different types of experiments were carried out. Hydatid cysts were implanted simultaneously in different viscera, mainly the liver and brain. It was found that in the rabbit the cyst grows much faster in the brain than in the liver. Cysts were also implanted into the vertebrae and the lungs. In this way, clinical effects similar to those found in humans could be reproduced.

The experimental hydatid cyst of the brain, produced by direct implantation, permits several different investigations.

First, the time required for biological tests to turn positive can be studied. Moreover, once a hydatid vesicle has been implanted in the brain serial blood serum tests can be performed.

Alterations produced by the vesicle in the surrounding nervous tissue can also be studied; identical phenomena to those observed in man were found; namely, a slight microglial reaction (Schroeder and Medoc, 1951).

Finally, the experimental hydatid cyst produced by direct implantation of a vesicle permits two different types of studies. First, it offers a means of observing the development of intracranial hypertension. Secondly, it enables one to precisely locate a chronic lesion within the nervous system.

These methods also afford the surgeon the opportunity of testing different surgical procedures used in treatment, as in the technique of saline irrigation for the removal of cerebral cysts (San Julián, and Arana-Iñiguez, 1954).

CEREBRAL HYDATID CYST

The hydatid cyst of the brain is usually solitary. For the difficult route to the brain is traversed by a single hexacanth embryo which becomes implanted there and undergoes transformation into a single cyst. The concept of primary hydatidosis is basic since it imolies that, if a cyst can be removed intact, the patient will recover.

Only in 2 per cent of our cases were there multiole brain cysts, secondary hydatidosis resulting from dissemination of scolices from a ruptured cardiac hydatid cyst. Another explanation for secondary encephalic hydatidosis is rupture of a primary brain cyst by trauma, infection, or in the course of surgery.

The clinical aspects of the disease in children and adults will be described separately below.

Cerebral Hydatid Cyst in Children

Symptomatology

Bearing in mind what has already been stated, the clinical picture in most cases is the consequence of a single, large-sized hydatid cyst. The most frequent location is the temporo-occipital area (Schroeder and Medoc, 1951).

The two main features of the disease are intracranial hypertension and ill-defined focal symptoms.

Intracranial hypertension entails headache, vomiting and papilloedema. It is frequently revealed by inattention at school in a child who has hitherto shown normal behaviour.

The disease sometimes presents two clearly defined stages due to the separation of cranial sutures. The child may suffer from headache and vomiting for 2 or 3 months, after which intracranial hypertension apparently recedes. Radiology shows separation of sutures and ophthalmoscopy reveals secondary optic atrophy. This is most often encountered between the ages of 3 and 7 years.

The focal syndrome is usually poorly defined. Due to the slow growth of the hydatid vesicle, the cyst is well tolerated by the brain. When the cyst attains a large size, which occurs quite often, diffuse, bilateral symptoms are observed with dysmetria of the upper limbs. These symptoms are apparently caused by dysfunction of basal structures and not by any particular location of the cyst. The general condition of the child is good until the final stage, when there is often blindness.

In countries such as Uruguay, the disease is most common in rural areas. In a series of 145 cases only three patients had never left Montevideo.

We often refer to 'Schroeder's four points' (Schroeder, 1941)—a child from a rural area, in good general condition, with marked intracranial hypertension, and with ill-defined focal signs.

Local examination of the cranium is important. Due to its slow growth the hydatid cyst often achieves a large size and modifies the consistency of neighbouring bone. Occasionally it becomes so thin that it produces a craniotabes. MacEwen's 'cracked pot' percussion sign results from thin bone and a large fluid accumulation close to it.

The vibrations of a tuning fork (Arana-Iñiguez, Azambuja, Dighiero, and García Guelfi, 1958) placed in the midline are better transmitted through the liquid mass of the cyst. This may be observed in a number of patients by auscultation of these vibrations at symmetrical points of the skull.

Neurological examination may disclose drowsiness (25 per cent of cases), papilloedema (85 per cent; 18 per cent with optic atrophy), homonymous hemianopia (50 per cent), mild facial paresis, hemiparesis—the most frequent sign according to Morquio (Morquio, 1929, 1932) and to our own observations.

Bilateral pyramidal signs are relatively common. In a series of 61 children, only nine had no pyramidal signs. Cerebellar signs were present in 32 per cent of patients; convulsions in 17 per cent.

In only two cases in our series was the cyst in the posterior fossa.

Diagnosis

Clincially, there is no diagnostic symptom or sign of cerebral hydatid cyst. Schroeder's 'four points' are thus the most important guide to diagnosis. We must not forget, however, that other cystic tumours found in children may be misleading, as in a patient with a cystic astrocytoma who presented with Schroeder's 'four points', the nature of which was established only during surgery.

The recognition of hydatid cysts in other organs is obviously very important. In our experience they are most frequently found in the liver and lung. The association of hepatic and pulmonary hydatidosis is not in our experience as frequently found as was pointed out by Dew (1928) in his classic book. He stated that 80 per cent of cerebral cysts were associated with hepatic cysts. In 1955 we published (Arana-Iñiguez and San Julián, 1955 *b*) a study of 13 intracranial cysts of which two also had pulmonary cysts; there were no hepatic cysts.

The main clinical differential diagnosis is from posterior fossa tumour, as intracranial hypertension and few focal signs are also found in this condition. In studies conducted 10 or 15 years ago air cystography was mentioned as a diagnostic tool, but it carries the hazard of brain contamination. Whenever a posterior fossa tumour is suspected in countries where hydatidosis exists, carotid angiography will assist in distinguishing between a supratentorial and infratentorial mass.

Paraclinical studies

Biological Tests. The following tests must be performed in all patients suspected of hydatid infestation: Cassoni's test, eosinophilia, Weinberg's test, haemo-agglutination, immuno-electrophoresis and immuno-fluorescein. The first three—when performed together —offer 83 per cent of positive results (Gurri, Bozzola, and Piquinela, 1963). When the last three are added, almost 100 per cent positivity is achieved. When all tests are negative the disease is very unlikely.

Electroencephalographic Studies. These have been conducted at the Laboratory of Electroencephalography and Clinical Neurophysiology of the Instituto de Neurologia of Montevideo. Fúster, Castells, and Gastaut (1955) and Bianchi Saus (1963) have made detailed studies of EEG changes in the pre- and postoperative stages.

Epileptic activity is observed in 71 per cent of preoperative and in 89 per cent of postoperative recordings. These findings are striking because epilepsy was considered to be seldom found in hydatid disease. In 17 per cent of the cases, however, epileptic seizures appear during the course of the disease. The EEG is useful in localizing a mass but not in determining its nature. EEG signs, as described by Fúster (1963) may point to a superficial or deep location of the cyst. The former are accompanied by polymorphous theta and delta waves and a depression of local voltage. The latter show bilateral, symmetrical and synchronous delta activity, and occasionally rhythmic, paroxysmal activity with similar topography. Deformation and unilateral 14 c/s spindles may appear, as in sleep recordings.

X-rays. These are of major importance. Simple X-rays may provide useful data, such as a thinning and erosion of the cranial vault, especially in oblique films.

Cerebral Angiography. As we consider with San Julián (Arana-Iñiguez and San Julián, 1955 *a*), this is the method of choice for diagnosing a hydatid cyst. We mentioned four characteristics:

1. Marked vascular displacement.
2. Absence of tumour vascularity.
3. No changes in vessels surrounding the tumour area.
4. Peritumoural arteries may show a circumferential disposition.

Displacements are usually greater than those observed in other tumours. The circumferential arrangement may be observed in lateral or AP views and also in oblique films.

Although none of these features is pathognomonic, being only indicative, according to Tolosa (1953), of a benign cystic tumour, we have found that these four points when clearly present are pathognomonic of hydatid disease [PLATE 38a].

Scintillography. In nine patients with brain hydatid cysts submitted to a scintillography, eight were supratentorial. Of these, the scan was positive in six and negative in two. In one case of an infratentorial location, the scan was negative.

Positive brain scintillography were of two types: in five the cyst showed as an abnormal hyporadioactive area [PLATE 38a]; in 1 case a slightly hyporadioactive area surrounded by a more intensively radioactive band was visualized.

In all positive cases a contralateral displacement of normal radioactive midline structures was present (Touyá *et al.*, 1968 *a* and *b*).

Cerebral Hydatid Cyst in the Adult

At the Instituto de Neurologia we have records of 31 cases of cerebral hydatidosis in adults. Cerebral hydatidosis of the child and the adult are considered separately because of their different clinical characteristics (Arana-Iñiguez and Gurri, 1963). Clinical and angiographic aspects in the adult are much less clearly defined.

In our series the proportion of hydatid cysts in the child and in the adult is 2·45 to 1. Other series show a lower frequency for adults: Schroeder and Medoc (1951) and Thomas (1884) have found a proportion of 4 to 1 and Dew (1928) 7 to 1.

Symptomatology

The condition predominates in young adults (Arana-Iñiguez and Maslenikov (1959). Ages varied between 16 and 61; 25 patients were under 40.

The course of the disease is short in the child; in 50 per cent it was less than 6 months; Carrillo, Matera, and Insausti (1951) cited similar figures. In the adult, however, the course is even more rapid: the shortest was 1 month, the longest, $2\frac{1}{2}$ years.

Cases of multiple cysts were found more often in adults, while only one case of multiple cysts was observed among our 76 children. The explanation for this may be that cardiac infestation is necessary for the development of secondary hydatidosis, and according to Di Bello (1956) this is more frequent in adults. In 12 cases all were over 15 years (Dumont, 1928).

Intracranial hypertension is a cardinal feature. In one case there were convulsive seizures for 3 years before the onset of intracranial hypertension. Fits occurred in nine out of 31 patients. In five cases there was a gradual onset of focal symptoms, both irritative and inhibitory, before intracranial hypertension developed.

Clinical signs are more varied in the adult than in the child.

Psychic symptoms are present, especially alterations of the level of consciousness, and marked depression. Particularly striking is the psychic improvement after removal of small cysts weighing 60 to 80 g. Papilloedema was present in 70 per cent of our patients. Hemiparesis was slightly more frequent than hemianopia (14 and 12 cases respectively).

Diagnosis

Diagnosis is more difficult in adults than in children. We usually suspect brain tumour, but sometimes in a patient from a rural area, with positive biological tests or identification of a cyst in another organ, the clinical diagnosis may be straightforward.

Paraclinical Studies

Angiography. The four characteristics described in children seldom appear in adults. This may be due to the larger size of the cyst in children or to the alteration of the cyst in adults. An angiogram showing an ordinary space-occupying lesion does not exclude the possibility of finding a hydatid cyst at surgery.

Electroencephalography. Similar conclusions obtain here. Adults rarely show the characteristics described by Fúster (1963).

Treatment of Brain Hydatid Cyst

The treatment is surgical.

The possibility of this disease must always be kept in mind by neurosurgeons working in areas where hydatidosis occurs. Craniotomy should be a delicate procedure. A rough technique may result in rupture of the cyst membrane and lead to surgical failure.

Schroeder's (1935) and da Gama Imaginario's (1952) procedures of puncturing the cyst are dangerous as they may cause further brain infestation; these methods have been abandoned.

Viale (1938) and Dowling and Orlando (1939) introduced the modern technique for complete removal of these cysts. It requires painstaking manoeuvres and compression with cotton pledgets, in a long, tedious and dangerous operation.

We have described two procedures (Arana-Iñiguez, Rodríguez Barrios, and San Julián, 1951, 1952; San Julián and Arana-Iñiguez, 1954). The first requires the injection of air into the contralateral ventricle; the second, saline irrigation into the space between the brain tissue and the cyst. In both there is an increase of intracranial pressure (with the patient's cranium opened), and the cyst is expelled without instrumental contact with the cyst's wall.

We now systematically employ the saline irrigation procedure [PLATES 38b and c; 39a, b and c], a very simple and effective one which does not require a contralateral burr-hole or a ventricular tap. This technique has been adopted by several neurosurgeons.

CRANIAL HYDATIDOSIS

Involvement of the skull is rare. Dévé (1948), in 637 cases of bone echinococcosis collected from the literature, found only 22 cases of skull involvement, or 3·4 per cent. The spine was affected in 44·2 per cent of bone echinococcosis.

Our experience is based on 11 cases. There was skull involvement in 7·5 per cent of patients with hydatidosis of the central nervous system, and in 10 per cent of the cases of brain hydatidosis. Sarni and Zadek (1965) cite similar figures.

The Pathology of Bone Echinococcosis

To understand neurological hydatid disease caused by the larvae of *Taenia echinococcus* lodging in cranial and spinal bones, it is well to recall the features of bone infestation in general. These differ from those of brain involvement.

The hexacanth embryo forms the microscopic vesicle of primary infestation, and as we have seen it develops by penetrating areas of least resistance within bone tissue, taking a multilocular form from the start. Two different phenomena occur, according to Dévé: a diverticular growth, and exogenous vesiculation. By means of these two mechanisms, the parasite gradually invades *de proche en proche* the neighbouring bone tissue.

In this way multivesicular hydatidosis develops, with considerable invasive power. Bone becomes rarefied, the subperiosteal space is invaded, the periosteum separates and ruptures, and the vesicles grow outwards. This multivesicular invasive process produces an aseptic inflammatory reaction with the formation of a fluid containing cells, fat corpuscles and tissue debris, resembling a 'pea soup'. There is no real periosteal inflammatory reaction and cold hydatid abscesses are formed in the course of its rupture and outward growth. This process most often occurs in the porous tissue of epiphyses, vertebrae, skull base, pelvis and, rarely, in large diaphyses.

The unilocular cyst, typical of brain and other visceral locations, is never seen in bone. Bone hydatidosis should never be considered a localized form of the disease but a diffuse, multivesicular invasive process.

Macroscopically the bone appears swollen, with a thin cortical layer, and infiltrated by multiple vesicles of varying size, either clustered together and deformed or separated by bone tissue of normal appearance. Vesicles are translucent or else they may contain turbid liquid. As the disease progresses, cavities become larger, with ragged walls containing microvesicles surrounded by a purulent fluid, parasitic debris and bone sequestra.

In cranial hydatidosis, infestation takes place primarily in the diploë either of the calvarium or the base. From there, by multiplication and growth, the cortical layers are perforated and the process grows outwards. In the calvarium the internal layer is more frequently pierced. One vesicle may grow within the cranial cavity and is then surrounded by daughter vesicles which usually leave the dura mater intact. These, in turn, give birth to new daughter vesicles. Usually, as the dura mater is displaced, a large-sized vesicle may simulate a brain cyst; that is, a large sphere within the cranium between the internal aspect of the bone and the dura mater.

The outer layer of the bone may be the first to be pierced and in this case a large vesicle will grow, pushing up the scalp (Sarni and Zadak, 1965). Such a vesicle may even pierce the scalp. If the process takes place at the skull base, the infiltrate will destroy various bone structures—the sella turcica, the clivus, the foramina and the orbital cavity—and involve the cranial nerves and the orbit.

Symptomatology

The disease is seen more often in the young; in our series there were three cases aged 2 to 10 years, six cases aged 10 to 20 years and two cases aged 40 to 50 years. Six of our 11 patients were under 16 years. On the other hand, vertebral hydatidosis, like bone hydatid disease in general, is more frequent among adults. Two of our cases presented cysts in other areas; one in the liver and another in subcutaneous tissue.

The course of cranial hydatidosis is slow. Symptoms are chronic; when patients are seen early the slow evolution of signs, for example blindness, can be observed. At the onset of the disease there are often no symptoms.

At the skull base hydatidosis most frequently presents with cranial nerve paresis.

In eight of our cases there was involvement of the inner table of the skull with intracranial hypertension and focal symptoms. There was external spread in five cases.

Intracranial hypertension of insidious onset dominates the clinical picture and was present in nine out of 11 patients with headache, vomiting, papilloedema and secondary optic atrophy. Optic atrophy was found in five cases; blindness in two.

The cranial nerves are commonly affected, especially the optic. One of our patients had been previously operated on for orbital hydatidosis and presented a Foster Kennedy syndrome. Optic atrophy resulted from orbital compression of the optic nerve. There was also paresis of the third nerve. Another case presented with involvement of the right sixth nerve. Among oculomotor symptoms we may find paretic nystagmus on lateral and vertical gaze as a consequence of brain stem dysfunction. Trigeminal neuralgia and paresis occur. Seventh, eighth, ninth, eleventh and twelfth cranial nerves may be involved and occasionally a pontocerebellar angle syndrome may develop.

A pyramidal syndrome was noted in four of our cases. Two cases presented a cerebellar syndrome, in both of which the echinococcosis was in the posterior fossa. Impaired gait with a tendency to deviate, but without clear-cut cerebellar signs, is sometimes a consequence of intracranial hypertension.

Speech disturbance was met only once. Psychic disorders are caused by intracranial hypertension and usually comprise confusion, depression and mental retardation. Convulsive seizures were not observed.

The general condition of these patients remained good until the final stages of the disease.

Paraclinical Tests

Plain X-rays play a very important role in these cases, as Schroeder has pointed out (1950, 1951). The findings of multiple round geodes may lead to a correct diagnosis [PLATE 40a]. These are usually situated in porous areas of bone at the skull base.

Carotid angiograms may be revealing in some cases. The abnormalities may resemble those seen in cerebral hydatid cyst when it develops between the dura mater and bone.

With regard to air studies, the same reservations that we made for brain hydatid cyst also apply here.

EEG was performed in three patients and showed lateralization from hemispheric disturbance, and in one case there were indications of a cerebral lesion. The electroencephalogram has a localizing value but does not assist differential diagnosis.

Biological reactions are as frequently positive in bone echinococcosis as in cerebral lesions.

Scanning has not been used in cranial hydatidosis.

Treatment

Treatment consists of the largest possible excision of affected bone tissue. Since in most cases the skull base is involved, it is almost impossible to achieve total excision of invaded bone tissue. In only two cases have we thought that excision was complete; one frontal and one parietal.

Involvement of the bones at the base of the skull is noteworthy; 50 per cent occurred in the temporal bones.

Six cases showed intracranial invasion with extradural, frontal, temporal or posterior fossa hydatidosis. In four other cases there was a tendency to exterior growth with perforation of the outer table. The dura mater was always intact. In only one case did we find hydatidosis inside the dura mater, a consequence of earlier surgery.

VERTEBRAL HYDATIDOSIS

Involvement of the spinal cord is nearly always a result of vertebral disease.

Dévé affirmed, 'There is no example of secondary osseous hydatidosis of metastatic origin arising from embolic dissemination from a primary hydatid cyst of the heart. Osseous echinococcosis is always primary.' This same author also said, 'The hexacanth embryo most frequently finds its way into short bones such as the vertebral bodies'. It is useful to recall, however, that different parts of the vertebral arch, the lamina, spinous process, pedicle and transverse process, may be initially involved and this may explain the varying course of lesions in different patients.

We have already seen that the vertebrae are the most frequent bone location; in 50 per cent of cases, according to Woodland (1949). Vertebrae are involved in 1 per cent of all cases of hydatidosis. Bearing in mind that brain hydatidosis comprises 2 per cent of the total, we have one case of vertebral for every two cases of cerebral hydatid cyst. However, our own figures differ slightly. We had 107 hydatid cysts of the brain and 27 of the vertebrae. It must be remembered that patients with cerebral hydatidosis are admitted to a neurology or neurosurgery unit, whereas vertebral hydatidosis may be seen in orthopaedic departments as well.

Although contrary opinions have been published by Dew (1928), Mills (1956), Acquaviva and Tamic (1964), Allende and Luque (1935), Ley and Martí (1970), and Boixadós (1961), we believe with Dévé that, 'contrary to general opinion, intraspinal echinococcosis has an exclusive osseous origin'. In 1948 Dévé stated that although the possibility of primary intraspinal lesion cannot be denied, no publication could be found in the literature fulfilling the necessary requisites to confirm its authenticity. Three recent reports, by Carrea and Murphy (1963), by Ley and Martí (1970) and by García Guelfi (1971) are undoubtedly genuine instances of intradural hydatid cysts.

Vertebral infestation—like bone echinococcosis in general—is more frequent in adults. In our 27 cases ages ranged from 5 to 60, with only three occurring in childhood and a maximum incidence between the ages of 41 and 50. The age-groups of 10 to 20, 21 to 30, and 51 to 60 included three cases each.

Dévé's figures were as follows: 16·7 per cent of cases occurred between 11 and 20 years, 30 per cent between 21 and 30, 22·6 per cent between 31 and 50, and 17 per cent between 41 and 50. As he pointed out, 40 per cent of all cases fall in the 30- to 50-year group, in contrast with what is observed in Pott's disease, where only 16 per cent of cases fall within this age-group. There is a higher incidence among males: 58 per cent.

As we have seen, hydatidosis tends to develop in porous bone, so that the vertebral body is most frequently involved. There seems to be a special predilection for the pedicle which is often destroyed; this led Dévé to describe a roentgenological sign visible in the anteroposterior view, which he called 'disappearance of the coffee bean' (pedicle) [PLATE 40b and c]. The spread from one vertebral body to another will follow Larghero Ibarz's concept (1939) of a subligamentous route, leaving the intervertebral disc intact for a long time. When it is finally invaded, the anterior part is first involved. In this passage from one vertebral body to another the rib is often involved. This is a typical lesional association of vertebral hydatidosis.

The cortical bone layer is eroded and hydatid vesicles spread beyond the vertebral body. Two types of clinical phenomena emerge: intraspinal and extraspinal. The latter gives rise to paraspinal abscess macroscopically quite polymorphous, due to the variety of tissues it may invade from the neck to the pelvis. On the other hand, intraspinal invasion consists of · independent vesicles which produce no reaction and which lodge between the dura mater and the wall of the spinal canal. Herein lies the neurological interest of vertebral hydatidosis.

Intraspinal invasion usually takes place by perforation of the posterior aspect of the vertebral body, either laterally or in the midline. The spinal cord is then compressed from the front, medially or laterally. In exceptional cases the dura mater is eroded and vesicles invade the spinal cord itself. This may be observed in the course of reoperations, when the dura mater has been opened in earlier surgery.

Vesicles emigrating beyond the spine will form a pouch, and the surrounding tissues then form a membrane. Thus, a cold abscess is produced as in tuberculosis. Tension is not raised within this abscess, nor does it elicit, as do inflammatory processes in general, any peripheral reaction. As the vesicles multiply, the abscess grows, compressing neighbouring tissues without invading or destroying them. The contents are hydatid cysts of varying sizes, floating in an opalescent fluid which is formed by the rupture of some of the vesicles. Some degenerate and create a 'pea soup' appearance which, on occasions, is brownish or infected. Although the abscess may track in different directions, the surgeon must appreciate that it remains in contact with the site from which the vesicles emerged. For this reason a well-explored abscess will always lead to the point where the vertebral hydatidosis pierced the periosteum and led to the abscess formation.

Symptomatology

The main feature is spinal cord compression, with onset of radicular pain, located according to the site of vertebral disease, in cervical, dorsal or lumbar regions. A cauda equina syndrome may also occur.

Although some authors believe there are not preferential sites, we know from Dévé's work that dorsal lesions are more frequent, and they form 58 per cent of our own observations. Lumbar, sacral and cervical lesions follow in that order of frequency. Dévé collected 262 cases from the literature and his figures are comparable with our own.

We agree with Benhamou and Goinard (1929) that the lower portion of the dorsal spine is most frequently attacked by the parasite.

Radicular symptoms are followed by the motor, sensory and sphincter disturbances of spinal cord compression. When there is localized vertebral pain, or signs of a cold abscess, a correct diagnosis is more likley to be made. This was the case in the majority of our patients.

Paraclinical tests

X-rays

There are four important signs which I described in 1948 with García Capurro and Caubarrére:

1. Disappearance of the 'coffee beans' or pedicles.
2. Erosion of the vertebral body and sometimes of the adjacent rib.
3. The intervertebral cartilage remaining intact.
4. An ossifluent abscess.

Whenever these signs appear together, simple roentogenology may allow a correct diagnosis to be made. Unfortunately these signs are not constant. In long-observed cases we did not once observe disappearance of a pedicle, as was the case in our first patient with vertebral hydatidosis. A plain roentgenogram is valuable when totally negative, since vertebral hydatidosis is then extremely unlikely. Since spinal cord compression develops, myelography is essential.

In the exceptional cases of intradural cysts, a characteristic myelographic picture is usually obtained.

Diagnosis

Little can be said on this subject as the clinical picture is one of spinal cord compression. Hydatidosis usually begins with radicular symptoms of slow onset, followed by the rapid development of spinal cord compression; but there is nothing typical about this evolution.

If the patient lives in an infested area and hydatidosis of other viscera is detected, diagnosis is facilitated. The age of the patient is important because the condition rarely occurs below the age of 15 years. Dorsal locations are more frequent. Roentgenology should be employed, therefore, when the above clinical picture exists. One of our cases was diagnosed at the radicular stage by this means. The patient was admitted with a diagnosis of cholecystitis, having pain in the right hypochondrium. An atypical clinical picture led to a neurological consultation, but there were no neurological signs except right radicular pain at T9. Compression and decompression of the jugular veins produced a positive Naffziger sign. Roentgenograms showed the four signs we have mentioned. The patient was operated on without myelography and a typical hydatid lesion was found.

Laboratory tests help if *all* of them are performed. As we have already stated, almost 100 per cent positivity is obtained.

The Course of the Disease and the Prognosis

As we have seen when studying cranial hydatidosis, bone hydatidosis can only be considered cured when all diseased bone tissue has been excised. Unfortunately this is very rarely possible in cranial or vertebral hydatidosis. For this reason vertebral hydatidosis is a severe affliction with a poor prognosis, although decompressive laminectomy may afford temporary relief of paraplegia. In the literature there are cases treated with several operations who have survived many years. But this is exceptional, and ultimately the majority of patients are paraplegic.

Treatment

The only possible treatment is surgery. The compressed spinal cord must be decompressed as quickly as possible.

The surgeon must appreciate that his aim should be total excision of diseased bone. Few cases, such as the one published by the author with García Capurro and Caubarrére in 1948, have been operated at the radicular stage, before cord signs have appeared. These exceptional cases are ideal for attempting the total excision of diseased bone tissue, since at this stage bone invasion is not extensive and may be limited to one vertebra. The importance of this type of excision was first underlined by Del Camp (1949) who excised the fifth lumbar vertebra through an anterior approach. Ivanesevich and Rivas (1961–62), Goinard and Descuns (1952), and Dévé (1933, 1948) consider that radical excision is an ideal but almost impossible form of treatment. Experience at our Institute and the standardization of a technique for total excision of one or more vertebrae, were demonstrated by Vigil Sóñora at the Fifth Uruguyan Congress of Medicine in 1962.

We believe that most patients should undergo a posterior or posterolateral approach, through wide transverse incisions, allowing an adequate view of the retro- and lateral-vertebral areas (Vigil Sóñora, Arana-Iñiguez, and Pérez Achard, 1961) [FIGS. 32.2 and 32.3].

There are some locations of bone echinococcosis in which prognosis is not so desperate, since pathological tissue may be radically excised. This is the case with the humerus and the femur (García Capurro and Pedemonte, 1951).

Biological Treatment

Surgical treatment of cranial as well as of vertebral hydatidosis must be followed by biological treatment. Injections of sterile total sheep hydatid liquid must be performed, first intradermally and then subcutaneously at a rate of three injections a week for not less than 1 year (Calcagno, 1939).

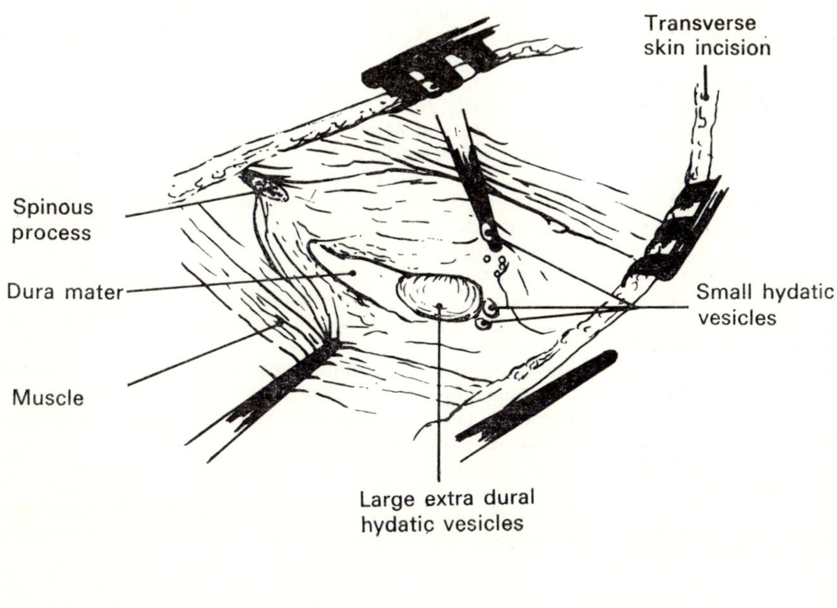

FIG. 32.2. Schematic representation of the spinal dura mater, covered by chronic hydatid granulation tissue. The dura mater has been exposed and one large and several small vesicles can be seen.

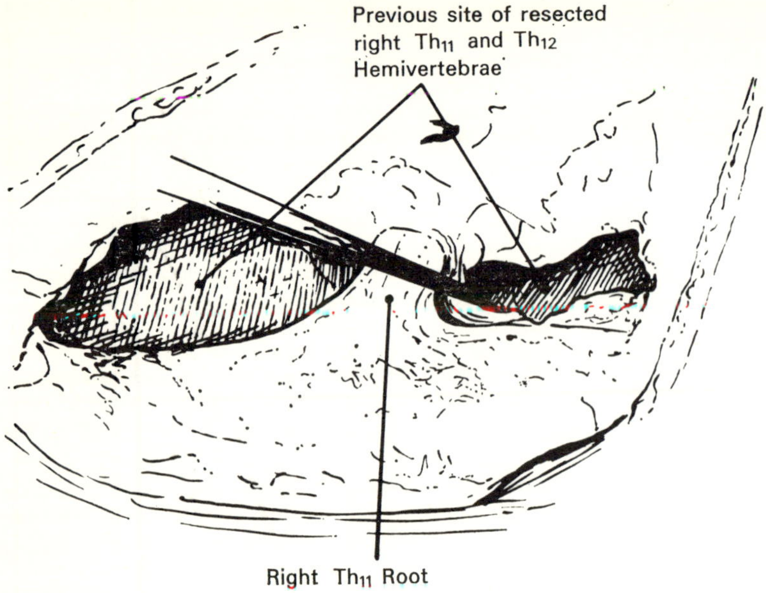

FIG. 32.3. Schematic representation of the site of the right half of T11 and T12 hemivertebrae after removal. The dural sheath of the right T11 root is thus fully exposed.

References

ACQUAVIVA, R., and TAMIC, P. M. (1964) L'échinococcose vertebromédullaire. A propos de 14 observations, *Neuro-chirurgie*, 10, 649–50.

ALLENDE, J. M., and LUQUE, O. (1935) Síndrome de compresión medular por quiste hidático intradural, *Bol. Trab. Soc. Cir. B. Aires*, 19, 283–95.

ARANA-IÑIGUEZ, R. (1961) Echinococcus cyst of the nervous system. Proceedings of the Second Internal Congress of Neurological Surgery, Washington, 1961, *Excerpta med.* (*Amst.*), *int. Congr. Ser.*, No. 36, Ch. 10.

ARANA-IÑIGUEZ, R. (1966) Hidatidosis del sistema nervioso, in *Grandes Síndromes Neurólogicos y Neuroquirurgicos*, eds. Asenjo, A., *et al.*, Buenos Aires, pp. 557–71.

ARANA-IÑIGUEZ, R., AZAMBUJA, N., DIGHIERO, J., and GARCÍA GUELFI, A. (1958) Sound transmission in cerebral hydatic cysts, *Acta neurol. lat.-amer.*, 4, 294–9.

ARANA-IÑIGUEZ, R., GARCÍA CAPURRO, R., and CAUBARRÉRE, N. (1948) Hidatidosis vertebral, *Día Méd. Arg.*, 20, 704–10. Also published in *Arch. int. Hidatid.* (1948), 7, 243–55.

ARANA-IÑIGUEZ, R., and GURRI, J. (1963) Echinococcosis of the nervous system, in *Tropical Neurology*, Buenos Aires, pp. 91–111. Also published in *Rev. neurol. B. Aires* (1962), 20, 155–75.

ARANA-IÑIGUEZ, R., and LÓPEZ FERNÁNDEZ, J. R. (1967) Parasitosis of the nervous system with special reference to echinococcosis, *Clin. Neurosurg.*, 14, 123–44.

ARANA-IÑIGUEZ, R., and MASLENIKOV, V. (1959) Contribución al estudio del quiste hidático cerebral en el adulto, in *Libro de Homenaje Alfonso Asenjo Gómez*, Lima, p. 241.

ARANA-IÑIGUEZ, R., RODRÍGUEZ BARRIOS, R., and SAN JULIÁN, J. (1951) Nueva técnica para la extirpación del quiste hidàtico cerebral. Nota previa, *Pren. méd. argent*, 38, 891–7.

ARANA-IÑIGUEZ, R., RODRÍGUEZ BARRIOS, R., and SAN JULIÁN, J. (1952) Surgical treatment of hydatid cysts of the brain, *Trans. Amer. neurol. Ass.*, 77, 210–11.

ARANA-IÑIGUEZ, R., and SAN JULIÁN, J. (1955 *a*) Angiografía quiste hidático cerebral, *Med. contemp.*, 73, 155–73.

ARANA-IÑIGUEZ, R., and SAN JULIÁN, J. (1955 *b*) Hydatid cysts of the brain, *J. Neurosurg.*, 12, 323–35.

ARANA-IÑIGUEZ, R., SAN JULIÁN, J., GORLERO, A., and FÚSTER, B. (1953) Contribución al diagnóstico y tratamiento del quiste hidático cerebral, *Arch. Pediat. Urug.*, 24, 631–53.

BENHAMOU, E., and GOINARD, P. (1929) Kyste hydatique intrarachidien à forme pseudopottique, *Rev. neurol.*, 51, 46–50.

BIANCHI SAUS, A. (1963) *Evolución Electroencefalográfica de los Pacientes Operados de Quiste Hidático Cerebral*, Tesis del Curso de Graduados de Neurología,

BOIXADÓS, J. R. (1961) Hidatidosis raquimedular, *Acta neurochir.* (*Wien*), 9, 157–70.

CALCAGNO, B. N. (1939) Terapéutica biológica de la hidatidosis, *Bol. Trab. Soc. Cir. B. Aires*, 23, 1481.

CARREA, R., and MURPHY, G. (1964) Primary hydatid cyst of the spinal cord, *Acta neurol. lat.-amer.*, 10, 308–12.

CARRILLO, R., MATERA, R. F., and INSAUSTI, T. (1951) Hidatidosis del sistema nervioso. Experiencia del Instituto de Neurocirguía en los últimos 10 años, *Pren. méd. argent*, 38, 3383–9.

DEL CAMPO, J. C. (1949) Equinococcosis vertebral. Resección total de la 5a. lumbar, *Bol. Soc. Cirug. Urug.*, 20, 211–31. Also published in *Arch. urug. Med.* (1950), 36, 337–57.

DÉVÉ, F. (1928) L'échinococcose vertébrale. Son precesus pathogénique et ses lésions, *Ann. Anat. path.*, 5,841–59.

DÉVÉ, F. (1933) *Trente-deux Années d'Étude de l'Échinococcose*, Buenos Aires.

DÉVÉ, F. (1946) *L'Échinococcose Secondaire*, París.

DÉVÉ, F. (1948) *L'Échinococcose Osséuse*, Montevideo.

DÉVÉ, F. (1949) *L'Échinococcose Primitive* (*Maladie Hydatique*), París.

DEW, H. R. (1928) *Hydatid Disease*, Sydney.

DI BELLO, R. (1956) *Contribución al Estudio de la Equinocosis Cardiaca*, Tesis de Agregación.

DOWLING, E., and ORLANDO, R. (1939) Quiste hidático del lóbulo frontal derecho, *Rev. Espec. Asoc. méd. argent.*, 4, 209–17.

DUMONT, M. (1928) *Echinococcose Cerebral Metastasique*, Thesis, Toulouse.

FÚSTER, B. (1963) The EEG in hydatid cysts of the brain, in *Tropical Neurology*, Buenos Aires, pp. 128–39.

FÚSTER, B., CASTELLS, C., and GASTAUT, H. (1955) The electroencephalographic study of hydatid cysts of the brain, *Electroenceph. clin. Neurophysiol.*, 7, 415–20.

GAMA IMAGINARIO, J. M. DA (1952) A propos du traitement neurochirurgical des kistes hydatiques, *Rev. neurol.*, 86, 489–90.

GARCÍA CAPURRO, R., and PEDEMONTE, V. (1951) Hidatidosis del Femur. Reposición Total de un Femur, in *Proceedings of the Second Uruguayan Congress of Surgery*, Vol. 2, Montevideo, pp. 471–81.

GARCÍA GUELFI, A. (1971) Personal communication.

GOINARD, P., and DESCUNS, P. (1952) Les kystes hydatiques du nevraxe, *Rev. neurol.*, 86, 369–15.

GURRI, J., BOZZOLA, J. L., and PIQUINELA, J. A. (1963) Diagnóstico biológico de la hidatidosis, *Tórax*, 12, 92–8.

IVANISEVICH, O., and RIVAS, C. I. (1961–62) *Equinococosis Hidática*, Ministry of Education and Justice, Buenos Aires.

LARHGERO IBARZ, P. (1939) Patogenia de la hidatidosis biepifisaria de las articulaciones, *Arch. urug. Med.*, 15, 545–54.

LEY, A. J., and MARTÍ, A. (1970) Intramedullary hydatid cyst, *J. Neurosurg.*, 33, 457–9.

LÓPEZ FERNÁNDEZ, J. R. ARANA-IÑIGUEZ, R., VELUTTI, R., and VARELA, J. C. (1966) Hidatidosis experimental del sistema nervioso, *Acta neurol. lat.-amer.*, 12, 106–13.

LÓPEZ FERNÁNDEZ, J. R., ARANA-IÑIGUEZ, R., VELUTTI, R., VARELA, J. C., and VILLAR, J. I. (1966) Implantación heterológica vesícula hidáticas, *Rev. urug. Pat. clin.*, 4, 9–17.

MILLS, T. (1956) Paraplegia due to hydatid disease, *J. Bone Jt Surg.*, 38, 884–91.

MORQUIO, L. (1929) Le kyste hidatique de cerveau chez l'enfant, *Arch. Méd. Enf.*, 32, 377–94; 456–75.

MORQUIO, L. (1932) L'hemiplegie du kyste hidatique cerebral chez l'enfant, *Rev. sud.-amér. Med. Chir.*, 3, 39–58.

SAN JULIÁN, J., and ARANA-IÑIGUEZ, R. (1954) Nevou método para la extirpación del quiste hidático cerebral, *Bol. Soc. Cirug. Urug.*, 25, 722–8. Also published in *Arch. urug. Med.* (1956), 48, 290–6.

SARNI, E., and ZADEK, F. (1965) Cranial and intracranial hydatidosis, *J. Neurosurg.*, 22, 425–33.

SCHROEDER, A. H. (1935) Quistes hidáticos del cerebro. Nueva técnica quirúrgica, *Bol. Soc. Cirug. Urug.*, 6, 141–51.

SCHROEDER, A. (1941) Diagnóstico del quiste hidático cerebral y su tratamiento, *An. Inst. Neurol. Montevideo*, 3, 11–38. Also published in *An. Fac. Med. Montevideo* (1941), 26, 793–820.

SCHROEDER, A. (1947) Diagnóstico del quiste hidático cerebral, *Arch. int. Hidatid.*, 7, 195–218.

SCHROEDER, A. H. (1950) Hidatidosis ósea craneana, *Arch. neurosurg.*, 7, 96–102. Also published in *Arch. int. Hidatid.* (1953), 13, 189–94.

SCHROEDER, A. H., and MEDOC, J. (1950) Hidatidosis vertebral, *An. Inst. Neurol.* (*Montevideo*), 9, 31–54. Also published in *J. nerv. ment. Dis.* (1952), 116, 1025–45.

SCHROEDER, A. H., and MEDOC, J. (1951) Quiste hidático del cerebro, in *Proceedings of the Third Panamerican Congress of Pediatrics*, Montevideo, pp. 687–708. Also published in *Arch. Pediat. Urug.* (1953), 24, 559–80.

THOMAS, D. (1884) *Hydatid Disease*, p. 84. Quoted by Dew, H. R. (1928).

TOLOSA, E. (1953) *Angiografía Cerebral*, Madrid.

TOUYÁ, J. J., and TOUYÁ, E. Personal communication.

TOUYÁ, E., TOUYÁ, J. J., BEKERMAN, C., FERRARI, M., OEHNINGER, C., GARCÍA GUELFI, A., OSORIO, A., and BENEDEK, P. (1968 *a*) Valor de la centellografía encefálica. A propósito de 240 observaciones, *Acta neurol. lat.-amer.*, 14, 325–39.

TOUYÁ, J. J., OSORIO, A., TOUYÁ, E., BEKERMAN, C., PAEZ, A., and FERRARI, M. (1968 *b*) Scintillography of the liver, lung, spleen, kidneys, brain, heart and bone in the diagnosis of hydatid disease in these organs, in *I.A.E.A. Symposium on Medical Isotopes Scanning*, Vienna.

VIALE, J. (1938) *Tratamiento quirurgico de los quistes hidáticos del encéfalo*, Buenos Aires, p. 65.

VIGIL SÓÑORA, E., ARANA-IÑIGUEZ, R., and PÉREZ ACHARD, L. (1961) Tratamiento de la equinococosis raquídea, *Bol. Soc. Cirug. Urug.*, 32, 514–22.

VIGIL SÓÑORA, E. (1962) Equinococcosis vertebral, in *Proceedings of the Fifth Uruguayan Congress of Medicine*, Vol. 1, Montevideo, pp. 155–212.

WOODLAND, L. J. (1949) Hydatid disease of vertebrae, *Med. J. Aust.*, 2, 904–10.

Part Six

WEST INDIES

33 Neurological Disorders in Jamaica

E. K. CRUICKSHANK

Jamaica is an island some 140 miles long and at the maximum 50 miles across, tapering at both ends. It lies between latitudes 17° 14′ and 18° 32′ N, and longitudes 76° 11′ and 78° 21′ W. There are several mountain ranges with some peaks rising to over 7000 feet in the eastern end of the island. The temperature at sea-level varies from 76° to 87·6° F. Much of the island is steep, hilly, relatively inaccessible country where more than half the population of about 2 million exist by subsistence-level peasant farming with, in some areas, seasonal employment on the sugar estates. The population is largely black or coloured with a small number of East Indians, Chinese, Syrians and Europeans. Over the last 20 years there has been the familiar mass movement towards the towns, and particularly Kingston, the only city in the island, which now has a population of over half a million. The majority of the patients at the University Hospital near Kingston are city-dwellers, but many of the chronic sick of the whole island—particularly those with neurological disorders—sooner or later find their way there. Hence, since the opening of the University Hospital nearly 20 years ago it has been possible to obtain a reasonably accurate picture of the types and prevalence of neurological disorders in the island community.

The commonest crippling chronic neurological disorder of adults, if cerebrovascular disorders are excluded, is a syndrome which has been termed 'Jamaican neuropathy'. Over 400 patients have been observed during the last 17 years and the findings will be discussed later in detail. The pattern of neurological disease does not otherwise differ significantly from that of Europe and North America; but there are some interesting features which are worthy of emphasis and it is with these that this chapter will be primarily concerned.

ACUTE INFECTIONS

1. *Bacterial*: acute bacterial meningitis is relatively uncommon. In children under 12 years of age, over 75 per cent of cases are due to *Haemophilus influenzae* while pneumococcal and streptococcal infections make up the residue. Only one or two sporadic cases of meningococcal infection occur per annum (Grant, Been, Bezjak, and Belle, 1965).
2. *Viral*: poliomyelitis has become a rare disease since the initiation of an extensive vaccination programme some years ago, and vaccination with live virus continues to be a routine public health measure at children's clinics and schools.

Viral encephalitis and encephalomyelitis occur sporadically both in adults and children, although the diagnosis is usually a clinical one (Irvine, Grant, and Belle, 1963) as viral isolation from the blood or CSF is rare and indirect blood tests for viral antibodies are not often helpful. In Irvine's series of 25 cases the age range was from 2 to 69 years with 12 children and 13 adults. A virus was isolated but not identified from one case. In three cases there was a significant rise in the titre of antibodies to St. Louis virus: there were four deaths, two children and two adults. Antibodies to St. Louis virus have been found in the blood of up to 80 per cent of a random sample of the rural population, 40–50 per cent showing immunity in the 10–19-year group and 70–80 per cent in older age-groups (Downs and Grant, 1962). Nevertheless, this virus has not been recovered from patients with encephalitis. A proportion of animals and wild and domestic birds also have positive antibody titres. It is therefore probable that the virus is either endemic in the island or is constantly being reintroduced by migrant birds, as there is a large migrant population and young birds can maintain a viraemia sufficiently long to get them from the American mainland to Jamaica. As a result of the banding of birds, some of the species are known to use the mississippi 'flyway' although the majority come down the East Coast. The virus is endemic in Texas, at times producing epidemics there; the most recent one occurred in Dallas in 1966 when there were over 545 cases reported with 20 deaths (*Lancet*, 1969).

In Jamaica in November 1962, there was a brief outbreak of Eastern equine encephalitis with 11 human cases and nine deaths. 79 animals (mules, horses and donkeys) were affected and 70 died. The outbreak occurred at a time when a large number of myrtle warblers were known to have recently arrived from the American continent. No virus, however, was recovered from the birds captured (Belle *et al.*, 1963).

Herpes simplex virus has been recovered from the brains of two fatal cases of encephalitis—one a hospital nurse. There has been one classical case of Behçet's syndrome which presented with the involvement of the nervous system described by Evans, Pallis, and Spillane (1957). The patient eventually died; unfortunately virus isolation from the brain was not attempted.

CHRONIC INFECTIONS

1. *Tuberculosis*: tuberculous meningitis and cerebral tuberculoma are now rarely seen, as an effective BCG

campaign was carried out some years ago and the incidence of acute or fulminant disease has dropped dramatically since. A radiographic survey of over 6000 subjects in a rural area in 1962 (Miall and Rerrie, 1962) showed a prevalence of 3·1 per 1000 males and 6·7 per 1000 females for both quiescent and active disease. These figures have possibly fallen since.

2. *Treponematosis*: neurosyphilis in its classical forms is surprisingly uncommon considering the high incidence of positive treponemal serology in certain sections of the community, as random sampling of the population has given figures of over 40 per cent positivity in the adult population, particularly in rural areas. However, in these areas as many as 25 per cent of the children under 15 have positive treponemal serology compared with under 1 per cent in the Kingston area (Ashcroft *et al.*, 1967). It can be assumed that a high proportion of these positives result from subclinical yaws infection, as the highest figures are obtained for areas where clinical yaws used to be prevalent before the introduction of penicillin. One injection of this drug is sufficient to produce rapid disappearance of the skin lesion but even prolonged treatment may not convert the positive serology. As the *Treponema* immobilization test (TIT), the most sensitive and specific of all tests for treponemal infection, is positive in both yaws and syphilis it is impossible to distinguish between the two by means of serological tests. A characteristic neurological involvement in yaws has never been described and it is generally accepted that there is no such entity as 'neuroyaws' (Gutierrez *et al.*, 1941). It is also possible that yaws infection in childhood gives some immunity to syphilis later.

Menigovascular syphilis, usually presenting with a sudden onset of hemiplegia in a relatively young and normotensive adult, is the commonest unequivocal syphilitic lesion of the CNS seen in Jamaica. In these patients the blood and usually the CSF tests for syphilis are positive and, if they come to post-mortem, syphilitic endarteritis of the cerebral arteries is seen. The majority, however, respond well to antisyphilitic therapy with only a minor residual disability.

General paralysis of the insane and classical tabes dorsalis are now relatively rare, although they were reputedly fairly common in the past. This may be because penicillin and other antitreponemal antibiotics are extensively used for all types of infection without a microbiological diagnosis being made, particularly as frequent skin infections are very common in rural areas and penicillin is available in all the government clinics. The dosage may be insufficient to convert the blood serology from positive to negative but it may prevent late neurological complications. Other neurological manifestations of syphilis and the possible role of the *Trepnoema* in tropical amblyopia and the Jamaican neuropathy will be discussed later under 'Diseases of Uncertain Origin' [p. 426].

3. *Other infections*: infections of the nervous system with other agents such as protozoa, helminths and moulds are exceptionally rare in Jamaica. Malaria was eradicated over 10 years ago. Bilharziasis, trypanosomiasis, trichinosis, cysticercosis and paragonimiasis have not been recognized and neurological manifestations attributable to ascariasis, a common infestation in children, occur very occasionally. Histoplasmosis and coccidioidomycosis, although they occur in parts of the adjacent American mainland, have not been identified. Chromoblastomycosis is occasionally seen but does not involve the nervous system.

NEOPLASMS

Malignant Tumours

The incidence and type of neoplasms of the nervous system in Jamaica follow the conventional pattern for other areas where accurate data are available. The Jamaican Cancer Registry, which has a full record of proven malignant disease in the island since 1958, does not place primary malignant disease of the nervous system on its list of the 30 commonest cancers (Bras and Watler, 1967).

In the under-15 age-group there have been 33 primary malignant cerebral neoplasms in this period, the great majority being in the posterior fossa with nine of them medulloblastomas (Miller and Ragbeer, 1971). In adults gliomas were the most common tumour, 36 having been proved by exploration. This is contrary to the observation of Trowell (1960) that the glioma is rare in the Bantu in South Africa. Primary malignant tumours of the cord are rare but, as elsewhere, compression of the cord from secondary disease of the vertebrae is common, although intracerebral metastases seem to be infrequent. It is also of interest that in five patients with malignant lymphomas the initial features were neurological with signs of cord compression in four and an equina lesion in one (Irvine, 1970).

Simple Tumours

Of the simple tumours, meningiomas are much commoner than neurofibromata. Some 30 have been explored and proven histologically, but only three of these have involved the spinal cord. Neurofibromatosis is a relatively common condition in Jamaica but it rarely affects the central nervous system. Only five cases of acoustic neuroma have been seen in 10 years and two of these were incidental post-mortem findings.

CEREBROVASCULAR DISEASE

As this is the commonest certified cause of death in Jamaican adults (12 per cent of all deaths over 15 years of age) it is a major problem, but there are few features which are specific for Jamaica. Of some 3000 autopsies on adults done at the University Hospital during the last 15 years, in nearly 300 (10 per cent) death was attributed to cerebrovascular disease (Cole and Cole,

1969). In nearly 70 per cent of these hypertension was a predisposing cause, the criteria being a diastolic of over 100 mm of mercury with a heart weight of over 400 g in the male and 350 g in the female. Thirty per cent were under the age of 50. Seventy-seven per cent were attributable to haemorrhage, mostly in the hypertensives, and 23 per cent were due to infarction with thrombosis in one-third and atherosclerosis without infarction in a quarter. Subarachnoid harmorrhage was present in 23 per cent, and in 80 per cent of these a berry aneurysm was identified, two-thirds of these occurring at the junction of the internal carotid artery and its branches; this is a much higher percentage than that reported from Europe and the United States. Multiple aneurysms were found in 10 per cent.

The important difference in these findings is that haemorrhage is a three times more frequent cause of stroke than infarction, while in the United Kingdom and the United States infarction is slightly more common than haemorrhage (Yates, 1964). This is in keeping with the observation that although the atherosclerotic indices are measured on the aorta, coronary and cerebral arteries were almost identical with similar measurements carried out on a group in New Orleans, only 2·4 per cent of the Jamaicans suffered myocardial infarction compared with 16·1 per cent on the New Orleans group (Robertson, 1959). In addition, we have not seen hemiparesis or hemiplegia due to thrombosis of the extracranial portion of the internal carotid artery, although for the last 10 years arteriograms have been done on most patients who rapidly develop a hemiplegia especially in the younger age-group. It is possible, therefore, that the factor or factors responsible for this difference occur in the coagulative processes of the blood rather than in the diseased vessel wall.

DEFICIENCY DISEASES

Vitamins

In spite of the marginal dietary levels in many of the poorer areas of Jamaica, neurological disease unequivocally attributable to specific vitamin deficiency in the diet has not been seen, but there may be a dietary component in two of the relatively common neurological disorders—retrobulbar neuropathy (tropical amblyopia) [p. 431] and the Jamaican neuropathy, which is discussed on page 427.

Pellagra has only occurred in patients with severe malabsorption resulting from hyperinfestation with *Strongyloides stercoralis*, 12 cases having been seen over the last 10 years. The skin and mucosal lesions have dominated the picture and apart from marked lethargy there have been no neurological features. Thiamine deficiency, manifesting itself in the acute form of Wernicke's encephalopathy or the more chronic peripheral neuropathy, has not been recognized.

Vitamin B_{12} Deficiency

Pernicious anaemia was considered to be a rare disease in Jamaica and in people of Negro extraction, but Stuart and MacIver (1961) described 10 cases discovered in a period of 30 months. Seven of them had signs of peripheral neuropathy and five of these were also judged to have cord involvement. In a further period of 30 months Milner (1965) diagnosed 15 more cases, and since that time 5 to 6 new cases per annum are seen. The majority show some evidence of peripheral nerve damage with some cord involvement but rarely enough to produce serious disability. A few patients have also shown some initial disorder of cerebral function which cleared rapidly with therapy. It is of interest that three patients have been in their early twenties—all satisfying rigid criteria for the diagnosis of pernicious anaemia, and one of them presented with signs of cord damage without anaemia.

Protein Deficiency

Recently, careful follow-up studies have been carried out on children in Jamaica who have been in the University Hospital with kwashiorkor. Special attention has been paid to their intellectual development, and preliminary assessment of data suggests that there has been significant permanent retardation compared with siblings and controls from an identical environment, *but only in the children from the rural areas* (Birch, 1971). It would appear that the child in the urban environment can 'catch up', which would not support the view that cerebral damage had occurred. There is good evidence, however, that severe protein malnutrition, particularly during the first 6 months of life when the brain cells are still multiplying, produces serious intellectual impairment (Cravioto, de Licardie, and Birch, 1966; Monckeberg, 1969; Fishman and Pransky, 1969; Champakan, Srikantia, and Gopalan, 1968; Winick and Rosso, 1969).

Work is also in progress on the chemistry of muscle protein in severe protein malnutrition. Picou, Alleyne, and Seakins (1966) have shown that sarcoplasmic proteins are reduced whereas collagen is relatively increased, and Waterlow (1959), using labelled methionine, demonstrated that the 'essential' organs, especially the liver and brain, lost very much less nitrogen proportionately than muscle. This suggests a 'built-in' protective mechanism for these organs so that after the critical growth period with rapid cell proliferation, even severe depletion of protein does not appear to produce significant nervous system damage. However, it may be recalled that Strom *et al.* (1962) reported a late progressive meningomyelopathy in Norwegians who had been interned in concentration camps.

EPILEPSY AND CONVULSIVE DISORDERS

In developing countries epilepsy is frequently a very common and important neurological problem. This is particularly so in certain parts of Africa, and in Nigeria the incidence has been reported to be as high as 3 to 10 per 1000 for different areas (Dada, 1969). This is attributable to the high incidence of infections with brain damage in infancy and childhood and to inadequate antenatal and obstetrical services. In Jamaica, where preventive and curative services are still seriously deficient in many areas, epilepsy commonly occurs. It is always difficult to get accurate figures on the prevalence of this disorder because of the stigma and even social ostracism attached to it in primitive communities. Hall (1964), reporting on his experience at the Kingston Public Hospital, found that in the 4-year period 1958–61 there were 825 patients admitted for epilepsy, more than half being under 16 years of age. In this latter group over 30 per cent were associated with acute infections, especially bronchopneumonia. Only 7 per cent had clinical evidence of prior intracranial damage and in the remainder no specific factor was demonstrable. It is of special interest that in none was a convulsion the presenting feature of a cerebral tumour or congenital syphilis, in spite of the high prevalence of positive treponemal serology in the adult female population: 14·7 per cent of the women attending the antental clinic at that hospital between the years 1943–54 (Grant, 1956). Petit mal and psychomotor epilepsy were very rare but this is probably because the minor presenting features of these disorders would not lead to admission to hospital, and at that time EEG investigations were not done—hence these conditions could have been overlooked.

Ackee Poisoning (Vomiting Sickness)

As the presenting feature of this syndrome in children is frequently convulsions with vomiting of a cerebral type, and as it is an interesting, if not unique, disorder seen in Jamaica, it is appropriate to discuss it here.

The medical literature of Jamaica contains accounts going back nearly 100 years of an acute illness characterized by the onset of vomiting, usually 2 to 3 hours after meals, rapidly followed by weakness, prostration and often convulsions, coma and death. The commonest victims are young children between the ages of 2 and 5 years, but cases occurred in all age-groups. The first published account of the syndrome came from J. J. Bowrey in the *Jamaica Gazette* in 1887, when he described 31 cases of 'vomiting sickness' with several deaths; 10 of these cases he attributed directly to the prior ingestion of ackee (a local fruit). Further accounts appeared over the years, the most comprehensive and detailed being that of Scott (1915), who reviewed 257 cases 242 of which he regarded as ackee poisoning, particularly when the unripe fruit was eaten. One of the puzzling features, however, was that very many people had eaten and still ate ackee in large quantities with no ill effects, and there was much speculation by various observers as to the reason for this, some claiming that the ackee was not the responsible agent, but that other foodstuffs, particularly certain yams which when immature contain toxic glycosides, could be incriminated (Barrett, 1943). It was well recognized, however, that the great majority, if not all, cases occurred in poorly nourished communities, particularly at times when drought or temporary unemployment reduced the dietary to submarginal levels, and that many patients had the classical clincal syndrome of ariboflavinosis—glossitis, angular stomatitis and nasolabial dermatitis. Clinical examination otherwise revealed little of note and the postmortem findings showed nothing specific, except that extensive fatty change in the liver was invariable and most marked in those who had died rapidly. As the disease had an acute onset, ran a rapid course with death or recovery and nearly always occurred in more remote parts of the island, biochemical studies of the disease had not been undertaken. In January 1951, an outbreak of 151 cases with 32 deaths occurred and a joint University and Government team moved in to investigate, but by the time they got there the majority of the patients were dead or recovered. Clinical examination again revealed only undernutrition and evidence of ariboflavinosis. A variety of haematological, serological and biochemical tests including blood urea and glucose gave no useful lead to the aetiology.

The breakthrough, as is so often the case, came by chance nearly a year later. A child arrived in the casualty department of the University Hospital semicomatose and with the usual history of 'vomiting sickness'. The clinical picture suggested hypoglycaemia to the alert casualty officer on duty; the blood glucose was under 10 mg per 100 ml and intravenous 20 per cent glucose produced a dramatic and rapid recovery of full consciousness. The diagnostic key had been found. This was acute toxic hypoglycaemia and from then on treatment with large doses of intravenous glucose was successful, unless the hypoglycaemia had been present for a long time and irreversible central nervous system damage had occurred.

The ackee (*Blighia sapida*) was brought from West Africa to Jamaica by Captain Bligh of the *Bounty* in 1793, although there is evidence that it had been already introduced by a Dr. Thomas Clarke in 1778 who was then the island botanist (Broughton, 1794). It is a tree of medium height with light-green shiny leaves attactively hung with red pear-shaped fruit when these are ripening. The fruit itself contains three smooth black seeds each with a large fatty arillus or placenta, and it is this which is eaten. It has a high fat content and is thus a valuable source of calories, particularly for undernourished people as it ripens in the 'lean' months of the year. In spite of its reputation, it still remains an important dietary item for the Jamaican, especially in the lower income groups, but one of the favourite dishes of the Jamaican family at all social levels is 'salt fish and ackee' —and this is not surprising as once the taste has been acquired, it is a delicious dish when properly prepared. The fruit is only eaten in other West Indian islands and in Central America where an occasional tree is found near the odd Jamaican who has emigrated to several of these countries as a labourer and taken this favoured fruit with him. There is at present a profitable export trade of canned ackees to the large Jamaican populations in the United Kingdom, Canada and the United States of America. It has been intensively studied by our botanists and pharmacologists and the outcome of this research can be summarized as follows:

1. The hypoglycaemic agent is found in the nut or seed in higher concentration than in the arillus, and in spoilt or unripe fruit concentration in the arillus is generally increased.
2. The agent has been identified as occurring as two closely related compounds, hypoglycin A and B. These are unusual amino acids, A being amino-methylenecyclopropylanepropionic acid and B is a dipeptide of A with glutamic acid (von Holt, von Holt, and Bohm, 1966).
3. In the experimental animal, the hypoglycaemic action of these agents is the result of their transformation in the body to methylenecyclopropane-acetyl-CoA or an oxidation product of this, which inhibits the mitochondrial fatty acid–oxidation system, thus preventing the utlization of fatty acids as a 'fuel' for the provision of energy from the high energy bonds of ATP (von Holt, von Holt, and Bohm, 1966) [FIG. 33.1]. Hence glycogen stores, which are low in the under-nourished child anyway, are quickly depleted and glucose is rapidly metabolized, leading to a disastrous fall in the blood level with the clinical features of severe hypoglycaemia. Of interest is the observation that in the rat riboflavine can alleviate the toxic effects of hypoglycin although the biochemical mechanism of this protective action is not fully understood (Fox and Miller, 1960). Thus, if a large evening meal of ackees or the 'soup' from boiled ackees is consumed by a child with high energy demands, who already has depleted liver glycogen stores and riboflavine deficiency from undernutrition, there may be a sufficient concentration of hypoglycin to produce major symptoms during the night, a frequent time for the onset of 'vomiting sickness'.

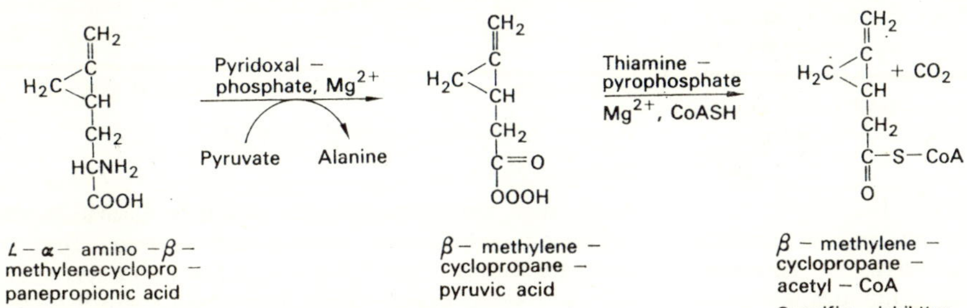

FIG. 33.1. Hypoglycaemic action of hypoglycin A and B, inhibiting mitochondrial fatty acid–oxidation system and preventing utilization of fatty acids as 'fuel' for provision of energy.

PERIPHERAL NEUROPATHIES AND MYOPATHIES

Diabetic Peripheral Neuropathy

The commonest cause of damage to the peripheral neurone in Jamaica is diabetes mellitus, as the prevalence of glycosuria in the population over 15 years of age is 1·26 per cent, with 0·94 per cent male and 1·5 per cent female (Tulloch, 1962). In a survey of 1000 cases attending the diabetic clinic at the University Hospital from 1955 to 1961, Tulloch (1962) found objective evidence of peripheral neuropathy in 31·4 per cent of cases. In this series three patients had third cranial nerve lesions, two retrobulbar neuritis, one a neurogenic bladder, one a Charcot's knee joint, and only one amyotrophy. Of 107 male patients 63·5 per cent complained of partial or complete impotence and this symptom was commonly the first one to draw attention to the diabetes. As with the peripheral neuropathy, the occurrence of this symptom sometimes preceded the appearance of established diabetes mellitus by months and occasionally years. This high incidence of neurological complications is in keeping with the evidence that poor control over a long period of time leads to increased frequency of complications. The average Jamaican diabetic, whose diet is often, of necessity, high in carbohydrate and low in protein and fat, varying in quantity with the changing fortunes of the patient, and whose insulin administration is either sporadic or cut off abruptly for long periods of time, is invariably poorly controlled.

The fundamental lesion responsible for neural damage in diabetes mellitus is still not fully understood. There is good evidence that, in the mononeuritides, occlusion of the vasa nervorum is a major factor (Raff, Sangalang, and Ashbury, 1968), but in the much commoner peripheral neuropathy the lesion is more likely to be a biochemical one and marked slowing of conduction velocity in peripheral nerves may precede the appearance of clinical features. The earliest demonstrable pathological change is segmental demyelination (Thomas and Lascelles, 1966). Gabbay and O'Sullivan (1968) reported that sorbitol was present in excess in the Schwann cells of diabetic nerves and was possibly responsible for the cell damage and demyelination. More recently, Beaumont, Hollows, Schofield, and Williams (1971) have put forward the hypothesis, based on a valid biochemical argument, that excessive secretion of growth hormone (GH) inhibits glucose metabolism and results in the accumulation of sorbitol in cells whose membranes are impermeable to the polyol, and the subsequent osmotic imbalance produces tissue damage generally throughout the body, especially in the capillaries.

Experience in the diabetic clinic over the last 10 years confirms Tulloch's observations. The commonest single nerve to be involved is the third cranial, and single or bilateral seventh nerve palsies come next in order. Lesions of the ninth, tenth and twelfth nerves have also occurred. Less often, individual peripheral nerves in the arms or legs are affected. Neurogenic bladder disturbances are also relatively common, and occasionally we see the full picture of diabetic pseudotabes—although in this community it is impossible to exclude syphilis even with negative serology.

Diabetic Myelopathy

Occasionally a diabetic patient presents with evidence of pyramidal tract, posterior column and minor spinothalamic tract damage with muscle wasting of a root distribution and fasciculation. However, it is again impossible to attribute this picture solely to diabetes, as the 'Jamaican neuropathy' can have all these features. As both disorders are common they may merely be two separate entities occurring in the same patient. The same can be said of retrobulbar neuropathy and eighth nerve deafness, when they are present in a diabetic.

Diabetic Myopathy (Amyotrophy)

Marked weakness and selective wasting of muscle groups, often fasciculation, are relatively common complications of diabetes mellitus in Jamaica and over 100 patients with these features have been seen during the last 15 years. This would appear to be a very much higher incidence than elsewhere. Richards and Haynes (1964) analysed the features of 26 patients whom they had seen over an 18-month period. All had marked wasting of the small muscles of the hands and feet. The degree of wasting was rarely symmetrical. Seven showed, in addition, proximal muscle wasting which is regarded as the characteristic presentation of this syndrome (Garland, 1960). Muscle biopsy showed only patchy degeneration of muscle bundles without cellular infiltration. Other causes of muscle wasting were excluded. The cause again remains speculative but the lesion probably lies in the peripheral motor neurone, as Gilliatt (1965) has demonstrated marked slowing of the conduction in the peripheral nerve which is not a feature of anterior horn cell disease such as poliomyelitis or amyotrophic lateral sclerosis. Gilliatt also reports—as did Garland— that marked improvement can occur with strict control of the diabetes. This we have not been able to achieve in our patients.

Thyrotoxic Myopathies

Muscle wasting and weakness which is out of proportion to the general weight loss in thyrotoxicosis in Jamaican patients is a relatively common finding, and this is in agreement with the observations of Ramsay (1966), who reviewed 54 consecutive patients with a proven diagnosis of thyrotoxicosis in Belfast. He found that half gave a history of muscle weakness, especially in the thighs on going up stairs and in the proximal muscles of the arms. Wasting was most marked in the supraspinatus and related shoulder girdle muscles. Although exact figures are not available our experience would be comparable to Ramsay's. Muscle biopsies in our patients also show the changes described by Ramsay—degeneration of isolated fibres with macrophage and lymphocytic infiltration, focal perivascular lymphorrhages, connective tissue proliferation and fat infiltration between the muscle fibres. The clinical features and muscle changes resolve in most patients with satisfactory therapy.

Carcinomatous Neuromyopathies

These are relatively uncommon but cortical cerebellar dysfunction, myelopathy and mixed peripheral neuropathy have occurred. It is of interest that two cases of carcinoma of the penis—relatively common in Jamaicans —developed myelopathies.

DISEASES OF UNCERTAIN AETIOLOGY

Where Auto-Immunity may play a Role

Multiple Sclerosis

As in most tropical areas this is a rare disease in the indigenous population. During the 10 years 1951 to 1961 the author (Cruickshank and Montgomery, 1961) saw only seven cases—three Europeans, two of whom had their first symptoms before leaving Europe and one who developed them 2 years after arriving in Jamaica; and four indigenous Jamaicans, three of whom had never left the island while the fourth developed his first symptoms while in Buffalo, in the United States (at the age of 38), after he had been living there for several years. The natural history and presenting features of these patients were classically those of multiple sclerosis. Two patients have since died from the disease but unfortunately in neither was a post-mortem examination obtained. Approximately 10 further cases have been diagnosed during the last 10 years but none of these has died. Ultimate proof of the disease requires pathological confirmation as even cases with classical histories may turn out to be something else at autopsy (Poser, 1968). The aetiology of multiple sclerosis remains obscure in spite of an enormous amount of investigative work. There is some evidence to support the case that auto-immunity plays a role (Zilkha, 1968), but its rarity in most tropical areas and the Southern hemisphere, its increasing frequency towards the higher Northern latitudes, and its incidence in Israeli Jews following that of their country of origin (Halpern, 1961), cannot be explained, particularly as diseases such as systemic lupus erythematosus and polyarteritis nodosa—accepted as being the result of auto-immunity—appear to be much commoner in Jamaica than in temperate climates. It is for this reason that the possibility of it being due to a 'slow' virus is considered (Poskanzer, Schapira, and Miller, 1963) and Cosnett (1966) has produced an ingenious hypothesis to support such an aetiology and to explain some of the puzzling features. He suggests that when myelin is laid down on the outer extremity of the helical path which it is believed to follow to reach the axon, it may be focally damaged by a virus or other agent. The progress to the core and axon takes years, the speed varying with the site. It is not until the damaged myelin reaches the axon that disordered function occurs.

Guillain–Barré Syndrome

Contrary to the opinion expressed by Haymaker and Kemohan (1949) the Guillain-Barré syndrome occurs quite commonly in Negroes, and 3 to 4 cases are seen per annum in the University Hospital. There has been one death from respiratory failure. The presenting features meet the accepted criteria for this syndrome although it is not always possible to get a history of a recent infection or fever.

Myasthenia Gravis

During a 5-year period, Hall (1967) reported 12 cases out of 6000 admissions to the Kingston Public Hospital. The age range of his patients was 10 to 79 years and 10 of them were female. Four had localized non-progressive disease mainly involving the cranial nerves. Four presented with acute fulminating disease, one of whom died, and four had generalized myasthenia. None was operated upon and in the fatal case no thymoma or thymus hyperplasia was found. Rodgers (1971) at the University Hospital has seen over 70 patients since 1962. She has analysed 50 of these observed between 1962 and 1969. The incidence is 1 per 38 000 which is more than twice the number in the United Kingdom where the figure is 1 per 100 000. The sex incidence was 31 females and 19 males—a ratio of 3:2. Nineteen were under the age of 20, which is a considerably higher proportion than reported from elsewhere. Seventy-four per cent were seen within a year of onset of symptoms, and in 82 per cent the presenting feature was diplopia. Thymectomy was carried out on 16 because of severity of symptoms and failure to respond adequately to drug therapy. There was one death in a patient with a malignant thymoma, but only three failed to make a dramatic response to surgery. Seven are now on no drug therapy and all have been able to return to normal life. The pathological changes in the thymus were hyperplasia with germinal centre formation. The case who died was the only patient with a thymoma.

Aetiology Unknown

Jamaican Neuropathy

Strachan (1897) published an account of 510 patients seen at the Kingston Public Hospital in Jamaica with a neurological syndrome which he termed 'malarial multiple peripheral neuritis'. The main features were pain, numbness and paraesthesiae of the palms and soles, dimness of vision, impairment of hearing and girdle pains. There was soreness and excoriation of the mucocutaneous junctions and evidence of polyneuritis —weakness, wasting, loss of sensation and reduction of reflexes. The gait was ataxic and the retinae showed hyperaemia and optic neuritis. The majority recovered but some died of respiratory paralysis. Again, in 1918, Scott described an illness which affected Jamaican sugar-cane workers. It was often ushered in by stomatitis, conjunctivitis and diarrhoea followed shortly by pains and paraesthesiae in the feet and legs, ataxia, deterioration of vision and deafness. Knee and ankle reflexes were lost and the plantar responses remained flexor. The only objective sensory loss was some impairment of temperature sense; position sense was said to be normal. Vibration sense was not recorded. Some patients died in 4 to 6 weeks, and in others there were residual neurological defects. These were mainly loss of vision, deafness and ataxia. The latter is hard to explain if position sense was normal, and there is nothing in the clinical reports to suggest it was cerebellar in type—perhaps residual muscle weakness was responsible. At autopsy, degeneration in the fibres of olfactory, optic and auditory nerves was found. The pyramidal tracts largely escaped, but considerable degeneration was found in the posterior root ganglia and in the posterior and spinocerebellar tracts of the spinal cord. Scott did not think the disease was of nutritional origin but considered a toxaemia more likely. Both of these accounts point to a sensory type of neuropathy with a tendency to residual ataxia and impairment of vision and hearing. Since then the numerous reports already referred to, of similar or related syndromes from different parts of the world, have accumulated. These are drawn from three broad groups:

1. Undernourished populations in tropical countries —Africa, India, the Far East and Jamaica.
2. Prisoners of war in the Middle and Far East (1941–45).
3. The besieged population of Madrid during the Spanish Civil War (1936–39).

These disorders are not seen in Europe (with the exception of Spain) and North America, and did not occur in the European concentration camps of the last war. Over 400 cases have been seen at the University

Table 33.1

Jamaican Neuropathy Cases.
Age and Sex Distribution per cent
(Age at Onset of Symptoms)

Age Distribution	*Ataxic Group (25 cases)*	*Spastic Group* (76 cases) VDRL + Neg.	(105 cases) VDRL or KW + Pos.
Years			
0–13	0	0	0
14–24	44	14	2
25–34	28	26	20
35–44	24	25	46
45–54	4	20	25
55–64	0	15	7
65+	0	0	0
Age range	14–53 yr	15–59 yr	20–61 yr
Sex: Male	48	39	67
Female	52	61	33

* VDRL = Standard cardiolipin slide test of the United States Veneral Diseases Reference Laboratory.
† KW = Kolmer–Wassermann complement-fixation test.

Table 33.2

Features of the Ataxic Group
(25 Cases)

	Total Cases
Presenting symptoms:	
Deafness	11
Weak legs	9
Failing vision	5
Clinical findings:	
Posterior column lesion	25
Nerve deafness	20
Retrobular neuropathy	18
Mild pyramidal tract lesion	11
Bilateral peroneal muscle wasting	6
Treponemal serology:	
VDRL and KW negative	16
VDRL or KW positive	6
VDRL positive 1:1–1:2	3
Dietary assessment (21 cases):	
Poor or very poor	19
Fair	2
Good	0
Gastric acidity (18 cases):	
Normal acid	8
Free acid after 1 ml histamine	5
Histamine-fast achlorhydria	5
Spinal fluid:	
Protein and cells normal and serology negative in all cases	

Hospital, Jamaica, in the last 15 years and 210 of these were reviewed in detail by Montgomery, Cruickshank, Robertson, and McMenemey in 1964. However, the great majority (over 80 per cent) had evidence of pyramidal tract damage compared with the small proportion with this lesion in the cases reported by Strachan (1897) and Scott (1918). Their findings are summarized in TABLES 33.1, 33.2 and 33.3.

Table 33.3

Features of the Spastic Group
(181 *Cases*)

	Cases per cent of Total	
Presenting symptoms:		
Weakness, pain or numbness of legs	97	
Deafness	3	
Gradual onset	81	
Sudden onset	19	
First symptoms in one leg only	32	
Lumbar backache	39	
Bladder dysfunction (later)	66	
Treponemal serology:		
VDRL and KW negative	40	
VDRL weakly positive, or history of positive	24	} 60
VDRL positive 1:1	22	
VDRL positive 1:2	9	
VDRL positive 1:4–1:16	5	

	VDRL Negative Cases	*VDRL Positive Cases*
Clinical findings:		
Pyramidal tract lesion	100%	100%
Posterior column lesion	50%	51%
Retrobulbar neuropathy	15%	15%
Nerve deafness	7%	7%
Peripheral nerve or root lesion	11%	15%
Spinal fluid:		
Cells 0–9 lympho per cmm	76	73
10–49 lympho per cmm	24	24
50– lympho per cmm	0	2
Protein 10–44 mg per 100 ml	65	67
45–74 mg per 100 ml	19	24
75– mg per 100 ml	16	9
Lange paretic	19	20
Lange luetic	5	6
VDRL only positive	—	1
KW only positive	—	3
VDRL and KW positive	—	2
Gastric acidity (147 cases):		
Normal acid	39	59
Free acid after 1 ml histamine	30	11
Histamine-fast achlorhydria	31	30

The circumstantial evidence suggests that malnutrition, using this term in its broadest sense, is mainly responsible. Many of the Jamaican patients, however, appeared to be in good health, and their histories indicated an adequate and balanced diet. Many were employed in heavy labour. Frank signs of known vitamin deficiency were not encountered. In other parts of the world evidence of malnutrition in these syndromes has often been obvious and it has usually taken the form of the mucocutaneous lesions of riboflavine deficiency This was also true of the earlier Jamaican cases of Strachan and Scott, and these differed in many respects from the present series—notably in the absence of pyramidal tract involvement—and resembled more closely the syndromes described elsewhere. In the prisoner-of-war camps, on the other hand, the neurological features often developed against a background of apparently fair general health despite loss of weight and energy. In other words, we must not necessarily expect to find the classical signs of vitamin deficiency. Since Addison's time we have known that the patient with pernicious anaemia or subacute combined degeneration may appear well-nourished. His deficiency manifests itself in a very selective way; and from the neurological point of view vitamin B_{12} deficiency more closely resembles the syndromes under discussion than any other common disease of the nervous system.

In the Jamaican cases a normal bone marrow was found in over 20 with a histamine-fast achlorhydria, and the great majority of the patients had normal blood pictures. This, and a normal Schilling test in four typical cases, make it very unlikely that B_{12} deficiency is an important aetiological factor. In addition, studies of blood pyruvate and glutathione have proved negative, although cases in the early acute state were not available for these estimations. A megaloblastic marrow was found in two women aged 22 and 29 years at the time of onset of the neurological symptoms, one of whom developed bilateral eighth nerve deafness. The diet of one was fair and her marrow rapidly returned to normal with B_{12} taken orally. The other patient's diet was very poor and her blood picture returned to normal with hospital diet alone. In neither was there any improvement in the neurological symptoms. In the circumstances they cannot be regarded as true cases of pernicious anaemia with subacute combined degeneration. The latter has, however, been described in patients assumed to have B_{12} deficiency from inadequate intake. The two patients referred to were more likely to be folate deficient, responding to the folate in the ward diet. No serum folate or B_{12} estimations were possible at that time.

Heredity does not appear to play a part in the syndrome. Cases arise in all parts of the island with no evidence of interbreeding and only once has a familial incidence been observed—in two sisters.

Of particular importance in these cases is the apparently high incidence of serological tests for syphilis and yaws. Excluded from the series were all cases showing serological abnormality in the cerebrospinal fluid. The incidence of a positive blood Wassermann or Kahn reaction in Jamaican adults varies from 12 to 41 per cent in different parishes, with averages of 23 per cent for farm labourers and 40 per cent for male industrial workers (Grant, 1956). There is no means of differentiating between yaws and syphilis by means of serological tests, but it is thought that latent yaws, which is endemic in Jamaica, may be responsible for a large number of positive serological findings, particularly in the hilly country areas where clinical yaws used to be common. As already noted [p. 422], 25 per cent of prepubertal children in one parish had positive serology compared with less than 1 per cent in urban Kingston (Ashcroft *et al.*, 1967). Of the 206 cases the blood Wassermann or VDRL test was positive in 48 per cent, the spastic group having a higher positive rate (60 per cent) than the ataxic group (36 per cent). This is more than the average for the populaion, but 40 per cent had no clinical or serological evidence of syphilis, except for two patients with negative serology, one of whom had aortic incompetence and a dilated ascending aorta, and the other a fusiform dilatation of the descending aorta, A very high proportion of the patients was born and brought up in the country—a much higher percentage than in all other chronic sick in the medical wards of the University Hospital. It is of interest that yaws was, until recently, common in the same areas and is not found in the town-bred population; a few patients in this series with negative serology gave a history of yaws. At the same time, the country population has much readier access to a wide variety of bush teas. Yaws and syphilis may be capable of producing such neurological damage, and yaws is also prevalent in other countries where unusual neurological syndromes occur. However, neurological sequelae of yaws have never been recognized (Hackett, 1953). Rodgers (1965) carefully reviewed 125 cases of Jamaican neuropathy, and 43 of these had been included in the series reported by Montgomery, Cruickshank, Robertson, and McMenemey (1964). She personally took a detailed history with special emphasis on possible previous infection with yaws or syphilis, injections for 'bad blood' (a positive treponemal serology) and penicillin therapy for any reason. A wider range of tests (Wassermann, Reiter, PCFT, VDRL) was carried out on the blood and CSF of the patients. X-rays of the pelves of some of the patients who denied previous 'bad blood' and who had negative serologies, had bismuth deposits in the buttocks suggesting that a positive serology had been suspected or diagnosed and treated in the past. A careful neurological examination was carried out. Rodgers classified 103 as spastic and 22 as ataxic. Her findings were as follows in the spastic group of 103 patients:

History of yaws	32 per cent
syphilis	47 per cent
Blood tests for treponematosis	72 per cent
CSF tests for treponematosis	26 per cent (compared with 6 per cent in Montgomery's *et al.* series)

In addition, Rodgers considered that 40 per cent of the patients had ptosis or some pupillary changes. She concludes that, 'the findings are all compatible with syphilis. This is supported by the presence of ptosis and abnormal pupillary reactions, deafness and optic atrophy as definite features in some patients. The varied clinical findings—myelitis, wasting, ataxia, peripheral neuritis, are all recognized as occurring in neurosyphilis and as all these patients fit into a basic pattern, there is no reason to postulate several diseases. The clinical syndromes into which these patients can be put are: Erb's paraplegia, syphilitic amyotrophy and neuritis, myelitis, encephalomyelitis, pachymeningitis cervicalis hypertrophica, and arachnoiditis. These names are used by some neurologists, but others prefer to avoid specific names and to use the general terminology. It is essential, however, to keep an open mind as 20 per cent of patients had no serological evidence of syphilis in the tests used, although the clinical features are the same as in the 80 per cent who do.'

However, there still remains the intriguing question that if syphilis alone is the cause of the Jamaican neuropathy, why should there be such a high incidence of this particular pattern of neurosyphilis in Jamaica compared with other parts of the world, and why should an almost identical clinical picture occur in some parts of the world where syphilis as a cause is very unlikely, such as Bangalore, India (Mani, Mani, and Montgomery, 1969). I prefer at present to regard the case against the spirochaete to remain 'not proven', although this or its products may be the trigger that initiates a complex auto-immune reaction within the nervous system of sensitized individuals.

Comparison of the Jamaican cases with those reported from West Africa (Money, 1959) shows a very much higher incidence of upper motor neurone damage, which is frequently the earliest and only feature in our patients, occurring in 94 per cent of our cases compared to 3 per cent in West Africa. A predominantly spastic syndrome was seen in prisoners of war in the Far East but not the Middle East, and has also been reported in Eritrea (Ferro-Luzzi, 1958), Iraq (Al-Witry, Shaby, and Kantarjian, 1950) and South India (Mani, Mani, and Montgomery, 1969). Other differences in our cases include the very low incidence of paraesthesiae which was an initial symptom in 99 per cent of Money's cases. Differences of this kind suggest that the syndrome in different parts of the world may well be due to a variety of factors producing closely related lesions. There seems little doubt that the neurological picture in Nigeria and elsewhere has been complicated by the presence of thiamine deficiency, which is evident in few, if any, of our cases.

In addition to the possibilities discussed above, consideration has been given to the questions of auto-immunity, toxic factors in cooking oils, trace metal deficiency, or toxicity due to selenium, molybdenum or cyanide, which may be present in excess in bushes, grasses, yams and cassava as cyanogenetic glycosides. The cyanide radical is neurotoxic to experimental animals (Hartmann, Lalich, and Akert, 1958), and there is good evidence that vitamin B_{12} in the form of hydroxocobalamin plays an intricate part in cyanide metabolism (Wokes, Badenoch, and Sinclair, 1955), and it can protect mice against cyanide poisoning to a remarkable extent (Muschett *et al.*, 1952). Cyanide may be the toxic agent in tobacco amblyopia of which there is a high incidence in smokers with pernicious anaemia (Smith, 1962; Freeman and Heaton, 1961; McLaren, 1962). Blood cyanide levels in the Jamaica patients have been within normal limits when tested but they may have been raised at the initial stage of the disease, and Mani, Mani, and Montgomery (1969) also found low thiocyanate levels in cases reported from South India. Monekosso and Wilson (1966), however, demonstrated raised thiocyanate levels in Nigerian patients with this type of neurological disorder. Not only are many tropical diets deficient in B_{12} but undernutrition is often associated with gastric hypo- or achlorhydria which hinders absorption; as a result the serum B_{12} is frequently at a low level in undernourished persons.

Spinal Arachnoiditis

This is possibly related to the syndrome just described and is generally regarded as uncommon. In Jamaica, however, it is the commonest cause of spinal cord compression if bony lesions of the vertebral column are excluded. Rodgers and Cruickshank (1962) reviewed 20 cases seen during the first 10 years of the University Hosptial and since that time more than double that number have been seen. The features have not changed significantly. Elkington (1951) reviewed the published work on this disorder and noted that with the development of myelography and neurosurgery it had become an established clinical and pathological entity. There is low-grade inflammation in the arachnoid and associated membranes, which may lead to the formation of cysts and fibrous bands that can cause direct compression of, or interference with, the blood supply to the cord or nerve roots.

The aetiology in most cases cannot be determined, although a wide range of factors has been suggested as responsible. These are low-grade infections—sometimes possibly by direct spread from the pleura and other adjacent tissues or along perineural spaces—larval infestations, subarachnoid bleeding, local trauma, disease of the spinal column or the introduction of foreign material into the subarachnoid space for diagnostic or therapeutic purposes. The age range is from 18 to 60 years, averaging 40 years, and the sex distribution is equal.

The earliest feature is usually weakness and 'deadness' in the affected limbs associated with pain which may be varied, both in site and character, and it is not as definitive as root pain due to compression by tumour.

Disturbances in micturition are not reported as common, but 50 per cent of the Jamaican patients complained of such symptoms. The physical signs depend on whether the lesion is primarily compressive or a polyradicular inflammation. The pyramidal tracts are invariably the most severely affected, but posterior column and more frequently spinothalamic sensation is also involved, and about half the patients have lower motor neurone wasting at the level of the lesion. Sensation to touch, pin-prick and temperature shows a definite level when the lesion is primarily obstructive, but if numerous roots are involved at various levels there are scattered areas of impaired sensation of root distribution. The cerebrospinal fluid usually shows a rise in protein and some increase in cells and there is often evidence of partial or complete block confirmed by myelography, or there may be fragmentation of the contrast medium and failure to show up the normal subarachnoid root sleeve, indicating radiculitis.

The pathological changes already described are demonstrated at laminectomy, and sometimes there is calcification and even ossification of the arachnoid membrane. The latter was present in one case.

The results of treatment are very varied and in most cases there is little to be gained by laminectomy, except when there is complete block and it is necessary to exclude tumour. The results, as might be expected for the treatment of long-standing cases, are poor with any form of therapy, but in patients with recent onset the use of steroids seems justified.

It is probable that arachnoiditis is much commoner than was previously believed, and in certain parts of India it is said to be the commonest cause of cord compression (Wadia, 1961; Mani, 1961, see pp. 81, 31) and there have been reports from other tropical countries (Ramirez, 1959; Monekosso, 1962).

It is tempting to speculate that there is a common aetiology for arachnoiditis and the neuropathies in Jamaica, the spectrum ranging from a relatively acute inflammatory process presenting the picture just described, through the spastic paraplegias with some increase in protein and cells in the cerebrospinal fluid and pathological evidence of some inflammatory change, to those without cerebrospinal fluid abnormalities indicating dominantly a degenerative process. The picture presented by a given case may depend on the type and degree of tissue response to the damage, whether it be the result of defective metabolism, an infectious or noxious agent, or an allergic reaction to exogenous or even endogenous factors.

Retrobulbar Neuropathy

In 1936 Clark, in Jamaica, reported a condition leading to defective vision, mainly in children. Usually, the parents or teachers noticed that the child was not seeing well and on examination it was impossible to improve vision with glasses. The optic discs appeared normal early in the disease but later temporal pallor often developed. Syphilis and septic foci were excluded. The children mostly came from poor homes with a poor dietary history, and many had angular stomatitis. Clark treated them with cod-liver oil and a good diet with eggs and milk where possible, as he knew retrobulbar neuritis had been described in pellagra and regarded it as identical with the 'central neuritis' described by Scott (1918). Generally, the children responded well, but when the defective vision had been of long standing or the patient was over 16 years of age the response was poor, probably because of irreversible damage to the optic nerve. In 1947, Whitbourne described her experiences with 1069 patients, seen over a period of 12 years, and she had the assistance of Carroll who carried out detailed ophthalmological assessment of some of these patients. He found that visual acuity varied from 20/40 to 20/200 when the patient was first seen. The discs were normal but later often showed marked temporal pallor even when the child had made an apparent complete recovery. Where visual fields could be tested satisfactorily the common finding was a relatively small central or caecocentral scotoma. In addition, he noted that approximately 10 per cent of the children had partial eighth nerve deafness. He regarded it as identical to the picture seen in prisoners of war who developed visual defects, and attributed it to riboflavine deficiency as most of the children had the typical skin or mucous membrane changes. Degazon (1956) described a similar syndrome in 289 outpatients at the Kingston Public Hospital but called it 'tropical amblyopia' as he considered that malnutrition played 'little or no part' in the aetiology and that treatment with vitamin B complex was only beneficial in early cases. This retrobulbar neuropathy is now well recognized in most parts of the tropical world and it is frequently reported from underprivileged areas with a poor diet, but the specific factor, whether a vitamin deficiency or a toxic one of a combination of both, has not been pin-pointed.

The condition was found in 15 per cent of patients of the spastic group of Jamaican neuropathy and over 70 per cent of the ataxic group.

In a recent neurological survey of 576 persons of a low-income suburban community in Kingston, randomly sampled, 25 (4·8 per cent of females and 4 per cent of males) had neurological signs possibly representing manifestations of the Jamaican neuropathy. Sensorineural hearing losses and retrobulbar neuropathy were more common in these than in normal subjects (26 per cent and 16 per cent respectively). The overall incidence for the 576 subjects was sensorineural hearing loss, 7·3 per cent, and retrobulbar neuropathy, 2·1 per cent.

Sensorineural Hearing Loss

As noted, this syndrome is frequently associated with the Jamaican neuropathy and it has been reported from various parts of the world where retrobulbar neuropathy and cord syndromes occur. In the survey already referred to, sensorineural hearing loss was more common than conductive deafness which was present in only 1·6 per cent of the subjects. Sensorineural hearing impairment at conversational frequencies in one or both ears is defined as a mean hearing threshold in excess of 25 dB at frequencies of 500, 1000 and 2000 Hz. The prevalence was greater among women than in men at all age levels, especially in the 55 to 64-year age-group in which 5·0 per cent of men but 21·3 per cent of women had impairment in one or both ears; at that age 14·7 per cent of women but no men had impairment in both ears. The cause of this nerve deafness is unknown. The prevalence rises with age, and presumably ageing is important, but only two men and six women (all of them over 55 years) had a sloping audiogram (higher thresholds at higher frequencies) which is typical of presbycousis. A valid history was difficult to obtain from these deaf subjects but none had been born deaf. The onset was usually described as having been gradual and was not attributed to a definite cause; the hearing loss had been progressive. The age of onset varied; in general the younger the patient, the younger the age of onset was said to be, a feature which may be due to a tendency to underestimate the length of time for the development of a chronic disorder. The answers to questionnaires showed no relationship between sensorineural hearing loss and a history of meningitis, encephalitis, yaws, malaria, quinine medication, typhoid, alcohol intake, smoking or parity. Reactive VDRL or RPCF tests were no commoner in those with hearing loss than in those of normal hearing. No significant differences were found in prevalence between those brought up in Kingston and those brought up in rural areas. Of the 49 cases of sensorineural hearing loss, 43 were of predominantly African origin, a proportion which was rather more, but not significantly so, than would be expected. At all ages mean blood pressure, both systolic and diastolic, was higher in females with sensorineural hearing loss than in those without such a loss; the same phenomenon was not found in males. It is possible that women with hearing defects were more apprehensive during the examination than were those with normal hearing and, as a result, their blood pressure rose. On the other hand, the two conditions may be related more directly. Vascular lesions in the labyrinth are believed to account for the giddiness associated with hypertension, and similar lesions in the auditory apparatus may account for hearing losses.

The tropical neuropathies, then, still present a fascinating problem to the epidemiologist and neurologist. There may be many contributing factors to the damage that occurs to what are probably the most susceptible neurones of the nervous system. The first sensory neurone for proprioception and the upper motor neurone have the longest, largest, and most heavily myelinated tracts of the spinal cord. As Osuntokun (1968) points out, the phylogenetically primitive bipolar neurones of the visual and auditory pathways and the pseudo-unipolar neurones of the posterior root ganglia may make them differentially susceptible to deranged metabolism.

Much more detailed information is required of the environments in which these disorders occur in different areas of the world. Until similarities and differences are established and until there is some clue on which to base experimental work, speculation as to the exact aetiology must continue to range over a wide field.

References

AL-WITRY, H., SHABY, J. A., and KANTARJIAN, A. D. (1950) Nutritional paraplegia in Iraq, *J. Fac. Med. Baghdad*, 14, 143.

ASHCROFT, M. J., CRUICKSHANK, E. K., HINCHCLIFFE, R., JONES, W. I., MIALL, W. E., and WALLACE, J. (1967) A neurological, ophthalmological and audiological survey of a suburban Jamaican community, *W. Indian med. J.*, 16, 233.

BARRETT, W. L. (1943) *Med. Dept. File 1 H.B.* 517, No. 31.

BARRETT, W. L. (1953) *Report of Investigations into Vomiting Sickness of Jamaica*, Island Medical Office, Jamaica.

BEAUMONT, P., HOLLOWS, F. C., SCHOFIELD, P. S., and WILLIAMS, J. F. (1971) Growth hormone, sorbitol and diabetic capillary disease, *Lancet*, **i**, 579.

BELLE, E. A., GRANT, L. S., URQUHART, K. D., McDONNOUGH, L. M., and BENT, P. (1963) Equine encephalitis in Jamaica, *W. Indian med. J.*, 12, 139.

BIRCH, C. (1971) Unpublished data.

BRAS, G., and WATLER, D. C. (1967) The five most frequent cancers in Jamaica, *W. Indian med. J.*, 16, 200.

BROUGHTON, A. (1794) *Hortus Eastebus*, Spanish Town, Jamaica.

CHAMPAKAN, S., SRIKANTIA, S. G., and GOPALAN, G. (1968) Kwashiorkor and mental development, *Amer. J. clin. Nutr.*, 21, 844.

CLARK, L. M. (1936) Retrobulbar neuritis, *Trans. Brit. med. Ass. Jamaica*, 5, 25.

COLE, I. M., and COLE, H. L. (1969) A pattern of fatal cerebrovascular disease in Jamaica, *W. Indian med. J.*, 18, 202.

COSNETT, J. E. (1966) Incubation period of multiple sclerosis, *Brit. med. J.*, 2, 702.

CRAVIOTO, J., LICARDIE, E. DE, and BIRCH, C. (1966) Nutrition, growth and neurointegrative development; an experimental and ecologic survey, *Pediatrics*, 38, 319.

CRUICKSHANK, E. K., and MONTGOMERY, R. D. (1961) Multiple sclerosis in Jamaica, *W. Indian med. J.*, 10, 211.

DADA, T. O. (1969) *Personal Communication and Report of the Scientific Group on Neurology, 1969* (restricted), World Health Organization, Geneva.

DEGAZON, D. W. (1956) Tropical amblyopia in Jamaica, *W. Indian med. J.*, 5, 223.

DOWNS, W. G., and GRANT, L. S. (1962) Arthropod-borne encephalitis viruses in the W. Indies area, Part III, *W. Indian med. J.*, 11, 253.

ELKINGTON, J. ST. C. (1951) in *Modern Trends in Neurology*, 1st Series, London, p. 149.

EVANS, A. D. PALLIS, C. A., and SPILLANE, J. D. (1957) Involvement of the nervous system in Behçet's syndrome, *Lancet*, ii, 349.

FERRO-LUZZI, G. (1958) Dietologia dietoterapia (Rome). Atypical nervous manifestations of vitamin B deficiency, *Trop. Dis. Bull.*, 56, Suppl., 203.

FISHMAN, M. A., and PRANSKY, A. L. (1969) Malnutrition and mental behaviour, *Nutr. Rev.*, 27, 191.

FOX, H. C., and MILLER, D. S. (1960) Ackee toxin—a riboflavine antimetabolite, *Nature* (*Lond.*), 186, 561.

FREEMAN, A. G., and HEATON, J. M. (1961) The aetiology of retrobulbar neuritis in Addisonian pernicious anaemia, *Lancet*, i, 908.

GABBAY, K. H., and O'SULLIVAN, J. B. (1968) The sorbitol pathway in diabetes and galactosemia-enzyme, and substrate localization and changes in kidney, *Diabetes*, 17, 239.

GARLAND, H. (1960) Neurological complications of diabetes mellitus: clinical aspects, *Proc. roy. Soc. Med.*, 53, 137.

GILLIATT, R. W. (1965) in *Biochemical Aspects of Neurological Disease*, 2nd ed., eds. Cumings, J. N., and Kremer, M., Oxford, p. 131.

GRANT, L. S. (1956) An analysis of interpretation of some public health laboratory reports Jamaica B.W.I. (1940–54), *W. Indian med. J.*, 5, 97.

GRANT, L. S., BEEN, T. E., BEZJAK, V., and BELLE, E. A. (1965) The microbiology of disease in Jamaican children, *W. Indian med. J.*, 14, 63.

GUITERREZ, P. D., NAVERRO, R. J., MORALLES, S. B., LOZANO, A. A., and GOMEZ, F. B. (1941) *Acta med. philipp.*, 3, 1. As quoted in *Stitt's Diagnosis, Prevention and Treatment of Tropical Disease* (1945), 7th ed., ed. Strong, R. P., London, o. 392.

HACKETT, C. J. (1953) First International Symposium on Yaws Control, *Wld Hlth Org. Monogr. Ser.*, No. 15, p. 129.

HALL, J. (1964) A pattern of convulsions in childhood, *W. Indian med. J.*, 13, 224.

HALL, J. (1967) Myasthenia gravis in Kingston, Jamaica (1967), *W. Indian med. J.*, 16, 51.

HALPERN, L. (1961) *Multiple Sclerosis. Studies in Various Ethnic Groups in Israel*, Paper presented at the International Congress of Neurology, Rome.

HARTMANN, H. A., LALICH, J. J., and AKERT, K. J. (1958) Lesions in the anterior horn cells or rats after administration of B cyanoethylamine—study of a nitrile closely related to the lathyrus factor, *J. Neuropath. exp. Neurol.*, 17, 298.

HAYMAKER, W., and KEMOHAN, J. W. (1949) The Landry–Guillain–Barré syndrome. A clinicopathologic report ot fifty fatal cases and a critique of the literature, *Medicine* (*Baltimore*), 28, 59.

HOLT, C. VON, HOLT, M. VON, and BOHM, H. (1966) Metabolic effects of hypoglycin and methylenecyclopropaneacetic acid, *Biochim. biophys. Acta* (*Amst.*), 125, 11.

IRVINE, R. A. (1970) Personal communication.

IRVINE, R. A., GRANT, L. S., and BELLE, E. A. (1963) Acute viral encephalitis in Jamaica. *Amer. J. trop. Med. Hyg.*, 12, 916.

LANCET (1969) Annotation, *Lancet*, ii, 1346.

MCLAREN, D. S. (1962) Malnutrition and eye disease in Tanganyika, *Proc. Nutr. Soc.*, 19, 89.

MANI, K. S. (1961) Personal communication.

MANI, K. S., MANI, A. J., and MONTGOMERY, R. D. (1969) A spastic paraplegic syndrome in South India, *J. neurol. Sci.*, 9, 179.

MIALL, W. E., and RERRIE, J. I. (1962) The prevalence of pulmonary tuberculosis in a rural population in Jamaica, *W. Indian med. J.*, 11, 145.

MILLER, C. G., and RAGBEER, M. M. (1971) Personal communication.

MILNER, P. F. (1965) Modern laboratory methods in clinical haematology. The assay of serum B_{12}, *W. Indian med. J.*, 14, 230.

MONCKEBERG, F. (1969) Malnutrition and mental behaviour, *Nutr. Rev.*, 27, 191.

MONEKOSSO, G. L. (1962) A clinical comparison of obscure myleopathies in Jamaica and W. Nigeria, *W. Indian med. J.*, 11, 230.

MONEKOSSO, G. L., and WILSON, J. (1966) Plasma thiocyanate and vitamin B_{12} in Nigerian patients with degenerative neurological diseases, *Lancet*, i, 1062.

MONEY, G. L. (1959) Clinical aspects of tropical ataxic neuropathies related to malnutrition. *W. Afr. med. J.*, 8, 3.

MONTGOMERY, R. D., CRUICKSHANK, E. K., ROBERTSON, W. D., and MCMENEMEY, W. H. (1964) Clinical and pathological observations on Jamaican neuropathy, a report on 206 cases, *Brain*, 87, 425.

MUSCHETT, C. W., KELLEY, K. L., BOXER, G. E., and RICHARDS, J. C. (1952) Antidotal efficacy of vitamin B_{12a} (hydroxo-cobalamin) in experimental cyanide poisoning, *Proc. Soc. exp. Biol.* (*N.Y.*), 81, 234.

OSUNTOKUN, B. O. (1968) An ataxic neuropathy in Nigeria; a clinical, biochemical and electrophysiological study, *Brain*, 91, 215.

PICOU, D., ALLEYNE, G. A. O., and SEAKINS, A. (1965) Hydroxyproline and creatinine excretion in infantile protein malnutrition, *Clin. Sci.*, 29, 517.

POSER, C. M. (1968) Clinical diagnostic criteria in epidemiological studies of multiple sclerosis, *Ann. N.Y. Acad. Sci.*, 122, 506.

POSKANZER, D. C., SCHAPIRA, K., and MILLER, H. (1963) Epidemiology of multiple sclerosis in the counties of Northumberland and Durham, *J. Neurol. Neurosurg. Psychiat.*, 26, 368.

RAFF, M. C., SANGALANG, V., and ASHBURY, A. K. (1968) Mononeuropathy multiplex-ischaemia associated with diabetes, *Arch. Neurol.* (*Chic.*), 18, 48.

RAMIEREZ, A. A. (1959) Circumscribed and cystic adhesive arachnoiditis, *Arch. Col. méd. El Salvador*, 12, 14.

RAMSAY, I. D. (1966) Muscle dysfunction in hyperthyroidism, *Lancet*, ii, 931.

RICHARDS, R., and HAYNES, J. (1964) Peripheral diabetic amyotrophy, *W. Indian med. J.*, 13, 135.

ROBERTSON, W. B. (1959) Atherosclerosis and ischaemic heart-disease: observations in Jamaica, *Lancet*, i, 444.

RODGERS, P. B. (1965) Jamaican neuropathy, *W. Indian med. J.*, 14, 244.

RODGERS, P. B. (1971) Personal communication.

RODGERS, P. B., and CRUICKSHANK, E. K. (1962) Spinal arachnoiditis, *W. Indian med. J.*, 11, 64.

SCOTT, H. H. (1915) *Report on Vomiting Sickness, Kingston Jamaica*, Island Medical Office, Jamaica.

SCOTT, H. H. (1918) Investigation into acute outbreak of central neuritis, *Amer. J. trop. Med. Parasit.*, 12, 109.

SMITH, A. D. M. (1962) Veganism: a clinical survey with observations on vitamin B_{12} metabolism, *Brit. med. J.*, 1, 165.

STRACHAN, H. (1897) On a form of multiple neuritis prevalent in the West Indies, *Practitioner*, 59, 477.

STROM, A., REFSUM, S. B., BITINGER, L., GRUNUIK, O., LONNUM, A., ENGESET, A., OSVIK, K., and ROGAN, B. (1962) Examination of Norwegian ex-concentration camp prisoners—progressive meningo-encephalopathy resulting from internment in concentration camps, *J. Neuropsychiat.*, 4, 43–62.

STUART, K. L., and MACIVER, J. E. (1961) Pernicious anaemia in Jamaica, *Brit. med. J.*, 1, 236.

THOMAS, P. K., and LASCELLES, R. G. (1966) The pathology of diabetic neuropathy, *Quart. J. Med.*, 35, 489.

TROWELL, H. C. (1960) *Non-infective Disease in Africa*, London, pp. 243, 244, 253.

TULLOCH, J. A. (1962) *Diabetes Mellitus in the Tropics*, Edinburgh, p. 9.

WADIA, N. (1961) Personal communication.

WATERLOW, I. C. (1959) Effects of protein depletion on the distribution of protein synthesis, *Nature* (*Lond.*), 184, 1875.

WHITBOURNE, D. (1947) Nutritional retrobulbar neuritis in children in Jamaica, *Amer. J. Ophthal.*, 30, 169.

WINICK, M., and ROSSO, P. (1969) The effect of severe early malnutrition on cellular growth of human brain, *Pediat. Res.*, 3, 181.

WOKES, F., BADENOCH, J., and SINCLAIR, H. M. (1955) Human dietary deficiency of vitamin B_{12}, *Amer. J. clin. Nutr.*, 3, 375.

YATES, P. O. (1964) A change in the pattern of cerebrovascular disease, *Lancet*, i, 65.

ZILKHA, K. J. (1968) Auto-immune demyelinating disorders, in *Biochemical Aspects of Neurological Disorders*, 3rd eds. Cumings, J. N., and Kremer, M., Oxford, p. 37.

Index

Abdominal paralysis, 213, 216, 218, 219
Abscess, 38, 137, 144, 145, 227, 250, 254–5, 263, 265, 269, 301, 304, 305, 306, 309, 414
  cerebral, 144, 145, 157, 165, 227, 239, 254–5, 266
  cold, 59, 65, 411
  cranial, 200
  dental, 270
  'dysenteric liver', 255
  epidural, 245, 267, 304
  extradural, 147, 305
  fluid, 58
  intracerebral, 304
  intracranial, 79, 200
  intramuscular, 171
  lung, 262, 266
  nerve, 329–30, 332
  paraspinal, 58, 414
  subdural, 239
  vertebral, 170
Achlorhydria, 84, 139, 140, 173, 181, 220, 221, 429, 430
Adenoma, pituitary, 167, 315
Addisonian pernicious anaemia, 28, 148, 201
Agranulocytosis, 305
Air encephalography, 242, 243
Albuminuria, 158, 181
Alcoholism, 25, 28, 138, 148, 191, 195, 202, 261, 266, 267, 269, 299, 310, 340, 432
Allergic disorders, 79
Alzheimer's disease, 362, 382
Aminoaciduria, 33
Amoebiasis, 34, 144, 150, 254–5
  cerebral, 255
  intestinal, 255
  liver, 255
Amoebic cerebral abscess, 144, 145, 157, 165, 227, 239, 255, 266
  prognosis, 255
  symptomatology, 255
  treatment, 255
Amok, 289
Amyelination, 15
Amyloid disease, 325
Amyloidosis, 170
Amyotrophic lateral sclerosis, 17, 81, 84, 106, 127, 134, 138, 148, 168, 212, 303, 355–75, 379, 426
  clinical appearances, 359–64
    ALS, 359–61
    bradykinesia, 361, 362, 369, 370
    dementia, 359, 361, 362, 365, 369, 370, 371, 372
    'parkinsonism', 363–4, 369, 370
    PD, 361–4
    rigidity, 361, 362, 369, 370
    tremor, 361, 362–3, 369, 370
Amyotrophic lateral sclerosis—*contd.*
  epidemiology, 356–9
    age, 357–8
    area, 358–9
    sex, 358
  Guamanians in the continental United States, 370–1
  historical background, 355–6
  neuropathology, 364–5
    ALS, 364
    macroscopic observations, 364
    microscopic observations, 364–5
    neuropathology of Guamanian controls, 365
    PD, 364–5
Amyotrophy, 31, 129, 425, 426, 430
  neuralgic, 170, 203, 212
  syphilitic, 199, 430
Anaemia, 73, 74, 78, 84, 92, 98, 116, 117, 155, 182, 192, 194, 221, 223, 305, 387, 388, 389
  Addisonian, 28, 148, 201
  aplastic, 158
  dimorphic, 95
  haemolytic, 250, 388
  hypochromic, microcytic, 95, 403
  iron-deficiency, 299, 300
  megaloblastic, 73, 78, 116, 166, 220, 221, 309
  pernicious, 28, 148, 171, 186, 201, 220, 309, 340, 423, 429, 430
  sickle-cell, 149–51, 156, 157, 159, 164, 166, 204, 210
André-Thomas technique for motor assessment, 15
Anencephaly, 108, 109
Aneurysm, 12, 28, 29, 32, 84, 92, 96, 120, 122, 137, 209, 232, 233, 296, 338, 345, 423
  aortic, 11, 157
  berry, 12, 28, 29, 120, 166, 296, 338, 423
  bleeding intracranial, 17, 29, 38, 80, 89, 120, 158, 283, 284, 285
  congenital intracranial, 308, 320, 338
  mycotic, 308, 338
Angiitis, 389
Angiography, 12, 29, 32, 44–5, 55–6, 89, 92, 95, 97, 106, 121, 123, 144, 152, 154, 159, 169, 210, 211, 241, 243, 244, 264, 265, 296, 302, 305, 306, 308, 311, 337, 338, 392, 408, 410, 411, 413
Angioma, 12, 17, 29, 69, 80, 81, 84, 137, 158, 159, 166, 233, 283, 285
Angiostrongyliasis, 343–4
Anidrosis, 327, 328
Ankylostomiasis, 5, 78
Anterior encephalocele, 12–13, 108–13
  aetiopathogenesis, 109–10
  classification, 109
  clinical features, 110–11
  differential diagnosis, 111

Anterior encephalocele—*contd.*
  incidence, 12–13, 108–9
  investigations, 111
  pathological anatomy, 110, 111
  prognosis, 112
  treatment, 111–12
Aortic arch syndrome, 29, 87, 90, 92–8
  aetiology, 29, 92, 97
  clinical syndrome, 94–5
  course and prognosis, 97
  incidence, 93–4
  laboratory data, 95–6
  pathology, 96–7
  radiology, 96
  treatment, 97–8
Aortitis, 92, 93, 95, 96
  luetic, 84
Apoplexy, 7, 87
Arachnoiditis, 38, 40, 48, 61, 63, 64, 65, 66, 68, 70, 79, 81, 138, 147, 148, 201, 211, 227, 229, 307–8, 338, 393, 430–1
Arboviruses, 135, 145, 150, 164, 307, 339, 346
Ariboflavinosis, 424
Arnold–Chiari malformation, 99, 105, 106, 209, 302
Arteriography, 226, 227, 232, 241, 242, 283, 285, 296, 394, 395, 423
Arteriopathies, 89, 337
Arteriosclerosis, 159, 195, 211, 299, 308, 387
Arteritis, 8, 28, 29, 40, 41, 43, 48, 58, 88, 89, 90, 92, 93, 95, 96, 97, 137, 210, 239, 338
  giant cell, 310
  temporal, 34, 122, 234
Arthritis, 64, 66
  rheumatoid, 64, 66, 104, 105, 121, 171, 221, 270
Ascariasis, 308, 422
Astereognosis, 101
Astrocytoma, 211, 303, 313, 314, 339
Astrogliosis, 117
Ataxia, 29, 56, 101, 106, 122, 139, 179, 180, 203, 204, 212, 221, 243, 245, 246, 304, 378, 427, 430
  cerebellar, 37, 210, 221, 243, 245, 269, 376
  Friedreich's, 29, 144, 203, 243, 271, 303–4
  heredofamilial, 269, 271, 371
  nutritional spinal, 221
  sensory, 28, 173
  spinocerebellar, 209, 220
Atheroma, 28, 88, 93, 95, 264, 296
Atheromatosis, 92, 93
Atherosclerosis, 8, 28, 29, 88, 90, 94, 97, 137, 152, 153, 154, 158, 159, 165, 224, 239, 241, 242, 244, 264, 269, 337, 423
  of cerebral vasculature, 232–3
Athetosis, 147, 234, 399, 400
  congenital, 270
Autosomal dominant trait, 30, 367

Babinski's sign, 162–3, 263, 378
Babinski–Froehlich syndrome, 315
Bacteraemia, 39
Bacterial endocarditis, 157, 165, 210, 262, 264, 304, 308
Basilar invagination, 103, 104, 105, 106
Behavioural disorders, 135, 204, 249, 289, 301
Behçet's syndrome, 421
Bell's palsy, 32, 123, 144, 170, 203, 209, 244, 319
Beriberi, 5, 6, 13, 16–17, 138, 148, 283, 340
Biochemical lesion, 16–17, 18
Bilharzia, 5, 136, 159, 223, 231, 234, 241, 256–8, 268, 422
  urinary, 256
Bilharzial effect on nervous system, 241, 256–8
  bilharziasis of spinal cord, 256–7
    bilharzial paraplegia, 256–7
    bilharzial radiculitis, 257–8
    transverse myelitis, 257
  cerebral bilharziasis, 256
Bilharzial myelopathy, 268
Bitot's spots, 83
Blindness, 29, 48, 56, 94, 100, 149, 166, 185, 202, 209, 269, 304, 312, 318, 343, 344, 410, 412, 413
  night, 74, 75, 76
Blood–brain barrier, 47, 75, 136, 201, 253, 400
Blood dyscrasias, 338
Bone-marrow changes, 28, 84, 140
  examination, 116
Bradyphrenia, 74, 75
Brain, infestation of, 230–2
  'acute brain syndrome', 194–5
  'chronic brain syndrome', 195
  injuries to, 144, 145–7, 195
  in tuberculous meningitis, 41–2, 43, 49
Bronchitis, 13, 216
Bronchopneumonia, 424
Brucellosis, 137, 305
Bulbar paralysis, 127, 168, 212, 213, 216, 217, 218, 244
Bulbospinal paralysis, 213, 216, 217–19, 220
Burkitt's lymphoma, nervous system in, 18, 144, 145, 147, 164, 170, 200–1
  disturbance of consciousness and mental state, 200–1
  myelopathy, 200
  multiple cranial neuropathy, 200
  treatment, 201
Burkitt's neoplasm, 167, 169, 170

Cachectic states, 17, 253
Cachexia, 74, 94
Calcification, 49, 53, 55, 96, 228, 339, 395, 431
  intracranial, 49, 53, 339
  pineal gland, 80, 339
Cancer, 97, 137, 194, 209, 365, 422
Cannibalism, 18, 377, 379–80
Carcinoma, 81, 120, 138, 144, 145, 168, 209, 211, 243, 262, 266, 269, 270, 287, 318, 340, 341, 365, 426
Carcinomatous neuromyopathy, 34, 245, 426
Cardiomyopathy, 137, 144, 157, 263, 265
Cardiopathy, 401, 404
Cardiovascular disease, 365
Carditis, 203, 263, 403
Cassava, 14, 15–16, 82, 139, 140, 143, 148, 161, 173, 178, 182, 185, 186, 191, 201, 220, 309
Causalgia, 234, 247
Central paralysis, 215–16, 217
Cerebellar ataxia, 37, 210, 221, 243, 245, 269, 376
Cerebellar disease, 269
Cerebellar lesions of unknown aetiology, 245–6
Cerebral embolism, 8, 87, 88, 153, 157, 241–2, 264–5, 290, 297, 337, 404
Cerebral haemorrhage, 12, 137, 149, 153, 157–9, 165, 166, 232, 241, 264, 289, 290, 291, 294–6
Cerebral hydatid cyst, 408, 409–12, 413
  in the adult, 411–12
    diagnosis, 411

Cerebral hydatid cyst in the adult—*contd.*
paraclinical studies, 411
symptomatology, 411
treatment, 411–12
in children, 409–11
diagnosis, 410
paraclinical studies, 410–11
symptomatology, 409–10
Cerebral lesions, 137
Cerebral malaria, 136, 144, 145, 165, 195, 196, 203–4, 219, 232, 240–1, 247–51, 256
clinical features, 248–50
treatment, 250
Cerebral palsy, 32, 79, 80, 106, 193, 204, 234, 243, 245
Cerebral tumour, 7, 8, 211, 221, 225–6, 256, 260, 368, 371, 411
Cerebroside, 14–15
Cerebrospinal fluid, 41, 43–4, 45, 47, 61, 64, 67, 68, 70, 75, 81, 84, 92, 104, 106, 111, 112, 116, 117, 118, 122, 129, 135, 139, 148, 153, 163, 164, 167, 169, 170, 197, 200, 201, 202, 203, 204, 210, 211, 212, 219, 221, 226, 227, 229, 231, 238, 240, 242, 244, 245, 247, 248, 249, 251, 253–4, 255, 256, 257, 265, 266, 267, 268, 269, 287, 288, 291, 297, 304, 305, 307, 308, 309, 318, 319, 338, 339, 340, 341, 342, 343, 344, 345, 349, 369, 372, 378, 380, 381, 388, 392, 394, 403, 404, 405, 421, 422, 429, 431
Cerebrovascular accidents, 7, 37, 38, 133, 134, 137, 152, 153, 165, 166, 211, 241, 289, 290, 291, 294, 295, 297, 308, 336, 337, 338
Cerebrovascular disease, 8, 27, 28, 37, 38, 88, 137, 144, 148, 152–60, 165, 168, 221, 239–40, 241–2, 264–5, 269, 283, 289–97, 299, 308, 320, 336–8, 421, 422–3
Cerebrovascular disorders in South India, 28, 86–91
epidemiology, 86–7
stroke in the young adult, 87–90
Cervical spondylosis, 64, 65, 83, 105, 125, 144, 148, 170, 201, 211, 212, 239, 270, 320, 340
lumbar, 144, 148
Chagas' disease, 397–407
aetiology and life-cycle, 397–8
invertebrate host, 398
life-cycle, 398
vertebrate host, 398
incidence and geographical distribution, 397
laboratory diagnosis, 397, 399
nervous system in, 399–407
autonomic, 401–2
central, 399–401
chronic form, 403–5
cerebral complications of chronic Chagas' cardiopathy, 404
laboratory diagnosis, 404–5
clinical picture in involvement of nervous system, 403–4
acute form, 403
exacerbation form, 403–4
mechanism of neuronal damage, 402–3
pathogenesis, 397, 398–9, 402
peripheral, 401
treatment and prophylaxis, 405
Charcot joints, 328, 332, 425
Chikungunya virus, 339, 346
Childhood, 43, 266, 280
cerebral malaria in, 247, 248
Childhood—*contd.*
disorders of, 42, 114–19, 135
neurological disorders of, 203–5
Chloroquine, 250, 255, 275, 331, 342
Cholaemia, 195
Cholecystitis, 414
Cholera, 3, 4, 5, 6
Chorea, 7, 135, 144, 147, 203, 210, 212–13, 245
Huntington's, 29, 144, 147, 203, 210, 212–13, 271, 382
rheumatic, 221
Sydenham's, 144, 147, 203, 210, 245, 270
Choreo-athetosis, 169, 204, 212, 243, 245
Choriocarcinoma, 167
Choroid plexus, 40, 315, 389, 394
Choroidoretinitis, 170
Claudication, 95
Climate, 133, 143, 161, 191, 207, 223, 259, 299, 321, 335, 387
Clioquinol, 34
Coccidioidomycosis, 422
Collagen diseases, 4, 97, 123, 309–10
lupus erythematosus, 123, 171, 309, 342, 427
polyarteritis, 170, 171, 310, 427
Coma, 43, 133, 135, 136, 148, 149, 154, 158, 166, 193, 197, 202, 232, 247, 248, 249, 250, 253, 256, 289, 294, 295, 305, 307, 311, 345, 348, 388, 403, 424
Complement-fixation test, 44, 84, 382, 392, 394, 399, 404, 405
Congenital anomalies, 37, 100, 101–2, 104, 105, 288, 342
Congenital atlanto-axial dislocation, 17, 27, 29, 81, 99–107
differential diagnosis, 105–6
investigations, 102–4
classification, 103–4
myelography, 104
radiology, 99, 102–3, 105
pathology, 104–5
maldevelopment, 105
mechanism, 104–5
spinal cord, 105
prognosis, 99, 106
symptomatology, 99–102
cervical symptoms, 99
neurological manifestations, 99–102
treatment, 99, 106
Congenital auditory imperception, 172
Congenital disorders, 79, 209–10
Congenital, hereditary and degenerative diseases, 243–4
Congenital malformations, 12–13, 38, 92, 99, 104, 108, 112, 167, 209–10, 283–6, 287–8, 302–3, 320
geographical variations, 108, 110
Consanguineous marriage, 33, 109, 243
Convulsions, 42, 43, 48, 56, 89, 100, 135, 136, 138, 144, 149, 162, 166, 201, 204, 242, 247, 249, 253, 288, 343, 345, 348, 388, 390, 391, 399, 403, 411, 413, 424
Corneal ulceration, 332–3
Cor pulmonale, 365
Corticosteroids, 32, 47, 70, 71, 121–2, 135, 164, 169, 197 341, 342, 344, 345, 346, 349
Costotransversectomy, 60
Cranial hydatidosis, 408, 412–13, 415
paraclinical tests, 413
pathology of bone echinococcosis, 412
symptomatology, 412–13
treatment, 413, 415

Cranial nerve palsies, 43, 48, 80, 101, 105, 106, 122, 163, 166, 209, 243, 244, 265, 266, 287, 314, 319, 338, 340–1, 388
Cranial suture, 410
  diastasis, 14
Craniopharyngioma, 38, 79, 167, 211, 315
Craniotomy, 226, 227, 230, 343, 345, 392, 411
Craniovertebral anomalies, 27, 29, 81, 99, 101–2, 106, 127, 129
Cranium bifidum, 12, 108, 109
Creutzfeldt–Jakob disease, 18, 376, 382
Cryptococcosis, 65, 67, 68, 70, 338
Cryptococcus neoformans, 64, 65, 137
Cyanide intoxication, 182–7, 430
Cysticercosis, 34, 38, 80, 136, 147, 151, 172, 223, 230–1, 240, 242, 265, 308, 339, 390–5, 422

Deafness, 31, 48, 125, 129, 165, 173, 179, 427, 430, 431–2
  and dumbness, 173
  eighth nerve, 209, 245, 426, 429, 431
  nerve, 245, 432
  sensorineural, 173, 180, 431–2
Decompression, 228, 229, 231, 345, 415
  anterior cervical, 228
  anterolateral, 60, 71, 228
  posterior, 415
  posterolateral, 415
  transthoracic, 228
Deficiency diseases, 79, 118, 163, 187, 202, 340, 423, 425
  protein deficiency, 14, 28, 173, 423
  protein-calorie deficiency, 173, 185
  riboflavine, 427, 429, 431
  vitamin B12 deficiency, 28, 34, 75, 78, 83, 118, 139, 186, 212, 267, 269, 309, 340, 399, 423
  vitamins, 75, 78, 83, 115, 139, 223, 340, 387, 423, 429, 431
Degeneration, 70, 180, 325, 401, 426, 427
  brain, 18, 84
  cerebellar, 269, 340
  Nissl, 394
  olivopontocerebellar, 304
Degenerative disorders, 37, 38, 79, 80, 127, 138, 168, 173, 224, 234–5, 304, 340, 380, 401
Degenerative vascular disease, 337
Dementia, 12, 155, 165, 168, 172, 180, 195, 199, 240, 312, 359, 361, 362, 365, 369, 370, 371, 372, 378, 382, 422
Demyelinating conditions, 210, 212–13
Demyelinating diseases, 79, 80, 82, 138, 169, 202, 244, 246, 267, 270, 286, 320
Demyelination, 31, 70, 84, 181, 187, 318, 340, 349, 365, 368, 378, 388, 394, 425, 426
Dendrites, 15
Dengue, 299, 339, 346
Dental caries, 126
Depressed skull fracture, 265
  in infants, 233–4
Depression, 233–4
Development of human nervous system, 14, 15
Diabetes, 28, 32, 87, 88, 120, 122, 138, 144, 153, 154, 158, 159, 170, 266, 292, 299, 309, 337, 349, 372, 426
  mellitus, 97, 155, 165, 168, 171, 173, 192, 232, 268, 425, 426
Diarrhoea, 76, 78, 115, 139, 249, 345, 346, 427
Diet, 25, 73, 78, 82–3, 133, 139, 140, 143, 152, 161, 163, 178, 186, 187, 191, 208, 222, 223, 232, 235, 260–1, 268, 335, 337, 379, 387, 424, 425, 428, 431
Diplegia, 400
  spastic, 106, 399
Disc syndromes, 65, 68, 138, 148, 170, 268, 336
  prolapsed intervertebral disc, 244–5, 270
  protrusion, 147, 201, 245, 320
  and spondylosis, 270
Diseases of the cranial nerves, 146, 148, 209, 244–5
Diseases of the extrapyramidal system, 168–9, 270
Diseases of the muscles, 37, 129, 137, 147, 148, 171–2, 196, 212, 222
Diseases of the peripheral nerves, 27, 146–7, 148, 170–1, 211–12, 244–5
Diseases of uncertain aetiology, 7, 73, 79, 117, 127, 426–32
Disorder of eye movement, 29, 30
Disorder of sleep, 33
Disorders of the spinal cord, 14, 31–2, 38, 79, 146, 201–2, 267–9
Down's syndrome, 243
Drug overdosage, 245
Dysarthria, 94, 101, 204, 304, 378
Dysentery, 78, 144, 150, 267
  amoebic, 263, 365
  bacillary, 263
Dysraphic lesions, 12, 302
Dysraphism, cranial, 12
  craniospinal, 302, 303
  spinal, 12, 302
Dysrhythmia, 75

Echinococcosis, 308, 408–17
Eclampsia, 159
Electroencephalography, 33, 44, 49, 73, 75, 87, 89, 116, 135, 136, 137, 138, 144, 149, 192, 209, 231, 242, 287, 288, 301, 305, 318, 339, 344, 345, 362, 382, 394, 395, 404, 410, 411, 413
Embolism, 8, 137, 210, 389
  cerebral, 87, 88, 153, 157, 241–2, 264–5, 290, 297, 337, 404
  pulmonary, 337
Encephalitis, 4, 34, 37, 79, 114, 118, 134, 135, 137, 145, 158, 164, 195, 203, 204, 210, 212, 216, 217, 226, 231, 240, 243, 247, 252, 253, 254, 286, 287, 338–9, 388, 389, 394, 399, 400, 403, 432
  arbovirus, 144, 164
  cysticercous, 393
  Eastern equine, 421
  von Economo's, 309
  granulomatous, 400, 401
  herpetic, 307
  Japanese, 307, 338–9
  measles, 145, 164, 210, 219
  postmumps, 219
  postvaccinial, 135, 204
  subacute sclerosing, 134, 136
  viral, 145, 164, 240, 253, 256, 301, 307, 338, 421
Encephalocele, 12, 13, 108–13, 167, 243, 283, 302
  anterior, 12–13, 108–13
  basal, 109, 110
  frontal, 108, 109, 110, 111, 112
  fronto-ethmoidal, 109, 110, 111, 112
  nasal, 108, 302
  nasofrontal, 109, 110, 111, 112
  naso-orbital, 109, 110, 112
  nasopharyngeal, 108
  occipital, 13, 108, 109, 111, 302

Encephalocele—*contd.*
orbital, 110
parietal, 109
parieto-occipital, 109
sincipital, 109
temporo-orbital, 109
Encephalomeningocele, 80, 109
fronto-ethmoidal, 342–3
Encephalomyelitis, 246, 342, 421, 430
rabies, 348, 349
Encephalomyelopathy, 401
Encephalopathy, 4, 43, 51, 134, 144, 149, 193, 195, 204, 231, 232, 247, 248, 253, 254, 256, 265, 399, 400, 401, 404
of bacterial origin, 135–6
'boxing', 342
mink, 382
subacute, 256
subacute spongiform virus, 382–3
trypanosomic, 400
Udorn, 345–6
Endarteritis obliterans, 54
syphilitic, 422
Endemic fluorosis, 6, 27, 31, 38, 81, 124–6
Endocarditis, 197
Endocrine ophthalmopathy, 122
Enteritis, 170
Enteroviruses, 135, 164, 339
Environment, 14, 15, 86, 276, 278, 280, 368–9, 372, 432
Eosinophilia, 83, 121, 123, 202, 231, 255, 256, 257, 267, 268, 344, 345, 392, 410
Ependyma, 40, 389, 394
Ependymitis, 40, 393, 394
Ependymoma, 312, 313, 318
Epidemiology, 263–4, 271, 289, 336, 356–9, 378–80
epidemiological studies, 27, 152, 185–6, 263, 320, 323, 336, 340, 345, 355
Epilepsies, the, 133, 209
Epilepsy, 7, 33–4, 42, 79, 134, 136, 144, 148, 155, 158, 165, 166–7, 194, 195, 199, 221, 226, 231, 232, 240, 242, 243, 256, 262, 265, 266, 270–1, 283, 284, 301–2, 336, 339, 342, 344, 392, 394, 400, 410
centrencephalic, 301
and convulsive disorders, 423–5
ackee poisoning, 424–5
focal sensory or motor seizures, 209, 242, 301–2, 339
grand mal, 34, 83, 148, 199, 209, 270, 301, 339
'hot-water', 34, 79
Jacksonian, 209, 227
petit mal, 148, 166, 199, 209, 242, 265, 270–1, 301, 339, 424
psychomotor, 424
Erythrocyte parasitosis, 389
Erythrocyte sedimentation rate, 43, 55, 59, 83, 95, 121, 123, 129, 251, 310, 341, 378, 380
Expanding intracranial lesions, 266
Experimental study, 41, 52, 380–2, 399, 400, 402
Extradural spinal tuberculoma, 61
Extrapyramidal syndromes, 146, 147, 168–9, 270, 342, 359, 361, 362, 363–4, 370, 371, 372, 378

Facial palsy, 56, 129, 134, 170, 209, 217, 244, 329, 330, 332, 349
paresis, 410
Fibrosarcoma, 311
Fibrosis, 53, 66, 69, 157, 268, 328, 329, 331, 332, 393, 404
Filariasis, 308
Fluorescent treponema antibody test (FTA), 84, 338, 348
Fluorosis, 6, 27, 31, 38, 81, 124–6
Foot-drop, 329, 331–2
Foster Kennedy syndrome, 413
Fowl paralysis, 16
Fungus granuloma, 38

Gastroenteritis, 144, 192
intestinal disease, 379
General paresis, 11–12, 79, 86, 100, 136, 244, 338, 346, 413
Genetics, 222, 322, 367–8, 372, 380, 382
Geography of medicine, 6–7
of neurology, 7–12
Gesell Infant Scale, 15, 114
Ghana, neurological disorders in, 143–60
Glia, 15, 393
Glioblastoma, 311, 314, 339
Glioma, 8, 17, 38, 55, 69, 79, 111, 137, 199, 225–6, 256, 266, 270, 303, 311, 312–13, 314–15, 339, 422
Gliosis, 54, 365, 389, 393
Glomerulonephritis, 159
Gnathostomiasis, 308, 344, 345
Goitre, 186, 299
Gonorrhoea, 192
Graft, 112
Granuloma, 54, 65, 93, 96, 147, 148, 169, 170, 227, 231, 241, 244, 248, 255, 256, 257, 305, 306, 308, 326, 327, 328, 388, 389
Griffiths Infant Scale, 15
Growth of the brain, 14–15, 28
Guam, neurological disorders, in, 371
Guillain–Barré syndrome, 32, 122, 170, 202, 245, 309, 319, 427
Guinea-pig inoculation, 44, 70, 398

Haemagglutination, 44
Haemangioblastoma, 38, 303, 316
Haemangioma, 209
Haematoma, 38, 158, 172, 239, 242, 266, 310–11, 342
extradural, 266, 310–11
intracerebral, 306, 310, 311
subdural, 37, 138, 144, 145, 149, 195, 211, 234, 241, 256, 264, 265, 266, 288, 311
Haematomyelia, 29, 106
Haemoglobinopathy, 149–51, 156, 163, 166, 170
Haemophilia, 311
Haemorrhage, 149, 153, 165, 195, 248, 283, 311, 314, 318, 346, 348, 387, 423
capillary, 256
gastro-intestinal, 365
hypertensive intracerebral, 89
petechial, 250, 311
subependymal, 389
Haemorrhagic leuco-encephalopathy, 41
Hartnup's syndrome, 80
Hashimoto's disease, 171
Head circumference, 14, 233
Head injury, 38, 79, 145, 162, 167, 195, 241, 243, 262, 265, 266, 310, 336, 342
sequelae, 38, 167, 227, 242
Head trauma, 210, 227
Heart disease, 97, 337, 365, 401
degenerative, 232

Helminthiasis, 134, 136–7
Hemianopia, 410, 411
Hemiballismus, 211, 270
Hemiparesis, 56, 115, 117, 232, 240, 243, 255, 296, 297, 305, 306, 309, 345, 410, 411, 423
Hemiplegia, 29, 43, 48, 86, 90, 95, 135, 138, 155, 158, 173, 204, 210, 219, 232, 239, 240, 241, 242, 243, 249, 256, 262, 264, 296, 306, 310, 312, 342, 422, 423
  infantile, 32, 86, 87, 89, 209
Hepatitis, 136, 140, 144, 150, 164, 342
Hepatoma, 243
Hereditary disorders, 243, 303–4
Heredofamilial diseases, 33, 34, 80, 168, 210, 401
Heredofamilial spinocerebellar degeneration, 29–30, 80, 168
Hernia, 109, 110, 111, 112, 331
Herniated lumbar intervertebral disc, 229
Herpes virus, 136, 164, 170, 307
  Ramsay Hunt syndrome, 170
  simplex, 421
  zoster, 144, 219, 240, 270, 372
Herxheimer reaction, 325
von Hippel–Lindau disease, 303, 317
Histoplasmosis, 422
Hodgkin's disease, 147, 372
Homocystinuria, 80
Hookworm, 3
Horner's syndrome, 101
Hydatid cyst, 211, 408–17
Hydatid disease, 34, 408–17
  general concepts on, 408–9
Hydatid echinococcosis, 408–17
  diagnosis, 410, 411, 414–15
  paraclinical tests, 410, 411, 413, 414
  symptomatology, 409–10, 411, 412–13, 414
  treatment, 411–12, 413, 415
Hydatidosis, 408–17
  of bone, 412, 415
  cerebral, 408, 409–12, 413
  cranial, 408, 412–13, 415
  experimental, 408, 409
  hepatic, 410
  life-cycle, 408–9
  primary, 409, 412
  pulmonary, 410
  secondary, 409, 411
  vertebral, 408, 413–16
Hydranencephaly, 283, 287–8
Hydrocephalus, 4, 12, 41–2, 44, 45, 47, 48, 80, 108, 110, 111, 112, 134, 137, 167, 204, 209, 233, 235, 240, 243, 288, 302, 305, 306, 307, 311, 313, 314, 315, 392, 395
Hydrocortisone, 70, 164, 250
Hydrophobia, 347
Hypercholesterolaemia, 28, 88, 156, 158
Hyperemesis gravidarum, 17
Hyperkalaemia, 346
Hyperkalaemic periodic paralysis, 341–2
Hyper-reflexia, 127, 139, 229, 240, 267, 333, 362
Hypertension, 8, 28, 56, 87, 88, 97, 135, 144, 152, 153, 154, 155, 156, 157, 158, 159, 165, 168, 210, 212, 213, 214, 220, 232, 242, 249, 264, 269, 285, 290, 292, 294, 295, 296, 299, 308, 337, 338, 345, 391–2, 394, 409, 410, 411, 412, 413, 423
Hypertensive encephalopathy, 87, 89–90, 154, 159, 242
Hyperthyroidism, 341–2
Hypocalcaemia, 74, 171, 209
Hypoglycaemia, 195, 250, 424–5
Hypoidrosis, 327
Hypokalaemia, 74, 75, 76, 297
Hyponatraemia, 75, 76
Hypoproteinaemia, 74
Hypotension, 296
Hypothermia, 219
Hypovitaminoses, 195
Hysteria, 7, 106, 144, 149, 173, 213, 219, 222, 269, 289
Hysterical conversion syndrome, 173

Idiopathic aortitis, 8
Immigrants, 9, 10
Immigration, 25, 277–80
Impotence, 124, 149, 194, 257, 425
Inborn errors of metabolism, 32–4
Infantile tremor syndrome, 17, 27, 32, 114–19
  aetiopathogenesis, 117
  clinical features, 32, 114–16
    age incidence, 32, 114
    birth history, 114
    family history, 114
    past illness, 114
    physical examination, 115–16
    post-natal history, 114
    presenting symptoms, 115
    seasonal incidence, 114, 118
    sex, 114
  course of the disease, 116
  laboratory investigations, 116–17
    brain biopsy, 117–18
  prognosis, 117
  treatment, 117
Infarction, 41, 159, 165, 195, 204, 248, 423
  cerebral, 265, 296, 338
  cerebral thrombosis, 87, 88, 89, 90, 158, 241, 423
  cystic, 95
  embolic, 165
  ischaemic cerebral, 93, 95, 97, 154, 155, 158, 165, 166
  ischaemic vascular, 404
  non-embolic, 166
Infection, 37, 70, 105, 117, 118, 127, 133, 134–7, 159, 166, 263, 343, 368, 391, 421, 430
  bacterial, 263, 421
  cross-infection, 219
  gastro-intestinal, 114, 117, 266, 279
  guinea-worm, 144, 147, 150, 172
  mycotic, 308
  paracervical, 104, 105
  pulmonary, 97
  pyogenic, 43, 54, 71
  respiratory, 114, 115, 117, 144, 216, 263, 309
  skin, 422
  syphilitic, 121
  tuberculous, 88, 95, 105, 123, 127
  urinary, 83, 182, 191
  urinary tract, 97
  virus, 136, 164–5, 200, 276, 279, 280, 338, 421
  worms, 192, 265
Infections and infestations, 5, 134–7
  fungal, 307
Infections of the nervous system, 27, 37, 145, 146, 163–5, 221, 238–41, 338
Infective disorders, 304–8
Inflammatory disorders, 79

Intracerebral haemorrhage, 12, 89, 137, 157, 185, 195, 241, 285, 294, 295, 296, 308, 336–7, 338, 345
  intracranial, 153, 283, 285
Intracranial arteriovenous malformation, 87, 89, 283–6, 296, 301, 308–9, 338, 345
Intracranial calcification, 49, 53, 339
Intracranial tuberculoma, 8, 27, 38, 40, 41, 47, 51–6, 63, 65, 68, 79, 137, 167, 200, 211, 221, 226, 234, 256, 269, 305, 338, 421–2
  aetiology, 52
  angiography, 55
  clinical picture, 54–5
    age incidence, 54
    sex incidence, 54
    site, 54
    symptoms and signs, 54–5
  extracranial, 52–3
  incidence, 51–2
  laboratory investigations, 55
  pathogenesis, 52–3
  pathology, 53–4
  prognosis, 56
  treatment, 56
Intracranial tumour, 8, 37, 61, 79, 137, 167, 195, 199–200, 242–3, 266
Intradural spinal tuberculoma, 61, 64
Intramedullary tuberculoma of the spinal cord, 61–2
  clinical picture, 61
  incidence, 61
  laboratory investigations, 61
  pathogenesis and pathology, 61
  prognosis, 62
  treatment, 61–2
Intraspinal tuberculous granuloma, 38, 59, 61–2, 64
  extradural spinal tuberculoma, 61
  intradural spinal tuberculoma, 61, 64
  intramedullary tuberculoma, 61–2
Ischaemia, 53, 59, 127, 201, 241, 290, 329, 388, 389
  cerebral, 87, 94, 154, 166, 296–7
  cerebrovascular disease, 154–7, 165, 166
  heart disease, 88, 94, 95, 96, 156, 165, 264, 296
  transient ischaemic attacks, 289, 291, 296–7
Ischaemic lesions, 41, 48, 137, 331
Isotope cisternography, 41, 45, 46, 111

Jamaica, neurological disorders in, 421–34
Jamaican neuropathy, 84, 140, 421, 422, 423, 426, 427–30, 431
Jaundice, 94, 249, 253
Juvenile motor neurone disease, 27, 31, 127–30
  clinical features, 31, 129
  epidemiology, 127–9
  family history, 129
  laboratory data, 127

Katayama syndrome, 255–6
Kenya, neurological disorders in, 207–22
Kernig's sign, 343
Kleine–Levine syndrome, 33, 167
Klippel-Feil anomaly, 99, 106
Kogaisantampa, 379
Koro, 289
Kugelberg–Welander–Wohlfart disease, 168
Kuru, 17, 18, 118, 307, 376–83
  aetiology, 380–2
Kuru—*contd.*
  clinical laboratory findings, 378
  clinical picture, 377–8
  epidemiology, 378–80
  pathological picture, 378
Kwashiorkor, 14, 28, 74, 114, 138, 185, 191, 195, 249, 423
  neurological disorders in, 138

Lagophthalmos, 332, 333
Laminectomy, 59, 60, 61, 64, 66, 69, 70, 71, 126, 148, 170, 201, 209, 229, 243, 257, 415, 431
Landry-Guillain–Barré syndrome, 67, 68, 80
Landry's paralysis, 219
Langhans giant cells, 53, 54, 326
Lassa virus, 164
Latah, 289
Lathyrism, 5, 6, 13, 15, 27, 31, 38, 84, 148, 268
Lathyrus sativus, 13, 31, 82
Laurence–Moon–Biedl syndrome, 303
Lepromatosis, 322
Leprosy, 4, 6, 27, 80, 88, 133, 144, 150, 170, 171, 194, 196, 211, 239, 267, 305, 309, 321–34, 340, 379
  'borderline', 322, 323, 324, 327, 328
  borderline lepromatous, 309, 322, 323–4, 329
  borderline tuberculoid, 322, 323, 326
  classification, 322–3
  clinical appearance, 323–4
  diffuse, 324
  geographical incidence, 321–2
  historical background, 321
  indeterminate, 322, 323
  lepromatous, 321, 322, 323, 324, 325, 326–7, 328, 329, 330, 331, 332, 333
  neural, 267, 323, 327, 330, 331
  neurological involvement, 323, 324, 325–30
  nodular, 324
  primary polyneuritic, 327
  tuberculoid, 196, 267, 309, 321, 322, 323, 325, 326, 327, 328, 329, 330, 331, 332
Leprosy of the central nervous system, 80, 333
  spastic paralysis in, 333
Leptomeninges, 53, 69, 307, 389, 393, 400
Leptomeningitis, 66, 68, 70, 399, 400
Leptospirosis, 307, 319, 338
Leucocytosis, 163, 171, 344, 392, 403
Leukaemia, 158, 201, 241, 371, 403–4
Lhermitte's sign, 100
Lipidoses, 80
  cerebral, 303
Lipids, 14–15, 93, 155, 156, 346
Lipoma, 302
Lupus erythematosus, 123, 171, 309, 342, 427
Lymphadenopathy, 253 341
Lymphoma, 18, 144, 145, 147, 164, 170, 200–1, 422

McArdle's syndrome, 171
Madarosis, 324
Malabsorption syndrome, 73, 74, 75, 170, 173, 181, 191, 423
Malaria, 4, 5, 6, 12, 78, 134, 135, 143, 145, 149, 150, 173, 192, 200, 210, 223, 234, 240, 247, 249, 250, 253, 254, 263, 275, 289, 311, 342, 379, 422, 432
Malaysia, neurological disorders in, 299–320
Malformations of the nervous system, 7, 12–13, 38, 92, 99, 104, 108, 112, 167, 209–10, 283–6, 287–8, 302–3, 320

Malnutrition, 13–17, 27–8, 42, 78, 110, 115, 117, 118, 173, 180, 195, 204, 223, 260, 263, 266, 267, 269, 289, 300, 387, 399, 428, 429, 431
in the adult, 15–17
and brain development, 14–15, 28
in the infant, 14–15, 110, 115, 117, 138, 195
neurological complications, 27, 138
protein-calorie, 14–15, 28, 42, 78, 118, 138, 144, 173, 181–2, 191, 200
vitamin, 173, 182
Marasmus, 28
Measles, 136, 137, 144, 150, 163, 164, 216
Medical practice in Ghana, 144
in Kenya, 208–13
in Kuala Lumpur, 301–20
in Natal, 261–3
in Nigeria, 162–3
in Senegal, 133–4
in S. India, 78–82
in Uganda, 192–6
Medical schools, 4, 26, 37, 133, 143, 162, 192, 208, 223, 261, 283, 335, 387
Medical services, 37, 78, 133, 143, 161–2, 172, 192, 208, 223, 261, 299–300, 335–6, 356
Medical treatment of leprosy, 330–2
treatment of neurological complications, 331–2
anaesthesia, 331
nerve abscess, 332
nerve pain, 331
paralyses, 331–2
trophic problems, 332
treatment of reactions, 330–1
acute exacerbation, 330
erythema nodosum leprosum, 330–1
treatment of uncomplicated leprosy, 330
Medulloblastoma, 313, 422
Melanoma, 169, 243
Ménière's syndrome, 17, 144, 149, 167, 203, 270, 319
Meninges, 40, 53, 54, 63, 64, 66, 69, 70, 71, 117, 255, 256, 307, 389, 392
Meningioma, 8, 17, 38, 55, 79, 81, 137, 145, 169, 199, 211, 226, 266, 270, 303, 312, 339, 422
Meningismus, 307, 319–20
Meningitis, 58, 65, 66, 68, 79, 122, 134–5, 137, 144, 158, 166, 195, 201, 203, 204, 210, 227, 240, 243, 247, 249, 250, 256, 260, 265, 283, 302, 338, 343–4, 379, 421, 432
amoebic, 192
aseptic, 163, 164, 339, 379
bacterial, 134, 170, 195, 196, 304, 305, 338, 379, 421
basal, 239, 338
benign lymphocytic, 210, 219
carcinomatous, 170
cerebrospinal, 7
cryptococcal, 198, 221, 239, 305, 306–7
eosinophilic, 308, 343–4, 345
inflammatory caseous, 40
meningococcal, 164, 196, 197, 238, 239, 263
pachymeningitis, 58
pneumococcal, 149–51, 163, 164, 166, 172, 196–8, 203, 205, 219, 239, 242, 263
pyogenic, 37, 64, 65, 144, 145, 210, 238, 239, 265–6, 338
and subdural effusions, 234
tuberculous, 27, 34, 37, 38, 39–51, 53, 54, 56, 58, 63, 66, 67, 68, 69, 70, 120, 122, 127, 133, 134, 135, 137, 144,
Meningitis, tuberculous—*contd.*
145, 163–4, 197, 198, 210, 221, 226, 250, 253, 263, 264, 26,5 304–5, 307, 338, 421
viral, 134, 135, 239
Meningocele, 109, 209, 243, 302
Meningo-encephalitis, 41, 118, 133, 196, 198, 253, 349, 379, 388, 389, 400, 403, 404, 405
Meningo-encephalocele, 109
Meningo-encephalomyelitis, 340, 349, 388, 400
Meningomyelitis, 81, 388
Meningomyelocele, 209–10, 243, 302–3
Meningomyelopathy, 84, 423
Mental deficiency, 209, 265, 269, 361, 395
disease, 11, 149
disturbance, 48, 149, 179, 204, 391, 392
retardation, 80, 114, 117, 136, 204, 239, 243, 301, 400, 413, 423
Metabolic bone disorders, 74
Metastatic lesions, 81, 138, 287, 317
Microcephaly, 110, 112, 243, 301, 368
Migraine, 17, 79, 122, 149, 166, 209, 234, 245, 270
Monkeys, 231, 342, 346, 398
experimental study in, 41, 52, 380–2
Monoplegia, 48, 155, 249
Mortality rates, 7, 8, 10, 45, 47, 90, 134, 135, 136, 143, 152, 153, 157, 164, 165, 166, 197, 204, 219, 220, 277, 286, 289–90, 291, 292, 294, 295, 296, 297, 307, 310, 311, 339, 343, 345, 349, 357–8, 365–7, 377, 390
Motor neurone disease, 7, 8, 31, 37, 80, 127–30, 144, 148, 168, 180, 181, 196, 203, 212, 244, 264, 340, 359, 360, 361, 371, 372, 379
Multiple sclerosis, 7, 8–10, 17, 34, 64, 80, 81, 83, 84, 106, 109, 134, 138, 144, 148, 202, 203, 205, 210, 213, 222, 237, 244, 246, 261, 264, 267, 269, 270, 283, 286–7, 304, 339–40, 349, 371, 372, 426–7
and migration, 10
prevalence, 9, 10, 277, 340
in South Africa, 273, 277–80
Muscular dystrophy, 34, 80, 138, 144, 148, 168, 171, 203, 212, 244, 310, 371
dystrophia myotonica, 171, 203, 371
Myasthenia gravis, 80, 134, 138, 144, 148, 171, 196, 203, 212, 244, 310, 341, 371, 427
Mycoses, 137
Mydriasis, 403
Myelin, 14–15, 41, 69, 84, 117
Myelin content of brain, 15
Myelination, 14–15
Myelitis, 64, 68–9, 134, 137, 256, 338, 430
ascending, 64, 67, 68–9, 345
transverse, 27, 32, 67, 68–9, 169, 202, 211, 219, 257, 267, 286, 304, 307, 318–19, 340, 349
Myeloencephalitis, 345
eosinophilic, 345
Myelography, 32, 58, 70, 81, 83, 102, 104, 106, 129, 138, 148, 170, 201, 210, 227, 245, 257, 267, 268, 414, 415, 430, 431
Myelomatosis, 170, 171
Myelopathy, 17, 29, 31, 37, 70, 74, 100, 104, 105, 106, 165, 170, 180, 200, 201, 245, 340, 426
bilharzial, 268
cervical, 138
compressive, 99
diabetic, 426
ischaemic, 70

Myelopathy—*contd.*
nutritional, 69, 267
obscure, 202, 205
spastic, 268
subacute, 34, 82
toxic, 267
tropical, 69
Myocardial infarction, 93, 94, 97, 264, 299, 337, 365
disease, 181
Myocarditis, 164, 253, 401, 402, 403–4
Myopathies, 33, 34, 74, 80, 134, 171, 212, 310, 425–6
diabetic, 426
metabolic, 172
proximal, 76, 171
thyrotoxic, 212
Myositis, 134, 164, 171, 212
dermatomyositis, 171, 212
Myxoedema, 270
Myxoviruses, 135–6

Natal, neurological disease in, 259–72
Necrosis, 40, 53, 61, 70, 87, 93, 96, 172, 187, 202, 255, 309, 310, 314, 328, 332, 346, 348, 368, 394
Neoplasia, 287
Neoplasms, 8, 79, 147, 166, 171, 200, 201, 225–6, 227, 266, 303, 311–18, 338, 339, 340, 422
malignant, 225, 311, 314, 422
simple, 422
Neoplastic disease, 239
Nephritis, 164, 342
Nephrosis, 159
Nerve entrapment syndrome, 270
Nerve lesions, 15, 244, 325–6, 326–30
Nerve palsy, 257, 342, 426
Neuralgia, 7, 166, 336
Horton's syndrome, 166, 234
Sluder's, 234
Neurinoma, 303, 316
Neuritis, 169, 170, 202–3
brachial, 170
bulbar, 169
interstitial, 401
optic, 121, 202–3, 244, 304, 319, 340, 343, 349, 427
retrobulbar, 10, 32, 169, 170, 179, 202, 244, 246, 286–7, 288, 304, 319, 425, 431
syphilitic, 430
'Neurobartonellosis', 388, 389
Neuroblastoma, 243
Neurocysticercosis, 390–5
aetiology, 390–1
frequency and geographical distribution, 390–1
modes of infestation, 391
parasite, 391
clinical manifestations, 391–2
cerebral cysticercosis, 391–2
clinical pathology, 392
radiology, 392, 394
diagnosis, 392, 394–5
history, 390
pathogenesis, 394
pathology of cerebral cysticercosis, 392–4
histology, 393–4
macroscopic anatomy, 393
prognosis and treatment, 390, 395
spinal cysticercosis, 392, 395
Neurodermatitis, 347
Neurofibroma, 38, 63, 69, 81, 102, 169, 211, 266, 267, 422
Neurofibromatosis, 8, 168, 243, 266, 422
Neurofibrosarcoma, 243
Neurogenic atrophy, 129, 181
Neurological complications of haemoglobinopathies, 149–51
in tropical sprue, 73–7
Neurological manifestations of systemic diseases, 342
of verruga peruana, 387–90
blood, 388
clinical manifestations, 388
pathogenesis, 389
pathology, 388–9
ependymal-choroidal lesions, 389
glial lesions, 389
meningovascular lesions, 389
neuronal lesions, 389
presence of *Bartonella* in brain, 389
verrucomas, 389
prognosis and treatment, 389–90
Neurological practice,
in Ghana, 144
in Kenya, 208–13
in Kuala Lumpur, 301–20
in Natal, 261–3
in Nigeria, 162–3
in Senegal, 133–4
in S. India, 78–82
in Uganda, 192–6
Neurology of leprosy, 325–30
complications of leprosy involvement in nerves, 327–30
anaesthesia, 325, 326, 327–8, 331
nerve abscess, 329–30, 332
nerve pain, 328–9, 331, 332
paralysis, 329, 331–2
direct involvement of nerves in leprosy, 326–7
borderline leprosy, 327
lepromatous leprosy, 326–7
neural leprosy, 327
tuberculoid leprosy, 326
nerve lesions, 325–6
Neurology in the tropics, 17–18
Neuroma, 8, 137, 168
acoustic, 422
Neuromyelitis optica (Devic's disease), 10, 80, 138, 148, 169, 202, 246, 270, 286, 287, 304, 340
Neuromyelopathy, 75
nutritional, 75
vitamin B12, 28, 75
Neuromyopathy, 4
carcinomatous, 34, 245, 426
Neuropathy, 7, 131, 144, 148, 170, 181, 309, 310, 431, 432
alcoholic, 148
ataxic, 15, 139, 168, 169, 170, 173–87, 196, 201, 202, 203, 268
autonomic, 404
cranial, 200, 201
peripheral, 3, 28, 37, 45, 74–5, 76, 80, 83, 138, 148, 168, 170, 172, 173, 181, 220, 245, 266–7, 304, 309, 318, 340, 423
retrobulbar, 15, 423, 426, 431, 432
tropical, 148, 201, 202, 203
vitamin B12, 283
Neuropraxia, obstetric, 170–1
Neurosarcoidosis, 34

Neurosis, 144, 149, 167, 269, 289
  anxiety, 167, 172, 194, 269
  obsessive-compulsive, 269
Neurosurgery, 26, 37, 78, 82, 144, 145, 223–36, 283, 332, 342–3, 430
Neurosurgical lesions, 8
  procedures, 224–34
Neurosyphilis, 11–12, 145, 148, 165, 195, 196, 198–9, 205, 264, 265, 338, 422, 430
  meningovascular form, 11–12, 265, 338
  parenchymatous form, 11–12, 265
Neurotuberculosis, 27
Neutrophilia, 403
Nigeria, neurological disorders in, 161–90, 196
Nigerian tropical ataxic neuropathy, 15, 139, 168, 169, 170, 173–87, 196, 201, 202, 203
  clinical features, 178–80
    age and sex distribution, 178, 179
    dietetic history, 178
    family history, 178
    intermittency, 179
    mode of onset, 179
    natural history, 180
    socio-economic status, 178
    symptoms and signs, 179–80
  epidemiological studies, 185–6
  investigations, 180–5
    cerebrospinal fluid, 180
    cyanide metabolism, 182–5
    electrocardiographic, 181
    electromyographic, 181
    histological, 181
    Kahn or VDRL, 181
    nutritional status, 181–2
Nutritional amblyopia, 16
Nutritional disorders, 27, 110, 186, 202, 212, 220–1, 245, 299
Nutritional myelopathy, 267
Nutritional neuropathy, 133, 134, 138–40, 144, 168, 170, 187, 212, 245
  clinical features, 139
  investigations, 139–40
  pathology, 140
Nutritional osteomalacia, 28

Obesity, 155–6, 158, 171
Occlusion, 88, 89, 94, 149, 152, 264, 310, 342
  anterior spinal artery, 81
  carotid, 338
  coronary, 337
  middle cerebral artery, 88
  vascular, 269, 336, 337, 404
Occlusive disease, 45, 137, 153, 264, 336, 337
  vascular disease, 92, 165, 337
Ocular leprosy, 332–3
Ocular palsy, 120, 135
Oculomotor neuritis (cranial polyneuritis), 27, 32
Oligodendroglioma, 211, 243, 313
Onchocerciasis, 144, 151, 202
Ophthalmoplegia, 17, 32, 42, 120–3, 212, 249
  diabetic, 120, 122
Optic atrophy, 28, 43, 80, 83, 121, 127, 144, 148, 149, 170, 173, 179, 180, 187, 199, 202–3, 209, 242, 244, 263, 312, 315, 344, 410, 413, 430
Optic neuritis, 121, 202–3, 244, 304, 319, 340, 343, 349, 427
Oroya fever, 387–90
Osteitis, 239
Osteoarthritis, 94, 148, 270
Osteomalacia, 37, 74, 171
Osteomyelitis, 219, 305, 328
Osteophytosis, 125, 126
Osteoporosis, 180, 268–9, 328
Osteosclerosis, 124, 125, 126
Otitis media, 39, 145, 209, 244, 266

Pachymeningitis, 308, 430
Painful ophthalmoplegia, 17, 32, 42, 120–3
  aetiology, 123
  clinical features, 120–1
    onset of symptoms, 120
    physical signs, 120–1
    sex and age incidence, 120
  course, 121
  differential diagnosis, 122
  investigations, 121
  pathology, 122–3
  treatment, 121–2
    corticosteroid therapy, 121–2
Panencephalomeningitis, 392
Papilloedema, 56, 122, 202, 211, 243, 263, 310, 312, 391–2, 395, 410, 411, 412
Papilloma, 315
Paragonimiasis, 148, 422
Paralysis agitans, 7, 270, 362, 363, 371, 372
Paraparesis, 170, 200, 229, 246
Paraplegia, 15, 17, 43, 48, 57–60, 63, 66, 67, 80, 82, 125, 137, 138, 139, 144, 145, 147, 148, 167, 200, 201, 209, 228, 229, 230, 231, 237, 239, 240, 246, 256–7, 267, 268, 302, 305, 307, 318, 345, 415
  ataxic, 15
  classification of, 58
  Erb's, 430
  hypotonic, 67
  spastic, 13, 15, 63, 81–2, 127, 212, 220–1, 243, 245, 371, 399, 431
  spinal, 135
  traumatic, 162
  tropical, 17
  tuberculous, 228, 229
Parasitaemia, 247, 342
Parasitic infections, 5, 34, 159, 223, 226, 234, 240, 263, 267, 299, 300, 338, 343–6, 379, 390
  infestation of the central nervous system, 34, 137, 226, 230–2, 247–58, 399
Parasitism, 398, 402–3
Parasitosis, 397
Parenchymal reaction, border-zone, 41
Parenchymatous lesions, 40, 41, 117, 118
Parkinsonism, 80, 118, 127, 144, 147, 168, 172, 203, 244, 253, 270, 340, 356, 363–4, 369, 370, 382
    parkinsonism-dementia syndrome, 17, 127, 168, 303, 355–75
Parkinson's disease, 7, 134, 138, 168, 180, 212, 221, 224, 234, 235, 270, 362, 363–4, 369–70, 371, 372, 379
Parotitis, 97
Paroxysmal disorders, 79, 147, 166–7
Pattern of neurological disease, 26, 223, 224
  in Natal, 264–9
  in Nigeria, 162–3
  in Singapore, 283–9

Pattern of neurological disease—*contd.*
in S. India, 78–81
in Thailand, 336–42
in Uganda, 192
Pellagra, 5, 13, 16, 27, 28, 34, 148, 195, 202, 212, 220, 221, 245, 260, 267, 423, 431
Periarteritis, 69, 400
Periodic paralysis, 172
Periostitis, 122, 123
Peripheral nerve, 73, 134, 181, 187, 323, 324, 325–6, 329, 333, 339, 341, 347, 348, 388, 401, 423, 425
lesions, 138, 212, 244, 325–6, 390
Peripheral neuritis, 106, 273, 275, 430
Peripheral neuropathy, 3, 28, 37, 45, 74–5, 76, 80, 83, 138, 148, 168, 170, 172, 173, 181, 220, 245, 266–7, 304, 309, 318, 340, 423
and myopathy, 245, 425–6
Peru, neurological disorders in, 387–96
Petit mal, 148, 166, 199, 209, 242, 265, 270–1, 301, 339, 424
Phenylketonuria, 32–3, 80, 303
Phlebitis, 40
Pick's disease, 362, 382
Pinealoma, 79, 167, 318
Plague, 3, 4, 5, 6
Plasma thiocyanate level, 84, 173, 182–3, 184, 185
Platybasia, 209
Pleocytosis, 164, 201, 204, 239, 240, 267, 268, 297, 343, 380, 392
Pneumoencephalography, 44, 116, 117, 121, 123, 167, 169, 227, 301, 302, 392, 394, 395
Pneumonia, 13, 192, 195, 197, 234, 243, 250, 263, 370, 378
Poisoning, 149, 193, 209, 210, 283, 309, 340
ackee, 424–5
cyanide, 430
Poliomyelitis, 129, 134, 135, 145, 164–5, 168, 198, 210, 240, 263, 279, 299, 319, 339, 421, 426
acute, 134, 137, 198, 213–20, 263, 388
diagnosis, 215–16
differential diagnosis, 219
distinctive features, 216
life-threatening, 213–15, 216, 219, 220
respiratory, 213, 215, 217, 218
treatment, 216–19
Polyarteritis nodosa, 170, 171, 310, 427
Polycythaemia, 98, 317
Polymyositis, 80, 138, 166, 171, 193, 212, 246, 310
Polyneuritis, 16, 129, 144, 147, 148, 211, 427
acute infective, 202
cranialis, 122, 167, 170
infective, 211
Polyneuropathy, 127, 138, 181, 196, 202, 211, 245, 341, 342
alcoholic, 138, 202, 245
diabetic, 138, 202, 245
INH-induced, 202
Polyradiculoneuropathy, 349
Polyradiculopathy, 167
Population, 25, 26, 38, 73, 78, 86, 109, 124, 133, 138, 143, 161, 162, 173, 191, 207, 223, 225, 226, 229, 248, 252, 259–60, 263, 275, 277, 280, 283, 290, 299, 310, 335, 339, 343, 355, 366, 372, 379, 387, 421, 426, 427
hospital, 163, 172, 223, 234–5, 237, 270, 275, 289, 365
studies in, 370
Pacific, 371
Porphyria, 170, 211–12, 267, 340
Porphyria variegata, acute, 267, 273, 275
coproporphyria, 275, 276
cutanea tarda, 267, 268
hepatic, 267
intermittent acute, 273–5, 276
prevalence, 275
in South Africa, 273–7
treatment, 275–7
Porter's neck, 229–30
Pott's disease of the spine, 63, 133, 134, 227–9
Pott's paraplegia, 38, 57–60, 81, 211, 221
aetiopathogenesis, 58
age, 58
clinical picture, 58–9
incidence, 57–8
laboratory investigations, 59
pathology, 58
prognosis, 58, 60
treatment, 59–60
Prednisolone, 70, 71, 121, 122, 169, 170, 330, 332
Pregnancy, 78, 138, 139, 140, 164, 170, 171, 178, 179, 212, 216, 233, 242, 247, 275, 343
Presenile dementia, 37, 80, 195, 376
Prevalence and incidence, 7, 8, 9, 86, 90, 93–4, 152, 163, 185, 263, 271, 273, 275, 277–8, 283, 289, 291, 336, 340, 355, 359, 365–7, 372, 376–7, 379, 380, 397, 414, 421, 422, 424, 425, 426
Primary cerebral tumours, 8, 81, 138, 144, 145, 167, 199, 200, 242–3, 263, 266, 267, 269, 270, 422
Prisoner-of-war camps, 15, 186, 423, 427, 429
neuropathy in, 174–7
Protein deficiency, 14, 28
Pseudoathetosis, 101
Pseudomyotonia, 74, 76
Pseudotabes, 426
Pseudotumour, 122
Psychiatric disorders, 149, 193, 269, 391, 413
psychoneurosis, 149, 245, 269
Psychogenic and psychiatric disorders, 147, 149
Psychoses, 149, 269, 342, 394
manic-depressive, 149
schizophrenia, 149, 269
Ptosis, 120, 121, 430
proptosis, 121, 122, 167, 212
Pulseless disease, 28, 29, 88, 92
Pyelonephritis, 94, 97, 159
Pyomyositis, 171, 172, 193, 195, 196

Quinine, 249, 250, 342, 432

Rabies, 144, 145, 164, 196, 338, 346–9
neurological sequelae of vaccination, 349
Radial nerve palsy, 212, 244
Radiculomyelopathy, 27, 31–2, 61, 63–72
aetiology, 63, 64
aetiopathology, 64–6
chronic form, 67
clinical features, 66–7
differential diagnosis, 65, 68–9
idiopathic agents, 64, 66
infective agents, 64–5
lumbar puncture, 64, 65, 67–8
myelography, 68
non-infective agents, 65–6
pathology, 64, 69–70

Radiculomyelopathy—*contd.*
prognosis, 69, 70
subacute form, 66–7
treatment, 69, 70–1
Reactions in leprosy, 324–5, 330–1
acute exacerbation, 324–5, 330, 331
erythema nodosum leprosum, 325, 329, 330–1, 332, 333
Lucio phenomenon, 325
von Recklinghausen's disease, 102, 211, 303, 311, 313, 315, 316, 320
Rehabilitation, 230
Relapsing fever, 5, 12, 150
Religion and witchcraft, 223–4, 260, 269, 299, 300, 335
Renal disease, 97, 156, 195
failure, 170, 250, 266
Respiratory disease, 379
obstruction, 219–20
paralysis, 213, 216, 217, 218, 276, 346, 427
Reticulosis, 69
Retrobulbar neuritis, 10, 32, 169, 170, 179, 202, 244, 246, 286–7, 288, 304, 319, 425, 431
neuropathy, 15, 423, 426, 431, 432
Rheumatic carditis, 263
heart disease, 157, 165, 241–2, 262, 264
Rheumatism, 148
Rhodesia, neurological disorders in, 237–46
neurosurgery in, 223–36
Rich's foci, 39, 40, 52
Rickets, 16, 33
Rickettsial infection, 319
Rinderpest, 4
Romberg's sign, 83, 221

St. Louis virus, 421
Sarcoidosis, 65, 170, 306–7, 308, 319
Sarcoma, 38, 311, 318
cerebellar, 318
primary, 318
Scabies, 4, 379
Schilder's diffuse sclerosis, 80
Schistosomiasis, 144, 148, 151, 156, 202, 211, 307, 319
Schwann cell, 325, 333, 425–6
Schwannoma, 79, 145, 169
Sciatica, 134, 138, 170
Scintillography, 411
Sclerosis, 31, 180, 328, 394
hypertrophic, 394
posterolateral, 106
primary lateral, 127, 168, 244, 286
Schilder's diffuse, 80
tuberous, 243, 303
Scotomata, 179
Scrapie, 118, 380, 382
Scurvy, 16, 268–9
Senegal, neurological disorders in, 133–42
Senility, 74
Sensorineural hearing loss, 431–2
Sensory impairment, 74, 83, 84, 101, 106, 120, 139, 169, 179, 180, 210, 221, 243, 245, 256, 266, 267, 331, 349, 427
Sequelae, 14, 38, 48, 49, 86, 138, 167, 227, 242, 304, 331, 338, 339, 349
Serum B12 level, 84, 92, 116, 183, 184, 220, 429, 430
Sickle-cell disease, 149–51, 156, 157, 159, 164, 166, 204, 210
trait, 249
Siderosis, 268
pancreatic, 268
Singapore, neurological disorders in, 283–98
Sinusitis, 121, 270, 304
Sleeping sickness (African trypanosomiasis), 3, 6, 192, 196, 232, 251–4
acute case, 251, 252
clinical features, 6, 252–4
Gambian, 251, 252, 254
healthy carrier, 252
nervous system in, 253–4
Rhodesian, 251, 252
subacute case, 251, 252
treatment, 254
Slow virus infection, 118, 280, 368, 376, 427
Smallpox, 4, 6, 150
Snake-bite, 144, 151, 346
Space-occupying lesions, 38, 51–2, 54, 55, 56, 122, 134, 226, 227, 242, 243, 306, 307, 311, 411
Spastic diplegia, 106, 399
Spastic myelopathy, 267–8
Spastic paraparesis, 245
Spastic paraplegia, 13, 15, 63, 81–2, 127, 212, 220–1, 243, 245, 371, 399, 431
nutritional, 220–1, 333
tropical, 27, 31, 81, 82–4
clinical features, 31, 82–3
investigations, 83–4
natural history, 84
Spasticity, 31, 34, 83, 100, 127, 139, 229, 243, 305, 360, 362
Spina bifida, 12, 80, 108, 167, 204
Spinal atrophy, 129, 168
Spinal block, 47, 48, 58, 68, 70
Spinal caries, 39, 58, 65, 67
tuberculous, 67
Spinal cord disorders, 14, 31–2, 38, 79, 146, 201–2, 267–9
lesions, 57, 58, 59, 61, 67, 124, 137, 211, 227
regeneration, 229
syndromes, 169–70
trauma, 65, 148, 229
tumours, 227, 228
Spinal injuries, 270, 311
Spinal meningitis, 27, 31–2, 61, 63, 64, 65, 66, 68, 69, 70, 71
Spinal respiratory paralysis, 213, 216, 217, 218
Spinal tumour syndrome, 59, 60, 61, 65, 66, 68
Spinocerebellar degeneration, 27, 29–30, 80, 127, 138, 188
Steatorrhoea, 73
Streptomycin, 41, 42, 45, 46, 47, 56, 59, 64, 65, 66, 67, 164, 226, 245, 260, 304
Stroke, 8, 13, 27, 79, 93, 94, 97, 144, 153, 154, 155, 156, 157, 159, 166, 264, 297, 308, 337, 345, 423
in the young adult, 8, 27, 28, 86, 87–90
Studies of amine metabolism, 369
Sturge–Weber disease, 166, 303
Subacute combined degeneration, 17, 28, 74, 75, 138, 144, 148, 187, 201, 212, 220, 309, 340, 376, 429
neuronal degeneration, 389
progressive degeneration, 382
Subacute myelo-optico-neuropathy, 34
Subacute sclerosing panencephalitis, 80, 134, 136, 164, 339
Subacute spongiform virus encephalopathies, 382–3
Subarachnoid haemorrhage, 12, 28, 66, 84, 87, 89, 149, 153, 154, 157, 158–9, 165, 166, 201, 211, 232, 241, 283, 285, 286, 289, 290, 291, 295–6, 337, 338, 342, 345, 423
and berry aneurysms, 12, 28, 29, 166, 338, 423

Subarachnoid space, 39, 41, 45, 65, 157, 201, 255, 393, 430
block, 67, 68, 70
Subclavian steal syndrome, 337
Subdural empyema, 304
Subdural haematoma, 37, 138, 144, 145, 149, 195, 211, 234, 241, 256, 264, 265, 266, 288, 311
extradural, 266, 310–11
Synaptic connexions, 15
Syncope, 242
Syphilis, 4, 6, 11–12, 32, 64, 65, 67, 70, 82, 84, 88, 92, 95, 122, 134, 136, 137, 154, 173, 191–2, 195, 198–9, 201, 202, 209, 239–40, 241, 242, 261, 263, 265, 267, 283, 308, 337, 422, 424, 426, 429, 430, 431
cerebral, 79
meningovascular, 147, 265, 269, 337, 338, 422
of nervous system, 133, 136, 239
spinal, 201
vascular, 394
Syringobulbia, 201
Syringomyelia, 101, 104, 106, 201

Tabes dorsalis, 7, 11–12, 17, 79, 136, 145, 165, 199, 201, 265, 338, 422
Takayasu's disease, 8, 29, 92, 97, 337
Tapeworm, 230, 390, 394
Temporal arteritis, 34, 122, 234
Teratoma, 167, 318
Tetanus, 7, 27, 136, 144, 145, 165, 166, 167, 193, 195, 240, 289
Tetany, 74, 76
Tetraparesis, 59, 169
Tetraplegia, 17, 48, 66, 124, 125, 229, 230
Thai haemorrhagic fever, 339
Thailand, neurology in, 335–52
Therapeutic trials with L-Dopa, 369–70
Thiacetazone, 45–6, 56
Thiamine, 16–17, 28, 139, 173, 182, 220
deficiency, 16–17, 139, 173, 186, 202, 423
Third nerve palsy, 32, 209, 244
Thrombosis, 8, 28, 58, 87, 88, 90, 137, 149, 157, 158, 219, 232, 250, 304, 337, 342, 389, 423
carotid artery, 87, 88–9, 404
cerebral, 8, 87, 88, 89, 90, 232, 240, 241, 289, 290, 291–4, 308, 337
coronary, 232, 235, 264, 278, 296, 337
occlusive, 69, 137
sinus, 166, 242, 310, 337
Thyrotoxic periodic paralysis, 297, 341
Thyrotoxicosis, 171, 212, 297, 341–2, 421
Tomography, 59, 102, 103, 111
Tongue wasting, 129
Toxaemia, 251, 427
Toxic disorders, 79, 311
myelopathy, 267
Toxocariasis, 151
Toxoplasmosis, 150, 170, 308
Toxins, 97, 127, 148, 340, 343, 346, 392
and other environmental exposures, 368–9
Tracheostomy, 217, 219, 220, 276, 294, 342
Transmissible presenile virus dementia, 382
Transverse myelitis, 27, 32, 67, 68–9, 147, 148, 169, 202, 211, 219, 257, 267, 286, 304, 307, 318–19, 340, 349
Trauma, 92, 97, 114, 127, 134, 137, 145, 147, 148, 158, 166, 170, 193, 195, 201, 242, 265, 300, 301, 310–11, 328, 332, 342, 343, 365, 379
Traumatic disorders, 79
Trends in ALS and PD, 365–7
Treponematosis, 422, 429
Trichinosis, 308, 422
Trigeminal neuralgia, 17, 79, 144, 148, 170, 203, 209, 234, 244, 270, 413
Trophic changes, 328, 332
of bone, 328
of joints, 328, 332
of skin, 328, 332
ulcers, 328, 332, 379
Tropical amblyopia, 183, 187, 203, 422, 423, 430, 431
Tropical medicine, 3, 4–6, 11
Tropical sprue, 5, 73–7
neurological complications in, 73–5
coma, 74, 75
disturbance of higher cerebral function, 75
incidence, 73–4
night blindness, 73, 75, 76
peripheral neuropathy, 74–5, 76
prognosis and treatment, 75–6
proximal muscle weakness and wasting, 74
subacute combined degeneration, 75
tetany, 74, 76
Trypanosomiasis, 5, 133, 134, 136, 144, 149, 150, 172, 192, 196, 198, 210, 221, 223, 232, 250, 251–4, 422
American, 397–407
clinical features, 252–4
treatment, 254
Tuberculoma of the brain, 8, 27, 38, 40, 41, 47, 51–6, 63, 65, 68, 79, 137, 167, 200, 211, 221, 226, 234, 256, 269, 305, 330, 421–2
extracranial, 52–3
Tuberculosis, 4, 13, 38, 39, 42, 53, 54, 56, 64–5, 78, 97, 121, 133, 134, 135, 137, 138, 192, 201, 203, 223, 226, 234, 261, 263, 266, 268, 283, 299, 304, 305, 307, 338
clinical features, 42–3, 54–5, 58–9
complications, 47, 64–5, 66
glandular, 135, 268
infective, 64–5
meningeal, 39
mental subnormality and psychiatric disturbances, 48
miliary, 39, 51, 163, 263, 305
non-infective, 65–6
pathology, 39–42, 53–4, 58
primary spinal variety, 64–5
prognosis, 47–9, 56, 58, 60
pulmonary, 61, 67, 121, 135, 145, 167, 268, 300, 338
secondary extension from caries of the vertebrae, 65
secondary involvement of the spinal meninges, 65
treatment, 45–7, 56, 59–60
Tuberculosis affecting the central nervous system, 37–62, 63, 64–5
Tuberculosis of the spine, 57–8, 59–60, 63–72, 137, 147, 169, 193, 201, 227–9, 237, 238, 240, 267, 268, 305
Tuberculous encephalopathy, 41
Tuberculous meningitis, 27, 34, 37, 38, 39–51, 53, 54, 56, 58, 63, 66, 67, 68, 69, 70, 120, 122, 127, 133, 134, 135, 137, 144, 145, 163–4, 197, 198, 210, 221, 226, 250, 253, 263, 264, 265, 304–5, 307, 338, 421
aetiology, 39
clinical features, 42–3
age incidence, 42–3
course, 43

Tuberculous meningitis—*contd.*
diagnosis, 42
incidence, 39, 42–3
laboratory investigations, 43–5
pathogenesis, 39
pathology, 39–42
prognosis, 47–9
complications in, 47
treatment, 45–7
Tumours, 32, 38, 92, 137, 145, 146, 158, 169, 170, 199–200, 211, 225–6, 234, 242–3, 256, 257, 263, 264, 266, 270, 283, 301, 339, 368, 391, 394, 411, 430
benign, 311
cerebral, 8, 211, 221, 225–6, 256, 260, 266, 368, 371, 411
epidural, 169
hemisphere, 211
intracranial, 79, 195, 199–200, 242–3
metastases, 79, 170, 199, 200, 226, 243
nasopharyngeal, 120, 122
pituitary, 38, 79, 137, 145, 170, 211, 242–3
secondary, 266, 267
Typhoid, 3, 134, 135, 137, 144, 149, 150, 172, 173, 195, 247, 249, 263, 267, 432
encephalitic forms of, 135
Typhus, 173

Uganda, neurological disorders in, 191–206
Ulnar nerve palsy, 212, 239, 244, 309
Uraemia, 159, 170, 195, 245
Uveomeningo-encephalitis, 318

Vascular change, 40–1, 348, 411
lesions, 389, 392, 394, 404, 432
Vascular diseases of the brain and spinal cord, 17, 79, 144, 155, 158, 159, 195, 196, 204, 210–11, 232, 233, 235, 265, 308–9
Vascular diseases—*contd.*
of the nervous system, 165–6, 336–7
peripheral, 95
Vasculitis, 45, 310, 325
Vegetation, 143, 207, 251
Venereal disease, 83
Ventriculography, 44, 55, 56, 144, 227, 394–5
Vertebral collapse, 268–9
Vertebral hydatidosis, 412, 413–16
course of disease and prognosis, 415
diagnosis, 414–15
paraclinical tests, 414
X-ray, 414
symptomatology, 414
treatment, 415
biological, 415
Vestibular neuronitis, 172, 319
Viraemia, 347, 421
Viral infections, 136, 164–5, 200, 276, 279, 280, 338, 421
Vitamines, 16

Wassermann reaction, 240, 242, 269, 405, 429
Wernicke's encephalopathy, 16–17, 340, 423
Whip-lash injury, 320
Whooping cough, neurological manifestations of, 135
Wilson's disease, 33, 34, 271, 303, 340
Wrist-drop, 329, 331–2
Writer's cramp, 172, 213

Xeroderma, 328, 332
Xerosis, 97

Yaws, 165, 180, 299, 379, 422, 429, 432
Yellow fever, 4, 5, 135